Veterinary Technician and Nurse's Daily Reference Guide

Canine and Feline

Fourth Edition

Veterinary Technician and Nurse's Daily Reference Guide

Canine and Feline

Fourth Edition

Edited by:

Mandy Fults
Liberty Hill Texas, USA

Kenichiro Yagi
Veterinary Emergency Group, New York, USA

WILEY Blackwell

This fourth edition first published 2022

Edition History
Candyce M. Jack and Patricia M. Watson (1e, 2003); Candyce M. Jack and Patricia M. Watson (2e, 2008); John Wiley & Sons Inc (3e, 2014)

Registered Office
John Wiley & Sons, Inc., 111 River Street, Hoboken, NJ 07030, USA

Editorial Office
111 River Street, Hoboken, NJ 07030, USA

For details of our global editorial offices, customer services, and more information about Wiley products visit us at www.wiley.com.

Wiley also publishes its books in a variety of electronic formats and by print-on-demand. Some content that appears in standard print versions of this book may not be available in other formats.

Library of Congress Cataloging-in-Publication Data

Names: Fults, Mandy, 1979– editor. | Yagi, Kenichiro, 1977– editor.
Title: Veterinary technician and nurse's daily reference guide : canine and feline / edited by Mandy Fults, Kenichiro Yagi.
Other titles: Preceded by (work): Veterinary technician's daily reference guide.
Description: Fourth edition. | Hoboken, NJ : Wiley-Blackwell, 2022. | Preceded by Veterinary technician's daily reference guide / editors, Candyce M. Jack and Patricia M. Watson ; consulting editor, Valissitie Heeren. Third edition. Ames, Iowa : John Wiley & Sons Inc., 2014. | Includes bibliographical references and index.
Identifiers: LCCN 2021050528 (print) | LCCN 2021050529 (ebook) | ISBN 9781119557203 (paperback) | ISBN 9781119557197 (adobe pdf) | ISBN 9781119557180 (epub)
Subjects: MESH: Veterinary Medicine–methods | Animal Technicians | Cat Diseases | Dog Diseases | Handbook
Classification: LCC SF748 (print) | LCC SF748 (ebook) | NLM SF 748 | DDC 636.089–dc23/eng/20211101
LC record available at https://lccn.loc.gov/2021050528
LC ebook record available at https://lccn.loc.gov/2021050529

Cover Design: Wiley
Cover Images: © Micaela Hinojosa; Leslie Semegran

Set in 10/12pt Berling by Straive, Pondicherry, India

SKY10035059_072722

Contents

Figures

Chapter 4: Diagnostic Imaging

Chapter 14: Patient Care Skills in Clinical Practice

Chapter 16: Medical Procedures

Chapter 17: Nutrition

Chapter 18: Pain Management

Preface

The *Veterinary Technician and Nurse's Daily Reference Guide, Fourth Edition*, continues to provide relevant information as a primary source for the veterinary profession. This book has evolved since the first edition in 2003 and since the previous edition in 2014; many new developments in veterinary medicine have occurred and this new edition provides updates, using veterinary technician specialists in their field of study. Their specialized knowledge obtained in practice takes the text to a new level. Evidence-based guidelines and consensus statements published to standardize best practices have been incorporated. Specific areas of updates include: RECOVER CPR guidelines, novel therapeutics in the field of dermatology, updated vaccination standards, stress-free handling and nursing care strategies, newly gained knowledge in pain assessment and management, advancement in diagnostic capabilities, regenerative medicine and updates in pharmacologic agents used to treat and manage disease states. A new section detailing the various credentials and certifications veterinary technicians and nurses can obtain, together with a new chapter discussing nursing theory and science and how it relates to veterinary nursing has been incorporated. The expansion of the title to include "nurse" allows for inclusion of members of our profession around the world.

Acknowledgments

We would like to express our heartfelt thanks to all of the contributors and the Wiley team for facing the challenges and adjustments made through the pandemic alongside us. To those who continue to work for our patients, pet owners, and veterinary teams in all capacities and roles in the veterinary practice through the new norms – thank you. You are not alone.

Summary of Key Features

Comprehensive Guide

This book was written as a quick reference guide. Its purpose is to assist an already trained and credentialed veterinary technician throughout the work day – providing a refresher for a seldom-taken radiograph, for example, or a pharmacology reminder to help answer a client's question. The veterinary technology/nursing student will also find this book useful as a supplement to more in-depth textbooks as they finish training and join the workforce.

Unique Chart and Table Format

The format of this book uses charts and tables and short passages for the efficient retrieval of pertinent information. This format leads veterinary technicians and nurses straight to the answers they need to perform a task quickly.

Extensive Set of Figures

More than 300 illustrations and photographs will provide visual assistance to the veterinary technicians and nurses performing laboratory tests, dentistry, client education, and much more.

Expansive Indexing

A comprehensive table of contents at the beginning and throughout each chapter will ease the movement through this information-rich text.

Companion Website

A collection of over 75 fully editable client education and training documents, together with over 600 vocabulary flash cards and a selection of review questions available online.

Contributors

Current Contributors

Megan Brashear, BS, RVT, VTS (ECC)
Small Animal Veterinary Nursing Manager
Purdue University Veterinary Hospital, West Lafayette, Indiana, USA

Marg Brown, RVT, BEdAdEd

Danielle Browning, LVMT, VTS (Surgery)
Large Animal Operating Room Technician
University of Tennessee Veterinary Medical Center Knoxville, TN

Kara M. Burns, MS, MEd, LVT, VTS (Nutrition)
Academy of Veterinary Nutrition Technicians

Ed Carlson, CVT, VTS (Nutrition)
Director of Veterinary Nursing Education
VetBloom

Jenny Cassibry Fisher, RVT, VTS (Oncology)
Director of Education
PractiVet, Tempe Arizona

Wendy Davies, BS, CVT, CCRVN, VTS (Physical Rehabilitation)
University of Florida Small Animal Hospital
Integrative Medicine Service-Physical Rehabilitation, Acupuncture, Nutrition and Hyperbaric Medicine
Gainesville, Florida 32610

Tina DeVictoria, BS, CVT, VTS (Clinical Practice C/F)
NorthStar VETS, Robbinsville, NJ, USA

Kathleen Dunbar, BA, RVT, VTS (Clinical Practice C/F)
Carnegy Animal Hospital, Nova Scotia, Canada

H. Edward Durham Jr, CVT, RVT, LATG, VTS (Cardiology)
Senior Cardiology Technician
Southwest Florida Veterinary Specialists
Bonita Springs, FL USA

Monique Feyrecilde, BA, LVT, VTS (Behavior)
Teaching Animals
Washington, USA

Mandy Fults, MS, LVT, CVPP, VTS (Clinical Practice C/F)
Director of Veterinary Nursing
Liberty Hill Texas, USA

Stephanie Gilliam, RVTg, MS, CCRP, VTS (Neurology)
Director of Veterinary Technology
Moberly Area Community College
Mexico, Missouri

Mary Ellen Goldberg, LVT, CVT, SRA, CCRVN, CVPP, VTS (Lab Animal), (Physical Rehabilitation), (Anesthesia and Analgesia-H)
Independent Consultant
Examination Coordinator Canine Rehabilitation Institute
Boynton Beach, Florida USA

Sandy Gregory, M.Ed, RVT, VTS (Physical Rehabilitation), CCRA
Associate Professor Foothill College, CA
Animal rehabilitation - Beacon Veterinary Specialists, CA

Kristen L Hagler, BS(An.Phys), RVT, VTS (Physical Rehabilitation), CCRP, CVPP, COCM, CBW, VCC
Head of Canine Programs Circle Oak Rehabilitation - Equine and Canine Center
Petaluma, USA

Chantelle Hanna, BS, CVT, VTS (Dermatology)-Charter Member

Natalie Herring, LVT, VTS (Ophthalmology)
Veterinary Technician Manager
BluePearl Christiana, Delaware, USA

Nicole LaForest, MPH, LVT, RVT
Locum Veterinary Technician Surgery and Anesthesia
Greater Seattle Area, Washington

Caitlin Lewis, RVT
Career Consultant
Evolve Veterinary Consulting
Adjunct Instructor, Veterinary Technology Program, Tulsa Community College,
Oklahoma, USA

Tami Lind, BS, RVT, VTS (ECC)
Emergency/Critical Care Veterinary Technician Supervisor
Purdue University Veterinary Hospital, West Lafayette, Indiana, USA

Ella Mitelberg, LVT, VTS (SAIM)
Lead Internal Medicine Technician
Austin Veterinary Emergency and Specialty Center, Austin, Texas, USA

Barbie M. Papajeski, MS, LVT, RLATG, VTS (Clinical Pathology)
Senior Instructor, Veterinary Technology/Pre-Veterinary Dept.
Murray State University, Murray, Kentucky, USA

Paula Plummer, LVT, VTS (ECC), (SAIM)
Texas A&M University Veterinary Teaching Hospital, Texas, USA

Heidi Reuss-Lamky, LVT, VTS, (Anesthesia/Analgesia),(Surgery), CFVP
Fear Free Elite Certified Professional
Surgery Technician
Oakland Veterinary Referral Services, Michigan, USA

Liza W. Rudolph, BAS, RVT, VTS (Clinical Practice- C/F),(SAIM)
Owner and Consultant
East Coast Veterinary Education, Maryland, USA

Heather A. Sidari, RVT, VTS (Anesthesia & Analgesia)
Anesthesia Supervisor
North Carolina State University - College of Veterinary Medicine
Veterinary Teaching Hospital, Raleigh, NC

Cristall Short, BSN, RN, CEN, CCRN, RVT, AAS
New Mexico Veterans Affairs Medical Center, Emergency Department
AirCare1 International, Critical Care Flight RN

Tammi Smith, MEd, CVT, VTS (Dentistry)
Chief Instructor at Veterinary Dental Education Services, Inc.

Rebeccah Vaughan, CVT, VTS (Anesthesia/Analgesia), (Clinical Practice-C/F)
Anesthesia Technician
VCA Aurora, Aurora, IL

Courtney Waxman, MS, CVT, RVT, VTS (ECC)
Distance Learning Instructional Technologist
Purdue University, Indiana, USA
Veterinary Nursing Development Manager
Veterinary Emergency Group, New York, USA

Kenichiro Yagi, MS, RVT, VTS (ECC), (SAIM)
Chief Veterinary Nursing Officer
Veterinary Emergency Group, New York, USA

Previous Contributors

Dina Andrews, DVM, PhD, Dip. ACVP
Gary Averbeck, MS
Byron Blagburn, MS, PhD
Richard Bowen, DVM, PhD
Dana Brooks, DVM, DACVIM
Daniel Chan, DVM, DACVECC, DACVN, MRCVS
John Chandler, DVM, MS, DACVS
Markiva Contris, LVT, CCRP
Mikki Cook, LVT
Kimberly Coyner, DVM, DACVD
Cindy Elston, DVM
Jay R. Georgi, DVM, PhD
J. Michael Harter, DVM
Peter Hellyer, DVM, MS, DACVA
Teri Hermann, RVT
Joyce Knoll, VMD, PhD, Dip. ACVP
Brita Kraabel, DVM
Bob Kramer, DVM, DACVR

Sally Lester, DVM, MVS, DACVP
Jody Lulich, DVM, PhD, DACVIM
Veronica Martin, LVT
James H. Meinkoth, DVM, DACVP
Kathryn Michel, DVM, MS, Dip. ACVN
Jeb Mortimer, DVM
Richard Panzer, DVM, MS
Anne Rains
Tara Raske
Patrick Richardson, DVM
Robert K. Ridley, DVM, PhD
Narda Robinson, DO, DVM, MS, FAAMA
Nancy Shaffran, CVT, VTS (ECC)
Stuart Spencer, DVM
Cheryl Stockman, MT (ASCP)
Sandy Willis, DVM, MVSc, DACVIM
DentaLabels
MILA International, Inc.
Laura Tautz-Hair, LVT, VTS (ECC)
Animal Emergency and Trauma Center
Hill's Pet Nutrition
International Veterinary Association of Pain Management
Iowa University Press
Phoenix Central Laboratories
David Stansfield/Novartis

About the Companion Website

This book is accompanied by a companion website:

www.wiley.com/go/fults/veterinary

The website includes:

- Figures
- Study guide questions and answers
- Supplementary Material
- Vocabulary
- Online Resources
- Glossary
- Abbreviations

Section One

Anatomy

Chapter 1

Anatomy

Sandy Gregory, M.Ed, RVT, VTS (Physical Rehabilitation), CCRA

Veterinary Technician and Nurse's Daily Reference Guide: Canine and Feline, Fourth Edition. Edited by Mandy Fults and Kenichiro Yagi.

Companion website: www.wiley.com/go/fults/veterinary

Abbreviations

AV, atrioventricular
CNS, central nervous system
PNS, peripheral nervous system
SA, sinoatrial

For a veterinary technician to be able to accurately complete many of their daily tasks, a clear understanding of the anatomy of the canine and feline body is needed. The following diagrams show the basic layout of the body systems.

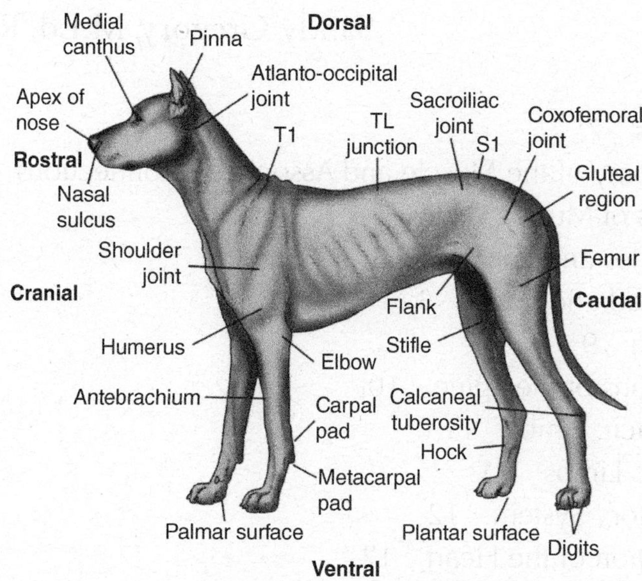

Figure 1.1 Overall anatomy.

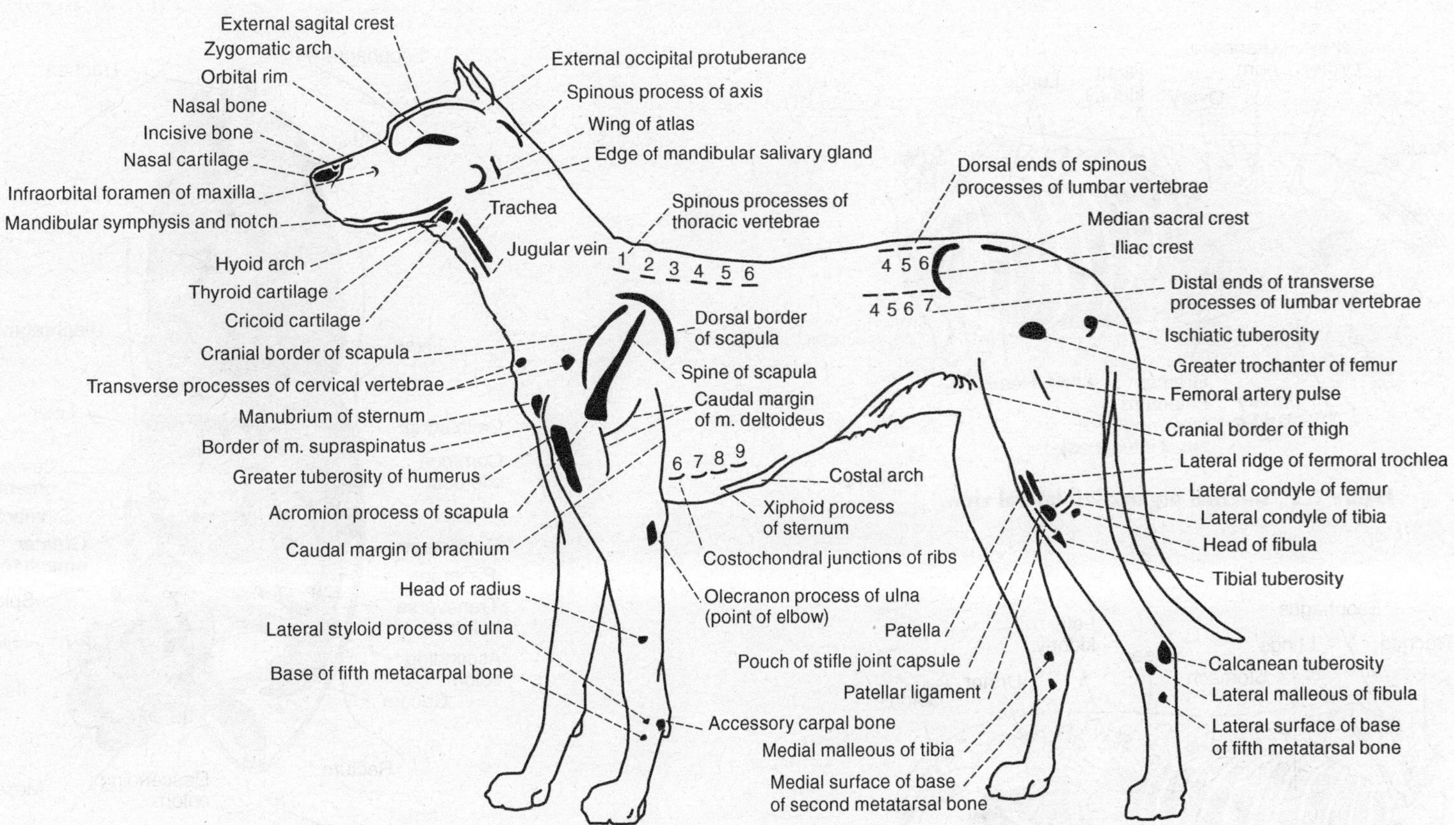

Figure 1.2 Palpation landmarks.

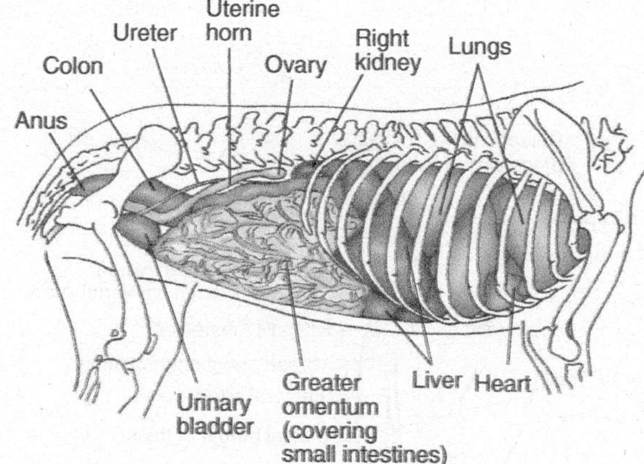

Figure 1.3 Internal organs: left lateral view.

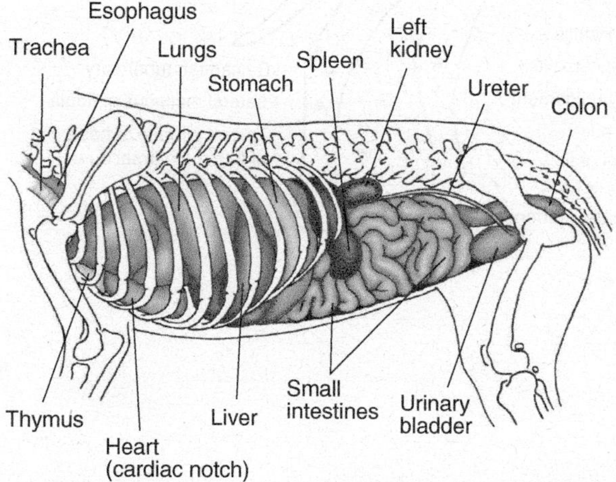

Figure 1.4 Internal organs: right lateral view.

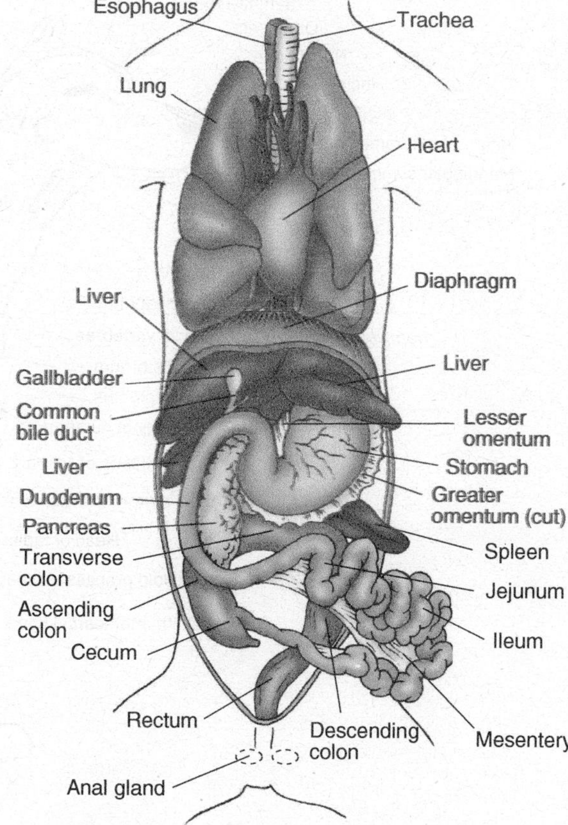

Figure 1.5 Internal organs: ventral view.

MUSCLES

The muscular system is closely connected to the nervous system. Animals can consciously or voluntarily control certain muscles. While other muscles are involuntarily controlled. There are three main types of muscles found in animals:

- Smooth—non-striated and involuntary (found in the visceral, intestines, and blood for example).
- Cardiac—striated and involuntary (found in the heart).
- Skeletal—striated and voluntary (skeletal muscles).

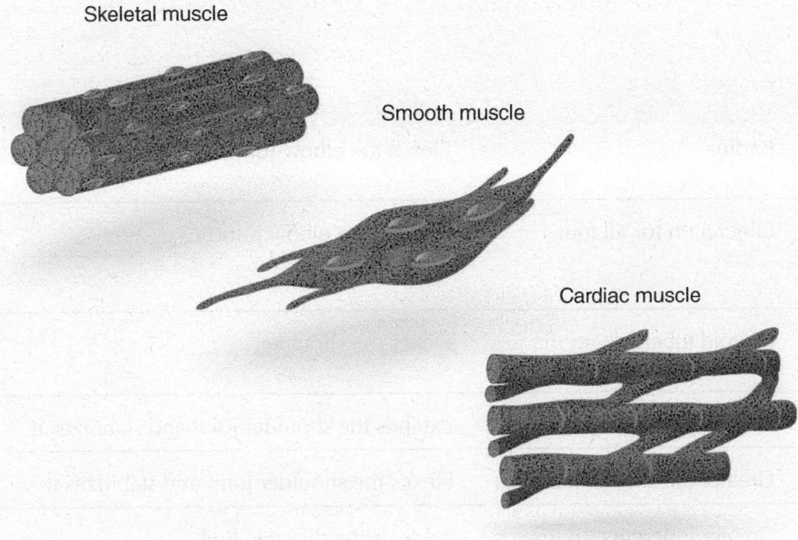

Figure 1.6 Three types of muscle tissue.

Skeletal muscles work essentially based on what is called the "sliding filament theory". The muscle has a stimulus to the nerve to begin the contraction. The muscles have striated muscle fibers that have elongated, striped dark and light bands. These functional groups of the striped muscles are arranged in a pattern called sarcomeres. Each of the striated muscle fibers have many threadlike fibers called myofibrils, which are made up of parallel filaments called *myosin* (thick) and *actin* (thin). The interaction and overlapping of these myofilaments create a separation of these units and shortens the sarcomere. The fibers then bind to create a cross-bridge. This shortens the muscle or creates a contraction.

Anatomy of the Muscle and Associated Connections

- Belly: the thickest, most fleshy central part.
- Head: where the belly tapers to at each end. It is here that the connective tissue of the tendon attaches muscle to the bone.
- Origin: the starting point of where the muscle attaches to the bone, which does not move when the muscle contracts.
- Insertion: the opposite end of the origin, where the muscle inserts and the movement occurs.
- Tendon: attaches muscle to bone.
- Ligament: attaches bone to bone.
- Bursa: a sac filled with synovial fluid between bony prominences and a tendon, ligament, or muscle.

Exceptions:

- A muscle can have a number of heads, such as the biceps brachii, which has two heads.
- The length of the tendon attaching to a bone can vary. There are flexors and extensors that attach to the digits, which are much longer than the muscles themselves.
- Some muscles can be more flat or sheath like, such as the tensor fasciae latae muscle on the lateral thigh or a sheath on the abdominal wall.
- Circular muscles, such as the sphincter muscles, control the entrance or exit of that structure, such as the anal sphincters.

Types of Muscle Action

- Flexion: the movement of closing the joint angle or decreasing it.
- Extension: the movement of opening the joint angle or increasing it.
- Abduction: the movement of the body limb away from the midline.

- Adduction: the movement of the body limb toward the midline.
- Circumduction: the movement can be a combination of the above in a circular motion.
- Contracture: pathological, by which the muscles are fixed in a shortened position.

Muscles are always under some type of tension. The tension decreases when the muscle is relaxed or increased when there is movement or stress. Each muscle has a specific action based on the location and the function of that animal's everyday activity.

Muscles and Location

Head and Spine

Temporalis: the largest muscle of the head; closes the jaw. It covers much of the lateral and dorsal surfaces of the skull.

Epaxial: lie above the vertebral column. If over the lumbar area, they are called the paralumbar muscle group. They support the spine and provide extension and lateral flexion.

Table 1.1 / Muscles

Muscle	Location	Origin	Insertion	Action
Biceps brachii	Craniomedial surface of the humerus	Scapula	Radius	Flexes the elbow joint
Triceps brachii	Caudal aspect of the humerus	4 heads with separate origins: 3 originate from the proximal humerus, 4th from the scapula	Olecranon for all four	Extends the elbow joint
Deltoid	Lateral scapula and shoulder	Spine of the scapula and acromion	Deltoid tuberosity of the humerus	Flexes the shoulder
Supraspinatus	Cranial to the spine of the scapula	Supraspinatus fossa of scapula	Greater tubercle of humerus	Extends the shoulder joint and stabilizes it
Infraspinatus	Caudal to the spine of the scapula	Infraspinatus fossa of scapula	Greater tubercle of humerus	Flexes the shoulder joint and stabilizes it
Pectorals	Ventral thorax	Sternum	Greater tubercle of humerus	Adducts the thoracic limbs
Muscles of the Pelvic Limbs				
Bicep femoris	Lateral most muscle of the hamstring group on the thigh	Ischiatic tuberosity of pelvis	Patella, proximal tibia and calcaneus of the hock	Extends the hip, flexes stifle and extends tarsus
Semitendinosus	Caudal thigh more lateral	Ischiatic tuberosity of pelvis	Tibia and calcaneus	Extends the hip, flexes stifle and extends tarsus
Semimembranosus	Caudal thigh most medial of the hamstrings	Ischiatic tuberosity of pelvis	Femur and tibia	Extends the hip

(Continued)

Table 1.1 / Muscles (Continued)

Muscle	Location	Origin	Insertion	Action
Gluteal (3 muscles: superficial, middle, and deep)	Lateral thigh at hip	Ilium and superficial is at the sacrum	Greater trochanter of femur	Abducts the pelvic limb and extends the hip
Sartorius	Craniomedial surface of the humerus (has 2 heads)	Crest of ilium	Cranial tibia and patella	Flexes the hip/extends the stifle
Quadriceps (4 muscles)	Cranial surface of the thigh	Ilium and proximal femur	Tibial tuberosity	Extends the stifle and flexes the hip (tendon of this muscle contains the patella)
Cranial tibialis	Cranial surface, proximal to the stifle	Cranial border of tibia	Proximal metatarsus	Flexes the tarsus
Gastrocnemius	Caudal surface, proximal of the stifle	Medial and lateral supracondylar tuberosities of femur	Proximal dorsal surface of calcaneus	Extends the tarsus/flexes the stifle

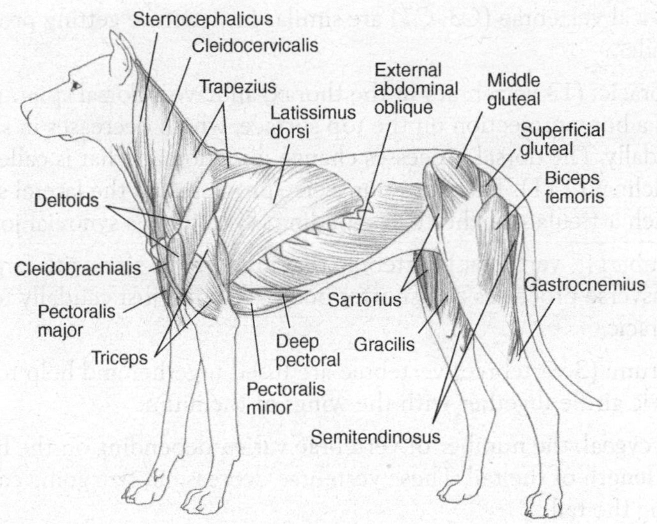

Figure 1.7 Musculature: lateral view.

SKELETON

The skeletal system is the support structure for the dog and cat. This base is what gives the animal its structure for movement, protection for soft tissues, storage of essential minerals, and production of red blood cells.

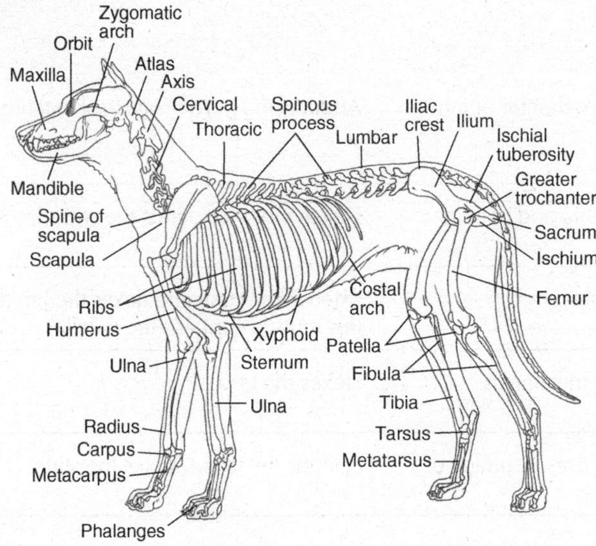

Figure 1.8 Skeletal: lateral view.

Bones are classified by their shape:

- Long bones: longer than they are wide, these bones are the main supporting bones of the body, such as femur, humerus, tibia, and fibula.
- Short bones: short, cube shaped, provide stability and some movement, such as carpal and tarsal bones.
- Flat bones: thin, flat bones with a protective function such as the ribs, pelvis, skull, and scapula.
- Irregular bones: asymmetrical, without a paired bone, and lie in the midline of the body such as the vertebrae.
- Sesamoid bones: sesame seed-shaped bones associated with joints, and often within a tendon, to reduce the stress and further protection.

The skeleton can be broken down into two general sections. The axial skeleton includes the skull, vertebrae, sternum, and ribs. The appendicular skeleton includes the appendages of the thoracic and pelvic limbs.

The skull is made up of the cranium and the mandible. It protects the brain and provides attachment for such muscles involved in chewing, facial expression, and swallowing. The hyoid apparatus, or hyoid bone, sits in the intermandibular space. It provides a suspension mechanism for the tongue and the pharynx and holds the larynx in place.

The vertebral column consists of sections starting at the base of the skull, extending to the tail. Depending on their position in the body, they have different shapes and numbers. The functions of the vertebrae are to provide protection for the spinal cord; they interlock to provide movement and support.

Sections of the Spine

- Cervical: (7 vertebrae) known as the neck region. The first cervical vertebra (C1) is called the atlas; it has a unique lateral bony process called the wings of the atlas. C2 is called the axis. The remaining cervical vertebrae (C3–C7) are similar in structure getting progressively smaller.
- Thoracic: (13 vertebrae) in the thorax; all have a dorsal spinous process and a bony projection on the top surface, which decreases in size going caudally. The dorsal processes change direction at what is called the anticlinal (T11). There are transverse processes on the lateral surface, which articulate at the corresponding rib to form a synovial joint.
- Lumbar: (7 vertebrae) vertebrae that are large in size, with larger transverse processes and shorter bodies, located just caudally to the thoracic.
- Sacrum: (3 vertebrae) vertebrae are fused together and help to form the pelvic girdle together with the wings of the ilium.
- Coccygeal: the number of vertebrae varies, depending on the breed and the length of the tail. These vertebrae decrease in size going caudally along the tail.

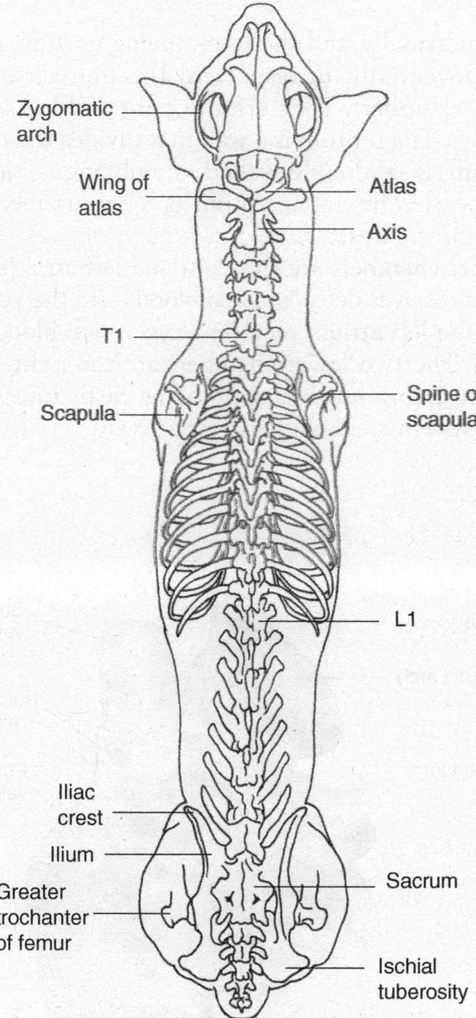

Figure 1.9 Skeletal: dorsal view.

Thoracic Limbs

- Scapula or shoulder blade: a large, flat bone with a bony ridge (spine of the scapula) down the center. The distal point of this ridge is another bony projection called the acromion. Just distal to this is a divot. It is here that the shoulder joint is palpable.
- Greater tubercle: forms the shoulder joint where the neck of the scapula narrows. The greater tubercle is a palpable prominence on the lateral surface of the proximal humerus.
- Humerus: the long bone forming the brachium of the thoracic limbs. This is the bone proximal to the elbow.
- Ulna: the long bone distal to the humerus. Just proximal on the edge of the bone is the olecranon. The olecranon is what is known as the elbow.
- Radius: the other long bone next to the ulna but shorter, which is the weight-bearing bone. This is considered the antebrachium, together with the ulna, meaning before the brachium, and is known as the forearm.
- Carpus: seven cube-shaped bones that make up the wrist.
- Metacarpus: five long bones distal to the carpus. The most medial is shorter and non-weight-bearing.
- Digits: made up of long bones called phalanges. The proximal phalanx articulates with the corresponding metacarpal bone.

Pelvic Limbs

- Pelvis: connects the hind limbs to the body. The pelvis is formed by three bones – the ischium, ilium, and pubis. All three meet at the acetabulum, which is a cup-shaped socket in which the femur sits. The wings of the ilium are a formed ridge or crest on the ilium that is palpable.
- Acetabulum: forms the "socket" for the femur to sit in, making up the ball-and-socket hip joint.

- Femur: the long bone that makes up the thigh of the pelvic limbs just distal to the hip joint.
- Greater trochanter: a palpable prominence on the lateral surface of the proximal femur.
- Patella: a small sesamoid bone that sits in a groove on top of the femur at the distal end, located within the tendon at the insertion of the main thigh muscle.
- Tibia: one of two long bones that make up the distal part of the hind limbs. This bone is more medial and proximally makes up the joint called the stifle. This is part of the tarsal bone, palpable on the medial surface, which is called the medial malleolus.
- Fibula: the second of the two long bones of the distal pelvic limb, more lateral and the smaller of the two. This is the part of the tarsal bone, palpable on the lateral surface, called the lateral malleolus.
- Tarsus: seven cube-shaped bones that make up the ankle; also known as the hock.
- Metatarsus: long bones distal to the tarsus. Most dogs and cats have four metatarsal bones with some breeds having five.
- Digits: made up of long bones called phalanges. The proximal phalanx articulates with the corresponding metatarsal bone.

CIRCULATORY SYSTEM

The heart is a muscular four-chambered organ, which works as a pump to deliver blood around the body by a series of rhythmic contractions.

Function of the Heart

1. To deliver oxygen, nutrients, cellular waste and hormones to all the organs and tissues.
2. To deliver metabolic waste and carbon dioxide to organs for excretion.

The heart lies in the thoracic cavity, slightly to the left of the midline and within the mediastinum, the space formed between the two pleural cavities of the thorax. The portion of the heart, termed the base, is positioned dorsocranially, and the free-moving portion, called the apex, is positioned caudoventrally, in respect to the transverse plane. The heart consists of four chambers. They are the right and left atria and the right and left ventricles. The septum is a wall that divides the right and left sides. The pericardium is a double-walled membranous sac protecting and enclosing the heart. The endocardium is a serous membrane lining the inner chambers of the heart.

The two upper chambers are the right and left atria (singular is atrium). The right atrium receives deoxygenated blood from the veins of the systemic circulation and the left atrium receives oxygen-rich blood from the pulmonary circulation. The two lower chambers are the right and left ventricles. They function to pump out blood from the heart into the arteries of the pulmonary and systemic circulations, respectively.

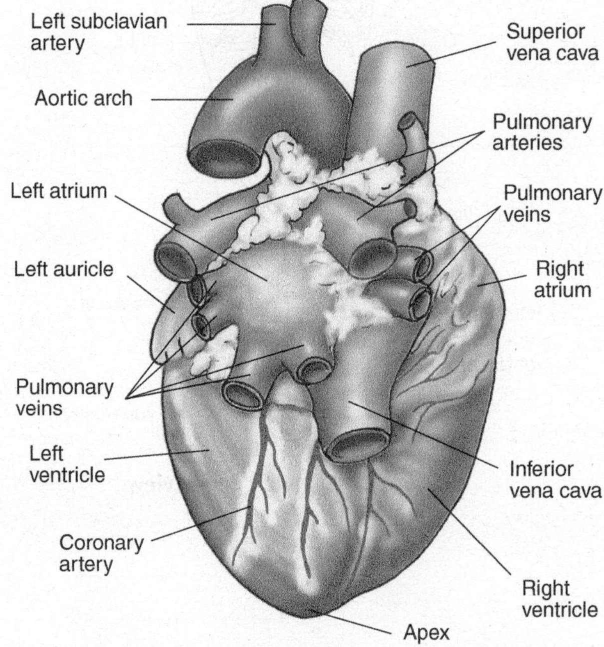

Figure 1.10 Circulatory: dorsal view of heart.

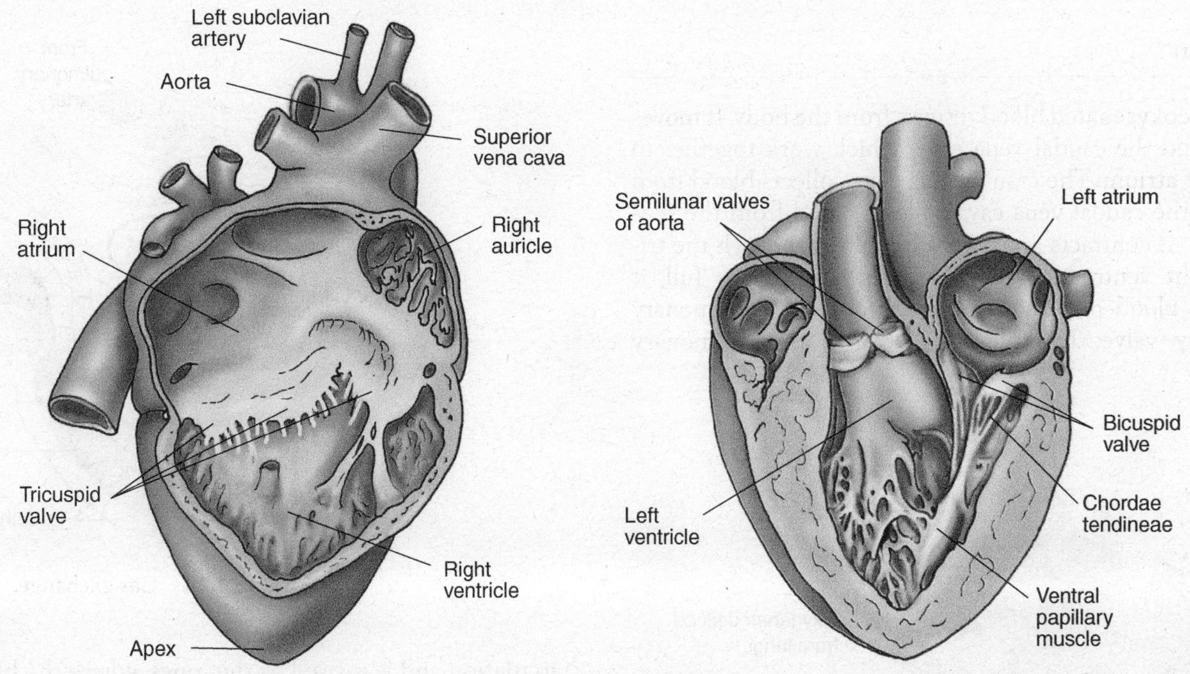

Figure 1.11 Circulatory: Internal view of heart.

Structure of the Heart Wall

- Inner layer: the endocardium is continuous with all the blood vessels.
- Middle layer: the myocardium is a single layer of the cardiac muscle and is capable of rhythmic contractions. Control of this muscle is involuntary because of the autonomic nervous system. The myocardium is thickest in the left ventricle because it must pump the blood into the aorta and all around the body.
- Outer layer: the epicardium is a double layer of epithelial cells on the outside.

- Heart valves:
  - Right atrioventricular (AV) or tricuspid valve lies between the right ventricle and right atrium, which can be identified by its three fibrous flaps or cusps. These fibrous rings encircle the opening of the right ventricle.
  - Left AV, bicuspid, or mitral valve lies between the left ventricle and left atrium, and can be identified by its two cusps.
  - Pulmonary valve lies at the base of the pulmonary artery as it leaves the right ventricle.
  - Aortic valve lies at the base where the aorta leaves the left ventricle.
- The chordae tendineae are threadlike cords that connect the bicuspid and tricuspid valves to the walls of the ventricles.

Pulmonary Circulation

Circulation occurs when deoxygenated blood returns from the body. It moves to the cranial vena cava and the caudal vena cava, which work together to empty blood into the right atrium. The cranial vena cava collects blood from the head and neck, while the caudal vena cava collects blood from the thoracic limbs. When it is full, it contracts and forces the blood through the tricuspid valve into the right ventricle. When the right ventricle is full, it contracts and pumps the blood out of the heart through the pulmonary artery via the pulmonary valve. The blood is now in the pulmonary circulation and is carried to the lungs, where the blood becomes oxygenated before returning to the heart via the pulmonary veins.

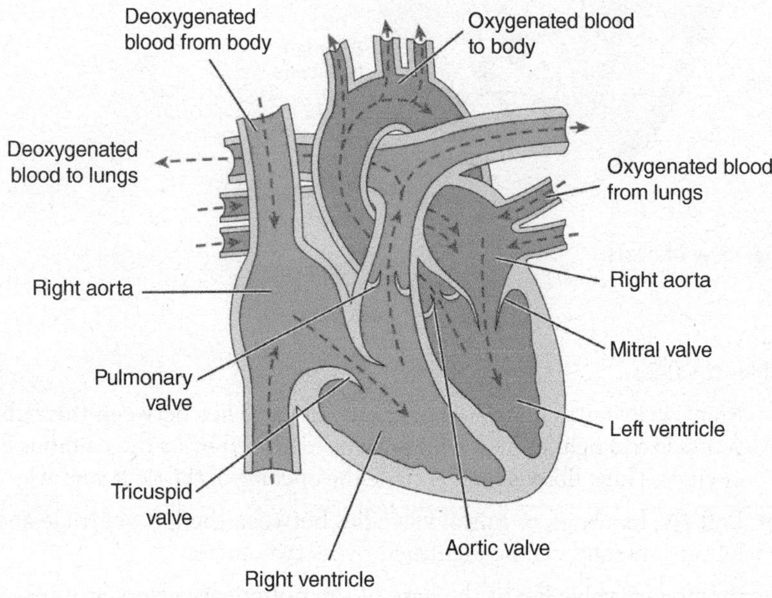

Figure 1.12 Route of deoxygenated to oxygenated blood.

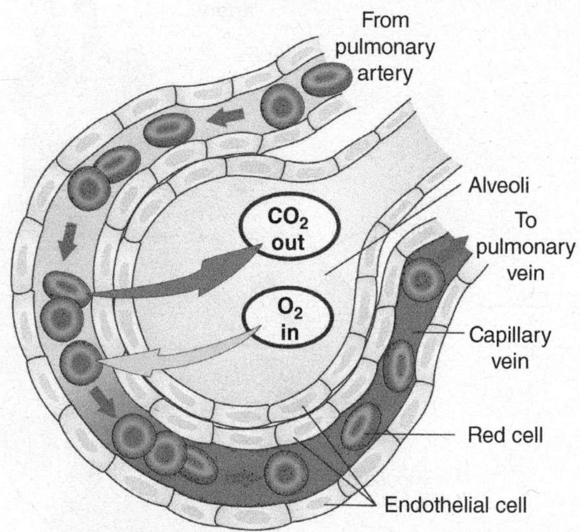

Figure 1.13 Gas exchange.

Systemic Circulation

The richly oxygenated blood from the lungs is carried into the pulmonary veins back to the left side of the heart. Blood enters the left atrium, contracting when it is full, forcing the blood through the bicuspid valve into the left ventricle. When the left ventricle is full, it contracts and is forced to pump blood out of the aorta to all parts of the body.

Blood Flow Sequence

→capillaries → venules → systemic veins → cranial and caudal vena cava → right atrium → tricuspid valve → right ventricle → pulmonary valve → pulmonary artery → lung → pulmonary vein → left atrium → bicuspid valve → left ventricle → aortic valve → aorta → systemic arteries → arterioles → capillaries

Blood Vessels

- Arteries carry oxygenated blood away from the heart to the body. They are more muscular and thicker than veins. Located usually deeper within the body.
- Arterioles are small arteries that travel to the capillaries and help to regulate the blood flow.
- Capillaries are branching blood vessels between the arterioles and the venules.
- Venules are smaller blood vessels that return deoxygenated blood from the capillaries into the veins.
- Veins are larger than arteries but have thinner walls. Blood pressure is low within them, although blood maintains a forward flow toward the heart due to backflow prevention valves.

Cardiac Cycle

One complete cycle of the heart consists of the atria contracting, known as systole, followed by the ventricle relaxing, known as diastole. This rhythmic cycle happens without input from the nervous system, unless there is a stressful event requiring stimulation from the autonomic nervous system for physiologic control.

Conduction System

The conduction system serves to coordinate the spread of the electrical activity and thus coordinates a contraction of the heart muscle, which results in effective filling and ejection of blood. Electrical activity initiated in one part of the heart readily spreads to adjacent regions, causing a wave that will spread through the heart muscle.

- Sinoatrial (SA) node: known as the pacemaker of the heart, setting the sinus rhythm. It is where the heartbeat begins. The SA node is found in the wall of the right atrium near the entrance of the inferior vena cava. The autonomic nerves can affect the contraction here. As the contraction starts, blood is pushed through the bicuspid and tricuspid valves and then into the ventricles.
- Depolarization of the SA node results in potential activity throughout both atria and triggers a contraction. Sodium and calcium ions move through channels from the exterior to the interior of the cell causing a contraction. Potassium ions do the reverse and move from the interior of the cell to the exterior.
- AV node: located at the top of the septum above the tricuspid valve. The AV node causes a slight delay before going to the ventricles. This delay helps to give time for the atria to completely contract before the ventricles contract.
- Bundle of His is where this potential activity travels to next. It lies in the cranial portion of the septum. The activity moves toward the apex of the heart from there.
- Purkinje fibers: specialized neurons that branch out and spread to the ventricular muscle walls. They pick up the impulse and carry them from the bundle of His and up to the myocardium of the ventricles. The conduction is complete, causing a contraction that travels from the apex to the base of the heart.

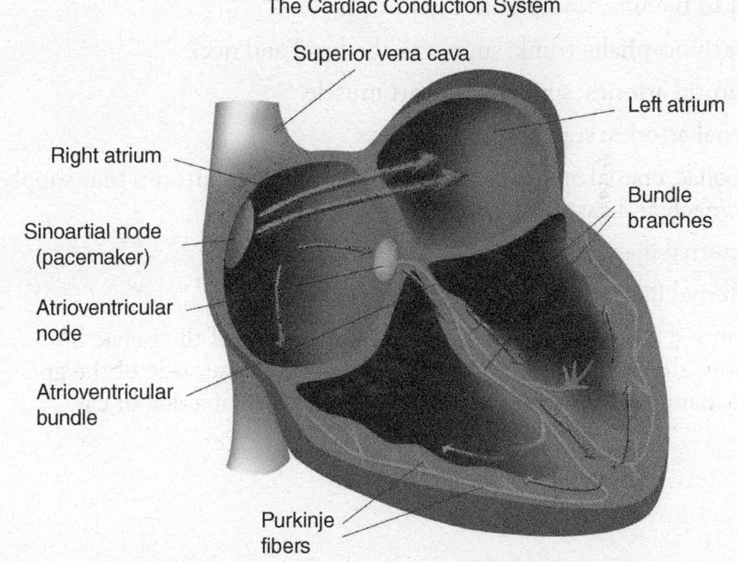

Figure 1.14 Cardiac conduction system.

Cardiac Conductive System Sequence

→ SA node → Atrium → AV node →> bundle of His → bundle branches → ventricular contraction

When auscultating or listening to the heart, you will hear a "lub-dub" and then a pause. The first sound is the "lub", a longer sound made when the AV valves close. The "dub" is the quicker sound made when the semilunar (pulmonary and aortic) valves close.

Arterial Circulation

When oxygenated blood leaves the left ventricle through the major artery, the aorta, it goes through multiple branches. Arteries carry blood away from the heart.

- Subclavian artery, left: supply to the left thoracic limb.
- Subclavian artery, right: supply to the right thoracic limb and branches off to the brachiocephalic trunk.
- Brachiocephalic trunk: supply to the head and neck.
- Carotid arteries: supply the heart muscle.
- Renal arteries: supply to the kidneys.
- Coeliac, cranial and caudal mesenteric: unpaired arteries that supply the stomach and gastrointestinal tract.
- External iliac arteries: supply the pelvic limbs.
- Internal iliac arteries: supply the pelvic viscera.
- Femoral artery: lies deep on the medial surface of the pelvic limbs at about the midpoint of the thigh itself on the other side of the greater trochanter. This is the site for feeling the pulse of a dog or cat.

Venous Circulation

Veins carry blood to the heart.

- Cranial vena cava: collects blood from the head and neck via the jugular veins and the subclavian veins.
- Caudal vena cava: collects blood from the pelvic viscera, pelvic limbs, and organs of the abdomen via parallel patterns of arteries.
- Azygous vein: collects blood from the thoracic body wall.
- Cephalic vein: a superficial vein that runs between the elbow and carpus on the craniomedial surface.
- Saphenous vein: a superficial vein that runs laterally and medially on the pelvic limbs between the tarsus and the stifle.
- Femoral vein: a superficial vein along the medial surface of the pelvic limbs between the stifle joint and the inguinal area.

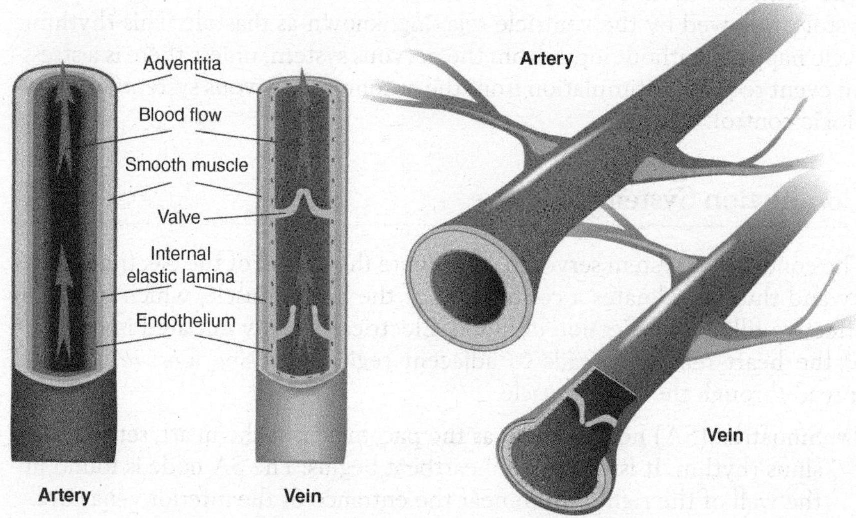

Figure 1.15 Artery and vein comparison.

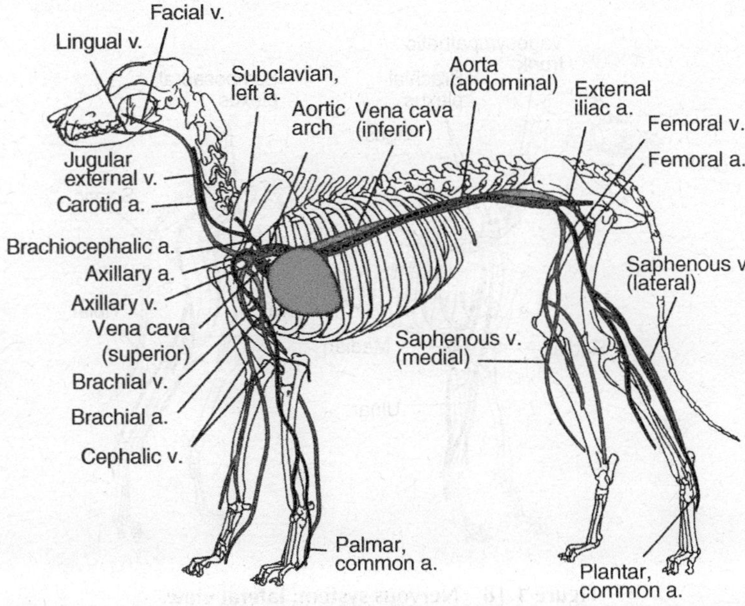

Figure 1.16 Circulatory: lateral view.

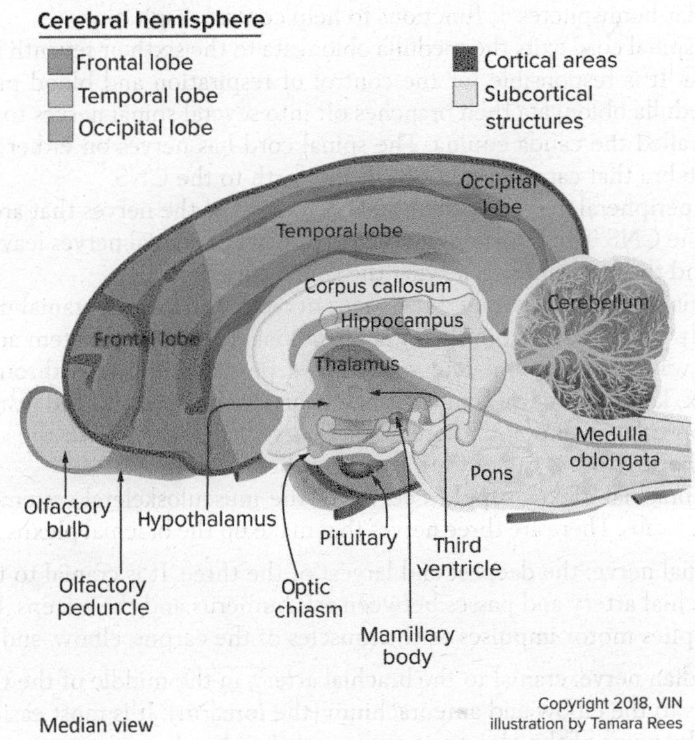

Figure 1.17 Canine brain.

NERVOUS SYSTEM

The nervous system can be divided into two sections. The central and peripheral nervous systems make up this well-integrated unit.

The central nervous system (CNS) consists of the spinal cord and the brain. The function of the brain is to control and regulate movement of the body. Control of the CNS is conscious or voluntary. This is when the animal can feel pain or is aware of making a movement.

There are three main sections to the brain for many mammals

- Forebrain: comprising the cerebrum, thalamus, and hypothalamus.
- Midbrain: the passage between the forebrain and hindbrain in either direction.
- Hindbrain: comprising the cerebellum, pons, and medulla oblongata.

The cerebrum has a right and left hemisphere, which consists of 90% of all neurons in the body. The corpus callosum links the right and left sides. The gyri are folds in the tissue like peaks and the sulci are like a valley; both help nutrients to reach the neuron cell bodies. The function of the thalamus is to process information from the sense organs and to relay that information to the cerebral cortex. The hypothalamus is the connection between the endocrine and the nervous system. Even though it is small, it has a large role. It controls most of the endocrine glands by secreting the releasing hormones and stores them in the pituitary gland. Importantly, it helps to regulate homeostasis.

In the forebrain, the cerebellum controls balance and coordination. It also has two hemispheres covered with deep crevices. It is here that information is received from the semicircular canals of the inner ear. The cerebellum will coordinate the final modifications for voluntary movements that are initiated in the cerebrum. The pons is the bridge for the nerve fibers between the cerebellar hemispheres. It functions to help control respiration.

The spinal cord exits the medulla oblongata to the sixth or seventh lumbar vertebra. It is responsible for the control of respiration and blood pressure. The medulla oblongata then branches off into several spinal nerves to form a group called the cauda equina. The spinal cord has nerves on either side of the vertebra that carry impulses back and forth to the CNS.

The peripheral nervous system (PNS) consists of the nerves that are given off by the CNS. The PNS consists of the 12 pairs of cranial nerves leaving the brain and the spinal nerves leaving the spinal cord.

Cranial nerve X, also called the vagus nerve, is the longest cranial nerve in the body. It originates from the medulla oblongata of the brainstem and runs all the way to the colon. The vagus nerve provides impulses through the pharynx, larynx, trachea, tongue, lungs, heart, esophagus, and the rest of the digestion tract. The point where cranial nerve XII merges with the cervical sympathetic trunk is called the vagosympathetic trunk.

The brachial plexus supplies nerves of the musculoskeletal system in the thoracic limbs. There are three nerves that make up the brachial plexus nerves:

- Radial nerve: the deepest and largest of the three. It is cranial to the brachial artery and passes between the humerus and the triceps. It supplies motor impulses to the muscles of the carpus, elbow, and digits.
- Median nerve: cranial to the brachial artery, in the middle of the three runs to the elbow and antebrachium (the forearm). It is most easily seen at the point of the olecranon process of the ulna. It carries sensory impulses to the brain from the footpads.
- Ulnar nerve: located very superficially near the olecranon process of the ulna. It is comparable to the human "funny bone", which gives that tingly feeling when it is bumped hard. It carries impulses from the skin of the caudal antebrachium.

In the pelvic limbs, the nerve supply goes through the lumbosacral plexus. The biggest nerve that originates here is the sciatic nerve. This plexus is made up of the last four lumbar nerves and the three sacral nerves. It is well protected under the bicep femoris muscle but can have iatrogenic trauma such as improper injections into this muscle. Starting midpoint between the greater trochanter and the ischial tuberosity, it goes distally to branch at the stifle, then divides into the tibial and peroneal nerves to the digital flexors.

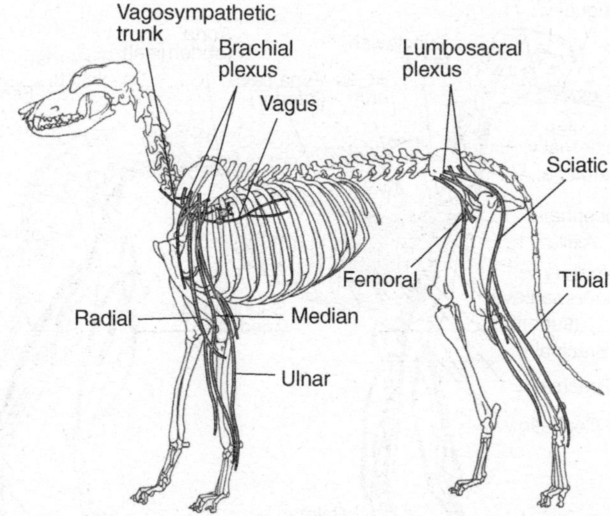

Figure 1.18 Nervous system: lateral view.

DIGESTION

Sequential Stages of Digestion

The function of the digestive system includes four sequential stages:

- Ingestion: food is taken in through the mouth.
- Digestion: food is broken down through the stomach and small intestine.
- Absorption: small units of food go into the bloodstream and the liver via the small intestine.
- Metabolism: food is converted into energy.

Dog and cat stomachs consist of a single chamber, and their digestion is termed "monogastric" because of the simple stomach. The digestive system starts working as soon as food enters the mouth. The main parts of the digestive system are:

- Mouth: including the lips, tongue, teeth.
- Pharynx.

- Esophagus.
- Stomach.
- Small intestine: duodenum, jejunum, ileum.
- Large intestine: cecum, transverse colon, ascending colon, descending colon, rectum, anus.
- Accessory glands: salivary glands, pancreas, gallbladder, liver.

How Digestion Works

Food is picked up with the lips and tongue. The teeth will start to cut and grind the food, turning it into a bolus. This formed food ball then gets lubricated with saliva by the salivary glands.

Next, the food passes the pharynx, which is the crossroad between the digestive and respiratory systems. The systems are separated from each other by the soft palate. The soft palate divides the pharynx into the nasopharynx and oropharynx. The epiglottis helps to keep food from entering the wrong places, such as the larynx and the trachea.

The esophagus is a continuation of the pharynx, which is a long tube transporting food to the stomach. It moves by what is called peristalsis. Peristalsis is an involuntary movement of the muscles that line the esophagus to create a wave-like movement advancing the food along the digestion process.

The stomach is a C-shaped organ in dogs and cats. Their stomachs lie mostly on the left side of the cranial abdomen. It is here that mucus is produced. The true body of the stomach produces gastric juices. The greater curvature is the outer, larger surface of the stomach. The lesser curvature is the innermost curve. The spleen has a loose attachment to the greater curvature. Its function is to help fight off infections and remove the non-functioning red blood cells. Inside are folds called rugae, which allow for expansion of the stomach and help mix the food with the digestive enzymes. When the stomach is full, these folds will flatten to allow for expansion.

There are sphincters in the stomach that help to control the rate at which food enters and leaves the stomach. The structure called the greater omentum is a fatty-tissue apron-like structure which hangs down over the greater curvature. It passes in front of the small intestine to the transverse colon. The lesser omentum hangs from the liver to the lesser curvature.

The small intestine is the main site for digestion and absorption. There are three divisions of the small intestine; they are similar in appearance but are hard to differentiate without using a microscope. The first part of the small intestine is the duodenum, which makes a U-shaped loop. Just medial to the duodenum and sitting within the loop is the pancreas. The two ducts (pancreatic and common bile duct) are routes of secretions for the pancreas. These secretions are bicarbonates and digestive enzymes. The largest and second part of the small intestine is the jejunum. The third and last is the ileum, which ends at the cecum. The junction where they meet is called the ileocecal junction.

The large intestine is appropriately named due to its larger diameter. It is here that water and electrolytes are absorbed from whatever is left from this breakdown. Mucus is added to help with elimination. The cecum is at the end of the ileocecal junction. It is considered a blind sac with very little function. The colon is divided into three sequential sections, starting with the ascending to the transverse and finally the descending colon. There is no clear distinction between the three parts of the colon other than their location.

Waste products move through the rectum and exit the anus.

Accessory Organs

The salivary gland is an accessory gland that provides minimal digestive enzyme activity. The primary function is to lubricate food and protect the oral mucosa. As food enters the mouth, it is mixed with amylase from this gland. Amylase breaks down into starch. To be used as a source of energy, it must be further broken down into soluble molecules to be absorbed into the bloodstream.

When food enters the stomach, it is mixed with the gastric juices, which are made up of protein-digesting enzymes called hydrochloric acid and mucus. The three sources of these digestive juices are pancreatic, bile, and intestinal secretions.

The pancreas is a mixed gland, with exocrine and endocrine parts. The endocrine contains the islets of Langerhans, which secrete the hormone insulin and glucagon. The exocrine portion releases bicarbonate and digestive enzymes into the duodenum and neutralizes acidic chyme.

The liver is the largest gland. It lies in the cranial abdomen close to the diaphragm. It has many functions, from carbohydrate metabolism to protein and fat metabolism. Amino acids and simple sugars are absorbed through the blood and are carried to the liver via the hepatic portal vein. The hepatic portal vein is a branch that carries deoxygenated and prefiltered blood from the digestive tract, spleen, pancreas, and gall bladder back to the liver.

The gall bladder is a small sac within the lobes of the liver that collects bile. Bile contains bile salts that emulsify fat during digestion. It is secreted into the duodenum by the common bile duct.

The whole process of digestion results in products that are carried around the body where they are metabolized and used by tissues. Any indigestible or unnecessary food is excreted in the feces.

INTEGUMENT

The largest organ in the body is the skin. Skin is the common integument system and includes the hair, footpads, nose pad, and claws. Accessory organs also included are the mammary, sweat, and sebaceous glands. The skin creates a barrier over the body where it meets with the mucous membrane lining at various openings such as the anus and mouth.

Functions

There is a contrast with the location and layers of the skin that determine its function. The functions include:

1. Protection from the environment: thicker cells, such as on the footpads, help to create a physical barrier against temperature and harmful microorganisms. Pigmentation helps against ultraviolet radiation.
2. Sensation: with many nerve endings that help to recognize temperature, pain, pressure, and touch. This sensation is then transferred through the CNS to the brain for information.
3. Secretion: glands under the skin provide various excretions. Sebum from the sebaceous gland keeps the skin waterproofed and lubricated. Sweat glands in cats and dogs are found primarily in the footpads; they are activated when the animal is too hot and help to regulate the temperature.
4. Storage of adipose tissue under the skin: serves as an insulating layer and a fat–energy storage. This adipose layer is also known as the subcutaneous layer or hypodermis.
5. Thermoregulation: keeps the core body temperature within the necessary limits. It prevents heat loss through vasoconstriction, diverting blood away from the surface. One way this happens is that the hair stands up, called piloerection, trapping the air underneath the hairs to keep in the warmth. Cooling happens mostly through panting, but some will happen through the sweat glands on the pads of the feet.
6. Production: this very important The process of absorption of vitamin D2 through ultraviolet rays starts in the skin.
7. Communication: provides a visual means to convey a message. When the hackles go up on a dog or cat, it is as a warning. Pheromones are released naturally through the skin itself or through the glands of the anal sacs.

Layers of the Skin

The actual integument layers consist of the epidermis and dermis. The outermost layer is the epidermis and is composed of three to five layers, depending on where it is located. The layers from deep to superficial are:

- Stratum basale: consists of the dividing cells in a single layer. This basement layer provides parent cells to all the other cells in the epidermis. Merkel cells help to provide sensory information to the animal at this level. Melanocytes supply the pigment melanin and carotene.
- Stratum spinosum: known as the spiny layer; there is some cell division in this layer. It is a relatively thick layer.
- Stratum granulosum: a granular layer where keratinization begins. The cells are starting to die at the upper border and continue to move superficially. Found only in the thick layer of the skin, not thin skin.
- Stratum lucidum: a translucent layer that is the thinnest of all the layers. Cells start to lose their nuclei. There are no real borders and this layer is only present in thick skin, not thin skin.
- Stratum corneum: the most superficial and toughest layer of the epidermis. These cells are essentially dead and fully keratinized. There are as many as 30 cell layers, which helps to provide thickness. This is seen on dogs and cats on their paw pads and their nose because of the increased protection needed at these sites.

Blood, lymphatic vessels and sensory nerve endings are found in the dermal layer just deep to the epidermis. The sebaceous glands, sweat glands, and hair follicles lie here.

The hypodermis or subcutaneous layer is not part of the integument system but is loose connective tissue below the dermis.

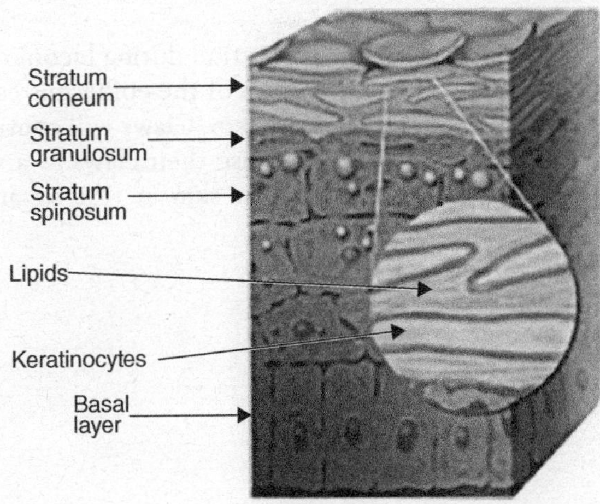

Figure 1.19 Structures of the skin. Source: Zoetis Inc. 2014.

Hair Formation

Hair covers almost the entire body of dogs and cats except for such places as the nose and paw pads. The hair is produced by individual hair follicles. The hair bulb is at the base of the follicle, with blood capillaries, known as dermal papilla, providing nutrients to the hair cells. They are formed from epidermal cells coming through the dermal layer. The cells within the bulb divide to produce a hair shaft. Dogs can have a group of three of these hair shafts per follicle. There are three main types of hairs:

- Guard hairs: thick, stiff, and long hairs that provide the outer, protective coat. They can give the waterproofing effect that help to repel water. Guard hairs primarily help to protect the dog or cat from such things as injury and maintaining normal body temperature. Each guard hair comes from the follicle with an arrector pili muscle attached to it. When this muscle contracts, it causes the hair to stand up.
- Wool hairs: form the innermost coat or undercoat. These hairs are thinner, shorter, and softer than guard hairs. There can be numerous wool hairs that grow from one follicle.
- Tactile hairs: surrounded by sensory cells such as Merkel cells to provide stimulus about the environment. Whiskers, also known as vibrissae, are tactile hairs on almost all mammals that allow an animal to feel. Usually found on the snout, above the eyes, but also on the feet, legs, and other parts of the body. They are stiffer and much longer than normal hair.

Hair grows continuously in a cycle, which includes a shedding or molting period. These cycles usually are based on the seasons. Hormones, seasons, nutrition, and health can all affect the growth cycle.

Foot Pads

Feet need the most protection and insulation from the environment than any other part of the skin. The pads are very thick, with more layers of the stratum corneum. They are composed of roughened conical papillae. These papillae give extra support and traction while walking or running. Adipose

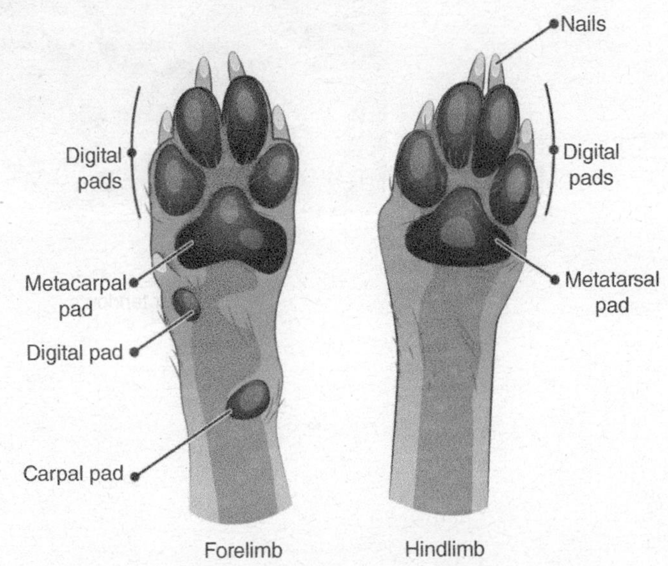

Figure 1.20 Forelimb and hindlimb paw pads.

tissue gives added insulation in the stratum corneum layer of the feet. These specialized pads cover the bottoms of the feet located appropriately at the ends of the digits and the joints.

Claws

The distal end of the phalanx on each digit has a bony extension called an ungual process. Covering this process is the claw, which is composed of keratinized cells. Their function is to give protection during locomotion and to provide extra grip. Each claw grows from part of the epidermis called the coronary border, which is under the fold of the skin. Claws will continuously grow through natural wear and tear. Cats can use their claws as a weapon, but they can also retract their claws into their skin at rest by an elastic ligament.

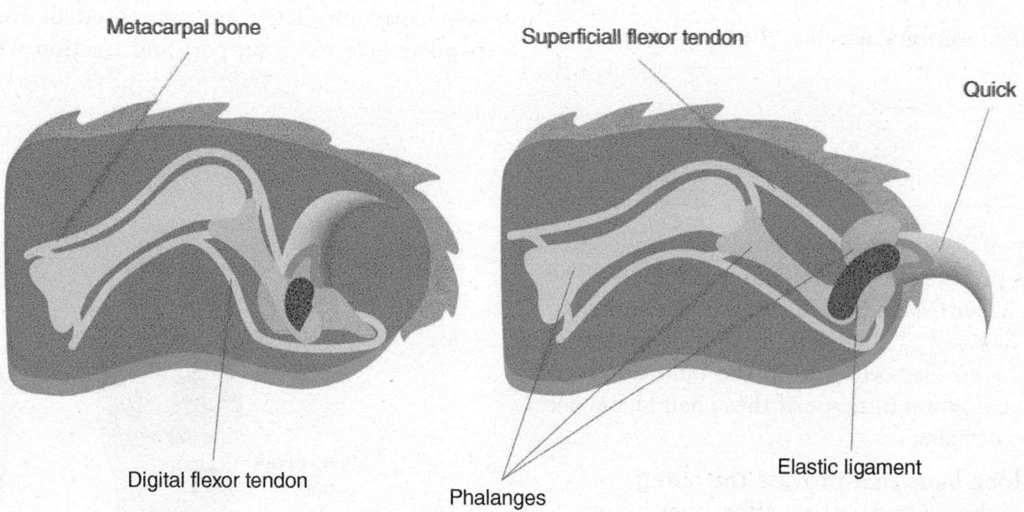

Figure 1.21 Claw.

RESPIRATORY SYSTEM

Respiration is the gaseous exchange between an organism and the environment. It is a system of tubes, held open by rings of cartilage, allowing air to flow in and out of the lungs. There are two stages of respiration:

- External respiration: gaseous exchange between air and blood, which occurs in the lungs.
- Internal respiration: gaseous exchange between the blood and tissues, together with getting rid of carbon dioxide, which occurs in the tissue.
- Ventilation: movement of air between the atmosphere and the lungs.

The upper respiratory tract, or upper airway, includes the nose, nasal passages, pharynx, larynx, and through to the cervical trachea. The lower respiratory tract includes extends from the thoracic trachea to the lungs.

The thoracic cavity is divided into the right and left pleural cavities by a double layer of pleura known as the mediastinum. Each pleural cavity is lined with a singular layer called the pleural membrane. The pleural membrane secretes a serous or watery fluid, which reduces friction between the pleural surfaces as the lungs move during respiration.

Structures of the Respiratory System

- Nose: opening to the nasal cavity.
- Septum: separates the right from the left side of the nasal cavity.
- Turbinate: multiple scroll-like, thin bones inside the nose, which are covered by mucous, which warm the air breathed, filters particles from entering and humidify the air as it passes through the nose.
- Pharynx: a short muscular tube located within the caudal aspect of the oral and nasal cavity, composed of three sections: oropharynx, nasopharynx, and laryngopharynx. The pharynx is the crossroads where the digestive tract and respiratory tract meet and is responsible for directing food and water into the esophagus and air into the larynx. The soft palate divides the pharynx further into the nasopharynx dorsally and the oropharynx ventrally. The nasopharynx helps direct the air breathed through the larynx.
- Larynx: lies between the pharynx and the trachea and is ventral to the esophagus. Its function is to help regulate the flow of gases from continuing on to the trachea and to prevent anything that is not a gas from getting into the respiratory tract. The hyoid bone (or hyoid apparatus) is a U-shaped structure that helps to suspend the larynx from the skull. The larynx houses the vocal cords.
- Epiglottis: a flap-like cartilage structure which helps to seal the cranial part of the larynx to prevent food from entering it. Most of the time, the epiglottis is in an open position to allow for breathing.
- Glottis: the opening of the larynx.
- Trachea: lies on the ventral surface of the neck. The trachea is kept open by C-shaped cartilaginous rings. It allows for the movement of food to pass in the neighboring esophagus and also withstands outside pressures. The inside is covered with ciliated mucus to assist in getting rid of unwanted particles through the pharynx.
- Bronchi: air enters the trachea that branches into two bronchi (one bronchus to each lung). The carina is where this branch of trachea bifurcates into the bronchi just cranial to the heart. This structure is similar to the trachea, except that now there are complete cartilaginous rings.
- Bronchioles: extending down the branch, the bronchi get smaller in diameter until the cartilage disappears. The autonomic nervous system controls the smooth muscle movement in the walls of both the bronchi and bronchioles.
- Alveolar ducts: the bronchioles branch into smaller structures known as alveolar ducts and end in the alveolar sacs, which have a grape-like appearance.
- Alveoli: essentially a receptacle where gas exchange occurs when in contact with the inspired air and blood. There are millions of alveoli in each lung.

Stridor is a term to describe an unusually loud breathing sound. A stethoscope is not needed to hear such sounds. Stridor is the result of air passing through an abnormally narrowed passageway. Usually there is a resistance to airflow because of partial blockage in the nasopharynx, pharynx, larynx, or the trachea.

Pathway of Respiratory System

→ nose → pharynx → larynx → trachea → bronchi → bronchioles → alveoli ducts → alveoli

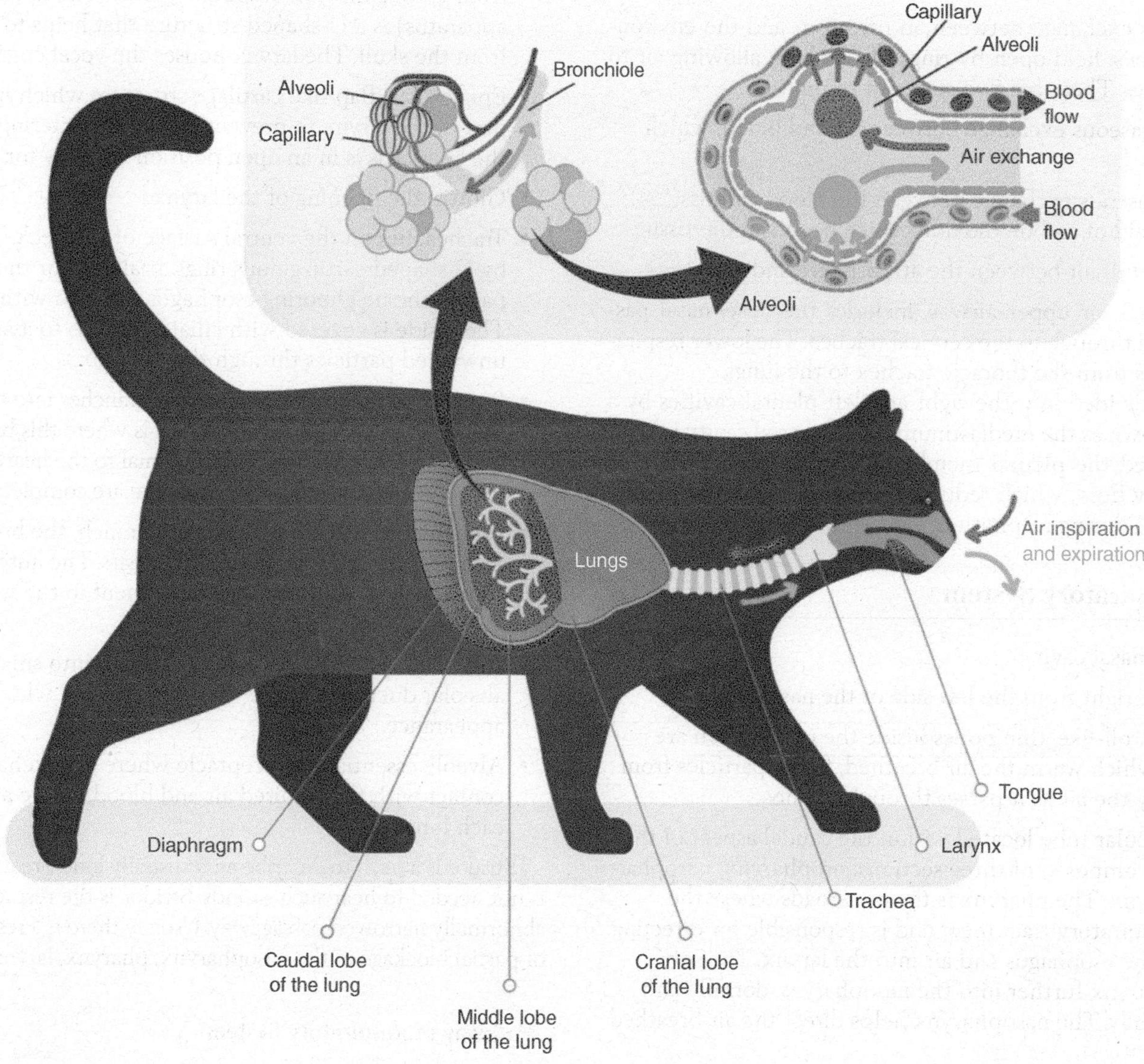

Figure 1.22 Respiratory system.

Lungs

The pulmonary pleura is a membrane that surrounds each lung, part of the bronchi, blood vessels, and connective tissue. The lungs are divided into lobes. The left has three lobes while the right has four. The lobes are identified by their location or direction, such as cranial or apical, middle or cardiac, caudal or diaphragmatic. The right side has an additional fourth lobe, called the accessory lobe, which is small and lies on the medial surface of the caudal lobe.

The thorax is divided into right and left pleural cavities. Inside are the pleural membranes, a lining that secretes a fluid that helps to lubricate the lungs during inspiration.

The lungs are suspended in the thorax. The pleural cavities have a type of vacuum that, with an increase of volume, will result in negative pressure. Air will be forced into the lung tissue. When the inverse happens and the volume decreases, the increase in pressure will push air out.

Muscles of Respiration

- Diaphragm: a large dome-shaped muscle that lies between the thorax and the abdomen.
- External intercostal muscles: lie in between the ribs. On contraction, they lift the ribs upwards and outwards so the thorax can expand.
- Internal intercostal muscles: lie between the ribs but deep to the external intercostal muscles. They work with the abdominal muscles to force air out.

Inspiration or inhalation is the action of the diaphragm and the external intercostal muscles working together to increase the volume of air in the lungs. The diaphragm contracts and flattens to move caudally. The pressure in the pleural cavity is reduced, the lungs expand, and air is moved through the trachea and into the lung tissue.

Expiration or exhalation is the action of the diaphragm and the external intercostal muscles relaxing and the ribs dropping downward. This is a passive movement. The pressure increases in the pleural cavity, the volume decreases, and air is pushed up and out of the trachea.

Respiratory Terms

- Tidal volume: the normal amount of air that is exchanged in the lungs during respiration.
- Inspiratory reserve: an additional amount of air that can be inhaled beyond the tidal volume.
- Expiratory volume: an additional amount of air that can be exhaled beyond the normal tidal volume.
- Residual volume: the air that is left in the lungs even beyond the forced expiratory volume amount; prevents the lungs from completely collapsing.
- Dead space: the parts of the respiratory tract that are not involved in the pathway of respiration.
- Vital capacity: the total amount of air that can be exhaled after the maximum inhalation.
- Total lung capacity: the total sum of the tidal volume, inspiratory reserve volume, expiratory reserve volume, and residual volume.

Section Two

Preventive Care

Chapter 2

Preventative Care and Vaccinations

Liza W. Rudolph, BAS, RVT, VTS (Clinical Practice- C/F),(SAIM)

Veterinary Technician and Nurse's Daily Reference Guide: Canine and Feline, Fourth Edition. Edited by Mandy Fults and Kenichiro Yagi.

Companion website: www.wiley.com/go/fults/veterinary

Abbreviations

AAFP, American Association of Feline Practitioners
AAHA, American Animal Hospital Association
bpm, beats per minute
CN, cranial nerve
ECG, electrocardiogram
FeLV, feline leukemia virus
IM, intramuscular
IN, intranasal
PO, orally
SQ, subcutaneous
USDA, United States Department of Agriculture
VPC, ventricular premature contraction

PHYSICAL EXAMINATION

A physical examination provides invaluable information in the assessment of an animal's health. Veterinary technicians are often called upon to assist the veterinarian to provide an orderly, precise, and timely examination. However, technicians should also be comfortable making observations during both initial patient presentation and as part of the continuing monitoring of inpatients. Physical examinations are an important part of the veterinary nursing process, which allows the veterinary healthcare team to effectively address changes in patient status.

Tables 2.1–2.5 cover methods and specific areas of the physical examination in both pediatric and adult patients.

Initial Examination

Table 2.1 / **Initial examination**

		Definition	Equipment and technique
History	Chief/presenting complaint	The current issue for which the owner is bringing the animal to the clinic	• Current history • Current appetite (vomiting), water intake, urination and defecation behavior (straining, diarrhea), coughing, sneezing, discharges, recent temperament, and current medications are noted • Travel history and recent activities to which the animal may have been exposed or changes in the home environment are also noted.
History	History	Previous medical conditions that may exacerbate the current complaint	• Presence of preexisting conditions are noted • Nutritional history including type of food, amount, feeding schedule, duration, and treats are noted • Immunization dates and current medical therapies (including supplements and heartworm/flea/tick preventative) are noted. • Housing and housemate status are noted
History	Signalment	Age, breed, sex, and reproductive status	• Not applicable

(Continued)

Table 2.1 / Initial examination (Continued)

		Definition	Equipment and technique
Vital signs	General appearance	The patient's overall health	• Visual evaluation of the condition of the animal's coat, skin, ambulation, and temperament
	Heart rate Cardiac function	Normal Canine: 60–160 bpm Feline: 140–220 bpm Abnormal Canine: < 60 and > 160 bpm Feline: < 140 and > 220 bpm	• Auscultation of thoracic cavity, direct palpation of chest wall, or pulse palpation (pulse rate/quality) • Smaller dog breeds may have higher rates • See Skill Box 2.1 • Electrocardiograph • See Chapter 6: Electrocardiogram, page 302
	Respiration Reflects proper oxygenation of the body's tissues Ability to eliminate carbon dioxide from the blood	Normal Canine: 16–32 breaths/minute Feline: 20–42 breaths/minute	• Visual assessment of respiratory rate and effort, presence of abdominal effort • Differentiate panting versus respiratory distress in the canine. • Auscultation of the thoracic cavity • See Skill Box 2.2
		Abnormal < 8 breaths/minute	• Pulse oximetry • Calculates the O_2 saturation of hemoglobin in circulating red blood cells. The probe is placed on an easily accessed non-pigmented capillary bed (e.g., tongue, lip fold, nasal septum, pinna, prepuce, vulva, skin folds, or toe web) • Normal: 99–100% • Abnormal: < 97%, 90% indicates hypoxemia and intervention is required

	Pulses
	Cardiac function
		Normal
		Match rate and rhythm of heart rate
		
		Abnormal
		Weak, bounding, thready, irregular, presence of deficits
			• Assess:
			  • Dehydration status (skin turgor, mucous membrane and eye position)
			  • Perfusion status (capillary refill time, heart rate, pulses, weight)
			  • See Skill Box 14.15: Hydration assessment, page 673
			• Direct palpation
			• Direct digital pressure over the left and right femoral or pedal artery
			• Evaluate pulse quality, strength, rate, and symmetry
			• Blood pressure measurement
			• Non-invasive blood pressure (Doppler vs. oscillometric)

(Continued)

Table 2.1 / Initial examination (Continued)

	Definition	Equipment and technique
Mucous membranes Evaluates for blood loss, anemia, and poor perfusion	Normal Pale pink to pink Abnormal • Pale, muddy, gray, white: poor peripheral perfusion, anemia, vasoconstriction, shock • Blue/purple (cyanotic): hypoxemia • Yellow: hyperbilirubinemia (hemolysis, liver disease, bile duct obstruction) • Red (hyperemic): carbon monoxide toxicity, vasodilation (sepsis, fever, anaphylaxis) • Brown: methemoglobinemia (feline acetaminophen toxicity)	• Visual observation • Observed at the gingiva, tongue, buccal mucous membranes, conjunctiva of the lower eyelid, mucous membrane lining the prepuce or vulva
Capillary refill time Reflects the perfusion of tissues with blood	Normal < 2 seconds Abnormal < 1 second > 2 seconds	• Direct palpation • Direct digital pressure is applied to the mucous membranes until blanched and then timed for blood (pink color) to return
Temperature Circulation	Normal 100.0–102.5°F (37.7–39.2°C) Abnormal < 100 – > 103°F (37.7–39.4°C)	• Rectal thermometer • Temperature probe (e.g., rectal or esophageal)
Weight	Normal/Abnormal See Figure 17.2: Body condition score system, page 755	• Recorded in kilograms and pounds • Note body condition score (5- vs 9-point scale) and dietary history
Pain assessment	Normal No pain symptoms noted Abnormal Changes in animal's behavior (lethargic, aggressive, restlessness, inappropriate urination, increased or decreased grooming), changes in posture, inappetence, hypersensitive reaction to touch, dilated pupils (photophobia), increased heart rate, respiratory rate, blood pressure, or temperature	• Owner input • Visual observation • See Chapter 18: Pain Management, page 775 • See Table 18.4: Various pain scales, page 794.

Table 2.2 Physical examination

Area	Specific Region	Examination	Findings	History
Head and neck	Head (general)	Visual	• Symmetry, alopecia, tumors or swellings, rashes, head tilt, ventroflexion, or uniformed muscle mass on skull	• Head tilt or shaking? • Seizures?
	Eyes (lids, eyeball, conjunctiva, sclera, pupil, cornea, lens)	Visual Ophthalmoscope	• Normal: bright, clear, uniform, responsive • Cysts, conformity, lash growth, third eyelid position and size, conjunctival edema, symmetry, ocular discharge, nystagmus, positioning within orbit: protruding versus sunken, color, vascularity, uniformity of pupils, scars, ulcerations, pigmentation, or opacities	• Pain? • Blinking, squinting, rubbing, or pawing? • Discharge? (e.g. quantity, consistency, color, uni- or bilateral) • Blindness?
	Muzzle	Visual	• Symmetry, inflammation, swelling, abscessed teeth, or pain on opening the mouth	• Rubbing or pawing?
	Nares	Visual	• Symmetry, patency, movement on inspiration (lateral movement), swelling, discoloration, or discharge	• Sneezing or heavy breathing? • Discharge? (e.g. quantity, color, consistency, color, uni- or bilateral)
	Oral cavity (lips, mucous membranes, teeth, hard and soft palate, tongue, pharynx, tonsils)	Visual	• Normal: symmetrical, pink, slightly moist • Halitosis, inflammation, tumors or papillomas, anatomic defects, excessive salivation, crusting, pigment changes, color and capillary refill time, tacky, periodontal status, ulcerations, erosions, or foreign bodies • See Chapter 21: Dentistry	• Excessive salivation or dripping water after drinking? • Inappetence or difficulty eating? • Changes? (e.g. gingival pigmentation, bark, meow)
	Ears	Visual Otoscopic	• Normal: clear and dry • Symmetry, debris, alopecia, thickening, crusting, exudate, odor, inflammation, foreign materials, masses, response to sound, or sensitivity to canal massage or palpation • See Skill Box 2.4	• Shaking head or scratching ears? • Discharge? (e.g. quantity, consistency, color, uni- or bilateral) • Hearing loss?
	Lymph nodes (submandibular)	Palpation	• Normal: firm, oval and freely movable • Symmetry and size • See Skill Box 2.5	• Increase in size?
	Salivary glands (mandibular, parotid)	Palpation	• Normal: irregular, bumpy texture • Symmetry and size (can be confused with submandibular nodes)	
	Neck (throat, trachea, larynx, thyroid, thoracic inlet)	Palpation Auscultation	• Coughing or sounds during examination (stertor or stridor), deviation, or displacement; tumors; swelling; thyroid slip; stridor; or jugular pulse waves	• Gagging, retching, difficulty swallowing? • If a cough is noticed, does the cough occur throughout the day? • Travel or exposure to other canines?

(Continued)

Table 2.2 / Physical examination (Continued)

Area	Specific Region	Examination	Findings	History
Trunk and limbs	Trunk (general)	Visual Palpation	• Normal: visible sheen and coat completeness • Body form and weight, symmetry, tumors, alopecia, inflammation, ectoparasites or their residues, crusts, scales, pustules, and hydration status	• Changes? (e.g. pigmentation, odor, hair loss, texture) • Allergen exposure? (e.g. type of bedding, feathers, carpets, indoor plants, tobacco smoke) • Pruritus? (e.g. behavior, frequency) • Scratching, biting, licking? • Did pruritus precede or coincide with lesions? • Bathing or grooming habits? • Changes in diet?
	Lymph nodes (prescapular, axillary, inguinal, popliteal)	Palpation	• Normal: firm, oval, and freely movable (axillary or disk shaped) • Size and consistency • See Skill Box 2.5	• Increase in size?
	Limbs (muscle, bone, joints, paws)	Visual Palpation	• Symmetry, inflammation, tenderness, tumors, range of motion, gait, atrophy, flexion and extension, interdigital, nails/nail bed, or knuckling	• Limping and/or favoring limb(s)? • Licking paws?
Thoracic cavity	Lungs	Auscultation Percussion	• Respiratory rate, effort, depth, and pattern of breathing (rales or rhonchi) and lung sounds (absence of lung sounds may indicate pleural effusion, and dull sound may indicate fluid-filled or solid lungs) • See Skill Box 2.2	• Fainting? • If cough is present, does it change throughout the day or worsen with exertion? • Frequency? • Recent travel?
	Heart	Auscultation	• Arrhythmias, murmurs, muffled heart sounds, verify pulses synchronous with heart rate (e.g., no pulse deficits) • See Skill Box 2.1	• Fainting, collapsing, or exercise intolerance? • Panting? • Coughing? (e.g. description, frequency)

(Continued)

Table 2.2 / **Physical examination (Continued)**

Area	Specific Region	Examination	Findings	History
Abdomen	Kidneys	Palpation	• Normal: oval shaped with indented side, firm, and smooth • Size, shape, and contours of surface, symmetry (between left and right kidneys), or pain	• Excessive water consumption or urinating?
	Liver	Palpation, lateral recumbency	• Normal: edges are smooth and well defined • Asymmetric or irregular surface? • Extension beyond costal arch may indicate hepatomegaly	
	Urinary bladder	Palpation	• Normal: palpable when urine-filled, thin wall with flexibility • Size, tone, and turgidity	• Urination (e.g. frequency, quantity, behavior, odor) • Foul odor, color change, or blood? • Straining? • Inappropriate urination?
	Small Intestine	Palpation	• Normal: not palpable or mildly gas filled • Tumors, foreign bodies, pain on palpation, or thickened/ firmness on palpation	• Vomiting, diarrhea, or constipation? (e.g., description, quantity, frequency, behavior) • Time since last bowel movement?
	Mammary glands	Visual Palpation	• Tumors, cysts, inflammation, temperature, and discharge	• If intact female, when did last birth occur? • When was ovariohysterectomy performed?
Perineal	General	Visual	• Tumors, fistulas, exudate, and hernias	• Reproductive status?
	Vulva	Visual	• Normal: vaginal discharge, lochia • Size, inflammation, and discharge from or between perivulvar folds	• Last heat cycle, mating, or birth? • Discharge (e.g. quantity, consistency, color, odor)
	Penis	Visual Palpation	• Normal: preputial discharge • Tumors, inflammation, or discharge	• Normal urination? • Blood or urine color change? • Discharge (e.g. quantity, consistency, color, odor)
	Scrotum	Visual Palpation	• Descended testicles, swelling, and symmetry	• Pain when sitting?

Pediatric Physical Examination

Table 2.3 is designed to show the specific areas to note on puppies and kittens. A full examination should be conducted following Table 2.2.

Table 2.3 / Pediatric physical examination

Region	Specific region	Exam method	Age	Normal		Evaluation
				Puppy	Kitten	
General appearance	Temperament	Visual exam	Birth–6 weeks	• First 3 weeks of life should consist of eating and sleeping. Nursing should be vigorous and active with a good "suckle reflex". Active playtime with mother and littermates from 3 weeks on		• Constant crying, restlessness, extreme inactivity, and failure to gain weight can be signs of inadequate milk consumption or illness • Separation from mother and littermates before 6 weeks of age can lead to numerous behavioral problems later in life
	Body weight	Weighing	Birth–4 weeks	• Toy: 100–400 g • Medium: 200–300 g • Large: 400–500 g • Giant: > 700 g • Birth weight should double in days 10–12	• 60–110 g • Birth weight should double in 14 days	• Failure to gain weight is often one of the first signs of illness • Body weight should be checked initially 12 hours after birth and daily for 2 weeks, then checked weekly
		Weighing	5 weeks–6 months	• Gain 1–2 g/day/lb of adult body weight • Obtained 50% of adult weight	• Gain 10–15 g/day on average	
		Weighing	Reached adult weight	• Small breed: 8–12 months • Medium breed: 12–18 months • Large–giant breed: 18–24 months • By maturity, most canines will gain 40–50 times their birth weight	• • 10 months	

(Continued)

Table 2.3 / **Pediatric physical examination (Continued)**

Region	Specific region	Exam method	Age	Normal: Puppy	Normal: Kitten	Evaluation
	Coat/skin	Visual exam, flea comb	Birth–6 months	• Complete hair coat		• State of hydration (skin turgor) difficult to determine, especially in young animals < 4 weeks of age • Completeness of hair cover, condition of foot pads, wounds, bacterial infections (e.g. omphalitis), external parasites, or dermatophytosis
	Temperature	Rectal thermometer	Birth–1 week	• 96–98°F (35.5–36.6°C). Cannot regulate own body temperature for first 3 weeks (puppy) or 1 week (kitten). Neonates should never be left unattended or warmed on electric heating pads because their neuromuscular reflexes are not present until 7 days of age		• Hyper- or hypothermia • Burns
			2–4 weeks	• 99–100.5°F (37.2–38°C)		
Head	Eyes	Visual exam, penlight, ophthalmoscope	Birth–6 months	• Eyes open around 5–14 days. Iris is blue-gray. Changes to adult color at approximately 4–6 weeks of age. Adult vision at 5–10 weeks of age. Pupillary light responses may not be evident until 21 days of age. Strabismus or deviation of eyes at 3–5 months of age		• Discharge, swelling, squinting or holding eye(s) closed, rubbing or pawing at eye(s)
	Ears	Visual exam, otoscope	Birth–6 months	• Complete hearing at 4–6 weeks of age. External ear canals open between 6 and 14 days and are completely open by 17 days. Canals may be full of desquamative cells and some oil droplets		• Size and position • Exudate and odor for possible bacterial or yeast infection or mites

(Continued)

Table 2.3 / Pediatric physical examination (Continued)

Region	Specific region	Exam method	Age	Normal		Evaluation
				Puppy	Kitten	
	Mouth	Penlight, tongue depressor or cotton swab	Birth–3 months	• Sucking reflex is present at birth and disappears at 3 weeks of age. Deciduous tooth eruption: • Incisors: 2–4 weeks • Canines: 3–5 weeks • Premolars: 4–12 weeks		• Hairlip, cleft palate, sucking reflex, occlusion, or malfunction of jaw bones (malocclusion)
			4–6 months	Permanent tooth eruption: • Incisors: 3–5 months • Canines: 4–7 months • Premolars: 4–6 months • Molars: 4–5 months		• Occlusion or malfunction of jaw bones (malocclusion)
	Nose	Visual exam	Birth–6 months	• Normal adult appearance		• Obstruction, stenosis, discharge, abnormal shape, or swelling
	Skull	Visual exam	Birth–4 weeks	• Normal adult appearance		• Open fontanel (soft spot on the forehead)
Thorax	General appearance	Visual exam	Birth–6 months	• Symmetrical chest wall		• Wounds and rib fractures • Congenital sternal or spinal abnormalities
	Heart	Visual examination, stethoscope with 2-cm bell and 3-cm diaphragm	Birth–4 weeks	• Heart rate 200–220 beats/minute • Heart rhythm is a regular sinus rhythm		• Heart rate and pattern • Murmurs (should be noted and veterinarian consulted, as some can be normal/physiological)
			5 weeks–6 months	• Heart rate: 70–180 beats/minute	• Heart rate: 140–220 beats/minute	
	Lungs		Birth–4 weeks	• Respiratory rate: 15–35 breaths/minute	• Respiratory rate: 25–35 breaths/minute	• Breathing rate and pattern • Asymmetrical or absent lung sounds

(Continued)

Table 2.3 / **Pediatric physical examination (Continued)**

Region	Specific region	Exam method	Age	Normal: Puppy	Normal: Kitten	Evaluation
			5 weeks–6 months	• Respiratory rate: 10–30 breaths/minute	• Respiratory rate: 25–40 breaths/minute	
Abdomen	General appearance	Visual exam	Birth–4 weeks	• Umbilical cord falls off in 2–3 days		• Umbilical hernia, inflammation, or infection/ulceration
	Internal organs	Palpation	Birth–4 weeks	• Kidneys are palpable in kittens and in some puppies • Normal spleen will sometimes be palpable in an older puppy if the foreleg is extended, allowing organs to fall caudally; the spleen is only palpable if enlarged in kittens • Liver margins should not extend past the ribs • Stomach will feel like a large fluid-filled sac if full. Intestines are soft and freely movable without pain and may be fluid or gas filled • Thickened/"ropy" feel may indicate endoparasitism • Urinary bladder should have resistance to urine outflow		• Enlarged or abnormally small organs, pain on palpation, or masses • Intussusception—a sausage-like mass and very painful
Limbs	Forelimbs, hindlimbs	Visual exam, palpation	Birth–6 months	• Normal adult appearance (breed influenced)		• Wounds, bruises, or swelling • Deformities or ↑ or ↓ range of motion in joints
Perineum, genitals	Genitalia	Visual exam, palpation	Birth–6 months	• Normal adult appearance • Descended testicles by 4–6 weeks of age (diagnose cryptorchid after 16 weeks)		• Cryptorchidism, vaginitis, or congenital abnormalities
	Anus	Visual exam, palpation	Birth–6 months	• Normal adult appearance		• Rectal prolapse, inflammation, irritation, congenital abnormalities • Defecation/urination on their own usually occurs between 2 and 3 weeks

Normal Parturition

In late term pregnancy (58–63 days), the bitch or queen should be observed for signs of labor. These signs may include a rectal temperature drop to < 100°F (37.7°C), vulvar discharge, and leaking milk. Once labor starts, the female should be left alone but should be observed occasionally for progression or signs of complications.

Table 2.4 / Normal parturition

Stage	Time	Observations	Complications
1	6–12 hours, up to 24 hours	• Early changes may not be noticed by the pet owner • Restless, getting up and down, nervous, panting • Nesting behavior (e.g., arranging bedding, chewing up paper) • Reduced body temperature (97–99°F; 36.1–37.2°C)	• Black, green, or red vaginal discharge • Failure to progress to stage 2 within 24–36 hours after a decrease in rectal temperature or progesterone levels
2	3–6 hours, up to 12–24 hours in the dog, up to 36 hours in the cat; up to 1 hour between the birth of each neonate	• Strong contractions; in lateral recumbency or posturing • Clear vaginal discharge • Delivery of first fetus should be within 1 hour of active labor or 2 hours of intermittent labor	• > 60 minutes of strong contractions with no neonate produced • > 2 hours between pups or > 1 hour between kittens is considered an emergency • Fetal distress (heart rate < 160 or stillbirths) • Maternal distress: lethargy, pain, green discharge, hemorrhage • Queen: if stressed may stop and restart labor the next day
3	Often occurs in conjunction with stage 2	• Placenta will be passed after each fetus; if multiple fetuses are passed within a short time the placentas will follow together • Mother will chew the placenta to free the neonate, sever the umbilical cord, and lick the neonate for stimulation • Placenta should be seen within 5–15 minutes • The next neonate should follow in 1–2 hours	• Mother may not release the neonate and sever the umbilical cord • Eating multiple placentas may lead to indigestion and diarrhea
Postpartum	1–2 months	• Bitch: 8–10 weeks of bloody discharge • Queen: 3 weeks of black or red discharge	• Mastitis (e.g. fever, lethargy, swollen glands) • Metritis (e.g. foul-smelling discharge) • Retained placenta (e.g. green discharge) • Eclampsia (e.g. tremors, excitation)

Geriatric Physical Examination

Table 2.5 is designed to show the specific areas to note in geriatric animals. A full examination should be conducted, following Table 2.2. However, geriatric animals go through additional changes as a result of the natural aging process and a physical is recommended every six months. Many of these changes cannot be visualized in a physical examination, but they may be inferred through the general examination and from discussion with the owner. These symptoms may contribute to or initiate more serious medical conditions, thereby making their determination valuable to the clinician.

Table 2.5 / Geriatric physical examination

Region	Specific region	Effects	Associated with
General appearance	Skin	↓ elastin and collagen ↓ blood flow to skin; thinning of skin and coat	• Ineffective barrier to pathogens • May be more difficult to assess hydration/skin turgor • May require more maintenance by owner
	Toenails	↑ length because of ↓ activity; more fragile, crumble when trimmed	• Difficulty walking • Wounds in foot pads
	Musculature	↓ strength; ↓ tone	• Muscle atrophy and coordination
	Eyes	Vision loss; ↓ pupillary light response; change in lens opacity; optic lens hardening	• Atrophy of the iris and ciliary muscles • Nuclear sclerosis
Head	Ears	Hearing loss	• Loss of cochlear hair cells
	Nose	↓ Sense of smell	• ↓ function of olfactory nerve endings, which can affect eating habits
	Neck	Thyroid nodules	• Hyperthyroidism (feline) • Tumor
Internal organs	Brain	Amyloid deposition; memory loss; personality changes	• Cognitive dysfunction disorder
	Lungs	Loss of lung elasticity; ↓ tidal volume; ↓ expiratory reserve; diminished cough reflex; ↑ density on lung radiography	• Rarely a cause of concern unless patient needs to undergo an anesthetic procedure
	Heart	Radiographic changes; ↑ sternal contact; tortuous, redundant aorta (feline)	• Rarely a cause of concern

(Continued)

Table 2.5 / Geriatric physical examination (Continued)

Region	Specific region	Effects	Associated with
	Kidney	↑ mineralization of renal pelvis; ↓ size, glomerular filtration rate, renal blood flow, ability to handle potassium	• Kidney disease
	Liver	↓ protein synthesis ↓ metabolic function	• Liver disease
Limbs	Joints/cartilage	↓ production of chondroitin sulfate, keratin sulfate, and hyaluronic acid; ↓ proteoglycan content	• Degenerative joint disease
Genitals	Urethral sphincter	↓ tone	• Primary urethral sphincter incontinence
Immune system		↓ function	• Chronic disease • ↑ susceptibility to infections
Blood		↓ ability to respond to red blood cell demand; hypertension	• Anemia • Renal or endocrine disease

Cardiac Examination

Skill Box 2.1 / Cardiac examination

Kristie Garcia

Technique

Perform auscultation in a quiet room with a calm patient. Place the patient in a standing or sitting position. Avoid listening to recumbent animals, as the change in heart position and configuration leads to errors. The flat diaphragm of the stethoscope is used to detect high-frequency sounds (e.g. normal heart and breath sounds, most murmurs), while the bell is used to detect lower-frequency sounds (e.g. third and fourth heart sounds, diastolic murmurs). The entire heart is examined, paying particular attention to the cardiac valves. Begin by placing the diaphragm gently but firmly at the left apex, where the first heart sound is best heard and also the location of the mitral valve (found on the left lateral thorax between the fourth and sixth intercostal space, behind the olecranon). From here, inch the stethoscope to the left base of the heart, which is approximately two rib spaces cranial and slightly dorsal. Note the second heart sound and possible basilar heart murmurs associated with the aortic and pulmonic valve. Next, palpate the same area on the right lateral thorax and move the stethoscope to this region. This is the tricuspid region and possible location of tricuspid regurgitation. Then move to the right base of the heart. Once an abnormality is noted, the surrounding region should be evaluated to find the point of the loudest sound. In this process, the entire heart region should be evaluated and a complete examination performed.

Rate

- Canine: 60–160 bpm
- Feline: 140–220 bpm

Heart Sounds

Normal

Heart sound	Location	Sound
First (S1)	Left apex of the heart	Low-frequency sound longer than S2
Second (S2)	Base of the heart	High-frequency sound shorter than S1
Third (S3)	Apex	Low-intensity sound shortly after S2
Fourth (S4)	Apex	Low-intensity sound slightly before S1

Abnormal

Murmurs

Characterized by their:

- Location (over which valve they are the loudest)
- Intensity (grades 1–6)
- Frequency (harsh, blowing, musical, honking, or grunting)

(*Continued*)

Skill Box 2.1 / Cardiac Examination (Continued)

- Timing (point in the cardiac cycle the murmur is best heard)
- Quality (character/ behavior).

Description of Intensity

Grade	Description
1	Very faint; requiring concentration and a quiet room to be heard
2	Soft; localized over one valve area, but easily auscultated
3	Moderate intensity; readily auscultable, usually radiating to another valve area
4	Loud; without precordial thrill, usually radiating to both sides of the chest
5	Very loud; with palpable thrill, audible with stethoscope barely touching the thorax
6	Very loud; with palpable thrill, audible when the stethoscope is removed from the thorax

Heart Valves

Normal

Valve	Location
Pulmonic	Left second to fourth intercostal space above the sternal border
Aortic	Left third to fifth intercostal space at mid-thorax
Mitral	Left fourth to sixth intercostal space just above the sternal border, the apex of the heart
Tricuspid	Right sixth to seventh intercostal space at mid-thorax, the apex of the heart

(*Continued*)

Skill Box 2.1 / Cardiac Examination (Continued)

Rhythms

Rhythm	Description
Gallop	The combination of sounds is similar to the sound of a horse galloping. It is abnormal in the small animal patient and is associated with ventricular stiffness. Hypertrophic cardiomyopathy and advanced dilated cardiomyopathy fall into this category.
Ventricular premature contraction	While a VPC cannot be ascultated per se, an arrhythmia with a pulse deficits can be ascultated. An ECG is necessary to determine the presence of VPC.
Atrial fibrillation	Rapid arrhythmia of varying intensity of the first and second heart sounds with pulse deficits and variable pule quality. An ECG is necessary to determine the presence of atrial fibrillation.

Artifacts

- Panting and excessive thoracic pressure in small patients sounds similar to murmurs.
- Skin twitching can sound similar to extra heart sounds.
- Friction from chest piece rubbing across fur can sound similar to crackles.

Tip: Ventilation artifacts can be discouraged by holding the mouth shut, whistling, or briefly obstructing a nare. Purring may be controlled with a visual distraction (e.g. visualization of water, another animal), blowing short bursts of air in their face, picking up the cat, or gently pressing over the larynx.
Tip: When locating heart valves, count the ribs from caudal to cranial.
Tip: The pulse and heartbeat should be synchronous. A heartbeat without a pulse is a pulse deficit and may indicate an arrhythmia.
Note: See also Figures 1.11, page 13, 1.12, page 14, and 1.13, page 14.

Pulmonary Examination

Skill Box 2.2 / Pulmonary examination

Technique

Begin the exam by observing the respiratory effort (quality) and pattern and any signs of respiratory distress (e.g. nostril flare, intercostal rib retraction). The normal inspiration to expiration is 1 : 2; meaning that expiration should take twice as long as inspiration. After the initial assessment, perform auscultation in a quiet room with a calm patient. Place the patient in a standing or sitting position. Avoid listening to recumbent patients as it leads to errors due to changes in thoracic conformation. Divide the thoracic cavity into quadrants to follow a sequential pattern. As each quadrant is auscultated, it is observed for respiratory rate and breath sounds.

Rate

- Canine: 16–32 breaths/minute
- Feline: 20–42 breaths/minute

(*Continued*)

Skill Box 2.2 / Pulmonary examination (Continued)

Breath Sounds

- Breath sounds should be heard equally on both sides of the thorax.
- Breath sounds heard outside the location defined as follows can indicate a medical problem.

Normal

Type	Location	Sound
Bronchial	Center of the chest over the caudal trachea and larger bronchi	Normal intense harsh sound head on both inspiration and expiration
Bronchovesicular	Bilateral bronchial and hilar region	Normal moderate sounds heard on full inspiration and short expiration
Vesicular	Peripheral lung fields	Normal soft sounds heard better on the slightly longer inspiratory phase

Abnormal

Type	Location	Sound	Cause
Stertor	Larynx or trachea	Discontinuous low-pitched snoring sound heard mainly on inspiration; sound radiates	Produced lower in the airway, most consistent with a partial airway obstruction
Stridor	Larynx or thoracic inlet; referred sounds maybe heard throughout the thorax	Intense continuous high-pitched wheezes heard on inspiration	Turbulent airflow at the pharynx or larynx, most consistent with a partial airway obstruction
Crackles (rales)	Lung fields	Popping sound heard mainly on inspiration; defined as fine, medium, or coarse	Fluid or exudate accumulation within airways or inflammation and edema in pulmonary tissue
Rhonchi (wheezes)	Isolated lung fields or variable	Continuous musical sounds, low or high pitched, heard at the end of inspiration or at the beginning of expiration; defined as high or low pitched	↓ airway lumen diameter
Muffled	Isolated lung fields or variable	↓ lung sounds	Pneumothorax, pyothorax, chylothorax, hemothorax

Tip: Listen to the lung sounds before listening to heart tones because the ear is much less sensitive to softer sounds once it has adjusted to louder sounds.

Abdominal Examination

Skill Box 2.3 / **Abdominal examination**

Technique

Gentleness when palpating an animal is essential, as internal structures may be damaged if handled roughly. Structure descriptions can be doughy (soft tissue that can be impressed with fingertips), firm (normal organ), hard (bones), or fluctuant (soft, elastic, and undulates under pressure). Abnormalities noted on palpation are pain, abnormal structures, and their size, consistency, shape, and location.

Large Canine

Place the patient in a standing position. Stand on either side or to the rear. Place one hand on either side of the abdomen in a flat and relaxed position. Begin at the spine and gently and slowly move ventrally, allowing the abdominal viscera to slip through the fingers. Repeat this process throughout the abdomen moving caudally.

Small Canine or Feline

Place the patient in a standing position. Stand next to the patient. Cup one hand around the abdomen with the thumb on one side and the fingers on the other side in a flat and relaxed position. Begin at the spine and gently and slowly move ventrally, allowing the abdominal viscera to slip through the fingers. Repeat this process throughout the abdomen moving caudally.

Internal Structure Location

Cranial Abdomen

- Palpation of the liver, spleen, and small intestine.
- Liver is difficult to palpate and extension past the costal arch may indicate hepatomegaly.
- Spleen is difficult to palpate and recognition may indicate splenomegaly.
- Normal stomach is rarely palpable, but with overeating (doughy or fluid filled) or gastric distention, it may be felt.

Mid-Abdomen

- Palpation of the small intestine, kidneys, and spleen.
- Right kidney is more cranial than the left kidney in felines and may be obscured by the ribs.
- Mesenteric lymph nodes are difficult to palpate unless enlarged.
- Caudal abdomen.
- Palpation of the colon, uterus, bladder, prostate, and small intestine.
- Feces can be discerned from a mass by its deformability with fingertip imprints.
- Prostate can occasionally be palpated central to the colon and caudal to the bladder.

Note: See also Figures 1.3, 1.4, and 1.5, page 6.

Otoscopic Examination

Skill Box 2.4 / Otoscopic examination

Technique

Examine the good ear first to avoid spread of infection and to decrease resistance to examination of the possibly more painful ear. Begin with an otoscope with the appropriate-sized cone for the patient. For ease of examination, the patient should be placed on a table or large canines in a sitting position. The head should be held in such a manner to avoid crushing the ear canal while directing the muzzle toward the thoracic inlet. Holding the pinna up and out from the base of the skull will allow straightening of the ear canal. Gently insert the otoscope into the external ear canal and slowly advance while observing the canal. As the cone enters the vertical canal, the pinna is pulled up and over the otoscope while the otoscope handle is rotated to a horizontal position. The tympanic membrane will then be visualized in a normal ear as a white translucent membrane. Any abnormalities such as inflammation, redness, exudate, foreign objects, mites, or tumors should be noted.

Note: See also Figure 23.2, page 1042.

Regional Lymph Node Examination

Skill Box 2.5 / Regional lymph node examination

Technique

Three pairs of lymph nodes are routinely palpated in a normal animal: submandibular, prescapular, and popliteal. Axillary and inguinal nodes can often only be palpated with enlargement. Peripheral lymph nodes should be palpated simultaneously to evaluate symmetry. Enlarged nodes may be an initial indicator of a problem. Lymph nodes are generally smooth and oval in shape and can be most easily felt by grabbing the skin and allowing it to slip through the fingertips while pulling the hands away.

Node	Location	Size
Submandibular	Ventral to the angle of the mandible, cranial to the parotid and submaxillary salivary glands	Group of two or three nodes of the size of a pea to a grape
Prescapular (superficial cervical)	In front of the cranial border of the scapula	Group of two or three nodes slightly larger than submandibular nodes
Popliteal	Caudal to the stifle	One node about the size of a pea, not always palpable in smaller animals
Axillary	Caudal and medial to the shoulder joint	One or two nodes, not palpable in normal animals (0.5–10 mm)
Inguinal	Furrow between the abdominal wall and the medial thigh	Two nodes, not palpable in normal animals

Neurological Examination

Skill Box 2.6 / Neurological examination

Brittany Laflen

A complete neurological examination consists of several tests, each evaluating different components of the nervous system. The results of all the various tests are considered together to determine what part of the nervous system is affected, which is called neurolocalization.

The neurological exam begins as the patient walks into the examination room. Notice should be paid to the patient's body posture (e.g. head tilt, leaning, circling), level of consciousness (e.g. normal, obtunded, comatose), and general movements. This portion of the exam also includes a thorough palpation of the animal's body to evaluate muscle mass, symmetry and tone. Additional neurological examination testing is as follows:

Gait Evaluation

Evaluation of gait to help differentiate a neurological disorder from an orthopedic problem.

Test	Positioning	Test	Reaction
Walking and trotting	Patient is handled on a leash or harness on a nonslip surface	The patient is walked toward, away from the assessor, and in a circle (both directions)	Paresis: weakness, ataxia

Postural Reactions

The patient's ability to recognize an abnormal position and to change its position to bear weight and be able to walk. These tests assess the integrity of the nervous system but do not localize the specific area of the nervous system involved. Postural reactions need to be evaluated in conjunction with all aspects of a patient's exam and diagnostics. As these tests are assessing the same pathways, it is the clinician's preference in the selection of which of these tests to perform, dependent on the animal's issues, temperament, and tolerance factors.

Test	Positioning	Test	Reaction
Extensor postural thrust	Support the patient under the thorax	Touch the hind limbs to the floor	Monitor for symmetric caudal walking motions
Hemi-standing/hemi-walking		A hind limb and front limb of the same side are lifted	Monitor for lateral walking movements
Hopping	Support the patient under the thorax	Lift three limbs and move the patient laterally and then medially; test all four limbs	Monitor for initiation and movement of hopping
Placing	Support the patient under the thorax	Bring the thoracic limbs into contact with the edge of a table; repeat this twice: once with the eyes covered and once with the eyes opened	Monitor for immediate placement of the limbs on top of the table

(Continued)

Skill Box 2.6 / Neurological examination (Continued)

Test	Positioning	Test	Reaction
Proprioceptive positioning	Support the patient under the thorax	Turn the hind foot over onto the dorsal surface	Monitor the length of time to turn it back to a normal position
Wheelbarrowing	Support the patient under the abdomen with the hind limbs lifted	Maintain the position until the animal starts walking forward	Monitor the length of time to start walking forward and the walking coordination

Sensory Evaluation

Evaluation of Deep Pain Perception

Test	Positioning	Test	Reaction
Spinal hyperpathia: recommended only when pain is not evident	Patient is in a standing or sitting position	Pressure is applied along the thoracic and lumbar regions to the spine and muscles at each vertebra	Monitor for a behavioral response to pain (e.g. guarding, tense abdominal muscles, crying out)
Sensory test for upper motor neuron issues: currently recommended only if the course of action will be affected by the prognosis and the patient is truly paralyzed; aggressive pain testing may result in broken digits	Patient is in a standing or sitting position	Pinch the toe to assess superficial pain or use a hemostat to pinch the toe to assess deep pain	Monitor for pulling back or behavioral response

Spinal Reflexes

Tests the sensory and motor components of a reflex arc (normal, hyporeflexia, hyperreflexia). Grading is typically:
0 (absent)
+ 1 (decreased)
+ 2 (normal)
+ 3 (exaggerated)
+ 4 (very exaggerated/clonus)

The following tests are the ones typically performed.

Test	Positioning	Test	Reaction
Hind limb and anal reflexes			
Patellar reflex	Patient in lateral recumbency and stifle gently supported in a flexed position	Percuss patellar tendon; test leg in both the recumbent and non-recumbent positions	Monitor for extension of the stifle

(Continued)

Skill Box 2.6 / **Neurological examination (Continued)**

Test	Positioning	Test	Reaction
Withdrawal (flexor)	Patient in lateral recumbency	Pinch digits with fingers; may need hemostat if no response is elicited	Monitor for flexion of the limb and pain recognition
Perineal reflex	Patient in standing position	Apply mild digital pressure on the anus or squeeze the anal tissue	Monitor the amount of contraction of the anal sphincter and tail flexion
Front limb reflexes			
Extensor carpi radialis response	Patient in lateral recumbency	Percuss the extensor carpi radialis muscle	Monitor for extension of the carpus
Triceps reflex	Patient in lateral recumbency with limb supported, elbow fully extended, and leg caudal	Percuss the triceps tendon	Monitor for slight extension of the elbow
Withdrawal	Patient in lateral recumbency	Pinch digits with fingers; may need hemostat if no response is elicited	Monitor for flexion of the limb and pain recognition

Cranial Nerves

The following tests assess the cranial nerves.

Test	Technique	Cranial nerve assessment	Assesses
Ophthalmoscopic exam		Optic nerve (CN II)	Pupillary light response
		Oculomotor nerve (CN III)	Pupillary restriction, size, and symmetry
		Trochlear nerve (CN IV)	Dorsal oblique eye muscle movement
Menace	Push the palm of the hand toward the eye in a short quick motion	Optic nerve (CN II)	Vision, menace response
		Trochlear nerve (CN IV)	Vision, menace response
		Trigeminal nerve (CN V)	Facial movements, blinking, lip retraction, nociception
		Abducent nerve (CN VI)	Dorsal oblique eye muscle, menace response
		Facial nerve (CN VII)	Menace response
		Vestibulocochlear nerve (CN VIII)	Eye movements

(*Continued*)

Skill Box 2.6 / Neurological examination (Continued)

Test	Technique	Cranial nerve assessment	Assesses
Strabismus	Move the head from side to side	Oculomotor nerve (CN III) Trochlear nerve (CN IV)	Ventrolateral strabismus
Palpebral	Gently touch the lateral medial canthus to see if the patient blinks	Trigeminal nerve (CN V) Facial nerve (CN VII)	Palpebral reflex
Sensory reflex	Cover the patient's eyes and stimulate the skin around the eyes, ears, and nose to stimulate facial movement	Facial nerve (CN VII)	Facial muscle movements (ears, eyelids, nose, lips)
Gait and postural	Refer to the gait evaluation in the previous section of this table	Vestibulocochlear nerve (CN VIII)	Equilibrium, posture
Examination and palpation of the head muscles		Trigeminal nerve (CN V)	Muscle mass, jaw tone
Examination of mouth and gag reflex		Glossopharyngeal nerve (CN IX)	Pharyngeal sensation, gag response, swallowing
		Vagus nerve (CN X)	Swallowing, gag response, laryngeal function, vocalization
		Hypoglossal nerve (CN XII)	Tongue movement and strength

Orthopedic Examination

Skill Box 2.7 / Orthopedic examination

Technique

Similar to the neurological examination, the orthopedic examination begins as the patient enters the examination room. Notice should be paid to the patient's conformation, stance, sitting, standing, rising, and gait. The examination should continue with a hands-on evaluation of the area of concern, including the alternate side. A systematic approach should be used to cover the entire limb, often beginning distally and moving proximally. Alterations in the range of motion and rotation should be noted, together with any crepitus, clicking, clunking, instability, swelling, muscle atrophy or overdevelopment, and pain. Begin the examination by evaluating the non-affected joint to assess the patient's normal response to manipulation and pressure.

Stifle

Cranial drawer motion:
- Patient in lateral recumbency; stabilize the femur proximal to the stifle with one hand.
- Place the second hand with the thumb behind the fibular head and the index finger over the tibial crest.
- With the femur stabilized, with the second hand move the tibia cranial and distal in a plane parallel to the tibial plateau.
- Monitor for the tibia sliding cranially or caudally in relationship to the femur, indicating cruciate ligament rupture or partial tear.
- Test should be performed with the stifle joint in extension, 90-degree flexion, and normal standing position.

Tibial compression test/tibial thrust:
- Holding the limb in a standing position, flex the hock to tense the gastrocnemius muscle, which compresses the femur and tibia together.
- Monitor for forward motion of the tibia in a ruptured cranial cruciate ligament.
- Patellar luxation—medial:
  - Hold the limb extended with the foot rotated internally.
  - Apply digital pressure medially.
  - Monitor for medial displacement indicating luxation.
- Patellar luxation—lateral:
  - Hold the limb slightly flexed with the foot rotated externally.
  - Apply digital pressure laterally.
  - Monitor for lateral displacement indicating luxation.

Pelvis

Barden's procedure:
- With the patient in lateral recumbency, grasp the femur with one hand.
- Place the thumb of the second hand on the greater trochanter of the femur, while resting the rest of your palm on the pelvis.
- With gentle pressure, attempt to lift the femur, keeping it parallel to the table.
- Monitor for subluxation of the femur through the thumb on the greater trochanter indicating hip laxity.

Barlow's sign:
- With the patient in dorsal recumbency with stifle flexed, place the left hand on the right stifle and slowly adduct.
- Monitor for luxation of the femoral head from the acetabulum indicating joint capsule stretching.

Hip luxation:
- With the patient in a standing position, place the thumb in the space caudal to the greater trochanter, externally rotate the femur.
- Monitor for the trochanter to roll over the thumb indicating luxation.

Ortolani maneuver—lateral recumbency:
- Hold the limb in a standing position parallel to the table surface.
- Place one hand over the hip joint, while cupping the stifle joint with the other hand to apply pressure, pushing the femoral head in a dorsal direction in relation to the acetabulum.
- Monitor for hip subluxation indicating hip laxity.

Ortolani maneuver—dorsal recumbency:
- Position the stifles parallel to each other and perpendicular to the table.
- Apply downward pressure on the stifles to subluxate the hip.
- Maintain pressure and abduct the stifle.
- Monitor for hip subluxation indicating hip laxity.

VACCINATIONS

Puppies and kittens receive 95% of their maternally derived antibodies via colostrum during the first four to six hours of nursing. Maternal immunity typically has a duration of between 8–16 weeks and is dependent upon multiple factors including the vaccine history of the mother and successful transfer to the neonate. Maternally derived antibodies provide initial protection against disease in young animals, but this temporary immunity can interfere in the effectiveness of the first immunizations by "blocking" the vaccine antigens. As the maternally derived antibodies wane, there is no longer sufficient protection, but there is still enough maternal protein present to prevent the young animal from its own response to a vaccine. This is known as the "window of susceptibility". The timing and duration of this window is highly variable between individual animals and even animals in the same litter. Multiple boosters are therefore recommended in young animals to provide the best opportunity for appropriate vaccine response and strong long-lasting immunity.

Vaccines must be refrigerated and need to be shaken well, but gently, before dispensing. As a general rule, vaccines should be used within 30–60 minutes of reconstitution; however, it is imperative to follow manufacturer recommendations as this is not true for all vaccines. Appropriate storage and handling of vaccines is imperative as incompatible diluents, heat, excessive cold, and light exposure can inactivate the vaccine and make them ineffective.

Guidelines to Follow When Vaccinating an Animal

- A complete physical examination and health evaluation is given by a veterinarian before any vaccination.
- Animals with a fever or in debilitated health should not be vaccinated until healthy.
- Vaccination during pregnancy should be avoided whenever possible to prevent potential injury to the fetus. However, vaccination may be considered in high-risk situations such as animal shelters where there is increased threat of exposure to highly pathogenic viruses. In this situation, the use of modified live virus (attenuated) vaccine in pregnant animals is discouraged.

To increase patient bonding and to improve client satisfaction, special steps can be taken to ensure patient and owner comfort. Taking the extra steps to make this a more enjoyable experience will benefit both the patient and staff in future visits. A few tips for making injections a more comfortable procedure include:

- Use two needles, the first to mix and draw out the vaccine and a smaller and a second new needle to deliver the vaccine into the pet.
- Distracting the pet with a high-value treat, tennis ball, petting, catnip, or anything else the pet likes.
- Gently dimple or pinch the skin a little bit in the spot you want the needle to puncture the skin.
- Deliver the injection slowly.

Vaccination Protocols

Vaccines are divided into two groups: core and non-core. Core vaccines, some of which are required by law, protect against diseases that have public health significance, are highly infectious, and pose risk of severe disease. These vaccines are considered high benefit and low risk to the patient population. Administration of non-core vaccines, those that protect against diseases of less frequency and risk, should be based on the risk associated with vaccine administration compared with the individual's risk of exposure, geographic location, and pet lifestyle. Regardless of the vaccine being administered, a minimum vaccination interval of two weeks is recommended.

Recommended small-animal vaccine protocols are charted below and are based on the American Animal Hospital Association (AAHA) 2017 *Canine Vaccination Guidelines* and the 2020 American Animal Hospital Association (AAHA)/American Association of Feline Practitioners (AAFP) *Feline Vaccination Guidelines*.

Canine Vaccination

Current canine vaccination guidelines do not specify injection-site recommendations. However, it is strongly encouraged to document the vaccination site and type in the patient's medical record.

Table 2.6 / Canine vaccination protocol

Vaccine	Route	≤ 16 weeks of age	> 16 weeks of age	Vaccine classification
Distemper: Adenovirus-2 Parvovirus ± canine parainfluenza (DAPPi) MLV/ recombinant • Canine distemper virus • Canine adenovirus • Canine parvovirus • ± Canine parainfluenza	SQ	• First dose as early as 6 weeks of age, then repeat every 2–4 weeks until at least 16 weeks of age • Dogs that are around 16 weeks of age when presented for initial vaccination should receive a second dose 2–4 weeks later • Dogs residing in a high-risk environment may benefit from receiving a final dose at 1–20 weeks of age • Revaccination: one dose within 12 months after the last dose of the initial vaccination series, then every 3 years or longer	• One or two doses of a combination vaccine • Dogs residing in a high-risk environment between 16–20 weeks of age may benefit from receiving a second dose 2–4 weeks later • Dogs residing in a high-risk environment and over 20 weeks of age when initially presented for vaccination are expected to develop protective immunity from a single dose • Revaccination: one dose within 12 months after the last dose of the initial vaccination series, then every 3 years or longer	Core
Rabies: Rabies virus	SQ/IM	• Single dose at no earlier than 12 weeks of age • Revaccination: one dose 12 months after the initial dose, then every 1–3 years, depending on vaccine type and local/state requirements	• Single dose • Revaccination: one dose 12 months after the initial dose, then every 1–3 years, depending on vaccine type and state/local requirements	Core; see rabiesaware.org for additional information on state-level rabies regulations and laws
Bordetella bronchiseptica: Canine infectious respiratory disease	SQ	• First dose as early as 8 weeks of age, then repeat in 2–4 weeks • Revaccination: one dose 12 months after the primary series, then annually	• Two doses, 2–4 weeks apart • Revaccination: one dose 12 months after the primary series, then annually	Non-core
	PO	• Single dose into the buccal pouch as early as 8 weeks of age • Revaccination: one dose 12 months after the initial dose, then annually	• Single dose into the buccal pouch • Revaccination: one dose 12 months after the initial dose, then annually	
Bordetella bronchiseptica: ± parainfluenza ± adenovirus	IN	• Single dose; generally administered ≥ 8 weeks of age, but may be considered as early as 3–4 weeks of age in high-risk environments • Revaccination: one dose 12 months after the initial dose, then annually	• Single dose • Do NOT administer parenterally or orally as severe adverse events can occur • Revaccination: one dose 12 months after the initial dose, then annually	
Canine influenza virus: Canine infectious respiratory disease	SQ	• First dose as early as 6–8 weeks of age, then repeat in 2–4 weeks • Revaccination: one dose 12 months after the primary series, then annually	• Two doses, 2–4 weeks apart • Revaccination: one dose 12 months after the primary series, then annually	Noncore

(Continued)

Table 2.6 / Canine vaccination protocol (Continued)

Vaccine	Route	≤ 16 weeks of age	> 16 weeks of age	Vaccine classification
Leptospira (quadrivalent): Canine leptospirosis	SQ	• First dose as early as 8–9 weeks of age, then repeat in 2–4 weeks • •Revaccination: one dose 12 months after the primary series, then annually	• Two doses, 2–4 weeks apart • Revaccination: one dose 12 months after the primary series, then annually	Noncore
Borrelia burgdorferi: Lyme borreliosis	SQ	• First dose as early as 8–9 weeks of age, then repeat in 2–4 weeks • Revaccination: one dose 12 months after the primary series, then annually	• Two doses, 2–4 weeks apart • Revaccination: one dose 12 months after the primary series, then annually	Noncore

Feline Vaccination

The AAFP recommends that subcutaneous administration of feline parvovirus, feline viral rhinotracheitis-1, and/or feline calicivirus vaccines be limited to the right forelimb below the elbow joint, rabies to the right rear limb below the stifle, and feline leukemia virus to be limited to the left rear limb below the stifle. Vaccine administration in the intrascapular space is not recommended.

Table 2.7 / Feline vaccination protocol

Vaccine	Route	≤ 16 weeks of age	>16 weeks of age	Injection site	Vaccine classification
Rhinotracheitis: Calicivirus Panleukopenia Feline parvovirus Feline calicivirus Feline herpesvirus-1	SQ/IN	• First dose as early as 6 weeks of age, then repeat every 34 weeks until at 16–20 weeks of age • Revaccination: one dose 12 months after the last dose of the initial vaccination series, then every 3 years	One to two doses Revaccination: one dose 6–12 months after the last dose of the initial vaccination series, then every 3 years IN: revaccinate 12 months after the primary series, then annually	SQ: below right elbow IN: is available	• Core • Cats entering high-risk situations (e.g. boarding) may benefit from revaccination 7–10 days prior to the event, particularly if they have not been vaccinated in the preceding year • Inactivated and attenuated live vaccines available
FeLV: Feline leukemia virus	SQ	• First dose as early as 8 weeks of age, then repeat in 3–4 weeks • Revaccination: one dose 12 months after the primary series, then annually	Two doses, 3–4 weeks apart Revaccination: one dose 12 months after the primary series, then annually	Below left stifle	• Non-core in adult cats; owing to susceptibility and environmental changes, FeLV should be considered a core vaccine in kittens (up to and including 1 year of age) • Retroviral status prior to vaccination is recommended • Recombinant and inactivated vaccines available
Rabies: Rabies virus	SQ	• Single dose at no earlier than 12 weeks of age • Revaccination: one dose 12 months after the initial dose, then every 1–3 years, dependent on vaccine type and local/state requirements	• Single dose • Revaccination: one dose 12 months after the initial dose, then every 1–3 years, dependent on vaccine type and state/local requirements	Below right stifle	• Core • See rabiesaware.org for additional information on state-level rabies regulations and laws. • Recombinant and inactivated vaccines available
Bordetella	IN	• For frequency and interval, follow label instructions	• For frequency and interval, follow label instructions		• Non-core; not recommended for the general cat population • Provides incomplete protection • May be used in a multi-cat household where infection is confirmed • Never administer parenterally
Chlamydophila: *Chlamydophila felis* virus	SQ	• For frequency and interval, follow label instructions	• For frequency and interval, follow label instructions	With other vaccines, can be in right lower shoulder	• Non-core; not recommended for the general cat population • Provides incomplete protection • May be used in a multi-cat household where infection is confirmed

Titers

Antibody testing for the purposes of determining protection from infection is valid only for canine distemper virus, canine parvovirus, canine adenovirus, and feline parvovirus. A positive antibody test result is indicative that immune memory exists and the patient, if exposed, is expected to mount a rapid, protective response. However, that result does not necessarily predict the duration of future immunity. Canine antibody testing algorithms can be found in the AAHA 2017 *Canine Vaccination Guidelines*.

Adverse Events

As with the administration of any drug, vaccine administration can result in an adverse event. The United States Department of Agriculture (USDA) considers a vaccine adverse event to be any undesirable or unintended effect (including lack of desired result) associated with the administration of a vaccine. Any suspected adverse event should be reported to the manufacturer and, if desired, the USDA. Possible reactions may range from minor to life threatening: sensitivity at the injection site, a small bump or knot at the injection site, slight fever, lethargy, and acute anaphylaxis (angioedema, urticaria, collapse, vomiting, diarrhea, dyspnea, shock, and death).

When possible, future vaccines should be avoided in those patients that have experienced an adverse event, but if they must be given, the following guidelines should be observed:

- A comprehensive risk assessment should be performed based on the patient's current health status, vaccination history, immune status (antibody testing), risk for exposure, as well as the number of vaccines deemed necessary at the time of the appointment.
- Patients with a history of a mild, acute post-vaccination reaction are commonly treated with a single dose of diphenhydramine prior to vaccination.
- Patients that have a mild post-vaccination reaction which requires treatment may receive a single anti-inflammatory dose of a corticosteroid.
- Patients with a history of having had a serious, acute vaccine-associated reaction (anaphylaxis) should not be revaccinated unless it is deemed absolutely necessary; the patient must be closely monitored for several hours post-vaccination.
- Patients that experience an anaphylactic reaction should be treated accordingly. Anaphylaxis is a rare adverse event to vaccination in veterinary medicine, but if a patient has been exposed to a potential allergen and has two compatible clinical signs (cutaneous signs, respiratory distress, hypotension, and/or persistent gastrointestinal signs), anaphylaxis is likely and the following interventions may be taken:
  - Obtain intravenous access
  - Epinephrine (drug of choice for life-threatening anaphylaxis)
  - Fluid resuscitation
  - Oxygen support
  - H1 blocker (i.e. diphenhydramine), ± glucocorticoids.

Feline Injection Site Sarcoma

Clients should be educated to monitor vaccination sites for lump formation and to contact their veterinarian if a lump is found. The International Society of Feline Medicine and AAFP recommends following the three-two-one rule and an incisional (vs excisional) biopsy should be performed if the lump:

- Has been present for three months or longer; or
- Becomes ≥ 2 cm in diameter; or
- Continues to increase in size one month after injection.

ANIMAL CARE

Together with medical care provided by the veterinarian, owners must take an active role in the day-to-day health of their animals. Dental care, grooming, and basic medical procedures can help provide the animal with increased health and longevity. Besides providing the basic care, it also allows the owners to be more aware of other health problems that might otherwise be missed (e.g. gum inflammation, tumors, pruritus, otitis externa).

Skill Box 2.8 / Client education: home dental care

Home dental care should be a daily part of each animal's life. The commitment to time, energy, and resources from the owner will impact the quantity and quality of their animal's life.

Supplies

- Toothbrush (e.g. finger brush, pet toothbrush, human toothbrush), gauze, washcloth.
- Veterinary enzymatic toothpaste.

Age

- Home dental care should begin between 8 and 12 weeks of age. Brushing is not critical until the adult teeth erupt, but starting early allows the animal to become accustomed to the procedure during an impressionable period of development.

Introduction

- Regardless of age, introduce brushing slowly and gradually, allowing the animal to determine the amount of time at each stage.
- As each step is begun, observe for the animal's reaction and only advance to the next step once the animal is comfortable.
- Choose a quiet time and place to begin.
- Start by rubbing your finger or a soft cloth over the outer surfaces of the animal's teeth, using a back-and-forth motion motion.
- For the first few lessons, it is a good idea to rub the cloth along only a few teeth rather than the whole mouth, especially if your pet is unsure or nervous about the process.
- Once the animal is comfortable with you rubbing their teeth, let them taste a little bit of pet toothpaste from your finger. Do not use human toothpaste, as it is not designed to be swallowed.
- Once your pet has accepted the taste of pet toothpaste, apply a small amount to the cloth and rub it over the teeth.
- Once your pet is completely used to you rubbing their teeth with a cloth, it is time to start using a toothbrush.
- Introduce a pet toothbrush held at a 45-degree angle to the tooth surface, brushing in an oval motion.
- Introduce the toothbrush with veterinary toothpaste.
- Be careful to stay on the outside surfaces of the teeth to avoid being bitten by accident. As the animal accepts the procedure, brushing of the lingual surfaces can begin.
- Place the non-brushing hand over the muzzle and tilt the head backward to open the animal's mouth.
- Brush the visible teeth (opposite side) and then repeat on the other side.

Maintenance

- Brush daily, at a minimum of every other day.
- Oral examination.
- Gums: redness, swelling, bleeding, pus.
- Teeth: loss, instability, broken, change in color.
- Mouth: halitosis, growth.

Adjuncts to Brushing

- Dental diets or treats. Check the Veterinary Oral Health Council website (vohc.org) for a list of recommended products.
- Yearly dental examinations and cleanings, if needed.

Tips for Successful Brushing

- Select the same time each day to brush so the animal expects it (routine and repetition).
- Brushing in the evening is often preferred, as everyone is in a quieter mood.
- Sessions should be short, roughly two to three minutes.
- Offer praise and reassurance during and following the brushing.

Avoid

- Human toothpaste, baking soda, or hydrogen peroxide.
- Heavy restraint.
- Brushing aggressively.
- Brushing if the procedure may cause pain (e.g. recent thorough oral examination, existing cervical line lesion, exposed pulp cavities, gingivitis, ulcerations, tooth mobility).
- Natural bones, cow hooves, hard nylon toys, as they may fracture teeth.

Note: see Chapter 21: Dentistry for further information.

Grooming

Skill Box 2.9 / Grooming

Grooming is a segment of veterinary care that is limited and typically presents itself as client education. Even though staff may not routinely provide grooming services, clients often have questions regarding the general care of their pets. Brushing, bathing, and toenail trims are the most basic of grooming procedures. There are also certain procedures that may be performed during periods of medical conditions that must be continued routinely to avoid reoccurrence of the problem, such as anal gland expression and ear cleaning and flushing.

Brushing should be a routine part of pet care to remove dead fur and dirt and to prevent matting. Besides providing the animal with a shinier and healthier coat and a chance to look and feel for abnormalities, brushing also allows bonding between the animal and the owner. There are many types of brushes and combs available for specific types of coats; a variety of options can be helpful. Applying a detangler spray before beginning may help with tangled or slightly matted fur. Using a systematic approach, begin at the head and work toward the tail. Use a gentle stroke, as ripping or pulling at the fur is painful and will make brushing a negative experience. For animals with long, thick coats, brush the fur against the natural lay of the fur and then finish with brushing the fur down. Following up with a comb may help remove the extra loose fur.

Bathing

Skill Box 2.10 / Bathing

Location

- A safe place for both owner and animal to stand, a mixture of hot and cold water available and an area able to withstand water (e.g. shaking wet canine).
- Place a towel or mat at the bottom of the tub to supply traction for the animal.
- Have a leash hook fastened to the wall so the animal can be secured without having to always have a hand on the animal.

Supplies

Multiple towels, appropriate shampoo, plastic apron, gloves (depending on the type of shampoo) and protective eyewear.

Technique

1. Comb, brush, and de-mat to remove excess fur, which allows better penetration of shampoo as detailed earlier.
2. Wet down the animal completely, making sure to get water down to the skin.
3. Apply the shampoo and lather the entire animal, including the face. If using a medicated shampoo, do not rinse until the appropriate amount of time has elapsed as directed.
4. Rinse the animal completely, making sure to remove all soapy residue.
5. Dry the animal's hair coat and ear canals with a combination of shaking (removes 95% of the water) and towels.
6. Comb and brush out the animal after the bath to remove all the hair that was loosened.

Note

- Keep the animal in a warm place until completely dry to avoid the animal becoming chilled.
- Do not place an animal in a heater/dryer cage without direct supervision and access to water to prevent overheating and death of the animal.
- If drying an animal with a blow dryer, be sure to keep the dryer on the lowest setting and continuously moving to prevent burns to the animals.

Nail Trimming

Skill Box 2.11 / Nail trimming

Nail trimming is another routine part of pet care. Failing to trim the nails may lead to the nails growing into the pad of the paw, difficulty or inability of the pet to walk, pain, and pad injuries. Most animals are adverse to nail trimming and may need some coaxing. Choosing a time when the pet is tired and comfortable may make the experience more tolerable. When trimming, it is best to hold the trimmer perpendicular (cutting top to bottom) to the nail; when held parallel (cutting side to side), crushing and splintering of the nail may take place.

When trimming nails, it is important to avoid cutting the quick, which is the blood vessels and nerves that supply the toenail. In canines, light-colored nails are easy to trim as the blood supply is easily seen and avoided (Figure 2.1). Dark-colored nails can be difficult to trim and should be done in small cuts (Figure 2.2). As small cuts are made, the white to pink crescent shape will begin to appear in the middle of the nail. This represents the quick and continuing to cut will eventually lead to bleeding. Remember to cut all nails including the dewclaws on both front and rear feet. The rear feet nails are typically shorter and require less trimming. In cats, the paw is gently squeezed to expose the nails and then they are trimmed to within 2 opmm of the quick.

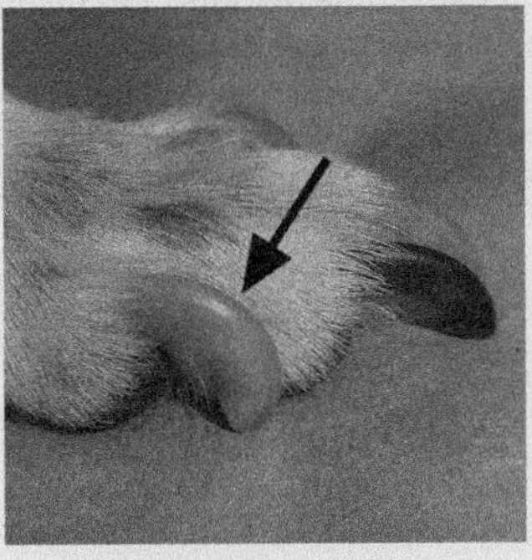

Figure 2.1 Toenail trim; (arrow) the change in color indicates the end of the blood supply, which is easily visualized in a white toenail. The nerve runs on the far end of this blood supply; thus, the trimming should be no closer than 1–2 mm of the blood supply.

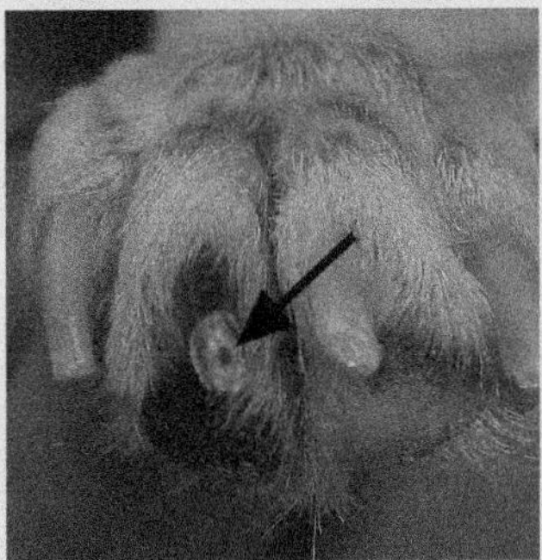

Figure 2.2 Toenail trim; (arrow) the small black circle indicates the beginning of the quick where further cutting will cause pain and bleeding. In black toenails, where the end of the blood supply is not visible, a slow approach of small trimming will reveal the end of the quick and a stopping point.

Anal Sac Expression

Skill Box 2.12 / Anal sac expression

Supplies

Gloves, water-soluble lubricant, absorbent material (e.g. rolled cotton, paper towels, baby wipes, gauze), and deodorizer.

Technique

1. Put all absorbent material into the gloved hand doing the expression to catch the expressed material; insert the forefinger into the rectum and immobilize the sac between the forefinger and the thumb on the outside of the rectum.
2. Gently apply pressure to the sac (located at 4 and 8 o'clock when looking at the anus) with the thumb and the forefinger, milking from the bottom of the sac upward toward the duct opening.
3. Note the amount and character of the material expressed. Normal secretions are a clear to slightly greenish, foul-smelling (similar to a dead fish) substance that is a liquid to a paste in consistency. Material that is very thick and pasty, purulent, or very dark should be brought to the attention of the veterinarian.
4. Clean the perianal area of the animal with absorbent material or baby wipe and then spray with a deodorizer.

Tips:

- If having difficulty expressing a gland, try rolling the skin outward with the finger outside the rectum to better expose the duct.
- If having trouble with positioning, switch and use the thumb on the inside and the forefinger on the outside or teach yourself to be ambidextrous and express the right gland with the left hand and vice versa.

Ear Cleaning and Flushing

Skill Box 2.13 / Ear cleaning and flushing

Ear Cleaning

Equipment

- Cotton balls
- Cleaning solution approved for aural use
- Syringe without the needle
- Towel

Technique

- Verify that the patient has an intact tympanic membrane.
- Using either a syringe without the needle filled with ear cleaner or a cotton ball soaked with the cleaner, fill the ear canal with a cleaning solution. Be careful not to form a seal between the instrument and the ear canal, and do not use a direct stream on the tympanic membrane.
- Put a towel or a piece of roll cotton at the entrance of the ear canal and begin gently massaging the ear canal from the bottom up. This will work the solution from the bottom of the ear canal to the opening. With a cotton ball, gently wipe out any debris. Do not push the cotton ball in the ear any further than your finger will go easily.
- Repeat steps 1 and 2 until the ear canal and solution on the cotton ball comes out clean (5–10 times).
- To dry the ear canal, use either a flushing solution or suction via an infant feeding tube attached to a syringe.

(*Continued*)

Skill Box 2.13 / Ear cleaning and flushing (Continued)

Ear Flushing

Equipment

- Cotton ball
- Cleaning solution
- Ear irrigator (filled with warm water)
- Video scope or endoscope
- Anesthetized patient
- 5 Fr red rubber feeding tube (cut to about one-half of its length)

Technique

- Take a picture of the ear canal.
- If cytology has not been done, take a sample of the ear debris.
- Insert the ear cleaner or saline and massage gently for three to four minutes.
- Wipe out any excess at the entry of the ear.
- Insert the feeding tube into the ear irrigator nozzle and turn on the machine, verifying that the pressure gauges are registering as prescribed in the manual.
- Position the video scope or endoscope into the ear and then insert the feeding tube into the port and watch on the monitor screen to see the tip protrude from the scope.
- Depress the water button on the trumpet, release, and then depress the suction button and suction out debris and liquid. Repeat several times. Remove the feeding tube if debris is clogging the tip and clean.
- A reapplication of the ear cleaning solution may be necessary in ears with a lot of debris.
- Be sure to remove all of the ear cleaner or saline.
- Take a second picture of the clean canal.
- Insert any medicines if needed.

Note: See also Figure 23.2, page 1042.

Section Three

Diagnostic Skills

Chapter 3

Clinical Pathology

Barbie M. Papajeski, MS, LVT, RLATG, VTS (Clinical Pathology)

Veterinary Technician and Nurse's Daily Reference Guide: Canine and Feline, Fourth Edition. Edited by Mandy Fults and Kenichiro Yagi.

Companion website: www.wiley.com/go/fults/veterinary

Abbreviations

AATG, anti-thyroglobulin antibodies
AChR, acetylcholine receptor
ACTH, adrenocorticotropic hormone
ALP, alkaline phosphatase
ALT, alanine aminotransferase
AST, aspartate aminotransferase
CAMP, Christie–Atkinson–Munch–Peterson
CBC, complete blood count
Cl, chloride
CSF, cerebrospinal fluid
DEA, dog erythrocyte antigen
DIC, disseminated intravascular coagulation
DTM, dermatophyte test medium
eACTH, endogenous adrenocorticotropic hormone
EDTA, ethylenediaminetetraacetic acid
ELISA, enzyme-linked immunoassay
FeLV, feline leukemia virus
FIP, feline infectious peritonitis
FIV, feline immunodeficiency virus
fT4, free tetraiodothyronine
GFR, glomerular filtration rate
GGT, gamma glutamyl transpeptidase
GLDH, glutamate dehydrogenase
GTT, gray-top tube
HCO_3, bicarbonate
HDL, high-dose lipoprotein
IgE, immunoglobulin E
IgG, immunoglobulin G
IM, intramuscular
IV, intravenous
K^+, potassium
LDDS, low-dose dexamethasone suppression
LDL, low-dose lipoprotein
LTT, lavender-top tube
MAC, MacConkey agar
MCH, mean corpuscular hemoglobin
MCHC, mean corpuscular hemoglobin concentration
MCV, mean corpuscular volume
mEq, milliequivalent
Na, sodium
NEFA, non-esterified fatty acids
NH_3, ammonia
nmol, nanomole
PCR, polymerase chain reaction
PCV, packed cell volume
PDH, pituitary-dependent hyperadrenocorticism
RBC, red blood cells
RDW, red cell distribution width
rpm, revolutions per minute
rT3, reverse triiodothyronine
RTT, red-top tube
SDH, sorbitol dehydrogenase
SGOT, serum glutamic oxaloacetic transaminase
SGPT, serum glutamic pyruvic transaminase
SST, serum separator tube
T3, triiodothyronine
T4, tetraiodothyronine
TPP, total plasma protein
TRH, thyroid-releasing hormone
TSH, thyroid-stimulating hormone
VLDL, very low dose lipoprotein
WBC, white blood cells

Each veterinary technician must be proficient in laboratory diagnostic skills. Knowing typical values for dogs and cats will make recognition of abnormalities in a patient clearer. This chapter encompasses many aspects of the veterinary laboratory. Included in each section are details of sample collection, preparation, and a brief overview of testing methods. It is important for each clinic to develop standard operating procedures and to follow test and equipment instructions where provided.[1]

BLOOD COLLECTION, HANDLING, STORAGE, AND TRANSPORT TIPS

Collection[1–5]

- Minimize fear and excitement during collection process by using low-stress and fear-free techniques.
- Minimize trauma at collection site and formation of hemolysis:
  - Use fresh needles with each attempt and avoid tissue contamination.
  - Use larger veins.
  - Collect sample quickly.
- Fast animals to minimize lipemia.

Handling[1–5]

- Handle samples gently to avoid hemolysis:
  - Allow gentle vacuum to fill tubes.
  - Never force blood into tubes.
  - Never shake tubes when mixing.
- Adequately fill tubes:
  - Follow tube guidelines for adequate fill rates.
  - Use microtainer tubes for smaller volumes.
- Avoid contamination of clot tubes with anticoagulant:
  - Fill the tubes in the correct order to prevent contamination of tubes with anticoagulant (Figure 3.1).
  - If anticoagulated tubes must be filled first to achieve accurate fill ratios, remove needle and top to fill plain tubes or serum separator tubes.
- Prepare blood smears immediately at time of collection to minimize changes in cellular morphology.
- Allow blood to clot in serum separator and red-top tubes (RTT) in an upright position for 15–30 minutes prior to centrifugation to minimize hemolysis.
- Remove serum or plasma from cells for chemistry testing to prevent alteration of values.
- Properly label each sample with the patient's full name, date, and time of collection and clinic or doctor for samples sent out.

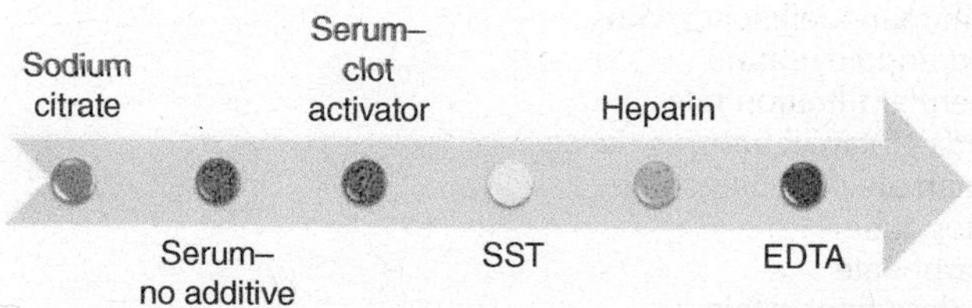

Figure 3.1 Order of draw when using a vacutainer or syringe for blood collection. Source: image courtesy of Barbie Papajeski.

Storage[1–5]

- Refrigerate serum/plasma samples if evaluation is delayed four to six hours and whole blood samples within one hour.
- Perform complete blood count within 1 hour and no longer than 24 hours post-collection.
- Complete chemistry panels within 24–48 hours of collection.
- Store unstained slides at room temperature to avoid condensation and subsequent hemolysis of cells.
- Whole blood must not be frozen, only serum or plasma is frozen for certain tests.

Transport[2]

- Use proper packaging and labeling to protect samples and personnel.
- Keep sample tubes cool to minimize artifacts and ensure sample viability.
- Package blood tubes with ice packs and protect both with paper towels.
- Further protect tubes with cushioning material and seal in secondary containers.

Table 3.1 / Blood collection tubes[2–4]

Tube	Contents	Uses	General information
Anticoagulated tubes	Whole blood/plasma	CBC, coagulation, toxicology, chemistry enzymes	• Invert immediately upon filling with at least 10 gentle inversions • Never freeze whole blood; separated plasma can be frozen
Green-top tube (GRNTT; Figure 3.3)	Lithium heparin	Blood chemistries, modified Knott's, heartworm, toxicology tests such as, lead, zinc, copper, iron,	• Heparin whole blood/heparinized plasma • Not suitable for CBC and cell morphology • Promotes platelet and WBC clumping • Interferes with staining characteristics of cells • Can be used for most chemistries panels if lithium heparin is used
Lavender-top tube (LTT; Figure 3.2)	EDTA	CBC, PCR, heartworm modified Knott's test, fluid analysis, toxicology tests, ACTH and insulin	• EDTA whole blood/plasma • Minimal changes to morphology • PCR samples must not contact formalin fumes • Underfilling tube dilutes sample and alters RBC morphology and indices due to hypertonicity • Overfilling (insufficient EDTA) the tubes may lead to clot formation • Preferred anticoagulant for most hematology tests
Light-blue-top tube(BTT)	Buffered sodium citrate	Coagulation determinations	• Yields citrated plasma when centrifuged • Chelates calcium in a gentler way than EDTA • Tubes are filled at a 1 : 9 ratio (10% dilution) • Not suitable for platelet evaluation • Plasma must be removed from cells immediately for coagulation studies
Red-top tube (RTT)	Plain	Blood chemistries, serologic testing, endocrinology except ACTH and insulin	• Yields serum when centrifuged • Missing fibrinogen proteins • Blood must fully clot before centrifugation • Remove serum from cells and place in new container to reduce glucose metabolism by RBC
Serum separator tube, SST), red/gray swirl, yellow, or brown top (Figure 3.4)	Clot activator polymer gel	Blood chemistries and serologic testing	• Once centrifuged, serum cannot mix with cells • Avoid use in some endocrine and clinical pathology tests • Check with reference laboratory regarding use
Gray-top tube (GTT), uncommon	Potassium oxalate with sodium fluoride	Glucose determinations	• Yields plasma when centrifuged • Potassium oxalate prevents clotting • Sodium fluoride stabilizes glucose • Sodium fluoride tubes alone will yield serum • Not suitable for other blood chemistry determinations

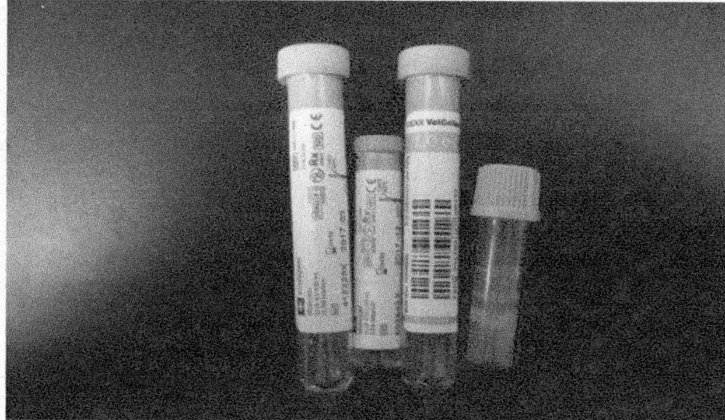

Figure 3.2 Various types of EDTA tubes. Source: image courtesy of Barbie Papajeski.

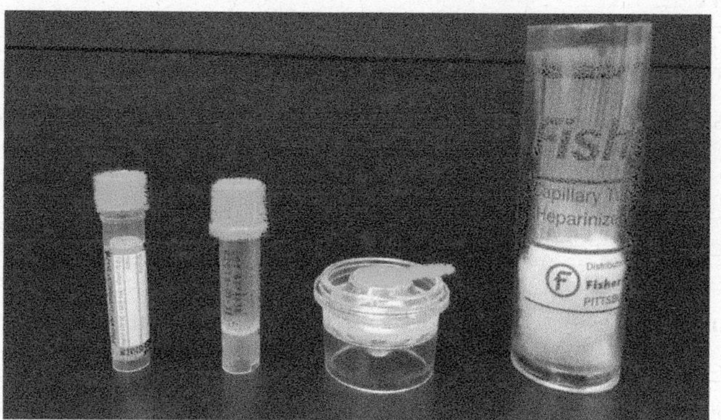

Figure 3.3 Various types of heparinized blood collection devices. The packed cell volume tubes are coated with heparin. Source: image courtesy of Barbie Papajeski.

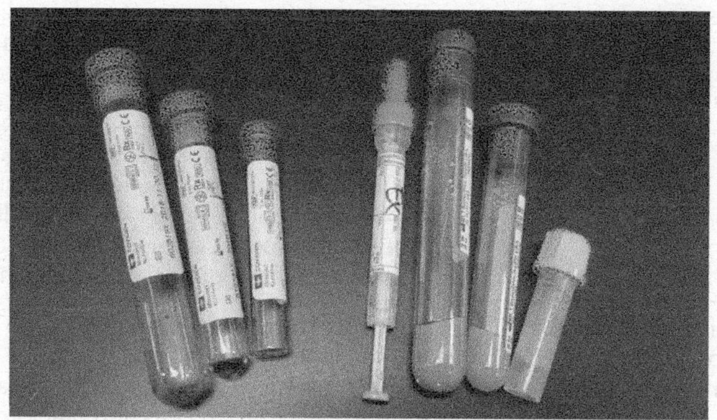

Figure 3.4 Various types of serum separator tubes. Source: Image courtesy of Barbie Papajeski.

ACID–BASE BALANCE EVALUATION

Acid–base analysis is often performed on analyzers in conjunction with electrolyte determinations and with samples already collected for these values.[4]

- Care should be taken with samples collected for acid–base evaluation.
- Limit exposure to room air.
- Cap samples immediately.
- Expel any bubbles in collection syringe.
- Use special syringes designed for electrochemical analysis.

Table 3.2 / Acid–base evaluations[2,4,6]

Chemistry	Definition	Use	Typical ranges	Associated conditions	Terminology/interferences
pH	Negative log of hydrogen ions	Measurement of blood acidity by ion selective electrode (potentiometry)	Canine: 7.31–7.42 Feline: 7.24–7.40	• Together with HCO_3, is the most useful in evaluating acid–base abnormalities	↑ alkalemia, ↓ acidemia
PCO_3	Partial pressure of carbon dioxide	Controlled by ventilation	29–42 mmHg	• Affected by respiratory conditions • Hypoventilation leads to respiratory acidosis • Hyperventilation leads to respiratory alkalosis • Disturbances develop rapidly	↑ hypercapnia, ↓ hypocapnia; measured in either venous or arterial blood
HCO_3	Bicarbonate	Major extracellular acidic buffer within the body	17.0–24.0 mEq/l	• Affected by metabolic factors: ↓ = metabolic acidosis ↑ = metabolic alkalosis • Dehydration, lactic acid production, renal failure, diabetes mellitus	Metabolic acidosis is most common cause of elevation; hemolysis, lipemia, icterus; aged samples may have falsely lowered values
PO_2	Partial pressure of dissolved oxygen in blood		85–95 mmHg	• Indicates blood oxygenation • Not accurate in certain conditions such as methemoglobinemia	Requires arterial blood; confirm oxygenation with pulse oximeter
Anion gap	Difference in measured cations and anions (Na^+, K^+, minus Cl^-, and HCO_3^-)		Canine: 12–24 mEq/l	• Indicates causes of metabolic acidosis • ↑ with lactate, ketones, and hyperalbuminemia • ↓ Hypoalbuminemia, acidemia	Calculated using measured electrolytes

BLOOD CHEMISTRY

Blood chemistry panels are an important tool in evaluating patient health status.[2,4] Correct collection methods and appropriate sample processing are critical in delivering reliable test results. Identifying and minimizing outside interferences is an important aspect of quality assurance and control. Preanalytical factors include patient preparation, sample collection and sample handling prior to testing. Analytical factors include precision and accuracy of test results. Post-analytical factors include data transmission and storage of samples for no longer than testing is valid for a particular analyte. Minimizing outside errors at each stage will ensure that any changes or atypical values are the result of a disease or condition occurring within the patient. Reference intervals are used to compare patient results. Each analyzer or laboratory will have varying reference intervals and even animals which fall within reference intervals may not be healthy. Analysis of multiple results and establishing baselines will aid in identifying atypical patterns.

Table 3.3 / Blood chemistries

Chemistry	Definition	Typical ranges	Associated conditions	Interferences/storage
Electrolyte				
Chloride	• Major anion of extracellular fluid • 1 : 1 ratio with sodium • Correct for water imbalance by dividing normal sodium by measured sodium, then multiply by measured chloride	Canine: 110–124 mg/dl Feline: 115–130 mg/dl	• ↑ Dehydration, anticonvulsant drugs, metabolic acidosis • ↓ metabolic alkalosis, diuretics, emesis	• Urine, serum or plasma (heparinized or EDTA) • Lipemia falsely ↓ • Hemolysis and icterus are not known to interfere • Separate cells from serum or plasma as soon as possible • Store at 2–8°C
Potassium	• Major cation of intracellular fluid • Important in resting potential of muscles and nerves • Balanced between ingestion and excretion through urine and feces	Canine: 3.9–5.1 mEq/l Feline: 3.7–6.1 mEq/l	• ↑ Renal diseases and aldosterone deficiency (Addison's) • ↓ Decreased dietary intake, vomiting, diarrhea, chronic renal failure	• Urine, serum or plasma (heparinized) • Separate cells from serum or plasma as soon as possible • Lipemia falsely ↓ • Hemolysis falsely ↑ • Icterus has no known effect
Sodium	• Major cation of extracellular fluid • Levels maintained by kidneys, antidiuretic hormone, aldosterone • Evaluated in light of hydration status	Canine: 142–152 mEq/l Feline: 146–156 mEq/l	• ↑ Renal tubular disease, water imbalance, water deprivation, heat stroke, vomiting, diarrhea • ↓ Increase in body water, hyperproteinemia, hyperlipidemia	• Urine, serum or plasma (Heparinized) • •Separate cells from serum or plasma as soon as possible • Lipemia falsely ↓ • Hemolysis falsely ↑ • Icterus has no known effect • Store 2 weeks at 2–8°C
Endocrine				
Thyroid hormone, free (free T4)	• Aids in definitive detection of thyroid changes • Radioimmunoassay	Canine: 9–39 pmol/l Feline: 10–53 pmol/l	• ↓ Suggests hypothyroidism	• Samples with severe hemolysis, lipemia, or warm will interfere with testing
Thyroid hormone, total T4	• Used to rule out canine hypothyroidism • Rules in hyperthyroidism in cats • Methods include radioimmunoassay, chemiluminescent enzyme immunoassay, ELISA	Canine: 11–60 nmol/l Feline: 10–47 nmol/l	• ↓ total T4 & fT4 = primary or secondary hypothyroidism • ↓ fT4 with increased TSH = primary hypothyroidism	• Samples with severe hemolysis, lipemia, or warm will interfere with testing

(*Continued*)

Table 3.3 / **Blood chemistries (Continued)**

Chemistry	Definition	Typical ranges	Associated conditions	Interferences/storage
Thyroid hormone, T3	• Not as diagnostic as other thyroid tests • rT3 is rarely used in dogs with euthyroid sick syndrome	Total T3: Canine: 0.8–2.1 nmol/l Feline: 0.6–1.4 ng/ml fT3: Canine: 1.2–8.2 pmol/l Feline: 0.3–2.9 pmol/l	• ↑ rT3 with ↓ total T4, fT4, TSH within reference interval indicates euthyroid sick canine	• Samples with severe hemolysis, lipemia, or exposed to elevated temperatures, will interfere with testing
Thyrotropin or TSH	• Used in conjunction with total T4 and fT4 to evaluate thyroid function • Differentiates primary, secondary hypothyroidism and euthyroid sick syndrome	Canine: 0–0.58 ng/ml Feline: 0–0.38 ng/ml	↑ primary hypothyroidism Within reference interval = euthyroid sick syndrome ↓ Secondary hypothyroidism	• Serum separated from cells • Store at 2–8°C • Samples with severe hemolysis, lipemia, or exposed to elevated temperatures, will interfere with testing
Kidney				
SDMA	• Amino acid which is used as an early indicator of decreased GFR and azotemia	0–14 µg/dl	↑ azotemia or hyperthyroidism	• Serum, plasma • Hemolysis, lipemia, icterus not known to interfere • Store 14 days at 2–8°C, 1 year at –20°C
Urine creatinine: urine protein ratio	• Method of quantifying protein loss in urine	< 0.5	↑ glomerular disease, glomerulonephritis, or amyloidosis	• Centrifuged urine • Test is invalid with hematuria, infection, inflammation • Corticosteroids mildly ↑ values
Function: cystatin C	• Indicator of GFR in dogs but not cats	Canine: 0.4–1.6 mg/l Feline: 0.58–1.59 mg/l	↑ prerenal azotemia, hypothyroidism in cats, kidney injury	• Serum, urine • Store 2 days at 2–8°C, 1 month at –20°C
Function: creatinine	• Byproduct of muscle catabolism • Measurements indicates GFR	Canine: 0.5–1.7 mg/dl Feline: 0.9–2.2 mg/dl	↑ decreased GFR ↓ decreased muscle mass, cachexia or starvation	• Urine, serum or plasma (EDTA or heparinized) • Hemolysis falsely ↑ • Icterus falsely ↓ • Lipemia has no known effect • Store 7 days at 2–8°C, 3 months at –20°C

(*Continued*)

Table 3.3 / **Blood chemistries (Continued)**

Chemistry	Definition	Typical ranges	Associated conditions	Interferences/storage
Function: BUN	• Produced by hepatocytes as a byproduct of amino acid catabolism • Measurement indicates GFR	Canine: 8–28 mg/dl Feline: 19–34 mg/dl	↑ severe icterus, ammonia contamination, increased protein catabolism, or decreased GFR ↓ decreased dietary protein, hyperadrenocorticism, diabetes mellitus, or liver disease	• Urine, serum or plasma (EDTA or heparinized) • Hemolysis falsely ↑ • Icterus falsely ↑ • Lipemia falsely ↓ • Store 7 days at 2–8°C, 1 year at –20°C
Liver				
Damage: ALT or SGPT	• Hepatic leakage enzyme • Liver specific enzyme for dogs and cats • Small amounts found in cardiac and skeletal muscle and RBC of cats • Half-life is 59 hours (canine), 3–4 hours (feline)	Canine: 10–109 u/l Feline: 25–97 u/l	↑ hypoxia, hepatic lipidosis, inflammation, neoplasia, toxins, hepatocyte injury, canine hyperadrenocorticism, feline hyperthyroidism, drugs such as corticosteroids and anticonvulsants ↓ insignificant	• Serum or plasma (heparinized or EDTA) • Hemolysis may falsely ↑ values in feline samples but not in canine samples • No significant interference with lipemia and icterus • ↑ differentiated from severe muscle disease with ↑AST • Store 3 days at 15–25°C, 7 days at 2–8°C, > 7 days at –60 to –80°C
Damage: GLDH	• Major source is mitochondria within hepatocytes • Sensitive for canine hepatic disease • Small amounts found in kidney, intestine, muscle, salivary glands • Half-life is 8 hours (canine)	Canine: 2–11 u/l Feline: 0–4 u/l	Hepatic injury, canine hyperadrenocorticism, anticonvulsants	• More stable than SDH • No known interferences from hemolysis, lipemia, or icterus • Store 2 days at 15–25°C, 1 week at 2–8°C, 6 months at –60 to –80°C
Damage: SDH or iditol dehydrogenase	• Major source is liver • Highly liver specific for hepatocellular damage • Superior to ALT in detecting hepatic injury • Half-life is 5 hours (canine), 3–4 hours (feline)	Canine: 0–8 u/l: 0–10 u/l	↑ hepatic injury ↓ delayed testing, otherwise insignificant	• Only available at reference labs • Delayed testing falsely ↓ • Hemolysis and lipemia may falsely ↑ values • Store 4 hours at 15–25°C, 1 week at 2–8°C, 1 month at –60 to –80°C

(*Continued*)

Table 3.3 / **Blood chemistries (Continued)**

Chemistry	Definition	Typical ranges	Associated conditions	Interferences/storage
Damage/ cholestasis: GGT	• Major source in serum is liver • Found in kidney and pancreas • Indicates cholestasis • Used with ALP to indicate hepatic disease	Canine: 0–6 u/l Feline: 0–2 u/l	↑ hepatic lipidosis in cats, biliary hyperplasia, toxins (xylitol in dogs), neoplasia, cholestasis; in renal disease, GGT is shed in urine	• Urine, serum or plasma (heparinized or EDTA) • Hemolysis and icterus may falsely ↓ values • Underfilled heparin tubes falsely ↓ values • Store 7 days at 15–25°C, 1 week at 2–8°C, 1 year at –20°C
Function: NH_3	• Formed as a byproduct of digestion • Liver is responsible for clearing by converting to urea • Not affected by cholestasis • Must perform assay within 1–3 hours	Canine: 0.0–98.0 µmol/l Feline: 0.0–95.0 µmol/l	↑ hepatic dysfunction, hepatic blood flow abnormalities, strenuous exercise, high-protein meals, inherited disorders	• Fast animals for 8 hours EDTA or ammonia-free heparin • Place in ice bath and separate plasma within 10 minutes with minimal exposure to air • Testing delays ↑ values
Function: bile acids	• Steroids produced in the liver from cholesterol • Liver function test • Fasting and post-prandial samples are tested	Canine and feline 0–13 µmol/l Canine postprandial: 0–30 µmol/l Feline postprandial: 0–25 µmol/l	↑ hepatic insufficiency, portosystemic shunt, cholestasis, cirrhosis, necrosis, hepatic lipidosis, neoplasia, glucocorticoid hepatopathy (canine)	• Serum or plasma (heparinized or EDTA) • Lipemia falsely ↑ • Hemolysis falsely ↓ values
Damage/ cholestasis/ cortisol: ALP	• Non-specific enzyme found attached to cell membranes in liver, bone, kidney, intestine, pancreas, and placenta • Half-life dependent on tissue; liver and bone is 2–3 days (canine), 6 hours (feline), intestinal, kidney, placental is < 6 minutes (canine) and < 2 minutes (feline)	Canine: 1–114 u/l Feline: 0–45 u/l	↑ in cholestasis, osteoblast activity in young animals or bone disorders, mammary tumors, corticosteroids, hyperadrenocorticism, anticonvulsants ↓ insignificant	• Serum or heparinized plasma • Hemolysis may falsely ↑ values • No significant interference with lipemia and icterus • Store 7 days at 15–25°C, 7 days at 2–8°C, 2 months at –60 to –80°C
Hemolysis: bilirubin	• Formed as a byproduct of hemoglobin degradation • Liver is responsible for conjugation (Direct bilirubin)	Canine: 0.0–0.3 mg/dl Feline: 0.0–0.1 mg/dl	↑ unconjugated in hemolytic diseases and hepatic injury or defect ↑ conjugated in cholestasis (also see bilirubinuria)	• Serum or plasma (heparinized or EDTA) • Hemolysis and lipemia may falsely ↑ values • Exposure to light oxidizes bilirubin and falsely ↓ values • Store at 2–8°C or freeze at –20°C

(Continued)

Table 3.3 / **Blood chemistries (Continued)**

Chemistry	Definition	Typical ranges	Associated conditions	Interferences/storage
Muscle damage: AST or SGOT	• Major source is skeletal muscle, then liver, then cardiac muscle and RBC • Parallels ALT elevations • Used to indicate hepatic or muscle injury • Half-life is 4–12 hours (canine), 77 minutes (feline)	Canine: 13–15 u/l Feline: 7–38 u/l	↑ hepatic injury (less change than ALT), muscular trauma, hyperthyroidism in cats, anticonvulsant drugs, corticosteroids which cause hepatocellular damage, and hemolytic diseases CK is used to confirm muscle trauma	• Serum or plasma (heparinized or EDTA) • Hemolysis may falsely ↑ values • Lipemia & icterus may ↑ values • Ketoacidosis may ↑ • ↑ differentiated from severe muscle disease with ↑ AST • Store 24 hours at 15–25°C
Metabolic				
Cholesterol	• Most common steroid, ingested from diet and produced in liver • Small amounts produced by intestines, adrenal glands and reproductive organs • Building block of lipoproteins (LDL, HDL, VLDL) and bile acids	Canine: 135–278 mg/dl Feline: 71–156 mg/dl	↑ hypothyroidism, cholestasis, diabetes mellitus, hyperadrenocorticism, pancreatitis, lipid metabolism disorders ↓ malabsorption, maldigestion, hepatic disease, altered metabolism, neoplasia	• Serum or plasma (heparinized or EDTA) • Fast animals for 12 hours • Hemolysis and lipemia may falsely ↑ values • Icterus may falsely ↓ values • Store 5–7 days at 2–8°C, 3 months at –20°C, several years at –60 to –80°C
Glucose	• Sources include dietary, glycogen breakdown, and glucose production by liver	Canine: 76–119 mg/dl Feline: 60–120 mg/dl	↑ postprandial, stress, pregnancy, drugs (e.g. xylazine, detomidine, propranolol, megestrol acetate, ketamine), diabetes mellitus, hyperadrenocorticism, hyperthyroidism ↓ liver disease, or increased insulin	• Serum, plasma (EDTA, heparinized or citrated), urine, and body cavity fluids • Separate cells from serum or plasma as soon as possible • No known interferences with hemolysis, lipemia, icterus
Lipids/triglycerides	• Lipid compounds which contain glycerol and three long-chain fatty acids	Canine: 22–125 mg/dl Feline: 25–133 mg/dl	↑ Pancreatitis, diabetes mellitus, postprandial, corticosteroid, hepatic lipidosis, hyperadrenocorticism, hypothyroidism, or cholestasis ↓ Insignificant	• Serum, plasma (EDTA or heparinized), peritoneal or pleural fluid) • No known interferences with hemolysis and lipemia • Icterus may falsely ↓ values
Fructosamine	• Glycosylated protein (glucose + albumin) • Indicates glucose levels over 2–3-week span	Canine: 222–348 μmol/l Feline: 174–294 μmol/L	↑ persistent hyperglycemia, diabetes mellitus ↓ Hyperthyroidism, insulinoma	• Serum or plasma (EDTA or heparinized) • Hemolysis may ↑ or ↓ • Hyperproteinemia falsely ↓ • Levodopa falsely ↑

(*Continued*)

Table 3.3 / Blood chemistries (Continued)

Chemistry	Definition	Typical ranges	Associated conditions	Interferences/storage
NEFA	• Hydrolyzed triglycerides	Canine: 0.1–1.2 mEq/l Feline: 0.13–1.32 mEq/l	↑ Exercise, excitement, stress, diabetes mellitus	• Serum or plasma (EDTA) • Heparin falsely ↑ • Hemolysis may ↑ or ↓ • No known interference with lipemia and icterus • Separate from cells as soon as possible • Place samples on ice
Ketones: β-hydroxybutyrate	• Ketone produced from NEFA metabolism • Indicates ketosis	Canine: 0–1 mg/dl Feline: 0–2 mg/dl	↑ Diabetes mellitus, ketoacidosis, starvation, lactation	• Serum or plasma (heparinized) • Separate from cells as soon as possible • No known interferences with hemolysis, lipemia, icterus
Mineral				
Phosphate	• 80–88% in bone • Major intracellular anion • Released by parathyroid hormone	Canine: 0.9–1.7 mg/dl Feline: 1.0–2.0 mg/dl	↑ Decreased renal excretion, increased dietary intake, osteolytic lesions, metabolic acidosis ↓ Hormonal imbalance, decreased renal reabsorption, hyperparathyroidism, decreased intestinal absorption, insulin	• Urine, serum or plasma (heparinized) • Hemolysis and icterus may falsely ↓ values • Store 24 hours at 15–25°C, 4 days at 2–8°C, 1 year at –20°C
Calcium (total and free)	• 99% of calcium in bones • Regulated by kidneys and gastrointestinal tract • Released by parathyroid hormone • Balanced with dietary intake	Canine: 9.1–11.7 mg/dl Feline: 8.7–11.7 mg/dl	↑ Addison's disease, renal disease, osteolytic lesions, hyperparathyroidism, hypervitaminosis D, increased dietary uptake or neoplasias ↓ hypoalbuminemia, hypoparathyroidism, hypovitaminosis D, hypoadrenocorticism, toxins, decreased osteolysis, or dietary uptake	• Serum or plasma (heparinized) • Lipemia and icterus falsely ↑ values • No known interferences with hemolysis
Magnesium	• Major intracellular cation • 50% is found in bone, skeletal muscle and soft tissue • Balanced through intestinal absorption and urinary excretion	Canine: 1.6–2.4 mg/dl Feline: 1.7–2.6 mg/dl	↑ Decreased renal excretion, renal failure, obstruction ↓ in conjunction with hypokalemia, or hypocalcemia, hypoalbuminemia, malabsorption, or diarrhea	• Serum or plasma (heparinized) • Hemolysis ↑ values • No known interferences with lipemia or icterus • Store 7 days at 2–8°C, 1 year at –20°C

(Continued)

Table 3.3 / **Blood chemistries (Continued)**

Chemistry	Definition	Typical ranges	Associated conditions	Interferences/storage
Muscle				
Creatine kinase	• Leakage enzyme of skeletal cardiac muscle and brain	Canine: 48–261 u/l Feline: 73–388 u/l	↑ Muscle trauma or disease, anorexia, neurologic injury (CSF)	• Serum, plasma (heparinized or EDTA), cerebrospinal fluid • Hemolysis, icterus, lipemia ↑ values • Store 7 days at 2–8°C, 4 weeks at –20°C
Damage: lactate dehydrogenase	• Enzyme catabolizes lactate to pyruvate • Nonspecific test	Canine: 30–236 u/l Feline: 30–236 u/l	↑ Liver damage, muscle disease or injury, or neoplasia	• Serum, plasma (heparinized), CSF • Hemolysis ↑ values • Lipemia will ↓ values • Severe icterus also affects results • Store 4 days at 2–8°C, 6 weeks at –20°C
Damage: cardiac troponin	• Proteins released from damaged cardiac muscle	0–0.059 ng/ml[9]	↑ Cardiomyopathy, mitral valve disease, acute myocardial injury, renal failure	• Plasma (EDTA) in plastic tube • Marked hemolysis interferes with test • Store 7 days at 2–8°C
Pancreas				
Function: trypsin-like immunoreactivity	• Uses a species-specific antibody to detect trypsin and trypsinogen in plasma or serum	Canine: 5–35 μg/l Feline: 8.0 μg/l	↓ Pancreatic exocrine insufficiency ↑ decreased GFR	• Fast for 12 hours • Serum or plasma (heparinized or EDTA) • Lipemia falsely ↓
Lipase immunoreactivity	• Uses a species-specific antibody to detect pancreatitis • Specific for pancreatic lipase	Canine: 0–200 μg/l Feline: 0–3.5 μg/l	↑ moderate to severe pancreatitis Canine: > 400 μg/l Feline: > 5.4 μg/l	• Fast for 12 hours • Hemolysis will interfere with testing
Liver/intestinal: lipase	• Secreted primarily by pancreas • Process triglycerides • Useful indicator of pancreatitis in canines but not felines	Canine: 78–765 u/l Feline: 5–222 u/l	↑ Pancreatitis (dogs), neoplasia, hepatic disease, azotemia, decreased GFR, corticosteroids, intestinal obstruction	• Serum, plasma (heparinized) • No interferences with hemolysis, lipemia, icterus • 1 week at 15–25°C, 1 year at –20°C
Kidney/intestinal: amylase	• Secreted mainly by pancreas • Minor amounts in liver and small intestine • Process complex carbohydrates into maltose and glucose • Used in conjunction with lipase activity – not specific for pancreatic injury	Canine: 226–1063 u/l Feline: 550–1458 u/l	↑ Pancreatitis, renal insufficiency, decreased GFR, intestinal obstruction	• Serum, plasma (heparinized or EDTA), or urine • Do not use citrate or fluoride • Hemolysis, lipemia, icterus ↓ values • Corticosteroid, ↑ glucose, ascorbic acid ↓ values • Store serum/plasma 30 days, urine 7 days at 2–8°C, serum/plasma 7 days at 15–25°C, urine 2 days at 15–25°C

(Continued)

Table 3.3 / Blood chemistries (Continued)

Chemistry	Definition	Typical ranges	Associated conditions	Interferences/storage
Protein				
Albumin–globulin ratio	• Identifies causes of serum protein changes	Typical values are 1 : 1	Evaluate together with total protein value: ↑ protein with A/G ratio of 1 = dehydration ↑ protein with ↓ ratio = hyperglobulinemia ↑ protein with ↑ ratio = hyperglobulinemia	• Calculated by dividing albumin concentration by the globulin concentration
Total protein	• Includes albumin, globulin and fibrinogen in plasma samples • Fibrinogen is not measured in serum • Interpreted with PCV and specific albumin components	Serum protein: Canine: 5.4–7.5 g/dl Feline: 6.0–7.9 g/dl Plasma protein: Canine and feline: 6.0–7.5 g/dl	↑ Dehydration (with ↑ PCV), ↓ Acute blood loss (with ↓ PCV); see albumin and globulin changes	• Serum or plasma (heparinized or EDTA) • Separate from cells within 4 hours • Severe hemolysis and lipemia ↑ value • Icterus may ↓ values • Store 3 days at 2–8°C or 6 months at −20°C
Liver: fibrinogen	• Produced by hepatocytes • Forms fibrin in clot formation • Not present in serum • Plasma protein/fibrinogen ratio used to distinguish dehydration and inflammation • Used more commonly in large animals	Canine and feline: 150–300 mg/dl TPP : fibrinogen < 10 = inflammation[4] TPP : fibrinogen > 15 = typical or dehydration	↑ Inflammation, dehydration, neoplasia, pregnancy ↓ DIC, hepatic failure	• Plasma (EDTA) • Hemolysis and lipemia may falsely ↑ values
Liver/other: albumin	• Produced by hepatocytes • Carrier protein and antioxidant • 60–80% of hepatic function is lost before decrease • Influenced by factors outside liver	Canine: 2.3–3.1 g/dl Feline: 2.8–3.9 g/dl	↑ Dehydration, adrenal dysfunction, neoplasia ↓ Malnutrition, liver failure, hemorrhage, inflammation, neoplasia, protein losing enteropathy, exudates, protein rich effusions	• Serum or plasma (heparinized or EDTA) • Lipemia falsely ↑ • Hemolysis and icterus – no interference • Store 2.5 months at 15–25°C, 5 months at 2–8°C, 4 months at −20°C

(Continued)

Table 3.3 / **Blood chemistries (Continued)**

Chemistry	Definition	Typical ranges	Associated conditions	Interferences/storage
Liver/other: globulin	• Includes hundreds of different proteins • α & β globulins produced by hepatocytes • γ globulins produced by lymphocytes and plasma cells	Serum protein: Canine: 2.7–4.4 g/dl Feline: 2.6–5.1 g/dl	↑ Dehydration, inflammation, gammopathy, hepatic disease, neoplasia ↓ Overhydration, hemorrhage, protein losing enteropathy, immune deficiency, failure of passive transfer (colostrum intake)	• Calculated by subtracting albumin from total protein • Factors affecting total protein and albumin will affect globulin
Urine				
Cortisol: creatinine ratio	• Add-on test used in conjunction with LDDS and ACTH stimulation to identify hyperadrenocorticism	Canine: 8 : 24	≥ 34 hyperadrenocorticism	• Uncentrifuged, voided urine sample collected post-rest in home environment • EDTA will interfere with testing • Store 5 days at 2–8°C, 4 weeks at –20°C

CHEMISTRY FUNCTION TESTS

Function tests are used to force a system in the body to perform in a specific way (e.g. suppression or stimulation) to provide predictable results. Depending on values, resultant tests determine the system is functioning correctly. Most of these procedures require a specific protocol of fasting, injections, and blood draw times; however, individual laboratories must be consulted regarding specific protocols, collection tubes, and storage of specimens prior to testing.

Table 3.4 / **Function tests**[4,6–8,10,11]

Test	Definition	Typical Range	Protocols / Handling and Special Considerations
AATG autoantibodies test	• Identifies lymphocytic thyroiditis • Autoantibodies against thyroglobulin is detected by radioimmunoassay	Canine: 0–35%	• Collect 1–2 ml serum in RTT • Corticosteroid or immunosuppressant therapy will alter results
AChR antibodies	• Identifies an immune response specifically against muscle AChRs • Identifies myasthenia gravis, most common neurological disorder in dogs	Canine: < 0.6 nmol/l Feline: < 0.3 nmol/l	• Collect 2 ml serum in RTT • Corticosteroid or immunosuppressant therapy will alter results • Hemolysis and lipemia interfere with test
eACTH plasma concentration	• Distinguishes pituitary-dependent hyperadrenocorticism from adrenocortical tumors	Canine: 6.7–25.0 pmol/l	• Fast for 12 hours • Collect blood in LTT (adequately fill) • Centrifuge and separate plasma into a plastic tube • Freeze sample and submit to reference laboratory • Contact with red blood cells and heat affects values
ACTH stimulation or response test	• Screens for hyperadrenocorticism, hypoadrenocorticism and monitors therapy effectiveness	Canine: Pre-test: 2–6 µg/dl Post-test: 6–18 µg/dl Feline: Pre-test: 0.5–5.0 µg/dl Post-test: 5–15 µg/dl	• Collect 1 ml serum for a baseline cortisol • Administer ACTH (Cortrosyn®) 5 µg/kg IV or IM • Collect 1 ml serum 1 hour post-injection • Label samples as "pre", "post-1 hour" • Icterus, anticoagulants, and corticosteroids will interfere with test[11] • Other forms of ACTH include generic cosyntropin, Cortrosyn, Synacthen®, and Synacthen Depot®
ADH (antidiuretic hormone, vasopressin, desmopressin) response test	• Antidiuretic hormone is secreted by the hypothalamus • Evaluates renal ability to concentrate urine in water deprived animals • Differentiates central from nephrogenic diabetes insipidus	Canine/feline: central diabetes insipidus: ↑ urine specific gravity within 2–12 hours; nephrogenic diabetes insipidus: no response to vasopressin administration	• Used in lieu of water deprivation • Typical 24-hour water intake is monitored and urine samples collected for 2–3 days and urine specific gravity measured • 2–4 drops of desmopressin (DDAVP®) is administered in the conjunctival sac • Empty bladder at 2 hours and measure specific gravity of urine at regular intervals: 4, 8, 12, 18, and 24 hours
HDDST (dexamethasone suppression test, high dose)	• Differentiates between PDH and adrenocortical tumors in canines • Dexamethasone at a high enough dose will decrease release of ACTH • If IV route is used, inject slowly	PDH cortisol < 1.4 µg/dl or < 50% of baseline cortisol at 4 or 8 hours	• Collect 1 ml serum in plain RTT • Give 0.1 mg/kg (canines) dexamethasone IM or IV • Collect a blood sample at 4 and 8 hours post-injection • Separate serum from cells and label tubes as "pre", "4 hour", and "8 hour", together with patient identifiers • Icterus, anticoagulants, corticosteroid therapy, and phenobarbital can alter results

(Continued)

Table 3.4 / Function tests (Continued)

Test	Definition	Typical Range	Protocols / Handling and Special Considerations
LDDST (dexamethasone suppression test, low dose)	• Differentiates between pituitary-dependent hyperadrenocorticism and adrenocortical tumors in canines	PDH cortisol < 1.4 µg/dl or < 50% of baseline cortisol at 4 and 8 hours cortisol < 59% of baseline but > 1.4 µg/dl	• Collect 1 ml of serum in plain RTT • Give 0.01–0.015 mg/kg (canines) or 1.0 mg/kg (felines) dexamethasone IV (check reference laboratories for dosage recommendations) • Collect a blood sample at 4 and 8 hours post-collection • Separate serum from cells and label tubes as "pre", "4 hour", and "8 hour", together with patient identifiers • Icterus, anticoagulants, corticosteroid therapy, and phenobarbital can alter results
Folate and cobalamin	• Tests used to detect exocrine pancreatic insufficiency, distal small intestinal mucosal disease, and/or small intestinal bacterial overgrowth	↓ Cobalamin = exocrine pancreatic insufficiency, distal small intestinal mucosal disease, and/or small intestinal bacterial overgrowth ↑ Folate = exocrine pancreatic insufficiency and/or small intestinal bacterial overgrowth ↓ Folate = proximal small intestinal mucosal disease	• Fast for 12 hours. • Collect 1 ml serum in plain RTT • Separate serum from cells as soon as possible • Hemolysis ↑ folate value • Avoid prolonged exposure to light and heat
Liver function; ammonia tolerance test	• Evaluates animals for portosystemic shunts or decreased hepatic function • Contraindicated in animals with fasting hyperammonemia	Canine: typical increase from pre- to post-administration is 2.0–2.5 times; portosystemic shunts/severe hepatic insufficiency 3.0–10.0-fold increase	• Obtain a fasting plasma sample (heparin or EDTA), cool and separate from cells within 10 minutes with minimal exposure to air • Administer ammonium chloride solution (20 mg/ml) at 100 mg/kg via stomach tube (not to exceed 3 g) • Collect sample 30 minutes post administration and assay • Samples must be immediately cooled, separated, and tested within 3 hours • Lipemia, hemolysis, and icterus may ↑ values
T_3 suppression test	• Evaluates thyroid ability to suppress pituitary TSH secretion followed by a drop in T_4 secretion • T_3 ↑ over baseline indicates owner compliance	Canine/feline: Baseline: T_4: 0.8–4.0 µg/dl; T_3: 32.5–130 µg/dl Post: T_4: < 1.5 µg/dl	• On day 1, obtain blood in RTT and separate serum for T_4 and T_3 • Give 25 µg/cat of synthetic T_3 orally, three times a day, starting the next morning, for 2 days • Morning of day 3, give 25 µg orally of T_3 and redraw blood sample within 4 hours for T_3 and T_4 • Anticoagulants and some drugs interfere with test results

(Continued)

Table 3.4 / Function tests (Continued)

Test	Definition	Typical Range	Protocols / Handling and Special Considerations
Thyroid-releasing hormone response test	• Exogenous TRH causes release of TSH in euthyroid felines which stimulates total T4 • Adverse effects of vomiting, defecation, salivation, and tachypnea	Euthyroid = 60% ↑ from base total T4 Hyperthyroid = 0–50% ↑ from base total T4	• Collect blood in RTT and separate serum for total T_4 baseline • Administer 0.1 mg/kg (felines) and 0.2 mg/kg (canines) of TRH IV • Collect second sample 30 minutes later and third sample 4 hours later (canines) and second sample 4 hours later (felines) for total T_4 • Label samples for collection time and with patient identifiers
Thyroid-stimulating hormone test	• TRH is responsible for the release of TSH from the anterior pituitary and synthesis of thyroid hormone • Evaluates thyroid gland function by the degree of change after administration of TSH	Hypothyroid = < 1.5 µg/dl Post-TSH: euthyroid > 2.5 µg/dl	• Collect blood in RTT and separate serum for total T_4 baseline • Administer 75–150 µg of recombinant human TSH (Thyrogen®) IV • Collect second sample 6 hours later (canines) and second sample 4 hours later (felines) for TT_4 • Label samples for collection time and with patient identifiers
Water-deprivation test	• Evaluates body's ability to release ADH and concentrate urine • Used only in animals without azotemia, dehydration, and renal disease • Detects diabetes insipidus • Rules out problems with renal GFR • Performed after other diagnostic tests are inconclusive • Patients are weighed daily, accessed for hydration status, and biochemistry assays such as blood urea nitrogen and creatinine	Canine/feline: A urine specific gravity of 1.025 is considered an adequate response	• Collect random urine samples in a 24-hour period, with free access to measured water • Determine the average 24-hour water intake by allowing free access to measured water for three 24-hour periods • Empty urinary bladder and measure urine specific gravity and weigh the animal • Withhold food and water until the end of the test • Every 2–4 hours, empty the urinary bladder, measure the urine specific gravity, and weigh the animal until it has lost ≥ 5% of body weight, becomes ill, or urine specific gravity is > 1.030 in canines or > 1.035 in felines

Miscellaneous Diagnostic Tests – Therapeutic Monitoring and Toxicity

Other testing in veterinary medicine includes monitoring therapeutic drug dosages and detecting exposure to toxic substances.[6,8,10] Some of these tests can be monitored in-house with chemistry units or test kits and others are sent to reference laboratories for more specialized testing.

Table 3.5 / **Miscellaneous diagnostic tests, therapeutic drug levels and toxins**[6,8,10]

Test	Definition	Typical ranges	Associated conditions	Sample collection/storage
Aminopyridine (Avitrol®)	Toxin used as bird repellent	None	Convulsions	• Stomach contents are submitted for testing
Anti-Xa	Therapeutic: heparin therapy monitoring	Peak is 3–4 hours in dogs and 2–3 hours in cats	Thrombosis or thromboprophylaxis	• Collect samples in citrated, plasma vacutainer tubes • Exposure to glass causes factor activation
Arsenic	Toxin: heavy metal toxicities	None	Damages capillaries leading to hypovolemic shock	• Collect 50 ml urine or 5 ml heparinized whole blood • Needs to stay refrigerated
Bromethalin	Toxin: rodenticide	None	Neurotoxin	• Stomach contents are submitted for testing
Bromide	Therapeutic: antiepileptic drug	Canine: 0.8–2.0 mg/ml Feline: 1.0–3.0 mg/ml	Seizures	• None known
Carbon monoxide	Toxin: fatal gas	None	Internal tissues are bright pink	• Collect samples in EDTA or heparin, filling tubes full to minimize air
Carnitine	Deficiency: amino acid synthesized in the body	Screening for deficiency; supplementation 50 mg/kg in dogs	Dilated cardiomyopathy, diabetes mellitus, hyperlipidemia, hepatic lipidosis, and obesity	• Collect samples in heparinized plasma or submit a urine sample • Avoid collecting in EDTA
Cholinesterase	Toxin detection: neurotransmitter	Canine: 3401–9337 iu/l Feline: 2845–3919 iu/l	Organophosphate toxicity	• Collect serum samples; no known interference
Copper	Toxin: heavy metal toxicities	None	Gastroenteritis and hemolytic anemia	• Collected in royal-blue tubes or heparinized tubes without hemolysis, separate plasma from cells and freeze • Liver, kidney, feed, and feces may also be tested

(Continued)

Table 3.5 / **Miscellaneous diagnostic tests, therapeutic drug levels and toxins (Continued)**

Test	Definition	Typical ranges	Associated conditions	Sample collection/storage
Cyanide	Toxin found in plants, burning plastic, and cigarette smoke	None	Bright cherry red blood, and sudden death	• EDTA whole blood, liver, kidney, muscle, feed, water, muscle, stomach contents, and plants placed in paper bags
Cyclosporine	Therapeutic: immunosuppressant	12-hour level before administration of 250–600 ng/ml	Atopic dermatitis	• Collect samples in EDTA • Clotted samples
Digoxin	Therapeutic: cardiac glycosin	Samples collected 4–6 hours post-administration (through sample)	Heart failure	• Collect samples in RTT • Avoid using SST
Ethylene glycol	Toxin	Negative = 0.5 mg/dl Exposure > 20 mg/dl	Ethylene glycol toxicity within 12 hours of ingestion	• Medication/foods containing propylene glycol, glycerol mannitol, or sorbitol
Fluconazole	Therapeutic: antifungal medication	None, human ranges are used as reference	Fungal disease	• Collect samples in RTT • Avoid using SST • Separate and freeze serum
Gentamicin	Therapeutic: aminoglycoside antibiotic	For peak samples draw 1½–2 hours post dosing Collect second sample 4–6 hours after first for half life Ideal peak value is 10–12 minimal inhibitory concentration	Nephrotoxicity	• Collect samples in RTT • Avoid using SST and glass • Glass may falsely lower values
Glucose curve	Therapeutic: test to find insulin dosage	Collect samples every 2 hours for a 12-hour period, post-feeding and insulin administration (24 hours if dosed once a day) using whole blood with veterinary glucometer for in-hospital testing	Diabetes mellitus	• Separated serum • Avoid using GTT
Iron	Deficiency: important metal for hemoglobin transport	Normal reference ranges: – Canine 46–147 µg/dl – Feline 42–165 µg/dl	Iron deficiency anemia often from hemorrhage	• Collect serum free of lipemia or hemolysis

(Continued)

Table 3.5 / **Miscellaneous diagnostic tests, therapeutic drug levels and toxins (Continued)**

Test	Definition	Typical ranges	Associated conditions	Sample collection/storage
Lead	Toxin: heavy metal toxicities	< 10 µg/dl normal 60 µg/dl lead poisoning	Lead toxicity	• Collect 2 ml EDTA whole blood in plastic container • Clots, sunlight, hemolysis, other anticoagulants
Levetiracetam	Therapeutic: antiepileptic drug	Peak sample 2 hours post-dose and Trough samples 8 hours Therapeutic range: 5–45 µg/ml	Seizures	• Collect samples in RTT • Avoid using SST and anticoagulants
Marijuana	Toxin: plant based illicit drug with tetrahydrocannabinol	None	Depression, seizures, ataxia, hypothermia, bradycardia, urinary incontinence, vocalization, hypersalivation, emesis, diarrhea, and coma	• Urine, EDTA whole blood, EDTA plasma or serum separated into RTT • Store refrigerated
MDR1	Gene	Positive or negative	Ivermectin sensitivity	• Collect 2 ml EDTA whole blood
Mercury	Toxin: heavy metal toxicities	< 0.1 mg/kg	Respiratory signs (if inhaled) and neurological signs	• EDTA whole blood, liver kidney cortex, water, feed, urine. • Refrigerate blood and urine • Freeze tissues and source items in nonmetal container
Metaldehyde	Toxin: ingredient used in pesticides (snail bait); neurotoxin	None	Emesis, diarrhea, hypersalivation, muscle tremors, anxiety, hyperesthesia, ataxia, tachycardia, and hyperthermia, nystagmus, and mydriasis	• Stomach contents, urine, serum, other source material • Separate serum from cells • Freeze for storage
Nitrate/nitrite	Toxin: found in fertilizer, plants	None	Hypothermia, ataxia, dyspnea, tachypnea, anxiety, and frequent urination, hypersalivation, hypoxia, dyspnea, convulsions, and methemoglobinemia,(chocolate brown blood)	• Collect serum samples in a RTT, feed, heparin or EDTA plasma, or water • Avoid using SST
Organophosphate Screen	Toxin: insecticide	None	Hypersalivation, emesis, diarrhea, dyspnea, frequent urination, muscle tremors, weakness, and convulsions,	• EDTA whole blood collected in glass container • Avoid plastic • Stomach, intestinal contents, and liver • Freeze samples other than whole blood

(*Continued*)

Table 3.5 / Miscellaneous diagnostic tests, therapeutic drug levels and toxins (Continued)

Test	Definition	Typical ranges	Associated conditions	Sample collection/storage
Paraquat	Toxin: herbicide	None	Excitement, convulsions, depression, incoordination, anorexia, gastroenteritis, dyspnea, renal damage, and contact lesions	• Urine or serum, frozen
Phenobarbital	Therapeutic: antiepileptic drug	Subtherapeutic <15 μg/ml Therapeutic15–45 μg/ml Ideal 20–30 μg/ml Possible toxicity>30 μg/ml	Seizures	• Collect samples in RTT • Avoid using SST
Rodenticide anticoagulant screening	Toxins used as rodenticides	None	Hemorrhage	• Stomach contents are submitted for testing
Strychnine	Toxin: pesticide for gopher control	None	Nervousness, tenseness, tetanic seizures, hyperthermia, cyanotic MM, dilated pupils, and death from asphyxiation	• Gastrointestinal contents, liver, serum, heparinized whole blood urine, or source bait • Do not use SST • Freeze tissues and stomach contents
Taurine	Deficiency: amino acid	Plasma levels are used to identify deficient animals	Hepatic lipidosis, cardiomyopathy	• Heparinized plasma, separated from cells • High numbers of WBCs will falsely elevate values • Avoid EDTA and SST
Theophylline	Therapeutic: cardiopulmonary drug, bronchodilator	Peak samples are drawn 2 h after dosing	Asthma (cats) Bronchitis (dogs)	• Collect samples in RTT • Avoid using SST • Store at room temperature
Vitamin D	Deficiency or toxicity	Plasma levels indicate whether vitamin D is adequate, decreased, or elevated	Vitamin D toxicity due to supplements, rodenticides Deficiencies cause rickets.	• RTT, GTT, or SST • Separate plasma or serum • Avoid EDTA, hemolysis, lipemia, and light exposure • Fast animals overnight prior to collection
Zinc	Toxin: heavy metal toxicities	None	Anorexia, vomiting, diarrhea, hemolytic anemia, cardiac arrhythmias and death	• Collected in royal blue tubes or RTT without contact with rubber stopper • Avoid using EDTA
Zonisamide	Therapeutic: antiepileptic drug	Peak sample 2 hours post-dose; 10–40 μg/ml	Seizures	• Collect samples in RTT • Avoid using SST

CYTOLOGY

Cytology is a routine procedure often performed in clinics at the point of care. Educated technicians and nurses who have diverse diagnostic skill sets are invaluable to the veterinary team in performing preliminary assessments of the patient. Proper collection and processing of specimens, cellular identification, accurate description of structures and execution of further in-house tests are essential in aiding the veterinarian in their final diagnosis and ensuring diagnostic results.

Cytology Collection, Handling, Storage, and Transport Tips

Collection[5]

- Method of collection will depend on lesion location, size, and firmness (Skill Box 3.1).
- Rapid, negative pressure (pulling back at least three-quarters of the syringe) while various depths and locations within the mass are sampled to retrieve cells.
- Prolonged aspiration or using too large a gauge needle leads to peripheral blood contamination and cellular destruction (Skill Box 3.2).
- Several slides should be made to allow for different staining techniques.

Skill Box 3.1 / Collection techniques[2,5]

Technique	Uses	Supplies	Procedure	Comments
Imprints	**External lesions or fresh tissue samples from a surgical biopsy or necropsy**	**Gauze, clean microscope slides**	• Blot the lesion or area to be imprinted with a clean, dry gauze • Touch the lesion against a clean glass slide to make an imprint and lift slide/tissue straight up • Can repeat several times on one slide, moving over with each touch • Imprint ulcers before and after cleaning	• Yields fewer diagnostic cells • Contamination with inflammatory cells common
Scrapings	**External lesions or tissues from surgical biopsy or necropsy**	**Gauze, scalpel blade, clean microscope slides**	• Clean lesion and blot dry • Hold scalpel perpendicular to lesion • Pull the blade toward oneself several times in a scraping motion • Transfer the material to the middle of a glass slide with the scalpel blade and smear	• Yields larger numbers of cells • Contamination with bacteria and inflammatory cells common
Swabs	**Fistulous tracts, otic and vaginal collections and when other methods are impractical**	**Saline, sterile cotton swab**	• Moisten a sterile swab with saline for vaginal swabs and fistulous tracts which are not moist • Gently roll the swab against the inside wall of the tract or vagina • When collecting a vaginal swab, follow a cranial dorsal path to the cervix • Gently roll the swab across a slide to transfer material in a thin smear	• Only option for tract-like lesions • ↑ Cell damage with rough or improper handling • Contamination with external vaginal cells can interfere with proper evaluation of estrus timing • Avoid swiping the swab by using complete revolutions on the slide

(*Continued*)

Skill Box 3.1 / Collection techniques (Continued)

Technique	Uses	Supplies	Procedure	Comments
Fine-needle biopsy:				
Aspirate	**Lesions and masses**	**Needle and syringe (22 gauge, 12 ml for most samples), clean microscope slides**	• Isolate and firmly hold the mass/lesion • Insert the needle/syringe into the mass and apply strong negative pressure by pulling the plunger three-quarters of the way back and then releasing pressure • Redirect the needle to a different part of the mass and again apply pressure • Continue this several times in different locations • Quickly smear the contents, using one of the smear techniques (Skill Box 3.3) • If the mass is large enough, negative pressure may be maintained while the needle is being redirected	• Avoids superficial contamination, but with ↑ contamination of tissues surrounding the mass during aspiration • ↑ Blood contamination with certain types of masses, if blood enters syringe, release negative pressure immediately and withdraw needle • Allows for collection from multiple locations within the lesion
Non-aspirate	**Any mass or solid lesion that is of large enough size to isolate, ultrasound-guided biopsy of deep tissues, highly vascular lesions**	Needle and syringe Clean microscope slides	• Isolate and firmly hold the mass • Insert the needle and syringe with syringe filled with air into the mass and rapidly move the needle up and down while maintaining the same track ("woodpecker" technique) • Quickly expel the contents onto a clean glass slide • Smear the contents, using one of the smear techniques (Skill Box 3.3)	• Often yields the best quality of samples by causing the least amount of damage to cells • Especially useful for highly vascular masses and lymph tissues • Minimal cells are collected, which may not be enough to be diagnostic

Skill Box 3.2 / Fine-needle biopsy needle and syringe selection[5]

- Mass firmness determines needle gauge size, soft masses = 25 g, firmer masses = 22 g.
- 22 g is the largest size to use to maximize free cell yield and minimizing peripheral blood contamination.
- 3–12-ml syringes are used depending on mass firmness, 3 ml for lymph nodes, 5–12 ml for firmer masses, and 12 ml for tissues of unknown firmness.
- For non-aspiration techniques, any syringe capable of expelling needle contents is acceptable.

Handling[2,5]

- Use frosted-edge slides to ensure adequate labeling.
- Label slides with anatomic location and patient's information.
- Nearly touch slide with needle or syringe opening to prevent spraying of content in clusters.
- Transfer material and immediately spread on slide to prevent drying, thick areas, and sample clotting.
- Keep spread material away from edges of slide.
- Allow to completely air dry or using a blow dryer set on low.
- Stain and examine at least one slide to evaluate quality when submitting to outside reference laboratories.
- Prepare four to five unstained slides to send, together with one stained slide.
- Fluid samples should be sent with prepared slides in EDTA at the correct ratio of fluid to anticoagulant and properly labeled with patient information and anatomical location.

Cytological assessment is only possible if the sample is properly handled and prepared. An improperly prepared slide may contain ruptured cells, may be prepared too thick to assess individual cells, or may dry in clusters before being smeared.

Skill Box 3.3 / Slide preparation techniques[3,5]

Technique	Definition/uses	Procedure	Illustrations
Blood smear, direct, or wedge technique	• Produces a thin layer of fluid material across the slide • Used with fluid samples with similar thickness to peripheral blood	1. Expel material on slide near frosted edge, making sure needle is in contact with slide (Figure 3.6) 2. Place the second glass slide at a 30–40-degree angle to the first slide in front of the material. Use fingertips to stabilize slide 3. Pull the second slide back into the material and then gently, but swiftly, push across to the end of the first slide 4. Resultant smear should have a feathered edge which does not exceed the edge of slide	Figure 3.5
Line smear	• Concentrates cells • Used for diluted samples (urine)	• Follow steps 1–2 above as for blood smear • Stop about two-thirds of the way down the slide and lift straight up	Figure 3.6
Slide over slide, compression, or squash preparation	• Generally produces better slides with fine-needle biopsy • Used with thicker samples (e.g. bone marrow aspirates)	• Expel material near frosted edge • Place a second glass slide on top of the material at a right angle • Without applying any downward pressure, quickly and smoothly pull them apart by moving the top slide gently down the bottom slide • Resultant smear should have a "flame" shape which does not exceed edge of slide	Figure 3.7

(*Continued*)

Skill Box 3.3 / Slide preparation techniques (Continued)

Technique	Definition/uses	Procedure	Illustrations
Squash-modified preparation	• Decreased cell rupture then regular slide over slide method • Used with thicker samples (bone marrow aspirates)	• Follow steps 1 and 2 above • Rotate the top slide 45 degrees and then lift up	Figure 3.8
Starfish preparation	• Prevents destruction of fragile cells • Any sample	• Expel material onto center of a glass slide • Using the tip of the needle, gently spread the material out into various directions in the shape of a starfish	Figure 3.9

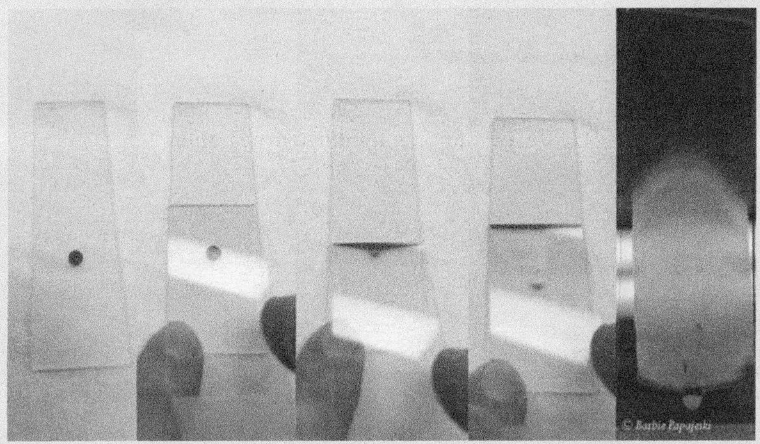

Figure 3.5 Blood smear, direct, or wedge technique.

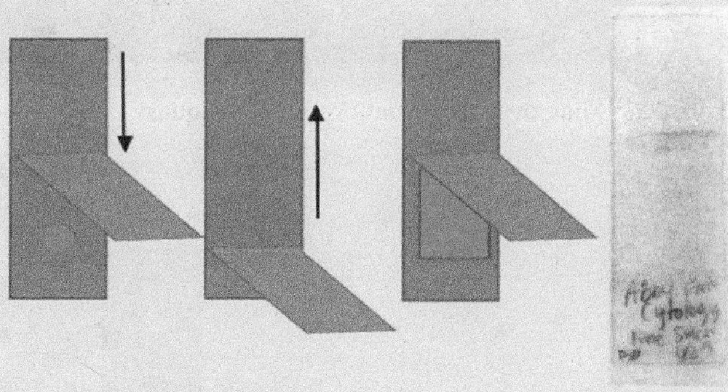

Figure 3.6 Line smear.

(*Continued*)

Skill Box 3.3 / Slide preparation techniques (Continued)

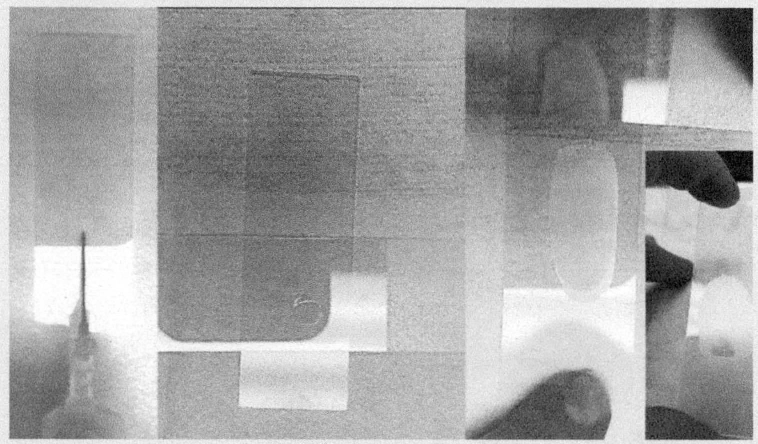

Figure 3.7 Slide over slide, compression, or squash preparation.

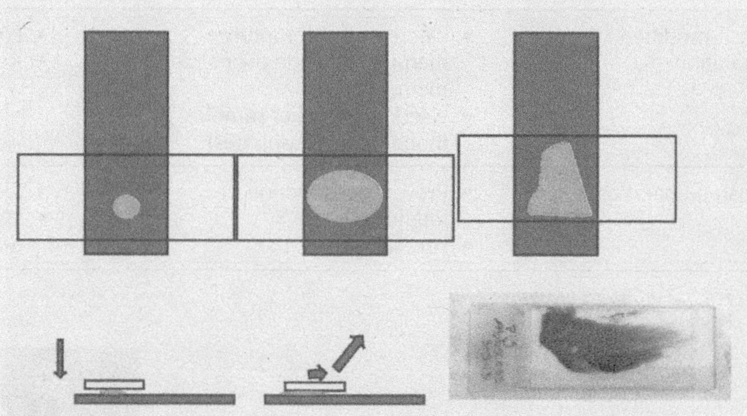

Figure 3.8 Squash-modified preparation.

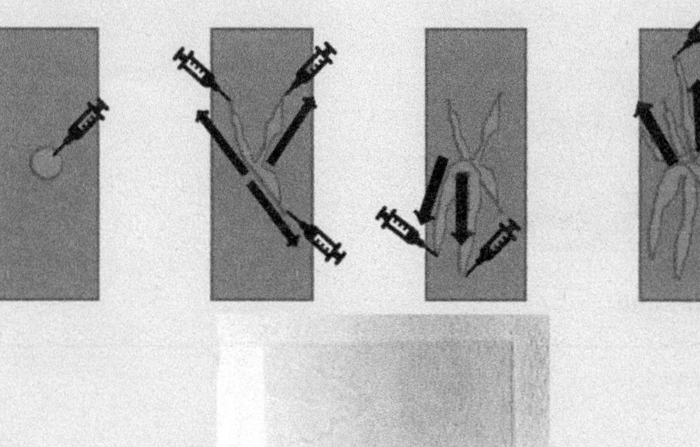

Figure 3.9 Starfish preparation.

Storage[3,5]

Slides must be completely air-dried before being placed in slide holders.

Transport[3,5]

- Cushion slides on all slides to prevent breakage (e.g. bubble wrap, padded envelopes).
- Slides must be kept separate from formalin, as formalin will partially fix cells on slides, altering staining characteristics.
- Protect unstained slides from moisture (do not place in the refrigerator or near ice packs, which will cause condensation).

Cytology Evaluation

Cytology is the examination of cells by microscopy.[3,5] This tool is often used in-house to determine whether a mass or lesion is neoplastic or inflammatory in nature. If neoplastic cells are noted, samples are often referred to a reference laboratory for further diagnostics.

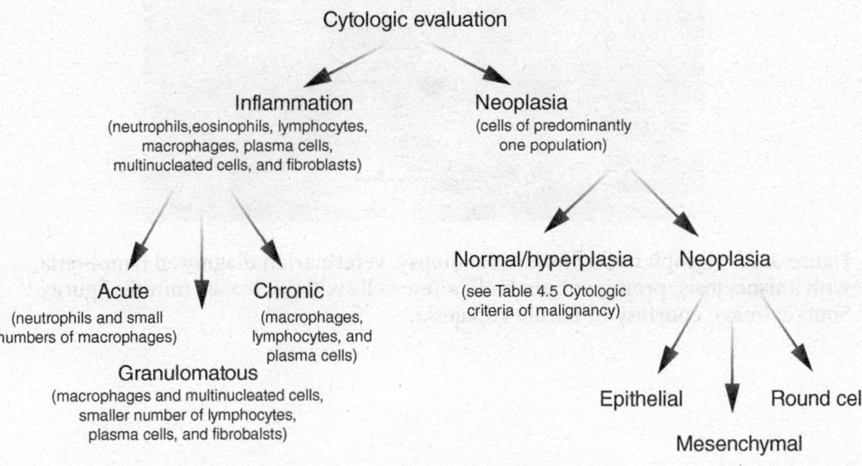

Figure 3.10 Cytology evaluation.

- Prepare the slide (Skill Box 3.3) and stain with Romanowsky-type quick stains or new methylene blue (Skill Box 3.13).
- Scan the entire slide using 10 × magnification:
  - Verify adequate staining
  - Access cellularity
  - Access cells for nuclear shape and cell size
  - Access viability of cells for identification (not ruptured, adequately stained)
  - Evaluate monolayer of cells.
- Examine the slide using oil immersion magnification:
  - Cell inclusions
  - Cell organisms (foreign bodies, parasites, bacterial, fungal hyphae, etc.)
  - Mitotic figures
  - Chromatin pattern
  - Nucleoli
  - Perform cellular identification (200-part differential; Table 3.7).

Ultimately, the veterinarian is responsible for determining the malignancy of a sample. Technicians must accurately identify, describe, and report any changes in cells observed.

Table 3.6 / **Cytological criteria of malignancy**[2–3,5]

Cytologic characteristics	Appearance
Nuclear	• Abnormal size, shape, and appearance of nucleoli (macronucleoli, angular nucleoli, anisonucleosis) • Anisokaryosis • Coarse, clumped chromatin pattern • Increased mitotic figures • Irregular nuclear membrane • Irregular nuclear pattern • Macrokaryosis • Multinucleation with anisokaryosis • Nuclear molding • Variation in nuclear/cytoplasmic ratio
Cytoplasmic	• Vacuolization • Variable cytoplasm among same cell types • Basophilia • Abnormal cytoplasmic boundaries
Structural	• Anisocytosis • Macrocytosis • Pleomorphic

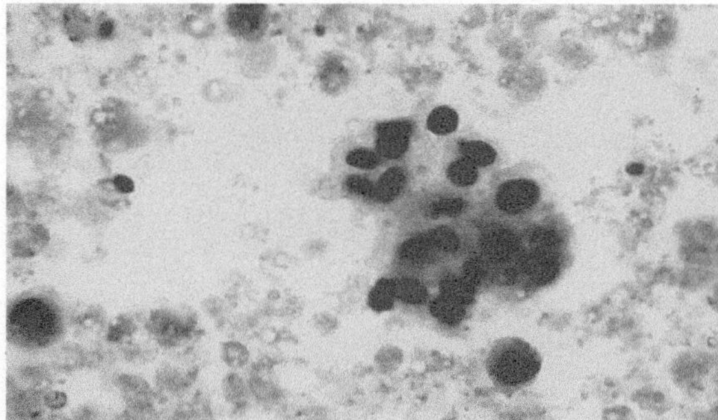

Figure 3.11 Fine-needle aspiration of a feline subcutaneous mass with cells showing malignant changes such as anisokaryosis, coarse, and clumped chromatin. Source: image courtesy of Barbie Papajeski.

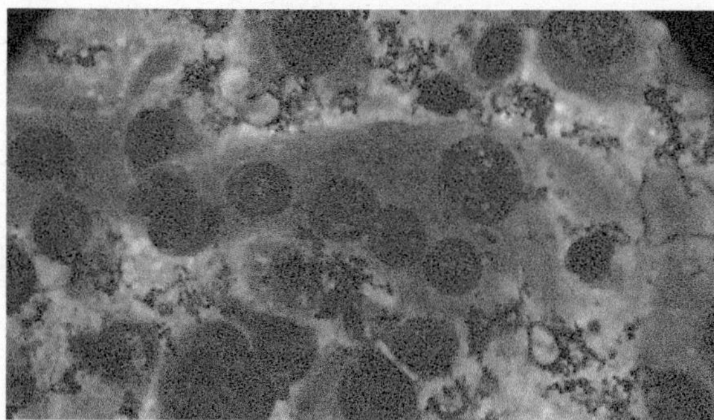

Figure 3.12 Osteoclast from canine osteosarcoma patient with multiple nucleation, nucleoli, anisokaryosis, and mitotic figures. Source: image courtesy of Barbie Papajeski.

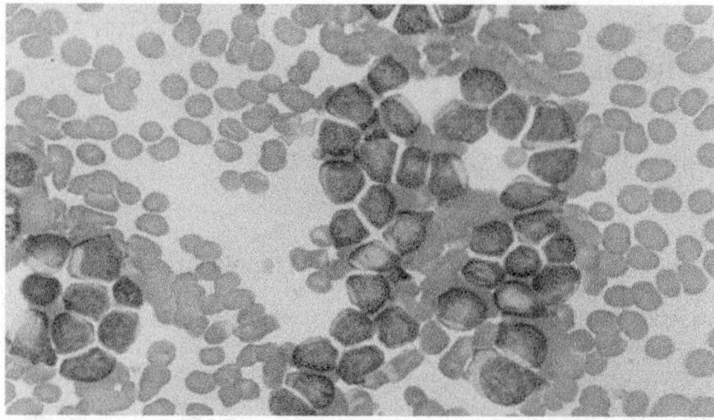

Figure 3.13 Lymph node fine-needle biopsy, veterinarian diagnosed lymphoma with anisocytosis, prominent nucleoli, a few cells with increased mitotic figures. Source: image courtesy of Barbie Papajeski.

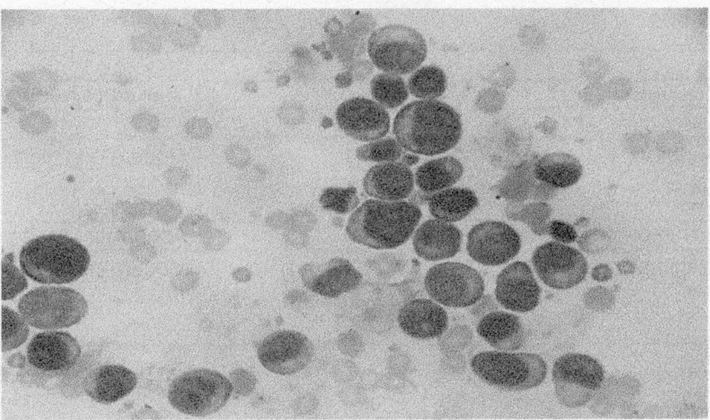

Figure 3.14 Lymph node fine-needle biopsy, veterinarian diagnosed lymphoma with anisocytosis, prominent nucleoli, cytoplasmic basophilia, and coarse chromatin. Source: image courtesy of Barbie Papajeski.

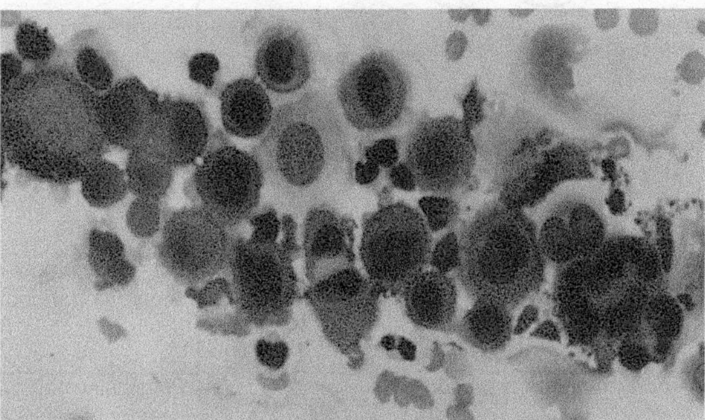

Figure 3.15 Pathologist-diagnosed case of mesothelioma. Mesothelial cells showing multinucleation, anisocytosis, and variable nuclear to cytoplasm ratio. Source: image courtesy of Barbie Papajeski.

Cytologic Criteria of Malignancy		
	Normal/Hyperplasia	Malignant Neoplasia
General or Population Criteria		
Cellularity	Low to moderate 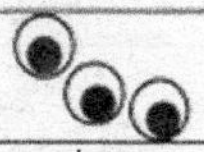	Moderate to high 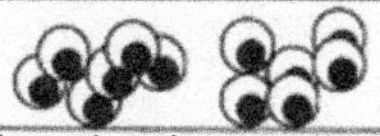
Location	Normal tissue present for tissue sample	Abnormal tissue present for tissue location
Pleomorphism Anisocytosis Macrocytosis	None to minimal 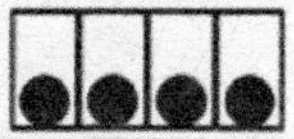	Moderate to marked 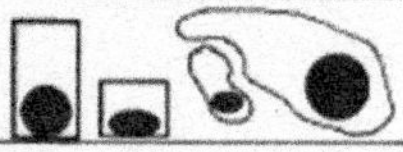
Nuclear Criteria of Malignancy		
Size (anisokaryosis)	Uniform 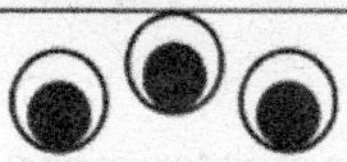	Variable 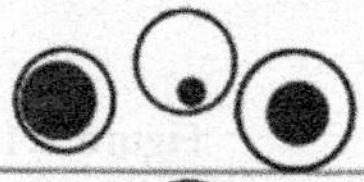
Nuclear/cytoplasmic ratios	Uniform 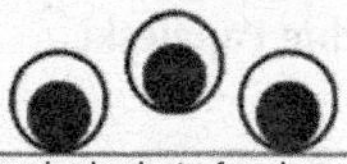	Variable 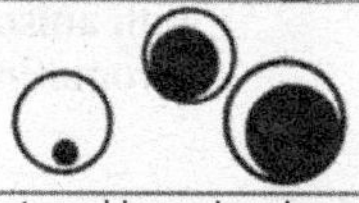
Nucleoli	Generally small and round, single to few in number 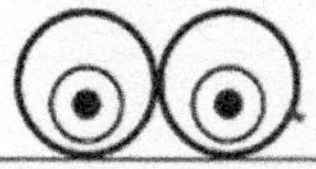	Large, multiple, prominent, and irregular shape 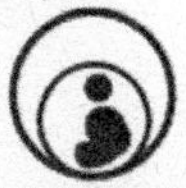
Nuclear chromatin	Uniform patterns 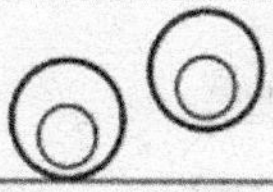	Abnormally clumped (around nucleoli, along nuclear envelopes) 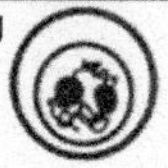
Mitosis	Few and normal 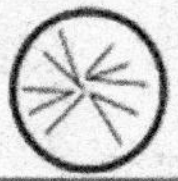	Increased in normal and abnormal configurations 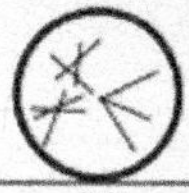
Nuclear shape	Uniform, round to oval 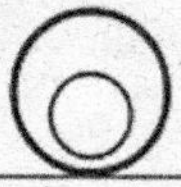	Potentially irregular, deeply indented, possible support for abnormal division 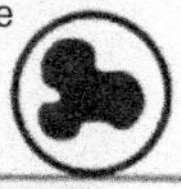
Nuclei number	Usually one or even numbers present 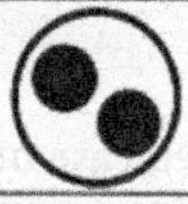	Potentially multiple with odd or even number of nuclei and variably sized nuclei in individual cells 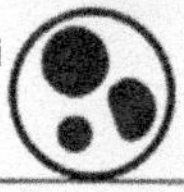
Cytoplasmic Criteria of Malignancy		
Basophilia	Minimal unless actively producing proteins	Potentially increased or deep blue
Vacuolization	Normal in phagocytic, secretory, or degenerating cells	Potential large and abnormal 'signet ring' morphology
Cannibalism	None	Potentially present

Figure 3.16 Cytologic criteria of malignancy.

Table 3.7 gives a general description of cells. Multiple variations can be seen because of location, duration, and malignancy. Each cell is evaluated, together with the rest of the slide and the general findings of the animal. The diagnosis of a particular condition must be made by the veterinarian.

Table 3.7 / Cytology cells[2–3,5]

Cell type	Cytology differentials
Inflammatory	
Neutrophils	Aging changes: hypersegmentation and pyknosis
	Degenerate changes = nuclear swelling (Figures 3.17 and 3.18)
	Often found in conjunction with endotoxin producing bacteria
Macrophages	Morphology similar to blood monocytes
	Abundant cytoplasm, vacuolated, with phagocytized material
	Multinucleated, large cells
	May be present in chronic inflammation (Figure 3.18)
Lymphocytes	Include small, medium, large (lymphoblasts), and plasma cells
	Mott (plasma) cells contain Russel bodies, large clear to basophilic vacuoles containing immunoglobulin
Eosinophils	Appearance is similar to those found in peripheral blood
	Variably sized and number of granules in dogs
	Cat eosinophil granules are rod shaped
	Nuclei may be round
	Free granules may be present in scrapings in high numbers (Figure 3.19)
Mesothelial cells	Larger cells with round shape
	Central, round nucleus unless reactive
	Eosinophilic fringe encircles periphery
	Cells which line pleural, peritoneal, pericardial and other visceral tissues (Figure 3.20)

(Continued)

Table 3.7 / Cytology cells (Continued)

Cell type	Cytology differentials
Round (discrete)	
Histiocytoma	Cells slightly larger than neutrophils, round to oval, irregularly shaped nuclei with finely stippled chromatin
	Vacuolated cytoplasm (small and uniform in size), anisocytosis, macrocytosis, variable N : C ratio, and multinucleation
Lymphoma (lymphosarcoma)	Lymphoblasts with high nuclear to cytoplasm ratio
	Profoundly basophilic cytoplasm
	Confirmed by molecular diagnostics and tissue histology (Figures 3.13 and 3.14)
Mast cell tumor	Cytoplasm contains numerous distinct, small reddish purple granules
	Degranulated mast cells may be present (Figures 3.21 and 3.28)
Plasmacytoma	Eccentric nucleus, often with clear Golgi zone
	Anisocytosis, anisokaryosis, multinucleation, and variable N : C ratio
Transmissible venereal tumor	Rare
	Smokey-gray to light-blue cytoplasm, numerous distinct vacuoles
	Vacuoles are also found in extracellular, proteinaceous material
	Anisokaryosis
	Coarse chromatin pattern
	Prominent nucleoli and atypical mitotic figures
Melanoma	Cells contain green to black melanin granules
	Pigmentation may be variable
	Malignant changes are difficult to view in heavily pigmented cells (Figure 3.22)

(Continued)

Table 3.7 / **Cytology cells (Continued)**

Cell type	Cytology differentials
Epithelial	
Cornified/keratinized	Small, pyknotic nuclei
	Angular areas of cytoplasm (Figures 3.35 and 3.36)
	Mature cells found on surface lesions
	Individual cells
Non-cornified	Variable cytoplasm with rounded edges
	Large nucleus with functional (non-pyknotic) chromatin (Figure 3.37)
	Less mature cells that may be mixed with cornified cells on scraping and swabs
	Found in clusters
Columnar cells	Elongated, columnar cells with cilia
	Found in respiratory and gastrointestinal tract
	Found in clusters of long rows
Endocrine epithelial cells	Cell nuclei are at periphery of cells in acinus formation
	High numbers of nuclei without cytoplasm
	Low nucleus to cytoplasm ratio
	Mature chromatin pattern
Mesenchymal	
Spindle cells	Fusiform, elongated shape
	Thin, rod-shaped nuclei
	Indistinct cytoplasmic borders (Figure 3.23)

(*Continued*)

Table 3.7 / Cytology cells (Continued)

Cell type	Cytology differentials
Osteosarcoma	Osteoclasts are multinucleated, irregularly shaped cells
	Dark-blue cytoplasm with clear vacuoles and pink cytoplasmic granules
	Karyomegaly, anisokaryosis, variably sized multi-nuclei, and large nucleoli (Figure 3.11)
Fibrosarcoma	Poorly exfoliate
	Large spindle cells with oval nuclei
	Reticular chromatin pattern
	Prominent, large nucleoli
	Atypical mitotic figures
Lipoma	Common tumor masses in dogs
	Adipocytes rinse off in stains, best viewed with new methylene blue (Figure 3.24)
	Free lipids may be present (Figures 3.24 and 3.25)

Interpretation[2–3,5]

Once a slide has been evaluated, the results should confirm an inflammatory or neoplastic process. The distinction of inflammation alone often will enable the veterinarian to determine an initial treatment plan. If the slide is found to have neoplastic cells, they are then reviewed against the criteria of malignancy. Often, the results are sent to a cytology laboratory for confirmation and staging.

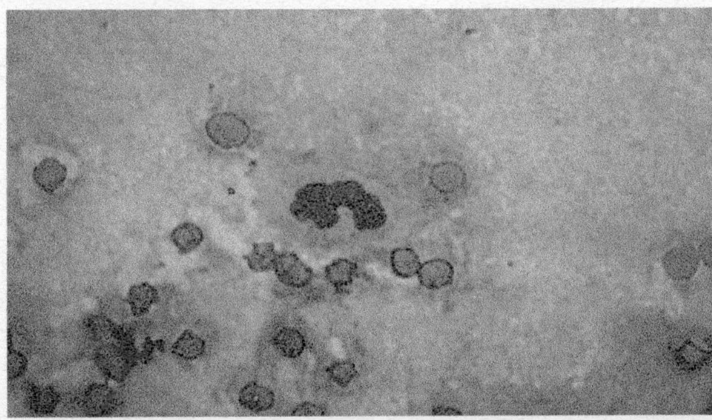

Figure 3.17 Degenerate neutrophil in synovial fluid with proteinaceous background and red blood cells. Source: image courtesy of Barbie Papajeski.

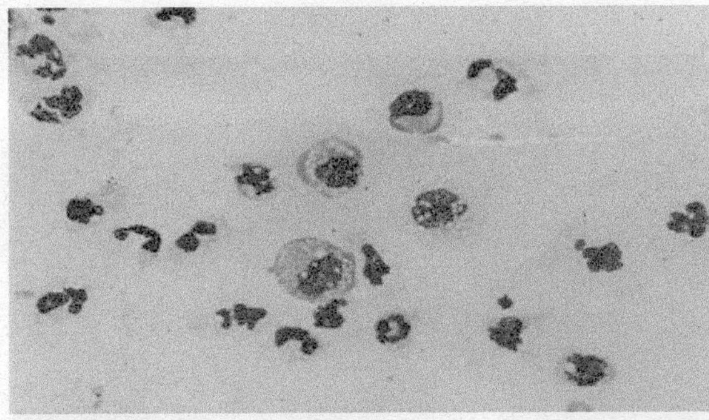

Figure 3.18 Neutrophils and vacuolated (foamy) macrophages in a thoracic fluid sample collected from a dog. Neutrophils made up 95% of this effusion. Source: image courtesy of Barbie Papajeski.

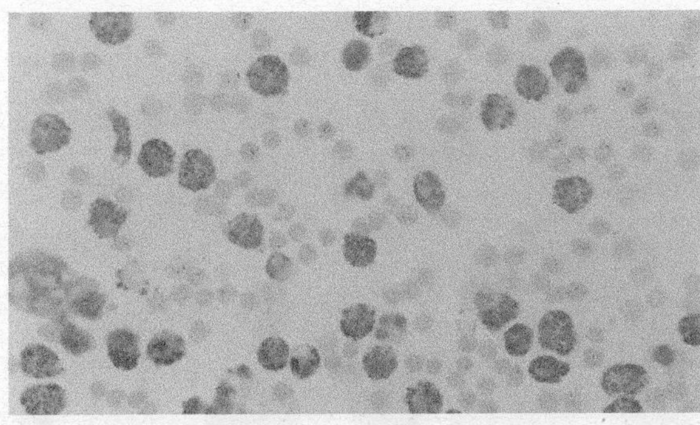

Figure 3.19 Eosinophil on canine peritoneal effusion. Source: image courtesy of Barbie Papajeski.

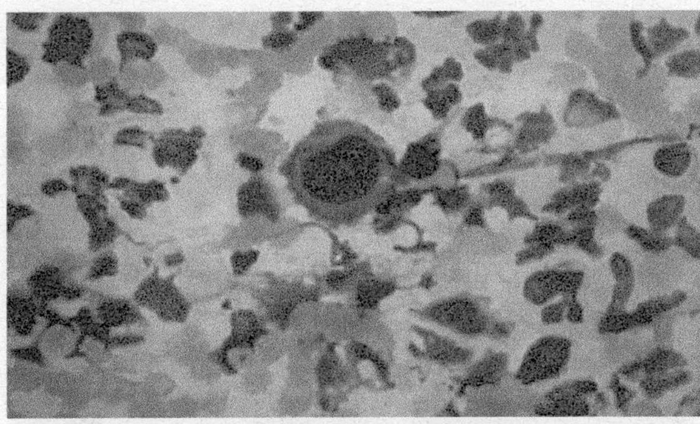

Figure 3.20 Reactive mesothelial cell in a canine thoracic effusion. Source: image courtesy of Barbie Papajeski.

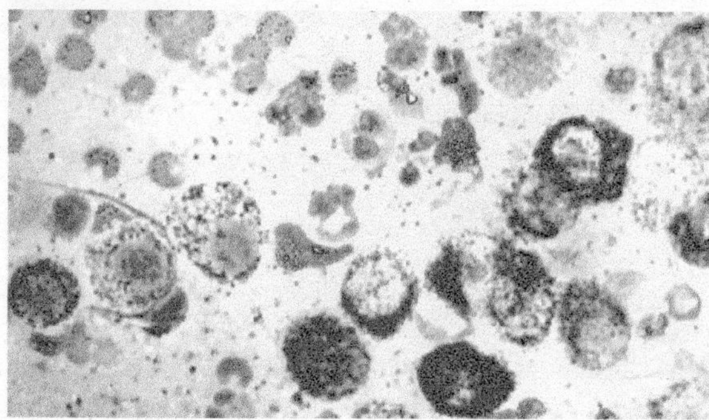

Figure 3.21 Mast cell tumor: anisocytosis, round to oval nuclei, stain palely, fine to coarse, reddish purple granules within the cytoplasm. Source: image courtesy of Barbie Papajeski.

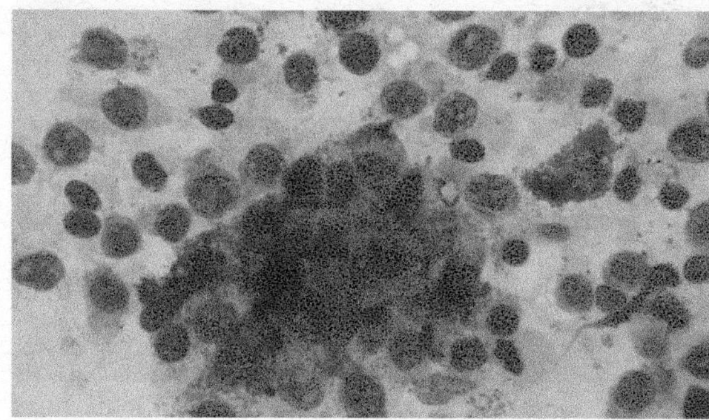

Figure 3.22 Melanocytes from a canine melanoma. Source: image courtesy of Barbie Papajeski.

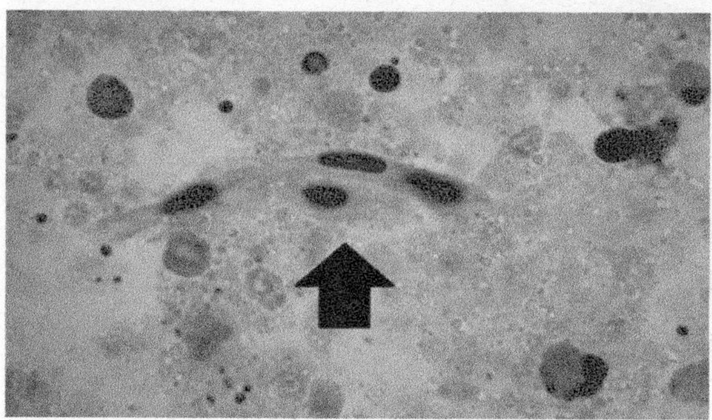

Figure 3.23 Spindle (mesenchymal) cells on a feline fine-needle biopsy of a cutaneous mass with lipid droplets in background. Source: image courtesy of Barbie Papajeski.

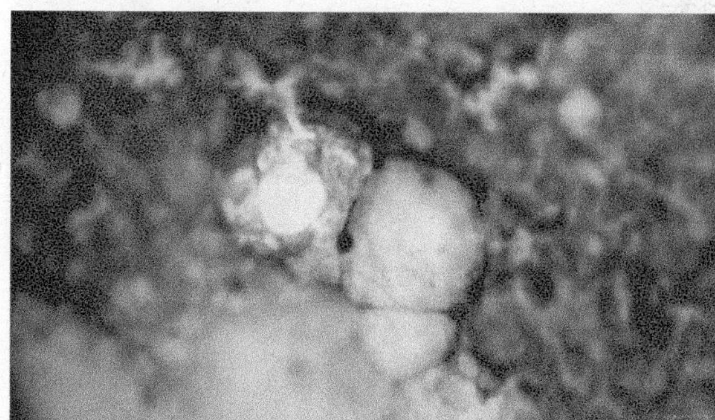

Figure 3.24 Adipocytes also known as lipocytes: cells with pyknotic nuclei and clear cytoplasm from a mammary mass and stained with new methylene blue. Source: image courtesy of Barbie Papajeski.

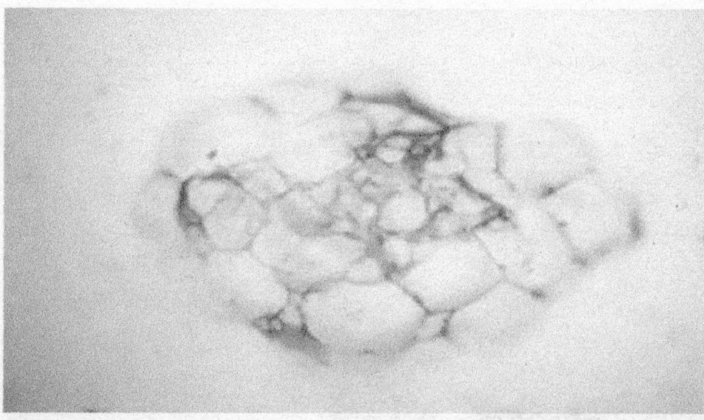

Figure 3.25 Lipoma: large and round fat cells with pyknotic nuclei pressed against the side of the cell by fat globules and clear cytoplasm. Source: image courtesy of Barbie Papajeski.

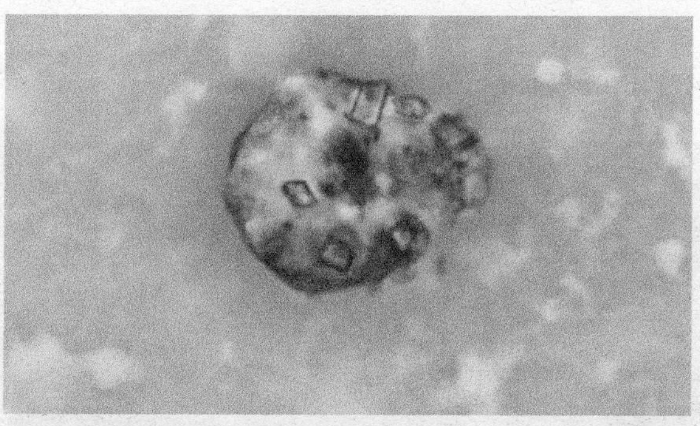

Figure 3.26 Hematoidin crystals in a macrophage from a fine-needle biopsy of a canine mass. Source: image courtesy of Barbie Papajeski.

Skill Box 3.4 / Buffy coat evaluation[2,3,5]

The buffy coat is typically a small, white layer found between plasma and red blood cells on a centrifuged sample of whole blood. The layer immediately above the red blood cells contains mostly WBC and some platelets. An additional white layer above the WBC contains the majority of platelets. Visualization of this layer is often only seen with a microscope. Evaluation of the buffy coat is useful for mast cell tumor staging, hematopoietic neoplasia, some infectious agents, and for concentrating WBC and abnormal cells. Buffy coat evaluation for mast cell tumor detection and staging is most accurately performed in cats, whereas dogs show variable and unreliable results.

Procedure

- Fill a capillary tube three-fourths full with well-mixed whole blood and plug one end
- Centrifuge the sample in a microhematocrit tube according to the manufacturer's directions
- Score and break the tube at the level right below the buffy coat (dedicated nail trimmers may be used)
- Place one drop of the buffy coat on a slide and smear using the direct technique
- Stain and examine
- See Cytology Evaluation section

Skill Box 3.4 / Buffy coat evaluation (Continued)

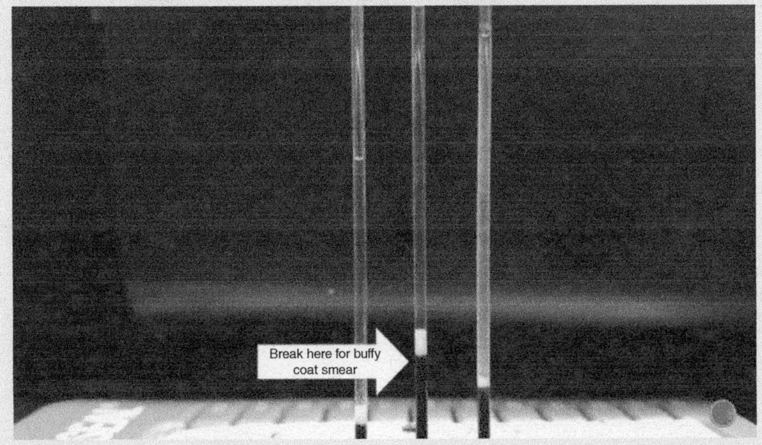

Figure 3.27 Buffy coat evaluation. Source: image courtesy of Barbie Papajeski.

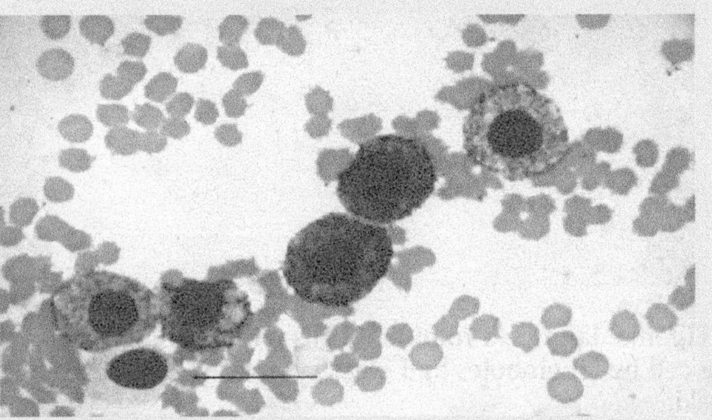

Figure 3.28 Buffy coat smear of a cat: mast cells with variable granularity are present, with the cell at the arrow exhibiting degranulation. Source: image courtesy of Barbie Papajeski.

Effusion Cytology

Effusions are excessive accumulations of fluid in a body cavity (pleural, peritoneal, pericardial). These cavities naturally have a small amount of fluid present, but with an increase in volume, they become an effusion and are classified as either transudate (non-inflammatory) or exudate (inflammatory). Normal fluid contains low numbers of mesothelial cells and few inflammatory cells. In effusions, neutrophils (canines) and lymphocytes (felines) are the most common cells found. Total nucleated cell counts may be performed with automated methods or manually by hemocytometer (Skill Box 3.6; Table 3.8).

Table 3.8 / Effusion cytology[2–3,5]

Effusion	Characteristics	Appearance	Specific gravity (g/dl)	Protein (g/dl)	Organisms	Total nucleated cell count/μl	Associated conditions
Transudate	• Low specific gravity, cellularity, and protein • Mesothelial cells, monocytes, macrophages, and lymphocytes (Figure 3.44)	Clear, yellow	< 1.018	< 2.5	Absent	< 1000	Congestive heart failure, liver failure, hypoalbuminemia, neoplasia
Modified transudate	• Transudate present long enough to signal an inflammatory response • ↑ Specific gravity, protein, and cellularity • Reactive mesothelial cells in ↑ numbers	Slightly cloudy	1.018–1.030	2.5–5.0	Absent	< 5000	Congestive heart failure, liver failure, hypoalbuminemia, pancreatitis, neoplasia

(Continued)

Table 3.8 / **Effusion cytology (Continued)**

Effusion	Characteristics	Appearance	Specific gravity (g/dl)	Protein (g/dl)	Organisms	Total nucleated cell count/µl	Associated conditions
Exudates	• Non-septic • Caused by nonmicrobial irritants • Non-regenerative neutrophils and macrophages • Serofibrinous or serosanguineous appearance	Clear to cloudy, yellow or pink	1.017–1.047	3.0–8.0	Absent	5000–300 000	Feline infectious peritonitis, diaphragmatic hernia, post-operative, bile peritonitis, trauma with ruptured bladder, sterile foreign bodies
	• Septic/inflammatory • ↑ Specific gravity, protein and cellularity • Reactive mesothelial, neutrophils • Pathogenic organisms	Cloudy, yellow/pink	1.020–1.050	2.5–9.0	Present	1000–20 000	Pyothorax, peritonitis, gastrointestinal perforation, foreign body migration
	• Chylous • Leakage of chyle from the lymphatic system • Moderate protein and low cellularity • Small lymphocytes, moderate numbers of reactive mesothelial and inflammatory cells	Opaque, white/pink	1.020–1.050	2.5–6.0	Absent	< 10 000	Thoracic duct trauma, neoplasia, cardiovascular disease, chronic coughing
	• Hemorrhagic • Rupture or ulceration of blood vessels • Predominantly red blood cells with a few leukocytes and possibly activated macrophages • Must be distinguished from a contaminated sample	Red, may clot	1.030–1.050	3.0–7.5	Absent	Similar to peripheral blood	Blunt injury, coagulation defect, lung lobe torsion, neoplasia, thrombocytopenia
	• Neoplastic • ↑ Protein • Difficult to distinguish cancer cells from mesothelial cells	Clear to cloudy, red	Variable	> 2.5	Absent	Variable	Thymic lymphosarcoma, adenocarcinoma, carcinoma

Ear Cytology

Ear cytology is a non-invasive technique which aids in diagnosis and treatment options for otitis externa.[2–3,5,12] Samples are collected separately from each ear and evaluated for presence of organisms, cells, and other structures. Separate quick stains must be used to prevent contamination of regular stains with excess bacteria and debris. Slides are evaluated for the following:

- WBC: inflammatory cells include neutrophils and macrophages and must be carefully examined for bacteriophages (Figure 3.29).
- Red blood cells
- Keratinocytes: keratinized epithelial cells
- Bacteria: identify whether rod or cocci and arrangement (i.e. chains, tetrads, clusters, etc.; Figure 3.30)
- Melanin granules are brown to yellow and may be mistaken for bacteria which stains blue to purple (Figure 3.31)
- Cerumen (ear wax)
- *Malassezia pachydermatis* (yeast; Figure 3.32).

Table 3.9 / Grading scheme for ear cytology[12]

Grade	Description
0	No bacteria/yeast/inflammatory cells
1+	Occasional bacteria/yeast/inflammatory cells present, but slide must be scanned carefully for detection
2+	Bacteria/yeast/inflammatory cells present in low numbers, but detectable rapidly without difficulties
3+	Bacteria/yeast/inflammatory cells present in larger numbers and detectable rapidly without any difficulties
4+	Massive amounts of bacteria/yeast/inflammatory cells present and detectable rapidly without difficulties

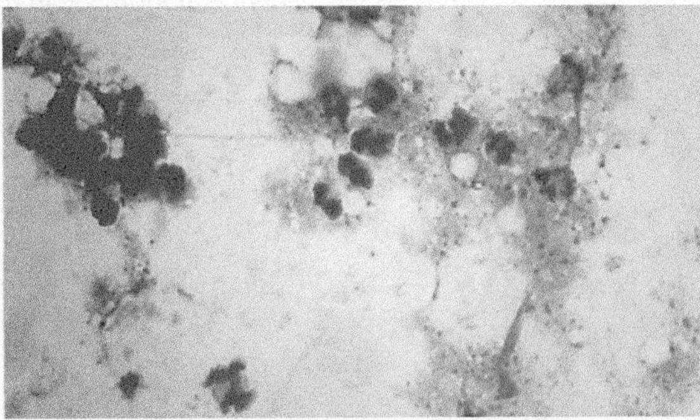

Figure 3.29 Canine ear cytology showing both rod and cocci bacteria in chains, clusters, tetrads, and pairs. Source: image courtesy of Barbie Papajeski.

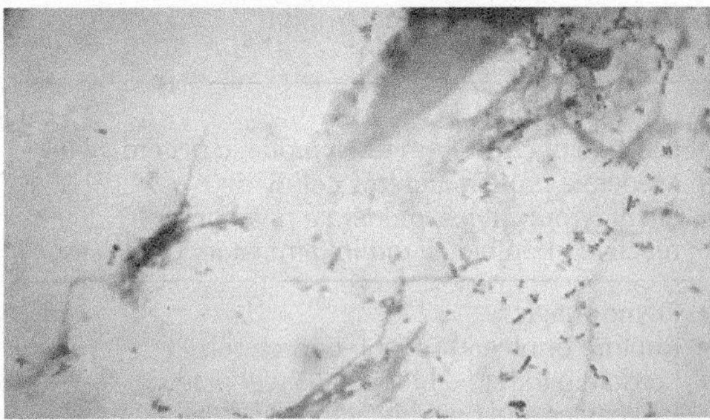

Figure 3.30 Canine ear cytology showing *Malassezia pachydermatis* and superficial epithelial cells. Source: image courtesy of Barbie Papajeski.

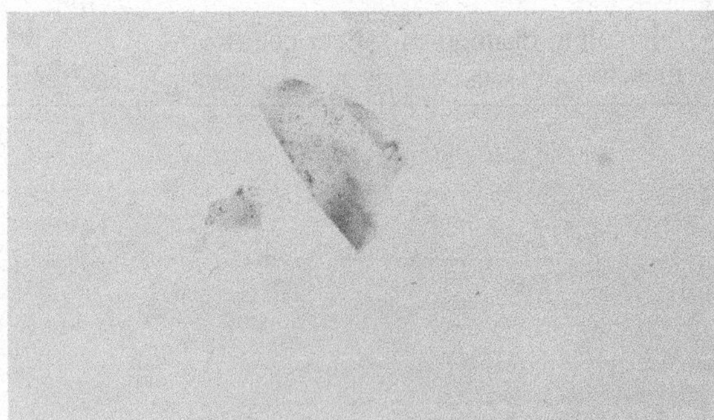

Figure 3.31 Feline ear cytology readily showing inflammatory cells and cocci bacteria. Source: image courtesy of Barbie Papajeski.

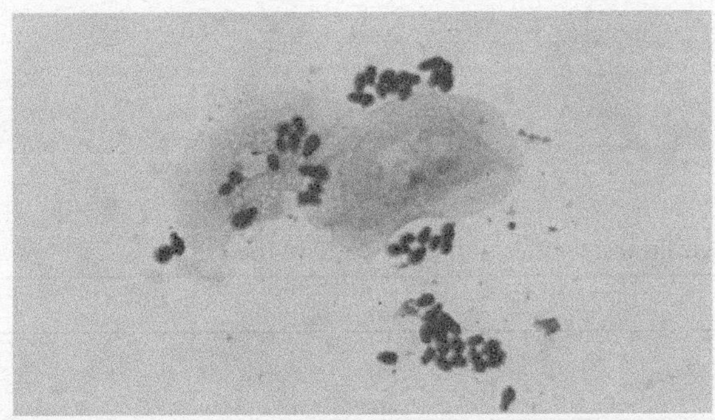

Figure 3.32 Melanin granules in a superficial cell on an ear cytology. Source: image courtesy of Barbie Papajeski.

Fecal Cytology

Fecal cytology is a diagnostic tool for identifying inflammatory cells and potentially pathogenic organisms of the gastrointestinal tract of animals with diarrhea.[2–3,5] The first step is to assess the presence and quantity of bacteria. Typical gut flora consists of various types of rod shaped bacteria. One predominant bacteria may indicate it as a pathogenic organism and warrant further microbial testing such as culture, or polymerase chain reaction (PCR). Some conditions may have more than one predominant bacteria (e.g. malabsorption, maldigestion). Large numbers of neutrophils or eosinophils may indicate inflammatory disease (e.g. *Salmonella*, *Campylobacter* sp., eosinophilic colitis). Fecal cytology may also reveal protozoal (e.g. *Giardia*) or fungal (e.g. *Histoplasma* sp.) organisms.

Fecal cytology may be collected by a swab of fecal material or by rectal mucosal scraping. Fecal material is removed and a swab is pressed and scraped against the intestinal wall to remove cells.

Table 3.10 / Fecal cytology[5]

Type	Appearance
Cells	• Nucleated cells are rare, clusters of columnar epithelia cells on rectal scrapings
Eosinophils, neutrophils, and/or lymphocytes	• Inflammation
Muscle fibers	• Cells with blunt ends and cross striations • Presence indicates pancreatic insufficiency (maldigestion)
Bacteria	• Should have a mixture of various sized rod-shaped bacteria (Figure 3.33)
Helicobacter (spirochete)	• Gram-negative • Motile "S" to "corkscrew" shaped
Campylobacter (spirochete)	• Gram-negative • Tiny, curved, gram-negative rods (not tightly spiraled) • Two attached together as a "seagull" or "W" shape • "Swarm of bees," rapid and darting motility • Size: 1.5–5 μm

(Continued)

Table 3.10 / **Fecal cytology (Continued)**

Type	Appearance
Clostridium sp.	• Large, Gram-positive rods • More easily recognized in the sporulated form • "Safety pin" appearance, which represents a non-staining spore within the sporangium (the body of the cell)
Protozoa:	
Cryptosporidium parvum	• Circular oocysts around 2–4 µm • Stain fuchsia with acid fast stains (Figure 3.89)
Entamoeba histolytica	• Eccentric nucleus, phagocytized red blood cells • Size: 12–50 µm
Giardia	Trophozoites: • Pear shaped with a concave ventral surface • Two outlined nuclei resembling eyes along with a nose and mouth, which are axonemes and median bodies • Forward or "falling leaf" motility • Size: 6–10 µm Cysts: • Crescent-shaped indentation when collapsing in fecal float solution • Nuclei, cyst wall, and axonemes seen • Size: 11–13 µm
Pentatrichomonas hominis	• Flagellated, 5 anterior and 1 posterior
Trichomonas spp.	• Single nucleus and undulating membrane • Rolling and erratic motility, flexing axostyle visible, jerky movement • Can be confused with *Giardia* (feline, diarrheic) • Special incubation pouches available to replicate for PCR testing
Yeast/fungi:	• See Figures 3.34 and 3.35
Candida spp.	• Oval to elongated, with hyphae • Size: 3–6 µm
Cryptococcus neoformans	• Refractile cell wall and narrow base budding • 5–25 µm
Cyniclomyes guttulatus	• Large elongated yeast with bipolar inclusions, sometimes see branching • Size: 5–7 x 15–20 µm
Histoplasma capsulatum	• Intracellular with half empty appearance, often in macrophages • Size: 3–6 µm
Prototheca spp.	• Algae surrounded by clear capsule
Pythium insidiosum	• Branching hyphae • Poorly stains

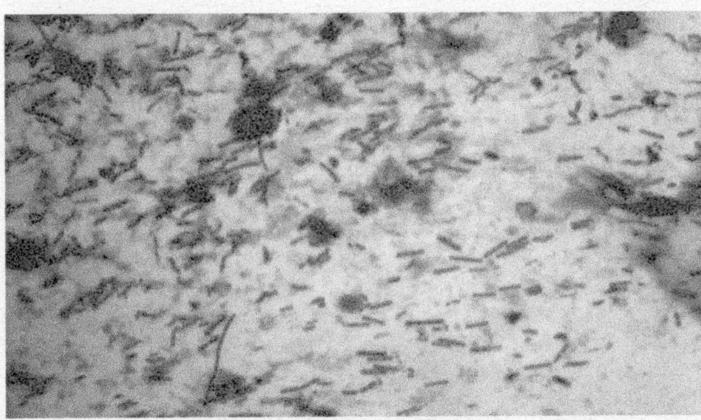

Figure 3.33 Rod-shaped bacteria and neutrophil on rectal mucosal smear. Source: image courtesy of Barbie Papajeski.

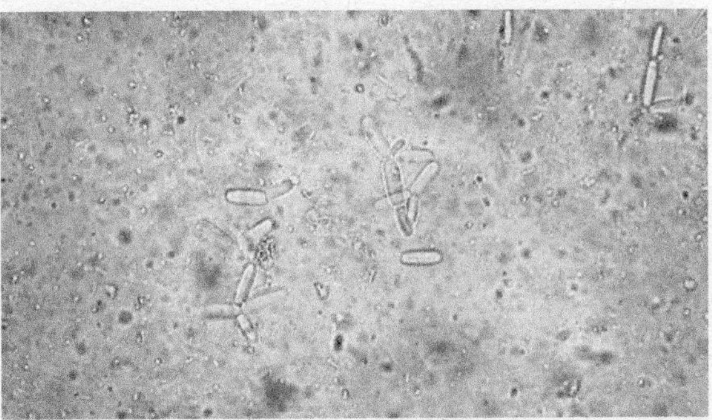

Figure 3.34 Budding yeast in a direct wet preparation of a canine sample. Source: image courtesy of Barbie Papajeski.

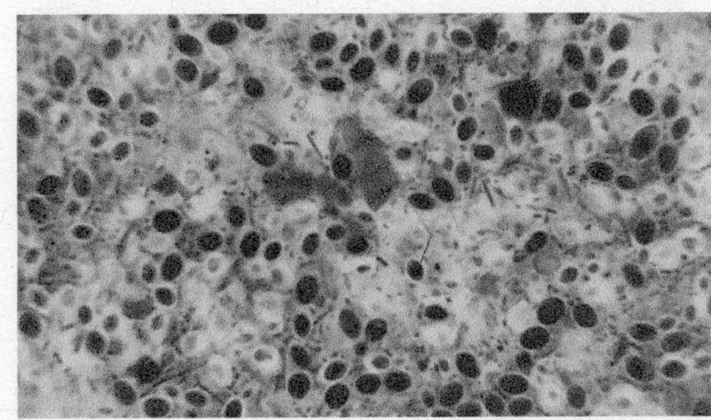

Figure 3.35 Large numbers of yeast and rod bacteria in fecal cytology of a diarrheic canine. Source: image courtesy of Barbie Papajeski.

Vaginal Cytology

Vaginal cytology is used in evaluating an animal's stage of estrus cycle.[2–3,5] Because of the constant changing of cellular structures during the estrus cycle, the evaluation of vaginal cells should be done every few days and in conjunction with a thorough medical history and examination (e.g. multiple, sequential samples increase accuracy of estrus stage estimation).

Table 3.11 / **Classifying vaginal cells**[2–3,5]

Squamous epithelial cell type	Appearance
Non-cornified:	
Parabasal (Figure 3.38)	• Small, round cells with a small amount of cytoplasm • Round, distinct nuclei • Uniform in size and shape
Intermediate (Figures 3.36 and 3.38)	• Large round cells with a large amount of cytoplasm • Round nuclei with stippled chromatin
Large intermediate (Figure 3.36)	• ↑ Cytoplasm that is irregular, folded, and angular • Smaller nuclei, pyknotic
Cornified:	
	• Large cells with a tiny, pyknotic nucleus or no nucleus
Nucleated superficial	• ↑ Cytoplasm, folded and angular
Anucleated superficial (Figure 3.37)	• Distinct edges

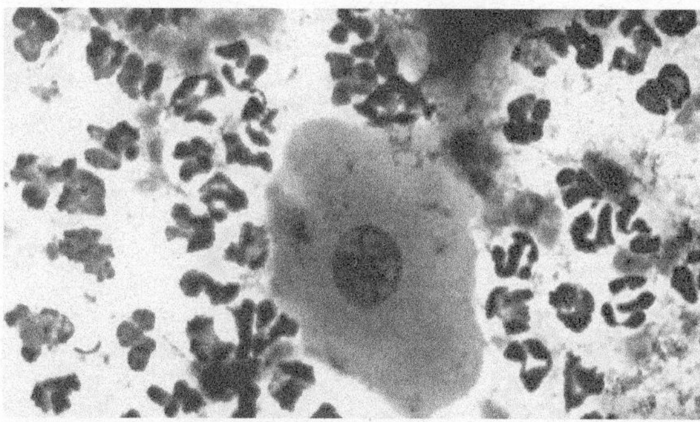

Figure 3.36 Large intermediate superficial cell and numerous white blood cells. Source: image courtesy of Barbie Papajeski.

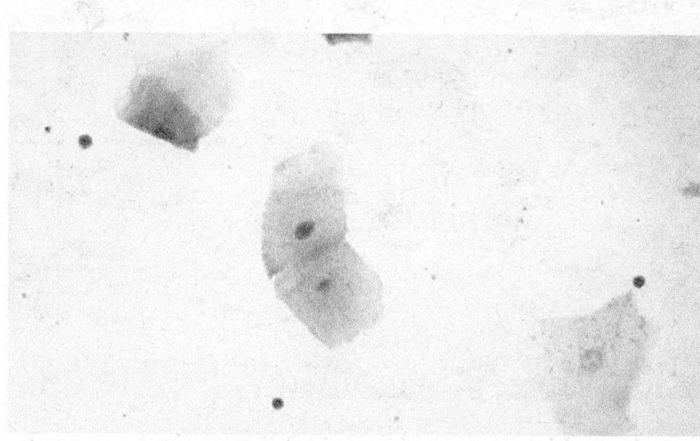

Figure 3.37 Superficial epithelial cell (cornified) with a few red blood cells. Source: image courtesy of Barbie Papajeski.

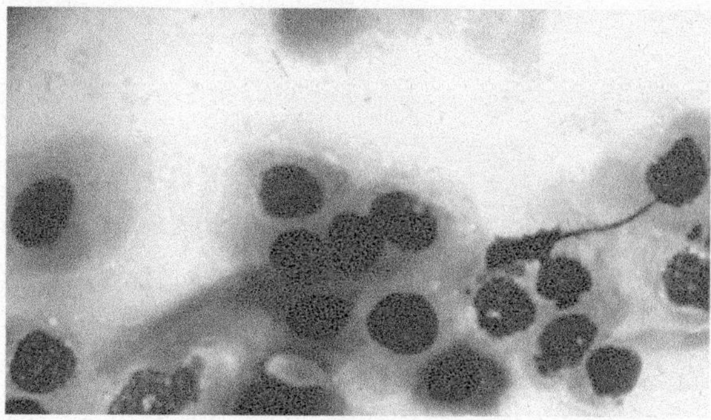

Figure 3.38 Small intermediate and parabasal epithelial cells (non-cornified). Source: image courtesy of Barbie Papajeski.

HEMATOLOGY

Even with the advent of automated modalities for complete blood counts (CBC), manual slide evaluation is still a vital factor in evaluating patient health.[13–14] Peripheral blood film evaluation is required to evaluate cellular morphology, locate and identify inclusions, parasites, and abnormal populations of cells as well as artifacts such as cellular aggregation or microclots, which will affect cell numbers. To date, analyzers have been unable to identify blood parasites such as microfilaria or trypanosomes.

Refer to Blood Chemistries, above. A CBC typically consists of evaluation of red and white cells, packed cell volume, hemoglobin concentration, WBC differential, platelet estimate, red blood cell indices, reticulocyte count and platelet indices. These tests require a whole blood sample from an anticoagulant tube, such as EDTA (Table 3.1). Total plasma protein is included in some practices. Morphology must be evaluated within the monolayer of an acceptably prepared blood slide. Cellular morphology and cell counts must be performed in a monolayer area of the slide.

Skill Box 3.5 / Complete blood count[1–4,6,15–17]

Procedure	Definition	Technique	Typical values	Associated conditions
Packed cell volume	Percentage of RBC in whole blood	1. Fill a capillary tube two-thirds to three-quarters with whole blood 2. Seal one end with a clay sealant 3. Centrifuge in microhematocrit centrifuge and read results as a percentage using a card reader 4. Record the color and transparency of the plasma	Canine: 35–57% Feline: 24–45% Plasma: clear to straw	↑ Polycythemia, dehydration, stress, neonates ↓ Anemia, overhydration, weanlings
Hematocrit	A calculated value on automated analyzers			
Hemoglobin concentration	Indicates oxygen carrying capacity of blood	1. Follow the manufacturer's guidelines for automated machines 2. Estimates are calculated by dividing PCV by 3 (if MCHC is within reference intervals)	Canine: 11.9–18.9 g/dl Feline: 9.8–15.4 g/dl	↑ (falsely) lipemia, Heinz bodies, ↓ Hypochromic anemias
RBC count	Cell responsible for transport of oxygen to tissues.[6] Automated analyzers are more accurate than manual methods	1. Follow the manufacturer's guidelines for automated machines 2. An estimate can be calculated by dividing PCV by 6 as a check of automated numbers (if MCHC is within reference intervals) 3. Main use is for indices calculation (PCV yields similar information)	Canine: 4.95–7.87 x 10^6/µl Feline: 5–10 x 10^6/µl	↑ Polycythemia, dehydration ↓ Anemia, overhydration

(Continued)

Skill Box 3.5 / Complete blood count (Continued)

Procedure	Definition	Technique	Typical values	Associated conditions
WBC count	Cell responsible for fighting infections and establishing immunity	1. Make a 1 : 20 dilution of whole blood and lysing diluent according to kit instructions 2. Load hemacytometer counting chamber 3. Count all 9 primary squares on both sides of hemacytometer under 10 × objective 4. Check that each sides count is within 10% of the other. Example: side 1 = 150, side 2 should be between 144 and 176 (160 × .10 = 16, then range is 160 ± 16) 5. If second side is outside this range, recharge hemacytometer with fresh, well-mixed fluid and begin count again 6. Count the entire grid on 10 × magnification 7. Calculate total WBC by averaging both sides, adding 10% and then multiplying by 100 If side 1 = 160 and side 2 = 155 160 + 165 = 315/2 = 157.5 157.5 + 15.75 x 100 = µl (Skill Box 3.6)	Canine: 5000–14 100/µl Feline: 5000–19 500/µl	↑ Leukocytosis ↓ Leukopenia Evaluation of specific WBC populations (differential) is required for determination of cause
WBC estimate	Provides a quick check of WBC numbers to verify automated cell counts	1. Prepare a thin blood smear and stain 2. Evaluate WBC in monolayer under 40 × objective 3. Count 10 different fields and average 4. Multiply average WBC/field by 2000	Same as for WBC count above	
Differential	Percentage of different types of circulating WBC. Absolute numbers are used to evaluate patients. Cellular morphology is evaluated in conjunction with manual differential cell counts	1. A quick scan is performed using 10 × objective to establish cellular distribution and approximate numbers 2. A systematic pattern is used to count up to 100 WBC (band neutrophils, BN, segmented neutrophils, SN, lymphocytes, L, monocytes, M, eosinophils, E, and basophils, B), and classify according to type under 100 × objective 3. Calculate the absolute differential (Skill Box 3.8)	Canine BN: 0–450/µl SN: 2900–12 000/µl L: 400–2900/µl M: 100–1400/µl E: 100–1300/µl B: 0–140/µl Feline BN: 0–300/µl SN: 2500–12 500/µl L: 1500–7000/µl M: 0–900/µl E: 0–800/µl B: 100–200/µl	Varies by type of cell, see Table 4.13 ↑neutrophils = neutrophilia ↓ neutrophils = neutropenia ↑ lymphocytes = lymphocytosis ↓ lymphocytes = lymphopenia ↑ monocytes = monocytosis ↓monocytes = monocytopenia ↑eosinophils = eosinophilia ↓eosinophils = eosinopenia

(*Continued*)

Skill Box 3.5 / Complete blood count (Continued)

Procedure	Definition	Technique	Typical values	Associated conditions
Nucleated RBC (nRBC; Figure 3.60)	Immature nRBC rarely found in circulation in healthy animals; nRBC counted as WBC on manual and automated cell counts; WBC counts are corrected when > 5 nRBC observed while completing a WBC differential	1. Track the number of nRBC observed while completing a WBC differential (100 WBC) 2. Calculate a corrected WBC count: WBC count/μl x 100 100 + number of NRBC/100 WBC = corrected WBC count/μl	< 1	Regenerative anemia, premature neonates, bone marrow injury, heat stroke, lead poisoning, dyserythropoiesis hemangiosarcoma, splenectomy, corticosteroids, immune-mediated hemolytic anemia
Platelet estimate	Verifies automated platelet numbers; platelets are important in maintaining hemostasis by clotting and preventing blood loss	1. Examine monolayer of a prepared blood smear using oil immersion, 100 × objective, where RBC are in close proximity but not overlapping (Figure 3.59) 2. Count 10 different fields and average 3. Multiply by 20 000 to obtain estimated platelets per microliter 4. If clumping is observed, all numbers are inaccurate. Platelets may be evaluated as appearing increased, decreased, or adequate	Canine: 211 000–621 000/μl Feline: 300 000–800 000/μl	↑ Thrombocytosis may be caused by bone marrow disease, chronic blood loss ↓ Thrombocytopenia may be caused by bone marrow disorder, immune mediate disease, drugs, toxins, acute blood loss
Slide evaluation	Morphological identification of cells by microscopy; used to verify automated cell counts; changes in cell morphology, presence of abnormal cell populations, hemoparasites, and inclusions	1. Examine monolayer of a prepared blood smear 2. Scan the slide using low magnification (10 × objective) for cellular distribution, approximate numbers and presence of larger parasites such as microfilaria 3. Evaluate morphology using the oil immersion 100 × objective (Skill Box 3.7)	(Tables 3.12–3.14, 3.16)	

(Continued)

Skill Box 3.5 / Complete blood count (Continued)

Procedure	Definition	Technique	Typical values	Associated conditions
Reticulocyte count (Figure 3.43)	Immature, macrocytic, anucleated RBC; indicates bone marrow response to anemia; reticulocytes contain blue aggregate material when stained with supravital stain, new methylene blue	1. Mix together an equal part of whole blood with NMB, agitate, and let it sit for 10 minutes 2. Prepare 2 thin smears, similar to blood smear 3. Examine under 100 × objective and count 500 RBC on each slide, keeping a tally of reticulocyte numbers 4. Add reticulocyte numbers from each slide, divide by 1000, and convert to a percentage 5. Calculate corrected reticulocyte percent by multiplying by patient's PCV and dividing by mean of PCV reference interval for species 6. Use CRP to calculate absolute values by multiplying CRP by RBC count to obtain reticulocytes/microliter	Canine: < 1% Feline: < 0.6%	↑ Regenerative anemia: Canine: > 95 000/µl Feline: > 60 000/µl ↓ Non-regenerative anemia
Mean corpuscular volume	RBC index indicating size and volume of RBC; measured on automated instruments	MCV (fl) = PCV x 10/RBC count[4]	Canine 60–77 fl Feline 39–55 fl	↑ Macrocytic – artifacts from clumping, agglutination and hypernatremia, hereditary, reticulocytosis, primary myelodysplasia, folate/ vitamin B12 deficiency ↓ Microcytic – artifact from excessive EDTA, hyponatremia, hereditary, young kittens/puppies, iron deficiency, liver disease
Red cell distribution width	RBC index indicating variation in RBC volume; electronic measurement of anisocytosis	RDW (%) = standard deviation of MCV/MCV	Canine: 10.6–14.3% Feline: 13.2–17.5%	↑ Macrocytosis
Mean corpuscular hemoglobin	Average weight of hemoglobin contained in individual RBC; not as useful as MCV and MCHC	MCH (pg) = hemoglobin × 10/RBC count[4]	Canine: 21.0–26.2 pg Feline: 13.0–17.0 pg	↑ Hemolysis, lipemia, Heinz bodies, agglutination ↓ Iron deficiency

(*Continued*)

Skill Box 3.5 / Complete blood count (Continued)

Procedure	Definition	Technique	Typical values	Associated conditions
Mean corpuscular hemoglobin concentration	Percentage of hemoglobin in each RBC	MCHC (g/dl) = hemoglobin × 100/PCV	Canine: 32.0–36.3 g/dl Feline: 30.0–36.0 g/dl	↑ Hemolysis, lipemia, Heinz bodies, agglutination ↓ Hypochromic, iron deficiency
Total protein concentration	Concentration of albumin and globulin proteins Interpreted together with PCV	1. Break a spun capillary tube above the buffy coat level 2. Place the plasma onto the prism of the refractometer and read	Canine: 6.0–7.5 g/dl Feline: 6.0–7.5 g/dl	↑ Hyperproteinemia, common cause of dehydration ↓ Hypoproteinemia, common cause anemia and overhydration

Skill Box 3.6 / Hemacytometer[15]

- Always follow manufacturer's instructions regarding sample preparation.
- Gently invert sample just before use to ensure consistent distribution of cells.
- Discard the first few drops out of the vial when using premeasured kits. This fluid is usually cell free.
- Avoid air bubbles.
- Clean cover glass and hemacytometer with alcohol and a soft cloth to remove any debris.
- Avoid under or overfilling area under cover glass.
- Use a moist or humidity chamber to reduce evaporation.
- Be consistent in counting cells on border lines. Count only those touching bottom and left or only those touching top and right each time.

Skill Box 3.7 / Blood smear evaluation[4]

Blood smears are used to evaluate morphology and numbers of white blood cells, red blood cells and platelets. While viewing in a monolayer area of the slide, any abnormalities are graded under 100 × oil immersion objective by degree of severity, occasional, slight, moderate, or marked.

1. Prepare a thin blood smear slide and stain with quick stains. (Skill Boxes 3.3 and 3.13; Figure 3.5).
2. Scan under 10 × objective for:
   - Platelet aggregation
   - RBC rouleaux
   - RBC agglutination
   - Approximate WBC numbers
3. Perform a WBC estimate under 40 × objective by remaining within monolayer of slide (Figures 3.39 and 3.40)
4. Examine slide, using oil immersion magnification (100 ×)
   - RBC size, shape, and color
   - WBC morphology: toxic changes, nuclear changes, cytoplasmic inclusions, other alterations
   - Platelet clumping, alterations

Skill Box 3.8 / Calculating a differential[16]

1. Differentiate 100 WBC to type on a blood slide and record totals of each.
2. Divide each number by 100 and multiply by the total white cell count to get absolute cell numbers of each type/μl or mm.
3. Example:
   - WCC = 9000/μl

Relative #s (%)	Calculation	Absolute value
Band neutrophils = 1	1/100 × 9000	90/μl
Segmented neutrophils = 60	60/100 × 9000	5400/μl
Lymphocytes = 30	30/100 × 9000	2700/μl
Monocytes = 3	3/100 × 9000	270/μl
Eosinophils = 5	4/100 × 9000	360/μl
Basophils = 0	2/100 × 9000	180/μl

4. As a check of numbers and calculations, each cell should add up to equal the total white blood cell count.

$$90 + 5400 + 2700 + 270 + 360 + 180 = 9000$$

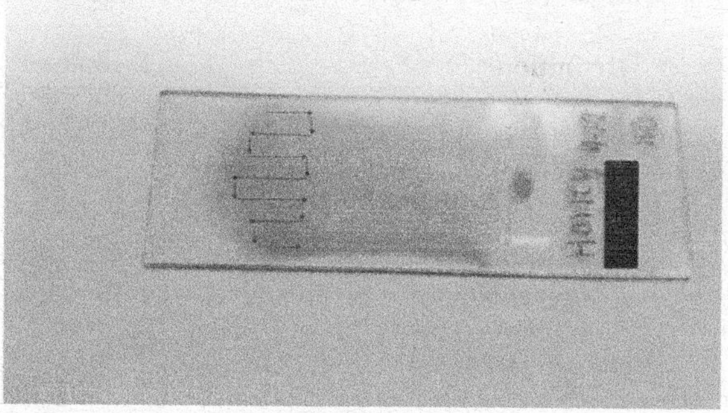

Figure 3.39 Slide evaluation showing consistent movement within monolayer of slide. Source: image courtesy of Barbie Papajeski.

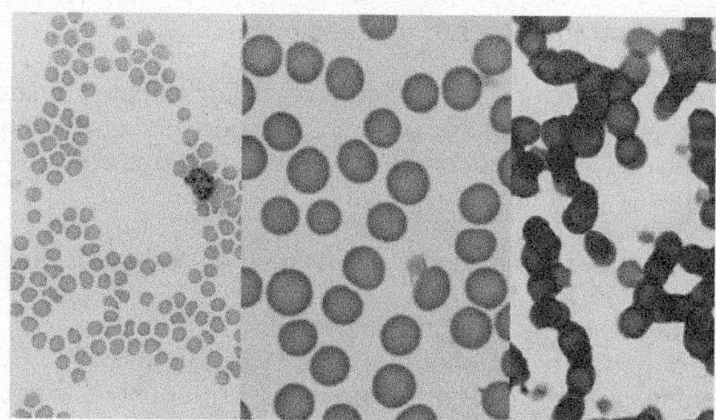

Figure 3.40 Area for cellular evaluation is monolayer (middle), feathered edge (left) shows cells too spread out and body (right) shows overlap of cells. Source: image courtesy of Barbie Papajeski.

Red Blood Cell Morphology and Alterations[5]

Typical, mature canine red blood cells are 7 µm while feline red blood cells vary between 5.5 and 6.0 µm. The biconcave shape of red blood cells causes an area of central pallor which fills one-third of canine red blood cells. Typical feline red blood cells have limited central pallor. Red blood cell morphology is evaluated for alterations in size, shape, color, and inclusions.

Table 3.12 / Red blood cell alterations and morphology[2–4,18]

Alteration	Definition	Appearance	Associated Conditions
Arrangement			
Agglutination (Figure 3.41)	• Clustering of RBC caused by antibody binding	Aggregation of RBC in three dimensional clusters	• IMHA, incompatible blood transfusion
Rouleaux	• Aggregation of RBC caused by ↑ in fibrinogen and immunoglobulins[4] • Slight rouleaux is common in felines • Any rouleaux is not typical in canines	Appearance of RBC in linear stacks	• Inflammation, renal disease in felines, B-cell neoplasia
Inclusions			
Basophilic stippling	• Residual RNA	Tiny dark aggregates scattered within RBC	• Regenerative anemia, lead poisoning
Distemper viral inclusions (Figure 3.42)	• Viral inclusion bodies	Variable sized round, oval, or irregular pink to magenta inclusions	• Canine distemper virus
Heinz bodies (Figure 3.44)	• Precipitation of oxidized hemoglobin[4] • Smaller forms seen in many felines	Rounded protrusion of RBC membrane; demonstrated by new methylene blue stain	• Inherited enzyme deficiencies, oxidative drugs, toxins, and other chemicals (acetaminophen, zinc, propofol, etc.)
Howell–Jolly bodies Figures 3.41 3.45	• Nuclear remnants left behind during nuclear extrusion • Low numbers common in cats	Perfectly round blue to black spherical inclusions	• Regenerative anemia, splenic dysfunction, erythroid dysplasia[2]
Morphology: color			
Hypochromasia (Figure 3.41)	• ↓ Hemoglobin in cells or ↓ MCHC • Graded as slight, moderate, or marked	↑ Central pallor, limited color in RBC	• Iron deficiency, copper deficiency, hemoglobin synthesis defects

(Continued)

Table 3.12 / Red blood cell alterations and morphology (Continued)

Alteration	Definition	Appearance	Associated Conditions
Polychromasia (Figure 3.45)	• Immature RBC released early from bone marrow • Reticulocytes	Darker purple in color with quick stains due to increased levels of RNA	• Regenerative anemia
Morphology: size			
Microcytosis	• ↓ Cell volume • MCV considered to be more accurate	RBC smaller than typical sizes for species	• Iron deficiency, cellular water loss, liver disease, hereditary
Macrocytosis	• ↑ Cell volume that may not correlate to MCV	RBC larger than typical sizes for species	• Immature erythrocytes, cellular water uptake, hereditary
Anisocytosis (Figure 3.47)	• Variation in cell volume[4] • Graded as slight, moderate, or marked	Variation in cell size; may include microcytic, macrocytic cells or both	• Liver disease, spleen disorders, regenerative anemia[2]
Morphology: shape[2–4,18]			
Acanthocytes (spur cells; Figure 3.46)	• Caused by either trauma or changes to cell membrane cholesterol and lipids	Spiculated RBC with projections of irregular length and a blunt tip	Fragmentation, lipid alterations in membrane, hemangiosarcoma, liver disease, DIC, and iron deficiency
Blister cells (prekeratocytes)	• Area devoid of hemoglobin often caused by oxidative injury	Blister or vacuole along edges of cell membrane	Fragmentation, oxidative injury, and liver disease
Crenation (Figure 3.46)	• Alteration in RBC membrane by changes in pH, reduced adenosine triphosphate, and water content	Even, uniform projections of equal distance and length around periphery of cells	Artifact from underfilled collection tube or aged sample (> 48 hours)
Dacrocytes	• Alteration in RBC shape due to fragmentation	Shaped like a hanging water or tear drop	Myelofibrosis Artifact in blood smear preparation if narrow ends point in same direction
Eccentrocytes (hemighost cells; Figure 3.47)	• RBC with displaced hemoglobin from oxidative damage (Heinz bodies)	Clear zone resembling half-moon shifted to edge of cell and no central pallor	• Oxidative injury causing cross-linkages of cell membrane
Echinocytes (burr cells; Figure 3.46)	• Alteration in RBC membrane by changes in pH, reduced adenosine triphosphate and water content	Even, uniform projections of equal distance and length around periphery of cells	• Artifact (see Crenation, above) • Renal disease, lymphoma, snake envenomation, chemotherapy drugs

(Continued)

Table 3.12 / **Red blood cell alterations and morphology (Continued)**

Alteration	Definition	Appearance	Associated Conditions
Keratocytes (helmet, bite cells)	• Form when a blister from an oxidative injury bursts	Spiculated cells with two or more projections Single projection is called an apple stem cell.	• Fragmentation, oxidative injury, and liver disease
Leptocytes (codocytes [target cells], knizocytes [bar cells])	• Larger RBC surface membranes with minimal contents in cells that tend to fold easily	Folded, bulls-eye target or "no" symbol	• Artifact in underfilled EDTA tubes • Iron deficiency, liver disease, lipid abnormalities
Nucleated RBC (metarubricytes, rubricytes; Figure 3.50)	• Immature RBC which still contain a nucleus[18]	Cytoplasm is dark purple to blue with a nearly black, pyknotic nucleus Rubricytes have blue cytoplasm and alternating light/dark chromatin pattern	• Regenerative anemia, premature neonates, bone marrow injury, heat stroke, lead poisoning, dyserythropoiesis, hemangiosarcoma, splenectomy, corticosteroids, immune-mediated hemolytic anemia
Poikilocytosis	• Generic term used to describe any variation in shape from typical biconcave disc	Changes in shape of RBC More specific descriptions should be used when possible (echinocytes, acanthocytes, schistocytes, etc.)	• Fragmentation, oxidative changes, surface lipid abnormalities, osmotic water loss/gain, energy loss, iron deficiency, liver, disease
Schistocyte (red blood cell fragments, schizocytes; Figure 3.47)	• Shearing of RBC without rupture[4]	Portions of red blood cells which appear as smaller, irregular fragments Often seen with acanthocytes	• Fibrin strands, DIC, hemangiosarcomas, liver disease, iron deficiency, vasculitis
Spherocyte (Figure 3.41)	• Partially phagocytized, spherically-shaped RBC with typical MCV values • Readily identified in dog but not cat	Intensely stained RBC without central pallor	• IMHA, incompatible transfusions, pyruvate kinase deficiency, zinc toxicity, snake envenomation, hemophagocytic syndrome, histiocytic sarcoma
Stomatocytes (mouth cells; Figure 3.41)	• RBC that are folded over in one direction	Central pallor is oval or elongated (mouth-shaped)	• Artifact in thick areas of slide, hereditary
Torocytes	• RBC with large areas of punched-out central pallor	Sharp demarcation from central pallor to hemoglobin within cell	• Artifact from improper spreading of cells on slide • Must be distinguished from true hypochromasia

(*Continued*)

Table 3.12 / **Red blood cell alterations and morphology (Continued)**

Alteration	Definition	Appearance	Associated Conditions
Parasites[4,11,18,19]			
Babesia spp. (Figure 3.48)	• Tick-transmitted protozoal hemoparasite of canines with worldwide distribution	Round to teardrop shaped piroplasms in RBC Size: 2.5–3.0 × 4–5 µm	• Causes hemolytic anemia, rare in healthy canines with intact splenic function
Cytauxzoon felis	• Tick-transmitted protozoal hemoparasite of felines • Bobcats serve as reservoir hosts	Signet ring merozoites in RBC Size: 0.1–5.0 µm	• Hemolytic anemia, DIC, shock, high morbidity and mortality
Mycoplasma spp. (Figure 3.49)	• Epicellular, bacterial hemoparasite transmitted by fleas • Detaches from EDTA stored RBC	Small cocci or rods found on surface of RBC individually, in chains or rings; chains may branch Size: < 1.0 µm	• Hemolytic anemia, causative agent of feline infectious anemia, common in felines, rare in healthy canines with intact splenic function

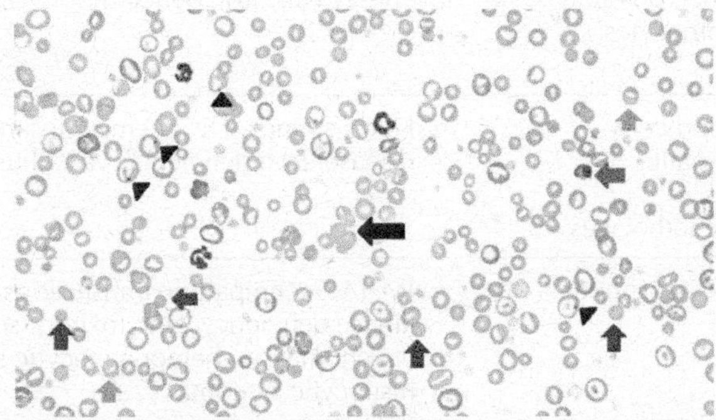

Figure 3.41 Red blood cell agglutination (black arrow), nucleated red blood cell (blue arrow), Howell-Jolly body (arrow heads), spherocytes (red arrows), stomatocytes (green arrows) marked hypochromasia and anisocytosis in canine sample with immune-mediated hemolytic anemia. Source: image courtesy of Barbie Papajeski.

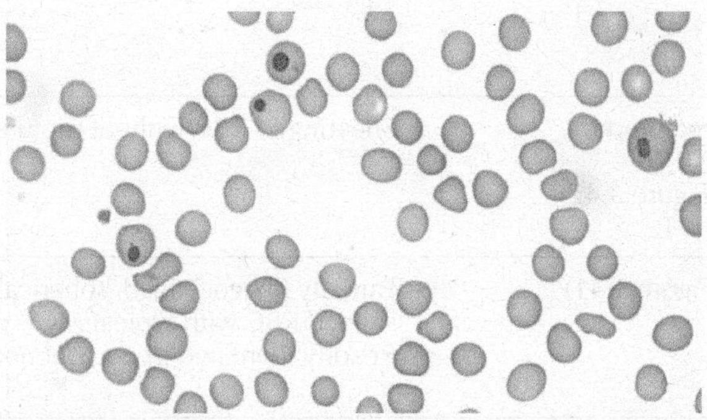

Figure 3.42 Canine red blood cells with variably sized distemper inclusion bodies. Source: image courtesy of Barb Lewis.

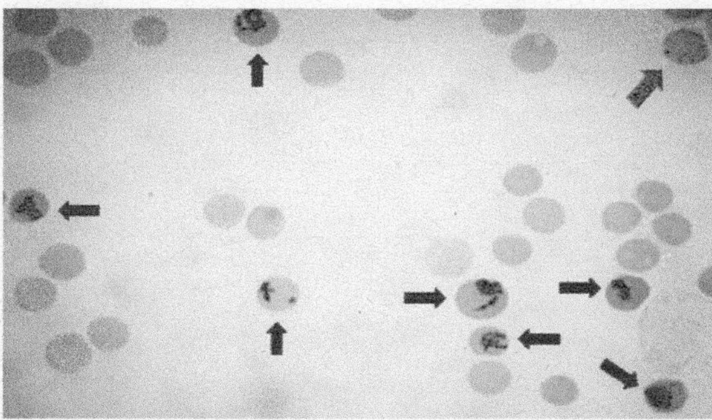

Figure 3.43 Feline aggregate (black arrows and punctate (red arrow) reticulocytes and mature red blood stained with new methylene blue. Source: image courtesy of Barbie Papajeski.

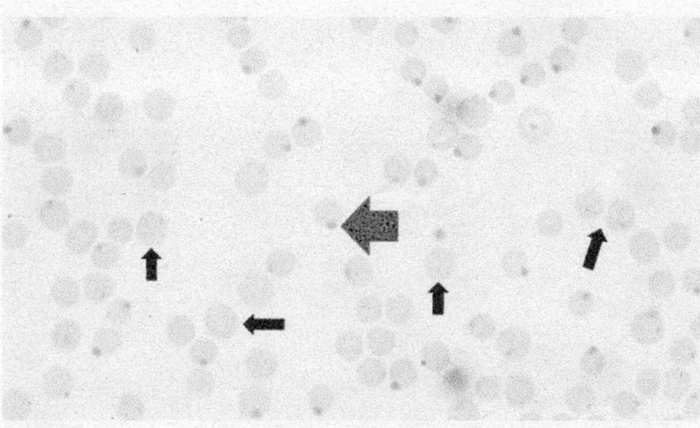

Figure 3.44 Heinz body inclusions (large red arrow) and punctate reticulocytes (black arrows) in a feline sample stained with new methylene blue. Source: image courtesy of Barbie Papajeski.

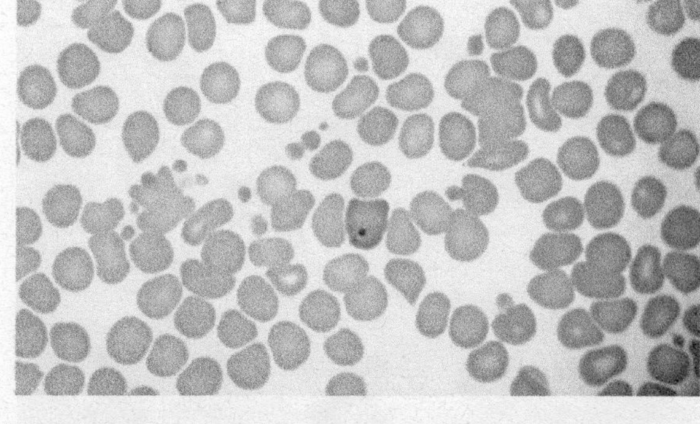

Figure 3.45 Canine blood smear showing a polychromatophil (center) and Howell–Jolly inclusion body. Source: image courtesy of Barbie Papajeski.

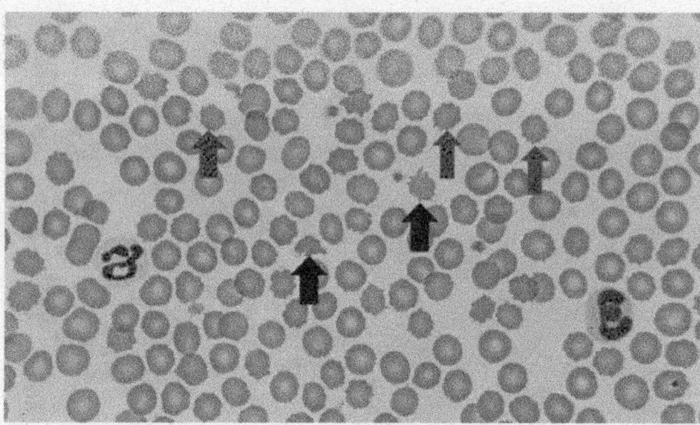

Figure 3.46 Canine blood smear showing acanthocytes (black arrows) and echinocytes (red arrows), segmented neutrophil (right) and basophil (left). Source: image courtesy of Barbie Papajeski.

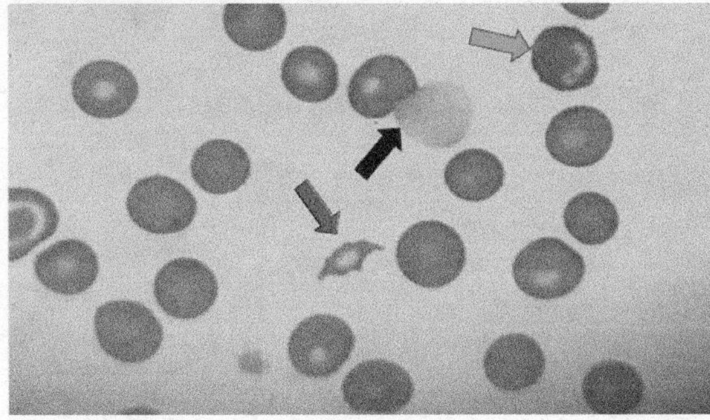

Figure 3.47 Canine blood smear showing anisocytosis, ghost cell (black arrow), schistocyte (red arrow), and eccentrocyte (blue arrow). Source: image courtesy of Barbie Papajeski.

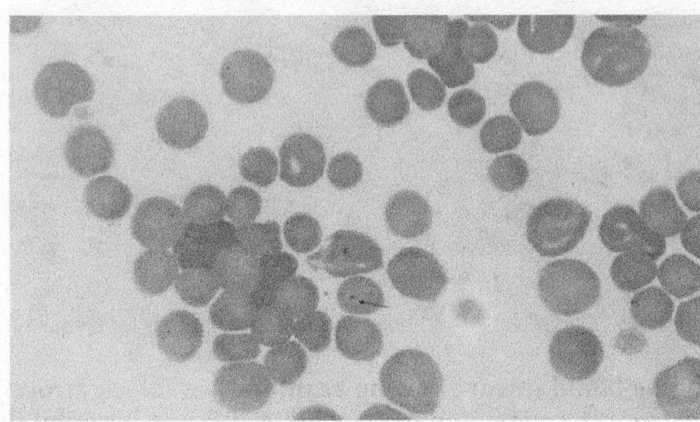

Figure 3.48 Canine blood smear showing anisocytosis, polychromasia and red blood cells infected with *Babesia gibsoni*. Source: image courtesy of Barbie Papajeski.

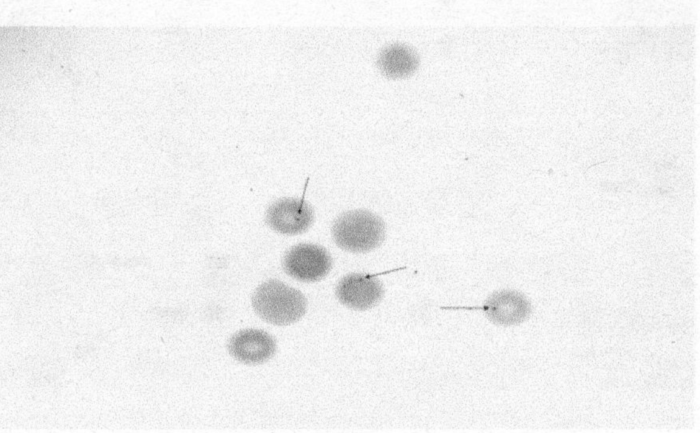

Figure 3.49 Feline blood smear showing anisocytosis, hypochromasia and red blood cells parasitized by *Mycoplasma haemofelis* (black arrow), schistocyte (red arrow), and eccentrocyte (blue arrow). Source: image courtesy of Barbie Papajeski.

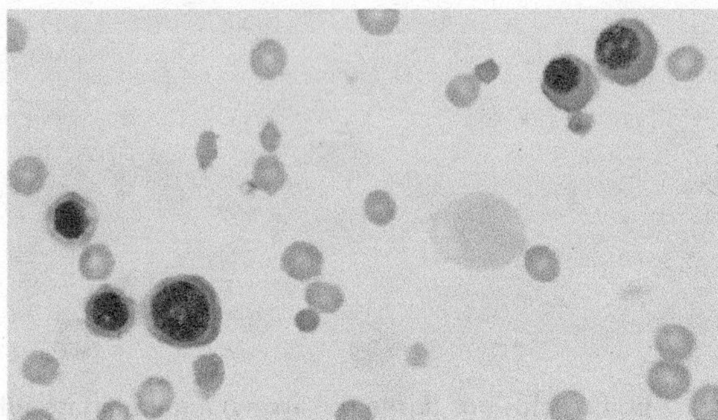

Figure 3.50 Feline blood smear showing anisocytosis, ghost cell and nucleated red blood cells including metarubricytes and rubricytes. Source: image courtesy of Barbie Papajeski.

White Blood Cell Morphology and Alterations[4]

Various WBC have specific functions within the body, primarily as a defense against viral, fungal, and bacterial infection. While neutrophil, monocyte, and lymphocytes functions are well known, exact functions of eosinophils and basophils have not been entirely discovered to date. Each cell has a specific cellular morphology and distinct terminology related to morphological changes.

Table 3.13 / White blood cell morphology[2,4,18]

Type	Definition	Appearance (stained)	Associated conditions
Band neutrophils	• Immature neutrophil • Low numbers to none in typical animals • Increased numbers called left shift	• Thick nucleus with parallel sides • No constrictions (indentations > 50% width of nucleus)	• ↑ during inflammation, bone marrow disorders, bone marrow injury or leukemia
Segmented neutrophils (polymorphonuclear or mature neutrophil; Figures 3.46, 3.51, and, 3.52)	• Most common WBC in dogs and cats[2] • Granulocytes with neutral staining granules • Phagocytic against bacteria • Remain in circulation 10–15 hours	• Nucleus with 3–5 constrictions and condensed chromatin pattern • Measures 10–12 µm • Clear, to faint blue or pink	• ↑ Inflammation, excitement/ epinephrine, fear, stress/ corticosteroids, • ↓ Acute inflammation, stem cell damage, viral diseases
Lymphocytes (B-cell and T-cell; Figures 3.51 and 3.52)	• Next most numerous cells in circulation of dogs and cats[2] • High nucleus to cytoplasm ratio • Produce antibodies and cytokines responsible for cell mediated immunity • Circulate longer than other WBC	• Nucleus is round with dense chromatin • Measures smaller than neutrophils • Scant light blue cytoplasm	• ↑ Excitement/epinephrine, fear, lymphocytic leukemia, ehrlichiosis • ↓ corticosteroids, acute viral diseases, immuno-deficiency diseases, damaged lymphoid tissue, loss of lymph fluid
Monocytes (Figures 3.51 and 3.52)	• Low numbers to none in typical animals • Phagocytes which enter tissues and mature to macrophages or dendritic cells • Phagocytize bacteria, protozoa, fungi, injured or aged cells, cellular debris, and foreign matter • Present antigen to lymphocytes	• Pleomorphic nucleus with lacy to fine granular chromatin pattern • Larger cell, measuring 15–20 µm • Blue-gray cytoplasm with fine, granular-looking material	• ↑ Inflammation, stress/corticosteroid response in canines, neoplasia, hypoadrenocorticism
Eosinophils (Figures 3.51 and 3.52)	• Low numbers to none in typical animals[18] • Granulocytes that fend off larval parasites • Participate in allergic inflammation and immune-complex reactions	• Segmented nucleus with condensed chromatin pattern • Slightly larger than neutrophils • Faint blue cytoplasm with orange-red granules • Granules are variably sized in canines and rod shaped in felines	• ↑ Parasitism, hypersensitivity, neoplasia, hypoadrenocorticism, eosinophilic leukemia • ↓ Stress/corticosteroids
Basophils (Figures 3.46, 3.51, and, 3.52)	• Rarely observed during differentials • Mechanisms of development and functions are unknown	• Poorly segmented, ribbon-like nucleus with condensed chromatin pattern • Granules are lavender in both canines and felines • Canine granules are indistinct and may not be noticeable • Feline granules are large and round, completely filling cytoplasm	• ↑ occurs with eosinophilia, neoplasia

Table 3.14 / **White blood cell alterations**[2,4,5,11,18,19]

Alteration	Definition	Appearance	Associated conditions
Inclusions			
Distemper	• Viral inclusion bodies[4] • May be found in any WBC	• Variable sized round, oval, or irregular pink to magenta inclusions	Canine distemper virus
Döhle bodies (neutrophils; Figures 3.53 and 3.54)	• Composed of swirls of rough endoplasmic reticulum[2] • Considered mild neutrophil toxicity	• Irregularly shaped blue to gray cytoplasmic inclusions	Inflammatory conditions
Chediak–Higashi	• Genetic disease observed in Persian cats of a blue smoke line • Autosomal recessive[4]	• Lysosomes fuse and stain lightly pink. • Appear as round to oval granules and measure 2.0 μm • Affect 25–33% of neutrophils	Chediak–Higashi syndrome; also affects platelets and causes prolonged buccal mucosal bleeding time
Morphology			
Cytoplasmic basophilia (neutrophils)	• Ribosomes and endoplasmic reticulum • Associated with marked neutrophil toxicity	• Streaky, blue coloration to cytoplasm	Inflammatory conditions
Cytoplasmic vacuolation (neutrophils)	• Prominent lysosomes become degranulated • Associated with severe neutrophil toxicity	• Foamy or frothy looking appearance to cytoplasm	Inflammatory conditions
Karyorrhexis	• Cellular degeneration	• Fragmented cell nucleus	Indicates cell death
Mitotic figures	• Cells undergoing cellular division	• Chromosomes within nucleus are visible	Neoplasia
Mucopolysaccharidoses (neutrophils and lymphocytes)	• Genetic, lysosome storage disorder • Affected animals are deficient in enzymes needed to break down glycosaminoglycans	• Dark purple to magenta granules (neutrophils) • Granules and vacuoles in lymphocyte	Mucopolysaccharidoses, lysosomal storage disorders
Nuclear hypersegmentation	• Prolonged circulating life	• > 5 nuclear lobes	Neutrophils retained in circulation > 10–15 hours
Pelger–Huët anomaly Figure 3.55	• Seen in heterozygotes for Pelger–Huët anomaly	• Hyposegmentation in mature granulocytes • Condensed chromatin pattern	Pelger–Huët anomaly
Pyknosis	• Densely stained nuclei • Indicates cell death	• Condensed nuclear chromatin	Indicates cell death
Reactive lymphocyte (immunocytes)	• Antigenically stimulated T and B lymphocytes	• Intensely blue cytoplasm with pale Golgi zone	Non-specific

(*Continued*)

Table 3.14 / White blood cell alterations (Continued)

Alteration	Definition	Appearance	Associated conditions
Vacuolated lymphocytes	• Nieman-Pick disease • Gangliosidosis • Mucopolysaccharidosis • Mannosidosis	• Cytoplasmic vacuoles	Lysosomal storage disease; artifact from prolonged storage
Azurophilic granules, granular lymphocytes	• T-lymphocytes or natural killer cells	• Reddish granules within cytoplasm of lymphocytes	Reactive conditions
Parasites			
Anaplasma phagocytophilum	• Tick-transmitted rickettsia bacteria of canines and felines	• Less organized blue to purple coccoid elementary bodies within neutrophils and eosinophils	Anaplasmosis
Cytauxzoon felis	• Tick-transmitted protozoal hemoparasite of felines • Bobcats serve as reservoir hosts	• Schizonts measuring 1–2 μm within lymphocytes or macrophages	Hemolytic anemia, DIC, shock, high morbidity and mortality
Ehrlichia canis	• Tick-transmitted rickettsia bacteria of canines and felines	• Morulae consisting of many small blue to purple coccoid elementary bodies within cytoplasm of monocytes and lymphocytes	Ehrlichiosis
Ehrlichia ewingii	• Tick-transmitted rickettsia bacteria of canines	• Morulae consisting of many small blue to purple coccoid elementary bodies within cytoplasm of neutrophils and eosinophils	Ehrlichiosis
Hepatozoon canis, Hepatozoon americanum	• Tick-transmitted protozoan of canines • Canines acquire by ingesting ticks	• Light-blue, large, oval gametocytes are found in neutrophils and monocytes • Measures 5–10 μm	Hepatozoonosis

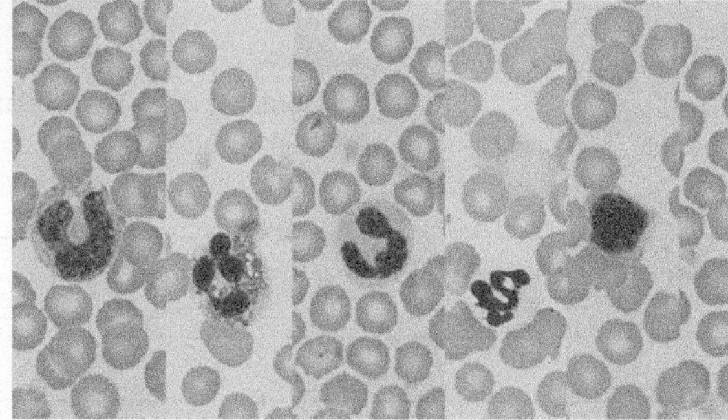

Figure 3.51 White blood cells in a canine blood smear as viewed under 100 × objective; left to right: monocyte, eosinophil, basophil, neutrophil, lymphocyte. Source: image courtesy of Barbie Papajeski.

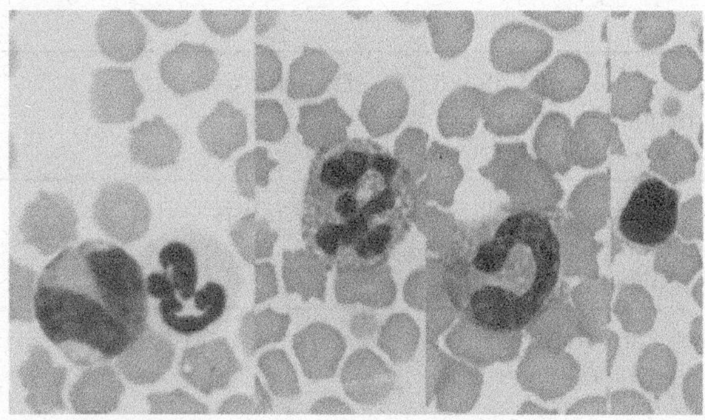

Figure 3.52 White blood cells in a feline blood smear as viewed under 100 × objective; left to right: monocyte, neutrophil, basophil, eosinophil, lymphocyte. Source: image courtesy of Barbie Papajeski.

White Blood Cell Alterations

During evaluation of a WBC differential, cellular morphology is evaluated and any deviations from typical WBC morphology must be notated. Morphological changes can occur with production problems, antigenic stimulation, infectious organisms, and in neoplastic conditions. Alterations in neutrophils often occur due to rapid proliferation and release of these cells to meet demands of inflammatory responses. These changes are termed "toxic", from a historical belief that bacterial endotoxins produced these changes within neutrophils. Toxic changes are the result of the expedited production process and are more of an indication of an increased demand and can indicate the magnitude of inflammatory response.

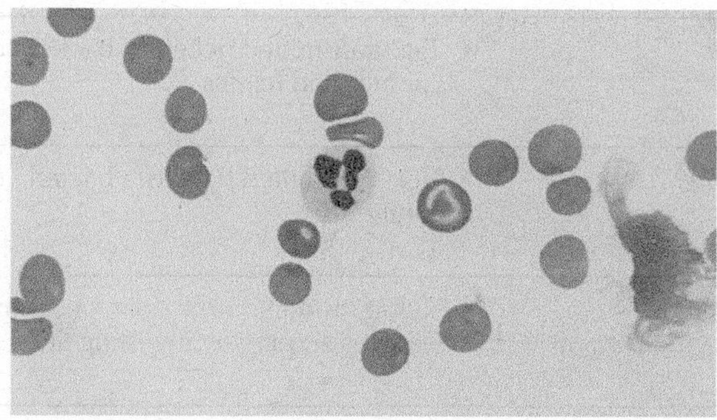

Figure 3.53 Canine toxic neutrophil exhibiting cytoplasmic vacuolation and Döhle body. Source: image courtesy of Barbie Papajeski.

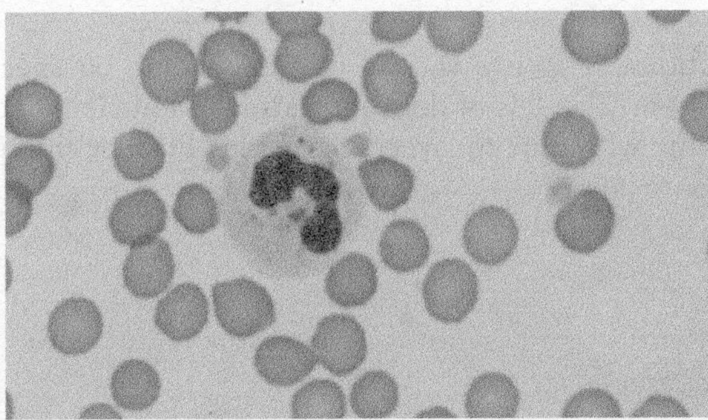

Figure 3.54 Feline toxic neutrophil exhibiting cytoplasmic granulation and Döhle bodies. Source: image courtesy of Barbie Papajeski.

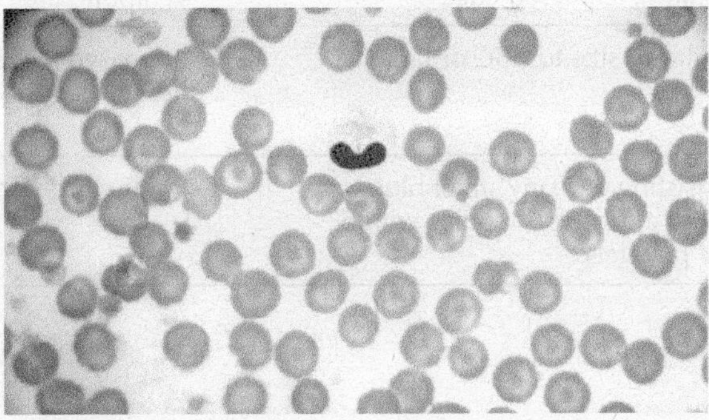

Figure 3.55 Pelger–Huët: hyposegmented mature neutrophils with a coarse chromatin pattern and many target cells (codocytes). Source: image courtesy of Barbie Papajeski.

White Blood Cell Population Changes

An increased number of circulating immature neutrophils indicates a left shift, so named due to the location of immature neutrophils on traditional cell counters. Bands are the most common immature neutrophil identified in left shifts, although earlier forms such as metamyelocytes, myelocytes, and myeloblasts are sometimes observed in extreme cases.

Table 3.15 / **White blood cell population changes**[2,4]

Change	Appearance
Left shift	• Immature neutrophils (bands) > 300 cell/μl • Other immature neutrophils
Regenerative left shift	• Mature segmented neutrophilia • Mature cells > immature cells • Lymphopenia • Monocytosis
Degenerative left shift	• Neutropenia or segmented neutrophils within reference intervals • Mature cells < immature cells • Leukopenia
Stress leukogram (corticosteroid response)	• Mature neutrophilia • Lymphopenia • Eosinopenia • ± monocytosis (canines)
Inflammatory leukogram	• Leukocytosis • Immature neutrophils • Neutrophilia ± toxic changes • Monocytosis
Inflammatory and stress leukogram	• Immature neutrophils • Neutrophilia • Lymphopenia • ± eosinopenia (canine)
Excitement/epinephrine leukogram (physiological leukogram, flight/fight response)	• Mature neutrophilia • Lymphocytosis • Eosinophilia/basophilia (feline)

Platelet Morphology and Alterations[2,4,18]

Platelets are also called thrombocytes; they carry plasma factors required in facilitating primary hemostasis and instigating secondary hemostasis. Platelets are important in maintaining vascular integrity and also are able to serve immune functions.[2] Platelets vary in size depending on species, generally measuring 2–4 μm. Platelets of dogs and cats lack a nucleus and stain a light pink to pale blue with blue to lavender granules. Platelet clumps render any count or estimate invalid.

Table 3.16 / Platelet alterations[2,18]

Alteration	Definition	Appearance	Associated conditions
Activated platelets (Figure 3.56)	Filopodia are threadlike extensions of glycoproteins from platelet surface	Platelets will have hair-like extensions of cytoplasm instead of discoid shape	Difficult venipuncture
Clumping (Figure 3.56)	Platelets adhere together	Two or more platelets in close proximity often found along feathered edge	Aged samples; difficult venipuncture
Macroplatelets (giant platelets; Figure 3.56)	Platelets larger than 5 μm May indicate immature platelets Common in felines	Platelets similar in size to RBC or larger	Increased platelet demand, hemorrhage
Anaplasma platys	Tick transmitted rickettsia bacteria of canines	Morulae consisting of many small blue to purple coccoid elementary bodies within cytoplasm of platelets	Cyclic thrombocytopenia

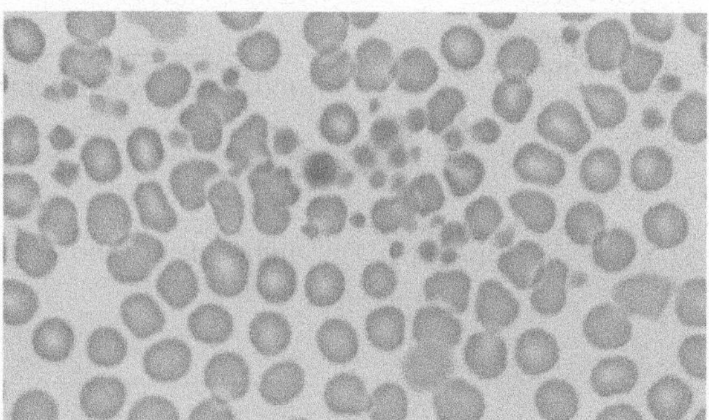

Figure 3.56 Clumped platelets, including macroplatelets, exhibiting anisocytosis and filipodia in a feline blood smear. Source: image courtesy of Barbie Papajeski.

Coagulation Tests[2,4]

Hemostasis is a natural cessation of bleeding and is the result of balanced interaction between proteins and cells. Any abnormality in this process can lead to excessive hemorrhage or excessive coagulation. Failure or deficiency in any factor or cellular component or combination thereof can lead to coagulopathy. Evaluation of coagulation abilities in patients with questionable ability involves proper collection and handling of samples for maximum results.

Some tips to remember include:

- Clean venipuncture on first attempt, using the largest vein possible.
- EDTA or citrate for anticoagulant, avoid heparin or heparin contamination from intravenous catheters.
- Fill tubes immediately to appropriate volume.
- Perform tests as soon as possible.
- Centrifuge citrated samples immediately and separate plasma.
- Redraw samples with hemolysis and visible clots with fresh needle.

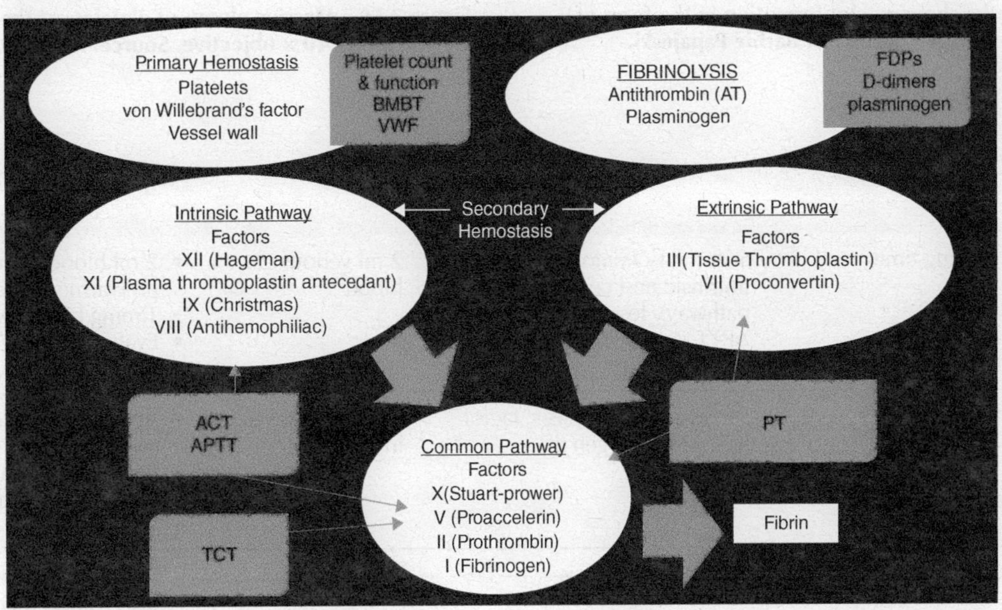

Figure 3.57 Coagulation overview.

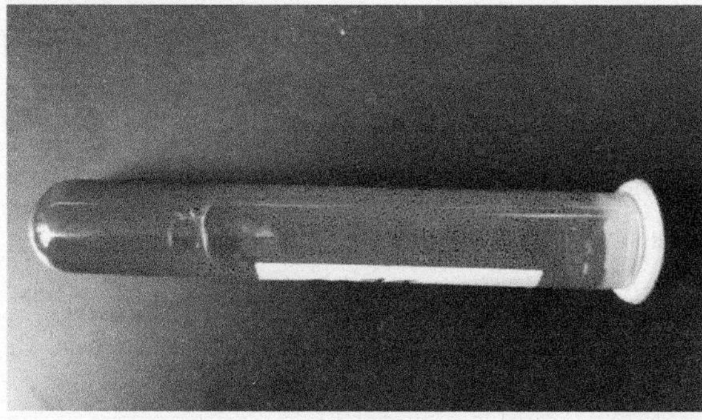

Figure 3.58 Activated clotting time tube showing clot formation in the form of tiny fibrin strands on the edge. Source: image courtesy of Barbie Papajeski.

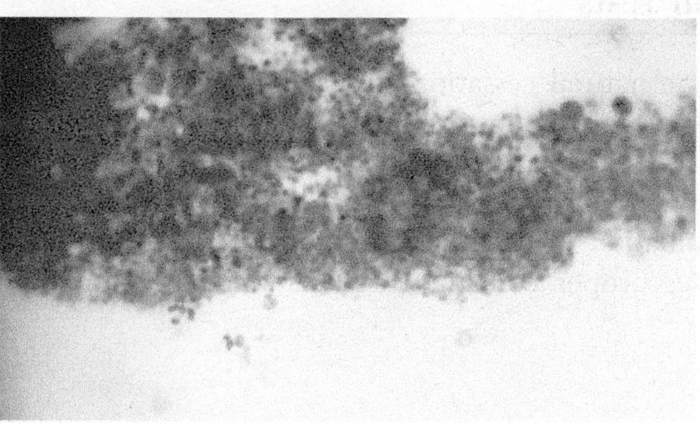

Figure 3.59 Massive clump of platelets at the periphery of a canine blood smear as viewed under 40 × objective. Source: image courtesy of Barbie Papajeski.

Table 3.17 / **Coagulation tests**[2,4]

Test	Definition	Evaluates	Sample required	General method
ACT (Figure 3.58)	Activated clotting time	Secondary hemostasis (intrinsic and common pathway); less sensitive than APTT	2 ml venous blood	• 2 ml blood collected and immediately placed into a prewarmed tube containing diatomaceous earth • Timing begins when blood enters syringe • Evaluate every 5–10 seconds for clot • Reference interval: 71.9–86.1 seconds (canine)
aPTT	Activated partial thromboplastin time	Secondary hemostasis; factor II, V, X; fibrinogen (I)	Citrated plasma in 1 : 9 ratio	• Activator is added to citrated plasma a repeated for average times • Reference interval dependent on activator • 9–11 seconds (canine) • 10–15 s (feline)
BMBT	Buccal mucosal bleeding time	Primary hemostasis	Live animal	• Incision in upper lip with lancet • Blot wound margins with filter paper every 30 seconds to evaluate clotting ability • Reference interval: 1–5 minutes
D-dimer determination	Plasmin mediated by-product of cross-linked fibrin	Fibrinolysis – fibrinogen degradation; thrombin	Citrated plasma in 1 : 9 ratio	• Commercial test kit detects neoantigen[4] • Reference interval: < 250 ng/ml
FDP	Fibrin degradation product	Fragments D, E; disseminated intravascular coagulation	Serum, citrated plasma	• Plasmin inhibitor is added to diluted serum • Latex agglutination indicates D and E fragments • Reference interval: < 10 μg/ml

(*Continued*)

Table 3.17 / **Coagulation tests (Continued)**

Test	Definition	Evaluates	Sample required	General method
Fibrinogen	Protein responsible for fibrin formation	Factor I (fibrinogen)	EDTA, citrated plasma	• Heat precipitation at 56–58°C • Clottable: modified thrombin clotting time • Fibrinogen antigen (ELISA or immunoturbidometric assay)
PLT	Platelet count	Primary hemostasis	EDTA whole blood	• Automated cell counts on fresh blood collected with minimal trauma • Reference interval: 211 000–641 000/µl (canine) • 300 000–800 000/µl
PT or OSPT	Prothrombin time or one-stage prothrombin time	Factor VII and common pathway	Citrated plasma separated from cells	• Activator is added and fibrin formation is measured by electrical impedance or optical endpoint • Reference interval: 6.4–7.4 s (canine) • 7.0–11.5 s (feline)
TCT	Thrombin clot time	Fibrinogen	Citrated plasma separated from cells	• Reference interval: 5–8 s (canine) • 5–9 s (feline)
Thromboelastography	Tests multiple pathways and platelets	Clot strength	Citrated plasma in 1 : 9 ratio	• Viscoelastic method requiring specialized equipment
Thrombotest	Protein induced vitamin K antagonism/absence (PIVKA)	Modified prothrombin test of factors II, VII, X	Citrated plasma separated from cells	• Diluted plasma is used • Test takes longer than PT and is rarely used
vWF	Von Willebrand factor antigen assay	Primary hemostasis; most common genetic defect	Citrated plasma	• ELISA • Immunoelectrophoresis

Blood Transfusions

Crossmatching

Performing a crossmatch prior to transfusion is critical in preventing severe reactions and death in recipient animals. Crossmatching indicates compatibility between donor and recipient blood by detecting previous sensitivities to prior exposure. Best practices are to perform both blood typing and crossmatch tests prior to transfusions, especially in cats which develop natural antibodies (Skill Box 3.9).

Skill Box 3.9 / Crossmatch slide agglutination[4]

Crossmatch test	Evaluates	Sample required	General method
Major	Checks for current antibodies in recipient serum against donor RBC	Donor and recipient blood in either EDTA or heparin	• Centrifuge both samples and separate plasma from packed RBC • Prepare a RBC suspension by pipetting 200 μl of packed RBC into a tube and adding 4.8 ml of phosphate buffered saline • On a glass slide, add 1 drop of donor RBC suspension to 1 drop of recipient plasma • Add a coverslip and examine for microscopic agglutination • If any agglutination is present, do not use donor for this recipient
Minor	Checks for current antibodies in donor which may destroy recipient cells	Donor and recipient blood in either EDTA or heparin	• Using samples prepared for crossmatch as outlined above, add 1 drop of recipient RBC suspension to 1 drop of donor plasma • Agglutination also contraindicates donor use for recipient
Major control	Checks for autoagglutination in donor	Donor blood collected in EDTA or heparin	• Using samples prepared for crossmatch as outlined above, add 1 drop of donor RBC suspension to 1 drop of donor plasma • Agglutination means all tests will be invalid with this donor
Minor control	Checks for autoagglutination in recipient	Recipient blood collected in EDTA or heparin	• Using samples prepared for cross match as outlined above, add 1 drop of recipient RBC suspension to 1 drop of recipient plasma • Agglutination means all tests will be invalid with this recipient

Blood typing

Blood groups are identified by antigens on the surface of red blood cells. When transfusing a patient, it is critical to identify blood type to avoid a fatal transfusion reaction. Commercial kits are available to determine either specific blood groups (felines) or to identify carriers of antigens which cause the most significant reactions (canines). Follow manufacturer's instructions for test kits (Figure 3.60).

Skill Box 3.10 / Blood typing[4]

Canine blood groups[2,4]

Type	Reaction
DEA 1.1	Acute hemolysis (illicit greatest reactions)
DEA 1.2	Acute hemolysis
DEA 3	Delayed hemolysis
DEA 4	None/unknown
DEA 5	Delayed hemolysis
DEA 6	None/unknown
DEA 7	Delayed hemolysis
DEA 8	None/unknown
Dal	Acute hemolysis
Kai-1	None/unknown
Kai-2	None/unknown

Feline blood groups[2–4]

Type	Reaction	Breeds
A	Most common	Domestic shorthair, domestic longhair, Siamese
B	Develop natural alloantibodies to A	Exotic breeds
AB	Rare	Domestic shorthair, Scottish fold, British shorthair, Birman
Mik	Requires crossmatch to detect	

(*Continued*)

Skill Box 3.10 / Blood typing (Continued)

Blood typing tests

Blood typing tests	**Format**	**Antigen detection**	**Limitation/advantages**
Blood typing cards	Lyophilized antisera	Agglutination indicates blood group	Kits only test for DEA 1.1 in canines
Immunochromatographic kit	Cell suspensions are used	Color line indicates antigen presence	Can be used in presence of autoagglutination
Gel tube	Cell suspensions	Cells appear together at top of column to indicate reaction	Test takes 10 minutes

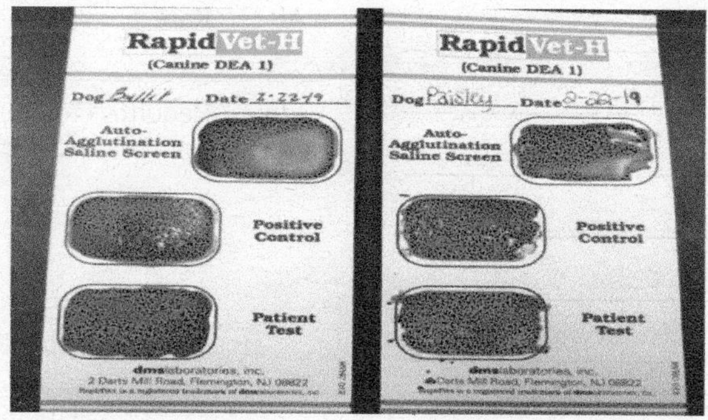

Figure 3.60 Blood typing card (left: dog erythrocyte antigen (DEA) 1.1 negative; right DEA 1.1 positive). Source: image courtesy of Barbie Papajeski.

IMMUNOLOGY AND SEROLOGY TESTS

Serological tests are used to detect either antigen or antibody to an infectious agent and may include serum, plasma, whole blood, feces, or saliva. Immunology is the study and function of the immune system and is used primarily to detect autoimmune disorders. To more accurately pinpoint a diagnosis, paired samples collected approximately two weeks apart may be warranted (acute and convalescent). Many types of in-clinic tests are available and an increasing array of testing is available at reference laboratories. It is prudent to check specific submission guides for individual laboratories.

See also Blood Collection, Handling, Storage, and Transport Tips.

Table 3.18 / Immunology and serology tests[6,10,20,21]

Test	Technique	Associated conditions
Complement fixation	Known antigen is added to the serum followed by specially sensitized RBC coated with antibody and a color change is observed; used to detect the presence of either a specific antigen or antibody in a patient's serum	Viral pathogens
Coombs test (direct antiglobulin test)	A species-specific Coombs reagent is added to the blood. RBC that are coated with antibodies will cause agglutination with the added reagent	Immune-mediated hemolytic anemia
Enzyme-linked immunosorbent assay (ELISA)	A tray with antibody coated wells is filled with the sample. If any antigen is present, it will bind with the antibody in the coated wells. A second enzyme-tagged antibody is added and binds to the antibody–antigen complex. A substrate that reacts with the enzyme is then added and results in a color change if antigen is present. The color change is proportional to the amount of antigen in the sample. The antigen may be actual viral/bacterial material or the host's antibody versus the pathogen	Anaplasma, distemper, Ehrlichia, Dirofilaria, canine parvovirus, feline immunodeficiency virus, feline infectious peritonitis, feline leukemia virus, Toxoplasma, progesterone, atopy, Neospora, allergies, Lyme disease
Hemagglutination assay	A virus and RBC dilution are added to the wells of a tray. The RBC bound by the virus will form a lattice and coat the well; a quick indicator of the relative quantities of the virus	Viral pathogens
Hemagglutination inhibition assay	A virus and RBC dilution are added to the wells of a tray. If sufficient serum antibodies are present, they will inhibit the virus attachment (hemagglutination)	Panleukopenia, parvovirus, and other viral pathogens
Immunodiffusion (agar-gel immunodiffusion)	Viral antigen and an antibody are placed into separate wells in agar. They diffuse through the agar and form a visible band of precipitation if any viral antigen is present	*Blastomyces*, *Histoplasma*, coccidiomycosis

(Continued)

Table 3.18 / **Immunology and serology tests (Continued)**

Test	Technique	Associated conditions
Immunofluorescence assay:		
Direct	An antibody for a specific pathogen is tagged with a fluorescent dye and combined with the sample. If the specific virus is present, the antibody will bind and appear fluorescent during microscopic examination	Antinuclear antibody, *Babesia*, *Brucella*, Coronavirus, *Ehrlichia*, distemper, *Leishmania*, Lyme, *Neospora*, Rocky Mountain spotted fever, and *Toxoplasma*
Indirect	An antiviral antibody (immunoglobulin) and a fluorescent tagged anti-antibody (against first) immunoglobulin are combined with a sample. The second antibody combines with the first antibody, which binds to any viral antigen present in the sample. The antibody–antibody–antigen complex will fluoresce during microscopic examination	
Immunoblot (Western blot)	Antigens are separated by electrophoresis and blotted to nitrocellulose sheets. The sheets are incubated with labeled antibodies and then observed for bound antibodies by using enzymatic or radioactive methods. Used to confirm ELISA results	FIV
Immunoperoxidase test (PAP)	A specific antibody is bound to the cell or tissue sample. The detection of specific antibody can be done through three different methods, all consisting of tagging the antibody and eventually generating a colored product	Distemper, FeLV, FIP, *Neospora*, and *Toxoplasma*
Intradermal tests	Allergenic extracts are injected intradermally and are observed for changes. A wheal formation indicates the presence of antibodies (IgE) and an allergic reaction	Allergies, insects, environmental, and Malassezia
Latex agglutination	Small, spherical antibody (or antigen)-coated latex particles are suspended in water. The sample is added, and any antibody–antigen complex will undergo agglutination. The water will be milky or contain clumps of latex particles	Canine rheumatoid factor, Brucella, Cryptococcus, DIC antigen complexes
Polymerase chain reaction (PCR)	A specific nucleic acid primer reacts with a portion of the genome from the microorganism in question. The combination is amplified to produce many fragments of the DNA sequence. Electrophoresis is then used to detect the combination and to measure its size and migration pattern. Often used to confirm results of other tests	Babesia, Brucella, canine influenza, leptospirosis, *Mycoplasma*, *Neospora*, *Salmonella*, *Toxoplasma*, *Trichomonas*, and many other bacteria, viruses, and parasites
Radioimmunoassay	An antibody for a specific virus or antigen is tagged with a radioactive element (e.g. iodine) and combined with the sample. A gamma counter is used to identify the antibody–antigen complex	Thyroid diseases, IgG
Serum antinuclear antibody (ANA)	Serum is serially diluted and added to a prepared slide with 10 areas of monolayer cell lines. If antinuclear antibodies are present, they bind to the nucleus and can be detected through immunofluorescence or immunoperoxidase techniques	Glomerulonephritis, immune-mediated thrombocytopenia, polyarthritis, polymyositis, systemic lupus erythematosus
Virus neutralization	A virus and a serum sample are mixed and are added to the wells of a tray. Cells are added and if they survive, then antibodies were present and have the ability to neutralize the biological activity of an antigen; a quick indicator of the relative quantities of the virus	Herpesvirus, calicivirus, adenovirus, distemper, parainfluenza, and other viruses

MICROBIOLOGY[22]

Basic microbiology can be performed in-house, while more specialized testing is often outsourced to a referral laboratory where access to a greater number of techniques and equipment is more cost effective. A basic in-house laboratory includes equipment and supplies such as an incubator, refrigerator, microscope, slides, and 3% hydrogen peroxide. Additional items needed are a heat source (e.g. incinerator, Bunsen burner or portable gas torch), inoculating loops, microbiologic media, Gram stain reagents and an oxidase reagent. Access to current books dedicated to the subject of microbiology should be available for consultation and for further discussion of alternative tests and techniques.

Skill Box 3.11 / Collection techniques[6,8]

Site	Collection
Abortion	Entire fetus or multiple specimens from a range of body parts should be obtained as soon as possible postmortem
Abscess/wound	Unruptured: sterile syringe with wide-bore needle
	Ruptured: swab near the edge of the wound and take scrapings from the inside wall of the abscess
Anaerobic bacteria	Sterile syringe with fine-gauge needle; expel all air out of syringe before obtaining a sample
Blood	5–10 ml of blood from at least two different sites and immediately placed in separate blood culture bottles; collect 3 consecutive samples (Skill Box 3.1)
Ear	Swabs of both ears canals and middle ear if needed
Eye	Corneal scrapings, swab of the conjunctival sac, or swab of lacrimal secretions
Fecal	1 g feces freshly voided or obtained from rectal examination; clean the anus before collection to avoid contamination with anal skin microflora
Genital	Swab of vulvar mucosa
Leptospirosis	20 ml midstream urine Wear gloves: zoonotic
Urine	5 ml urine via cystocentesis (see Skill Box 16.22: Urine collection: voided, manual expression, cystocentesis, page 730)

Microbiology Collection, Handling, Storage, and Transport Tips[6,8]

Collection[6,8,22]

- Collect the sample aseptically.
- Samples obtained from closed body compartments that have been aseptically prepared provide the best diagnostics with the least amount of contamination.
- Collect an adequate amount of the samples (> 1 ml body fluid or > 3 cm^3 tissue samples).
- Adequate quantities of submitted samples allow for smear preparations, inoculation of multiple culture media, and the ability to obtain quantitative results and avoids desiccation.
- Samples should ideally be obtained before starting antibiotic therapy.

Handling[6,8,22]

- Samples should be handled carefully to avoid cross-contamination from gloves, table tops, and so on.
- Separate multiple samples to avoid cross contamination.
- Maintain a clean environment in which the laboratory tests are run.
- Wood-shafted cotton-tipped swabs should not be used with samples of suspected Chlamydia.
- Samples must be clearly marked with patient's name, number, origin of the sample, time of collection, and whether it was refrigerated.

Storage[6,8,22]

- Avoid prolonged refrigeration of samples; freezing may be recommended for some samples.
- Swabbed samples need to be placed in a transport media if they are not immediately inoculated.
- Agar plates must be stored inverted to prevent condensation buildup on the surface.
- Samples for PCR analysis are *not* placed in charcoal or in agar.
- Do not use EDTA for sample collection or storage as it is bactericidal.

Table 3.19 / Specimen storage[8,22]

Test	Specimen	Storage
Acid-fast stain	Tissue	• RTT
	Slides	• Slide holder
Anaerobic bacteria	Fluid	• Anaerobic culture transport tube such as anaerobic transport systems, BBL™, Port-a-cul™ • Do not refrigerate transport tubes
Blood	Blood (5–10 ml)	• Blood culture bottle, e.g. VersaTREK™ Redox™
Culture and sensitivity (bacterial)	Swab	• Culturette swab, e.g. Amies bacterial transport medium and swab, with charcoal
	Fluid	• RTT
	Tissue	• Enteric transport media or RTT

(Continued)

Table 3.19 / Specimen storage (Continued)

Test	Specimen	Storage
Fecal culture	Feces	• Culturette swab/Para-Pak® • Enteric transport media • RTT • Clean, dry container
Fungal culture	Hair, scrapings, or swab (yeast only)	• RTT • Culturette swab, e.g. Amies bacterial transport medium and swab, with charcoal
	Fluid	• Screw-cap tube
Gram stain	Slides	• Slide holder
	Swab	• Culturette swab, e.g. Amies bacterial transport medium and swab, with charcoal
	Fluid or tissue	• RTT
Identification only	Swab	• Culturette swab, e.g. Amies bacterial transport medium and swab, with charcoal
	Fluid	• RTT
	Tissue	• Enteric transport medium • RTT
	Plate with growth	• Culture plate
Potassium hydroxide (KOH) preparation	Scrapings or clipped hair or nails	• RTT
Polymerase chain reaction analysis	Swab	• Dacron or other synthetic fiber, plastic handled • Place in sterile glass or plastic vials
Sensitivity only	Plate with growth	• Culture plate
Urine	Fluid	• Culture needs to be set up within 2 h to avoid overgrowth of insignificant bacteria or refrigerated for no longer than 18–24 hours
Tritrichomonas	Swab	• InPouch™ TF system • Do not refrigerate
Viral, *Mycoplasma, Ureaplasma*	Swab	• Viral transport media

Transport[8,22]

- Tape the lids and caps of inoculated tubes and plates before shipment.
- Tissue submitted for fungal cultures should be frozen.
- Empty the water that has accumulated on the lid to avoid it dropping onto the agar plate and mixing the colonies of bacteria.
- Do not use EDTA, cotton, wooden, or calcium alginate swabs.
- Avoid delays in getting samples to reference laboratory.

Most Commonly Used Culture Media

Various media types are available to selectively grow various pathogen(s) found in animals, but most clinics use only a few types. Samples are ideally inoculated onto both a solid and a liquid medium. A solid medium allows for isolation and differentiation of normal flora and pathogens and a rough count of bacterial numbers. Liquid media allow for the growth of small numbers of bacteria. More extensive cultures are sent to reference laboratories for growth and interpretation.

Table 3.20 / Most commonly used culture media[22,23]

Medium	Preparation	Uses	Interpretations
Blood agar (Figures 3.61 and 3.62)	• Tryptic soy agar • Sheep blood	All-purpose medium which supports growth of a wide array of bacteria to identify by rate of growth, morphology and hemolytic pattern	• Alpha: partial hemolysis = green halo (*Enterococcus faecalis*) • Beta: lysis of red blood cells, clear halo around bacterial growth (Includes most pathogens, *Staphylococcus aureus*, *Streptococcus* spp.; Figure 3.61) • Gamma: no lysis or color change
Brain–heart infusion (BHI) broth	• Calf brain and beef heart tissue • Available ± dextrose	General purpose enrichment media to increase the number of organisms	• Subcultures are made onto agar plates after incubation of 24 hours • 6.5% sodium chloride used as selective agent
Eosin methylene blue agar (Figure 3.63)	• Eosin Y • Methylene blue	Partially selective and differential agar for Gram-negative, enteric bacteria	• Large colonies with blue/black sheen (*Escherichia coli*) • Large colonies with mucoid appearance (*Enterobacter, Klebsiella*) • Large colorless colonies (*Salmonella, Proteus, Shigella*) • Irregular, colorless (*Pseudomonas*)
Fungal, yeast, mold, and dermatophyte test medium (DTM; Figure 3.64)	• Sabouraud BHI dextrose agar with antibiotics • Potato dextrose agar • DTM with chloramphenicol and phenol red	Selective growth of yeast, molds, and fungi	• After growing on Sabouraud agar, tape preparation and microscopic morphology examination performed • DTM: observable growth with a simultaneous red color change in 10–14 days
Hektoen enteric agar (HE)	• Bile salts • Bromothymol blue • Acid fuchsin	Selective growth of Gram-negative enteric bacteria	• Salmon colonies: carbohydrate fermenters (*E. coli*) • Blue-green colonies: non-fermenters (*Shigella* spp.) • Black or blue-green colonies with a black center: reduce sulfur to hydrogen sulfide (*Salmonella* spp.)

(*Continued*)

Table 3.20 / **Most commonly used culture media (Continued)**

Medium	Preparation	Uses	Interpretations
MacConkey agar (MAC; Figure 3.65)	• Crystal violet • Bile acids • pH indicator	Selective and differential agar in a variety of formulations; selectively grows Gram-negative bacteria	• Pink to red colonies: lactose fermenters (*E. coli*) • Colorless to light yellow colonies: non-lactose fermenters (*Salmonella* spp.)
Mannitol salt agar (MSA; Figure 3.66)	• NaCl • Mannitol • Phenol red	Selective for *Staphylococcus* spp. and inhibits most Gram-negative organisms	• Medium turns yellow: ferments mannitol and produces an acid (*S. aureus*) • Growth with no color change: does not ferment mannitol (*Staphylococcus epidermidis*)
Mueller Hinton agar (Figure 3.67)	• Casein • Sheep blood • Beef extract	A non-selective, nondifferential media used for antibiotic susceptibility	• Chocolate agar is supplemented with beef extract • Used for Kirby–Bauer test
Phenylethyl alcohol agar (**PEA**)	• Phenylethyl alcohol • NaCl	Selective for Gram-positive cocci such as *Staphylococcus* spp.	• Observable growth of colonies
Thioglycollate media	• Thioglycolic acid • Yeast extract • Dextrose	Supports growth of anaerobic and facultative anaerobic bacteria	• Turbid or streaks if turbidity is not disturbed • Used with other culture and collection media

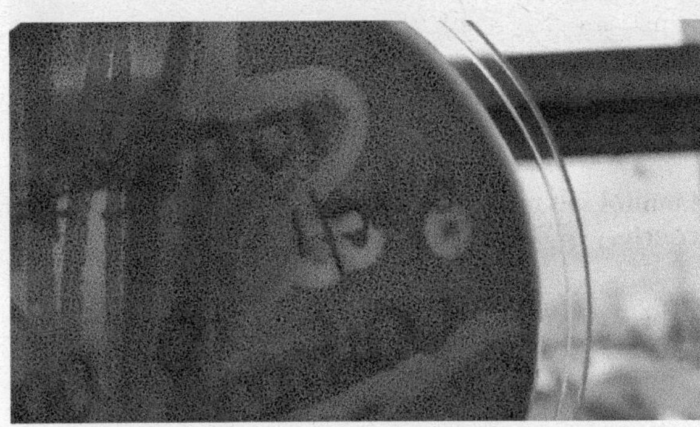

Figure 3.61 Blood agar plate showing bacterial colonies with β-hemolysis. Source: image courtesy of Barbie Papajeski.

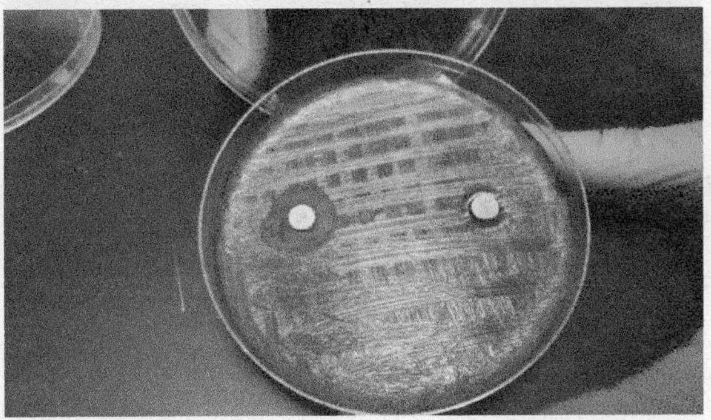

Figure 3.62 Sheep blood agar with antibiotic susceptibility discs. Source: image courtesy of Barbie Papajeski.

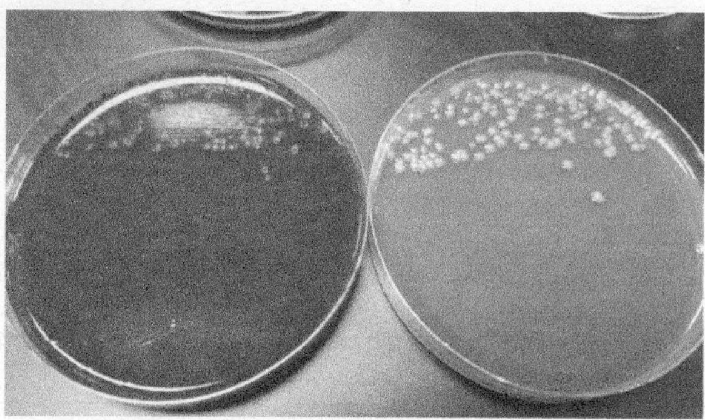

Figure 3.63 Eosin methylene blue plate with *Escherichia coli*, together with a special media plate called spirit blue which indicates lipolytic organisms. Source: image courtesy of Barbie Papajeski.

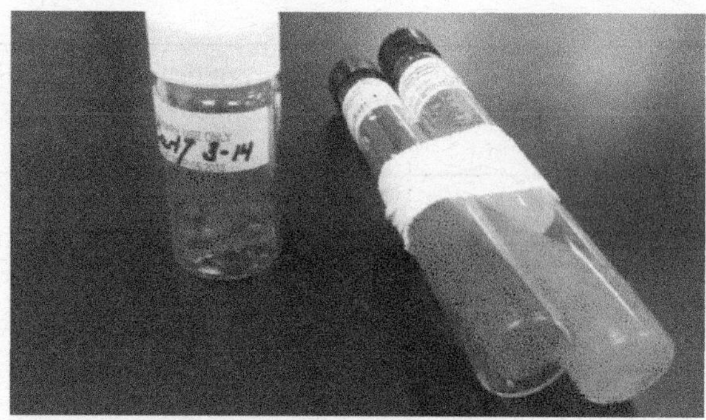

Figure 3.64 Dermatophyte test medium media showing red indicator for dermatophytes. Source: image courtesy of Barbie Papajeski.

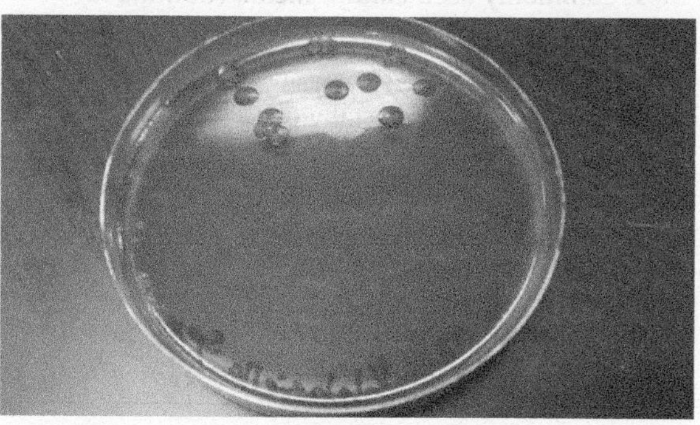

Figure 3.65 MacConkey agar with *Klebsiella* spp., a lactose fermenter. Source: image courtesy of Barbie Papajeski.

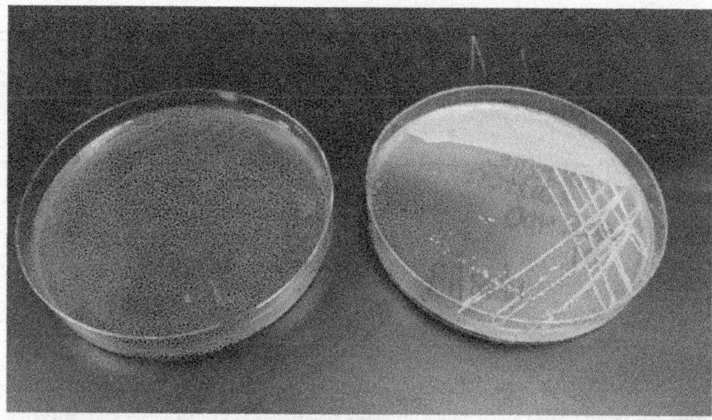

Figure 3.66 Mannitol salt agar plate showing *Staphylococcus* growth on right. Source: image courtesy of Barbie Papajeski.

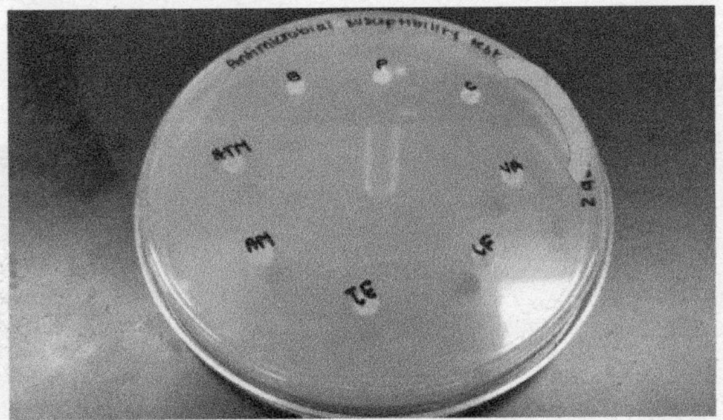

Figure 3.67 Mueller Hinton agar with antibiotic discs. Source: image courtesy of Barbie Papajeski.

Culture Media Inoculation and Incubation

Skill Box 3.12 / Culture media inoculation and incubation[22]

General Points for Proper Technique

- Media that is refrigerated should be allowed to warm to room temperature prior to use.
- Keep culture plates closed unless inoculating or transferring specimens.
- Do not set down the tube cap of the medium to avoid contamination.
- Flame the neck of the tube before and after transferring specimens.
- When flaming the inoculation loop or wire, place the end closest to the handle in the hottest portion of the flame, the blue portion, and then move toward the loop to prevent splattering.
- Be sure to cool loop before touching agar to prevent aerosol of bacteria.
- When transferring the sample to the agar, use a gentle touch to avoid tearing the surface of the agar.

Plate Inoculation

- Mentally divide the agar plate into four quadrants.
- Flame and cool the inoculation loop.
- Dip the loop into the specimen to be cultured.
- Streak the specimen in quadrant A by a gentle back and forth motion.
- Stab loop into clean area or flame and cool loop.
- Turn plate to next quadrant.
- Streak back and forth slightly overlapping previous quadrant.
- Turn plate slightly to next quadrant and repeat streaking steps.
- Remove the loop and flame.
- Be sure to only overlap the previous quadrant's streaks one to two times to prevent excessive numbers of bacteria in one area.
- Quadrant D is expected to grow isolated colonies (Figures 3.68 and 3.69).
- Plates for susceptibility testing will be covered with bacterial by rolling an inoculated swab across the agar (Figure 3.70).

Slant Inoculation

- Flame and cool the inoculation wire.
- Tip: Work with two inoculation loops; one can be cooling while the other is in use.
  - Dip the wire into the specimen to be cultured.
  - Types of slant inoculations:

(*Continued*)

Skill Box 3.12 / Culture media inoculation and incubation (Continued)

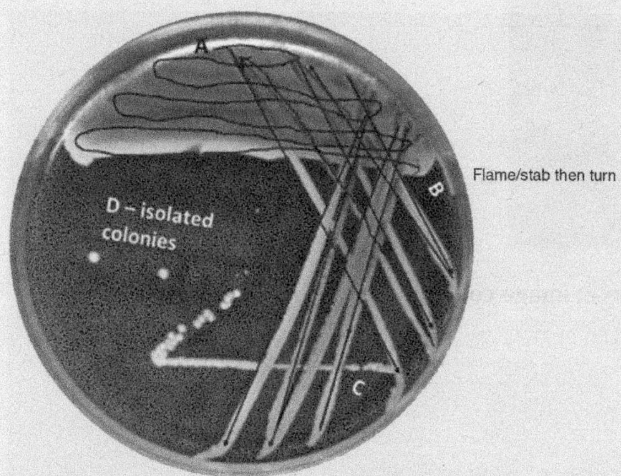

Figure 3.68 Illustration of streaking method. Source: image courtesy of Barbie Papajeski.

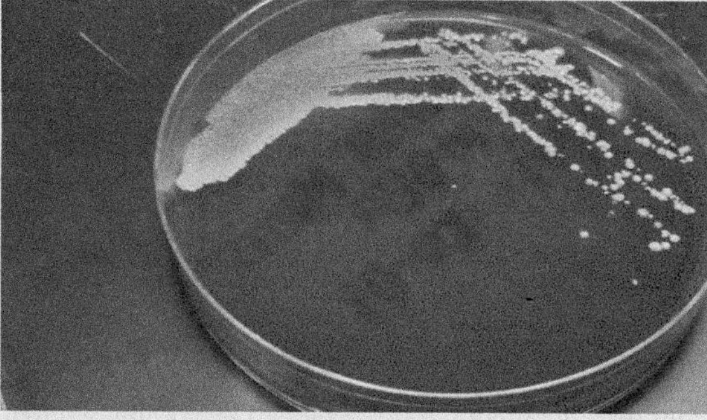

Figure 3.69 Sheep blood agar with isolated colonies. Source: image courtesy of Barbie Papajeski.

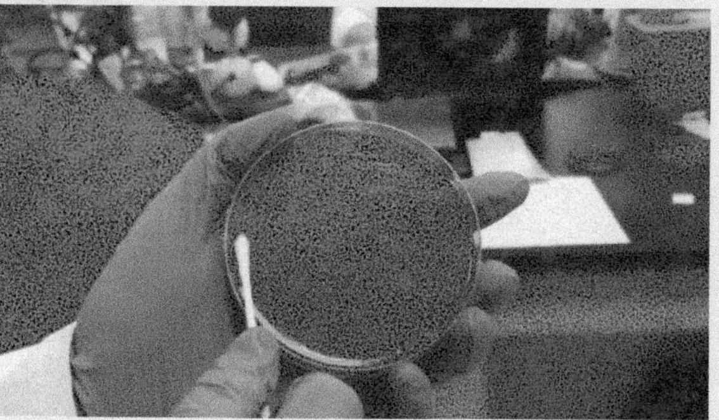

Figure 3.70 Inoculating a plate for microbial susceptibility. Source: image courtesy of Barbie Papajeski.

- Stab only: stab the wire through the agar and then slowly withdraw it along the same stab path (Figure 3.71).
- Slant only: make an "S" shape across the slant with the tip of the inoculation wire (Figure 3.72).
- Butt and slant: combine the above two methods, starting with the stab method and finishing with the slant method.
- Remove the wire and flame again (Figures 3.71 and 3.72).

Broth Inoculation

- Flame and cool the inoculation loop or wire.
- Dip the wire into the specimen to be cultured.
- Insert the loop or wire into the broth just below the surface and touch the side of the tube.
- Remove the loop or wire and reflame.

(Continued)

Skill Box 3.12 / **Culture media inoculation and incubation (Continued)**

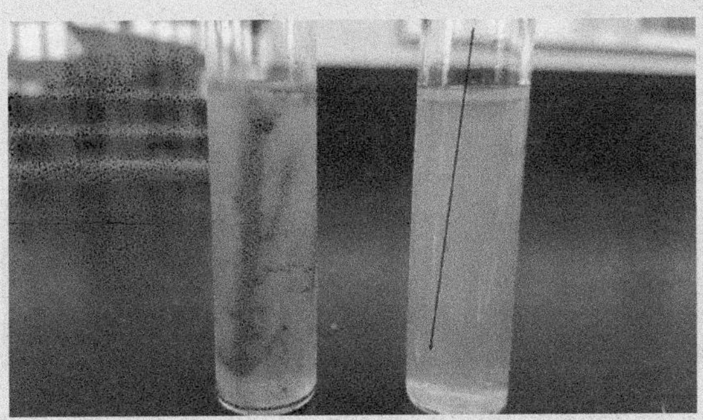

Figure 3.71 Tube media showing motility from stab technique with *Escherichia coli*. Source: image courtesy of Barbie Papajeski.

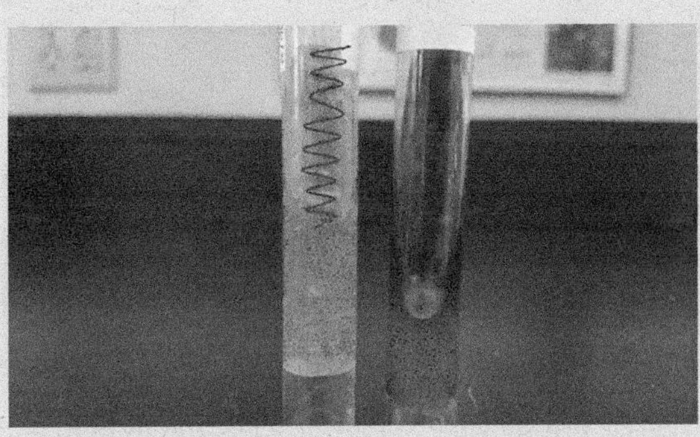

Figure 3.72 Tube media showing motility from stab technique. Source: Image courtesy of Barbie Papajeski.

Incubation of Cultures

- Maintain incubator temperature at 98.6°F and humidity of 70%.
- Plates should be placed upside down to prevent the accumulation of condensation on the surface of the agar plate.
- Tube media screw caps should be left loose during incubation.
- Cultures should be incubated for 48 hours and checked after 24 hours.
- Place a bowl of water in the bottom of the incubator to maintain a high humidity.

Culture Growth Evaluation[22]

1. Identify the source of the sample.
2. Grow the sample.

Significant	Not significant
Only one to two types of bacterial growth	> 3 types of scant bacterial growth
Circular colonies with clear edges, smooth, convex, or rounded	Large, irregular, and granular colonies and spreading edges
Opaque to gray	Heavily pigmented

3. Changes to the media
   a. Hemolytic pattern
   b. Color change
   c. Odor
4. Microscopic evaluation
   a. Simple stain
   b. Gram stain
   c. Acid-fast stain
   d. Negative stain (Skill Box 3.13)
5. Differentiation tests
   a. Catalase test
      - Differentiates between catalase-positive (staphylococci) and catalase-negative (streptococci, enterococci) bacteria
      - Positive test: formation of bubbles

   b. Coagulase test
      - Differentiates between coagulase producing staphylococci and non-coagulase producing staphylococci
      - Positive test: agglutination on slide card (Figure 3.73)

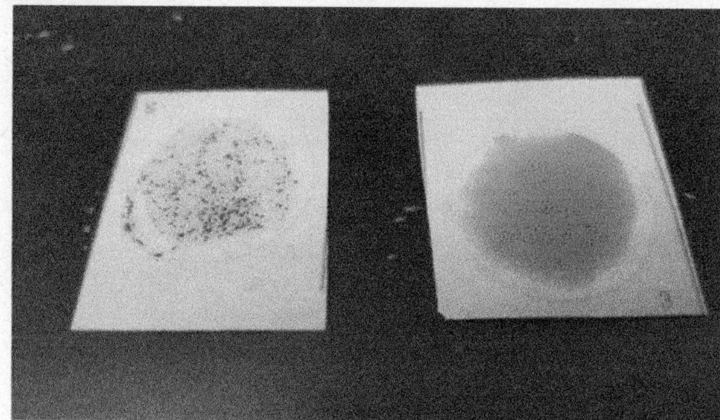

Figure 3.73 Coagulase test showing *Staphylococcus aureus* (left) and a non-coagulase producing bacterium on right. Source: image courtesy of Barbie Papajeski.

c. Oxidase test
- Differentiates between oxidase-positive (*Bordetella bronchiseptica, Pseudomonas aeruginosa, Pasterurella* spp.) and oxidase-negative (*Enterobacter* spp., *Escherichia* and *Salmonella* spp.) bacteria
- Positive test: pink to purple color change

d. Indole test
- Differentiates between indole-positive (*Escherichia coli, Proteus vulgaris*) and indole-negative (*Streptococcus pyogenes, Salmonella typhimurium*) bacteria
- Positive test: red color on the surface of the tube

e. Urease test
- Differentiates between urease degrading (*Proteus* spp., *Corynebacterium urealyticum, Helicobacter pylori, Ureaplasma, Nocardia, Cryptococcus, Staphylococcus* spp., *Brucella*) and non-urease degrading bacteria
- Positive test: hot pink color (Figure 3.74)

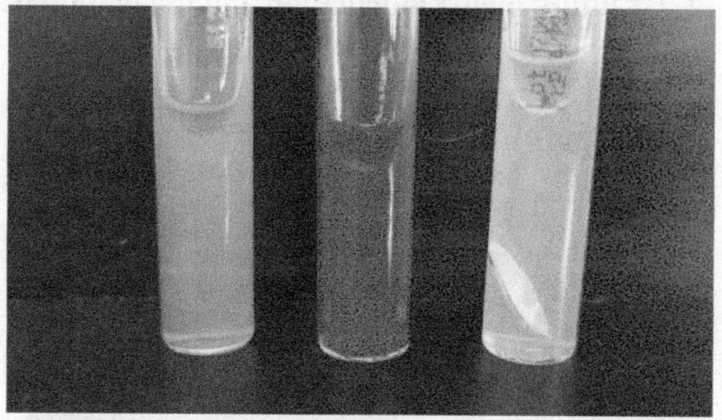

Figure 3.74 Urease test with positive in the middle and negative on right. Tube on the left is the original media color. Source: image courtesy of Barbie Papajeski

f. Multiple biochemical tests in one kit
- Enterotube™ test or analytical profile index (Figure 3.75)

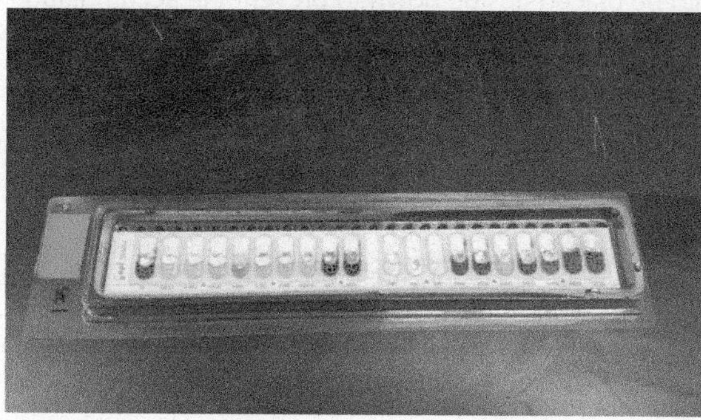

Figure 3.75 CAMP test showing enhanced hemolysis at arrow. Source: image courtesy of Barbie Papajeski.

g. Motility test
- Tube test supports growth and includes color indicators (Figure 3.71)
- Direct microscopic view of liquid cultures

h. CAMP test
   - Identifies interacting hemolysins and is used to confirm bacterial identification (*Streptococcus agalactiae*, *Corynebacterium renale*, *Listeria monocytogenes*) by streaking suspected bacteria near *Stapholoccocus aureus*
   - Enhanced hemolysis will indicate CAMP (Christie–Atkinson–Munch–Peterson)-positive isolates (Figure 3.76)

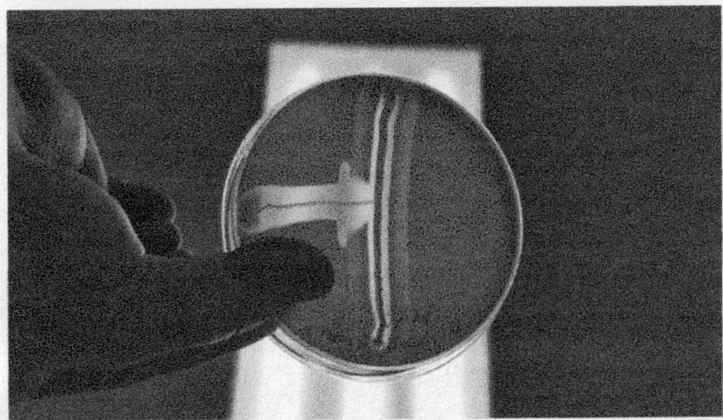

Figure 3.76 API strip inoculated with bacteria. Source: image courtesy of Barbie Papajeski.

i. Triple sugar iron
   - Identifies bacteria's ability to ferment glucose, sucrose, and lactose and whether gas production occurs in the process
   - Slant tube has color indicators and media lift at butt of tube indicates gas formation

j. Reference laboratory testing
   - PCR detects DNA of microorganisms
   - Matrix-assisted laser desorption/ionization time-of-flight mass spectrometry measures protein profiles

Staining Solutions and Procedures

The first step to identification of microbiology slides is to prepare the slide correctly. Be sure to follow specific manufacturer's guidelines when using stains. Slides are often stained on an air-dried or heat-fixed slide. To heat-fix a slide, make several rapid passes of the bottom of the slide over a flame source (incinerator, matches, lighter, or Bunsen burner). While the slide is immersed in staining solution, agitating it will allow the fresh stain to remain in contact with its surface.

Skill Box 3.13 / Staining solutions and procedures[22]

Staining technique	Uses	Preparation	Procedure	Interpretation
Differential stains				
Capsule stain	Detection of capsules (*Cryptococcus*)	• India ink • Maneval's method • Anthony's capsule stain	1. Apply 1 drop of stain to a clean slide and air dry 2. Add organism from tube or plate with a flamed loop and mix 3. Use the end of another slide to spread the sample across the slide with capillary action 4. Air dry 5. Saturate slide with India ink 6. Rinse with water 7. Air dry	Capsules (if present) will appear clear against the dark background. Bacterial cells will stain purple
Endospore stain	Detection of endospores (*Bacillus* and *Clostridium*)	• Dorner method: carbol fuchsin and nigrosine • Schaeffer–Fulton method: malachite green, safranin	1. Flood the prepared slide with carbofuschin or malachite green and heat over a flame until it steams and then let it sit for 5 minutes 2. Rinse with water 3. Counterstain with nigrosine or safranin for 2 minutes 4. Rinse with water and blot with blotting paper or dry over low heat	• Dorner method: Colorless parent cell and black endospore • Schaeffer–Fulton method: red parent cell and green endospore
Gram stain (Figure 3.77)	Distinguish between Gram-positive and -negative bacteria based on their cell wall structure (peptidoglycan layer)	• Primary stain: crystal violet • Mordant: Gram's iodine • Decolorizer: alcohol • Counterstain: dilute carbol fuchsin or safranin	1. Flood prepared slide with crystal violet for 30–60 seconds 2. Rinse with water for 5 seconds 3. Flood slide with Gram's iodine for 30–60 seconds 4. Rinse with water for 5 seconds 5. Decolorize until the purple color is gone for around 10 seconds 6. Rinse with water for 5 seconds 7. Flood slide with dilute carbol fuchsin or safranin for 30–60 s 8. Rinse with water for 5 s 9. Air-dry or blot between towels	• Purple-stained bacteria = Gram-positive • Red-stained bacteria = Gram-negative *Tip:* When working with an unknown organism, place and label a known Gram-positive and a Gram-negative organism on the slide for comparison and to ensure proper staining technique.

(*Continued*)

Skill Box 3.13 / Staining solutions and procedures (Continued)

Staining technique	Uses	Preparation	Procedure	Interpretation
Lactophenol cotton Blue (Figures 3.78 and 3.82)	Detection of fungi	• Lactophenol cotton blue	1. Apply 1 drop of lactophenol cotton blue to a clean glass slide 2. Apply tape to fungal colony 3. Place tape sticky side down on stain and examine	Visualization of hyphae, septae, and structure of spores
Romanowsky quick stains (modified Wright's and Giemsa stains; Figures 3.79 and 3.81)	General hematology, cytology, and demonstration of bacteria	• Fixative: methanol • Eosinophilic: eosin dye • Basophilic: thiazine or methylene blue dye mixture	1. Dip the prepared slide five times slowly in methanol fixative 2. Repeat above with eosinophilic stain and basophilic stain 3. Rinse with water 4. Air dry	Clear differentiation of cellular morphology Staining ranges from pale pink to dark purple Bacteria appear dark purple in color
Ziehl/Neelson or acid-fast stain	Detection of *Mycobacterium* spp., *Nocardia and Cryptosporidium*	• Primary stain: carbol fuchsin • Decolorizer: acid alcohol or acetic acid • Counterstain: methylene blue	Various types are available – refer to specific stain instructions	Acid-fast bacteria and Cryptosporidia stain red/fuchsia Non-acid-fast bacteria stain blue/green
Simple stains				
Negative staining	Detection of capsules and difficult to stain bacteria (spirilli) by providing a dark background	• India ink • Nigrosin	Technique 1: 1. Apply one to two drops of stain to the prepared slide 2. Apply coverslip and examine as a wet mount Technique 2: 1. Apply one drop of stain to a clean slide 2. Add organism from the tube or plate with a flamed loop and mix 3. Use the end of another slide to spread the sample across the slide with capillary action Air-dry and examine	Capsules appear clear and unstained, surrounded by dark particles

(*Continued*)

Skill Box 3.13 / Staining solutions and procedures (Continued)

Staining technique	Uses	Preparation	Procedure	Interpretation
Methylene blue, new methylene blue	Demonstration of bacteria and general morphology and shape arrangement	• Simple stain consisting of single stain methylene blue	Technique 1: 1. Place one drop on the coverslip and apply to the prepared slide 2. Place a paper towel over the coverslip and apply gentle pressure to absorb excess stain Technique 2: 1. Place one drop of stain next to the coverslip on a prepared slide and allow the stain to leak under the coverslip 2. Place a paper towel over the coverslip and apply gentle pressure to absorb excess stain Technique 3: 1. Saturate the smear with dye for one min 2. Rinse gently from the back with water 3. Blot dry with blotting paper	Visualization of cell shape and arrangement; reticulocytes, Heinz bodies, urine sediments, and oily preparations (suspected lipomas using new methylene blue)

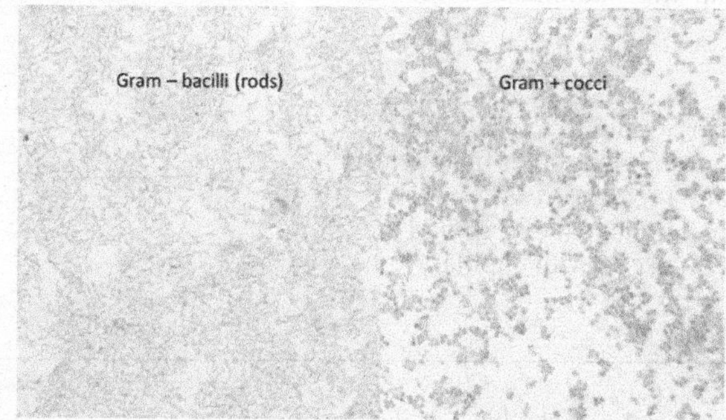

Figure 3.77 Gram stain, Gram-negative *Actinobacillus* spp. (left) and Gram-positive *Micrococcus* spp. (right). Source: image courtesy of Barbie Papajeski.

Staining Problems

To avoid staining problems, use fresh clean stains and slides. Do not touch the surface of the slide and immediately stain slides after air drying. Filter stains periodically to reduce precipitant formation and rinse slides well by placing the back side against the water stream to protect the sample. Use a blood filter attached to a stain-filled syringe for those stains that are not rinsed (simple stains).

Skill Box 3.14 / Staining problems[3,14,22]

Problem	Solution
Excessive staining	• ↓ staining time • Rinse adequately between stains and after staining • Prepare a thinner sample on the slide • Allow the slide to dry before applying a coverslip
Weak staining	• ↑ staining time • Change stains • Stain slides sooner after air-drying • Keep the caps tightly placed on the stain containers to prevent evaporation
Uneven staining	• Use only clean and dry slides, avoid use of previously cleaned slides • Do not touch the sample area of the slides before or after preparation • Place slides at an angle for drying to prevent liquid from drying onto the slide • Inadequate mixing of stains • Keep the caps tightly placed on the stain containers to prevent contamination and evaporation
Slide precipitate	• Rinse adequately between stains and after staining (Skill Box 3.13) • Use clean slides • Do not allow stains to dry onto the slide while staining • Change or filter stains periodically and regularly • Keep the caps tightly placed on the stain containers to prevent contamination and evaporation

Table 3.21 / Bacteria Identification[22]

Organism	General information	Associated conditions	Microscopic	Diagnostics
Bordetella bronchiseptica	Gram-negative	Upper respiratory infection and pneumonia, kennel cough	Small rods	• Blood agar: small, circular, dewdrop shape with ± β-hemolysis; slow grower • MAC: weak growth
Borrelia burgdorferi	Gram-negative	Lyme disease	Small spirochete, dark field microscopy	• Antibody titers used for diagnosis
Brucella canis	Gram-negative	Infertility, abortion, discospondylitis	Small, red coccobacilli in clumps	• Blood agar: round, smooth, glistening, and translucent • ELISA, indirect fluorescent antibody test, PCR also used

(Continued)

Table 3.21 / **Bacteria Identification (Continued)**

Organism	General information	Associated conditions	Microscopic	Diagnostics
Campylobacter spp.	Gram-negative; does not survive outside the host ≥ + 3 hours	Gastroenteritis, infertility, abortion	Tiny, spiral, curved rods (not tightly spiraled); two attached together as a "seagull" or W shape; "swarm of bees," rapid and darting motility; dark field microscopy	• Require microaerophilic conditions • Urease negative • PCR available at reference labs
Chlamydia	Resemble Gram-negative; obligate, intracellular parasite	Conjunctivitis, pneumonia	Small, red, pleomorphic coccobacilli in clumps	• Cytology samples with stained elementary bodies within macrophages • PCR
Clostridium	Gram-positive; obligate anaerobes, resistant to most disinfectants; requires 20 minutes of boiling or 121 °C in an autoclave	Botulism, gastroenteritis, otitis, tetanus	Large, spore-forming rods with rounded ends; "safety pin" appearance with a swollen, clear center and dark staining ends	• Blood agar: 1–3 mm in diameter, round to slightly irregular, raised, granular, transparent with a double zone of hemolysis • MAC: no growth • Spores stain with methylene blue or malachite green • PCR, FA, ELISA
Escherichia coli	Gram-negative facultative anaerobes, readily killed by disinfectants, sunlight, and desiccation	Genital tract infection, musculoskeletal infection, pneumonia, enteritis, abscesses, urinary tract infection, sepsis	Small, non-spore-forming rods	• Blood agar: large, smooth, gray, mucoid colonies with ± hemolysis • MAC: red growth, lactose fermentation, hemolytic pattern • HE: yellow to salmon-orange colonies • Indole positive • analytical profile index, PCR
Fusobacterium	Gram-negative, obligate anaerobes; opportunistic	Pleuritis and abscesses	Slender, long rods with pointed ends and long, beaded filaments	• Blood agar: small, smooth, convex and whitish-yellow in color colonies with a narrow zone of α- or β-hemolysis
Klebsiella	Gram-negative non-spore forming coliform	Gastrointestinal commensal; opportunistic urinary tract infection in canines	Slender, long rods with pointed ends and long, beaded filaments	• Blood agar: large mucoid colonies • MAC: pink colonies • Capsulated • TSI: no gas formation
Leptospira spp.	Gram-negative	Liver and kidney damage	Spiral rods	• Serology, FA, cytology

(*Continued*)

Table 3.21 / **Bacteria Identification (Continued)**

Organism	General information	Associated conditions	Microscopic	Diagnostics
Mycobacterium tuberculosis	Gram-positive	Pulmonary nodules (canine), gastrointestinal problems (feline)	Small, straight, or slightly curved acid-fast rods, singly or in clumps	• Culture may take up to 2 months • PCR, serological tests
Mycoplasma spp.	Gram-positive; lack a cell wall, so do not stain adequately enough to evaluate; readily killed by common disinfectants	Genital tract infection, arthritis, conjunctivitis (feline), pneumonia	Small, coccobacillus-like, non-spore-forming, no cell wall ± pleomorphic	• Incubation 4–5 days • Blood agar: Pin-point colonies • Hemotropic forms identified in blood smears • PCR
Nocardia spp.	Gram-positive aerobes; saprophyte in the soil, partially acid-fast	Pleuritis and abscesses in multiple tissues	Branching, filamentous rods, or coccobacilli	• Blood agar: irregularly folded, raised, smooth to rough with a dry granular texture; slow grower, needs 2 weeks • Grows on Sabouraud agar • MAC: no growth
Pasteurella spp.	Gram-negative facultative anaerobes, readily killed by most common disinfectants	Conjunctivitis, genital tract infection, upper respiratory infection, pneumonia, pleuritis, abscesses, and urinary tract infections	Small, non-spore-forming coccobacilli or rods	• Blood agar: round, smooth, gray colonies with ±hemolysis • MAC: no growth • Serotyping
Proteus spp.	Gram-negative facultative anaerobes, readily killed by common disinfectants, sunlight and desiccation	Cystitis, urinary tract infections, diarrhea, wounds, and otitis	Medium-sized non-spore forming, motile rods	• Blood agar: large, smooth, gray, swarming, mucoid colonies with ±hemolysis • HE: yellow-orange colonies • MAC: colorless growth that may spread • PEA: no growth • TSI: produce gas, turning black (Figure 3.69)
Pseudomonas spp.	Gram-negative; killed by most common disinfectants; ↑ resistance to high dilutions of quaternary ammonium compounds and phenolic compounds; can grow in chlorhexidine and saline	Conjunctivitis, otitis, musculoskeletal infection, abscesses, and urinary tract infections, opportunistic	Small, slightly curved, motile rods	• Blood agar: 3–5 mm in diameter, irregular, spreading, translucent, bluish-metallic sheen, β-hemolysis, and grapelike odor • MAC: yellow-green pigmented growth with a grapelike odor • PEA: no growth

(*Continued*)

Table 3.21 / Bacteria Identification (Continued)

Organism	General information	Associated conditions	Microscopic	Diagnostics
Rickettsia	Resemble gram-negative; obligate, intracellular parasite resides in endothelial cells; smallest organism able to reproduce on its own; cannot live outside the host	Rocky Mountain spotted fever, salmon poisoning disease, *Ehrlichia*	Small, pleomorphic coccobacilli	• Serological testing
Salmonella	Gram-negative; readily killed by common disinfectants, sunlight, and desiccation	Gastroenteritis, abortion, hepatitis, septicemia	Small non-spore-forming rods	• Blood agar: large, smooth, gray, mucoid colonies ± hemolysis • HE: green colonies with black centers • MAC: colorless growth • Indole negative
Staphylococcus spp.	Gram-positive; stable, surviving for months when dried in pus or other body fluids; resistance to common disinfectants	Conjunctivitis, genital tract infection, mastitis, pyoderma, otitis, osteomyelitis, musculoskeletal infection, pneumonia, abscesses, urinary tract infections	Cocci, often in grapelike clusters, non-spore forming, ± capsules	• Blood agar: 4 mm in diameter, round, smooth, glistening with a double zone of hemolysis and gold pigmentations • Catalase positive • MAC: no growth • MSA: agar color change to yellow • PEA: growth • ELISA
Streptococcus spp.	Gram-positive facultative anaerobes; remain living for weeks to months after being expelled from the body; readily killed by common disinfectants	Conjunctivitis, genital tract infection, otitis, pneumonia, abscesses, urinary tract infections	Cocci, singly or in chains of varying lengths and non-spore-forming	• Blood agar: 1 mm in diameter, round, smooth, glistening and resemble dewdrops with β-hemolysis (α- and γ-hemolysis are typically normal flora) • Catalase negative • Coagulase positive • MAC: no growth • PEA: growth

Table 3.22 / **Fungi identification**

Organism	Associated conditions	Microscopic	Culture
Aspergillus Figure 3.78	Nasal infections, common laboratory contaminant	• Preparation: clear cellophane tape with lactophenol blue or scrapings mixed with 10% sodium hydroxide • Identification: short pieces of thick, septate hyphae	• Medium: blood agar or Sabouraud dextrose agar • Additive: none • Incubation: 48 hours at 77–98.6 °F • Identification: flat, white, and floccose, then turns green to dark green and powdery
Blastomyces dermatitidis (Figure 3.79)	Pulmonary nodules, internal ulcers, abscesses	• Preparation: wet mount with 20% KOH • Identification: large, oval, or spherical, thick walled with a single bud that is connected to the mother cell by a wide base • Fine-needle aspiration/biopsy	• Highly zoonotic = cultures at reference lab • Cytology • Serology • PCR
Candida spp.	Mycotic stomatitis (canine), enteritis (kittens)	• Preparation: scrapings of lesions made as wet mounts with 20% KOH, India ink, or lactophenol cotton blue • Identification: thin-walled (no capsule) oval budding yeast cells ± pseudohyphae	• Blood agar or Sabouraud dextrose agar • Additive: none • Incubation: 2 days at 77–98.6°F • Identification: creamy, smooth colonies with yeast-like odor
Coccidioides immitis	Systemic and bone infections, extremely virulent fungal pathogen	• Preparation: scrapings of lesions made as wet mounts with 20% KOH, India ink, or lactophenol cotton blue • Identification: thick-walled sporangia	• Highly zoonotic = cultures at reference laboratory • Cytology/histology • Serology • PCR
Cryptococcus neoformans	Paranasal and central nervous system infections	• Preparation: impression smears stained with Romanowsky stains; sediment stained with India ink • Identification: narrow-base, budding, yeast-like cells with large capsules	• Blood agar or Sabouraud dextrose agar • Additive: none • Incubation: 14 days at 95–98.6°F • Identification: wrinkled, whitish granular colonies to mucoid, cream to brown colonies • Serology
Histoplasma capsulatum (Figure 3.80)	Systemic, pulmonary, and gastrointestinal infections, soil borne	• Preparation: Romanowsky stains • Identification: small oval (teardrop to eggplant shaped) cells surrounded by a halo seen intracellularly in monocytic cells	• Highly zoonotic = cultures at reference laboratory • Cytology/histology
Malassezia pachydermatis (Figures 3.30 and 3.81)	Chronic otitis externa (canine), pyoderma	• Preparation: wet mounts with 10% NaOH • Ear cytology swab • Identification: oval or bottle-shaped, small, budding cells	• Blood agar or Sabouraud dextrose agar • Additive: antibiotic • Incubation: 14 days at 77°F in a CO_2 incubator • Identification: greenish pigmentation • Cytology
Microsporum canis *Trichophyton* spp. (Figure 3.82)	Dermatophytosis	• Preparation: Place a few pieces of plucked hair, scales, or crust from skin scraping, 20% KOH, and India ink, or lactophenol cotton blue • Gently heat the slide and let it sit for 10–15 minutes. • Identification: spores and chains of highly refractile arthrospores	• DTM, modified Sabouraud dextrose agar • Additive: phenol red, pH indicator (Figure 3.62) • Incubation: 2 weeks at room temperature • Identification: flat colony, white surface, and silky in center, red color change to agar • Wood's lamp

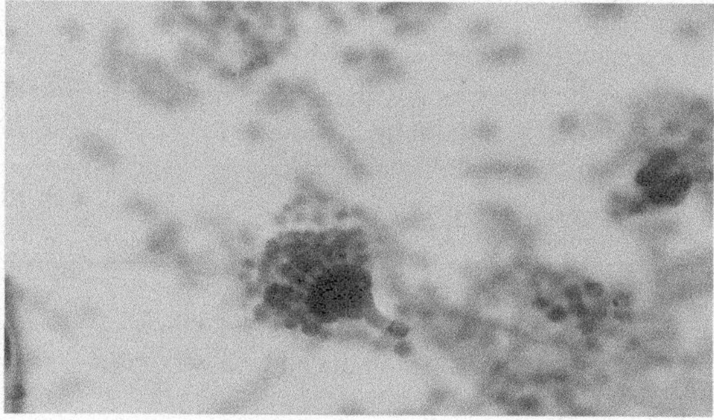

Figure 3.78 *Aspergillus* spp. stained with lactophenol cotton blue on a tape prep from a culture. Source: image courtesy of Barbie Papajeski.

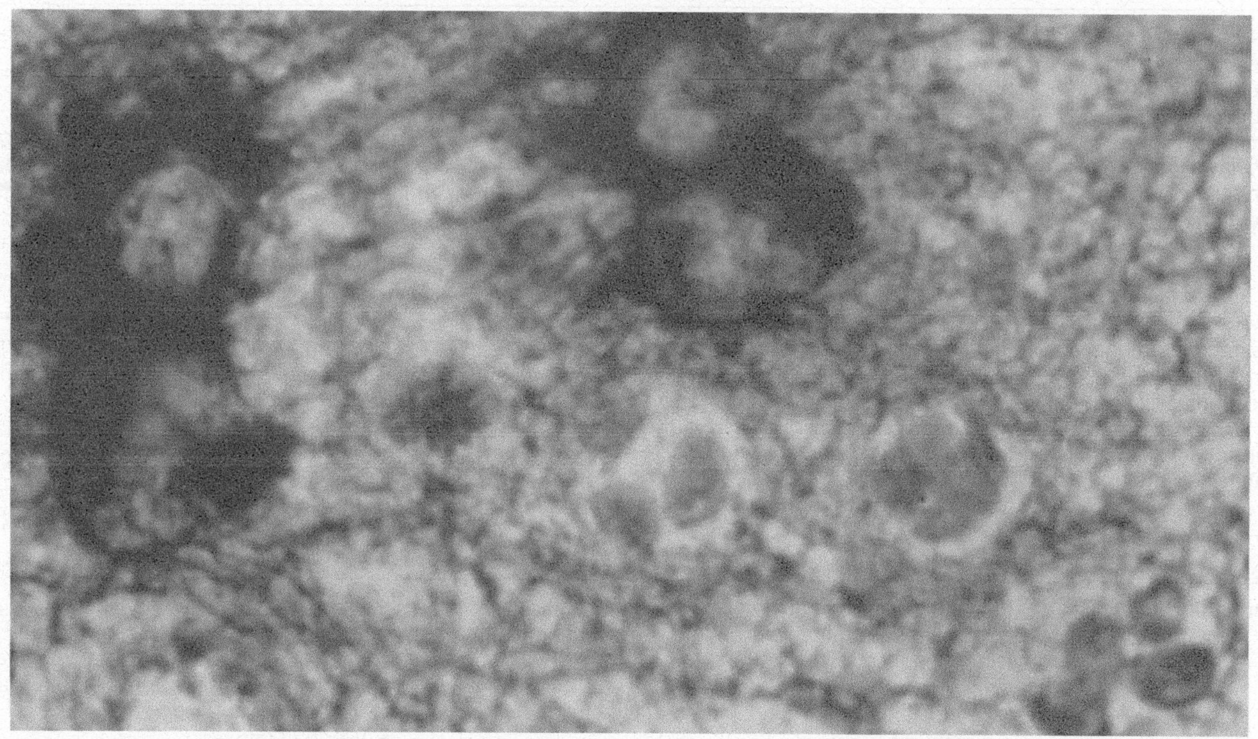

Figure 3.79 *Blastomyces dermatitidis* in a canine lymph node aspirate cytology, stained with Romanowsky stains. Source: image courtesy of Barbie Papajeski.

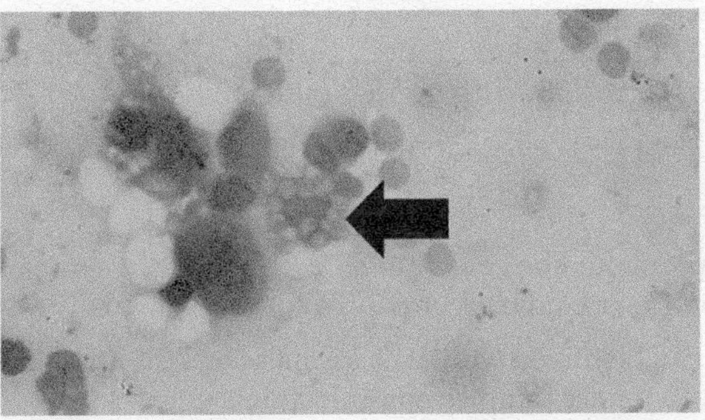

Figure 3.80 ***Histoplasma capsulatum*** **in liver impression smear stained with Romanowsky stains. Source: image courtesy of Barbie Papajeski.**

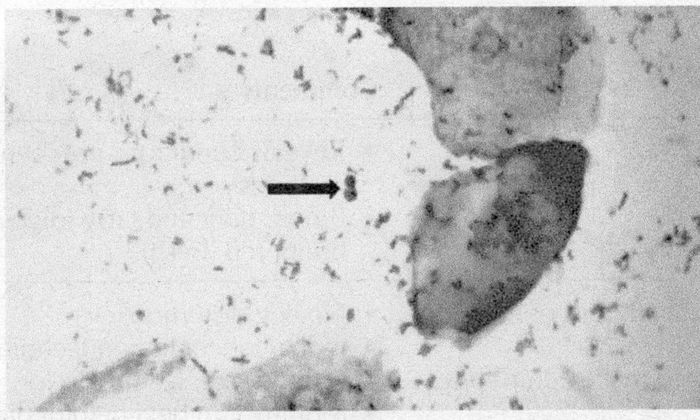

Figure 3.81 ***Malassezia pachydermatis*** **and numerous rod-shaped bacteria with a few cocci on an ear cytology swab stained with Romanowsky stains. Source: image courtesy of Barbie Papajeski.**

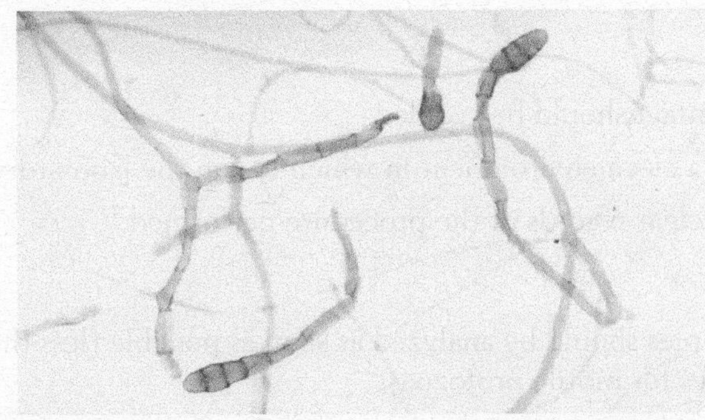

Figure 3.82 ***Trichophyton*** **spp. stained with lactophenol cotton blue on a tape prep from a culture. Source: image courtesy of Barbie Papajeski.**

PARASITOLOGY

Fecal analysis is one of the most common set of laboratory tests run by veterinary technicians and nurses in small-animal clinics. The majority of tests require competent skills in microscope use, cellular, and organism identification. Veterinary technicians and nurses also serve as client educators and play a vital role in the dissemination of information to protect human health.[24]

Fecal Collection, Handling, Storage, and Transport Tips[24,25]

Collection[24,25]

- Samples are collected manually (fecal loop, moistened swab, or gloved finger) or as a voided sample.
- The sample must be as fresh as possible because of the rapid deterioration of fragile organisms or development of eggs once passed.
- The owner should witness the animal defecating to ensure freshness and observe for any straining, fresh blood, or other problems.
- Fresh samples, not expected to be examined within 2 hours, should be refrigerated for no longer than 24 hours.
- Submit at least 10 g feces for analysis.
- Label sample with the patient's name and number, time of collection, and whether it was refrigerated.

Handling[24,25]

- Direct contact should be avoided.
- Maintain a clean environment in which to run the laboratory tests.
- Maintain clear records of the procedure performed.

Storage[24,25]

- Fecal samples should be analyzed as soon as possible (less than 30 minutes for motile protozoa).
- Fecal samples can be stored in sample bags, small plastic sandwich bags, plastic containers, or disposable laboratory gloves turned inside out.
- Samples can be stored indefinitely in 10% formalin (one part feces to three parts formalin), with minor limitations.
- Freezing samples is only appropriate for antigen-detection methods.

Transport[24,25]

- The sample should be cooled to 39.2°F in the refrigerator and then packed on ice or cold packs for 24–48 hours.
- Samples can be mixed with 10% formalin or 70% ethyl alcohol for transport to render samples non-infectious.
- Place important papers in a separate plastic bag in case of sample fluid leakage.

Fecal Evaluation

Skill Box 3.15 / Endoparasite examination methods[24,25]

Method	Uses	Technique	Comments
Gross examination	• Consistency • Color • Blood, mucus, or adult parasites	Visualize feces	• Reveals conditions not seen in other methods • Blood: dark and tarry (digested) and bright red (fresh)
Direct smear: wet preparation	• Protozoa (*Giardia*) • Parasite ova or larvae • Parasite burden • Bacteria (e.g. spirochetes, *Cryptosporidium*, *Campylobacter*) • See Table 3.10	1. Place a drop of saline or water with an equal amount of feces on a slide 2. Thoroughly mix feces and water and smear to make a thin film over slide 3. Remove any large pieces of feces and add a coverslip to examine 4. Examine under 10 × objective for parasite eggs, 40 × for protozoal organisms 5. Stain (methylene blue or Lugol's iodine) can be added to the side of the coverslip for clearer identification and to "freeze" protozoans	• No egg distortion • Not a concentration technique (small sample size) leading to low numbers • Motility can be a helpful diagnostic aid • Typical findings: polymorphic bacilli, small amount of amorphous material, plant material, yeast, and epithelial cells • Read immediately and do not store

(*Continued*)

Skill Box 3.15 / Endoparasite examination methods (Continued)

Method	Uses	Technique	Comments
Direct smear: dry preparation	• Protozoa (*Giardia*) • Parasite burden • Bacteria (spirochetes, *Cryptosporidium*, *Campylobacter*) • Spore-forming bacteria (*Clostridium* spp.) • Fungi (*Histoplasma*, *Aspergillus*, *Candida*) • Inflammatory and abnormal noninflammatory cells	1. Using a swab, roll a thin layer of feces across a slide and allow to air dry 2. Stain with Romanowsky stains for cytology or acid-fast stain for *Cyptosporidia* spp. examination 3. Examine under 10 × for parasite eggs, 40 × for protozoal organisms, and 100 × for bacteria	• No egg distortion • Does not concentrate sample • Not able to judge motility of parasites • Typical findings: polymorphic bacilli, small amount of amorphous material, plant material, yeast, and epithelial cells • Can be stored at room temperature • Protect from light and humidity
Standard, passive, or simple flotation	• Most parasites (ova, oocysts, and cysts) • Parasite burden	1. Place 1–2 g feces in a suitable container (paper cup) and add flotation solution (Skill Box 3.16) 2. Mix the contents thoroughly with a tongue depressor and strain through a tea strainer or cheesecloth into a second container 3. Pour this mixture into a test tube and add more flotation solution until a meniscus is formed 4. Place a glass coverslip over the meniscus for 10–15 minutes 5. Remove coverslip, place on a slide, and examine under 10 ×	• Concentrates parasites • Commercial fecal flotation kits available • Less efficiently recovers eggs than the centrifugal flotation method • Misses larvae that settle because of gravity
Centrifugal flotation	• Most parasites (ova, oocysts and cysts) • Parasite burden	1. Mix 1 tsp (2–5 g) feces in a paper cup with enough water or flotation solution to make a semisolid suspension 2. Place a tea strainer or cheesecloth over a second paper cup, and empty the contents on top of it 3. Push the liquid through the strainer with the tongue depressor and then discard the solid waste 4. Pour the strained mixture into a 15-ml centrifuge tube 5. Fill the tube with flotation solution to form a slight positive meniscus (swing-arm rotor); fill nearly full if using a fixed rotor 6. Place a coverslip on top of the tube(swing-arm rotor); cap tubes in a fixed rotor 7. Put the tube in a balanced centrifuge and spin at 1300 rpm for 5–6 minutes 8. Remove the tube (follow step 5 for fixed rotor) and let it stand for 10 min 9. Lift the coverslip directly upward and place on a glass microscope slide 10. Systematically examine the entire coverslip at 10 × and then review at 40 × to confirm findings	• Concentrates parasites • More efficiently recovers eggs than the standard flotation method • Requires a centrifuge with either a fixed or a swing-arm rotor capable of holding 15-ml tubes • Misses larvae that settle because of gravity

(*Continued*)

Skill Box 3.15 / Endoparasite examination methods (Continued)

Method	Uses	Technique	Comments
Baermann technique	• Nematode larvae (lungworm or *Strongyloides* spp.)	1. Fill the funnel in a ring stand with warm water or physiological saline (86°F) to cover the wire screen 2. Spread a piece of cheesecloth or gauze square over the wire screen in the funnel 3. Place 5–15 g feces, soil, or tissue on the cheesecloth and fold any excess cloth over the sample. Make sure that the warm water covers the sample 4. Leave the sample undisturbed overnight (> 8 hours) 5. Fill a 15-ml sediment tube with liquid and centrifuge as for centrifuge flotation 6. Pipette sediment to a clean glass slide 7. Apply a coverslip and examine	• Efficient recovery of larvae
Sedimentation technique	• Trematode eggs (*Nanophyetus samincola, Paragonimus kellicotti)*	1. Mix 5 g feces with 15–30 ml of water thoroughly in a cup 2. Filter the mixture into a centrifuge tube 3. Centrifuge for 5 minutes at 1500 rpm 4. Decant the supernatant (optional: add 1 drop new methylene blue) 5. Use a pipette to remove some of the sediment from the top layer and place on a slide 6. Examine the sediment with a microscope for large, operculated eggs	• Efficient recovery of trematode eggs
Fecal culture	• Hookworm larvae • To distinguish between parasites that have similar-appearing eggs and cysts	1. Place feces in a glass jar rinsed with 0.1% sodium carbonate solution or on a piece of filter paper in a Petri dish 2. Cover the container and place in a dark area for 7–10 days 3. Add water if condensation does not appear on sides 4. After 7–10 days, rinse the container with a small amount of water, collect liquid, and centrifuge 5. Examine the sediment microscopically	• Guaranteed identification

(Continued)

Skill Box 3.15 / Endoparasite examination methods (Continued)

Method	Uses	Technique	Comments
Wet mount/ fecal culture InPouch™	• *Tritrichomonas foetus*	Follow manufacturer's instructions: 1. Remove the pouch from the bag and confirm that around 1 ml of liquid is in the upper chamber 2. Open the pouch and insert an applicator stick with 0.03 g of fresh feces or a coated swab into the liquid of the upper chamber 3. Remove the feces by gently rubbing the stick between the thumb and forefinger and walls of chamber 4. Close the pouch and label 5. Store at room temperature in the dark Wet mount 1. Stand the pouch upright for 15 minutes to concentrate *T. foetus* at the bottom of the pouch 2. Place the viewing clip horizontally across the pouch and then lay the pouch across the microscope and examine, paying special attention to the edges Fecal culture 1. Squeeze all liquid into the lower pouch, close the pouch, and incubate for 18–24 hours 2. Mix the pouch up and down against an edge three to four times 3. Place the viewing clip horizontally across the pouch and then lay the pouch across the microscope and examine	• Addition of excess fecal material will make the medium too cloudy to view • If no *T. foetus* are seen, evaluate daily for 2–4 days and up to every other day for 12 days • 1–10 organisms are sufficient to result in a presumptive positive test • Pouches are often sent to reference labs for PCR
Proglottid exam/ tapeworm identification	• Used to differentiate between *Taenia*-type and *Dipylidium* tapeworms	1. Using gloved hand or forceps, transfer the proglottid to a clean glass slide 2. Using a blade, macerate the proglottid and then add a drop of saline, water, or float solution over the material and coverslip 3. Examine under 10 × to determine if the tapeworm ova is *Dipylidium* or a *Taenid*-type ova	• Guides client education

Fecal Flotation Solutions

Fecal flotation solutions are used to concentrate and enhance discovery of parasitic eggs in fecal material. The solution chosen must have a specific gravity that allows parasite eggs to float and the bulk of the fecal debris to sink. Because water has a specific gravity just slightly lower than many parasite eggs, sugar or salts are added to increase the solution's specific gravity and to allow the eggs to float. The desired specific gravity is between 1.2 and 1.25. Solutions with a specific gravity greater than 1.30 will allow both debris and parasite eggs to float, making egg identification more difficult. A specific gravity less than 1.10 will force both debris and parasite eggs to sink, resulting in failure of ova recovery. If left for longer than one hour, ova may sink after floating or become distorted.

Solutions that are purchased premixed are preferred because of quality control. Solutions mixed in the clinical setting tend to have less quality control and give variable results. A hydrometer is used to ensure an ideal specific gravity of float solutions. Almost all solutions will form crystals on the slide if left sitting.[24,25]

Skill Box 3.16 / Fecal flotation solutions[24,25]

Media	Preparation	Specific gravity	General information
Magnesium sulfate (Epsom salts)	• Magnesium sulfate: 350 g • Tap water: 1000 ml	1.20–1.30	• Readily available and inexpensive
Sodium chloride (table salt)	• Sodium chloride: 400 g • Tap water: 1000 ml • Stir while adding the sodium chloride to water • Heating is not necessary but speeds the dissolution • Add salt until no more goes into solution but starts to settle	1.18–1.20	• Readily available and inexpensive • Corrodes expensive laboratory equipment • Severely distorts eggs
Sodium nitrate (Fecasol™)	• Sodium nitrate: 315 g • Tap water: 1000 ml • Stir while adding the sodium nitrate to water. • Heating is not necessary but speeds the dissolution	1.20–1.25	• Floats the greatest percentage of eggs • Distorts *Giardia* cysts • Can be purchased in a ready-to-mix solution • Distorts the eggs after 15 minutes • May not be readily available and may be more expensive
Sugar solution, Sheather's solution	• Granulated sugar: 454 g • Tap water: 355 ml • Dissolve sugar in water by heating on low and stirring. Add 6 ml of 37% formaldehyde or phenol crystals to prevent bacterial growth	1.25–1.27	• Floats an adequate percentage of eggs • Readily available and inexpensive • Causes less damage • *Giardia* cyst wall collapses • Best if used with centrifugal flotation techniques • Sticky
Zinc sulfate	• Zinc sulfate: 386 g • Tap water: 1000 ml • Stir while adding the zinc sulfate to water • Heating is not necessary but speeds the dissolution	1.18–1.25	• Best for intestinal protozoa (*Giardia*) • Light must be ↓ and focused immediately under the coverslip. • Best when combined with centrifugal techniques

Endoparasites

Prevention of human infection from endoparasites involves proper hygiene (washing hands and properly cooking food), isolation of infected animals, and quarantine of newly acquired animals. All samples should be thought of as a zoonotic risk and treated appropriately.

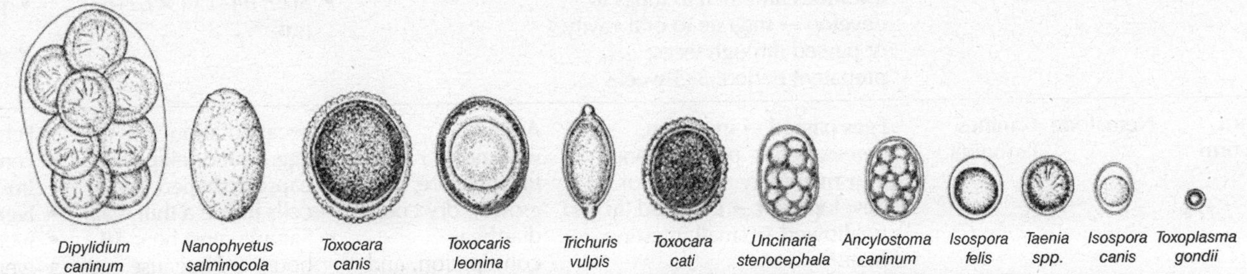

Figure 3.83 Relative size of parasite eggs. Source: Adapted from Veterinary Parasitology Reference Manual by William J. Foreyt.

Table 3.23 / Endoparasites[19,24,25]

Parasite	Common name	Type	Affected species	Transmission route	Clinical signs	Diagnostics	Common treatments/ disinfection
Aelurostrongylus abstrusus	Feline lungworm	Nematode	Felines	Eggs passed → intermediate host is infected (snail or slug) → ingested by paratenic host (mice, voles, birds, frogs, and lizards) → ingested by definitive host → migrate into bloodstream, then tissues, to lungs → migrate to small intestines to mature; prepatent period: 6 weeks	Chronic cough, dyspnea, pleural effusion (severe)	• Zinc sulfate fecal floatation • Baermann technique • Sputum sample or tracheal wash • Larva: 400 μm long, with an undulating tail	• Fenbendazole • Imidacloprid/moxidectin • Ivermectin

(Continued)

Table 3.23 / Endoparasites (Continued)

Parasite	Common name	Type	Affected species	Transmission route	Clinical signs	Diagnostics	Common treatments/ disinfection

Alaria spp. (Figure 3.84)	Stomach fluke	Nematode	Canines and felines	Eggs passed → first intermediate host is infected (snail or slug) → ingested by second intermediate host (mice, voles, birds, frogs, and snakes) → ingested by definitive host → migrate to small intestines and then to lungs to develop → migrate to oral cavity or passed through feces; prepatent period: 3–5 weeks	Asymptomatic or hemorrhage and respiratory compromise due to larval migration	• Sedimentation technique
						• Adults measure 2–6 mm
						• Ova golden brown, operculated
						• Size: 94–134 × 62–68 µm
							• No approved treatment
							• Veterinarians may choose to use the following off label:
							  • epsiprantel
							  • fenbendazole
							  • praziquantel

Ancylostoma caninum (Figures 3.84 and 3.102)	Southern hookworm	Nematode	Canines (zoonotic)	Eggs passed → ingestion, percutaneous, prenatal, and transmammary → lungs for development → coughed up and swallowed → small intestines to mature Prepatent period: 2 weeks	Anemia, weakness, inappetence, poor growth, dry cough, diarrhea, constipation, and dark, tarry stools	• Fecal flotation • Egg: oval or ellipsoid, capsule shaped, 8–16 cells inside a thin wall • Sample must be < 48 hours old because eggs larvate rapidly • Size: 56–75 × 34–47 µm • Fecal antigen	• Febantel/praziquantel • Fenbendazole • Imidacloprid/moxidectin • Ivermectin • Ivermectin/pyrantel • Ivermectin/pyrantel/ praziquantel • Mebendazole • Milbemycin oxime/ lufenuron • Milbemycin oxime/ lufenuron/praziquantel • Milbemycin/spinosad • Moxidectin • Praziquantel/pyrantel/ febantel • Pyrantel pamoate • Disinfect with bleach • Can live in cool, moist soil for several weeks

(Continued)

Table 3.23 / Endoparasites (Continued)

Parasite	Common name	Type	Affected species	Transmission route	Clinical signs	Diagnostics	Common treatments/ disinfection
Ancylostoma tubaeforme (Figures 3.86 and 3.91)	Feline hookworm	Nematode	Felines (zoonotic)	Eggs passed → ingestion, percutaneous, prenatal, and transmammary → lungs for development → coughed up and swallowed (or paratenic host ingested) → small intestines to mature; prepatent period: 3–3.5 weeks	Interdigital dermatitis, pulmonary lesions, anemia and poor hair coat	• Fecal flotation • Egg: oval or ellipsoid, capsule shaped, 8–16 cells inside a thin wall • Size: 56–75 × 34–45 µm • Sample must be < 48 hours old since eggs larvate rapidly in the external environment	• Eprinomectin/ praziquantel • Pyrantel • Selamectin
Aonchotheca putorii (Image: Figure 3.87)	Feline gastric capillarid	Nematode	Felines	Eggs passed → ingestion, → develop to adults in stomach mucosa	Rare gastritis with vomiting	• Fecal flotation • Eggs must be distinguished from *Eucoleus* and *Pearsonema* • Ellipsoidal with asymmetric poles • Deep longitudinal ridges on surface • Size: 53–70 × 20–30 µm	• No approved treatment • Veterinarians may choose to treat as for *Trichuris* spp.
Baylisascaris procyonis (Figure 3.88)	Raccoon roundworm	Nematode	Canines and felines (zoonotic)	Eggs passed → ingested via environment or paratenic host → hatch in small intestines and penetrate mucosa → migrate through the liver and heart until the lungs → develop in lungs → coughed up and swallowed → mature in the small intestines for 4–6 weeks	Enteric parasitism (canine), central nervous system and ocular symptoms (canine and feline)	• Fecal flotation • Egg: spherical, unembyronated • Deeply pigmented center with rough, pitted outer shell • Smaller than *Toxocara canis* • Size: 63–75 × 53–60 µm	• No approved treatment • Veterinarians may choose to treat as for other roundworm species

(*Continued*)

Table 3.23 / Endoparasites (Continued)

Parasite	Common name	Type	Affected species	Transmission route	Clinical signs	Diagnostics	Common treatments/ disinfection
Cryptosporidium (Figure 3.89)	Crypto	Protozoa	Canines and felines (zoonotic)	Oocysts passed → ingested by definitive host → develop in the ileum and cecum Prepatent period: 2–7 d	Asymptomatic or diarrhea	• Fecal flotation, acid-fast staining, negative staining, ELISA, and IFA tests • Oocysts: oval to spherical, thick walled, and sporulated • Size: 4–6 μm • Red to fuchsia pink when stained with acid fast stains • Note: difficult to distinguish from yeast cells on fecal flotations	• Azithromycin • Clindamycin • Nitazoxanide • Paromomycin • Tylosin • Disinfect by heating > 131°F for 15–20 minutes, thorough drying, 5% ammonia solution, and formaldehyde • Resistant for months
Cystoisospora canis/felis (Figures 3.90, 3.91 and 3.108)	Coccidia	Protozoa	Canines and felines	Eggs passed, usually by mother → sporulated oocyst ingested, often by puppy or kitten → develop to a trophozoite → sporozoites enter intestinal epithelial cells to replicate by schizogony and sporogony Prepatent period: 1–2 weeks	Asymptomatic or diarrhea progressing to vomiting, inappetence, and dehydration	• Fecal flotation • Egg: small, oval, and thin walled • Size: *C. canis* = 34–40 × 28–31 μm • *C. felis* = 38–51 × 27–29 μm • Sporulated: two sporocysts per egg • Unsporulated: one-cell stage inside egg	• Amprolium • Amprolium/ sulfadimethoxine • Diclazuril • Furazolidone • Ponazuril • Quinacrine • Sulfadimethoxine • Sulfadimethoxine • Ormetoprim • Sulfaguanidine • Toltrazuril • Trimethoprim/sulfonamide • Disinfection: incineration, steam cleaning, immersion in boiling water and 10% ammonia solution • Prevention: insect and rodent control and sanitation • Extremely resistant to environmental conditions

(Continued)

Table 3.23 / **Endoparasites (Continued)**

Parasite	Common name	Type	Affected species	Transmission route	Clinical signs	Diagnostics	Common treatments/ disinfection
Diphyllobothrium latum (Figure 3.92)	Broad fish tapeworm	Cestode	Canines and felines (zoonotic)	Eggs are passed in feces → hatch in water → embryos are eaten by water fleas (first intermediate) → water flea is eaten by fish of pike, perch or salmon family → larva (plerocercoid) develops in muscle of fish → fish is eaten by final host; prepatent period: 5–6 weeks	Asymptomatic	• Recovery of eggs by sedimentation • Light-brown eggs with rounded end and operculum at opposite end • Size: 67–71 × 40–50 µm	• No approved treatment • Veterinarians may choose to use praziquantel off label
Dipylidium caninum (Figure 3.92)	Flea tapeworm	Cestode	Canines and felines (zoonotic)	Proglottids passed and rupture to release thousands of eggs → ingested by intermediate host (flea and biting lice) → development → definitive host **ingests the intermediate host → attaches to lining of small intestines to mature** Prepatent period: 4 weeks	Anal pruritus, chronic enteritis, vomiting, nervous system disorders	• Fecal flotation or visual examination of feces, perianal area, or bedding • Egg: double-pored, rice or cucumber-seed appearance, oblong packets of 20 eggs or less • Packet size = 120–200 µm • Eggs = 35–60 µm	• Epsiprantel • Febantel/praziquantel • Nitazoxanide • Praziquantel • Praziquantel/emodepside
Dirofilaria immitis (Figure 3.94)	Canine heartworm, feline lungworm	Nematode	Canines and felines (zoonotic)	Intermediate host (mosquito) must carry the larva for 15–17 days with the temperature ≥ 58°F → intermediate host feeds on definitive hose and larvae crawl into subcutaneous tissues → larva passes from venous circulation to heart → resides in pulmonary arteries and right ventricle of heart → microfilaria circulate in blood and are picked up by intermediate host (mosquito); prepatent period: 6–7 months	Murmur, lack of stamina, weight loss, chronic cough, obstruction of pulmonary vessels, congestive heart failure	• Modified Knott's test • Filter test • Buffy coat examination • Direct blood smear • Millipore filtration of blood • Serological antigen tests of adult worm • Microfilaria: straight with one tapered end and one straight end • Size: 295–325 × 5–7.5 µm	• Adulticides • Melarsomine + doxycycline • Microfilaricides • Ivermectin • Levamisole • Milbemycin oxime • Moxidectin • Selamectin

(*Continued*)

Table 3.23 / Endoparasites (Continued)

Parasite	Common name	Type	Affected species	Transmission route	Clinical signs	Diagnostics	Common treatments/ disinfection
Echinococcus granulosus, *E. multilocularis* (Figure 3.95)	Canine and feline tapeworm	Cestode	Canines and felines (zoonotic)	Proglottids passed → ingested by intermediate host (cattle, swine, sheep, and rodents) → attaches to liver → definitive host ingests the intermediate host → attaches to lining of small intestines to mature; prepatent period: 4–5 weeks	Diarrhea, hydatid cyst disease in intermediate host	• Fecal flotation or purging the animal and collecting the clear mucus at the end to identify adults • Egg: ovoid containing a single oncosphere with three pairs of hooks • Size: 35–60 μm • Note: indistinguishable from *Taenia* spp. eggs • Coproantigen ELISA • PCR	• Albendazole • Praziquantel

Eucoleus aerophilus, *E. boehmi* (Figure 3.96)	Respiratory capillarid	Nematode	Canines and felines (zoonotic: *E. aerophilus*)	Ova passed in feces and sputum → larvate within egg in 30–50 days → hatch in intestine of new host → tracheal migration to lungs → larvae penetrate alveoli and migrate upwards as they mature → *E. aerophilus* adults live in trachea and bronchi and thread themselves into mucosal lining while *E. boehmi* lives in dog nasal passages → male and female adult worms mate and release eggs into lungs → coughed up, swallowed	Asymptomatic to cough, dyspnea, tracheitis, bronchitis, leading to pneumonia in young dogs and cats with *E. aerophilus*, rhinitis in dogs with *E. boehmi*	• Fecal floatation
						• Tracheal/nasal secretions
						• Differentiate from similar whipworm and other capillarid eggs
						• Asymmetrical poles
						• *E. aerophilus*:
						  • Size: 58–79 × 29–40 μm
						  • Network of interconnected ridges
						• *E. boehmi*
						  • Size:54–60 × 30–35 μm
						  • Pitted shell surface
						  • Morula do not completely fill egg
							• Fenbendazole
							• Imidacloprid/moxidectin
							• Ivermectin
							• Milbemycin oxime
							• Eggs viable up to 1 year

(*Continued*)

Table 3.23 / **Endoparasites (Continued)**

Parasite	Common name	Type	Affected species	Transmission route	Clinical signs	Diagnostics	Common treatments/ disinfection
Oslerus osleri	Tracheal worm, canine lungworm	Nematode	Canines	Eggs passed → ingested (passed from dam to pup through grooming or regurgitated meals) → migrate to small intestines and then to lungs to develop → migrate to oral cavity or passed through feces; prepatent period: 10 weeks for nodules, 6–7 weeks for larvae in feces	Coughing and chronic tracheobronchitis with nodule formation in large airways	• Fecal flotation • Baermann technique • Sputum smear • Larva: short, with an S-shaped tail • Size: 240–290 μm	• Doramectin • Fenbendazole • Ivermectin • Levamisole • Oxfendazole • Thiabendazole
Giardia Common name: *Giardia* (Figures 3.97 and 3.98)	Giardia	Protozoa	Canines (assemblages A1, C, D) and felines (assemblages A1, F) – zoonotic (assemblage A1)	Oocysts passed → ingested → migrate to small intestines; prepatent period: 5–7 days	Asymptomatic or diarrhea (appearing pale and greasy with a foul odor)	• Fecal flotation • Direct fecal smear • Active form: pear shaped with the anatomy resembling a face of crossed eyes, nose, and a mouth • Size: Trophozoites = 12-18x10–12 μm • Cysts = 8–12 × 7–10 μm • IFA • ELISA • PCR • Disinfect with bleach and quaternary ammonium	• Metronidazole • Fenbendazole • Febantel/pyrantel/ praziquantal

Nanophyetus salmincola	Salmon poisoning fluke	Trematode	Canines and felines (zoonotic)	Eggs passed by definitive host → ingested by intermediate host (snail) → larva passed → ingested by intermediate host (salmon) → salmon ingested by definitive host → develop in intestines; prepatent period: 1 week	Lymphadenopathy, depression, vomiting, hemorrhagic enteritis caused by the rickettsial agent (*Neorickettsia helminthoeca*) and carried by the fluke	• Fecal flotation or fecal sedimentation
						• Egg: gold, operculum at one end and blunt point at opposite end
						• Size: 52–82 × 32–56 μm
							• No approved treatment
							• Veterinarians may choose to use the following off label:
							  • epsiprantel
							  • fenbendazole
							  • praziquantel
							  • tetracyclines

(*Continued*)

Table 3.23 / **Endoparasites (Continued)**

Parasite	Common name	Type	Affected species	Transmission route	Clinical signs	Diagnostics	Common treatments/ disinfection
Paragonimus kellicotti (Figure 3.99)	Lung fluke	Trematode	Canines and felines	Eggs coughed up and passed by definitive host → enter water → miracidia enter snail intermediate host and develop → cercaria exit snail and enter crayfish → ingested by ingested by definitive host → develop in lungs; prepatent period: 1 week	Pulmonary hemorrhage, pneumothorax, or granulocytic pneumonia with heavy parasite load	• Fecal sedimentation • Tracheal wash • Thoracic radiographs • Egg is yellowish brown with distinct notches (shoulders) at operculum • Size: 75–118 × 42–67 µm	• No approved treatment • Veterinarians may choose to use the following off label: • epsiprantel • fenbendazole • praziquantel
Pearsonema plica, P. feliscati (Figure 3.100)	Bladder worm	Nematode	Canines and felines	Eggs passed in urine → earthworms ingests larvae → dog or cat ingests earthworms or bird paratenic host → larvae travel to bladder and mature; prepatent period: 4–5 months (canines), 2 months (felines)	Asymptomatic to cystitis	• Urine sediment by cystocentesis • Differentiate from similar whipworm and other capillarid eggs • Size: 51–65 × 24–32 µm • Outer shell appears globular	• No approved treatment • Veterinarians may choose to use the following off label: • fenbendazole • ivermectin
Physaloptera spp. (Figure 3.101)	Stomach worm	Nematode	Canines and felines	Eggs are passed in feces→ Intermediate host ingests larvae → animal ingests insect intermediate host or paratenic host → adults attach firmly stomach mucosa; prepatent period: 2–5 months	Chronic vomiting and peritonitis in heavy infestations	• Endoscopy • Direct smear • Gross examination of vomit • Embryonated eggs rarely recovered • Size: 42–53 × 29–53 µm	• Physical removal of adults • Pyrantel pamoate
Platynosomum concinnum	Liver poisoning fluke	Trematode	Felines	Eggs coughed up and passed by definitive host → first intermediate host is a land snail → cercariae emerge from the snails and infiltrate soil → isopods (pill bugs) ingest sporocysts → Insectivorous vertebrates such as frogs, lizards, and birds serve as paratenic hosts → cat is infected by ingesting paratenic host; prepatent period: 4–5 weeks	Enlarged bile ducts, hepatic hyperplasia, leading to renal failure	• Fecal sedimentation • Ultrasound • Eggs are brownish • Size 34–50 × 20–35 µm	• No approved treatment • Veterinarians may choose to use the following off label: • epsiprantel • fenbendazole • praziquantel

(*Continued*)

Table 3.23 / Endoparasites (Continued)

Parasite	Common name	Type	Affected species	Transmission route	Clinical signs	Diagnostics	Common treatments/ disinfection
Sarcocystis spp. (Figure 3.102)	Flesh cyst	Protozoa	Canines and felines	Oocysts are passed in the feces of carnivore host → herbivore intermediate host ingests oocysts from fecal contaminated water or feed → cyst stage in muscle tissues → animal ingests tissues of intermediate host → reproductive stages in small intestines	Non-pathogenic in dog and cat but causes severe disease in livestock intermediate host	• Fecal floatation • Sporulated oocysts • Must differentiate from pathogenic protozoans • Size: 7–24 × 3–15 μm • Non-pathogenic protozoa	• Not treated
Spirocerca lupi	Esophageal worm	Nematode	Canines	Egg passed by definitive host (canine) → ingested by intermediate host (beetle) → ingested by paratenic host (lizards, birds, rodents) or definitive host (dog) → larva penetrates stomach wall and migrates through the arteries to the esophagus → forms a fistula and releases egg in the feces; prepatent period: 5–6 months	Dysphagia, regurgitation, vomiting, esophageal neoplasia, hypersalivation, hypertrophic osteopathy	• Fecal sedimentation • Fecal flotation • Direct fecal smear • Egg: thick-walled, ellipsoid embryonated egg • Size: 30–38 × 11–15 μm	• Ivermectin
Spirometra spp. (Figure 3.103)	Zipper or sparganosis tapeworm	Cestode	Canines and felines (zoonotic)	Eggs passed by definitive host → come in contact with water → coracidium larvae ingested by intermediate host (copepod) → second intermediate host ingests first and sparganum forms in tissues (amphibians and fish) → ingested by definitive host → develop to adults in intestines	Diarrhea, weight loss, vomiting	• Fecal floatation • Fecal sedimentation • Necropsy/ histopathology • Proglottid identification • Non-motile with medial pore • Eggs are oval & yellow brown • Size 60 × 36 μm	• No approved treatment • Veterinarians may choose to use praziquantel at higher doses off label

(Continued)

Table 3.23 / **Endoparasites (Continued)**

Parasite	Common name	Type	Affected species	Transmission route	Clinical signs	Diagnostics	Common treatments/ disinfection
Strongyloides stercoralis (Figure 3.104)	Intestinal threadworm	Nematode	Canines and felines (zoonotic)	Eggs passed by definitive host → larvae follow one of three pathways: (1) Develop rapidly into infective third stage larvae while still in the intestine of the host, (2) reinfect mucosa and grow to adults without ever leaving the intestine of the host (autoinfection), (3) parthenogenic females release larvated eggs → passed in feces → develop into third stage larvae (free living males and females mate producing parasitic female larvae which are ingested or enter percutaneously → new host is infected by oral ingestion or by active skin penetration → carried via bloodstream to lungs → mature in intestine; transmammary route also occurs in newly infected dams; prepatent period: 8–14 days	Asymptomatic to respiratory illness and diarrhea in young puppies	• Baermann technique • Embryonated ova hatch quickly and are not often observed in fecal floatation • Feces must be fresh to differentiate from developed hookworm ova • Ova size: 50–58 × 30–34 μm • Larvae length: 150–390 μm	• No approved treatment
Taenia spp. (Figure 3.105)	Tapeworm	Cestode	Felines	Proglottids passed → ingested by intermediate host (rodent, rabbit and ruminant) → attaches and develops in peritoneal cavity or liver → definitive host ingests the intermediate host → develops in the small intestines; prepatent period: 8 weeks	Enteritis, diarrhea and intestinal blockage	• Fecal flotation or visual examination of feces, perianal area, or bedding • Adult Identification • Eggs are identical to Echinococcus • Egg: ovoid containing a single oncosphere with three pairs of hooks • Shell of egg has radial striations • Size: 35–40 μm • Each proglottid carries many eggs	• Epsiprantel • Praziquantel

(*Continued*)

Table 3.23 / **Endoparasites (Continued)**

Parasite	Common name	Type	Affected species	Transmission route	Clinical signs	Diagnostics	Common treatments/ disinfection
Toxascaris leonina (Figure 3.106)	Roundworm, ascarid	Nematode	Canines and felines	Eggs passed → ingested by definitive host or intermediate host (e.g. mice) → definitive host ingests intermediate host → attaches and develops in small intestines; prepatent period: 8–10 weeks	Chronic diarrhea, vomiting, constipation, and unthriftiness	• Fecal flotation or visual examination of feces • Egg: spherical to ovoid • Unembyronated • Light cytoplasm, • Smooth outer membrane • Size: 75–85 × 60–75 μm	• Fenbendazole • Imidacloprid/moxidectin • Ivermectin/pyrantel • Ivermectin/pyrantel/ praziquantel • Milbemycin oxime • Milbemycin oxime/ lufenuron/praziquantel • Milbemycin oxime/lufenuron • Milbemycin oxime/spinosad • Moxidectin • Piperazine • Praziquantel/pyrantel pamoate/febantel • Pyrantel pamoate • Pyrantel/praziquantel • Disinfect with bleach • Eggs can remain infective in the soil for months to years
Toxocara canis (Figure 3.107)	Canine roundworm	Nematode	Canines (zoonotic)	Eggs passed → ingested via environment or paratenic host → hatch in small intestines and penetrate mucosa → migrate through the liver and heart until the lungs → develop in lungs → coughed up and swallowed → mature in the small intestines; prepatent period: 3–5 weeks	Distended abdomen, weakness, unthriftiness, and diarrhea	• Fecal flotation • Fecal antigen • Egg: spherical, unembyronated • Deeply pigmented center with a rough, pitted outer shell • Size: 85–90 × 75 μm	• Fenbendazole • Imidacloprid/moxidectin • Ivermectin/pyrantel • Ivermectin/pyrantel/ praziquantel • Milbemycin oxime • Milbemycin oxime/ lufenuron/praziquantel • Milbemycin oxime/lufenuron • Milbemycin oxime/ spinosad • Moxidectin • Piperazine • Praziquantel/pyrantel pamoate/febantel • Pyrantel pamoate • Pyrantel/praziquantel • Disinfect with bleach • Eggs can remain infective in the soil for months to years

(Continued)

Table 3.23 / Endoparasites (Continued)

Parasite	Common name	Type	Affected species	Transmission route	Clinical signs	Diagnostics	Common treatments/ disinfection
Toxocara cati (Figure 3.108)	Feline roundworm	Nematode	Felines (zoonotic)	Eggs passed → ingested via environment or paratenic host → hatch in small intestines and penetrate mucosa → migrate through the liver and heart until the lungs → develop in lungs → coughed up and swallowed →mature in the small intestines; prepatent period: 3–5 weeks	Stunted growth and damage caused by migrations	• Fecal flotation • Fecal antigen • Egg: spherical, unembyronated • Deeply pigmented center with rough, pitted outer shell • Size: 75 × 65 μm	• Fenbendazole • Imidacloprid/moxidectin • Ivermectin/pyrantel • Ivermectin/pyrantel/ praziquantel • Milbemycin oxime • Milbemycin oxime/ lufenuron/praziquantel • Milbemycin oxime/ lufenuron • Milbemycin oxime/spinosad • Moxidectin • Piperazine • Praziquantel/pyrantel pamoate/febantel • Pyrantel pamoate • Pyrantel/praziquantel • Selamectin • Disinfect with bleach • Eggs can remain infective in the soil for months to years
Toxoplasma gondii	Toxoplasmosis	Protozoa	Felines	Oocysts passed → ingested via environment, intermediate host (most warm-blooded vertebrates) or transplacental → migrate to small intestines and extraintestinal dissemination elsewhere via blood and lymph Prepatent period: 3–10 d for ingestion of cysts and 20–40 d for oocysts	Asymptomatic or transient diarrhea, anorexia, depression, fever, and clinical signs dependent on site and extent of injury from migration (CNS, hepatic, pulmonary)	• Fecal flotation • ELISA • Agglutination procedures • Oocysts: oval and unsporulated and only shed for approximately 2 wk • Size: 10 × 12 μm	• Clindamycin • Pyrimethamine • Sulfadiazine + trimethoprim • Toltrazuril • Can live in the soil for months to > 1 year

(*Continued*)

Table 3.23 / **Endoparasites (Continued)**

Parasite	Common name	Type	Affected species	Transmission route	Clinical signs	Diagnostics	Common treatments/ disinfection
Trichuris vulpis (Figure 3.109)	Whipworm	Nematode	Canines	Eggs passed → ingested → penetrate and develop in small intestines → migrate to cecum and develop for 60–80 d Prepatent period: 9–12 wk	Weight loss, intermittent and chronic diarrhea, and typhlitis	• Fecal flotation • Egg: thick, brown-yellow symmetrical shell with clear polar plug at each end and unembyronated • Size: 72–93 × 35–58 µm	• Febantel/pyrantel/ praziquantel • Fenbendazole • Ivermectin • Mebendazole • Milbemycin oxime • Milbemycin oxime/ lufenuron/praziquantel • Milbemycin oxime/ praziquantel • Milbemycin oxime/spinosad • Moxidectin/ imidacloprid • Disinfect with diluted sodium chloride • Very resistant
Uncinaria stenocephala (Figure 3.85)	Northern canine hookworm	Nematode	Canines and felines (zoonotic)	Eggs passed → ingestion, percutaneous, prenatal, and transmammary → lungs for development → coughed up and swallowed → small intestines to mature; prepatent period: 2 weeks	Weakness, inappetence, poor growth, and diarrhea	• Fecal flotation • Egg: oval or ellipsoid, capsule shaped, 8–16 cells inside a thin wall • Size: 71–93 × 35–58 µm • Sample must be < 48 hours because eggs larvate rapidly in the external environment	• Febantel/praziquantel • Fenbendazole • Imidacloprid/moxidectin • Ivermectin • Ivermectin/pyrantel • Moxidectin • Praziquantel/pyrantel/ febantel • Pyrantel • Disinfect with bleach • Can live in cool, moist soil for several weeks

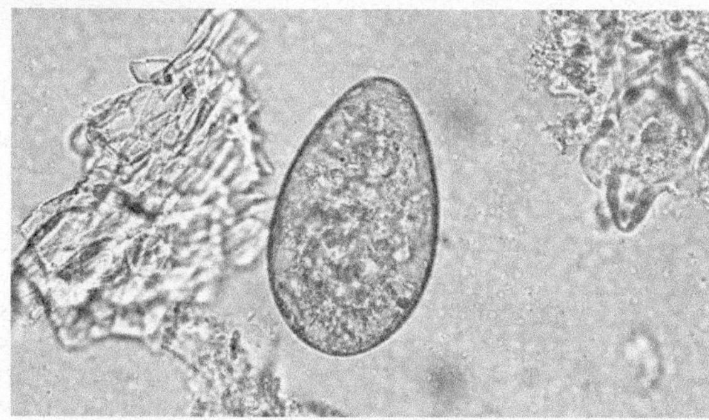

Figure 3.84 *Alaria* spp. Source: image courtesy of Barbie Papajeski.

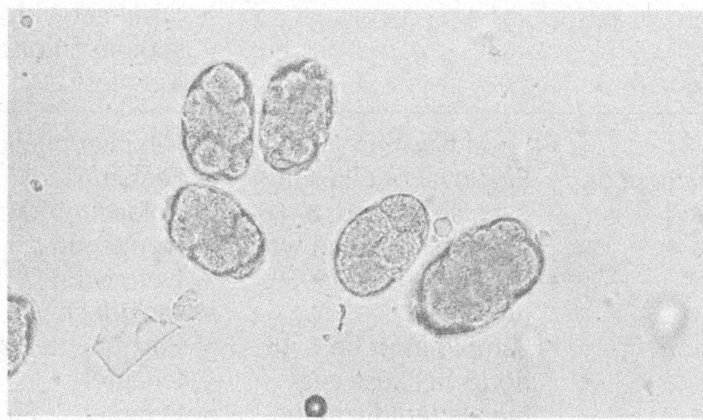

Figure 3.85 *Ancylostoma caninum* (smaller ova) and *Uncinaria stenocephala* (larger ova on right). Source: image courtesy of Barbie Papajeski.

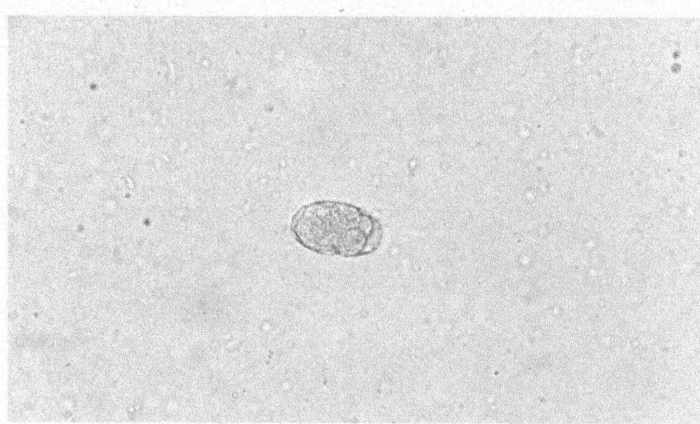

Figure 3.86 *Ancylostoma tubaeforme*. Source: image courtesy of Barbie Papajeski.

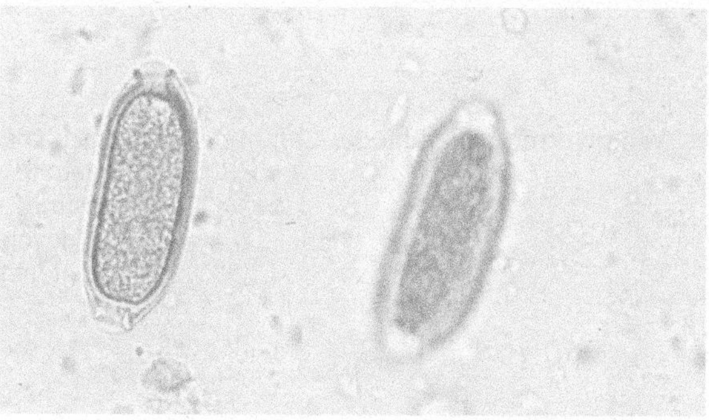

Figure 3.87 *Aonchotheca putorii*. Source: image courtesy of Barbie Papajeski.

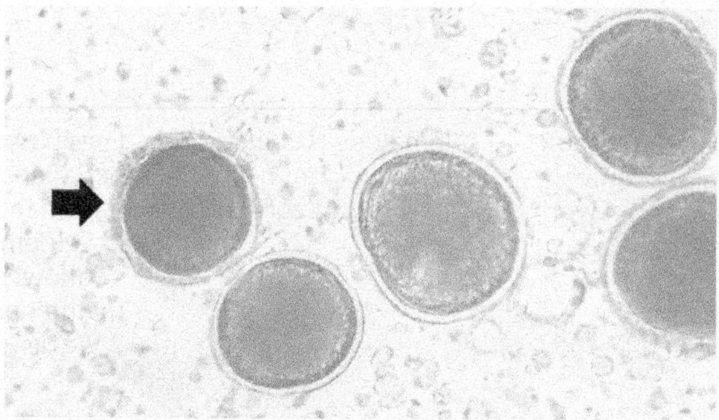

Figure 3.88 *Baylisascaris procyonis*. Source: image courtesy of Barbie Papajeski.

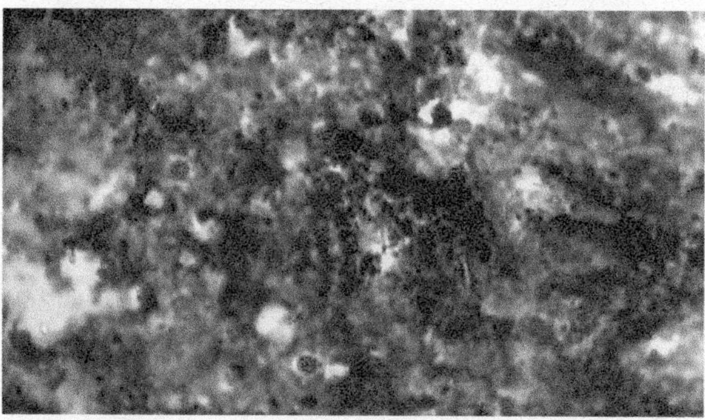

Figure 3.89 *Cryptosporidium* spp. (acid-fast stain). Source: image courtesy of Barbie Papajeski.

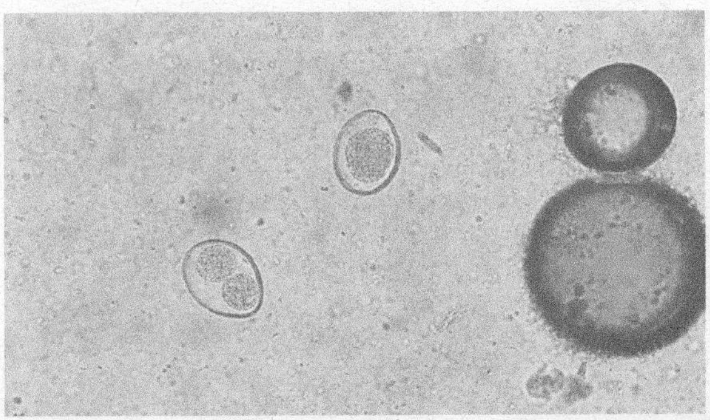

Figure 3.90 ***Cystoisospora*** **spp. (Formerly** ***Isospora*****). Source: image courtesy of Barbie Papajeski.**

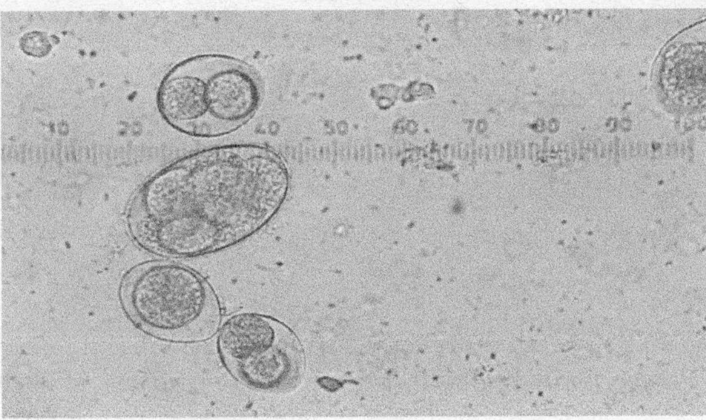

Figure 3.91 ***Cystoisospora*** **spp. (Formerly** ***Isospora*****) and** ***Ancylostoma tubaeforme*****. Source: image courtesy of Barbie Papajeski.**

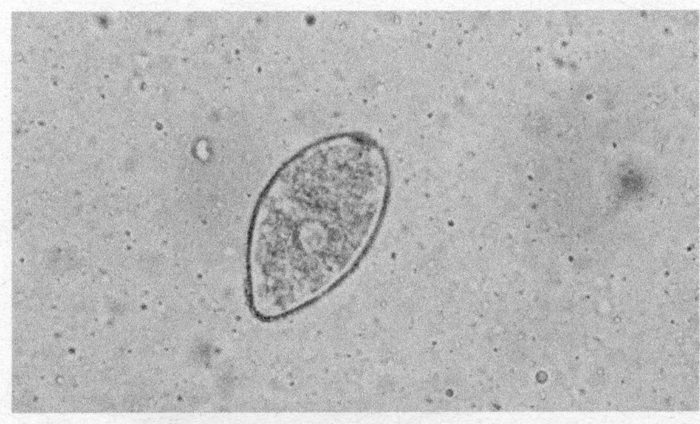

Figure 3.92 ***Diphyllobothrium latum*****. Source: image Courtesy of Barbie Papajeski.**

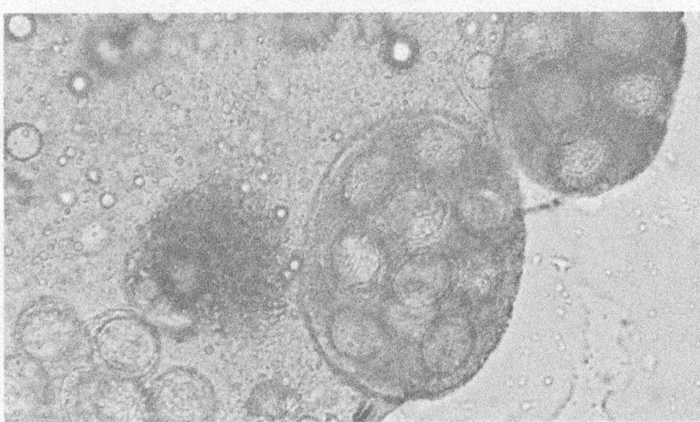

Figure 3.93 ***Dipylidium caninum*****. Source: image courtesy of Barbie Papajeski.**

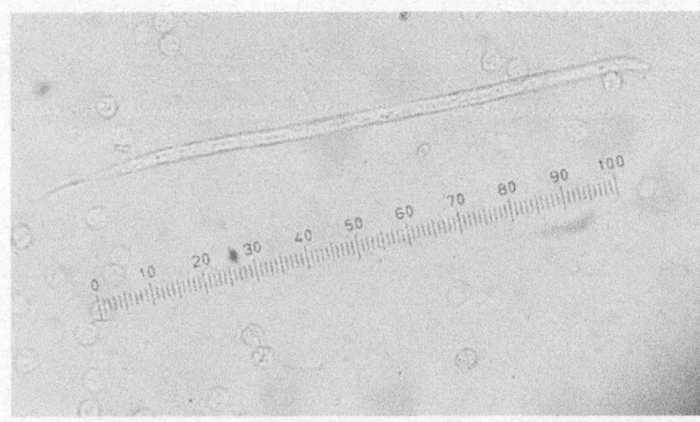

Figure 3.94 ***Dirofilaria immitis*****. Source: image courtesy of Barbie Papajeski.**

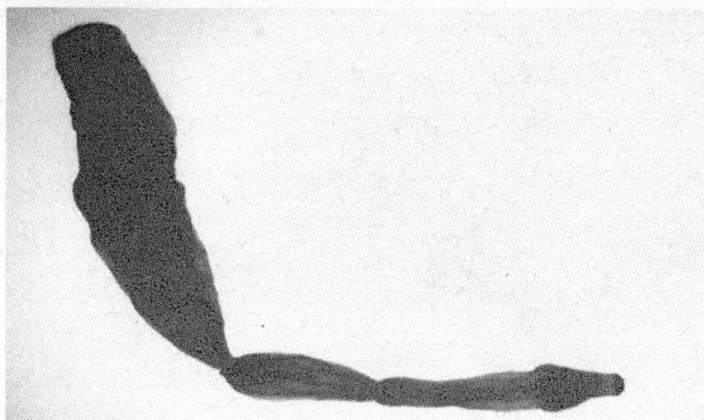

Figure 3.95 *Echinococcus granulosus* adult. Source: image courtesy of Barbie Papajeski.

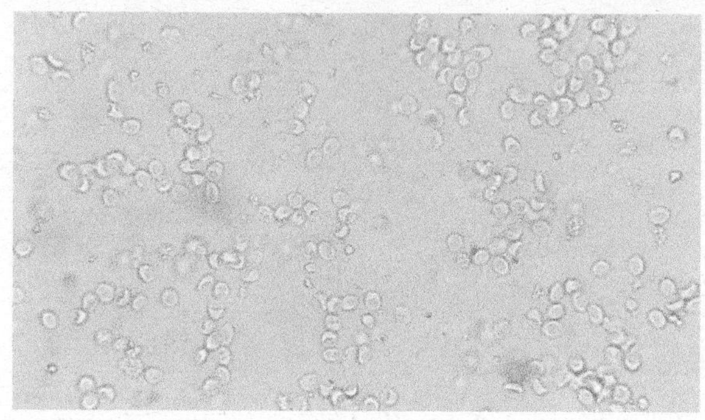

Figure 3.98 *Giardia* spp. Source: image courtesy of Barbie Papajeski.

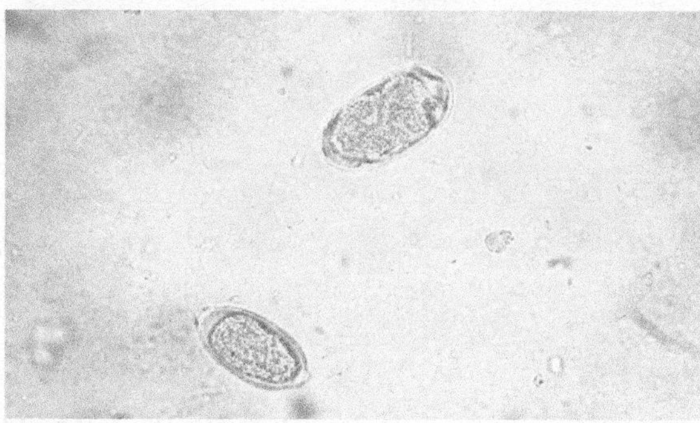

Figure 3.96 *Ancylostoma caninum* (top) and *Eucoleus boehmi* (bottom). Source: image courtesy of Barbie Papajeski.

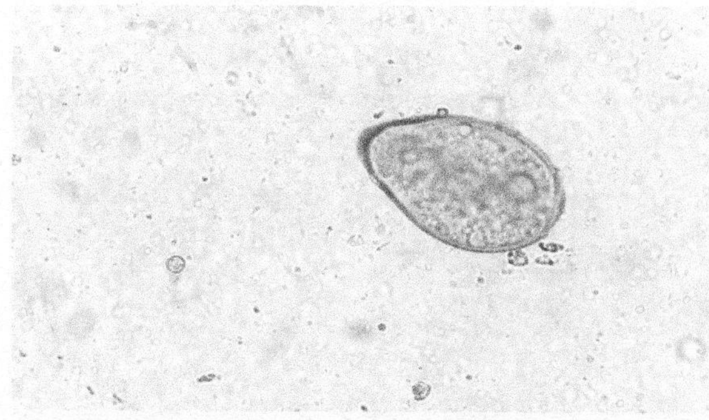

Figure 3.99 *Paragonimus kellicotti*. Source: image courtesy of Barbie Papajeski.

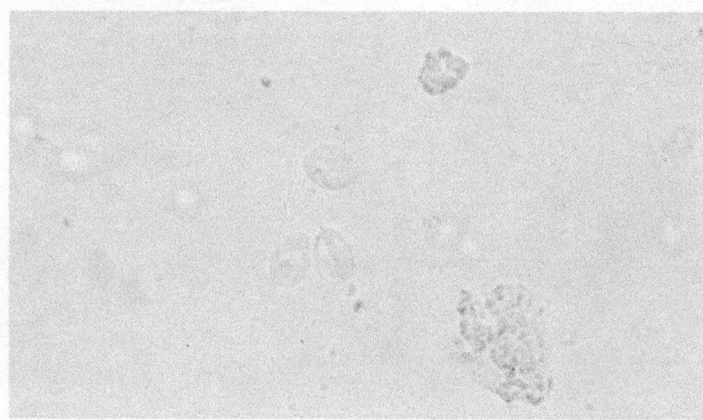

Figure 3.97 *Giardia* spp. Source: image courtesy of Barbie Papajeski.

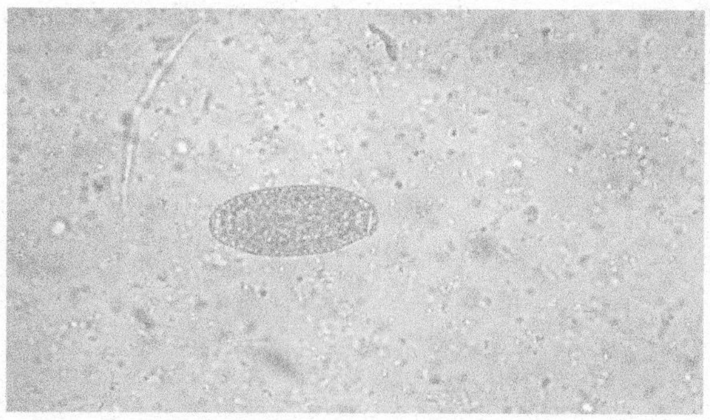

Figure 3.100 *Pearsonema feliscati*. Source: image courtesy of Barbie Papajeski.

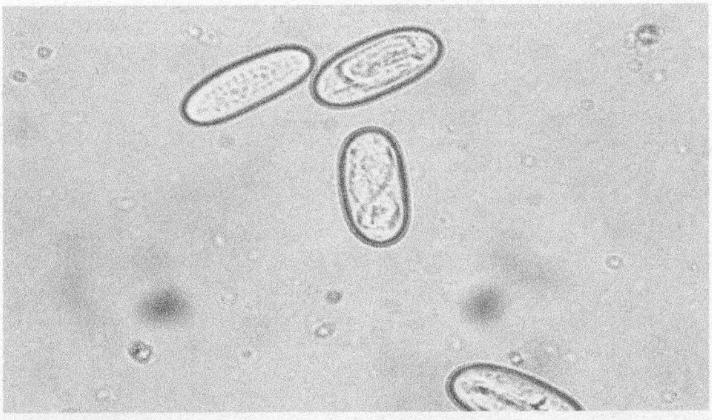

Figure 3.101 ***Physaloptera* spp. from an adult female worm. Source: image courtesy of Barbie Papajeski.**

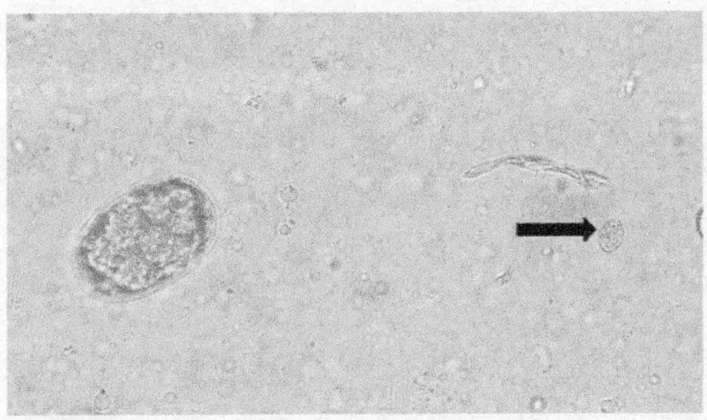

Figure 3.102 ***Sarcocystis* spp. and *Ancylostoma caninum* (left). Source: image courtesy of Barbie Papajeski.**

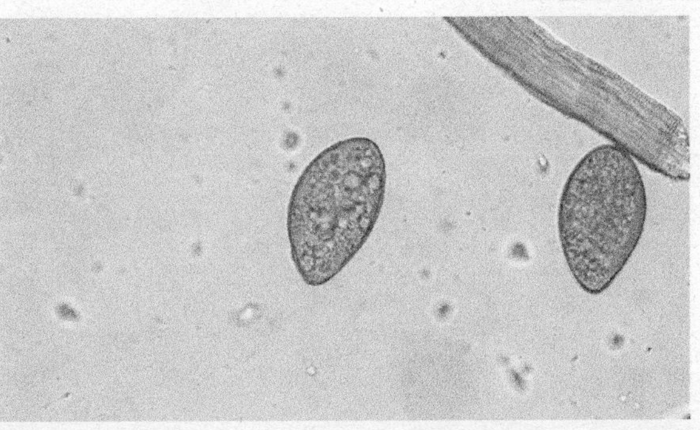

Figure 3.103 ***Spirometra* spp. Source: image courtesy Jean Miller, Breathitt Veterinary Center.**

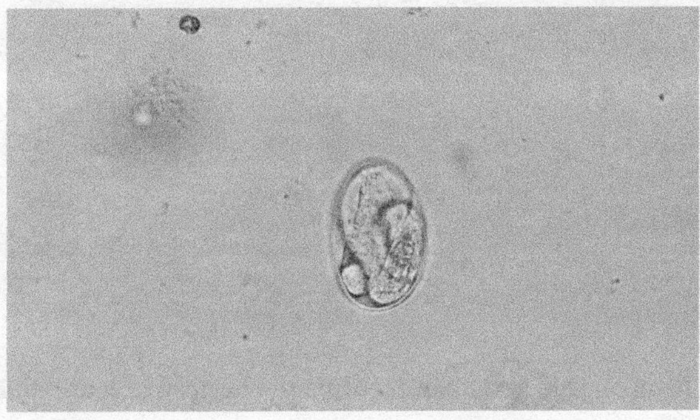

Figure 3.104 ***Strongyloides* spp. in a fresh fecal sample. Source: image courtesy of Barbie Papajeski.**

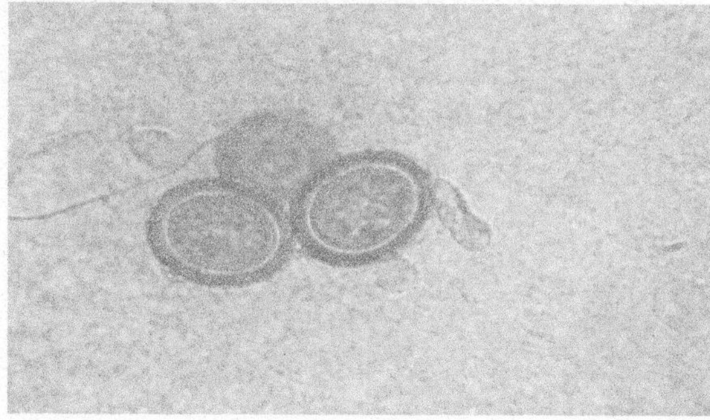

Figure 3.105 Taeniid-type ova. Source: image courtesy of Barbie Papajeski.

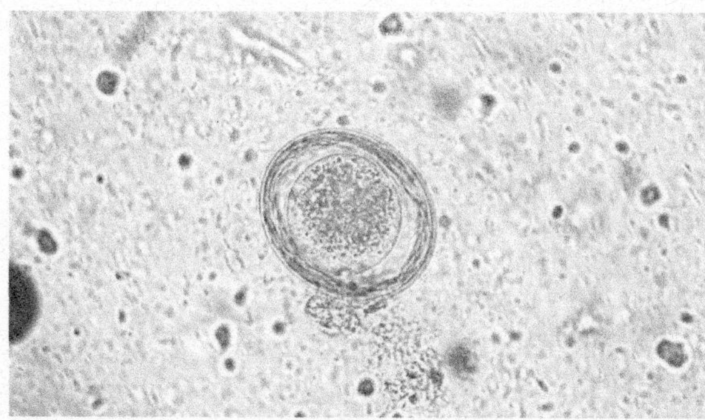

Figure 3.106 *Toxascaris leonina*. Source: Image courtesy of Jean Miller, Breathitt Veterinary Center.

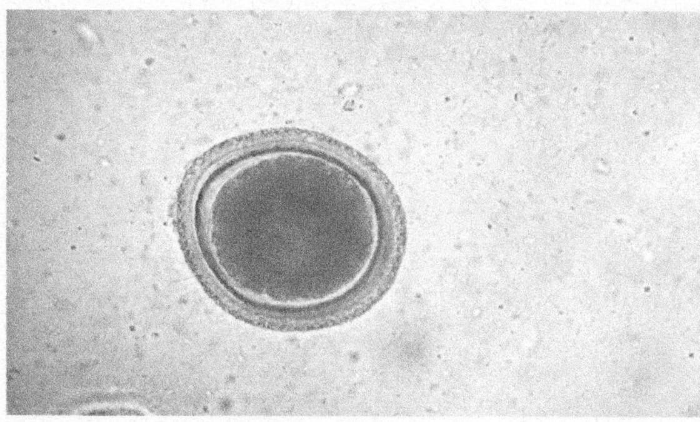

Figure 3.107 *Toxocara canis*. Source: image courtesy of Barbie Papajeski.

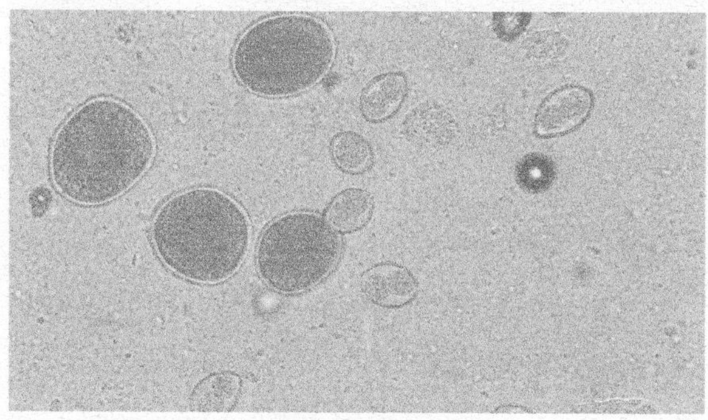

Figure 3.108 *Toxocara cati* (larger ova) and *Cystoisospora felis* (smaller, lighter ova). Source: Image courtesy of Barbie Papajeski.

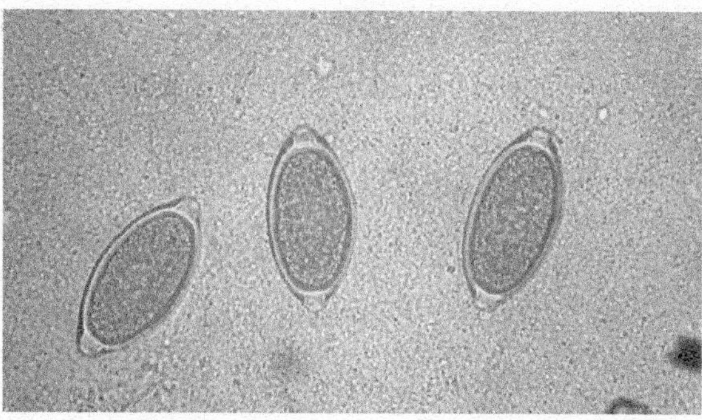

Figure 3.109 *Trichuris vulpis*. Source: image courtesy of Barbie Papajeski.

Skill Box 3.17 / Blood parasite examination methods[24,25]

Method	Uses	Technique	General Information
Direct examination	Microfilariae	• Add one drop of blood to a slide • Add a coverslip and examine for movement	Small sample volume owing to low sensitivity
Thin blood smear (Figure 3.110)	Trypanosomes, protozoans, and Rickettsia	• Place a drop of blood near one end with a glass slide laying on a flat surface • Place another slide at a 30–40-degree angle in front of the blood • Back the slide up until the blood runs along the edge of the second slide • Then gently and steadily push the slide forward and off the first slide, producing a smear with a feathered edge (Skill Box 3.3) • Air dry, stain with quick stains and examine	Small sample volume
Thick blood smear	Microfilariae, protozoa, and rickettsiae	• Place 3 drops of blood on a slide, then spread the drop out with a wooden applicator stick into a 2-cm circle • Air dry the slide • Place the slide in a slanted position in a container of distilled water • Once the smear losses its red color, remove it and allow it to air dry • Place the slide in methyl alcohol for 10 minutes • Add Giemsa stain for 30 minutes • Rinse the slide and examine[24]	Larger sample volume; placing the slide in distilled water will lyse the red bloods cells
Buffy coat (Figure 3.111)	Microfilariae	• Fill a PCV tube 75% full and centrifuge for 3 minutes • Break tube just below the buffy coat and snap apart • Tap the tube until the buffy coat drops onto a glass slide • Add a drop of saline and stain, place a coverslip on, and examine • Alternately place PCV tube on stage of microscope and view area immediately above the buffy coat	Does not allow differentiation of microfilariae species (Skill Box 3.4)
Knott's technique, modified (Figure 3.112)	Microfilariae	• Mix 1 ml whole blood with 9 ml 2% formalin in a test tube • Mix well to lyse red blood cells • Centrifuge at 1300–1500 rpm for 5 minutes • Pour off the supernatant and add two to three drops of stain to the sediment • With a pipette, mix the sediment and stain (new methylene blue) • Place 1 drop on a glass slide, apply a coverslip, and examine under 10 × objective	Allows differentiation of microfilariae species; mix whole blood sample well before adding formalin

(*Continued*)

Skill Box 3.17 / Blood parasite examination methods (Continued)

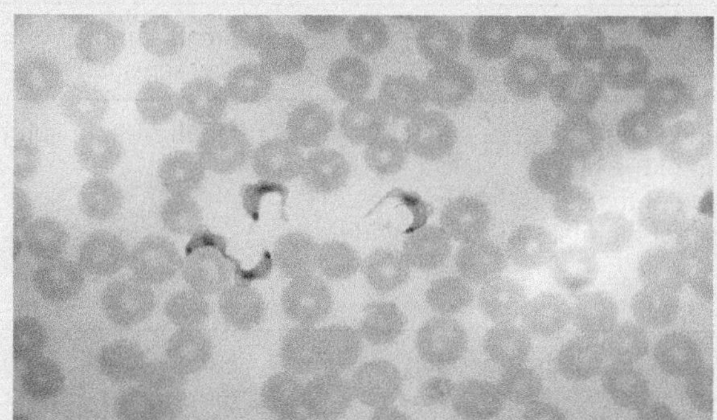

Figure 3.110 ***Trypanosoma cruzi*** **on a thin blood smear. Source: image courtesy of Barbie Papajeski.**

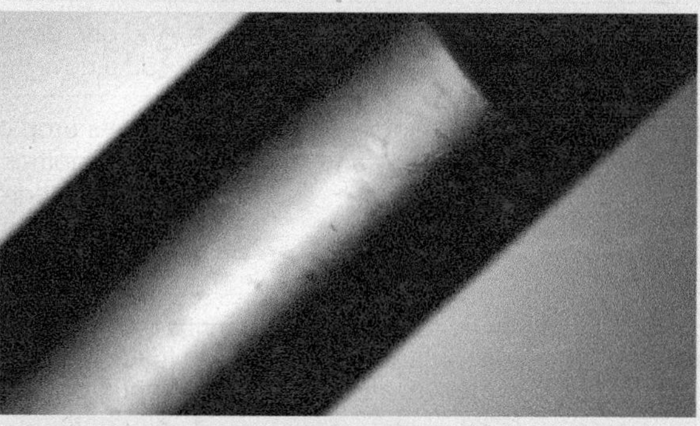

Figure 3.111 ***Microfilaria*** **concentrated just above the buffy coat layer in a packed cell volume tube. Source: image courtesy of Barbie Papajeski.**

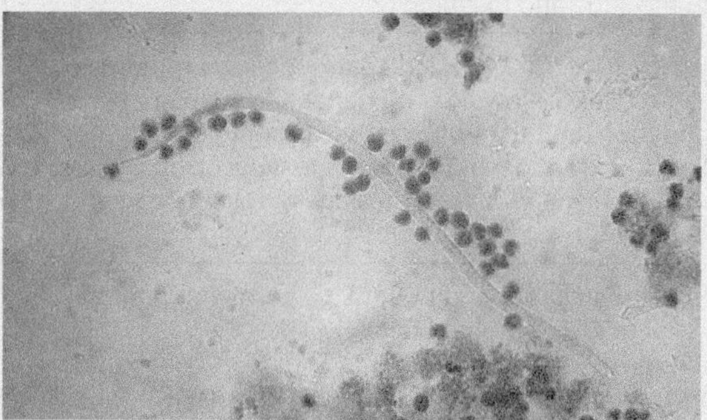

Figure 3.112 ***Dirofilaria immitis*** **modified Knott's stained with new methylene blue. Source: image courtesy of Barbie Papajeski.**

Skill Box 3.18 / Ectoparasite examination methods[24,25]

Method	Uses	Technique	General information
Gross examination	Lice, mites, ticks, flies, or fleas	• Visualize the ectoparasite on the animal or by using a flea comb	Limited number of parasites visible
Cellophane tape	Lice or mites	• Bend the cellophane tape into a loop with the sticky side out • Press the tape against the animal's skin • Put one drop of water on a slide and lay tape over it and press down. • Examine under a microscope.	Limited number of parasites visible
Microscopic examination	Most ectoparasites	• Collect a sample through skin scrapings, hair samples, or swabs • Place a drop of mineral oil on a glass slide • Roll the swab or material collected in the mineral oil to deposit any debris • Place a coverslip on the slide and examine with a microscope, using 4 × magnification	Most thorough technique for ectoparasite diagnosis

Ectoparasites

Table 3.24 / Ectoparasites[19,24,25]

Parasite	Common name	Type	Affected species	Transmission route	Clinical signs	Diagnostics	Common treatments
Amblyomma spp. (Figure 3.113)	Lone star tick, Gulf coast tick	Tick	Canines and felines (zoonotic: human risk high)	Ingest: blood Location: whole body Transmission: contact Lifecycle: 3-host tick Egg → larval → nymph → adult	Irritation, pruritus, anemia, inflammation, hypersensitivity, toxic reactions (paralysis); vector for *Cytauxzoon, Ehrlichia,* tularemia, Rocky Mountain spotted fever	Visual Adults: ornamented, long mouthparts, single white spot on scutum	Manual removal (wear gloves) Pyrethroid/pyrethrin spray + manual removal Afoxolaner Amitraz Etofenprox Fipronil Flumethrin Fluralaner Permethrin Sarolaner

(*Continued*)

Table 3.24 / **Ectoparasites (Continued)**

Parasite	Common name	Type	Affected species	Transmission route	Clinical signs	Diagnostics	Common treatments
Cheyletiella (Figure 3.114)	Walking dandruff	Mite	Canines and felines (zoonotic: human risk low)	Ingest: keratin debris and tissue fluid Location: skin Transmission: direct contact with other animals and indirect through inanimate objects Lifecycle: 3–5 weeks	Asymptomatic, mild alopecia, dandruff, pruritus	Scrape margins of lesions, flea comb, visual, or cellophane tape Adult: body shape resembles a shield or acorn, hook-like accessory mouth parts and comb like structures at the tip of each leg	No approved treatment; veterinarians may choose to use the following off label: ivermectin, milbemycin oxime, moxidectin, selamectin, fipronil, pyrethrin
Ctenocephalides canis/felis (Figure 3.115)	Flea	Insect	Canines and felines (zoonotic: human risk high from newly emerged fleas)	Ingest: blood Location: head and base of tail Transmission: direct contact or through contact with inanimate objects Lifecycle: 21 days to 1 year	Fleabite dermatitis, anemia, pruritus, red lesions, hair loss, ulcers	Visual and flea comb Adult: medium brown to mahogany in color, laterally flattened body, 2–8 mm long with pronotal and genal combs Transmit *Dipylidium* and *Hemobartonella* spp.	Afoxolaner Cyphenothrin Deltamethrin Dinotefuran Fipronil Flumethrin Fluralaner Imidacloprid Lufenuron Methoprene Moxidectin Nitenpyram Pyrethrins/pyrethroids Pyriproxyfen Selamectin Spinosad
Cuterebra (Figure 3.116)	Rodent botfly, warbles, wolves	insect larvae	Canines and felines (zoonotic: human risk low)	Ingest: host tissues Location: face and neck region, can be found on any furred area Transmission: contact with rodent burrow or eggs from an adult fly Lifecycle: 3–4 weeks	Cutaneous lump with a breathing hole, neurological and respiratory disease with migrating larvae	Visual Larval second stage: cream to white, toothlike spines, 5–10 mm long; third stage: large, coal-black, heavily spined, 3 cm long	Surgical removal of larvae; note: do not crush larva when removing – may cause anaphylaxis Wound treatment

(*Continued*)

Table 3.24 / **Ectoparasites (Continued)**

Parasite	Common name	Type	Affected species	Transmission route	Clinical signs	Diagnostics	Common treatments
Demodex canis (Figure 3.117)	Follicular mange mite, red mange	Mite	Canine (no human risk)	Ingest: unknown Location: hair follicles and sebaceous glands Transmission: direct contact from dam to pup; otherwise, not contagious between hosts Lifecycle: 21 days	Alopecia of muzzle, face, and forelegs; erythema, second-degree bacterial pyoderma, pruritus	Deep skin scrapings on squeezed skin or biopsy Adult: cigar-shaped, eight stubby legs at anterior end of body, 0.25 cm long	Amitraz 0.025% Veterinarians may choose other treatments off label: doramectin, ivermectin, milbemycin oxime, moxidectin
Dermacentor variabilis/ andersoni (Figure 3.118)	American dog tick, wood tick	Tick	Canines and felines (zoonotic: human risk high)	Ingest: blood Location: whole body Transmission: contact Lifecycle: 3-host tick 3 months to 2 years Tick must be attached for 5–20 hours to transmit disease	Asymptomatic or vasculitis, primary vector for Rocky Mountain spotted fever, tularemia, and other *Rickettsia* spp.	Visual Adults: ornate markings, short mouthparts, rectangular basis capitulum	Manual removal (wear gloves) Pyrethroid/pyrethrin spray + manual removal Afoxolaner Amitraz Etofenprox Fipronil Flumethrin Fluralaner Permethrin Sarolaner Selamectin
Ixodes spp.	Black-legged tick, deer tick	Tick	Canines and felines (zoonotic: human risk high)	Ingest: blood Location: whole body Transmission: contact Lifecycle: 3-host tick	Irritation, pruritus, anemia, inflammation, hypersensitivity, toxic reactions (paralysis); vector for Lyme disease, tularemia, Anaplasma	Visual Adults: long alps, anal groove surrounds anus	Manual removal (wear gloves) Pyrethroid/pyrethrin spray + manual removal Afoxolaner Amitraz Etofenprox Fipronil Flumethrin Fluralaner Permethrin Sarolaner

(*Continued*)

Table 3.24 / Ectoparasites (Continued)

Parasite	Common name	Type	Affected species	Transmission route	Clinical signs	Diagnostics	Common treatments
Linognathus setosus	Sucking louse of dogs	Louse	Canine (zoonotic: human risk low)	Ingest: blood Location: whole body Transmission: contact Life cycle: 3–4 weeks, live 7 days away from host	Skin irritation, itching, dermatitis, alopecia, anemia, roughened hair coat	Visual Adult: dorsoventrally flattened, red to gray in color; head narrower than widest part of thorax, first pair of claws smaller than second and third pairs	Fipronil Imidacloprid Permethrin Selamectin
Otobius megnini	Spinose ear tick	Tick	Canine (zoonotic: human risk high)	Ingest: blood Location: ear Transmission: contact Lifecycle: adults are free living; larval ticks remain on host until nymph molts to adult	Large numbers in ear canal can cause ulcerations and ear drum rupture	Visual: tiny backward facing spines; mouthparts are only visible from ventral side	Manual removal (wear gloves) Pyrethroid or pyrethrin spray + manual removal Afoxolaner Amitraz Etofenprox Fipronil Flumethrin Fluralaner Permethrin Sarolaner
Otodectes cynotis (Figure 3.119)	Ear mite	Mite	Canine (no human risk)	Ingest: epidermal debris Location: ear and base of tail Transmission: contact Lifecycle: 18–21 days	Shaking of head, irritation, otitis media, hematomas, head tilt, circling, convulsions	Visual or ear swab Adult: oval with eight legs, fused head and thorax, short unjointed pedicel with suckers on the end of some of the legs	Clean the ear of all crusty debris Moxidectin/imidacloprid Selamectin

(*Continued*)

Table 3.24 / **Ectoparasites (Continued)**

Parasite	Common name	Type	Affected species	Transmission route	Clinical signs	Diagnostics	Common treatments
Rhipicephalus sanguineus	Brown dog tick	Tick	Canine (zoonotic: human risk high)	Ingest: blood Location: whole body Transmission: contact Lifecycle: 6 weeks to 1 year	Irritation, pruritus, anemia; vector for *Anaplasma, Babesia, Ehrlichia, Hepatozoon,* Rocky Mountain spotted fever	Visual Adult: brown with prominent lateral extensions on head, giving a hexagonal appearance, ridged palps	Manual removal (wear gloves) Pyrethroid/pyrethrin spray + manual removal Afoxolaner Amitraz Etofenprox Fipronil Flumethrin Fluralaner Permethrin Sarolaner
Sarcoptes scabiei canis (Figure 3.120)	Mange mite, scabies	Mite	Canine (zoonotic: human risk low)	Ingest: interstitial fluid Location: ears, lateral elbows, and ventral abdomen Transmission: contact Life cycle: 2–3 weeks	Severe itching, dry and thickened skin, erythema, papular rash, scaling, crusting, excoriations	Deep skin scraping Adults: oval with eight legs, fused head and thorax, long unjointed pedicel with suckers on the end of some of the legs	Fipronil Flumethrin/imidacloprid Moxidectin/imidacloprid Selamectin
Trichodectes canis (Figure 3.121)	Biting louse of dogs	Louse	Canine	Ingest: skin and hair Location: whole body Transmission: contact Life cycle: 3–4 weeks; live 7 days away from host	Itching, rough hair coat, dermatitis	Visual Adult: dorsoventrally flattened, yellow, large rounded head; head wider than any other part of the body, 2–4 mm	Fipronil Imidacloprid Permethrin Selamectin

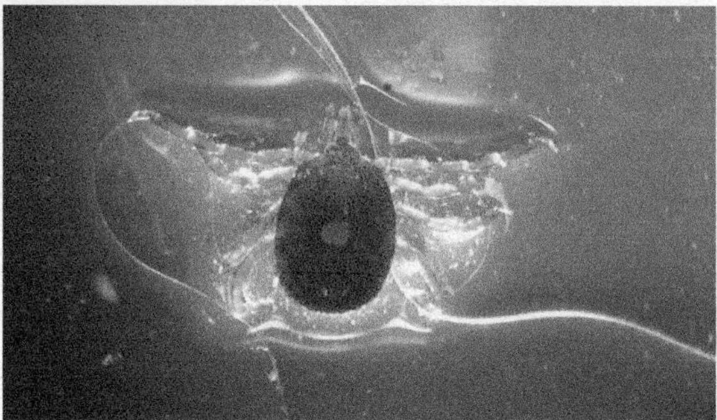

Figure 3.113 ***Ambylomas*** **spp. Source: image courtesy of Barbie Papajeski.**

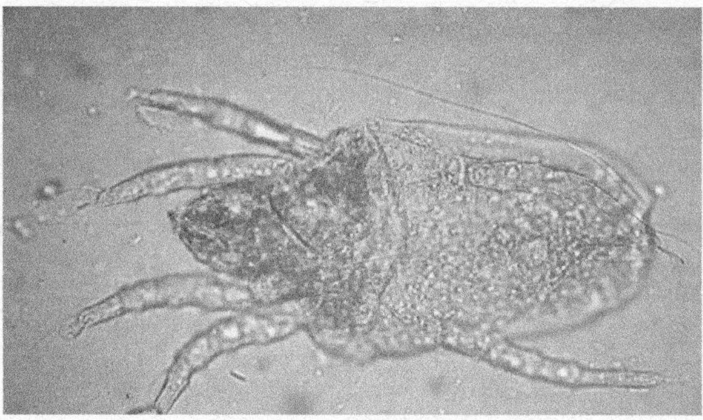

Figure 3.114 ***Cheyletiella*****. Source: image courtesy of Barbie Papajeski.**

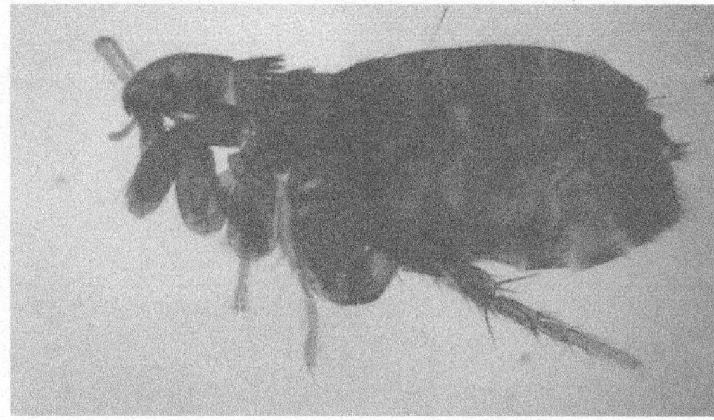

Figure 3.115 ***Ctenocephalides felis*****. Source: image courtesy of Barbie Papajeski.**

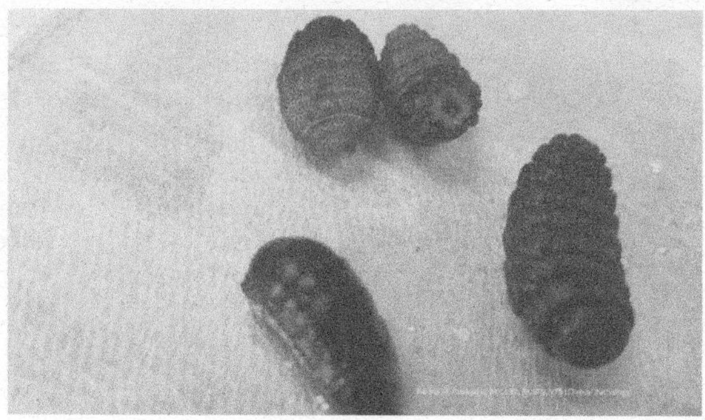

Figure 3.116 ***Cuterebra*****. Source: image courtesy of Barbie Papajeski.**

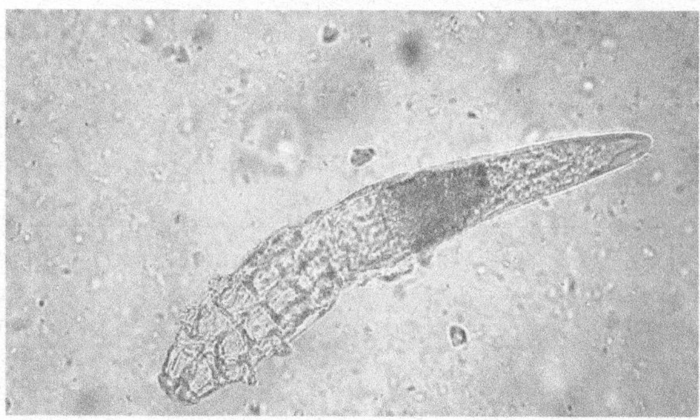

Figure 3.117 ***Demodex canis*****. Source: image courtesy of Barbie Papajeski.**

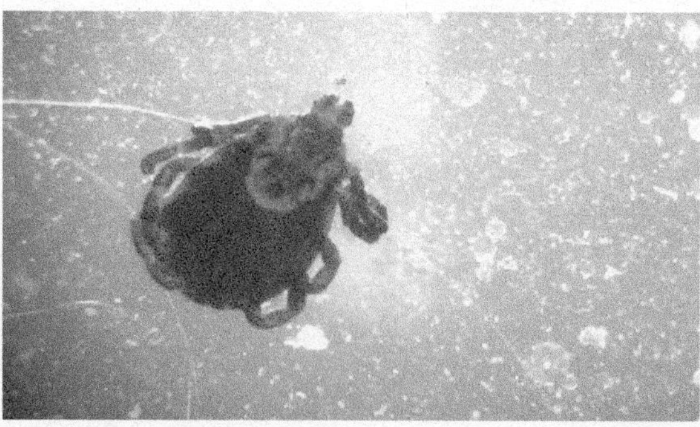

Figure 3.118 ***Dermacentor*** **spp. Source: image courtesy of Barbie Papajeski.**

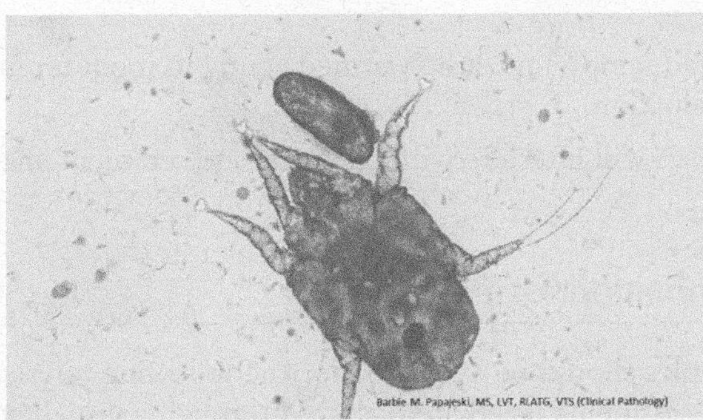

Figure 3.119 ***Otodectes cynotis*** **mite and egg. Source: image courtesy of Barbie Papajeski.**

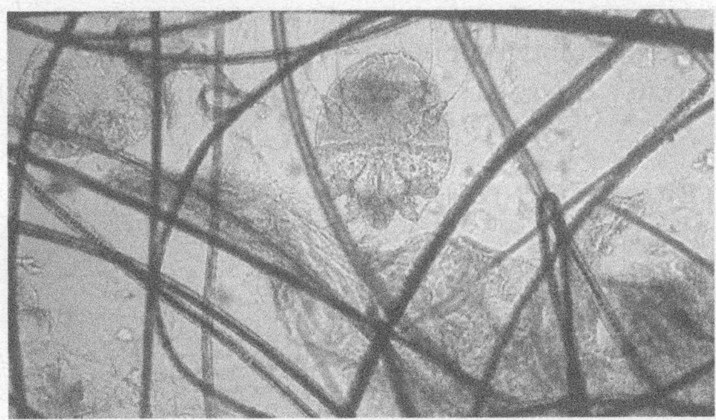

Figure 3.120 ***Sarcoptes scabiei canis.*** **Source: image courtesy of Barbie Papajeski.**

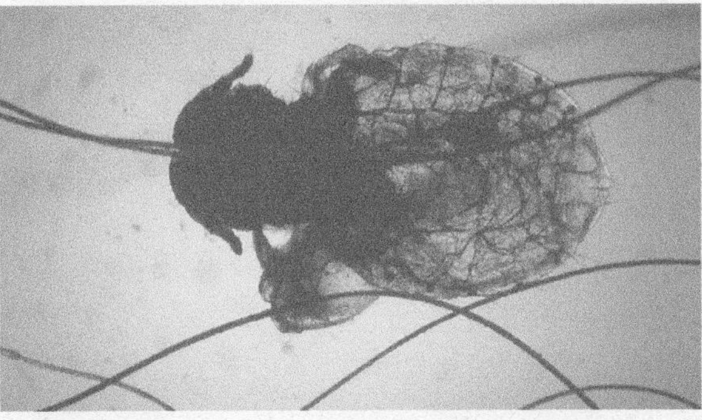

Figure 3.121 ***Trichodectes canis.*** **Source: image courtesy of Barbie Papajeski.**

URINALYSIS

Together with CBC, a urinalysis is one of the most frequently performed laboratory tests in small animal clinics. The collection and handling of the sample and the skill of the person performing the test directly affect the quality of the results. Considering all pre-analytical factors which affect urine and minimizing their effect is vital for obtaining valid results.[26]

Urine Collection, Handling, Storage, and Transport Tips

Collection[26]

- Collection before administration of any medication, if possible.
- Morning, preprandial samples offer the most accurate specific gravity, pH, and cellular components but allow for the degeneration of casts overnight in the bladder.
- Collection containers must have a tight fitting lid, be clean, well rinsed, and free of any disinfectant residue.
- Ideally, a new, sterile, opaque container is used to prevent photochemical breakdown of components and introduction of chemical and bacterial contamination.
- Collect a minimum of 5 ml of urine, if smaller volumes are collected partial urinalysis may be performed such as specific gravity and chemical analysis depending on analyzer, sedimentation requires a minimum of 5 ml.
- See Skill Box 16.22: Urine collection: voided, manual expression, cystocentesis, page 730, for procedural information on urine collection.

Handling[2,4,26]

- Samples should be covered immediately to avoid pH changes and contamination.
- Samples with a delay of examination of over one hour should be refrigerated.
- Avoid delays, which can lead to changes in all aspects of urinalysis: pH increases, bacteria proliferate, cells and casts deteriorate, and bilirubin and ketones degrade to low or undetectable levels.
- Thoroughly mix a sample before specific gravity is tested, chemical analysis, and transference to another container.

- Allow urine to cool down to room temperature after collection.
- Centrifuge the sample according to manufacturer's instructions, typically 1500–2500 revolutions/minute for three to five minutes.
- Avoid using the centrifuge brake to stop the centrifuge, as this may resuspend the sediment.
- Pipet or gently pour the off the supernatant to avoid disturbing the remaining pellet.
- Gently mix the pellet to avoid cellular damage.

Storage and transport[2,4,26]

- Samples at room temperature should be examined within 1 hour and no longer than 12 hours
- Samples can be refrigerated, but changes will occur, such as crystal formation and changes in specific gravity.
- Refrigerated samples must be warmed gently to room temperature before evaluation.
- Preservatives will interfere with chemical and sediment analysis.
- Ship urine on ice packs.

Urine Examination/Urinalysis[2,4,26]

All urine samples should be evaluated for the following physical properties. Each of the assessments listed are observed through a visual examination of the sample, except for specific gravity. Specific gravity is obtained with a refractometer that indirectly and accurately measures the amount of solids dissolved in a urine sample as compared with distilled water. Strip methods for specific gravity are inaccurate when measuring canine and feline samples. The refractometer should be checked daily to ensure correct calibration. Using distilled water, the specific gravity reading should be 1.000.

Table 3.25 / **Gross examination**[2,4,26]

Physical property	Observation	Common cause	Associated conditions
Color	Colorless to pale yellow	Dilute, correlates with low USG	Puppies < 4 weeks, renal failure, liver failure or extrarenal diuresis, drugs (diuretics, glucocorticoids), diabetes insipidus
	Light to medium yellow	Urochromes and urobilin give urine a natural yellow color	Considered typical coloration
	Dark yellow to amber	Concentrated urine	Variations are often attributable to changes in concentration
	Orange to orange-brown; yellow-brown to brown	Bilirubinuria	Liver disease
	Greenish yellow	Oxidation of bilirubin to biliverdin	Liver disease
	Red or red-brown	Hematuria: clears upon centrifugation, often cloudy, red blood cells in sediment Hemoglobinuria: red coloration persists after centrifugation and serum or plasma is hemolyzed, precipitates with ammonium sulfate, anemia present Myoglobinuria: red coloration persists after centrifugation and serum or plasma is clear, increased AST and creatine kinase values	UTI, trauma, cystitis, urolithiasis, neoplasia; intravascular hemolysis, muscle cell degradation
	Brown to black	Myoglobinuria Methemoglobin Animals given oxyglobin or metronidazole	Muscle cell degradation; hemoglobin in urine has been oxidized to methemoglobin
	Wine red to deep red color	Porphyrin will fluoresce under Wood's lamp	Will fluoresce under Wood's lamp
	White	Contains leukocytes, crystals, or mucous	UTI, cystitis, and heavy crystalluria
Odor	Ammonia	Breakdown of urease	UTI, cystitis, aged sample
	Sweet, fruity odor	Contains ketones and glucose	Diabetes mellitus

(Continued)

Table 3.25 / Gross examination (Continued)

Physical property	Observation	Common cause	Associated conditions
Urine specific gravity (USG)	Canine: 1.020–1.045 Feline: 1.025–1.050	Animal is able to concentrate urine if hydration is normal	Expected values; dehydrated and azotemic animals may still have renal problems with these values
	Canine: > 1.035 Feline: ≥1.040	Hypersthenuria; false ↑ cold urine, glucosuria, proteinuria	Dehydration; indicates adequate renal function
	1.007–1.013	Isosthenuria	Urine has same specific gravity as plasma; nephrons are unable to dilute or concentrate urine; potential renal failure in dehydrated or azotemic animal
	≤1.007	Hyposthenuria	Nephrons can dilute urine but have lost concentrating ability; liver disease, renal disease, diuretics, diabetes insipidus
Transparency/ turbidity	Clear to slightly cloudy	No or minimal suspended solids present	Typical finding in normal urine
	Cloudy, opaque, or flocculent (turbid)	Contains suspended solids such as cells, crystals, bacteria, lipids, mucus, semen, or fecal contamination; examine sediment	UTI, crystalluria
Volume	Polyuria	↑ Urine production, pale with a ↓ USG (≤ 1.020)	Nephritis, diabetes mellitus, diabetes insipidus, pyometra, liver disease, renal disease
	Oliguria	↓ Urine production	↓ Water intake, fever, shock, heart disease, dehydration
	Pollakiuria	Frequent urination	UTI, cystitis, urolithiasis, crystalluria
	Anuria	Complete lack of urine output No urine output in 12 hours	Urinary obstruction, urinary bladder rupture, death

Chemistry Strip Examination

Chemistry strip evaluation provides detection of elements present in a urine sample that may or may not be seen during visual or microscopic examination. Because chemistry strips provide many false results, both a visual examination and a microscopic examination should always be performed. Evaluation is performed on suspended urine samples prior to centrifugation.

Chemistry strip bottles should be kept at room temperature and away from intense light, moisture, and heat. Strips can be immersed in a urine sample for two to three seconds to allow saturation of the pads, or a pipette or dropper may be used to saturate each pad. Always consult the strip manufacturer's instructions for the correct technique. Extended time may lead to test reagents leaking into the urine sample or subsequent run-off into other reagent pads. The edge of the strip can be blotted with an absorbent material to collect excess urine or the strip can be withdrawn by sliding along the rim of the container to remove excess urine. The results are then read at the time indicated by the manufacturer in consistent artificial light to avoid the fluctuations seen with natural light. The color change can be subjective and also altered by the presence of urine pigments (bilirubin, hemoglobin). Automated readers are available, which eliminate inconsistencies in color evaluation times and human interpretation.

Table 3.26 / Chemistry strip examination[2,4,26]

Chemical property	Observation	Definition	Associated conditions
Bilirubin	Bilirubinuria	A by-product from the breakdown of hemoglobin Trace amounts found in dogs if USG is $\geq$ 1.030, but not common in cats False negative: exposure to light Confirmation tests: Ictotest®	Hemolytic anemia, bile duct obstruction, liver disease, fever, pancreatitis, neoplasia, prolonged fasting or starvation
Blood	A positive test pad indicates hematuria, hemoglobinuria, or myoglobinuria and should be evaluated with a microscopic exam False negatives: poorly mixed sample, large amounts of bacterial nitrites, and formalin used as a preservative False positives: contamination with bleach or other disinfecting agents and peroxidase from bacterial growth		
	Hematuria	Presence of intact RBC. After centrifugation, urine will appear clear with a red pellet. Sample should be well mixed to ensure no RBC settling. Alkaline urine will cause RBC to lyse showing a positive reagent pad but no microscopic RBC	UTI, cystitis, renal disease, strenuous exercise, trauma, coagulopathy, and genital tract contamination
	Hemoglobinuria	Presence of free hemoglobin, typically caused by intravascular hemolysis or alkaline urine. After centrifugation, urine will remain tinted red; may interfere with the interpretation of other chemistries	Hemolytic anemia, severe burns, incompatible transfusions, leptospirosis, babesiosis, systemic lupus erythematosus, metal toxicity
	Myoglobinuria	Presence of myoglobin typically due to muscle damage. Urine is dark brown to black; may interfere with the interpretation of other chemistries	Muscle damage or necrosis

(Continued)

Table 3.26 / Chemistry strip examination (Continued)

Chemical property	Observation	Definition	Associated conditions
Glucose	Glucosuria	Appears when blood glucose levels exceed renal threshold; canine: > 180 mg/dl; feline: > 300 mg/dl. Not detectable in the urine of normal animals False negatives: vitamin C, bilirubinuria, salicylates, tetracycline, cold urine, formaldehyde exposure False positives: oxidizing cleaning agents, baking soda, bleach, hydrogen peroxide	Diabetes mellitus, Cushing's disease, chronic liver disease, high carbohydrate meal, stress, fear, restraint, intravenous administration of glucose, Fanconi's syndrome
Ketones	Ketonuria	Formed from the rapid or excessive breakdown of fatty acids. Not detectable in the urine of normal animals. Produces a sweet, fruity smell False negative: delayed analysis, bacteriuria, or prolonged pad exposure False positive: pigmented urine, highly acidic urine Confirmation tests: Acetest®	Diabetes mellitus, liver disease, persistent fever, high-fat diets, starvation, fasting, late-stage pregnancy, and long-term anorexia
pH	Normal	Concentration of H+ ions, a measure of the degree of alkalinity or acidity Expected values 5.0–7.0	
	Alkaline	↑ Concentration of H+ ions; < 7.0 False increases: delayed analysis, contamination with detergents or disinfectants, postprandial sample Crystals: ammonium biurate, amorphous phosphate, calcium carbonate, calcium phosphate, struvite	Postprandial alkaline tide, plant diets, UTI, metabolic and/or respiratory alkalosis, crystalluria, distal renal tubular acidosis, urine retention, certain drugs (bicarbonate, citrate)
	Acidic	↓ Concentration of H+ ions; > 7.0 Crystals: calcium oxalate, amorphous urate, uric acid, leucine, tyrosine, cystine	Protein diets, metabolic or respiratory acidosis, fever, starvation, excessive muscular activity, chloride depletion, crystalluria, certain drugs (DL-methionine, furosemide)
Protein	Proteinuria	Measurement of albumin and globulins. Only found in trace amounts in normal, highly concentrated urine. Always interpret with USG and contents of urine sediment False positives: ↑ USG, ↑ pH, pigmented urine, detergent contamination Confirmation tests: sulfosalicylic acid test, microalbuminuria test	Glomerulonephritis, glomerular amyloidosis, multiple myeloma, parturition, estrus, UTI
Protein : creatinine ratio	Normal	Quantifies level of proteinuria as significant or not; not dependent on urine concentration Canine: ≤ 0.3 Feline: ≤ 0.6	
	Increased	↑ Urine protein loss; > 1 False positive: urogenital contamination of voided sample, traumatic cystocentesis	Chronic interstitial nephritis, glomerulonephritis, and amyloidosis

Sediment Examination[2,4,26]

Microscopic examination of the urine sediment should be a part of every routine urinalysis. Findings confirm gross examination and chemistry strip examination results. A significant amount of additional information can be gained from a microscopic examination that cannot be determined by any other method. Samples collected after a period of rest or water deprivation increase the likelihood of finding formed elements.

Each laboratory varies slightly in their protocols; however, a standard amount of 5 ml urine is centrifuged and poured off, leaving the pellet and approximately 0.3 ml urine in the tube. The remaining urine and pellet are mixed together, and one drop is placed on a slide. A coverslip is placed over the drop, and the sample is evaluated unstained first and then staining if cells are observed.

When examining an unstained sample, it is important to achieve proper light adjustment (lower stage and partially close diaphragm to increase contrast) of the microscope. A slide using cytology techniques can also be made to better evaluate cells, intracellular bacteria, and other organisms. A drop of sediment is placed on a slide, a line smear prepared and dried with a blow dryer, and then stained (Skill Box 3.3; Figure 3.5).

The entire slide is examined with low power (10 × magnification) to look for areas of cell clusters, casts, and cellularity, paying attention to the periphery. Casts and crystals are evaluated at low power and reported as #/lpf (low-power field). Red and white blood cells, and epithelial cells are examined with high power (40 ×) and are reported as #/hpf (high-power field). Bacteria and sperm are examined under high power and reported as rare through 4+ or by using another semiquantitative scheme such as occasional, few, moderate, marked, or many.

Reporting of Bacteria, Yeast, Mucus, Fat, and Other Urine Sediment Elements[2,4,26]

None observed		
Rare	1+	< 1/hpf
Small amount	2+	1–5/hpf
Moderate amount	3+	6–20/hpf
Large amount or many	4+	> 20/hpf

Table 3.27 / Sediment examination[2,4,26]

Type	Appearance	Definition	Associated conditions
Cocci	Circular bacteria in singles, pairs or chains; refract light and have Brownian movement. Confirm with Gram stain of an air-dried smear of urine; cocci will be Gram-positive	Acid pH: *Enterococcus* and *Streptococcus* spp. Alkaline pH: *Staphylococcus* spp.	UTI, cystitis, pyelonephritis, metritis, prostatitis, vaginitis
Bacilli (Figure 3.122)	Rod-shaped bacteria in singles, pairs, or chains; refract light and have Brownian movement	Acid pH: *Escherichia coli* Alkaline pH: *Proteus* spp.	UTI, cystitis, pyelonephritis, metritis, prostatitis, vaginitis

(*Continued*)

Table 3.27 / **Sediment examination (Continued)**

Type	Appearance	Definition	Associated conditions
Blood cells			
Blood cells are reported by number per high-power field (#/hpf). Blood cells are thought to always be significant unless reviewed against other factors affecting the animal. For example, an animal with only a few RBC and no other abnormalities may have received trauma through a catheterization or cystocentesis procedure. WBCs are always thought to be significant because they typically only appear with some level of an infection, unless contamination of infected genitalia takes place. WBCs do not need to be classified into type; by the time they reach the bladder, they have degenerated to an unrecognizable state. The presence of WBCs should always result in an in-depth evaluation of a cytology slide of sediment for bacteria and bacterial culture.			

RBC (Figures 3.123 and 3.137)	Smooth edges, small, biconcave; size: 6–7 µm.
	Unstained: pale, yellow to orange discs without nuclei
	Stained: varying color from light pink to dark red
	Crenated: ruffled edges and slightly darker
	Lysed: colorless rings of varying size
	Dilute urine may show larger, swollen and globular RBC
		• Normal:
		  • Voided: 0–8/hpf
		  • Catheter: 0–5/hpf
		  • Cystocentesis: 0–3/hpf
		• A traumatic technique will produce the above numbers, multiple attempts may ↑ the number of RBC
			Cystitis, neoplasia, calculi inflammation, necrosis, trauma, bleeding disorder

WBCs Figures 3.122, 3.123, 3.127, 3.136, 3.137, 3.139)	Round with granular appearance (distinct nuclei); size: 10–14 µm. WBCs may lyse in hypotonic or alkaline urine	• Normal: voided: 0–1/hpf • Neutrophils are the most common type of WBC seen	Nephritis, pyelonephritis, cystitis, urethritis, ureteritis
Casts			
Casts are cylindrical molds of the distal and collecting tubules of the kidney and are formed from mucoproteins secreted by epithelial cells lining this area. Any element in this area may be incorporated into the protein matrix of the cast. Casts may be destroyed by high-speed centrifugation, rough handling, and delayed analysis. Degradation occurs in highly alkaline urine or if a sample is aged. The presence of ↑ numbers of casts (cylindruria) may indicate tubular disease, but the quantity does not suggest the duration or severity of disease.			
Epithelial (Figure 3.122)	Nearly transparent, clear, and highly refractive with renal epithelial cells	• Originate from the loop of Henle, distal tubule, and collecting tubule • Never observed in normal urine	Nephrotoxicity, acute renal disease, ischemia, pyelonephritis
Fatty (Figure 3.124)	Coarsely granular with fat droplets within the protein matrix	• Signify degeneration of the renal tubules	Diabetes mellitus, renal disease
Granular (Figure 3.125)	Coarse to finely granular; orange: bilirubin, pink to red: hemoglobin or myoglobin	• Composed of particulate matter from renal tubular cell necrosis or degeneration • Hyaline casts containing granules, degeneration of cellular casts • Normal: 0–2/hpf	Exercise, acute renal disease

(Continued)

Table 3.27 / **Sediment examination (Continued)**

Type	Appearance	Definition	Associated conditions
Hyaline (Figure 3.126)	Nearly transparent, clear, and highly refractile. Rounded ends Stained: light pink to purple May contain a few inclusions such as fat	• Composed of pure protein precipitates (mucoprotein matrix) • Normal: 0–2/hpf • Difficult to see and easily confused with mucous strands (variable in size with irregular margins)	Fever, mild renal disease, general anesthesia, intravenous diuresis, strenuous exercise
RBC/WBC (Figure 3.127)	RBC: contains a few to many RBC; deep yellow to orange WBC: contains a few to many WBCs. Appearance changes to granular once the cells start to degenerate	• Formed from the aggregation of RBC and/or WBCs • Not normally observed in healthy animals	Intrarenal bleeding or infection, trauma, glomerulonephritis, renal tubulointerstitial inflammation, toxicity
Waxy	Highly refractive, homogenous, and translucent. Parallel side borders, blunted ends and cracks	• Final stage of granular cast degeneration	Chronic renal disease
Crystals			
Crystalluria does not always indicate disease and may be formed through sample handling (refrigeration). Urine pH, concentration, temperature, and solubility of the components all contribute to the type of crystal formed. Crystals form in urine from a super saturation of salts. They are reported as relative numbers per low power field or are reported as occasional, moderate, many or by using a 1–4+ scale.			
Amorphous phosphate (Figure 3.128)	Granular precipitate; dull brown in color	• Typically seen in neutral or alkaline urine • Seen in normal urine • Easily confused with bacteria	Liver disease, portosystemic shunts and breed predisposed (Dalmatians and English bulldogs)
Amorphous urate (Figure 3.129)	Granular precipitate (sodium, potassium, magnesium, and calcium salts); yellow or yellow-brown in color	• Typically seen in acidic urine • Dissolve in alkaline urine • Easily confused with bacteria	Liver disease, portosystemic shunts, breed predisposed (dalmatians and English bulldogs)
Ammonium biurate (Figure 3.130)	Round with long spicules; resemble a thorn apple; yellow to brown in color	• Seen in alkaline, neutral, or slightly acidic urine	Liver disease, portosystemic shunts, urate urolithiasis, breed predisposed (dalmatians and English bulldogs)
Bilirubin (Figure 3.131)	Fine elongated spicules; red-brown or golden-yellow in color	• May be seen in small amounts in normal canine urine	Liver disease, hemolytic anemia
Calcium carbonate (Figure 3.132)	Round with lines radiating out from the center; may resemble short dumbbells	• Typically seen in alkaline urine	N/A

(*Continued*)

Table 3.27 / Sediment examination (Continued)

Type	Appearance	Definition	Associated conditions
Calcium oxalate dihydrate (Figure 3.135)	Colorless, square with refractive lines forming an × across the surface (e.g., envelopes) Radiopaque with hard, sharp protrusions ± cuboid shape	• Typically seen in neutral or acidic urine • May be seen in normal urine	Ethylene glycol toxicity and oxalate urolithiasis
Calcium oxalate monohydrate	Small, flat, elongated structures with pointed ends (picket fence, spindles)	• Typically seen in neutral or acidic urine	Ethylene glycol toxicity, and oxalate urolithiasis
Cystine	Hexagon and flat; may appear as singles or in layers	• Typically seen in acidic urine	Renal tubular dysfunction
Struvite (triple phosphate, magnesium, ammonium, and phosphate; Figures 3.124 and 3.127)	Eight-sided prisms with tapered sides and ends; resemble coffin lids. ↑ Ammonia leads to fern leaf like appearance	• Typically seen in neutral or alkaline urine	Cystitis or struvite urolithiasis
Sulfonamide	Clear to brown, eccentrically bound needles in sheaves	• Rarely seen with the newer forms of sulfonamide drugs • Lignin confirmation test, 1 drop urine + 1 drop hydrochloride on newspaper will turn yellow if sulfa metabolites are present	Sulfonamide treatment
Tyrosine	Colorless or yellow, very fine needles in sheaves or clusters	• Typically seen in acidic urine • Not well understood	Acute liver disease and chloroform or phosphorus toxicity
Uric acid	Yellow-brown diamond, rosettes, or oval plates with pointed ends	• Typically seen in acidic urine	Liver disease, portosystemic shunts, breed predisposed (dalmatians and English bulldogs)
Epithelial cells			
Squamous and transitional epithelial cells are common in urine from apparently healthy animals. Squamous epithelial cells are the largest of the epithelial cells and are considered insignificant. Transitional epithelial cells only prove to be significant with a large increase in number. Renal epithelial cells, however, are typically only seen with renal disease and always thought to be significant. They are the smallest of the epithelial cells and are often confused with WBCs but are slightly larger.			

(Continued)

Table 3.27 / **Sediment examination (Continued)**

Type	Appearance	Definition	Associated conditions
Renal (Figure 3.122)	Round to caudate with a large eccentric nucleus displaced near the bottom; prominent nucleolus; often confused with WBCs	• Epithelial cells originating from the renal tubules • Rarely found and usually indicate renal disease	Renal disease
Squamous (Figures 3.125 and 3.136)	Very large, thin, and polygonal; tend to fold on to themselves and appear singularly or in sheets; small, round nucleus, close to the center	• Epithelial cells originating from the urethra, bladder, vagina, prepuce, and skin	Common in low numbers in voided samples and typically not significant
Transitional (Figures 3.136 and 3.137)	Round to caudate, granular with a small nucleus centrally located; varying size	• Epithelial cells originating from the ureter, renal pelvis, and mostly from the bladder	Catheterization, cystitis, pyelonephritis, neoplasia
Miscellaneous			
Hemoglobin cast	Yellow-red or pink-red to brown with a smooth texture and may contain granular material	• Rare cast formed from intravascular hemolysis or myoglobinuria	Hemolytic anemia or muscle degradation
Lipid droplets (Figures 3.123 and 3.124)	Variable size, round, light green, and highly refractive; seen in the plane of field just below the coverslip	• Often confused with RBC • Commonly seen in urine associated with no disease condition	Diabetes mellitus, obesity, and hypothyroidism, common finding in cats without lipemia
Mucus threads (Figure 3.138)	Resemble twisting ribbons	• Often confused with RBC • More commonly seen after catheterization • May be seen in normal animals	Urethral irritation and genital contamination
Parasites			
Fecal contamination may lead to finding an array of parasites in urine, but the following are the only ones that originate from the bladder in the dog and cat. In heartworm positive dogs, microfilaria may be observed in urine			
Pearsonema spp. (Figure 3.100)	Clear to yellow with flattened bipolar end plugs and a roughed shell	• Bladder worm of dogs and cats • Travels through the lungs and may cause coughing	Nonpathogenic
Dioctophyma renale	Barrel shaped, bipolar, yellow brown with a pitted shell	• Giant kidney worm of the dog • Largest nematode affecting domestic animals • Ingest the parenchyma of the right kidney, leaving only the capsule • Crayfish and fish are the intermediate hosts	Renal disease and peritonitis

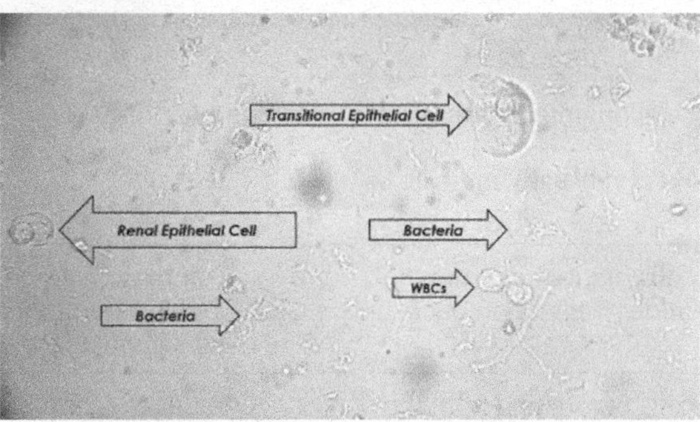

Figure 3.122 Bacteria, white blood cells, renal and transitional epithelial cell. Source: image courtesy of Barbie Papajeski.

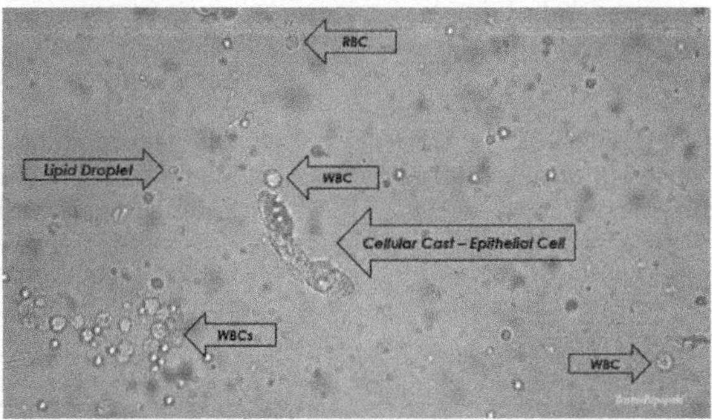

Figure 3.123 Epithelial cast, white blood cells, red blood cells, and lipid droplets. Source: image courtesy of Barbie Papajeski.

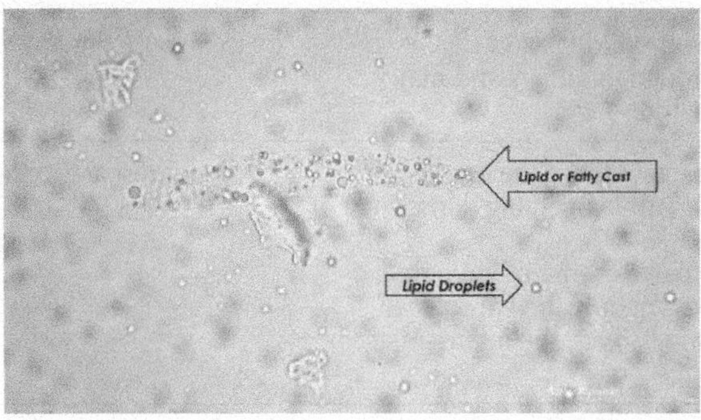

Figure 3.124 Fatty or lipid cast. Source: image courtesy of Barbie Papajeski.

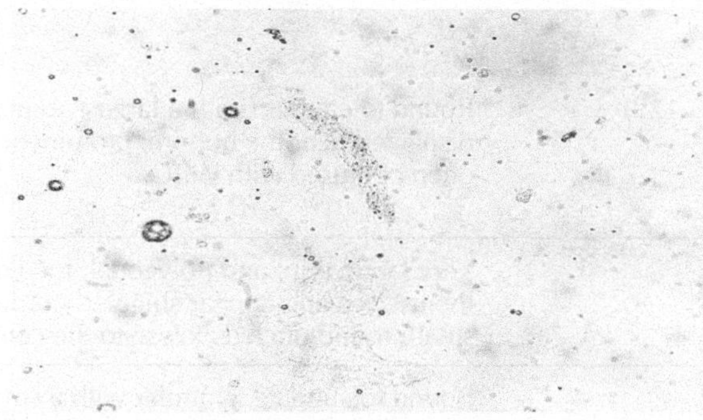

Figure 3.125 Granular cast (top) and raft of squamous epithelial cells (bottom). Source: image courtesy of Barbie Papajeski.

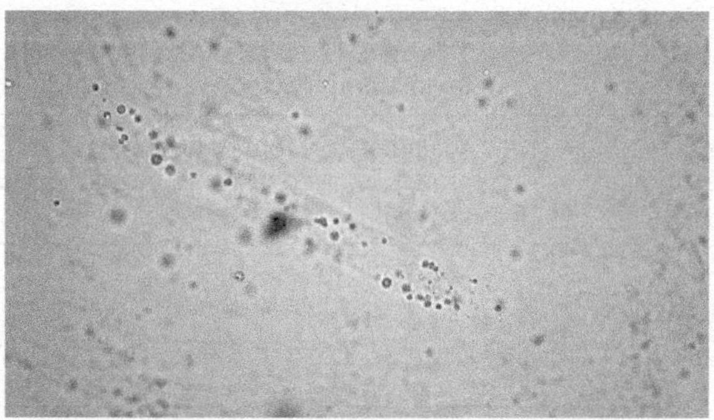

Figure 3.126 Hyaline cast. Source: image courtesy of Barbie Papajeski.

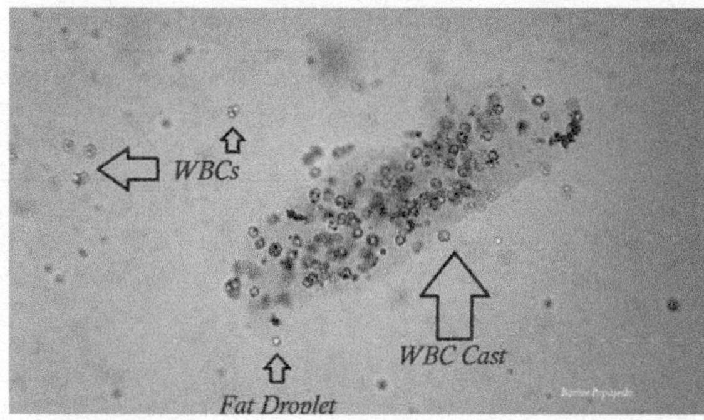

Figure 3.127 White blood cell cast stained with new methylene blue. Source: image courtesy of Barbie Papajeski.

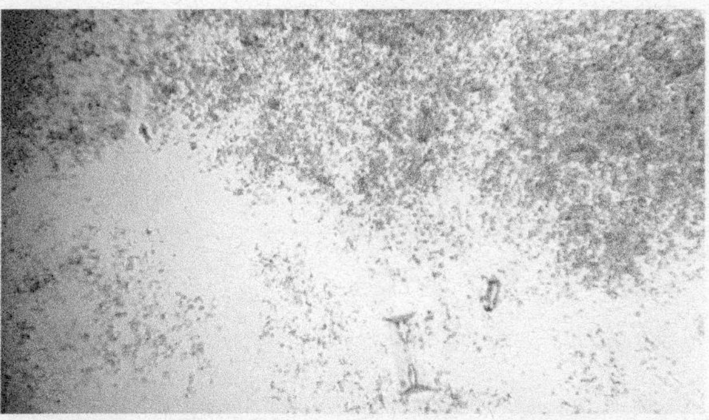

Figure 3.128 Amorphous phosphate and struvite crystals in alkaline urine. Source: image courtesy of Barbie Papajeski.

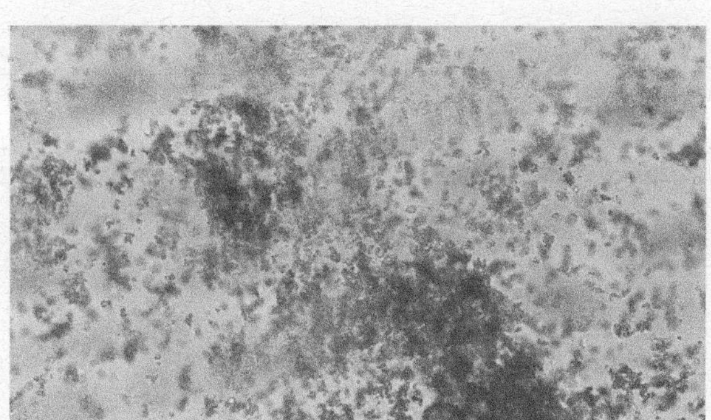

Figure 3.129 Amorphous urate in alkaline urine. Source: image courtesy of Barbie Papajeski.

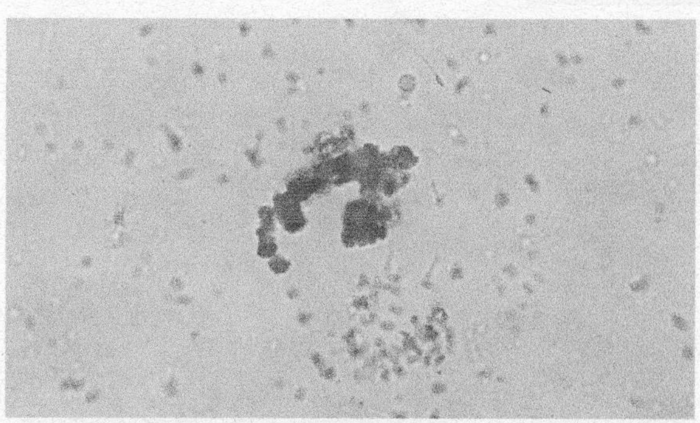

Figure 3.130 Ammonium biurate crystals and sperm cell. Source: image courtesy of Barbie Papajeski.

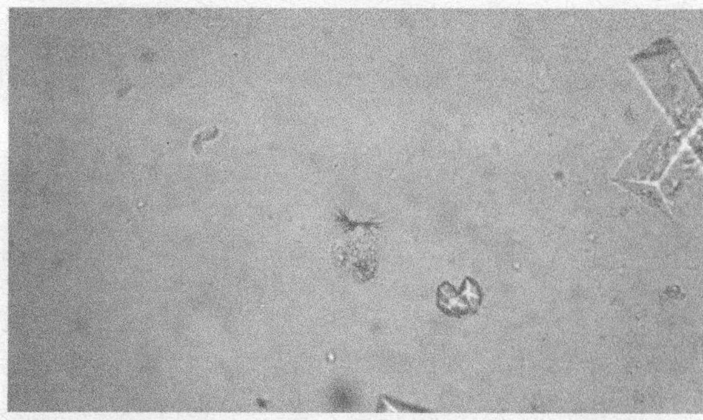

Figure 3.131 Bilirubin crystal, center. Source: image courtesy of Barbie Papajeski.

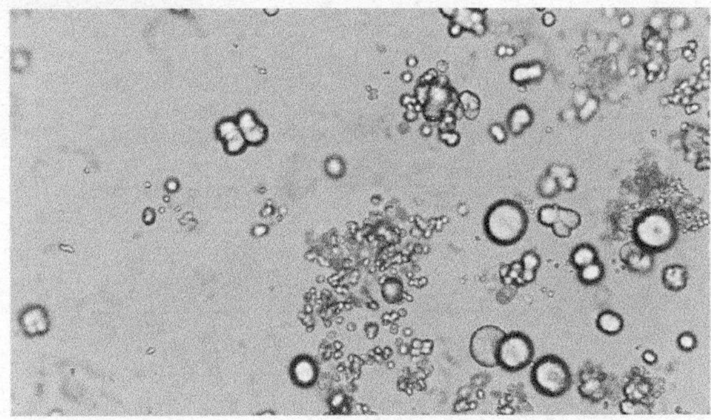

Figure 3.132 Calcium carbonate crystals. Source: image courtesy of Barbie Papajeski.

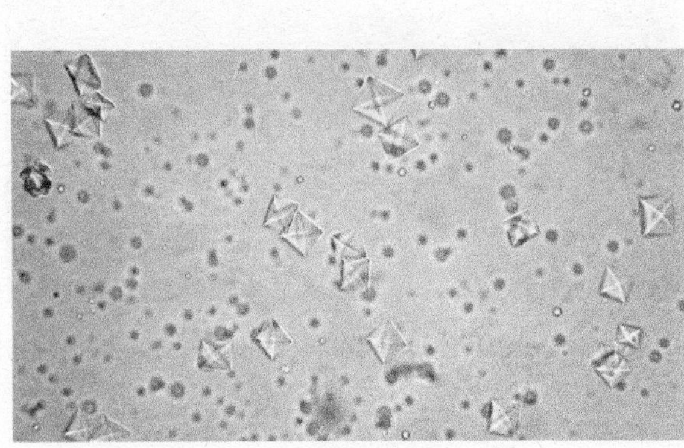

Figure 3.133 Calcium oxalate dihydrate crystals. Source: image courtesy of Barbie Papajeski.

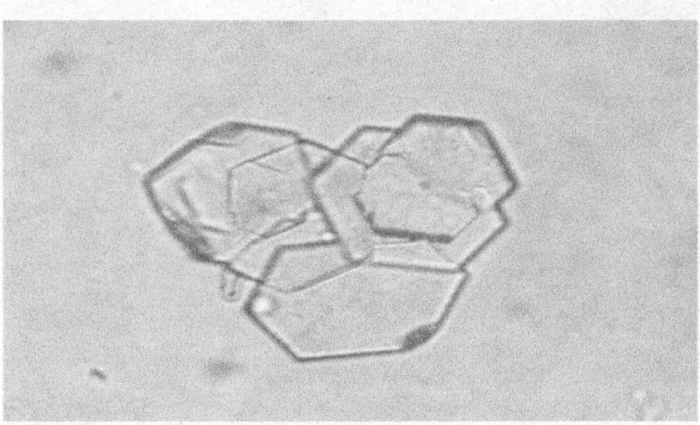

Figure 3.134 Cystine crystals and air bubbles. Source: image courtesy of Barbie Papajeski.

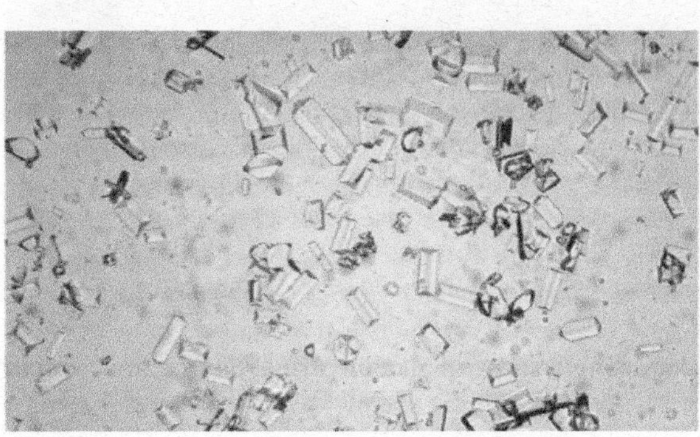

Figure 3.135 Triple phosphate crystals. Source: image courtesy of Barbie Papajeski.

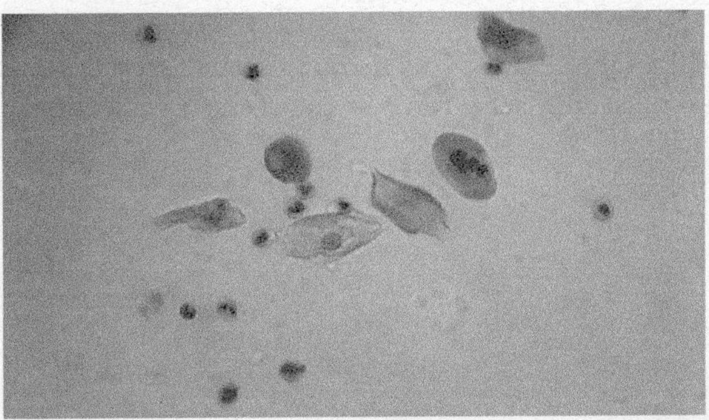

Figure 3.136 Squamous epithelials, transitional epithelials and white blood cells stained with new methylene blue. Source: image courtesy of Barbie Papajeski.

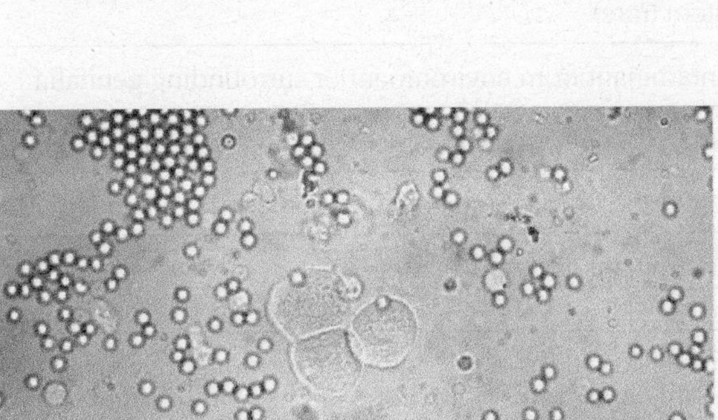

Figure 3.137 Transitional epithelial cells (center) with numerous red blood cells and a few white blood cells. Source: image courtesy of Barbie Papajeski.

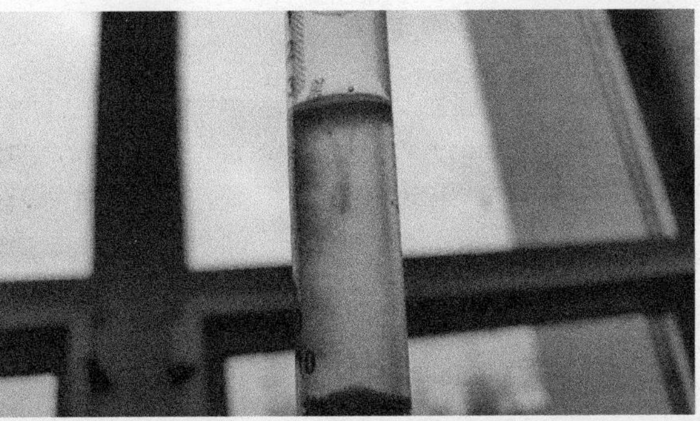

Figure 3.138 Mucus in canine urine sample. Source: image courtesy of Barbie Papajeski.

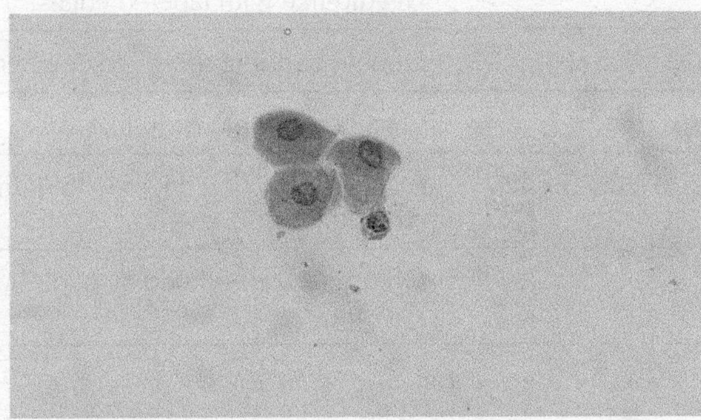

Figure 3.139 Urine cytology slide prepared from sediment and stained with quick stains showing transitional epithelial cells and a white blood cell that has phagocytized cocci bacteria. Source: image courtesy of Barbie Papajeski.

Urine Artifacts[2,4,26]

Many substances can contaminate a urine sample. They may arise from improper collection, the environment, or general anatomy. Besides the artifacts listed in Table 3.28, parasite eggs, fecal material, fungal spores, and fungi also may be seen. Please refer to the respective sections for identification of these items.

Table 3.28 / Urine artifacts

Artifact	Appearance	Definition
Air bubbles	Varying size, round, flat, refractive with a dark border	Result from the trapping of air during the application of the coverslip
Fungi	Aseptate or segmented hyphae	Contaminant; patients with systemic fungal disease affecting the urinary system (rare)
Hair	Needle-like with tapered edges	Contaminant from environment or surrounding genitalia
Pollen	Double budding spores resemble mouse ears	Contaminant from environment
Sperm (Figure 3.130)	Oval head with a whip like tail	Seen in the urine of intact males or recently mated females
Starch granules (Figure 3.140)	Faceted or scallop edges with indented or dimpled center Not refractive	Contaminant from gloves
Yeast	Oblong, colorless budding bodies with double refractive walls Varying size	Contaminant from environment or surrounding genitalia; certain species may infect the urinary tract of patients with resistant UTI (rare)

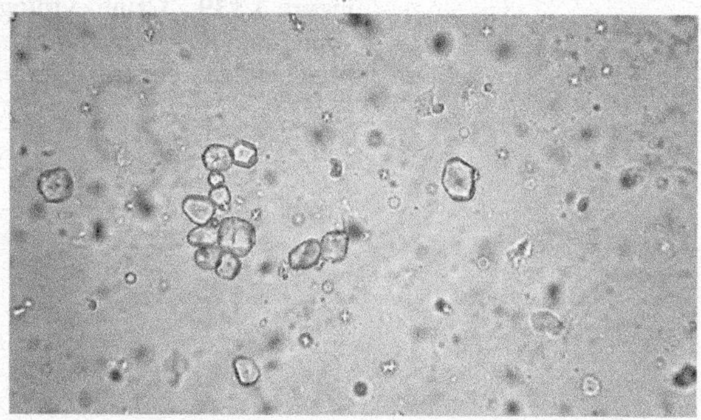

Figure 3.140 Starch granules with red blood cells and calcium oxalate dehydrate crystals. Source: image courtesy of Barbie Papajeski.

REFERENCES

1. Arnold, J.E., Camus, M.S., Freeman, K.P. et al. (2019). ASVCP Guidelines: Principles of Quality Assurance and Standards for Veterinary Clinical Pathology (version 3.0). *Veterinary Clinical Pathology* 48: 542–618.
2. Cornell University College of Veterinary Medicine. (2020). Hematology. *eClinPath* http://www.eclinpath.com/hematology (accessed 27 June 2021).
3. Sirois, M. (2015). Laboratory Procedures for Veterinary Technicians, 6e. St. Louis, MO: Elsevier Mosby.
4. Thrall, M.A. (2012). Veterinary Hematology and Clinical Chemistry. Ames, IA: Wiley-Blackwell.
5. Valenciano, A.C. and Cowell, R.L. (2014). Cowell and Tyler's Diagnostic Cytology and Hematology of the Dog and Cat, 4e. St. Louis, MO: Elsevier.
6. Fields, S.E. (2015). Hematologic reference ranges. *Merck Veterinary Manual.* Kenilworth, NJ: Merck Sharp & Dohme Corp. https://www.merckvetmanual.com/special-subjects/reference-guides/hematologic-reference-ranges (accessed 27 June 2021).
7. Michigan State University Veterinary Diagnostic Laboratory. (2021). Endocrinology Reference Ranges. Revision 20. https://cvm.msu.edu/vdl/laboratory-sections/endocrinology (accessed 27 June 2021).
8. Cornell University Animal Health Diagnostic Laboratory. (2019). Tests and submissions fact sheets. https://www.vet.cornell.edu/animal-health-diagnostic-center/programs/nyschap/modules-and-documents (accessed 27 June 2021).
9. Texas A&M University Gastrointestinal Laboratory. (2021). Cardiac troponin: reference intervals – canine. http://vetmed.tamu.edu/gilab/service/assays/cardiac-troponin (accessed 27 June 2021).
10. IDEXX Reference Laboratories. (2019). Directory of tests and services. https://www.idexx.com/en/veterinary/reference-laboratories/tests-and-services (accessed 27 June 2021).
11. Chandler, M.L. (2009). Practical matters: desmopressin is safer than water deprivation to identify the cause of polyuria and polydipsia in dogs. *dvm360.* http://veterinarymedicine.dvm360.com/practical-matters-desmopressin-safer-water-deprivation-identify-cause-polyuria-and-polydipsia-dogs (accessed 27 June 2021).
12. Budach, S.C. and Mueller, R.S. (2012). Reproducibility of a semi quantitative method to assess cutaneous cytology. *Veterinary Dermatology* 23: 426–e80.
13. Metzger, F.L. and Rebar, A. (2004). Three-minute peripheral blood film evaluation. *dvm360.* http://veterinarymedicine.dvm360.com/three-minute-peripheral-blood-film-evaluation-preparing-film (accessed 27 June 2021).
14. Papajeski, B.M. (August, 2018). Diagnostic blood smear preparation. *Veterinary Team Brief* August. 37–41.
15. Biomedical Polymers. (2012). Instructions for BMP Leukochek. https://www.corelabsupplies.com/assets/pdf/BMP-LeukoChek-Procedural-Instructions.pdf (accessed 27 June 2021).
16. Academy of Veterinary Clinical Pathology Technicians. (2015). AVCPT Formula Guide. https://avcpt.net/candidate_packet/resources (accessed 27 June 2021).
17. Paltrinieri, S., Paciletti V., and Zambarbieri, J. (2018). Analytical variability of estimated platelet counts on canine blood smears. *Veterinary Clinical Pathology* 47: 197–204.
18. Reagan, W.J., Irizarry, R.A., DeNicola, D.B.et al. (2019). *Veterinary Hematology: Atlas of common domestic and non-domestic species*, 3e. hoboken, NJ: Wiley Blackwell.
19. Companion Animal Parasite Council. (2020). General guidelines for dogs and cats. https://capcvet.org/guidelines/general-guidelines (accessed 27 June 2021).
20. Quinn, P.J., Markey, B.K., Leonard, F.C. et al. (2011). *Veterinary Microbiology and Microbial Disease*, 2e. Chichester: Wiley Blackwell.
21. Doan, T. Melvold, R., Viselli, S. et al. (2013). *Immunology*, 2e. Baltimore, MD: Lippincott Williams & Wilkins.
22. Vemulapalli, T.H. and Hammac, K.G. (2015). *Microbiology for Veterinary Technicians*. Bloomington, IN: Animalibris Publishing.
23. Zimbro, M.J., Power, D.A., Miller, S.M. et al. (2009). *DifcoTM & BBLTM Manual of Microbiological Culture Media*, 2e. Sparks, MD: Becton Dickinson & Company.
24. Hendrix, C.H. and Robinson, E. (2017). *Diagnostic Parasitology for Veterinary Technicians*, 5e. St. Louis, MO: Elsevier.
25. Zajac, A.M. and Conboy, G.A. (2012). *Veterinary Clinical Parasitology*, 8e. Chichester: Wiley Blackwell.
26. Sink, C. A., Weinstein, N., & Marlowe, A. (2012). *Practical Veterinary Urinalysis*. Chichester: Wiley Blackwell.

Chapter 4

Imaging

Marg Brown, RVT, BEdAdEd

Veterinary Technician and Nurse's Daily Reference Guide: Canine and Feline, Fourth Edition. Edited by Mandy Fults and Kenichiro Yagi.

Companion website: www.wiley.com/go/fults/veterinary

Abbreviations

ALARA, as low as reasonably achievable
BCS, body condition score
CHF, congenital heart failure
CRT, capillary refill time
CT, computed tomography
DV, dorsoventral
IV, intravenous
kV, kilovoltage
L-LAT, left lateral
LAT, lateral
ma, milliamperage
mAs, milliampere-seconds
MRI, magnetic resonance imaging
NCRP, National Council on Radiation Protection and Measurements
OBL, oblique
R-LAT, right lateral
R-VD, right ventrodorsal
SID, source–image distance
Sv, Sieverts
TMJ, temporomandibular joint
VD, ventrodorsal
w/v, weight per volume

RADIOGRAPHY

Radiographic imaging is an extremely useful diagnostic tool for the veterinarian, and veterinary technicians are a valuable resource in their production. An understanding of the anatomic layout of the species and the manner in which a radiographic image is taken is of great assistance to the production of a diagnostic image. This chapter contains basic information about radiographic equipment, imaging factors, positioning information, and contrast radiography.

The greatest risk associated with radiography is patient and staff safety. It has been scientifically proven that ionizing radiation causes damage to living cells (e.g. reproductive, growth, gonadal, cancer, metabolically active cells). There is no level of exposure that is non-damaging; therefore, caution should be taken to limit exposure to the lowest level possible.

Radiographic Equipment

Radiographic equipment is expensive and extreme care should be taken with its use and maintenance. Digital radiography is expanding in the veterinary field. Technically, there are different types of digital units. Computed radiography is any imaging system that relies on photostimulable luminescence to make a radiographic image. Direct digital radiography systems produce digital radiographs from the photoelectric interaction of x-rays with the detector itself. Indirect digital radiography systems are sensitive to the light produced by an intensification screen, while optically coupled direct radiography systems use optical components to focus fluorescence onto charge coupled detectors. In this chapter, digital radiography includes any radiographic image acquired without photographic film.

Similar ancillary radiography equipment is used for computed and digital radiography, and film systems, and similar concepts such as collimation and grids apply, although grids are not required in some digital systems because vendor software can manipulate the final image.

Classic technical errors such as malpositioning, patient motion, incorrect patient identification, incorrect examination, and double exposure still occur with digital radiography. Radiation is not lower in computed and digital imaging, so the same principles of radiation safety apply.

The advantages of digital radiography include increased time efficiency in processing, storing, and retrieving of radiographs, improved contrast resolution, allowing soft tissue and bone evaluation in one image, and the ability to use teleradiology. There is also the ability to change the contrast and density of the image to improve diagnostic sensitivity, so fewer retakes are required, but this technique can also add artifacts, leading to confusion and misdiagnosis. Provided positioning is correct, retakes should be minimized with computer manipulation and the increased efficiency of the digital radiography unit.

Table 4.1 / Ancillary radiographic equipment

Equipment	Description	Maintenance
Protective apparel	• Aprons • Thyroid shields, lead glasses • Gloves • Dosimeter (worn to monitor the amount of radiation exposure to the wearer); generally, a report is generated every 3 months to be posted at the clinic)	• Hang aprons vertically or lay flat • Gloves should be placed on vertical holders or over bottomless soup cans to allow air flow and to avoid cracks in the lead lining • Radiograph all apparel quarterly to assess protectiveness of shield and check for cracks, tears, or other irregularities
Positioning devices	• Tape, gauze, towels • Velcro strapping, sandbags, troughs, foam wedges	• Replace as needed • Clean after use
Film-screen radiography		
Processing tanks	• Develops the film • May be manual or automatic	• Clean routinely and replenish liquids as needed • Clean thoroughly every 2–3 months • Check the manufacturer's guidelines for your specific machine
Film	• Imprints the image (various types)	• Handle carefully • Store unused film in a vertical position in a cool, dry, dark place
Cassettes	• Houses the film and intensifying screens	• Do not drop or allow leaking liquids into the cassette • Clean the exterior regularly with mild soap and water • Clean the intensifying screens routinely with a commercial solution, mild soap and water, or dilute ethyl alcohol • Leave the cassette open and propped in a vertical position to dry • Store in a vertical position when loaded with film
Computed radiography		
Reader	• Reads the image from the image plate	
Image plate	• Imprints the image	• Erase the plates daily • Clean the plates once a week
Computer	• Manipulates and permits viewing of the image	
Direct digital radiography		
Image plate within the System	• Uses a direct energy conversion process to capture the image	• Offset calibration daily

Table 4.2 / Radiographic exposure and image factors

Factor	Definition	Application
Contrast	The difference between the lightest and darkest part of the film, reflecting two adjacent radiographic densities	• High kV (low contrast = more shades of gray) preferred for tissue • Low kV (high contrast = fewer shades of gray) preferred for bone
Density	The degree of blackness of a film	• To produce a darker film: ↑ mA, kV, or exposure time
Detail	The clarity of the image on the film	• For better detail, use a longer SID, have the patient closer to the film/image, and use a shorter exposure time
Distortion	The alteration of the original image causing penumbra due to factors such as magnification and incorrect angles	• For less distortion, avoid short SID, have the patient closer to the film/image, and use less angulation of the film or patient
Exposure time (second)	Measures the length of time electrons flow across the tube	• Longer exposure time = ↑ production of x-rays • mAs is the product of milliamperage and the exposure time. It indicates the number of x-rays being produced during an exposure • Using a high mA setting allows for the use of shorter exposure times because mAs and mA are inversely proportional
Grid	The ↑ in exposure required to compensate for absorption of the beam by the grid device	• Changes the exposure required when not used
Kilovoltage (kV)	Measurement of the electric potential difference between the cathode and anode in the x-ray tube	• ↑ kV = greater penetration power • Controls the quality of the beam • Directly proportional to film density and inversely proportional to film contrast • Sometimes referred to as kVp which is the peak voltage applied to the x-ray tube
Milliamperage (mA)	Measurement of the number of electrons that flow across the tube from cathode to anode	• ↑ mA = production of more x-rays • Directly proportional to film density
Milliampere-second (mAs)	The number of x-rays produced per second	• Controls the number and quantity of x-rays produced
Source–image distance (SID)	The distance between the source of x-rays on the target anode, known as the focal spot, and the radiographic film/image detector; formerly called focal spot to film distance	• ↑ SID = ↓ in number of x-rays reaching the film

Radiographic Technique Chart for Film Radiography

Technique charts are predetermined x-ray machine settings that are developed for a specific machine based on tissue thickness, anatomy, position, and factors such as source–image distance (SID), film type, cassette screen, and development process. If you change any of these factors within your practice, the technique chart will need to be updated. A basic knowledge is important so that any changes can readily be implemented to ensure optimal images. Technique charts are commonly set up with the use of a patient. The basic process is:

1. Choose an animal of respective size to reflect its species (e.g. canine: an animal around 50lb; feline: an animal around 9lb).
2. Accurately measure the animal laterally around the thickest part of the abdomen. Set standard SID as a constant (40 cm).
3. Calculate the kilovoltage (kV) requirement using Santes' rule:

$$(2 \times \text{tissue thickness in cm}) + \text{SID} + \text{grid factor} = \text{kV}.$$

Example:

$$(2 \times 15\,\text{cm}) + 40 + 8 = 78\,\text{kV}$$

4. Milliampere-seconds (mAs) setting will depend on the type of x-ray unit, speed of film, and screens used. If a faster system is used and the mAs is 7.5 for the abdomen, extremities will require about 2.5 (there will be no grid), the thorax about 5.0 mAs, the pelvis 10 and 1.5 mAs for a cat.
5. Depending on the anatomical tissue, a grid is often used for a thickness greater than 10 cm to absorb scatter radiation produced with higher kV settings.
6. Since the body is composed of about 80% water, a plastic flat-bottomed bucket can also be used to set up a technique chart. The amount of water in the bucket equates to the body measurement in thickness. Values similar to Sante's rule would be used. When the image is exposed and processed, the density should be a uniform light silver-gray.
7. Determine the milliamperage (mA) and exposure time with emphasis on the highest mA possible. Divide mA by mAs to get exposure time (seconds); for example:

$$300\,\text{mA} \div 5.0\,\text{mAs} = 1/60.$$

8. Take a trial radiograph using the calculated factors and assess its quality.
   a. There is a relationship between kV and mAs, so if the film density is too dark, either the mAs setting could be halved or the kV decreased by 15% (multiply the original by 0.85 between 55 and 95 kV). Table 4.3 determines which factor should be changed.
   b. If the film density is too light, either double the mAs or increase the kV by 15% (multiply the original kV by 1.15 between 55 and 90 kV). Table 4.3 indicates which factor should be changed.
9. The technique chart can be formulated once the correct exposure factors are determined. Subtract or add 2 kV for each centimeter decrease or increase from the original measurement up to 80 kV. Add 3 kV for each centimeter increase between 80 and 100 kV, and 4 kV for each centimeter increase up to 125 kV.
10. It is helpful to have your chart reviewed by a board-certified radiologist.
11. Factors may need to be modified and changes made from an operational technique chart for variations.
    a. An increase in exposure may be required if there is pleural fluid, ascites, obvious organ enlargement, obesity, heavily muscled dogs, positive contrast studies, or bandages, casts, and splints (Table 4.5).
    b. A decrease in exposure may be required with excessively thin patients, puppies or kittens.
12. It is usually better to change the mAs first assuming that you have enough penetration, rather than altering kV. mAs is directly proportional to image density while kV changes are logarithmic affecting both contrast and density.
13. If exposure factors are normally satisfactory but the film is too light, aging of processing chemicals or low temperatures may be the problem.
14. If a change in technique does not improve a dull gray image, assume fogging has occurred.

Digital Radiography Technique Charts

Technique charts for digital systems are less complicated, allowing mAs and kV to expose a wide range of body tissues and sizes. In digital units, program algorithms are used more than actual technique charts, often using the patient's weight rather than tissue thickness. Adjustments are made depending on patient variations.

Grids may be removed by vendors in digital units. Any scattered radiation is incorporated into the algorithm. Contrast will still be increased if grids are available.

Collimation is essential. All the exposed portion of the plate is used by the algorithm. There will be reduced contrast on the image if there is improper collimation because the uncollimated densities and the anatomy is averaged by the algorithm.

Digital Image Quality

Digital radiography has several further concepts that are not relevant in film radiography. The image is converted into an electronic form that is digitized and numerically encoded into tiny, discrete squares known as pixels. Each pixel only displays one shade of gray from a black to white intensity. The pixel size and spacing affects spatial resolution, which is the ability to separate two closely spaced objects. The smaller and more numerous the pixels, the better the spatial resolution. If there is magnification, pixilation and a loss of quality will result. Together with the algorithm, the histogram also affects how the image is produced electronically. The histogram or graphic display of the image takes into account how many times a pixel with certain brightness occurs.

Every image is a combination of spatial resolution and contrast resolution. Contrast resolution is expressed as the values of black and white. The highest contrast available is an image that is completely black and white with no intervening shades of gray. The descriptor for contrast resolution is dynamic range or many shades of gray. Digital detectors have a wider and greater linear dynamic range than film radiography, which means that images with good contrast characteristics can be produced over a wide range of exposure values. Exposure errors do not result in images with loss of contrast as with film. Wider dynamic range or wide latitude means that more attention needs to be paid to exposure indicator values rather than to brightness and contrast.

A wide latitude has many shades of gray, which permits both bone and soft tissues to be seen at the same exposure setting when the full exposure range is captured. Digital processing can then be used to enhance and optimize the contrast. Since digital systems automatically compensate for overexposures and underexposures, mAs is not related to image blackening in digital imaging, provided there is no severe underexposure, resulting in too few x-ray photons striking the imaging plate. Underexposure causes "quantum mottle" or "noise", which leaves a mottled, grainy image with poor resolution. Excessive quantum noise is a potential problem in digital radiography because it is possible to produce images with low exposures that will still produce good contrast. Noise is reduced with increased exposure and imaging processing.

Correct exposure produces an image with an acceptable noise level without unnecessary or excessive exposure to the patient and personnel. There is also the ability to convert very high doses into acceptable images, which means that the mAs can be much higher than necessary to produce an image. However, depending on the amount of post-processing alteration required, contrast and resolution can be compromised if acceptable technique is not initially applied. Dose "creep", or using more radiation than necessary, occurs if the patient is measured incorrectly, if parameters are set too high, or if one assumes that technical factors will compensate for increased exposure. Other factors that are significant in manipulating and viewing digital imaging quality are monitor resolution, pixel density, and brightness.

To produce images, the digital radiography device must be properly calibrated, configured, maintained, and operated. Every individual device must be calibrated for overall gain and uniformity.

Evaluating Radiograph Technique

To determine whether the image needs to be adjusted, one must first be able to evaluate the quality of a film. There are some basic guidelines to a properly exposed image, but there is also veterinarian preference. Begin by evaluating the overall appearance (e.g. too light or too dark) of the radiograph. If it is determined that an image is too light or too dark, further evaluations need to take place to find the cause.

Table 4.3 / Exposure evaluation

Area exposed	Underexposed (too light)	Good exposure	Overexposed (too dark)
Hand test for film radiographs	• Fingers, wrinkles, and creases all visible when held under the film while examining on a standard viewing box	• Fingers visible but not the wrinkles and creases when held under the film while examining on a standard viewing box	Fingers not visible when held under the film while examining on a standard viewing box
Thorax	• Visible: surrounding vasculature • Not visible: vasculature over the heart, lung over diaphragm	• Visible: caudal vena cava, descending aorta, bronchi, pulmonary vessels, cardiac silhouette, air-filled lungs • Taken on inspiration • Optimal: high kV and low mAs (low contrast and ↓ density)	Lungs are as black as the background
Abdomen	• Internal organs are washed out and are not distinguishable	• Visible: margins of the internal organs, stomach, diaphragm, small and large intestines, liver, spleen, bladder, ± kidneys, prostate • Taken on expiration • Optimal: high kV and low mAs (low contrast and ↓ density) ↓	Internal organs are dark and not distinguishable
Bony structures	• Bone is bright white with no detail	• Clear margins of compact bone with a radiolucent center) • Optimal: low kV and high mAs (high contrast and ↑ density)	Bone is dark with no detail

Density Evaluation

The density of a film is the degree of blackness and is mostly controlled by mAs in film radiography. mAs is directly proportional to image density, and does not appreciably alter image contrast if the density is correct. Begin evaluating the density by determining the degree of blackness. The area outside the patient's body and inside the collimated area should be black. Lighter shades would indicate an increase in density is needed.

SID is inversely proportional to image distance squared. A change in SID means a change in image density. SID does not alter image contrast if image density is correct. To compensate for the change in SID, use the equation:

$$\text{Old mAs} \times (\text{new distance})^2 / (\text{old SID})^2 = \text{new mAs setting}$$

Contrast Evaluation

The scale of contrast is the shades of gray or the degree of black and white, and is mostly controlled by kV. Kv is directly proportional to image density and inversely proportional to image contrast. Low kV provides low density and high contrast, known as a short scale, with large differences between each step (e.g. strong blacks and whites). A kV setting that is too high will give too much density with a lack of contrast (e.g. overall gray or dark appearance). There is a long scale of contrast with fewer differences between each step.

Once a radiograph has been evaluated and it is determined that alterations are needed, the decision needs to be made as to what settings need to be altered. Unfortunately, this is not an exact science and adjustments of one or more settings may be needed. However, there are some general starting points when adjusting the settings. In general, mAs is altered by 50% to make large overall changes to alter the density (degree of blackness). kV is altered by 10–15% to make small subtle changes to the density and to alter the scale of contrast.

Altering the kV by 10–15% is approximately the same change in exposure as altering the mAs by 50% (e.g. halving or doubling the mAs). Therefore, if there is proper exposure or film density, but the contrast needs to be changed, alter the kV and mAs together in the opposite direction (e.g. increased kV and lowered mAs for less contrast).

Table 4.4 / Scale of contrast evaluation

Film evaluation	Solution	Example
↑ film density • Film is too dark. You cannot see the soft tissue but still see bones so the contrast has not significantly been altered	↓ mAs • To ↓ the amount of x-rays and ↓ the blackness • The overall contrast will not change but film density will be lower	
↓ film density • Film is too light but anatomical parts are clearly visible	↑ mAs • To ↑ the amount of x -rays and ↑ the blackness • The contrast or differences between the tissues will not change but the film density will be darker	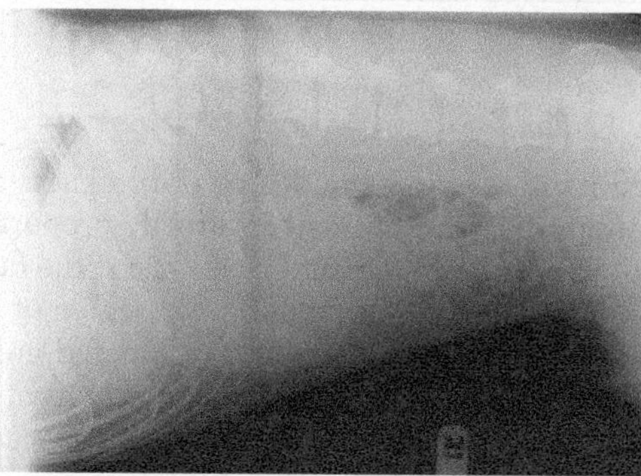

(Continued)

Table 4.4 / Scale of contrast evaluation (Continued)

Film evaluation	Solution	Example
↓ contrast • Film is washed out or has a gray appearance – both the bone and tissue are dark), the problem is over penetration (kV is too high); look in the cranial abdomen	↓ kV • To ↓ the penetrating power of the x-rays and to shorten the scale of contrast • There will be greater difference between tissue and bone and less gradations or steps • Film will be less dense or black	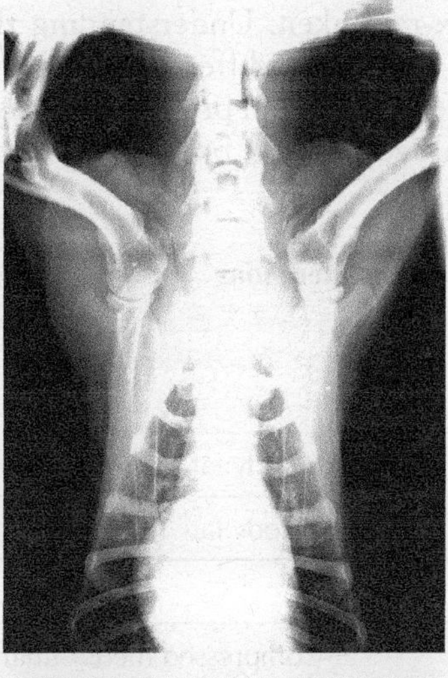
↑ film contrast • Film has strong blacks and whites; the anatomical parts are not clearly visible	↑ kV • To ↑ the penetrating power of the x-rays and to lengthen the scale of contrast so there are more graduations with fewer differences between tissues and bones • Together with decreased contrast, there will be more blackness or film density	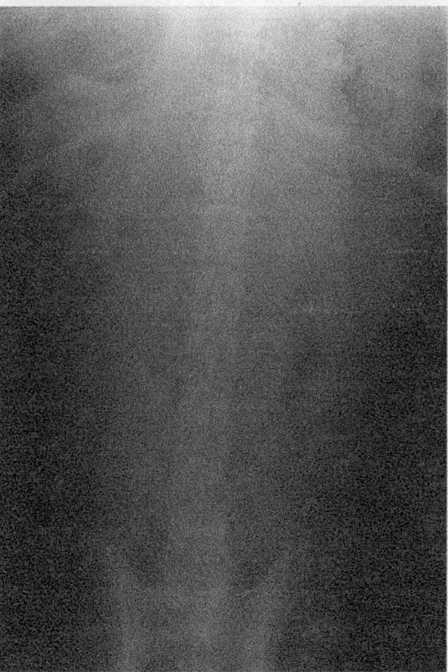

Radiographic Alterations and Artifacts

With radiology experience, adjustments to the mAs and kV can be made prior to the first x-ray taken. Understanding their relationship, together with the patient's individual differences based on body condition score, breed, and disease condition can produce the desired quality of radiograph. Certain anatomical factors (e.g. body weight, muscle mass, hair coat) are known to alter the image based on the technique chart. The technique chart is based on an 'average' animal and alteration from the average often require adjustments in the settings. The most important point to remember is that large changes are made with mAs and subtle changes are made with kV.

Table 4.5 / **Radiographic alterations**

Evaluation	Radiograph effect	Setting alteration	Comments
BCS			
BCS 1–2	↓ Body fat, muscle wasting	↓ mAs or kV	↓ Subject density
BCS 4–5	↑ Body fat	↑ mAs or kV	↑ Subject density
Breed and anatomy			
Achondroplastic dwarf	Compressed mediastinal area-short dense legs	↑ mAs or kV	↑ Subject density Use tape or strips to pull legs out of the view
Barrel-chested	↑ Thoracic size	↑ mAs	↑ Subject density Extend cervical region as far forward as possible
Brachycephalic	X-rays not taken on inspiration/expiration; motion artifacts	↓ mAs or kV to ↓ density	Blow on nose to briefly stop panting
Deep-chested	Deep cranial thorax and thin caudal thorax	↓ mAs or kV	Two views may be required to achieve proper exposure in both regions. True VD images required to avoid oblique images
Giant breeds	↑ Overall size	↑ mAs	↑ Subject density. Divide thorax into cranial and caudal to view the entire area
Hair coat	Excessive amount or mats Debris and foreign bodies	↑ kV	↑ Subject density. Move excessive hair out of view if possible. Verify that any imaged foreign bodies are not within the hair coat
Muscle	↑ Muscle mass	↑ mAs or kV	↑ Subject density. Ensure proper positioning of VD images (e.g. supportive devices) to avoid oblique images
Skin	↑ Skin folds	↑ mAs or kV	↑ Subject density. Pull skin folds out of view if possible
Disease			

(Continued)

Table 4.5 / **Radiographic alterations (Continued)**

Evaluation	Radiograph effect	Setting alteration	Comments
Any condition resulting in	Ascites/edema	↑ mAs and ±↓ kV	↑ kV along with free fluid = ↑ scatter
	Free air	↓ mAs or kV	↓ Subject density
	Foreign bodies	± mAs and kV alterations	Adjustments are made based on the opacity of the item
	Soft tissue swelling	↑ mAs or kV	↑ Subject density

Table 4.6 / **Radiographic artifacts**

Problems seen on film radiograph	Artifact	Solution
Blurred images	Motion double exposure	• Proper positioning and handling of patient • Do not trigger the foot pedal twice; remove the cassette after each exposure
Black or gray areas partially covering the film	Film fogging	• Proper handling and storing of the film
Clear areas on the sides of the radiograph	Mislocation of beam to film	• Verification that the beam and cassette are aligned and that the cassette is pushed all the way in
Dark line with mirror image of object	Film folded on itself	• Proper loading of cassette
Dark semicircle impression	Finger pressure mark	• Proper handling of film
Dark striations (sea lichen or dotted)	Static electricity	• Proper handling of film
Gray streaks	Wet animal fur	• Clean off and dry patient
White lines or objects visualized outside/inside the |patient's body that are unexplainable.	Foreign objects in or on the cassette (hair, paper, etc.)	• Proper cleaning of cassette and proper handling of film
White lines across the film	Scratches on the film	• Proper handling of film

Table 4.7 / Digital artifacts[2]

Problems seen with digital radiography	Artifact
Underexposure (if ¼–½ settings used	• Quantum mottle or noise showing as a grainy appearance
Overexposure that cannot be manipulated (if greater than 10 times exposure level)	• Disappearance of thin tissues or soft tissues surrounding bone • Loss of subject contrast • Poor contrast
Lucent halo around metal implants	• Uberschwinger artifact or rebound effect that may be mistaken for bone lysis
Nonuniform appearance of the image	• Improper use of heel effect • Contrast media on table or detector (seen mostly with contrast radiography systems)
Ghost images	• Previous high exposure remaining on digital radiograph detector panel and then taking an image quickly • Double exposures on contrast radiography cassette • Improper erasure of a contrast radiography plate in the reader
Fogging	• Extraneous radiation on contrast radiography plate from any source
White spots	• Scratches on contrast radiography imaging plate • Hair, dirt, or other particles trapped in the contrast radiography cassette
Planking artifact	• Linear striations in background of image caused by plate saturation, or overexposure

Radiographic Safety and Positioning

X-rays are forms of ionizing electromagnetic radiation that have wavelengths much shorter than that of visible light, causing penetration of some substances and energy absorption by other material. All tissues are sensitive to ionizing radiation, so attention to safety is absolutely essential when working with radiation.

Interaction between x-rays and tissues occurs at the atomic level, but visible injury results from ionizing effects of macromolecules (DNA) and water. Injury to cells, tissues, and organs occurs at the time of exposure, but may require time or a generation to show damage. Damage in the body includes both genetic damage and somatic cell damage. Genetic damage occurs to the DNA of reproductive cells, which may not be detected until later generations. Somatic cell damage manifests at some point but, because of tissue repair, the damage may not be obvious. The area of the cell that is most sensitive to ionization is the nucleus of proliferating somatic and genetic cells with greater sensitivity occurring in those tissues and organs with a higher metabolic rate and of growing individuals.

The National Council on Radiation Protection and Measurements (NCRP), under the recommendations of the International Commission on Radiological Protection, sets the maximum permissible dose of radiation measured in Sieverts (Sv) that a person may receive in a given period. The NCRP requires that dosimeters or personal exposure monitoring devices be properly worn by each individual involved in taking radiographs every time he or she is in the vicinity of the radiation. These are then sent to approved laboratories for evaluation. For more information, contact the radiation protection service of the department of health of your state or province or the International Commission on Radiological Protection (icrp.org).

Always keep the NCRP-developed ALARA ("as low as reasonably achievable") principle in mind when restraining patients and working with x-rays. It is essential to follow the essential components of radiation safety – minimum time, maximum distance and maximum shielding – consistently to achieve ALARA. As long as the maximum permissible dose of radiation is not reached, most provincial and state regulations allow occupationally exposed persons to restrain and position patients when absolutely necessary, but other states or provinces prohibit any manual restraint. Every staff member who is involved in taking radiographic images must wear an individual dosimeter badge. Remember there is no such thing as safe radiation.

There are many radiation safety practices that must be adhered to but the most important is not to be exposed at all. Distance is the best protection. Shielding includes protective apparel such as lead aprons, thyroid shields, gloves, and lead glasses. No positioner body part should ever be in the primary beam. Wear goggles and stay as far back from the primary beam and subsequent scatter radiation as possible. Avoid excessive and unnecessary exposure. Use the shortest exposure time possible making sure that the resulting image is ideal to avoid retakes. This is especially important in digital radiography, where there can be a tendency to take extra images.

Proper patient alignment is essential for high-quality images. These can easily be obtained with non-manual restraint, through the use of supports such as sandbags, nonradiopaque wedges, nonradiopaque "V" troughs, towels, Velcro (Figure 4.1), bungee cords, gauze tape, and chemicals. Every effort should be made so that the patient is not held during the exposure. Use calm, deliberate movements, be patient and use positioning devices so the patient has the illusion it is being held. See the Hands-Free Xrays website from the Safe Veterinary Radiography Initiative (handsfreexrays.com) for excellent suggestions.

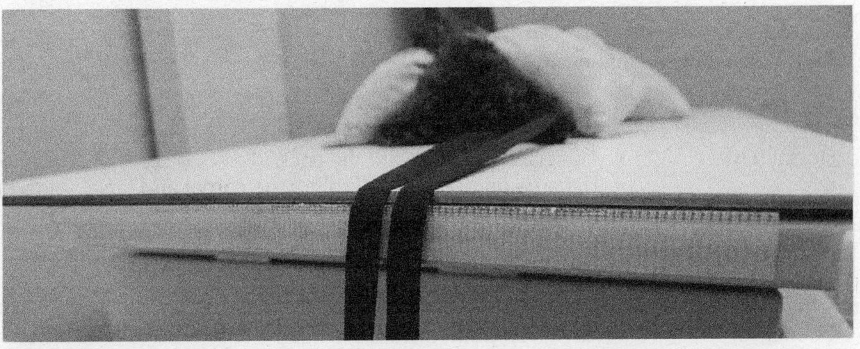

Figure 4.1 Velcro straps wrapped around the limbs and then secured to Velcro tape on the x-ray table, secures the patient and allows for quick removal.

Another important factor in positioning a patient for radiographs is to have a mental vision of the part of the body to be radiographed and a good understanding of its anatomic placement. Understanding directional terminology is critical to the proper positioning of every radiograph. Specific anatomical landmarks are identified in Chapter 1.

Table 4.8 / **Directional terms**

Directional term	Definition
Dorsal (D)	• Any given point toward the back • The area on or below (distal to) the carpal and tarsal joints on the limbs toward the head
Ventral (V)	• Any given point toward the lower area of the thorax and abdomen, closest to the ground
Cranial (C)	• Any given point toward the head • The area above or proximal to the carpal and tarsal joints on the limbs toward the head
Caudal (Cd)	• Any given point toward the tail • The area above the carpal and tarsal joints on the limbs toward the tail
Rostral (R)	• Any given point on the head toward the nose
Proximal (Pr)	• Any given point nearest the point of origin or attachment
Distal (Di)	• Any given point farthest away from the point of origin or attachment
Medial (M, Med)	• An area near the midline • The inside aspect of the limbs
Lateral (L, Lat)	• An area situated away from or opposite the midline • The outside aspect of the limbs
Palmar (Pa)	• Caudal portion of the forelimb on and distal to the carpal joint
Plantar (Pl)	• Caudal portion of the hindlimb on and distal to the tarsal joint

Positional Terms

The patient is positioned so that the x-ray beam enters and exits based on the positional term. For example, in a ventrodorsal position, the patient would be lying on their back so that the beam enters the abdomen and exits the patient's back. Additional examples include dorsoventral, craniocaudal, caudocranial, dorsopalmar, palmarodorsal, dorsoplantar and plantarodorsal.

Recumbent: the patient is lying down; in lateral (left or right) recumbency, the patient is lying on that particular side; sternal recumbency (the patient is lying on its abdomen), or dorsal recumbency (the patient is lying on its back).

Oblique: in small animals, the patient is generally placed in a slanted or inclined position so that the x-ray beam will enter the body at an angle. For large animal limbs, the beam will be angled less than 90 degrees to the axis.

The following skill boxes and images focus on correct positioning and imaging with the emphasis on non-manual restraint. Depending on the species, size, and condition of the patient being imaged, positioning guidelines may be adjusted accordingly.

Skill Box 4.1 / Abdomen

Anatomic area	Abdomen	
View	**Lateral**	**Ventrodorsal**
Positioning	• Right lateral recumbency is most common • Forelimbs extended cranially with use of Velcro and straps or sandbag • Hind limbs extended caudally with straps or sandbag • Support with one sandbag over the neck, adjusting the sand so that breathing is not constricted, and one sandbag over the pelvis out of the field of view. A small foam pad may be placed under the thorax to keep the vertebrae and sternebrae on the same plane	• Dorsal recumbency either placed in a foam V-trough or directly on table • Forelimbs extended cranially and parallel to each other with use of Velcro and straps • Hind limbs extended caudally with straps or sandbag and parallel to each other • With the patient in foam trough, place a sandbag just cranial to the stifle over the pelvis. A sandbag may also be placed over the neck adjusting the sand, so breathing is not constricted • The patient can also be placed directly on the table with foam pads and sandbags alongside for support • The vertebrae and sternebrae should be superimposed
Measurement	• Caudal aspect of the 13th rib or widest area	• Caudal aspect of the 13th rib or widest area
Beam center	• Caudal aspect of the 13th rib	• Caudal aspect of the 13th rib
Field of view	• 2–3-inches cranial to xyphoid process of sternum to the to the greater trochanter	• 2–3-inches cranial to xyphoid process of sternum to the greater trochanter
Notes	• Taken on expiratory pause • A left lateral may also be requested • Two images of the abdomen may be needed with large dogs	• Taken on expiratory pause • Two images of the abdomen may be needed with large dogs

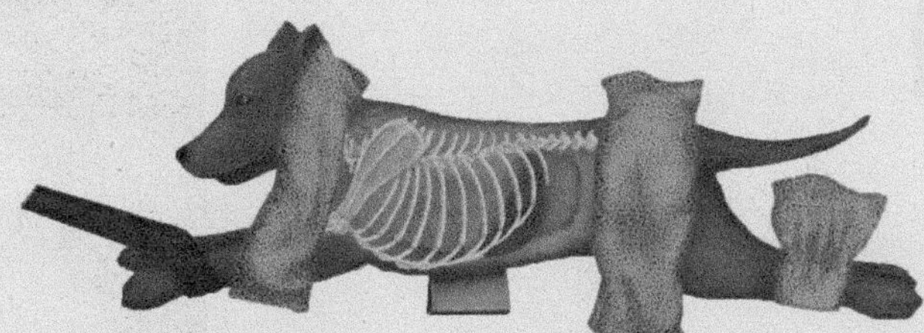

Figure 4.2 Universal positioning for lateral thorax, abdomen or spine. Strategic use of sandbags over the neck and pelvis as well as Velcro and straps to secure the limbs prevent movement. Source: courtesy of Julia Bitan (handsfreexrays.com).

(*Continued*)

Skill Box 4.1 / Abdomen (Continued)

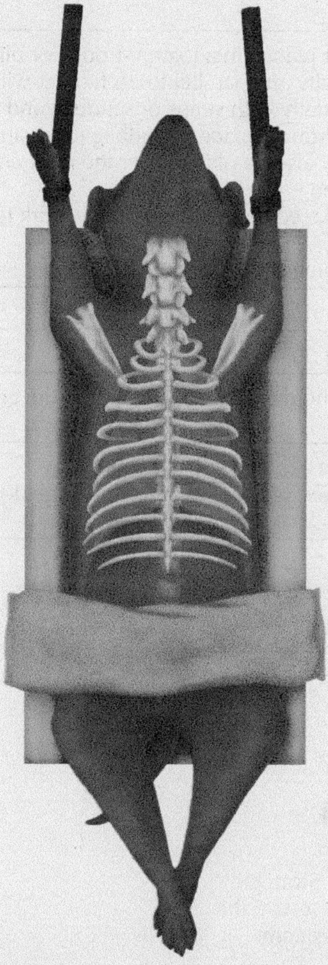

Figure 4.3 Universal positioning for ventrodorsal thorax, abdomen or spine. Placement in a foam trough and strategic use of sandbags as well as Velcro and straps to secure the limbs prevent movement. Source: Courtesy of Julia Bitan (handsfreexrays.com).

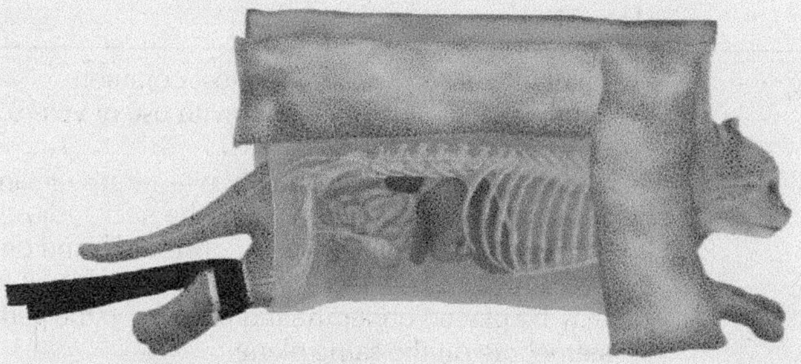

Figure 4.4 Untranquilized felines are best restrained with the use of a towel folded over the body with sandbags positioned along the patient's back and over the neck holding the towel edges. Velcro tape and straps support the limbs. Source: courtesy of Julia Bitan (handsfreexrays.com).

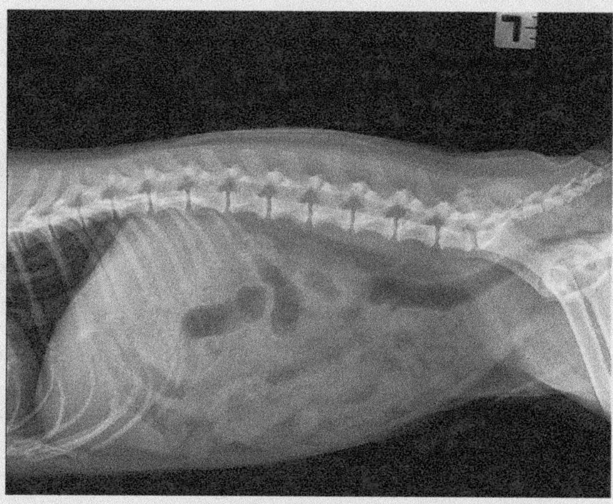

Figure 4.5 Abdominal radiograph in lateral positioning. Source: courtesy of Ashley Jenner, Toronto, ON.

(Continued)

Skill Box 4.1 / Abdomen (Continued)

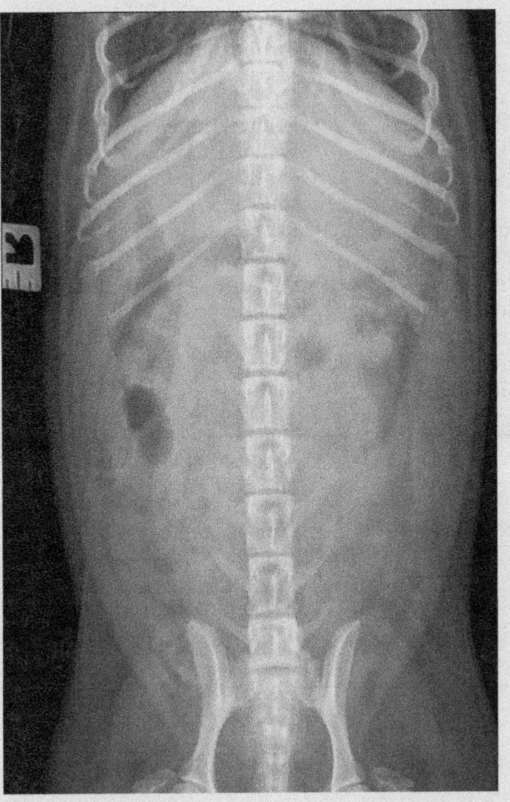

Figure 4.6 Abdominal radiograph in ventrodorsal positioning. Source: courtesy of Ashley Jenner, Toronto, ON.

Skill Box 4.2 / Thorax

Anatomic area	Thorax		
View	**Lateral**	**Ventrodorsal**	**Dorsoventral**
Positioning	• Left (for lungs) or right (heart) lateral recumbency • Forelimbs and head extended cranially with the use of Velcro tape and straps or a sandbag • Rear limbs extended caudally with use of straps or sandbag • Support with one sandbag over the neck, adjusting the sand so that breathing is not constricted and that it is out of the field of view. Place a sandbag over the pelvis. A small foam pad may be placed under the thorax to keep the vertebrae and sternebrae on the same plane • Feline patients can be restrained as shown in Figure 4.4	• Dorsal recumbency • Foam V-trough or directly on table supported with foam pads and sandbags along the sides • Forelimbs extended cranially with straps or sandbags • Rear limbs flexed • Sandbag over the pelvis region • The vertebrae and sternebrae should be superimposed	• Sternal recumbency • Forelimbs extended caudally and elbows abducted • Head lies low between forelimbs • Rear limbs in crouching position • The vertebrae and sternebrae should be superimposed
Measurement	• Widest area of ribcage or caudal border of the scapula.	• Highest point of thorax or over caudal border of scapula.	• Highest point of thorax or over caudal border of scapula.
Beam center	• Caudal border of scapula (5th–6th intercostal space)	• Caudal border of scapula (6th rib)	• Caudal border of scapula (6th rib)
Field of view	• Thoracic inlet to last rib	• Thoracic inlet to the last rib	• Thoracic inlet to the last rib
Notes	• Taken on peak inspiration	• Taken on peak inspiration	• Taken on peak inspiration • Preferred view for cardiac evaluation or for patient in respiratory stress

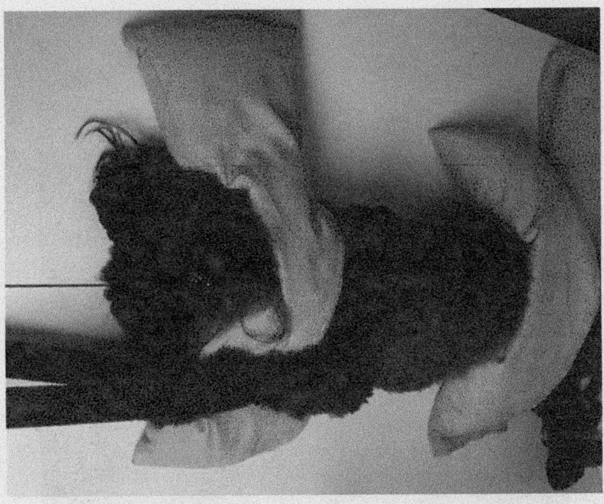

Figure 4.7 Canine positioning for lateral thorax with the use of Velcro straps and sandbags. Source: courtesy of Ashley Jenner, Toronto, ON.

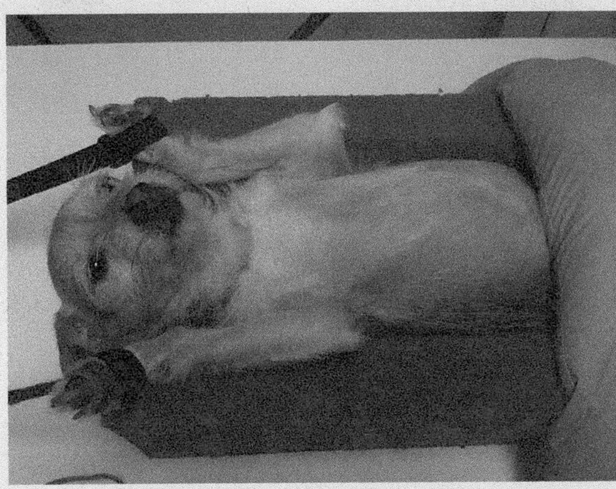

Figure 4.8 Canine positioning for ventrodorsal thorax with the use of foam trough and sandbags. Source: courtesy of Ashley Jenner, Toronto, ON.

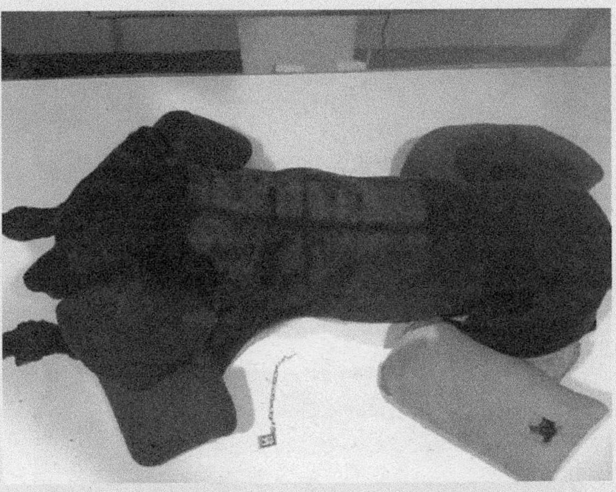

Figure 4.9 Proper positioning for dorsoventral. Extension of the front limbs and use of sandbags over the neck and pelvis will keep the patient in position. Source: courtesy of Ashley Jenner, Toronto, ON.

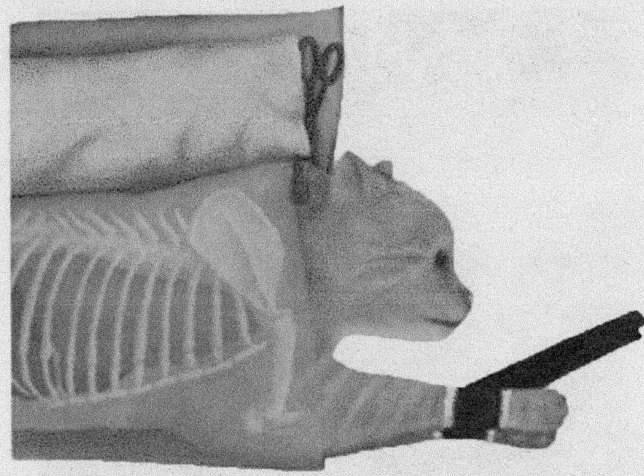

Figure 4.10 Feline positioning for lateral thorax with the use of Velcro straps, towel and sandbags. Source: courtesy of Ashley Jenner, Toronto, ON.

(Continued)

Skill Box 4.2 / Thorax (Continued)

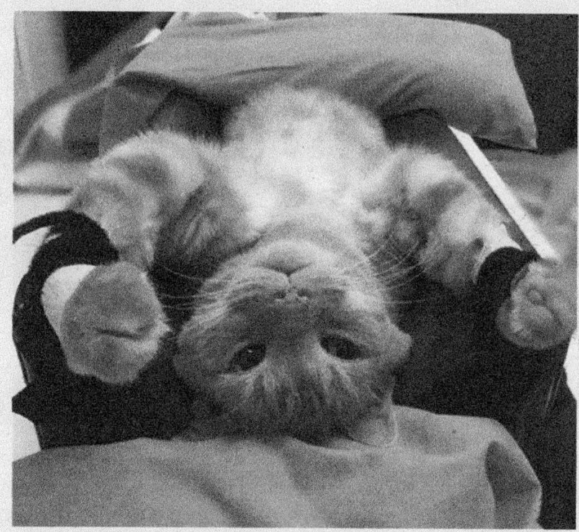

Figure 4.11 Feline ventrodorsal thorax positioning. Source: courtesy of Ashley Jenner, Toronto, ON.

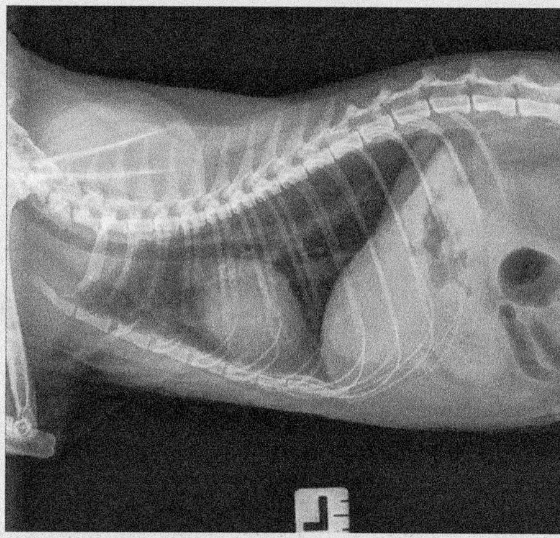

Figure 4.12 Thoracic radiograph in lateral positioning, thoracic inlet to the last rib. Source: courtesy of Ashley Jenner, Toronto, ON.

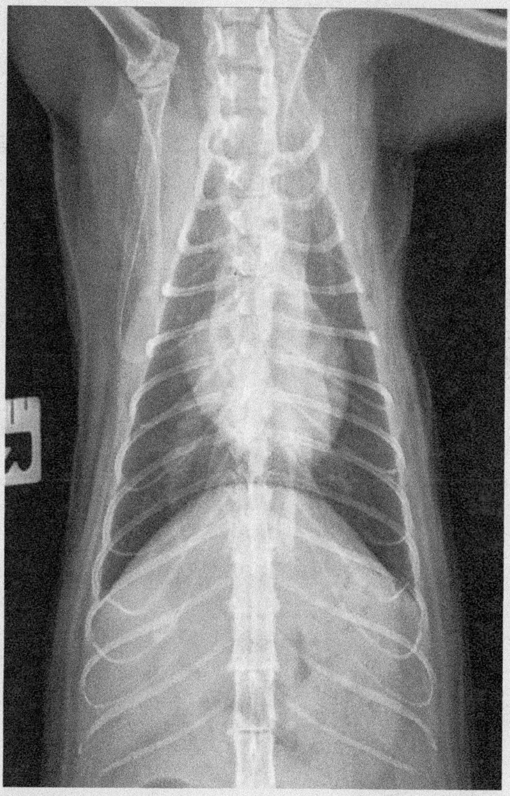

Figure 4.13 Thoracic radiograph in ventrodorsal positioning, thoracic inlet to the last rib. Source: courtesy of Ashley Jenner, Toronto, ON.

(Continued)

Skill Box 4.2 / Thorax (Continued)

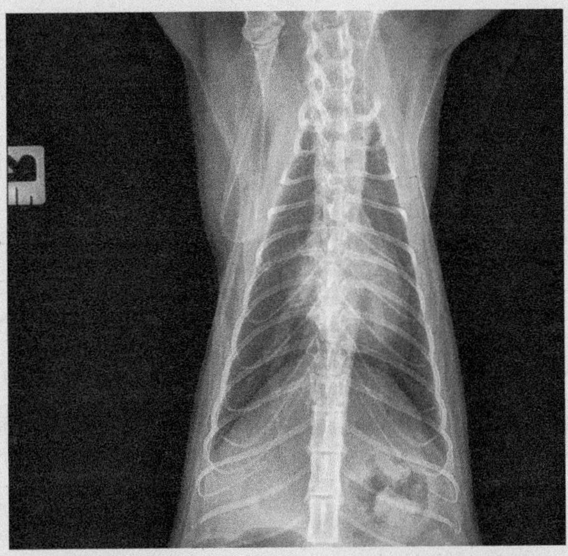

Figure 4.14 Thoracic radiograph in dorsoventral positioning, thoracic inlet to the last rib. Source: courtesy of Ashley Jenner, Toronto, ON.

Head Positioning

The skull must be precisely positioned to produce a diagnostic radiograph. Supports strategically placed under the muzzle, neck, or cranium and straps over the head or neck region will assist in achieving the correct position. Strong sedation or general anesthesia is highly recommended. It may be more difficult to obtain symmetry for brachycephalic dogs because of their wide skulls. Computed tomography (CT), if available, will provide more detailed information of the head than x-rays.

Skill Box 4.3 / Head: Routine Views

View	Lateral	Dorsoventral	Ventrodorsal
Anatomic area	• Skull – survey • Nasal cavities and frontal sinus • TMJ • Tympanic bullae • Zygomatic bone and orbit • Foramen magnum • Pharynx	• Skull – survey • Nasal cavities and frontal sinus • TMJ • Tympanic bullae • Zygomatic bone and orbit • Foramen magnum • Mandible	• Skull – survey • Nasal cavities and frontal sinus • TMJ • Tympanic bullae • Zygomatic bone and orbit • Foramen magnum • Maxilla
Positioning (avoid manual restraint; use strategically positioned devices to extend limbs and support the body and head)	• Lateral recumbency • Affected side down • Foam wedge placed under the mandible to keep the muzzle parallel to the cassette or table • Nasal septum parallel to the cassette or table • Forelimbs extended caudally via straps or sandbags • Position a sandbag over the neck and Velcro strap over the cranium • For true lateral the lateral canthi should be perpendicular to the table • Include opposite lateral for nasal cavity and frontal sinus • An open mouth lateral view is beneficial for nasal sinuses, mandible and maxilla • Pharynx: extend the neck, keeping head parallel to the table	• Sternal recumbency • Head is resting on the cassette or table with sandbag over the neck • Forelimbs are relaxed with carpi flexed and out of the beam supported with sandbags • Position a sandbag over the neck and Velcro strap over the cranium • For a true DV view, the lateral canthi should be parallel to the table	• Dorsal recumbency • The head is extended on the cassette or table with support under the mid-cervical region to keep proper alignment • The nose is parallel to the cassette or table • The skull is level on the cassette or table • Forelimbs extended caudally
Measurement: on area of interest	• Highest point of the zygomatic arch over the area of interest • Foramen magnum and pharynx: base of skull	• Highest point of the cranium on the area of interest • Foramen magnum: base of skull	• Highest point of the cranium on the area of interest • Foramen magnum: base of skull
Beam center: on area of interest	• Survey: lateral canthus of the eye midway between eye and ear • Nasal cavities and frontal sinus: lateral canthus of the eye midway between eye and ear • TMJ: rostral to the ears • Tympanic bullae: on midline between ears – palpate • Zygomatic bone and orbit: over the area of interest • Pharynx and foramen magnum: base of skull	• Survey: lateral canthus of the eye midway between eye and ear • Nasal cavities and frontal sinus: lateral canthus of the eye midway between eye and ear • TMJ: rostral to the ears • Tympanic bullae: center of ear – palpate • Zygomatic bone and orbit: over the area of interest • Mandible: lateral canthus of eye	• Survey: lateral canthus of the eye midway between eye and ear • Nasal cavities and frontal sinus: lateral canthus of the eye midway between eye and ear • TMJ: rostral to the ears • Tympanic bullae: center of ear – palpate • Zygomatic bone and orbit: over the area of interest

(*Continued*)

Skill Box 4.3 / Head: Routine Views (Continued)

View	Lateral	Dorsoventral	Ventrodorsal
Field of view: include area of interest	• Survey: tip of the nose to the base of the skull • Nasal cavities and frontal sinus: tip of the nose to the base of the skull • TMJ: cranial and caudal to the joint • Tympanic bullae: cranial and caudal to the ear • Zygomatic bone and orbit: tip of the nose to the base of the skull • Foramen magnum and pharynx: C3 to lateral canthus	• Survey: tip of the nose to the base of the skull • Nasal cavities and frontal sinus: tip of the nose to the commissure of the lips • TMJ: cranial and caudal to the joint • Tympanic bullae: cranial and caudal to the ear • Zygomatic bone and orbit: tip of the nose to the base of the skull • Foramen magnum: C_3 to lateral canthus	• Survey: tip of the nose to the base of the skull • Nasal cavities and frontal sinus: tip of the nose to the commissure of the lips • TMJ: cranial and caudal to the joint • Tympanic bullae: cranial and caudal to the ear • Zygomatic bone and orbit: tip of the nose to the base of the skull • Foramen magnum: C3 to lateral canthus
Notes	• There will be superimposition of tympanic bullae and TMJ	• Superimposition of the cranium makes views of tympanic bullae less than ideal, but this view does permit comparison of right and left in one view	• Often better for deep-chested dogs to reduce geometric magnification

Skill Box 4.4 / Head: Other Views

View	Ventrodorsal – open mouth	Lateral oblique open mouth	Frontal or rostrocaudal	Dorsoventral: occlusal
Anatomic area	• Nasal cavities and sinuses • Zygomatic bone and orbit • Maxilla	• Nasal cavities and sinuses • TMJ • Tympanic bullae • Zygomatic bone and orbit • Mandible and maxilla	• Nasal cavities and sinuses • Foramen magnum tympanic bullae • Zygomatic bone and orbit	• Nasal cavities and sinuses • Maxilla
Positioning (avoid manual restraint; use strategically positioned devices to extend limbs and elevate the body)	• Dorsal recumbency in V-trough • Forelimbs extended caudally • The head is extended on the cassette or table with support under the mid-cervical region • The nose is parallel to the cassette or table and may be taped in position with the mandible extended caudally with supports • The skull is level on the cassette or table	• Lateral recumbency with forelegs extended caudally and hind limbs in a natural position. If patient is anesthetized, secure endotracheal tube to maxilla • Nasal cavities, frontal sinus, zygomatic arch: cranium supported with wedge to achieve the oblique angle of the arch • Nasal septum perpendicular to the cassette or table. • Tympanic bullae: unaffected bullae toward the cassette or table • Skull slightly obliqued on table while resting in a natural position keeping mouth closed • TMJ, craniocaudal oblique, mandible raised about 20 degrees, keeping mouth closed • Maxilla: affected maxilla down • Head supported with wedge under mandible to create a 10°–30° angle depending on the breed so that superimposition is minimized. • Mouth opened wide with radiolucent speculum placed between the canines. • Mandible: affected mandible down. Raise maxilla 20–45 degrees depending on the breed. Keep mouth open as wide as possible • Feline tympanic bullae: foam positioning devices not needed as feline cranium naturally tilts 10′, separating the tympanic bull	• Dorsal recumbency • Forelimbs extended caudally • The base of the skull is resting on the cassette or table with the neck in a flexed position • Nasal and frontal sinus: the nose points straight up at 90 degrees to the table • Zygomatic bone and orbit: nose is slightly off perpendicular to x-ray beam • Foramen magnum: using tubing, pull the nose toward the thorax about 20–30-degrees, depending on the breed • Tympanic bullae: open the mouth with tubing or gauze so the nose is pulled about 10 degrees cranial and the mandible is relatively perpendicular; also referred to as a basilar view • Feline tympanic bullae: mouth is closed and tilted cranially about 20 degrees	• Sternal recumbency • Head is resting on the table. • Film/cassette placed between the maxilla and the mandible with the corner of the receptor into the mouth for better coverage • Forelimbs are relaxed with carpi flexed and out of the beam, supported with sandbags • Position a sandbag over the neck and Velcro strap over the cranium to support the patient

(Continued)

Skill Box 4.4 / Head: Other Views (Continued)

View	Ventrodorsal – open mouth	Lateral oblique open mouth	Frontal or rostrocaudal	Dorsoventral: occlusal
Measurement: area of interest	• Bridge of nose to third upper premolar • Maxilla: zygomatic arch • Zygomatic arch: slightly off center from the mid-cranium	• Frontal sinus/zygomatic arch: highest point of cranium • Tympanic bullae: level of tympanic bullae • Temporomandibular joint: lateral canthus of the eye	• Most caudal aspect of the muzzle (nose stop) frontal sinuses • Tympanic bullae: commissure of lips at level of maxillary premolar	• Caudal portion of maxilla
Beam center: on area of interest	• Angle beam 10–20 degrees (depending on the patient anatomy) from vertical into the open mouth between the upper third and fourth premolars • Zygomatic arch: At a 45-degree angle to the maxilla between the upper third and fourth premolars • Maxilla: lateral canthus of eye	• Zygomatic arch: slightly off center from the mid-cranium • Frontal sinus/lateral canthus of the eye • Tympanic bullae: center of tympanic bullae • TMJ: TMJ	• Between the eyes • Tympanic bullae: commissure of the lips over the bullae	• Caudal portion of maxilla
Field of view: include area of interest	• Tip of the nose to the pharyngeal area • Zygomatic arch: nasal cavities to the cranial temporal skull	• Zygomatic arch and frontal sinus: tip of the nose to the base of the skull • Tympanic bullae: lateral canthus of the eye to the base of the skull • Temporomandibular joint: medial canthus of the eye to the base of the skull	• Tip of the nose to the base of the skull • Tympanic bullae: nasopharyngeal region of cranium	• Tip of the nose to orbital bones
Notes	• Remove or tie the endotracheal tube to the mandible • This position can only be used if the x-ray tube head can rotate • Due to range of motion the x-ray tube will not likely need to be angled for feline patients	• For nasal sinuses: typically done only if trauma has occurred and fractures are suspected, or to visualize the mandibular arcade	• Remove or tie the endotracheal tube to the mandible	• A conventional intraoral view may not be possible with digital radiography

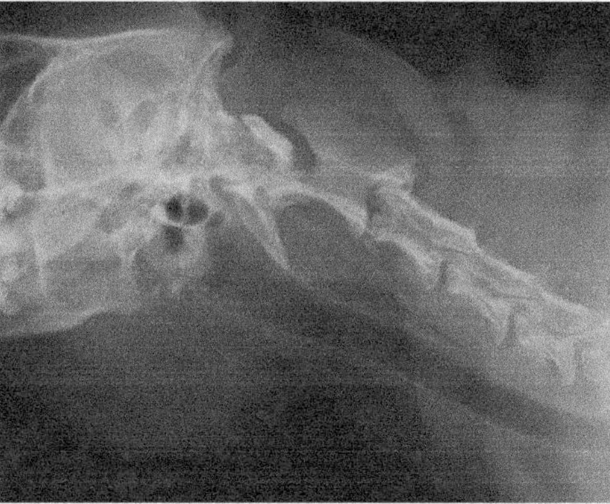

Figure 4.15 Pharynx in lateral positioning, lateral canthus to C3.

Spine Positioning

The spine must be kept level as images are taken. A misaligned spine will result in distortion on the image and therefore is nondiagnostic.

For laterals, the vertebrae and sternebrae should be on the same plane. Levelness can be accomplished with supports under the mandible, neck, thorax, or between the limbs. Strategically placed sandbags, tape or straps, and Velcro over the neck, limbs and pelvis are used to keep the patient supported. Keep sandbags out of the field of view. A towel can be used for felines (Figure 4.18).

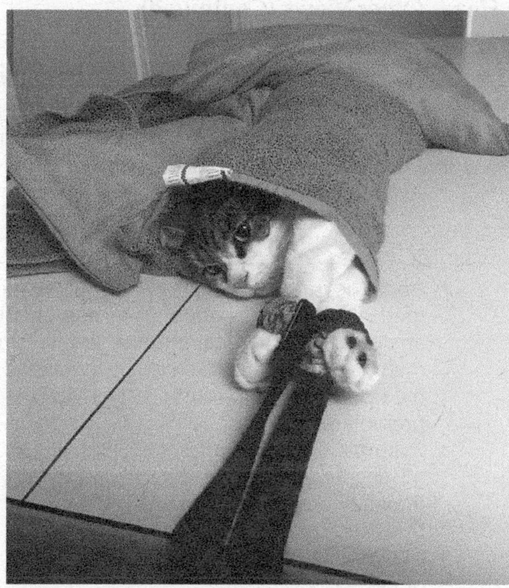

Figure 4.16 The standard position can also be used for the spine on an untranquilized patient.

In the ventrodorsal position, the vertebrae and sternebrae are superimposed. A "V" trough or wedges are recommended on all ventrodorsal views to stabilize patient's body. Use sandbags and straps/Velcro over the limbs as necessary, and support the neck with appropriately placed sandbags.

Some of these non-manual positions can be accomplished without sedation or general anesthesia; however, either may occasionally be required.

Always collimate in on either side of the spine to exclude the soft tissues. Minimize the number of vertebrae on an image when possible, to prevent the appearance of narrowing of the vertebral spaces at the outer edges due to image distortion and beam angle.

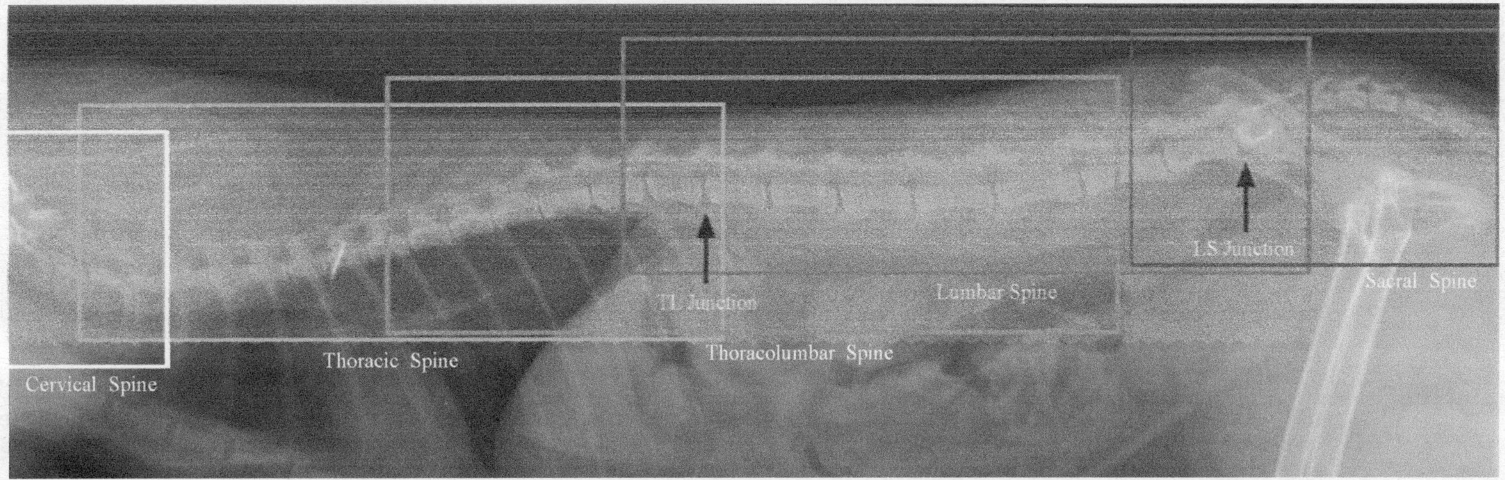

Figure 4.17 Spine in lateral positioning with boundaries for spinal radiographs. LS, lumbosacral; TL, thoracolumbar.

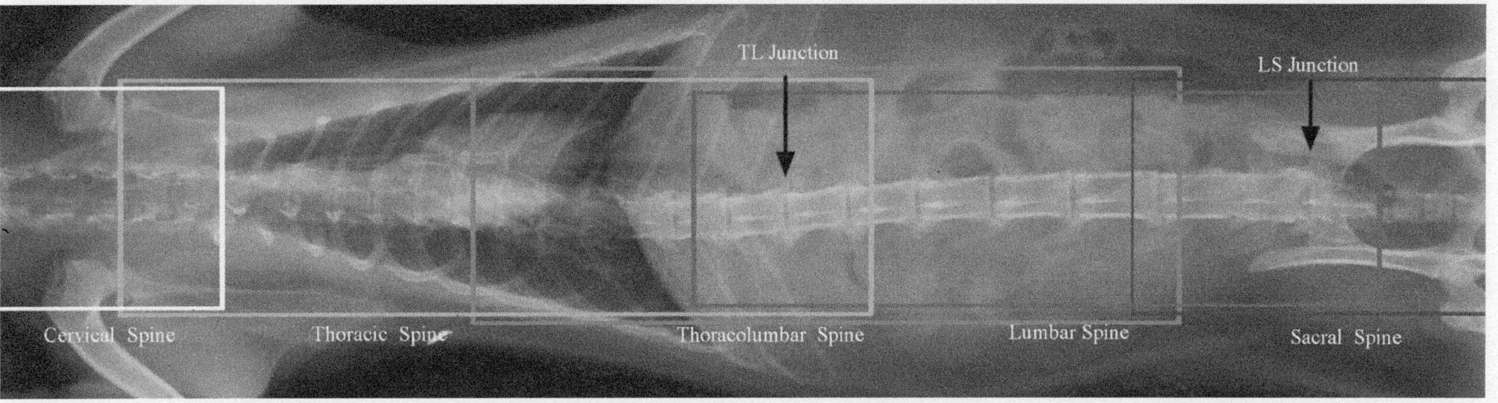

Figure 4.18 Spine in ventrodorsal positioning with boundaries for spinal radiographs. LS, lumbosacral; TL, thoracolumbar.

Skill Box 4.5 / Spine: Cervical

View	Lateral	Ventrodorsal	Extended lateral	Flexed lateral	Oblique lateral
Positioning (avoid manual restraint; use strategically positioned devices to extend limbs and elevate and support the body)	• Lateral recumbency • Forelimbs retracted caudally, atlanto-occipital joint is flexed at a 45-degree angle • Use a foam pad to elevate the mandible to be parallel to the table and secure with tape or straps. • Gauze may be needed around the mouth to keep the head pulled slightly forward	• Dorsal recumbency • Forelimbs extended caudally alongside the body • Spine parallel to the cassette or table • Support under the neck can minimize distortion caused by a misaligned vertebra	• Lateral recumbency • Forelimbs extended caudally • Extend the neck dorsally until resistance is met; gauze may be placed around the muzzle • Place support under the mandible and neck to maintain a level spine (especially with long-necked dogs)	• Lateral recumbency • Forelimbs extended caudally – atlanto-occipital joint is flexed at a 90-degree angle • Elevate the neck if necessary to keep it level with the spine • Pull the lower mandible open with gauze to maintain the 90-degree angle	• Lateral recumbency • Elevate the mandible to be parallel to table with support • Elevate the sternum 20 degrees above vertebral level/plane with support
Measurement	• Over C7	• C5/C6	• Thoracic inlet (C7)	• Thoracic inlet (C7)	• Thoracic inlet (C7)
Beam center	• Vertebral column over C4	• Vertebral column over C4	• Vertebral column over C4	• Vertebral column over C4	• Vertebral column over C4
Field of view	• Caudal skull to T1/T2	• Caudal skull to T1/T2	• Caudal skull to T1/T2	• Caudal skull to T1/T2	• Caudal skull to T1/T2
Notes	• Two images are recommended for large dogs	• Two images are recommended for large dogs	• Mainly used to evaluate for instability	• Be careful not to overflex the neck as tracheal damage may occur • Mainly used to evaluate for instability	• Mainly used to evaluate for instability

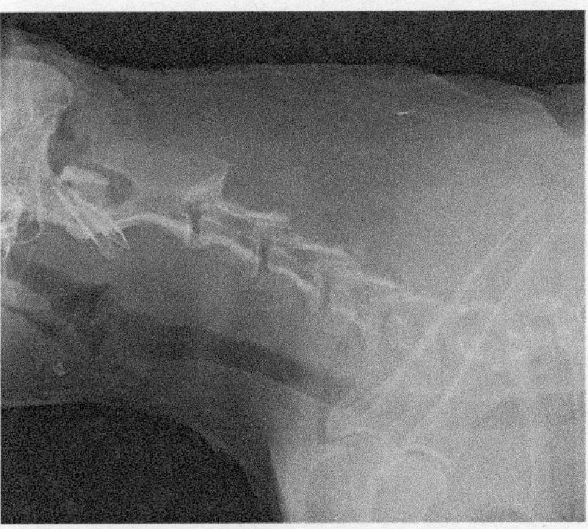

Figure 4.19 Cervical spine in lateral positioning, caudal skull to T1.

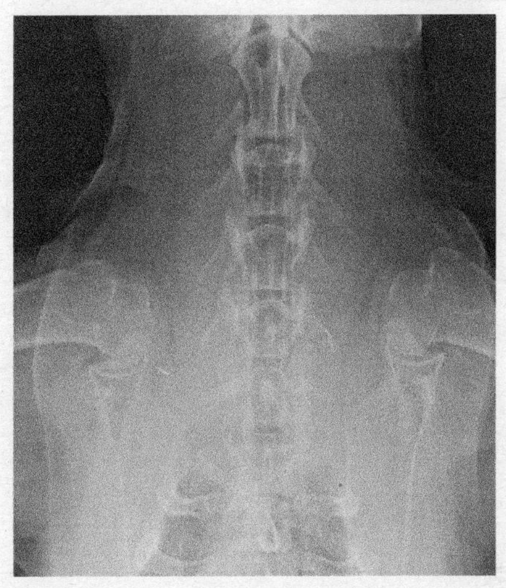

Figure 4.20 Cervical spine in ventrodorsal positioning, caudal skull to T1–T2.

Skill Box 4.6 / Spine: Thoracic–Lumbar

Anatomic area	**Thoracic**		**Thoracolumbar**		**Lumbar**	
View	**Lateral**	**Ventrodorsal**	**Lateral**	**Ventrodorsal**	**Lateral**	**Ventrodorsal**
Positioning (avoid manual restraint; use strategically positioned devices to extend limbs and elevate and support the body)	• Lateral recumbency • Forelimbs extended cranially • Hind limbs extended caudally • Elevate the sternum to thoracic vertebrae level to reduce rotational artifact	• Dorsal recumbency • Forelimbs extended cranially • Hind limbs are in a relaxed position	• Lateral recumbency • Forelimbs slightly extended cranially • Hind limbs slightly extended caudally	• Dorsal recumbency • Forelimbs extended cranially • Hind limbs are in a relaxed position	• Lateral recumbency • Forelimbs are in a relaxed position • Hind limbs are extended caudally with support between them to keep hips parallel to the table	• Dorsal recumbency • Forelimbs extended cranially • Hind limbs are in a relaxed position
Measurement	• 7th to 8th rib	• Highest point of the sternum	• Thoracolumbar junction	• Thoracolumbar junction	• Thickest area (L1)	• Thickest area (L1)
Beam center	• T6/T7	• T6/T7 (caudal border of scapula)	• Thoracolumbar junction	• Thoracolumbar junction	• L4	• L4

(Continued)

Skill Box 4.6 / Spine: Thoracic–Lumbar (Continued)

Anatomic area	Thoracic		Thoracolumbar		Lumbar	
View	Lateral	Ventrodorsal	Lateral	Ventrodorsal	Lateral	Ventrodorsal
Field of view	• C7 to L1	• C7 to L1	• T10 to L3	• T10 to L3	• Caudal T12 to S1	• Caudal T12 to S1
Notes	• Veterinarian may prefer two images for large dogs	• Veterinarian may prefer two images for large dogs	• May require support under the sternum and mid-lumbar region for prevention of axial rotation artifact		• May require support under the sternum and mid-lumbar region for proper alignment and prevention of axial rotation artifact (especially in chondrodystrophic dogs with elongated backs)	

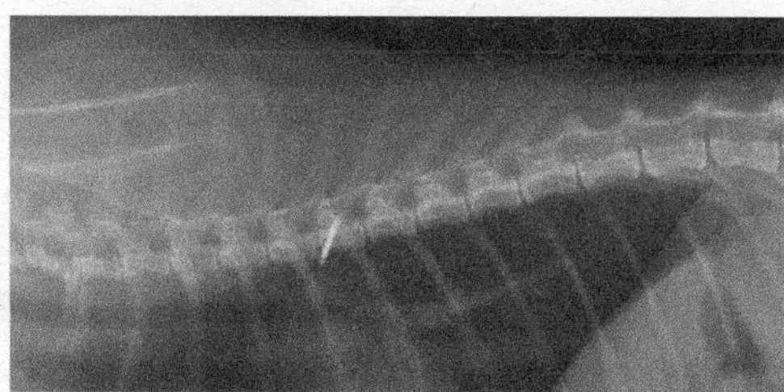

Figure 4.21 Thoracic spine in lateral positioning, C7–L1.

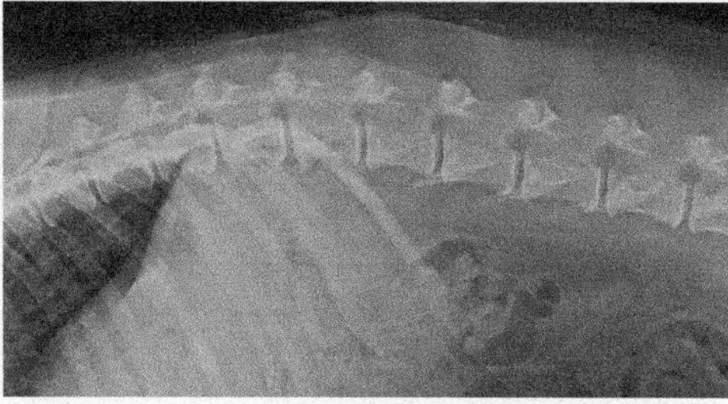

Figure 4.22 Thoracolumbar spine in lateral positioning, T8–L5.

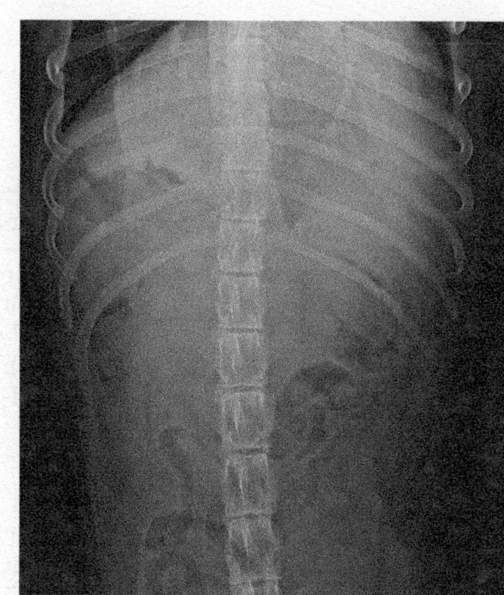

Figure 4.23 Thoracolumbar spine in ventrodorsal positioning, T8–L5.

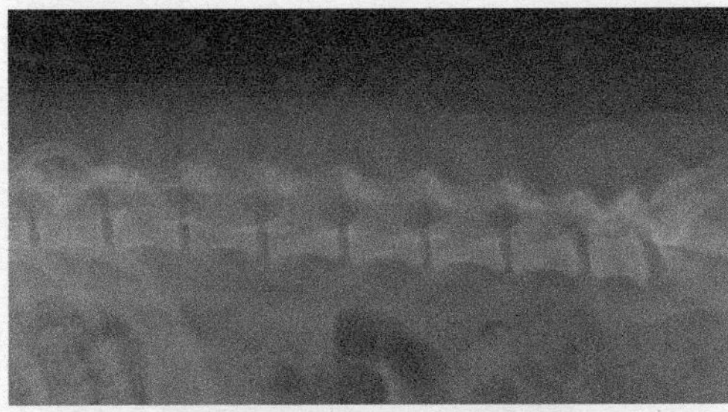

Figure 4.24 Lumbar spine in lateral positioning, T13–S1.

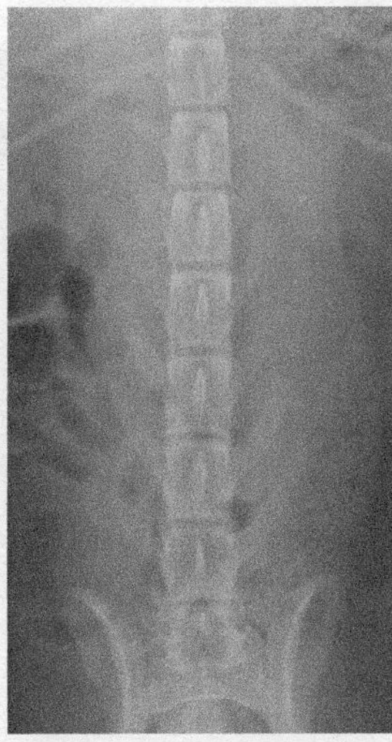

Figure 4.25 Lumbar spine in ventrodorsal positioning, T13–S1.

Skill Box 4.7 / Spine: Sacrum–Caudal

Anatomic area	Sacrum		Caudal	
View	**Lateral**	**Ventrodorsal**	**Lateral**	**Ventrodorsal**
Positioning (avoid manual restraint; use strategically positioned devices to extend limbs and elevate and support the body)	• Lateral recumbency • Hind limbs are slightly apart and relaxed with a support between them • Tail is extended caudally, not supported	• Dorsal recumbency • Hind limbs are relaxed in semiflexion	• Lateral recumbency • The tail is extended caudally and supported as needed to prevent excessive sagging or lateral flexion	• Dorsal recumbency • Hind limbs are relaxed in semiflexion • Tail is extended straight caudally and supported as needed to prevent excessive sagging or lateral flexion
Measurement	• Trochanters	• Mid-sacrum	• Area of concern	• Area of concern
Beam center	• Greater femoral trochanter	• At 30 degrees toward the pubis (if x-ray head rotates), centered over the lumbosacral junction	• Area of concern	• Area of concern
Field of view	• Pelvis to proximal caudal vertebral segments	• L6 to proximal caudal vertebra	• Includes area of concern plus several vertebra on either side	• Includes area of concern plus several vertebra on either side

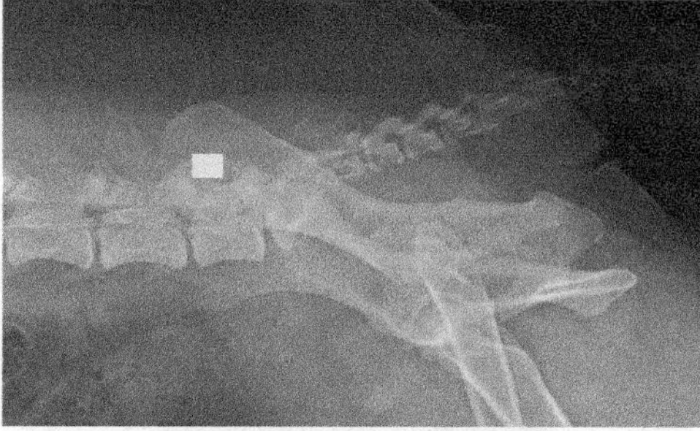

Figure 4.26 Sacral spine in lateral positioning, pelvis to proximal caudal vertebral segments.

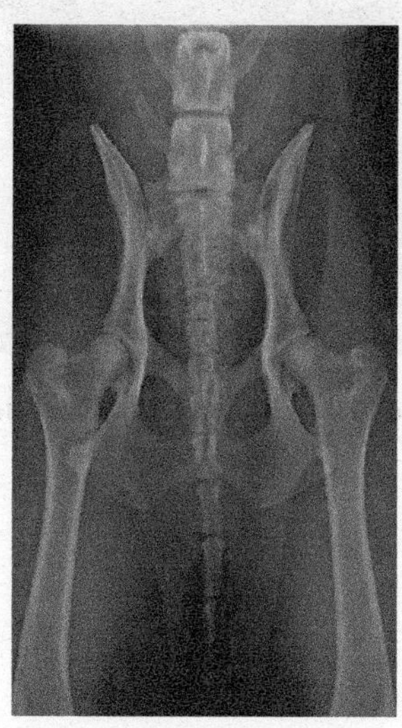

Figure 4.27 Sacral spine in ventrodorsal positioning, L6 to proximal caudal vertebra.

Shoulder and Forelimbs[1]

Skill Box 4.8 / Shoulder and Scapula[1]

Anatomic area	**Scapula**			**Shoulder**	
View	**Lateral with tension**	**Lateral without tension**	**Caudocranial**	**Mediolateral**	**Caudocranial**
Positioning (avoid manual restraint; use strategically positioned devices to extend limbs and support the body)	• Lateral recumbency with the affected side up • Position the skull and neck ventrally with a sandbag so the nose is pointing down • The affected forelimb is flexed at the elbow and secured with tape or Velcro and pulled dorsally placing the carpus above the skull • The shoulder joint will be at the level of the thoracic spinous processes and the scapula will be superimposed over the thoracic spinous processes so both are visualized • The unaffected forelimb is extended cranially and distally	• Lateral recumbency • The affected forelimb is down and pulled cranially and ventrally • The unaffected forelimb is extended distally	• Dorsal recumbency • Forelimbs are extended cranially and each secured separately • The sternum is rotated 10–12 degrees away from the scapula of interest (just opposite midline) to avoid superimposition	• Lateral recumbency with affected side down • Affected forelimb is extended cranially and distally • Unaffected forelimb is flexed caudodorsally, parallel to the thorax • Head is extended cranially about 135 degrees to thoracic spine	• Dorsal recumbency • Each thoracic limb taped separately and pulled cranially; tape at mid-antebrachii to pull elbows medially • Rotate the sternum slightly away from the shoulder of interest • Push the head and neck away from the shoulder of interest

(Continued)

Skill Box 4.8 / Shoulder and Scapula[1] (Continued)

Anatomic area	Scapula			Shoulder	
View	**Lateral with tension**	**Lateral without tension**	**Caudocranial**	**Mediolateral**	**Caudocranial**
Measurement	• Thickest area of the shoulder/cranial thorax	• Thickest area of the shoulder/cranial thorax	• Thickest area of the shoulder	• Over the manubrium	• Thickest area of the shoulder
Beam center	• Mid-scapula	• Mid-scapula	• Mid-scapula	• Shoulder joint	• Shoulder joint
Field of view	• Cranial aspect of the shoulder joint to the caudal scapular crest	• Cranial aspect of the shoulder joint to the caudal scapular crest	• Shoulder joint to T6	• Distal third of scapula and proximal third of humerus	• Distal third of scapula and proximal third of humerus
Notes	• This gives an unobstructed view of the scapula, dorsal to the vertebral column • Place marker dorsally to indicate affected limb • There will likely be slight geometric distortion as the torso is rotated dorsally	• Used when the patient is injured or in pain • This view visualizes the scapular neck	• Best method for viewing acromial process of scapular spine	• The shoulder joint should be cranial to the manubrium and ventral to the trachea	• Be aware of any rotation in the humerus that would result in an oblique view

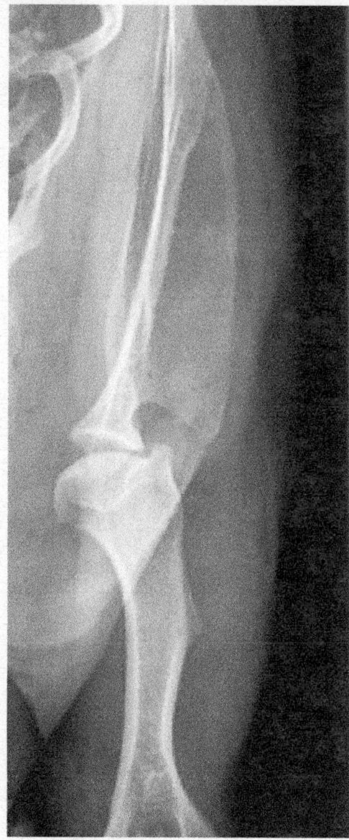

Figure 4.28 Caudocranial view of the right shoulder joint and scapula. Source: courtesy of Ashley Jenner, Toronto, ON.

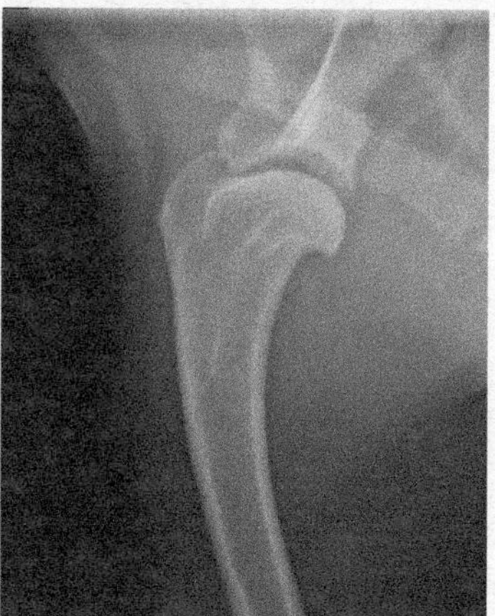

Figure 4.29 Shoulder in lateral positioning, mid-scapular to mid-humerus.

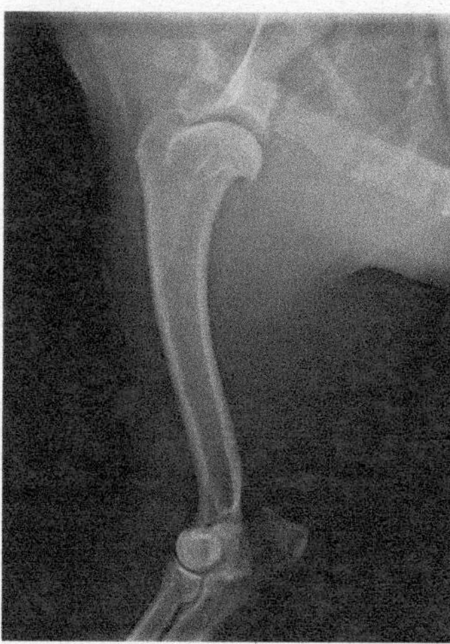

Figure 4.30 Humerus in lateral positioning, shoulder joint to elbow joint.

Skill Box 4.9 / Humerus

Anatomic area	Humerus		
View	**Mediolateral**	**Caudocranial**	**Craniocaudal**
Positioning (avoid manual restraint; use strategically positioned devices to extend limbs and support the body)	• Lateral recumbency • The affected forelimb is down and extended cranioventrally • The unaffected forelimb is extended caudodorsally • The head is extended dorsally	• Dorsal recumbency • Forelimbs extended cranially and held in place with tape at the mid-radius • The affected forelimb is parallel to the image receptor or table	• Dorsal recumbency • Affected forelimb extended caudally alongside the body but just clear of the thorax
Measurement	• Thickest area of the shoulder	• Thickest area of the shoulder	• Thickest area of the shoulder
Beam center	• Mid-humerus	• Mid-humerus	• Mid-humerus
Field of view	• Shoulder joint to elbow joint	• Shoulder joint to elbow joint	• Shoulder joint to elbow joint

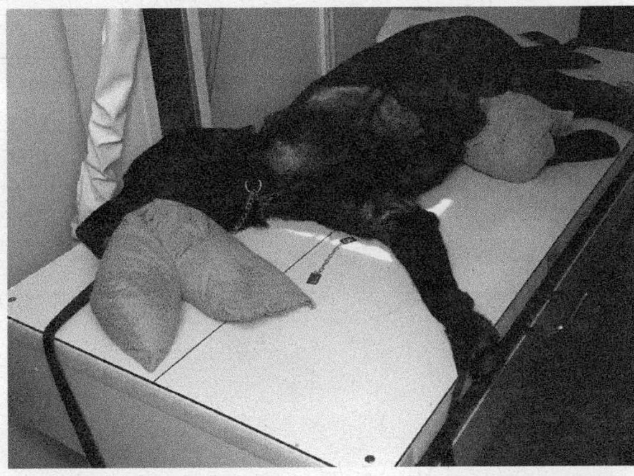

Figure 4.31 General positioning of the scapula, shoulder and radius/ulna with the affected limb down. Source: courtesy of Ashley Jenner, Toronto, ON.

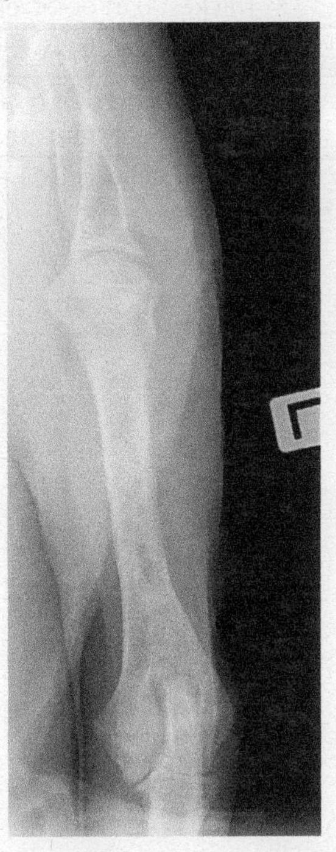

Figure 4.32 Craniocaudal scapula, shoulder, humerus. Source: courtesy of Ashley Jenner, Toronto, ON.

Skill Box 4.10 / Elbow

Anatomic area	Elbow		
View	**Mediolateral**	**Flexed Mediolateral**	**Craniocaudal**
Positioning (avoid manual restraint; use strategically positioned devices to extend limbs and support the body)	• Lateral recumbency • Affected limb down extended cranially and flexed up to 90° • Unaffected limb extended dorsally and caudally over the body • Cotton or foam wedge under the elbow enables true lateral through radiohumeral joint space • The head is extended dorsally away from the cassette or table	• Lateral recumbency • Affected limb hyperflexed at the elbow joint with carpus pulled toward neck and elbow flexed as much as possible and supported • Unaffected limb extended and taped caudodorsally • The head is extended dorsally • Keep the elbow in a true lateral position with no rotation	• Sternal recumbency • Affected limb extended cranially • The head is placed resting over the unaffected limb • Avoid rotation by placing a thin foam pad under the elbow • Keep humerus, radius and ulna in a straight line
Measurement	• Thickest part of the elbow/distal humerus	• Thickest part of the elbow joint during flexion	• Thickest part of the elbow joint
Beam center	• Center over elbow	• Elbow joint	• Elbow joint
Field of view	• Proximal third of humerus to distal third of antebrachium	• Proximal third of humerus to distal third of antebrachium	• Proximal third of humerus to distal third of antebrachium
Notes	• Oblique view may be needed in some cases	• This view is best for screening for elbow dysplasia (especially lesions of anconeal process of ulna) • Check requirements and submission information for Orthopedic Foundation for Animals dysplasia evaluation (https://www.ofa.org)	• Palpate so that the olecranon feels positioned midway between the humeral condyles for a true craniocaudal view

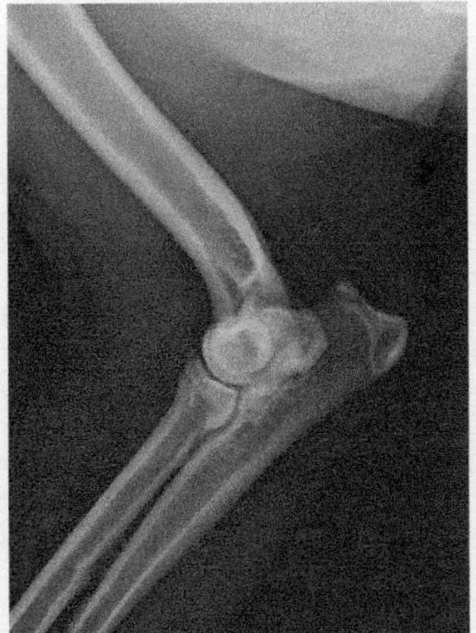

Figure 4.33 Elbow in lateral positioning, mid-humerus to mid-antebrachium.

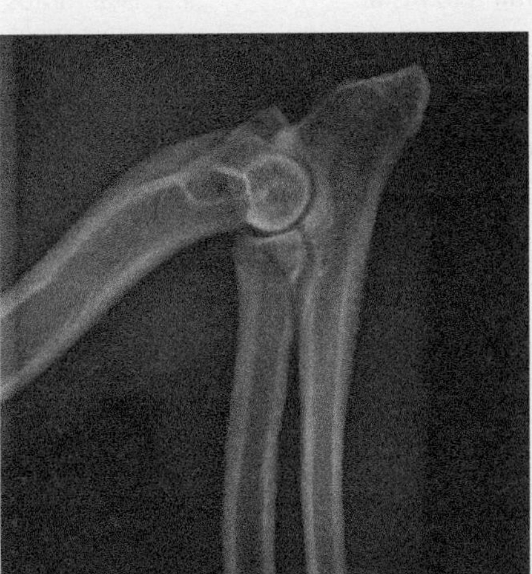

Figure 4.34 Elbow in flexed lateral positioning, mid-humerus to mid-radius/ulna.

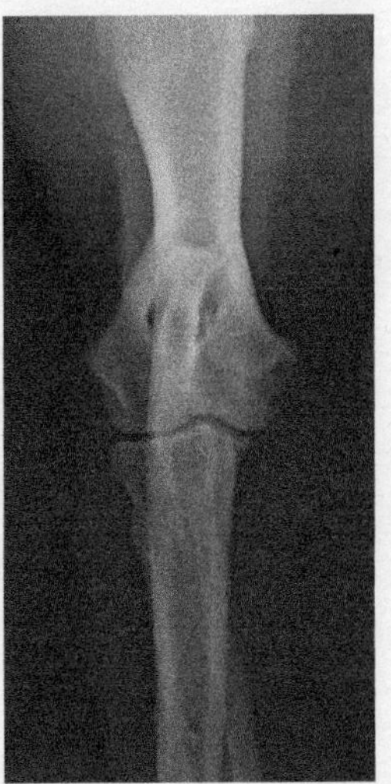

Figure 4.35 Elbow in craniocaudal positioning, mid-humerus to mid-radius/ulna.

Skill Box 4.11 / Radius, Ulna, and Carpus

Anatomic area	Radius and ulna		Carpus	
View	**Mediolateral**	**Craniocaudal**	**Mediolateral**	**Dorsopalmar**
Positioning (avoid manual restraint; use strategically positioned devices to extend limbs and support the body)	• Lateral recumbency • Affected limb extended cranially flexed at the elbow 45–90 degrees • Unaffected limb is extended dorsally and caudally • Head is extended dorsally away from the cassette or table	• Sternal recumbency • Both limbs extended cranially; a thin foam pad under the affected elbow may stabilize it and a small foam pad placed under the unaffected limb will prevent rotation or rolling • Head is placed resting over the unaffected limb	• Lateral recumbency • Affected limb extended cranially • Support under the elbow may assist in maintaining proper carpal positioning • Unaffected limb extended ventrally and relaxed • The head is extended dorsally away from the cassette or table	• Sternal recumbency • Affected limb extended and secured cranially • Support under the elbow may assist in maintaining proper carpal positioning • Unaffected limb extending cranially in a natural position • The head is placed resting over the unaffected limb
Measurement	• Elbow joint	• Thickest area of the elbow joint	• Mid-carpus	• Mid-carpus
Beam center	• Mid-radius/ulna	• Mid-radius/ulna	• Mid-carpus	• Mid-carpus
Field of view	• Distal humerus to mid-metacarpals	• Distal humerus to mid-metacarpals	• Distal radius/ulna to distal metacarpals	• Distal radius/ulna to distal metacarpals
Notes	• Avoid rotation of radius/ulna in cats	• Palpate so that the olecranon feels positioned midway between the humoral condyles for a true craniocaudal view	• Hyperextended or hyperflexed views under sedation or general anesthesia may be needed to show the presence of ligament laxity	• Oblique view at a 45-degree angle may also be required

Skill Box 4.12 / Metacarpus and Phalanges

Anatomic area	Metacarpus and Phalanges	
View	**Mediolateral**	**Dorsopalmar**
Positioning (avoid manual restraint; use strategically positioned devices to extend limbs and support the body)	• Lateral recumbency • Affected limb down and extended cranially • Affected phalange is isolated with gauze or tape and pulled dorsally • Unaffected limb extended caudally and relaxed • The head is extended dorsally away from the cassette or table	• Sternal recumbency • Both limbs extended cranially • The head is placed resting over the unaffected limb
Measurement	• If interest is the entire metacarpus, measure at the middle of the metacarpal bones • If interest is the digit, measure at mid-digit	• Mid-metacarpal or area of interest
Beam center	• Middle phalanges or affected phalanx	• Mid-metacarpal or area of interest
Field of view	• Distal radius/ulna to distal digits	• Distal radius/ulna to distal digits
Notes	• Support under the elbow may assist in maintaining proper carpal positioning • Oblique view may be needed in some cases	• Support under the elbow may assist in maintaining proper carpal positioning • Oblique view at 45-degree angle also may be required

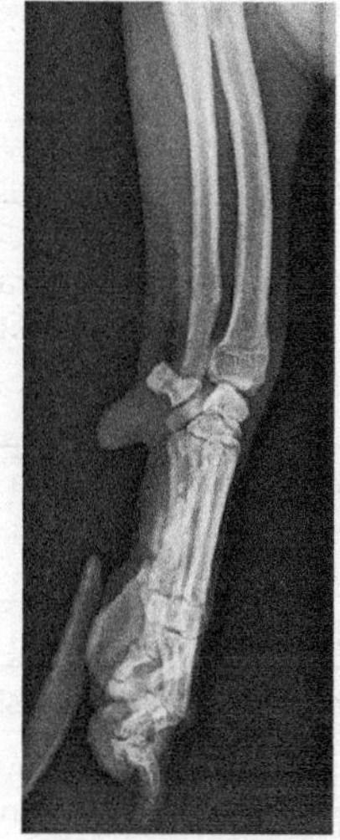

Figure 4.36 **Metacarpus and phalanges in lateral positioning, distal radius/ulna to distal digits.**

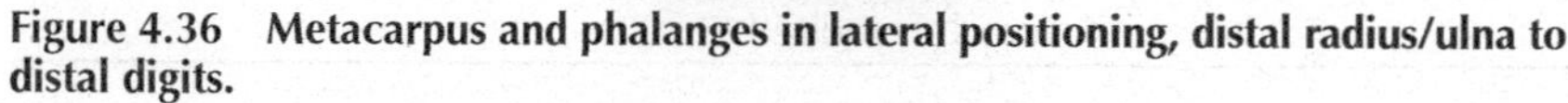

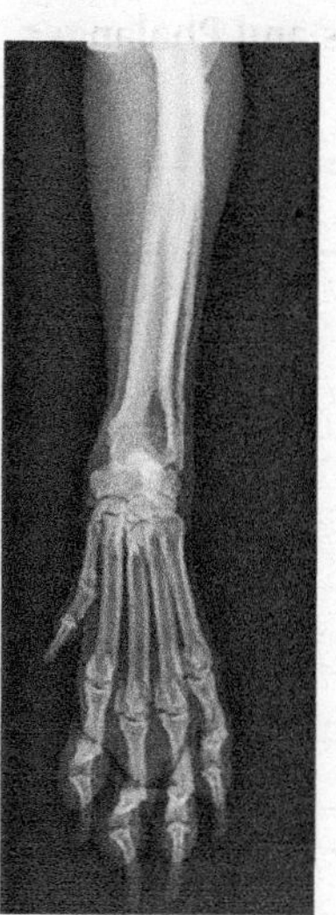

Figure 4.37 **Metacarpus and phalanges in dorsopalmar positioning, distal radius/ulna to distal digits.**

Pelvis and Hind Limb Positioning

Skill Box 4.13 / Pelvis

Anatomic area	**Pelvis**			
View	**Lateral**	**Lateral oblique**	**Ventrodorsal frog leg**	**Ventrodorsal extended**
Positioning (avoid manual restraint; use strategically positioned devices to extend limbs and elevate the body)	• Lateral recumbency • Hind limbs are extended down ventrally, slightly apart with the affected limb slightly cranial to the unaffected limb, separated with a support to avoid spine rotation	• Lateral recumbency • Affected hind limb is extended down ventrally and slightly cranially • The unaffected hind limb is elevated to a 20-degree angle dorsally	• Dorsal recumbency • Hind limbs should be abducted and flexed at a 45-degree angle to the spine, positioned identically	• Dorsal recumbency • Pelvis flat on the table • Hind limbs start in a flexed frog leg position. The area just above the hocks is grasped and limbs are rotated medially so stifles come within 1–2 inches of each other • While rotating the femurs, a second person uses a long piece of tape at the caudal proximal stifle, forcibly securing the ends to the opposite limb. • Both limbs extended caudally ending in a full straight extension of the hind limbs with the patella centered over the femurs • Place sandbags below and above the tarsus for further support

(Continued)

Skill Box 4.13 / Pelvis (Continued)

Anatomic area	Pelvis			
View	**Lateral**	**Lateral oblique**	**Ventrodorsal frog leg**	**Ventrodorsal extended**
Measurement	• Greater trochanter	• Greater trochanter	• Acetabulum (groin)	• Acetabulum (groin)
Beam center	• Greater trochanter	• Greater trochanter	• Pubis/acetabulum	• Pubis/acetabulum
Field of view	• Mid-lumbar spine to mid-femurs	• Mid-lumbar spine to mid-femurs	• Mid-lumbar spine to mid-caudal vertebrae	• Mid-lumbar spine to distal stifle
Notes	• Best view for lumbosacral bony changes if cauda equina pain is suspected • Requires high mAs to penetrate a large dog's pelvic bones	• Typically used if lesions are suspected or for further clarification	• Used if trauma to the pelvis is suspected • Sandbags and V-trough will assist in proper positioning	• Heavy sedation is necessary • Standard for assessment of hips • Correct positioning will result in parallel femurs, patellae centered between femoral condyles, and left and right pelvis displayed as a mirror image • If hip laxity is in question, sometimes the PennHIP method is also recommended, which requires special certification of the veterinarian • Check requirements and submission information for the Orthopedic Foundation for Animals dysplasia evaluation

The Orthopedic Foundation for Animals provides evaluation of radiographs to screen for hip and elbow dysplasias. These x-rays require absolute precision and are reviewed by three radiologists. The combined scoring system consists of normal (excellent, good, fair), borderline, or dysplastic.

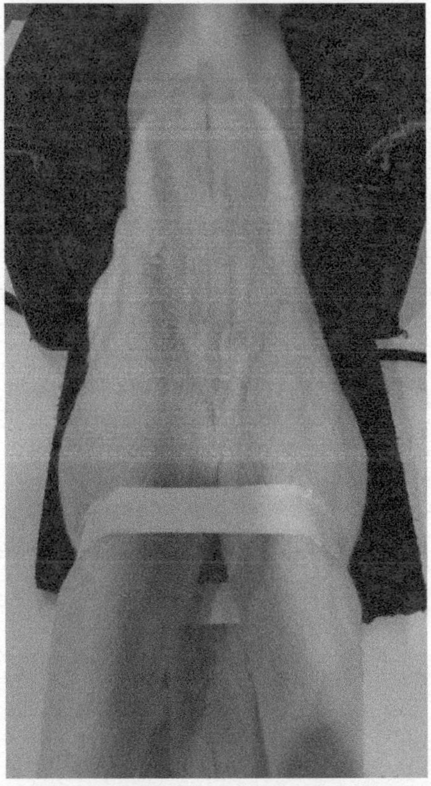

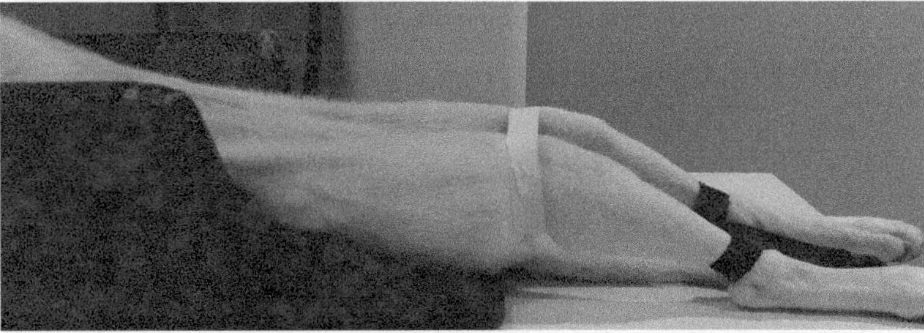

Figure 4.38 a,b Hands-free positioning with the use of foam pad, tape secured around the stifles so that the limbs are parallel with each other and limbs secured with Velcro secured to the end of the table. A small sandbag can be placed below the distal limbs so the full limbs are parallel to the table. A small sandbag can also be placed above the tarsus for further support. Source: courtesy of Ashley Jenner, Toronto ON.

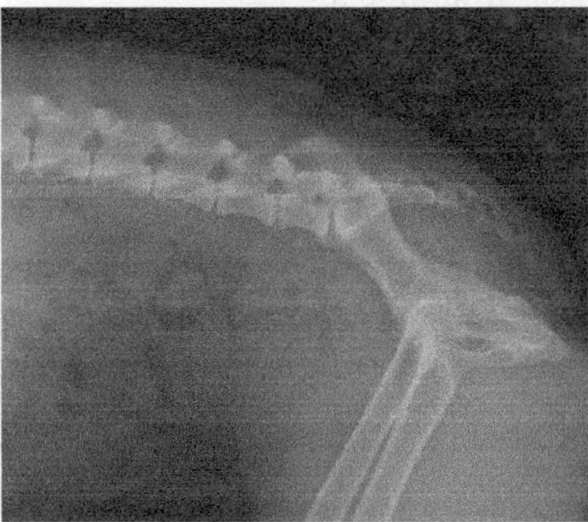

Figure 4.39 Pelvis in lateral positioning, mid-lumbar spine to mid-femurs.

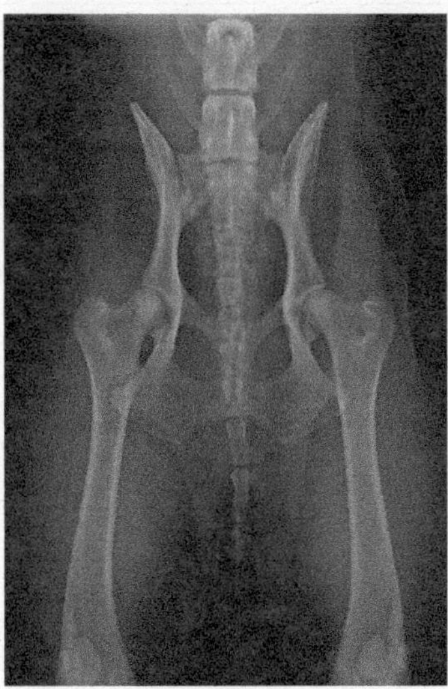

Figure 4.40 Pelvis in ventrodorsal positioning, mid-lumbar spine to distal stifle.

Skill Box 4.14 / Femur, Stifles, Tibia, and Fibula

Anatomic area	Femur		Stifles		Tibia and fibula	
View	**Mediolateral**	**Craniocaudal**	**Mediolateral**	**Caudocranial**	**Mediolateral**	**Caudocranial**
Positioning (avoid manual restraint; use strategically positioned devices to extend limbs and elevate the body)	• Lateral recumbency with affected limb down • Affected limb joints slightly flexed and relaxed • Unaffected limb extended dorsally or abducted out of the beam	• Dorsal recumbency • Affected limb extended caudally with slight abduction • The unaffected limb is relaxed • Keep tail out of the field of view	• Lateral recumbency with affected limb down • Affected limb slightly flexed and relaxed, with support under the hock if necessary to keep knee from rotating • Unaffected limb extended dorsally out of the beam	• Sternal recumbency • Affected limb extended caudally • Unaffected limb is relaxed, and supported with a foam pad under the limb to assist in true craniocaudal position of the affected limb	• Lateral recumbency with affected limb down • Affected limb slightly flexed and relaxed, with support under tarsus to keep tibia from rotating • Unaffected limb is extended cranially or dorsally out of the beam	• Sternal recumbency • Affected limb extended caudally resting on the patella • Unaffected limb is flexed, relaxed, and supported • Place a foam pad underneath to assist placement of affected limb
Measurement	• Mid-femur	• Mid-femur	• Thickest part of stifle	• Thickest part of stifle	• Mid-tibia/fibula	• Mid-tibia/fibula
Beam center	• Mid-femur	• Mid-femur	• Mid-stifle joint	• Mid-stifle joint	• Mid-tibia/fibula	• Mid-tibia/fibula
Field of view	• Coxofemoral joint to proximal tibia/fibula	• Coxofemoral joint to proximal tibia/fibula	• Proximal third of tibia/ fibula and distal third of femur	• Proximal third of tibia/fibula and distal third of femur	• Stifle joint to distal tarsus joint	• Stifle joint to distal tarsus joint
Notes	• Best view for bony neoplasia of femur or if trauma has occurred		• Slightly rotate affected limb to table to avoid rotation • Flex stifle and tarsal joints if cruciate ligament tear is suspected	• Support under the unaffected limb/ pelvis area will assist in proper alignment of affected patella • Skyline view may be required		• Depending on the size of the patient, elevation of the pelvic area will alleviate weight off the stifle

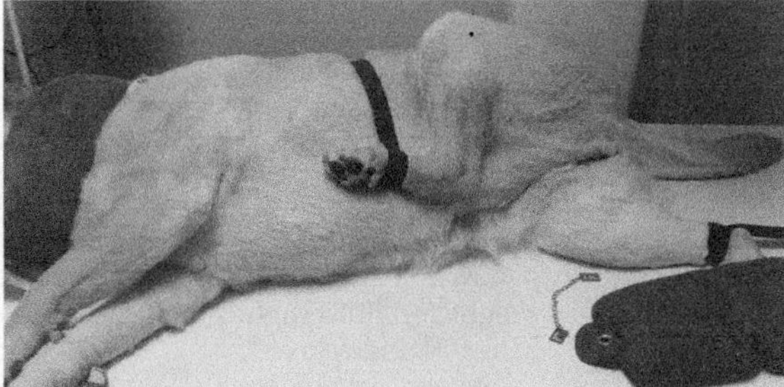

Figure 4.41 Patient positioned in lateral recumbency for stifle. Use of sandbag over the neck and Velcro and straps securing both limbs as shown with sandbag over affected limb maintains the position. The same technique can be used for any of the lateral hind limb positions. Source: courtesy of Ashley Jenner, Toronto, ON.

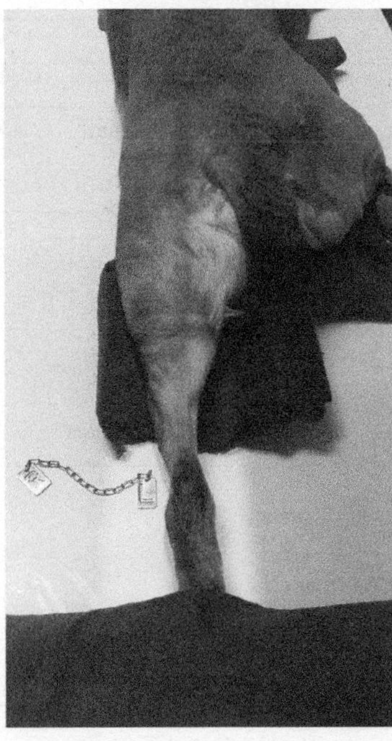

Figure 4.42 Positioning for craniocaudal rear limb. Patient is in ventral recumbency positioned in a foam trough. The affected limb is extended with Velcro and strap and a foam pad is placed under the stifle. The unaffected limb is slightly raised. A sandbag over the neck and cranial to pelvis will further support. Source: courtesy of Ashley Jenner, Toronto, ON.

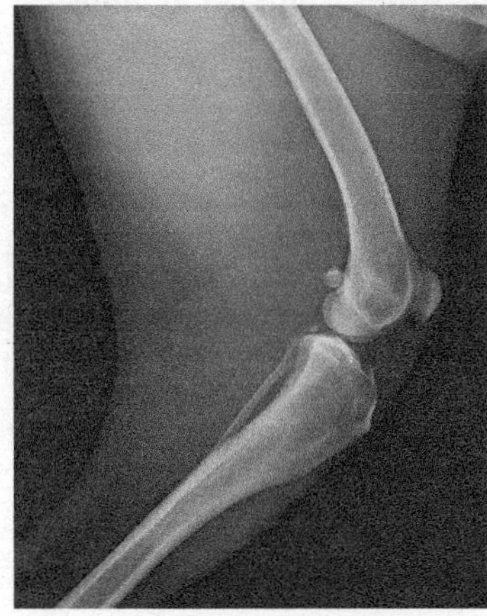

Figure 4.43 Stifle in lateral positioning, mid-femur to mid-tibia/fibula.

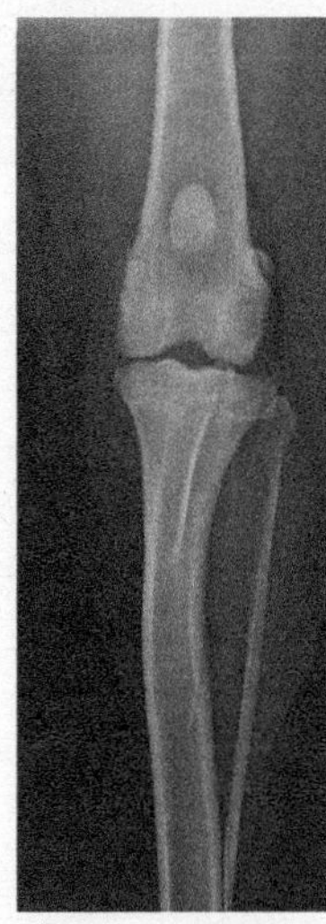

Figure 4.44 Stifle in caudocranial positioning, mid-femur to mid-tibia/fibula.

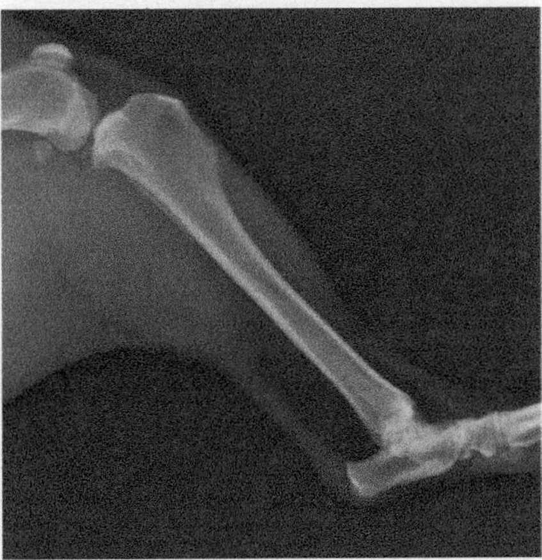

Figure 4.45 Fibula in lateral positioning, stifle joint to distal tarsus joint.

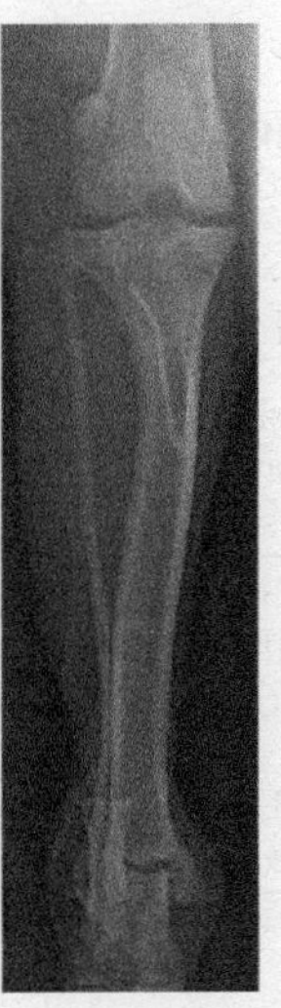

Figure 4.46 Tibia and fibula in caudocranial positioning, stifle joint to distal tarsus joint.

Skill Box 4.15 / **Tarsus and Metatarsals**

Anatomic area	**Tarsus**		**Metatarsus**		
View	**Mediolateral**	**Plantarodorsal**	**Mediolateral**	**Plantarodorsal**	**Dorsoplantar**
Positioning (avoid manual restraint; use strategically positioned devices to extend limbs and elevate the body)	• Lateral recumbency • Affected limb extended and relaxed with support under the tarsus • Unaffected limb extended cranially or abducted dorsally	• Sternal recumbency • Affected limb extended caudally with support under the stifle • The unaffected limb is relaxed and supported next to the body	• Lateral recumbency • Affected limb slightly flexed at stifle and tarsus with support under stifle • Unaffected limb extended cranially	• Sternal recumbency • Affected limb extended caudally with support under the stifle • Unaffected limb is relaxed and supported	• Sternal recumbency with the patient in a crouch-like position • Affected limb extended slightly laterally and cranially with support under pelvis so the plantar aspect of the foot is against the detector
Measurement	• Thickest area of tarsus	• Thickest area of tarsus	• Distal tarsal joint	• Distal tarsal joint	• Distal tarsal joint
Beam center	• Mid-tarsus	• Mid-tarsus	• Mid-metatarsals	• Mid-metatarsals	• Mid-metatarsals

(Continued)

Skill Box 4.15 / Tarsus and Metatarsals (Continued)

Anatomic area	Tarsus		Metatarsus		
View	Mediolateral	Plantarodorsal	Mediolateral	Plantarodorsal	Dorsoplantar
Field of view	• Distal third of tibia/fibula to proximal third of metatarsals	• Distal third of tibia/fibula to proximal third of metatarsals	• Distal tibia/fibula to distal digits	• Distal tibia/fibula to distal digits	• Distal tibia/fibula to distal digits
Notes	• If a flexed lateral is required, the tarsus is flexed 90 degrees and supported or taped in a figure-of-8 at the distal metatarsus	• A dorsoplantar view as described for the metatarsus can be completed • A flexed dorsoplantar may also be required	• Oblique views may be needed for the tarsus or metatarsus	• A foam pad under the unaffected limb will minimize rotation of the affected limb	• There is less distortion for this view than if the patient is in dorsal recumbency and the affected limb extended caudally

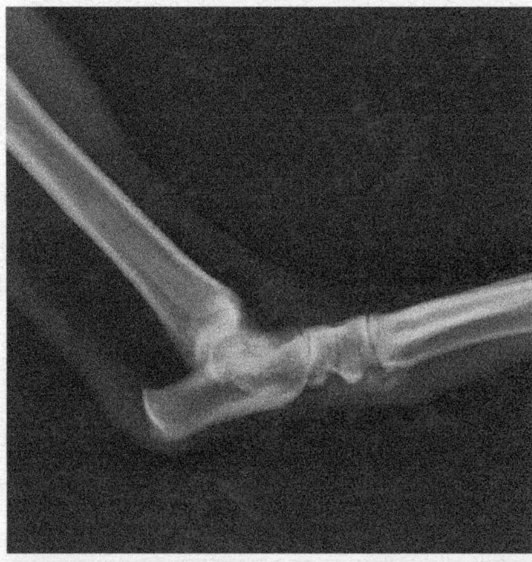

Figure 4.47 Tarsus in lateral positioning, mid-tibia/fibula to mid-metatarsals.

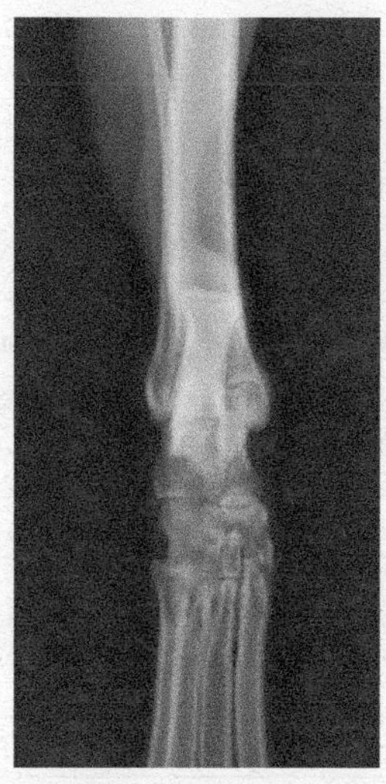

Figure 4.48 Tarsus in dorsoplantar positioning, mid-tibia/fibula to mid-metatarsals.

Skill Box 4.16 / Metacarpus and Phalanges

Anatomic area	Metacarpus and phalanges	
View	**Lateral**	**Dorsopalmar**
Positioning	• Lateral recumbency • Affected limb extended cranially • Affected phalange is isolated with gauze or tape and pulled dorsally • Unaffected limb extended caudally and relaxed • Head is extended dorsally away from the cassette or table	• Sternal recumbency • Affected limb extended cranially • Unaffected limb is extended cranially • Head is placed resting over the unaffected limb
Measurement	• If interest is the entire metacarpus, measure at the middle of the metacarpal bones • If interest is the digit, measure at mid-digit	• Mid-metacarpal
Beam center	• Middle phalanges or affected phalanx	• Mid-metacarpal
Field of view	• Distal radius/ulna to distal digits	• Distal radius/ulna to distal digits
Notes	• Support under the elbow may assist in maintaining proper carpal positioning • Oblique view may be needed in some cases	• Support under the elbow may assist in maintaining proper carpal positioning • Oblique view at 45-degree angle also may be required

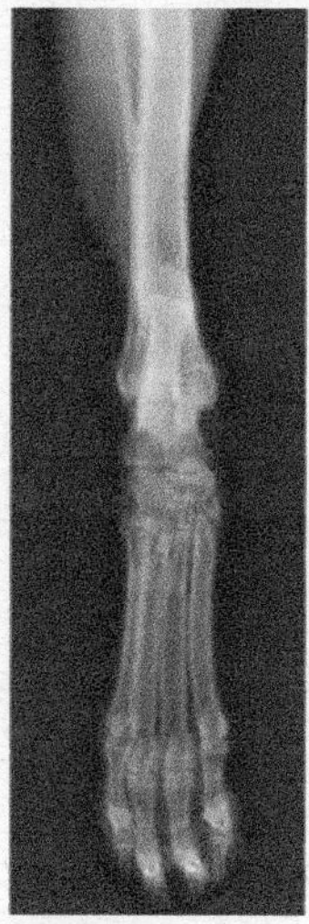

Figure 4.49 Metatarsals and phalanges in dorsoplantar positioning, distal tibia/fibula to distal digits.

RADIOGRAPHIC CONTRAST STUDIES

Contrast studies are performed when survey radiographs do not assist in the diagnosis of the area of concern. The addition of positive radiopaque and negative radiolucent media can provide the veterinarian with a more thorough observation of the affected area.

Modalities such as endoscopy, ultrasonography, magnetic resonance imaging and others, can replace contrast studies if they are available. Only common radiographic studies have been included in this section. Some of the procedures listed in the tables are to be performed by a veterinarian only.

Patient preparation is of extreme importance, and the animal should always be clean and dry for these procedures. In some cases, an enema and fasting may be required so that the gastrointestinal tract is clear of food or feces that could superimpose or distort the anatomic images. The technician should be aware of the possible adverse effects from the contrast medium and should be prepared for appropriate emergency procedures. Preparation for these procedures, as well as the dosage of the contrast medium, should always be reviewed with the veterinarian before the procedure.

Table 4.9 / Types of contrast media

Contrast media	Positive non-iodinated		Positive iodine	Negative
Classification	• Barium sulfate (micropulverized suspension)	• Ionic	• Nonionic	• Gases
Proprietary names	• Microtrast®, Esophotrast®, E-Z Paste®, Novopaque®, Barotrast®, Polibar Plus®, Esobar®, BIPS • Readi-Cat® 2, VoLumen®, HD 200®	• Conray® 420, 280, Urografin® 150 • Gastrografin® (oral only)	• Optiray® 240, 350 (Ioversol), Isovue® (Iopamidol), Omnipaque® (iohexol), Ultravist® (iopromide), Visipaque® (iodixanol), Oxilan® (Ioxilan)	• Room air
Indications	• Visualization of esophagus, stomach, small and large bowels	• Intravascular usage	• Intravascular and myelographic studies, fistulas, and gastrointestinal studies • Given IV, intraurethrally, into fistulas, intraperitoneally	• Visualization of the bladder, pneumocolon, pneumogastrogram

Table 4.9 / Types of contrast media (Continued)

Contrast media	Positive non-iodinated		Positive iodine	Negative
Contraindications	• Perforations or suspected ruptures	• Myelography and arthrography • CHF, dehydration, and renal failure	• CHF, dehydration, or hematuria	• Areas not able to tolerate a transient reduction or interruption in blood flow
Adverse effects	• Results in granulomas/lesions if leaks outside gastrointestinal tract, lung aspiration can be fatal	• Acute renal failure, transient pulmonary edema, urticaria, diarrhea, dehydration, and vomiting • Oral: (bitter tasting to cats; use gastric tube to administer), hypertonic	• Less frequently noted	• Gases may result in an embolism; possibly fatal if they access the vascular system
Monitoring	• Vomiting and apnea	• Vitals including pulse, CRT, mucous membranes, and temperature; watch for nausea, vomiting, skin erythema, facial swelling, pulmonary edema (respiration), dehydration, hypotension, hypovolemia		
Notes	• Radiopaque – shows white on radiograph • Has excellent mucosal-coating properties but can mask foreign bodies; do not use before ultrasound	• Radiopaque – shows white on radiograph • Patient must be well hydrated for any ionic contrast medium • Whenever an iodinated contrast is needed, a nonionic contrast should be used to reduce possible complications		• Radiolucent – shows up black on radiograph • May be combined with other contrast media for double-contrast images

Gastrointestinal Tract Contrast Studies

Skill Box 4.17 / Gastrointestinal Tract Contrast Studies: Esophagography and Gastrography

Procedure	Esophagography	Gastrography		
		Positive contrast study	**Negative contrast study (pneumogastrogram)**	**Double-contrast study**
Indications	• Vomiting of undigested food, gagging, or dysphagia	• Gastric masses/foreign body, or vomiting	• Gastric masses/foreign body, or vomiting	• Gastric masses/foreign body, or vomiting
Contraindications	• Rupture/perforation, or dyspnea	• Parasitic infection, rupture/perforation	• Presence of ingesta or fluid	• Rupture/perforation
Contrast media	• Barium sulfate or, if perforation is suspected, nonionic iodinated contrast (240–300 mg/ml) 10 ml/kg at a 1 : 2 dilution	• Barium sulfate 30–60% w/v • Organic iodide (diatrizoate solution 10%)	• Carbon dioxide, nitrous oxide, or oxygen	• Barium sulfate 30–60% w/v and room air
Equipment	• Large syringe • Wet towels • Optional: canned food or kibble	• Orogastric tube • Large syringe • Wet towels • Bite block	• Orogastric tube • Large syringe • Three-way valve • Bite block	• Orogastric tube • Large syringe • Wet towels • Three-way valve • Bite block
Patient preparation	• Fasting: not required • Survey radiographs • Conscious patient	• Fasting: 12–24 hours • Large bowel evacuation or enema • Survey radiographs • Conscious patient	• Fasting: 12–24 hours • Survey radiographs	• Fasting: 12–24 hours • Survey radiographs • Conscious patient
Technique	1. Mucosal assessment 2. Place patient in lateral recumbency 3. Administer positive contrast medium (5–20 ml of 60% w/v of barium or around 10–15 ml of non-ionic iodinated at a 50 : 50 mixture of water) into the buccal pouch 4. Radiograph as the patient swallows 5. Typically followed by 6. Stricture and motility assessment 7. Feed barium-coated kibble mix (this should not be used if a perforation is suspected) 8. Radiograph	1. Administer positive contrast medium (5–10 ml/kg 30% w/v barium of nonionic iodinated (240–300 mg/ml) 10 ml/kg at a 1 : 2 dilution orally with a syringe or through an orogastric tube 2. Radiograph immediately centering over the cranial abdomen	1. Insert an orogastric tube into the stomach; verify placement 2. Administer 20 ml/kg room air 3. Remove the orogastric tube and hold the muzzle closed while radiographing immediately	1. Insert an orogastric tube into the stomach; verify placement 2. Administer a positive contrast medium (2 ml/kg) 3. Follow with 20 ml/kg room air to achieve a tympanic stomach 4. Roll the patient to coat the stomach and radiograph immediately

(*Continued*)

Skill Box 4.17 / Gastrointestinal Tract Contrast Studies: Esophagography and Gastrography (Continued)

Procedure	Esophagography	Gastrography		
		Positive contrast study	Negative contrast study (pneumogastrogram)	Double-contrast study
Radiographic views	• Immediate: R-LAT, R-VD OBL of neck and thorax	• R- and L-LAT, DV, VD	• R- and L-LAT, DV, VD	• R- and L-LAT, DV, VD
Notes	• Monitor for aspiration of contrast • Fluoroscopy may aid in the evaluation of motility and function • General anesthesia is not recommended because of the risk of aspiration after vomiting • Double-contrast study may be used	• Monitor for aspiration of contrast • General anesthesia is not recommended because of inhibition of gastrointestinal motility and risk of aspiration after vomiting • If a perforation is suspected, iodine should be used. However, these iodinated contrast materials are bitter tasting and may result in vomiting; some are also hypertonic (if inhaled, could result in pulmonary edema)	• Slight sedation may be more comfortable for the patient • Effervescent carbon dioxide granules can be substituted for the air in both double and negative contrast studies	• Monitor for aspiration of contrast • Fluoroscopy may aid gastric lesion evaluation • Slight sedation may be more comfortable for the patient but vomiting must be clearly monitored

w/v = weight (of solute) per volume (of solvent).
Note: See Skill Box 16.10: Orogastric tube passage and gastric lavage.

Skill Box 4.18 / Gastrointestinal Tract Contrast Studies: Upper and Lower Gastrointestinal Study

Procedure	Upper gastrointestinal study		Lower gastrointestinal study
Medium	**Barium**	**Iodinated contrast**	**Double-contrast barium enema**
Area of study	• Small intestine morphology and functionality	• Small intestine morphology and functionality	• Large-bowel morphology
Indications	• Vomiting, diarrhea, neoplasias, obstructions, anorexia, melana, chronic weight loss, persistent abdominal pain	• Vomiting, diarrhea, neoplasias, or obstructions and a perforation is suspected	• Large-bowel obstruction, bloody diarrhea, other abnormal and painful defecation
Contraindications	• Perforated esophagus or stomach • Lower bowel obstruction, gastric dilatation/ volvulus, paralytic ileus	• Dehydrated patient • Hypertonic solutions (ionic e.g. Gastrografin®) should not be used in hypovolemic patients	• Rupture/perforation • Avoid procedure if proctoscopy completed within 12 hours
Contrast media	• Barium sulfate (30% w/v)	• Non-ionic iodinated contrast	• Barium sulfate diluted (10–20% w/v)
Equipment	• Orogastric tube • Wet towels • Large syringe • Bite block	• Orogastric tube • Wet towels • Large syringe • Bite block	• Examination gloves • Warmed barium sulfate • Enema syringe • Lubricant • Foley catheter • Three-way stopcock • Compression paddle • Wet towels
Patient preparation	• Fasting: 24 hours • Enema to evacuate the colon prior to the study • Conscious patient • Survey radiographs	• Fasting: 24 hours • Enema to evacuate the colon prior to the study • Conscious patient • Survey radiographs	• Fasting: 24 hours • Oral laxative and tepid water (or isotonic saline) enema • General anesthesia • Survey radiographs

(*Continued*)

Skill Box 4.18 / Gastrointestinal Tract Contrast Studies: Upper and Lower Gastrointestinal Study (Continued)

Procedure	**Upper gastrointestinal study**		**Lower gastrointestinal study**
Medium	**Barium**	**Iodinated contrast**	**Double-contrast barium enema**
Technique	1. Administer barium (5–10 ml/kg; non-ionic iodinated (240–300 mg/ml) 10 ml/kg at a 1 : 2 dilution) orally with a syringe or through an orogastric tube 2. Radiograph at times indicated	1. Administer iodinated contrast (around 1–5 ml/kg) orally with a syringe or through an orogastric tube 2. Radiograph	1. Place the patient in right lateral recumbency and insert the balloon catheter in the anus; inflate the balloon to completely occlude the anal canal 2. Slowly infuse the diluted, body temperature barium sulfate mixture into the large bowel and cecum (around 10–15 ml/kg) 3. lamp the catheter and radiograph (add more contrast medium if bowel distention is not sufficient) 4. After these radiographs have been completed, evacuate the barium (if a portosystemic shunt is suspected, place the patient in left lateral recumbency) and infuse gas to redistend the colon 5. Radiograph
Radiographic views	Canine protocol: • 0–5 minutes: R- and L-LAT, VD, DV (for stomach) • 15 minutes: R-LAT, VD • 60 minutes: R-LAT, VD • Hourly R-LAT, VD until most of barium has cleared the small intestine and the contrast medium is in the large intestines Feline protocol: • Same images taken at 0–5, 15, 30 and every 30 minutes as above	• For both dogs and cats, take the initial R- and L-LAT, VD, DV at 0–5 minutes(for stomach) • Then LAT, VD for canines every 30 minutes and felines every 15 minutes, until the contrast medium is in the large intestine	• R-LAT, VD abdominal after barium infusion and then again after gas infusion • Obliques may be required, especially in males
Notes	• Care must be taken on the choice of anesthesia/sedation, if needed, so as not to impede the motility of the gastrointestinal tract • barium-impregnated polyethylene spheres may be used to evaluate gastric dysmotility and intestinal transit time	• Care must be taken on choice of anesthesia/sedation so as not to impede the motility of the gastrointestinal tract	• If study is for diagnosis of obstruction or intussusception, no fecal evacuation is necessary • Elevation of the cranial two thirds of the body may assist removal of the contrast media

Urinary Tract Contrast Studies

Preparation of the patient is extremely important in producing quality contrast radiographs of the urinary tract. A warmed isotonic saline enema should always be done before the procedure to minimize superimposition of any colonic contents on the ureters and bladder. Hydration should be assessed and stabilized before beginning any of these procedures. The technician should note the special precautions and monitoring needed when completing excretory urography. Although rare, when complications do occur, they can be fatal, and being prepared for the possible emergency can make a difference.

With the increasing availability of ultrasound, radiographic contrast studies are not as frequently completed.

Another procedure to differentiate gas and material in the colon from the intestines and to define gas dilated loops of intestines from colon (possible obstruction) as well as colonic strictures is pneumocolon (placing room air in the colon).

Skill Box 4.19 / Urinary Tract Contrast Studies: Intravenous Urography

Procedure	**Intravenous urography (also called excretory urography , intravenous pyelography)**
Area of study	• Urinary system: kidneys and ureters
Indications	• Suspicion of calculi, strictures, or masses within the urethra
Contraindications	• Dehydration, urethral obstruction
Contrast media	• Iodinated contrast for intravascular injection, warmed
Equipment	• IV catheter; large bore, short (contrast is viscous) • Syringe • 22-gauge, 1-inch needle • Iodinated contrast • Compression bandage • Fluids ready to use • Resuscitation kit (epinephrine, Ambu bag, oxygen ready)
Patient preparation	• 24-hour fast but have water available • Enema (warm, isotonic saline, not a soapy enema): 4 hours prior • Hydration assessed, stabilized, and monitored • Urine sample obtained prior to procedure • IV catheter • Sedation or general anesthesia • Abdominal survey radiographs
Technique	1. Bolus intravenous infusion of a warmed non-ionic iodinated contrast media (600–800 mg/kg, 3 ml/kg, 90 ml maximum for dogs and 15 ml for cats) 2. Radiograph immediately and follow-up radiographs as listed next

(Continued)

Skill Box 4.19 / Urinary Tract Contrast Studies: Intravenous Urography (Continued)

Procedure	Intravenous urography (also called excretory urography , intravenous pyelography)
Radiographic views	**Minutes of exposure:**
	• 0 minutes: , LAT
	• 3–5 minutes: VD, ± LAT, ± VD OBL, ± R-LAT OBL • Compression bandage may be applied
	• 10–15 minutes: VD LAT, ± LAT OBL • Remove the compression bandage if applied
	• 30–120 minutes: VD, LAT, ± LAT OBL
Notes	• Monitor for hypotension, vomiting, urticaria, arrhythmia, cardiovascular collapse, anaphylaxis, and contrast medium-induced acute renal failure • Abdominal compression may be used to visualize the renal collecting system and proximal ureters • Oblique radiographs may be required to visualize the distal ureters
Complete urinary tract examination	
A complete urinary tract examination can be completed by combining the IV urography, cystography and urethrogram using both positive and negative contrast. Also known as the Rendano method, named after Dr. Victor Rendano.	
Indications, contraindications, contrast media, equipment and patient preparation	• As above • In addition, for equipment and patient preparation, place an urethral catheter in the bladder and use a three-way stopcock to infuse air and positive contrast • The amount of urine removed from the bladder should be noted
Technique	• Bolus intravenous infusion of a warmed non-ionic iodinated contrast media (600–800 ml/kg, 3 ml/kg, 90 ml maximum for dogs and 15 ml for cats)
Radiographic views	• VD radiographs within 20–40 seconds • Distend bladder with negative contrast media using three-way stopcock to keep air in bladder • Take ventrodorsal and LAT 5 minutes after distention; determine whether more air is needed • 20 minutes after IV injection VD, LAT, ± LAT radiographs • Inject 5–15 ml iodinated medium into the urethra and take LAT radiograph either during administration of the last few ml contrast medium or remove the catheter and take LAT radiograph when contrast agent is leaking from urethra

Skill Box 4.20 / Urinary Tract Contrast Studies: Cystography

Procedure	Cystography		
Type	**Positive contrast**	**Negative contrast (pneumocystography)**	**Double contrast**
Area of study	• Urinary bladder wall integrity and position	• Urinary bladder wall evaluation and aid in identifying strictures	• Urinary bladder mucosal detail
Indications	• Trauma, hematuria, or straining	• Bladder wall thickness, mural lesions and calculi	• Trauma or straining, abnormal urination, mucosal lesions, mural masses
Contraindications	• Enlarged bladder	• Enlarged bladder, hematuria	• Enlarged bladder, hematuria
Contrast media	• Iodinated contrast (one part contrast to three parts water)	• Gas (room air)	• Negative and positive non-ionic iodinated contrast media
Equipment for all three procedures	• Urinary catheter (Foley, tomcat, or soft flexible male catheter) • Large syringe • Three-way stopcock • Sterile saline • Lubricant • Wet towels • Bowl • 3–5 ml 2% lidocaine (to ↓ spasms)		
Patient preparation for all three procedures	• 24-hour fast • Give warm, isotonic saline enema four hours before to void colon of feces • Obtain urine sample before procedure • Sedation or general anesthesia • Survey radiographs		

(Continued)

Skill Box 4.20 / **Urinary Tract Contrast Studies: Cystography (Continued)**

Procedure	**Cystography**		
Type	**Positive contrast**	**Negative contrast (pneumocystography)**	**Double contrast**
Technique	1. Aseptic placement of a urinary catheter to the bladder neck 2. Empty the bladder and note the amount of urine removed to estimate the amount of contrast medium to use 3. Infuse 3–5 ml lidocaine to ↓ bladder spasticity 4. Infuse positive contrast medium 240 or 300 mg/ml at a dosage of 5–10 ml/kg for dogs and 2–5 ml/kg for cats (max 25 ml) into the urinary catheter 5. Monitor the bladder by palpation until distended 6. Radiograph	1. The patient should be in *left* lateral recumbency 2. Aseptic placement of a urinary catheter to the bladder neck 3. Empty the bladder and note the amount removed to estimate the amount of contrast medium to use 4. Infuse 3–5 ml lidocaine to ↓ bladder spasticity 5. Infuse gas (room air) at a volume sufficient to distend the bladder about 3–12 mg/kg (maximum of 25 ml for cats) into the urinary catheter, carefully monitoring the bladder by palpation until distended 6. Radiograph	1. The patient should start in *right* lateral recumbency. Aseptic placement of a urinary catheter to the bladder neck 2. Empty the bladder and note the amount removed to estimate the amount of contrast medium to use 3. Infuse 3–5 ml lidocaine to ↓ bladder spasticity 4. Infuse a small amount (canine: 1–10 ml depending on the size of the dog, feline: 0.5–1.0 ml) of non-ionic iodinated contrast into the urinary catheter 5. Roll the patient to coat the bladder wall and radiograph 6. Place the patient in left lateral recumbency. Infuse gas (room air) into the urinary catheter and monitor the bladder by palpation until distended 7. Radiograph
Radiographic views	• LAT, VD • If further radiographs are necessary, inject additional contrast media	• LAT, VD, ± OBL • If further radiographs are necessary, inject additional contrast media	• LAT, VD OBL
Notes	• Complications may include trauma due to improper catheterization, iatrogenic infection, or chemical cystitis	• Keeping the patient in left lateral recumbency minimizes the risk of formation of an air embolus • Complications may include trauma caused by improper catheterization, iatrogenic infection, or air emboli	• On infusion of air, keeping the patient in left lateral recumbency minimizes the risk of formation of an air embolus • Complications may include trauma caused by improper catheterization, iatrogenic infection, air emboli, or chemical cystitis • Gas bubbles that interfere with interpretation are less likely to occur if performed in this order
	• See Skill Box 16.23: Canine urinary catheterization, page 732, and Skill Box 16.24: Feline urinary catheterization, page 733.		

Urethra Contrast Studies

Skill Box 4.21 / Urethra Contrast Studies: Urethrography

Procedure	**Urethrography**
Area of study	• Urethra location and morphology
Indications	• Stranguria, hematuria, dysuria, suspected masses or lesions
Contraindications	• Uncontrolled hematuria
Contrast media	• Iodinated contrast medium (120 mg/ml, 5–15 ml; give only enough to distend the urethra)
Equipment	• Urinary catheter (Foley, soft polyethylene male catheter for canines and tomcat catheter for felines) prefilled with contrast media • Large syringe • Three-way stopcock • Sterile saline • Lubricant • Wet towels • Bowl • Lidocaine • Radiolucent paddle or wooden spoon
Patient preparation	• Fasting: 24 hours • Enema 4 hours before • Sedation • Survey radiographs • Lateral of perineal and penile regions with hind limbs extended cranially for males

(*Continued*)

Skill Box 4.21 / **Urethra Contrast Studies: Urethrography (Continued)**

Procedure	**Urethrography**
Technique	1. Retrograde urethrography (more common in males) 2. Aseptic placement of a urinary catheter to distal urethra 3. ± Infuse 2–5 ml of lidocaine to ↓ urethral spasms 4. Infuse undiluted contrast (10–20 ml) to fill the urethra 5. Radiograph during administration of the last few ml contrast medium. Repeat infusion for additional radiographs 6. Antegrade or voiding urethrography 7. Aseptic placement of a urinary catheter to distal urethra 8. ± Infuse 2–5 ml of lidocaine to ↓ urethral spasms 9. Infuse enough undiluted contrast to fill the bladder and induce urination 10. Radiograph during voiding; gentle pressure may need to be applied to the bladder 11. If it is difficult to catheterize feline and canine females, a voiding urethrogram can be completed after positive contrast cystography 12. Be prepared to catch voided urine 13. Vaginourethrogram (frequently performed to evaluate the urethra in a female canine or feline and vaginography
	14. To study vagina, cervix, and urethra morphology for strictures, vaginal or urethral tears, masses, or suspected ectopic ureter 15. General anesthesia may be required 16. Place a urinary catheter (Foley, soft polyethylene male catheter), prefilled with contrast media into the vulva and inflate cuff just inside the vaginal vault 17. ± Purse-string suture or Babcock forceps is used to keep the vulvar lips closed and the Foley catheter in place during the procedure 18. Infuse with undiluted iodinated contrast media to fill the vagina (e.g. back pressure felt on syringe) 19. Radiograph as the infusion is administered while the vagina is distended. Overdistention of the vagina forces the contrast medium up the urethra and into the bladder
Radiographic views	• Lateral (including perineal area), ventrodorsal (females), ventrodorsal oblique (male) • Repeat infusion for any additional radiographs
Notes	• See Skill Box Box 16.23: Canine urinary catheterization, page 732, and Skill Box 16.24: Feline urinary catheterization, page 733.

Spinal Contrast Studies

Skill Box 4.22 / Spinal Contrast Studies: Myelography

Procedure	**Myelography**
Area of study	• Spinal cord
Indications	• Clinical transverse myelopathies
Contraindications	• Myelitis and meningitis
Contrast media	• Positive non-ionic media only
Equipment	• Clippers, scrub solutions, drape, sterile gloves • 20–22-gauge spinal needle in various sizes: 1½, 2½, and 3½ depending on the breed and species • Two 10-ml syringes for dog, and two 5-ml syringes for cat • 3 ml syringe to collect cerebrospinal fluid
Patient preparation	• General anesthesia without phenothiazine derivative • Spinal survey radiographs • Aseptic preparation of appropriate spinal location • Withdraw and examine cerebrospinal fluid for systemic or local infection
Technique	• Aseptic spinal puncture of subarachnoid space at either cisterna magna or an interarcuate space of caudal lumbar spine (L5–L6) • Inject nonionic contrast media slowly to fill the subarachnoid space (200–300 mgl/ml at a dose of 0.45 ml/kg • The needle may be removed or left in place for lateral radiographs
Radiographic views	• Lateral, ventrodorsal, dorsoventral, oblique, extended/flexed lateral
Notes	• Myelography may cause intensification of preexisting neurological signs • There must be patient movement during placement of spinal needle and injection • Do not inject contrast media of there is blood in the tap • Tilting of the body may be necessary to assist in the coating of the contrast media • Elevate the head during recovery • Monitor for apnea and seizures

ULTRASONOGRAPHY

Ultrasonography is a cross-sectional computer-generated image created by the reflection of high-frequency sound waves. It is used to confirm or further evaluate abnormalities found on radiographs, primarily evaluating soft tissue structures of the head/neck region, thorax/heart, abdomen, and musculoskeletal (joints and tendons). The indications for the use of ultrasound are extensive and provide an additional level to diagnostics. This non-invasive, non-painful technique is used in the evaluation, diagnosis, and staging of many diseases. Ultrasound is a good modality for the evaluation of fluid-filled and soft-tissue organs. Doppler ultrasonography is an additional technique used to identify blood flow and velocity, and to calculate pressure of the heart and uterus. Owing to the minute complexities of ultrasound findings, it is often necessary to seek the opinion of a board-certified veterinary radiologist, when feasible and practical. An ultrasound machine, appropriate transducers (e.g. 5, 7.5-MHz transducers), and ultrasound gel are required.

Skill Box 4.23 / Basic Terminology

Terminology	Meaning
Echogenicity	The gray scale noted on the monitor
Hypoechoic	The structure indicated is darker than the surrounding tissue
Hyperechoic	The structure is brighter than the surrounding tissue
Anechoic	Image is black such as in fluid
Isoechoic	The structure is the same as compared to another organ
Near field	The part of the image that is closest to the probe at the top of the ultrasound monitor
Far field	The part of the image that is further from the probe at the bottom of the ultrasound screen
Echotexture	Describes the texture of each organ; a coarse texture is more heterogeneous or diverse with less of a uniform quality throughout than normal
B-mode	B refers to brightness mode where the echo data is depicted as dots or pixels on a screen as a two-dimensional image; the higher the intensity of the returning echo, the brighter the pixel
M-mode	M or motion mode is depicted as a two-dimensional display of reflector over a time oriented baseline, so that stationary objects are represented in straight lines and moving objects produce wavy lines
Doppler	A Doppler is used to detect the flow of blood or other fluids while measuring their velocity; the frequency heard is either lower or higher than that transmitted by the source
Reverberation	An artifact caused by the repeated reflection of the sound wave between two highly reflective interfaces such as between gas in the intestine and the ultrasound probe
Acoustic shadow	An artifact where no sound waves penetrate into deep tissue because the majority of the ultrasound beam is reflected or absorbed at an interface such as bone or gas

Skill Box 4.24 / Basic scanning technique and considerations.

1. Prepare the patient:
   a. Withhold food 8–12 hours for gastrointestinal tract scans.
   b. A full bladder is helpful for urinary studies.
   c. Because hair traps air, most of the beam is reflected prior to entering the body if the patient is not properly prepared.
      i. Closely clip (#40 if possible) and clean the full area of interest. For a full abdominal study, shave from the xiphoid to the pubis about the width of the costal arch.
      ii. Alcohol is sprayed on the skin last to remove superficial fats.
      iii. Apply liberal amounts of ultrasound gel to the skin and transducer to improve contact.
   d. Sedation or general anesthesia may be necessary for anxious patients and for ultrasound-guided needle aspirations or core biopsies.
   e. In abdominal examinations, small animals are generally placed in dorsal recumbency on a padded V trough or in lateral recumbency.
   f. If cardiac ultrasound is required, the patient is placed in sternal or lateral recumbency with the shaved area placed over a hole in the table to allow the transducer to be passed through it.
2. Dim the room lighting to reduce reflections from the screen and to enhance visualization of the image.
3. Enter the patient data after turning on the ultrasound machine. Choose the probe and preset for the particular patient.
4. Set the power setting as low as possible but ensure that the most distal structure in the field can be seen.
5. Position the patient in a consistent orientation on the scanning table (this will make learning and consistent orientation of images easier) and follow a similar sequence for each evaluation.
6. Choose the highest frequency transducer possible for the patient and area under examination.
   a. This provides the best resolution but also limits the depth of penetration of the sound beam. A 7.5 MHz transducer has a depth of 10 cm and wavelength of 0.21 mm which allows for better spatial resolution (0.42 mm). This can be used for small dogs and cats or superficial organs in larger dogs
   b. A lower frequency probe may be needed for deeper structures or larger dogs. A 5 MHz transducer will probe deeper to 15 cm but with the longer wavelength of 0.31 mm, the maximum spatial resolution is 0.62 mm, accounting for less detail than a higher-frequency transducer.
   c. It is common to switch between probes during an examination.
7. Orient the marker on the transducer toward the associated marker on the upper left corner of the US screen to assist in performing a standardized ultrasound.
8. It is usually easiest for a right handed person to hold the transducer in the right hand and to use the left hand to make control panel adjustments.
9. Hold the transducer perpendicular to the skin with the area of interest as close to the surface as possible. Do not press the transducer too hard against the patient as this may cause discomfort. Just use sufficient pressure to maintain good contact between the skin and the transducer.
10. Scan slowly and thoroughly to ensure complete examination of each structure, scanning organs in at least two planes to allow a three-dimensional impression to be built up from the cross-sectional images. Ensure that the each organ scanned is done so in entirety.
11. Each organ should be imaged in sagittal (mimics a lateral radiograph) and transverse planes (represents a VD image). In sagittal plane, the transducer is fanned from left to right while in transverse plane, fan the transducer cranial to caudal. For standardization, in sagittal scanning display the cranial aspect of the patient to the left side of the monitor, while in transverse planes, the patient's right side should be toward the left of the screen.
12. The two most common controls used for adjusting are depth and focal zone. The depth depends on the organ of interest. The focal zone is the depth at which the image has the highest resolution and should be set at or just below the organ of interest.
13. Use the time gain compensation control to adjust overall image brightness keeping in mind that since this is a post processing technique, there is no effect on the ultrasound waves.
14. The dynamic range controls the overall greyscale of the image and can be adjusted to better image lesions.
15. The major limiting factor for scanning is obstruction due to gas-filled organs or bony structures.
16. Artifacts on examination can lead to misleading information and an incorrect diagnosis or treatment (experience of operator critical).
17. Owners should be made aware that a large area of fur may be clipped.
18. Transducer care and cleaning:
    a. Avoid dropping or hitting probe so as not to damage the piezoelectric crystals.
    b. Wipe probe clean of gel as soon as possible after the procedure.
    c. Wash transducer probe with dry or moistened soft cloth.
    d. Check with manufacturer's service manual to use proper cleanser to remove contaminated fluids on the transducer.
    e. Never use alcohol beyond 2 cm from the tip of the transducer as damage can occur to the housing joint seals.
    f. Avoid contact with gels containing mineral oil, lanolin or lotions and never autoclave or use ethylene oxide gas sterilization transducers.

Skill Box 4.25 / Sonographic Appearance and Concerns

Organ	Transducer placement and imaging concerns	Appearance/location
Abdomen	• Dorsal or lateral recumbency • Scan entire ventral abdomen	• Note differences in echogenicity; note free fluid or unidentified masses (e.g. mesenteric tumors) • Liver and gall bladder
Liver and gall bladder (Figure 4.52)	• Directly caudal to xiphoid process • Image through 10th and 12th intercostal space • Depth of field should be adequate to image the dorsal-most aspect • In deep-chested dogs, the transducer needs to be moved a great distance along the costal arch to note portocaval shunts and venous congestion	• Normal parenchyma is echogenic, homogenous, and of medium texture which changes with focal and diffuse lesions • Hepatic and portal veins are round and tubular anechoic structures • Left liver lobe can be seen along the body wall • Gall bladder is located between right medial and quadrate lobes of the liver • Neck of the gall bladder extends to the cystic duct that continues as the bile duct, and terminates at the duodenum • Bile duct is ventral to the portal vein
Spleen (Figure 4.53)	• As for the liver, but extend further caudally; locate head of spleen on left then follow body and tail • To view the body and tail of the spleen, reduce depth of field • In large dogs, it may be necessary to switch between high and low frequency probes to fully evaluate the entire organ	• Homogeneous and finely textured parenchyma which is usually hyperechoic • Focal and diffuse lesions changes the texture
Kidney (Figure 4.54)	• Slightly beneath sublumbar muscles • Left: behind last rib • Right: over the last two intercostal space • Once the left kidney is visualized, adjust the depth of view to display the entire kidney and gently rock the transducer until the kidney has disappeared from the image • To find the right kidney, position the transducer along the right side of the cranial abdomen, just caudal to the costal arch in a sagittal plane • Slowly sweep the probe from left to right to find the right kidney	• Medullary tissue is hypoechoic and may be mistaken as hydronephrosis • Sagittally, there is echogenic cortical tissue surrounding hypoechoic medulla tissue • Left kidney is caudal to the stomach, dorsal and medial to the spleen along the left side of the abdomen • Right kidney is generally more dorsal and cranial than the left kidney and is medial and dorsal to the right lobe of the pancreas • Lateral recumbency is best to note local and diffuse lesions or hydronephrosis while dorsal recumbency best indicates pyelonephritis and renal calculi
Adrenal	• Left adrenal gland is located by scanning medial to the left kidney to the aorta • Normal adrenal gland is flattened and bilobed in dogs but appearance changes with hyperplasia • There is hyperplasia in Cushing's and atrophy in Addison's diseases	• Adrenal located medial to cranial pole of kidney • Adrenal gland is uniformly hypoechoic to the surrounding fat • Left adrenal gland is located between the cranial mesenteric artery and the left renal artery • Right adrenal gland is located medial to the right kidney, between the aorta and the caudal vena cava, just caudal to the liver • Adrenal gland is approximately 7 mm in a medium-sized dog, and 4 mm in cats

(*Continued*)

Skill Box 4.25 / Sonographic Appearance and Concerns (Continued)

Organ	Transducer placement and imaging concerns	Appearance/location
Stomach and duodenum (Figure 4.55)	• Dorsal or lateral recumbency • The stomach is directly caudal to the liver with the transducer at level of xiphoid • Canine stomach is viewed in transverse axis when in sagittal plane • To keep in a transverse plan, rotate the transducer clockwise as the stomach curves from body to pyloric antrum • To image proximal descending duodenum in cross-section, rotate the transducer counterclockwise	• Canine stomach centrally located with long axis perpendicular to spine while feline stomach is left of midline and parallel to spine • Fundus is to the left and body on midline • In dogs, the stomach extends further right, while in cats it is just to the midline • As the pylorus leads to the duodenum, the typical layered appearance of small intestine will be noted
Pancreas (Figure 4.56)	• Dorsal or lateral recumbency • Scan caudal to stomach and medial to duodenum but best to scan entire ventral abdomen from the xiphisternum to the umbilicus to note pancreatitis and tumors • Most difficult organ to determine if there is absence or presence of disease	• A poorly marginated hypoechoic organ that may be flat and thin and somewhat triangular or lobulated • Consists of right and left lobes • The two lobes are connected by the body in the angle of the pylorus and duodenum
Gastrointestinal tract (Figure 4.57–4.60)	• Dorsal or lateral recumbency • Entire ventral abdomen • Note bowel wall thickening, intussusception, intestinal tumors, foreign bodies, gastrointestinal obstruction, lymph nodes • Gas or feces may mask lesions	• Five layers (mucosal surface, mucosa, submucosa, muscularis, serosa) are noted in the wall of the intestinal tract • Whole jejunum will not be evident • Strong acoustic shadow and reverberation artifacts are evident in the colon • Important to scan Ileocolic junction in cats due to area of high pathology
Urinary bladder (Figure 4.61)	• Place the transducer in the caudal abdominal area cranial to the pubis for both sagittal and transverse planes of the bladder • The bladder should at least be moderately full • Patient may need to be imaged standing to rule out gravity-dependent echogenic sediment or calculi, adherent blood clots, and mass lesions	• An anechoic round or oblong structure with a thin, echogenic wall • Empty bladder wall appears artificially thickened that can mimic or mask various pathological conditions • Note cystic calculi, tumors, and cystitis
Ovary	• As for kidney • Used to diagnose polycystic ovaries and tumors • Located caudal and slightly lateral to caudal poles of kidney	• Appearance varies with stages of estrous cycle • In anestrus, ovaries are small, uniform with a homogenous echogenicity similar to the renal cortex • Follicles appear as focal hypoechoic to anechoic rounded structures making ovaries easier to identify as follicular development progresses
Prostate	• To one side of the prepuce just in front of the pubic brim; locate the bladder then move caudally • Can follow the urethra into the pelvic inlet	• Bilobed with a bright appearance as it surrounds the urethra • In an intact male, it is larger and more echogenic • Focal and diffuse lesions change appearance as does paraprostatic cysts

(*Continued*)

Skill Box 4.25 / Sonographic Appearance and Concerns (Continued)

Organ	Transducer placement and imaging concerns	Appearance/location
Uterus	• Ventral midline from umbilicus to pubis • An enlarged uterus is seen between the bladder and the colon in the transverse plane • Uterus bifurcates as the probe is moved cranially and would not show flow on Doppler	• Wall is hypoechoic • Optimal time for pregnancy detection is at 20 days of gestation • Gestational sacs with viable embryos can be identified though the number of fetuses may not be easily noted
Testicle and scrotum	• Considered part of the abdominal cavity • For cryptorchid testicle center on the pubis to umbilicus on appropriate side of midline; start in front of the pubis and work toward the bladder and then the kidney	• Scrotal hernia and tumors are evident • Normal testes characterized by a coarse medium echo pattern
Heart	• A table with a hole in the center allows for evaluation from beneath; this keeps the heart close to chest wall and the lung out of the way • Positioning is the cardiologist's preference but if starting in right lateral recumbency, the transducer can come from underneath • Ventral third of ribs 4–6 with the transducer placed in intercostal spaces • Both M-mode and two-dimensional B-mode are suggested with Doppler imaging useful to assess turbulence and velocity of blood flow • Should obtain both long- and short-axis directional views	• Heart walls and valves are echogenic • Normally the left ventricle is three to four times larger than the right ventricle when viewing the four chambers • Left and right atria are about the same size • Check for pericardial effusion, valvular disease, myocardial disease and congenital defects
Thorax	• Positioning is the cardiologist's preference as for the heart • Place transducer over the area of interest	• Note free fluid, masses (e.g. thymic lymphoma, chest wall masses), diaphragmatic rupture
Eye and orbit	• Use local anesthetic drops on cornea • Place the transducer directly on the cornea (can scan through closed eyelids but image not as clear)	• Most useful if direct visualization obscured • Note retinal detachment or intraocular masses in the eye and retrobulbar foreign bodies, abscesses, tumors in the orbit

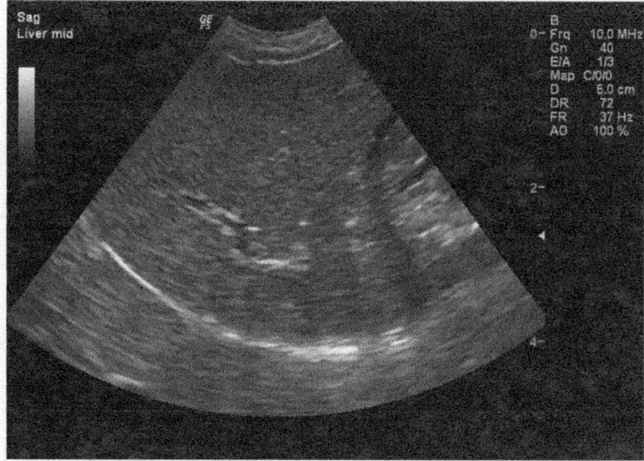

Figure 4.50 Sagittal scan of the mid-liver where the transducer is fanned from left to right. Source: image courtesy of Blair Animal Hospital, Ottawa, ON.

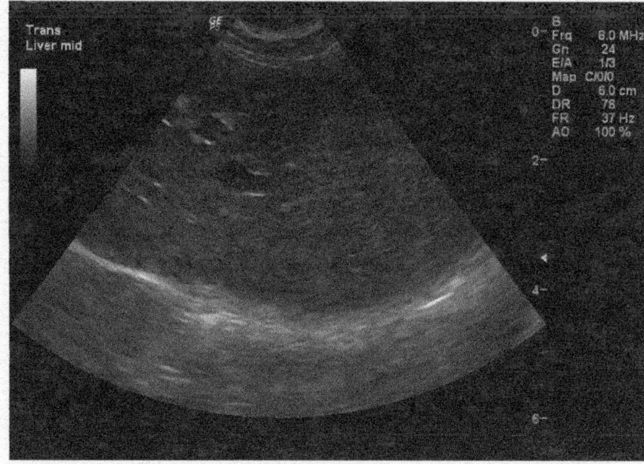

Figure 4.51 Transverse scan of the mid-liver where the transducer is fanned cranial to caudal. Source: image courtesy of Blair Animal Hospital, Ottawa, ON.

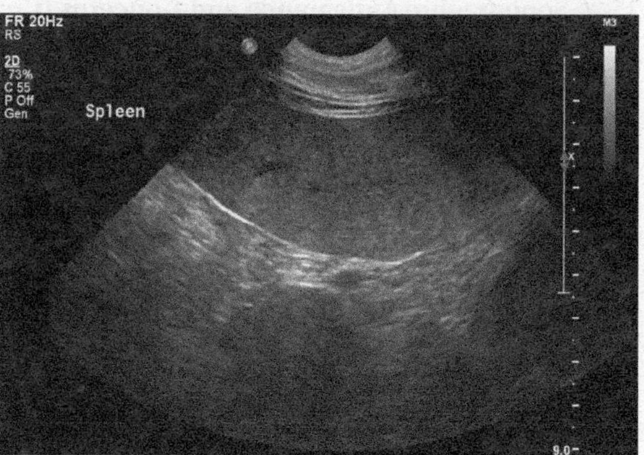

Figure 4.52 Ultrasound of the spleen. Source: image courtesy of Ashley Jenner, Toronto, ON.

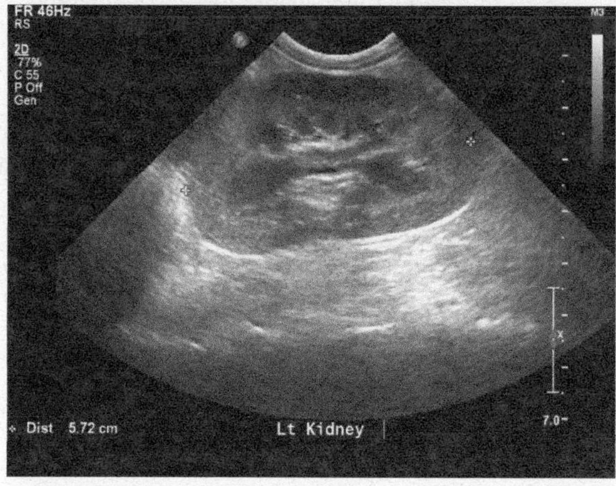

Figure 4.53 Ultrasound image of the left kidney. Source: image courtesy of Ashley Jenner, Toronto ON.

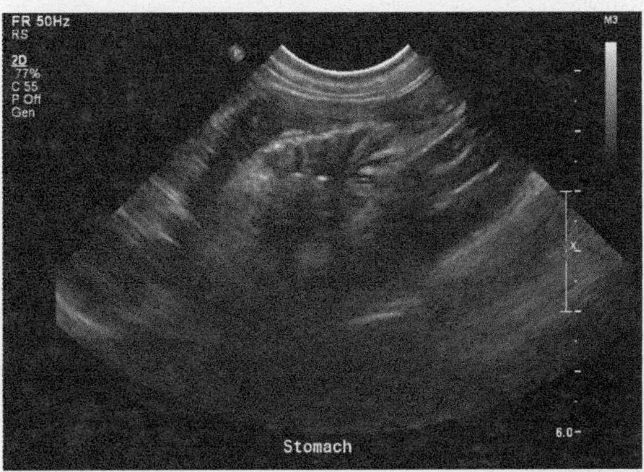

Figure 4.54 Ultrasound image of the stomach. Source: image courtesy of Ashley Jenner., Toronto, ON.

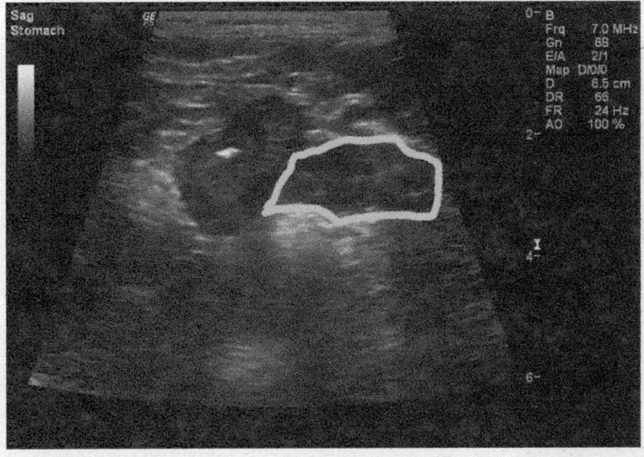

Figure 4.55 The lined area is the pancreas in a sagittal plane. Source: image courtesy of Blair Animal Hospital, Ottawa, ON.

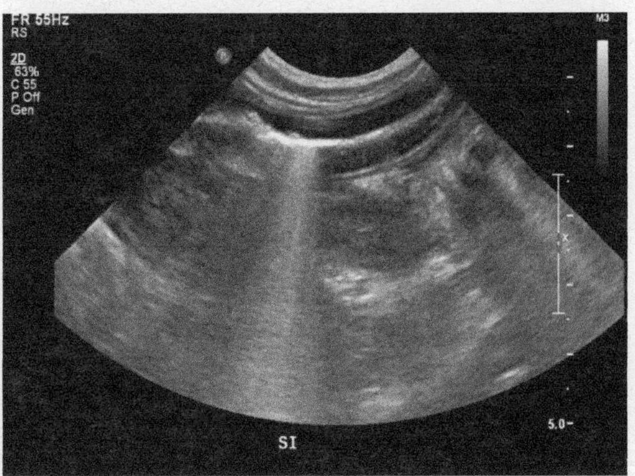

Figure 4.56 Sagittal plane of the small intestine. Source: image courtesy of Ashley Jenner, Toronto, ON.

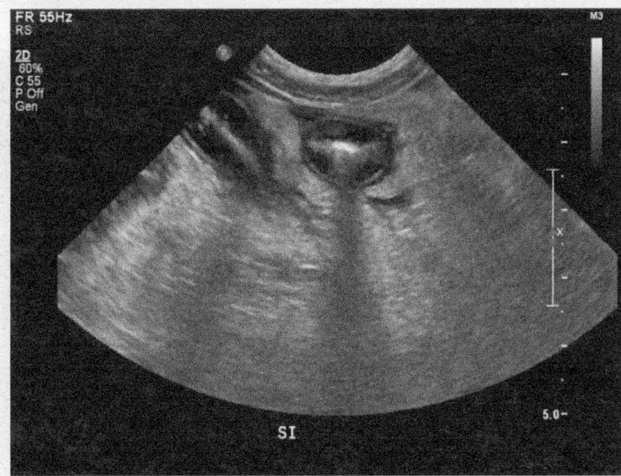

Figure 4.57 Transverse plane of the small intestine. Source: image courtesy of Ashley Jenner, Toronto, ON.

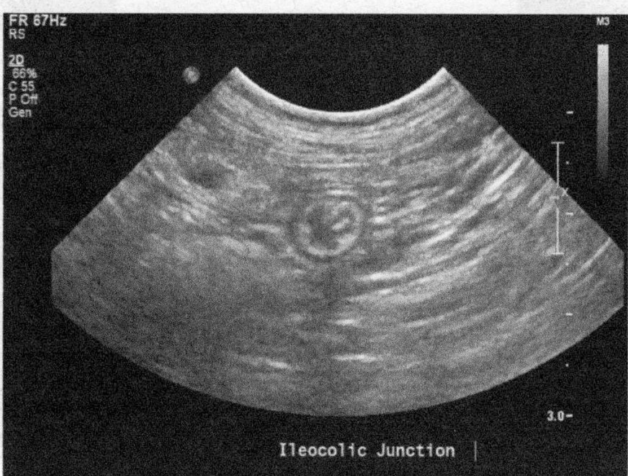

Figure 4.58 Ultrasound of the ileocolic junction showing the classic "pin wheel" image of the ileum. Source: image courtesy of Ashley Jenner, Toronto, ON.

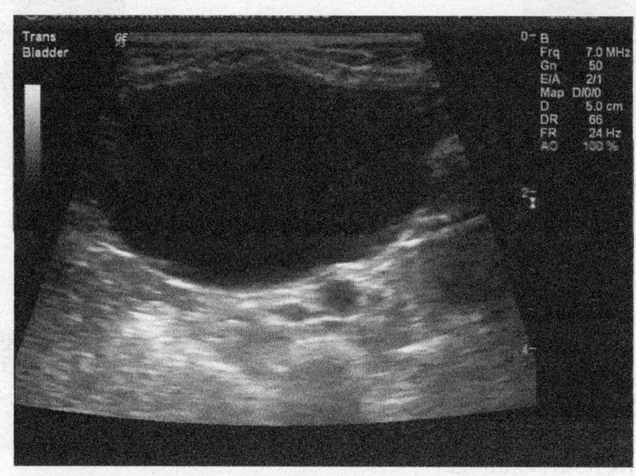

Figure 4.59 Transverse plane of the bladder. Source: image courtesy of Blair Animal Hospital, Ottawa, ON.

FURTHER IMAGING TECHNIQUES

In addition to, or as an alternative to radiographs, the following modalities can be used to further assist in the diagnosis of a patient's medical problem. Consider survey radiographs first.

Skill Box 4.26 / Computed Tomography and Echocardiography

Procedure	Computed tomography	Echocardiography
Definition	• A diagnostic imaging procedure creating cross sectional views of a body part incorporating x-rays and computers	• Noninvasive study of the heart and its structures (aorta, ventricles, atria, auricular appendages, and all the cardiac valves) using ultrasonography
Technique	• A thin rotating x-ray beam passes through the patient transaxially, and three views of the area of interest are reconstructed by a computer using the transmitted data onto a video screen to create, two- or three-dimensional images and volume rendering to assess and diagnose patients • Completed with or without iodine contrast media	• Ultrasound transducer is placed on a clipped and cleaned area with ultrasound gel • B-mode is used to view the cardiac structures and produce the image • Patient may be in lateral or dorsal recumbency, or standing if necessary
Indications	• Confirmation or further evaluation of radiographic results and ultrasound findings, surgical planning • Primarily for central and peripheral nervous studies in addition to musculoskeletal, nasal and vascular abnormalities, thoracic, and abdominal disorders	• Visualize internal cardiac structures • Evaluate cardiac function and size, defects (e.g. valvular lesions, shunts, myocardial abnormalities, masses, effusions, stenotic lesions)
Specialized equipment	• CT unit that directs a thin beam of radiation at a series of detectors	• Ultrasound machine with cardiac software and Doppler
Notes	• Performed under sedation only, especially for orthopedic concerns • Thoracic studies often require general anaesthetic to allow patients to hold their breath for less movement artifact • Inherent high contrast • Superimposition of overlying structures is eliminated thus clear indication of shape and location of organs, soft tissue and bones indicating only anatomy • Increased risk of radiation exposure	• Real-time movement of blood flow and velocity to detect both physiology cardiac output and structural abnormalities without invasive procedures

Skill Box 4.27 / Fluoroscopy

Procedure	Fluoroscopy
Definition	• X-rays are used for real-time radiographic viewing of moving anatomical parts
Technique	• X-rays pass through the patient's body to an image intensifier or detector that creates an image that is displayed on a monitor • The tube moves without patient repositioning
Indications	• Used in assessing the motility and function of the pharynx, esophagus, stomach, and bowel as well as angiography studies • Also useful in equine extremities to determine fracture reductions • Evaluation of respiratory and cardiac function • Interventional studies such as direct aspirates, biopsies or angiographic catheter placement
Specialized equipment	• Fluoroscopic x-ray tube • Image intensifier/detector • Mirror imaging or monitor for viewing the images • Radiopaque contrast medium • Protective apparel
Precautions	• ↑ risk of radiation exposure due to high doses of radiation for this procedure
Notes	• Bone appears black and gas appears white on image

Skill Box 4.28 / Magnetic Resonance Imaging and Nuclear Medicine

Procedure	MRI	Nuclear medicine (scintigraphy)
Definition	• A cross-sectional view of a patient's body using magnetic fields and radio waves without the use of ionizing radiation	• The use of radiopharmaceutical drugs to ascertain the functional status of an organ or body part of a patient often used in equine medicine • Images are plotted on the computer as a series of dots that indicate radioactive outbursts
Technique	• A powerful magnet surrounds the patient • This magnet aligns hydrogen atoms and with the use of radio frequencies, these alignments are systematically altered • This alteration is detected and recorded to produce a computer-generated image	• A radionuclide such as technetium-99m is administered IV • Gamma cameras capture radiation produced by the radiopharmaceutical and an image is generated as the radioisotope is carried to the area with the most blood supply • Technetium-99m is attracted to bone and will demonstrate hot spots or areas of osteoblastic activity showing increased bone metabolism. The pooling of the nuclide demonstrates tendons and ligaments injuries as well as bone
Indications	• Confirmation of further evaluation of radiographic results • Soft tissue contrast, brain, and spine	• Specific areas requiring more information on the functionality of specific organs for diagnostic assessment such as tendons, ligaments and lower limbs in equines • In small animals, indications are hyperthyroidism, lameness, and liver dysfunction, but due to cost, heavy regulations, etc., the procedure is not common
Specialized equipment	• MRI unit • Special room/building for unit • Non-ferrous contrast media • General anesthesia with mechanical ventilation	• Radiopharmaceutical drugs such as technetium-99m • Gamma scintillation camera • Protective lab coat • Specialized training in handling drug, patient, and patient's excretions
Precautions	• Patient and operator must be free of any metallic devices (pacemakers), metallic foreign bodies (bullets, shrapnel, skin staples, etc.), or ferromagnetic implants • The operator is in a separate area from the patient • Lungs are better imaged with CT as there are fewer hydrogen molecules in thorax	• Requires special handling of the patient's excretion and restricted contact time with the patient • The half-life of the radionuclides need to be considered
Notes	• Compared with CT, MRI has greater image resolution and ability to distinguish between tissue composition. Thus, it is much better for evaluation of the brain and spine • Both anatomic and functional information is given with many more obvious shades of gray compared with CT	• Nuclear-approved sites are required • The patient is the radiation emitter so the half-life of the radioisotope is essential when considering patient care and length of stay • Waste products are radioactive for a certain time period depending on the half-life, so precautions need to be taken

Skill Box 4.29 / Interventional Radiology

Procedure	Interventional radiology
Definition	• The use of fluoroscopy, ultrasound, CT, MRI, and endoscopy to access various organs or structures within the body to deliver chemical materials or support structures for therapeutic purposes
Technique	• Dependent upon the instruments
Indications	• Surgery is not an option • Urethral stenting, nasopharyngeal stenosis, blood clots, liver shunts, various tumors, kidney, urethral and bladder stones, canine incontinence
Specialized equipment	• Angiography suites • Lead gowns and shields • Fluoroscopy unit • Specialized training
Precautions	• Dependent upon procedure

REFERENCE

1. Mauragis, D., Berry, C.R. Small animal radiography of the scapula, shoulder and humerus. *Today's Veterinary Practice* 2012;May/June. https://todaysveterinarypractice.com/1475 (accessed 3 July 2021).

Section Four

Diseases and Conditions

Chapter 5

Dermatologic Diseases and Conditions

Chantelle Hanna, BS, CVT, VTS (Dermatology)-Charter Member

Veterinary Technician and Nurse's Daily Reference Guide: Canine and Feline, Fourth Edition. Edited by Mandy Fults and Kenichiro Yagi.

Companion website: www.wiley.com/go/fults/veterinary

Abbreviations

CBC, complete blood count
CT, computed tomography
ECG, electrocardiogram
EDTA, ethylenediaminetetraacetic acid
ELISA, enzyme-linked immunoassay
HCl, hydrochloride
IgG, immunoglobulin G
MRI, magnetic resonance imaging
PO, orally
SQ, subcutaneously

ACNE

Acne is a chronic inflammatory disorder most often seen in short-coated breeds. It is often associated with superficial and deep pyoderma. It is typically found on the chin and lips of young animals. Feline acne is often associated with the chin and lower lip. There may be a single episode or the animal may have a continual lifelong problem. Poor grooming is thought to be one cause for this condition.

Table 5.1 / **Acne**

Disease		Acne	
Species		Canines	Felines
Presentation	Presenting clinical signs	• Erythematous papules, swelling, exudates, and scarring	• Comedones, erythema papules, serous crusts, swelling, alopecia
Diagnosis	General	• Clinical signs	• Clinical signs
	Laboratory	• Culture, bacterial: bacteria isolation and identification	• Not applicable
	Imaging	• Not applicable	• Not applicable
	Procedures	• Skin scraping: parasites (*Demodex*) • Cytology: bacteria or fungal organisms • Biopsy: to confirm diagnosis • Allergy testing: food, flea, environmental	• Skin scraping: parasites (*Demodex*) • Cytology: bacteria or fungal organisms • Biopsy: to confirm diagnosis • Allergy testing: food, flea, environmental

(Continued)

Table 5.1 / Acne (Continued)

Disease		Acne	
Species		Canines	Felines
Treatment	General	• Symptomatic • Skin treatment	• Symptomatic • Skin treatment
	Medication	• Antibiotics: cephalexin, amoxicillin and clavulanate potassium (Clavamox®), clindamycin, erythromycin, cefpodoxime • Antibiotics (topical): mupirocin • Corticosteroids: prednisone, prednisolone, dexamethasone, methylprednisolone • Cleansing agents: benzoyl peroxide, salicylic acid, chlorhexidine–phytosphingosine • Medicated shampoo: benzoyl peroxide • Retinoids (topical): tretinoin gel (Retin-A®) • Immunotherapy: allergen-specific desensitization • Flea control • Novel protein diet	• Antibiotics: amoxicillin and clavulanate potassium (Clavamox), enrofloxacin, cefpodoxime • Antibiotics (topical): mupirocin • Antiparasitic: ivermectin • Corticosteroids: prednisolone, dexamethasone, methylprednisolone • Cleansing agents: benzoyl peroxide, salicylic acid, chlorhexidine-phytosphingosine • Medicated shampoo: benzoyl peroxide or sulfur–salicylic acid • Retinoids (topical): tretinoin gel (Retin-A) • Immunotherapy: allergen-specific desensitization • Flea control • Novel protein diet
	Nursing care	• Treated as outpatient • Prevent self-trauma: (e.g. rubbing of chin, chewing on bones that ↑ salivation)	• Treated as outpatient
Follow-up	Patient care	• Frequent cleaning/shampooing of chin • Warm compresses	• Shampoo once or twice weekly and then taper over a 2–3-week period • Physical examination monthly
	Prevention/ avoidance	• Maintenance: lifelong treatment may be necessary	• Maintenance: lifelong treatment may be necessary • Avoid the use of plastic feeding dishes
	Complications	• Deep pyoderma • Discourage owners from expressing the lesions; can lead to massive inflammation	• Deep pyoderma
	Prognosis	• Excellent	• Excellent
Notes		• English bulldogs, boxers, Doberman pinscher and great Dane • Medications should be tapered over 2–3 weeks	• Medications should be tapered over 2–3 weeks

ACRAL LICK DERMATITIS

Acral lick dermatitis (lick granuloma, acral pruritic nodule) is an area of a firm, raised, ulcerative, or thickened skin that is usually located on the dorsal aspect of the carpus, metacarpus, tarsus, or metatarsus. The area may have a history of trauma, foreign body reaction, neoplasia, allergy, endocrinology, or others. The problem is typically made worse by the constant licking and chewing of the patient.

ATOPY

Atopy is found in animals that have formed allergies to normally innocuous substances such as pollen, grass, fleas, molds, and mites. This disease is the cause of the majority of dermatologic problems.

FLEA ALLERGY DERMATITIS

The antigens in the saliva of fleas are the cause of a hypersensitivity reaction. Flea allergy dermatitis is the most common skin disease in most geographical areas, especially during the summer months. *Ctenocephalides felis* is the flea type that usually infests both dogs and cats.

Table 5.2 / Acral lick dermatitis, atopy, and flea allergy dermatitis

Disease		Acral lick dermatitis	Atopy	Flea allergy dermatitis
Presentation	Presenting clinical signs	• Alopecia, excessive licking, chewing	• Pruritis and skin lesions • Canine: alopecia, edema, face rubbing, foot chewing, hyperpigmentation • Feline: alopecia and miliary dermatitis	• Alopecia, pruritus, skin lesions • Feline: alopecia (head, neck, and dorsal lumbar) • Canine: alopecia (tail base, dorsal lumbar region, caudal thighs, groin, abdomen, head, and neck), broken hairs, chewing, dry hair, excoriations
	Exam findings	• Firm, hyperpigmentation, raised, thickened, ulcerative	• Canine: otitis externa, recurrent pyoderma, seborrheic dermatitis, malasseziasis • Feline: miliary dermatitis, eosinophilic granuloma complex, rodent ulcers	• Canine: erythema, otitis externa, papules, pustules, secondary infection, lichenification, hyperpigmentation, alopecia • Feline: lymphadenopathy, miliary dermatitis, eosinophilic granuloma complex, rodent ulcers

(Continued)

Table 5.2 / **Acral lick dermatitis, atopy, and flea allergy dermatitis (Continued)**

Disease		Acral lick dermatitis	Atopy	Flea allergy dermatitis
Diagnosis	General	• History/clinical signs	• History/clinical signs	• History/clinical signs • Presence of fleas or flea dirt is not indicative
	Laboratory	• Skin scraping: bacteria, demodex, dermatophytosis • Biopsy, skin: neoplasia • Culture, bacterial: bacteria isolation and identification	• CBC: eosinophilia (occasional) • ELISA and rapid simple tests: ↑ values (non-specific)	• CBC: hypereosinophilia (cats, variable) • Fecal flotation: *Dipylidium caninum* • Serology: + serum IgE anti-flea antibody titer
	Imaging	• Radiograph, lower limb: neoplasia, radiopaque foreign body, bony proliferation, and some forms of trauma	• Not applicable	• Not applicable
Treatment	Procedures	• Hypoallergenic test diet: food hypersensitivity	• Intradermal allergy test: most reliable specific test	• Flea combing • Intradermal skin test: + (reliable)
	General	• Intradermal skin test: atopy • Symptomatic • Laser ablation	• Symptomatic • Laser ablation	• Symptomatic • Laser ablation
	Medication	• Antibiotics: variable but often required for several months • Antihistamines: chlorpheniramine, hydroxyzine HCl, cetirizine, diphenhydramine, loratadine • Psychotropic drugs: clomipramine HCl, amitriptyline or fluoxetine HCl	• Antihistamines: chlorpheniramine, hydroxyzine, diphenhydramine, cetirizine, loratadine • Corticosteroids: prednisone or methylprednisolone	• Antihistamines: diphenhydramine, chlorpheniramine, cetirizine • Corticosteroids: triamcinolone, prednisolone, methylprednisolone • Fatty acid supplements • Insecticide: imidacloprid, selamectin, spinosad, nitenpyram, dinotefuran, fluralaner, spinetoram, sarolaner/selamectin combo • Insect growth regulator: lufenuron, pyriproxyfen, methoprene (not recommended as the sole method of flea control, only in conjunction with an adulticide)

(Continued)

Table 5.2 / Acral lick dermatitis, atopy, and flea allergy dermatitis (Continued)

Disease		Acral lick dermatitis	Atopy	Flea allergy dermatitis
	Nursing care	• Treated as outpatient	• Treated as outpatient	• Treated as outpatient
Follow-up	Patient care	• Monitor closely for licking and chewing. Elizabethan collar if necessary • Check CBC, biochemistry, and ECG every 1–2 months for those receiving tricyclic antidepressants • cytology of lesion prior to discontinuing antibiotic therapy	• Fatty acid supplementation • Frequent bathing in cool water to reduce pruritus • Examine patients every 2–8 weeks following treatment then every 3–12 months	• Flea comb regularly
	Prevention/ avoidance	• Determine the underlying disease when possible	• Avoidance is difficult with most allergens	• Maintain year-round flea control: flea comb, monthly oral medication, and "spot-on" medication
	Complications	• Deep pyoderma	• Superficial pyoderma • Flea allergy dermatitis • Malasseziasis • Food hypersensitivities	• Superficial or deep pyoderma • Acute moist dermatitis • Acral lick dermatitis
	Prognosis	• Guarded (not life threatening) if no underlying disease is found and psychogenic causes are suspected	• Good if allergen is determined	• Excellent
Notes		• E-collars, foul-tasting medications and sprays, or bandages may be used to prevent licking and chewing • Additional attention and exercise may help if psychogenic causes are suspected	• Do not use penicillins or tetracyclines for treatment of superficial pyoderma • Some types of treatment are often needed for life • It may take up to 6–12 months before results from immunotherapy are seen	• **A complete flea control plan includes treating the pet, other pets in the household, and indoor and outdoor environments** • Control may take 4–12 weeks to achieve • With many new alternatives to flea control, dips, sprays, and flea collars should be the last choice for control • Extra care should be taken when using insecticides to avoid overdose or misuse

FOOD HYPERSENSITIVITY OR ADVERSE FOOD REACTION

Food hypersensitivity is an immunologic reaction to food and food additives marked by non-seasonal skin and ear issues; often concurrent with atopy.

OTITIS EXTERNA

Otitis externa is the inflammation of the soft tissue of the external ear canal. Its causes are often multifactorial, signifying a generalized dermatologic problem. It can be either a primary or a secondary disease (e.g. hypothyroid, atopy, food allergy), making it difficult to treat.

Table 5.3 / Food hypersensitivity and otitis externa

Disease		Food hypersensitivity or adverse food reaction	Otitis externa
Presentation	Presenting clinical signs	• Alopecia, acral lick granulomas, crusts, diarrhea, flatulence, hyperpigmentation, lichenification, otitis, pustules, pruritis (feet, ears, face, neck, inguinal, or axillary areas, perineum), pyotraumatic dermatitis, seizures, urticaria, vomiting	• Behavioral changes (irritable, aggression), foul odor, head shaking, head tilting, hearing loss, pain, scratching, rubbing at the ears, aural hematomas
	Exam findings	• Erythema, otitis externa, *Malassezia* dermatitis, superficial pyoderma, papular rash, self-trauma, seborrhea, wheals	• Calcification/thickening of canal, debris, exudate, inflammation, swelling, ulceration
Diagnosis	General	• History/clinical signs • Nonseasonal occurrence and partial or incomplete response to corticosteroids or modified cyclosporine	• History/clinical signs • Otoscopic exam
	Laboratory	• Serum allergy tests are non-diagnostic	• Cytology: parasites, cells, bacteria, yeast, and fungi • Culture: bacteria recognition and identification
	Imaging	• Not applicable	• Radiographs, skull: only used in chronic cases to determine patency of the ear canal and to rule out otitis media. Not as sensitive as CT/MRI • CT/MRI: to determine middle ear involvement when considering total ear canal ablation or video otoscopy with deep ear flush, ± myringotomy
	Procedures	• Intradermal skin testing: inconsistent findings • Hypoallergenic test diet or novel elimination diet trial	• Intradermal skin tests: + results • Hypoallergenic test diet or novel elimination diet trial • Deep ear flush with myringotomy

(Continued)

Table 5.3 / **Food hypersensitivity and otitis externa (Continued)**

	Disease	Food hypersensitivity or adverse food reaction	Otitis externa
Treatment	General	• Symptomatic	• Symptomatic • Flush and dry ear canals; Tris-EDTA as pretreatment wash • Surgery: total ear canal ablation
	Medication	• If any, dependent on clinical signs • Antibiotics/antifungals: secondary infections	• Antibiotics: cephalexin, trimethoprim-sulfa, enrofloxacin, clindamycin, amoxicillin and clavulanate potassium (Clavamox®), ciprofloxacin, difloxacin, cefpodoxime • Antibiotics (topical): enrofloxacin, tobramycin, silver sulfadiazine, amikacin, florfenicol, orbifloxacin, neomycin, gentamicin, polymyxin B sulfate • Antifungals: ketoconazole, miconazole, terbinafine, posaconazole, clotrimazole • Corticosteroids: prednisone, dexamethasone, triamcinolone, mometasone, betamethasone, prednisolone acetate, fluocinolone, hydrocortisone • Ear cleaner • Parasiticides: ivermectin
	Nursing care	• Treated as outpatient	• Treated as outpatient
Follow-up	Patient care	• Feed the restricted diet exclusively for 10–12 weeks • A partial response indicates a possible other allergen (e.g. flea, environmental) • Avoid flavored chew toys, bones, treats, vitamins, and medications, including gelatin capsules	• Recheck ears frequently until resolved: do not treat prior to exam for better visibility
	Prevention/ avoidance	• Restrict the feeding of hypersensitive foods	• Clean ears regularly (see Skill Box 2.13: Ear cleaning and flushing, page 62). • Thoroughly dry ears after swimming and bathing • Lateral ear canal resection surgery vs. total ear canal ablation surgery
	Complications	• Pruritus: by other sources	• Vestibular complications, Horner syndrome (common in cats following ear flushing) • Ruptured ear drum • Otitis media or interna • Permanent ear canal changes: stenosis and calcification • Deafness • Vestibular disease
	Prognosis	• Good if offending food is determined	• Excellent if treated early and thoroughly

(Continued)

Table 5.3 / **Food hypersensitivity and otitis externa (Continued)**

Disease	Food hypersensitivity or adverse food reaction	Otitis externa
Notes	• Diet should consist of foods that the animal has not been previously exposed to (e.g. quinoa, oatmeal, potatoes, buffalo, venison, rabbit) and without additives or preservatives. Some novel OTC diets may be contaminated during production. (See Table 17.6: Disease nutritional requirements in disease, page 763) • If there is no improvement, review other food sources and other forms of allergens (e.g. fleas and inhalant) • Corticosteroids should only be used with severe pruritus and tapered off during the food trial to determine efficacy of the food trial; oclacitinib can be used similarly	• Enough topical medication must be used to coat the entire ear canal for effectiveness and then its use tapered once infection is resolved. • Debris in the middle ear can be a nidus for recurrent infection Possible reasons for certain exudates: • Dark, dry, and granular: ear mite infection • Moist, yellow, and odiferous: bacterial infection • Brown and waxy: yeast infection • Yellow and waxy to oily: keratinization disorders • Total ear canal ablation or lateral canal resection does not address the underlying cause of the recurrent infections (food hypersensitivity, atopy) • Use only warmed 0.9% saline to flush an ear canal with a ruptured tympanic membrane • Plucking hair from within the ear canal may cause irritation and predisposes the animal to otitis externa

PYODERMA

Deep

Deep pyoderma extends into the dermis and, in severe cases, into the subcutaneous tissue. This bacterial skin infection has many different forms, two of the most common being folliculitis and furunculosis. It is typically secondary to another disease process.

Superficial

In superficial pyoderma (superficial bacterial folliculitis or superficial pustular dermatitis), the epidermis is the target of a bacterial infection with superficial pyoderma. It can manifest itself in two ways: penetrating the stratus corneum of non-haired skin (impetigo) or invading the hair follicles and adjacent epidermis (folliculitis).

Surface

Acute moist dermatitis (hot spots) is a localized area of surface infection and inflammation caused by self-trauma. The infection does not invade the dermis.

Skinfold dermatitis (intertrigo) is a frictional dermatitis characterized by surface infection and inflammation that occurs where two skin surfaces are intimately apposed. It is often complicated by poor air circulation and moisture accumulation (sebum, tears, saliva, and urine).

Table 5.4 / **Pyoderma**

Disease		Pyoderma		
		Deep	Superficial (superficial bacterial folliculitis or superficial pustular dermatitis)	Surface: acute moist dermatitis (hot spots), skinfold dermatitis (intertrigo)
Presentation	Presenting clinical signs	• Alopecia, anorexia, depression, peripheral lymphadenopathy, and fever • Pustules: inguinal, ventral abdominal, and axillary areas extending to the whole body • Erythematous, discolored, painful, pruritic skin	• Dull hair coat, excessive shedding, scales • Impetigo: pustules, papules, and crusts (inguinal and ventral abdominal area especially in young animals), patchy alopecia	• Biting, licking, and rubbing by the patient • Acute moist dermatitis • Alopecia, thin exudate layer, erythema, surrounded by matted hairs, and thickened skin with excoriations • Skinfold pyoderma
	Exam findings	• Exudate, ulcer, and crust formation, drainage tracts, and hemorrhagic bullae, cellulitis	• Folliculitis: epidermal collarettes ("bull's-eye" lesions), erythema, possibly pruritic skin • Impetigo: papules, pustules, crusts, non-painful or pruritic	• Inflammation, exudate, fetid, alopecia, and erythema
Diagnosis	General	• History/clinical signs	• History/clinical signs	• History/clinical signs • Self-trauma, environmental irritant, or any pruritic skin
	Laboratory	• CBC: leukocytosis with a left shift (variable) • Chemistry panel: ↑ globulin (variable) • Cytology: neutrophils, macrophages, and bacteria • Skin scrapings: ectoparasites • Blood culture: bacteria • Culture: bacteria recognition and identification • Skin biopsy: to confirm folliculitis, perifolliculitis, or furunculosis	• CBC: depending on underlying condition (anemia, stress leukogram, eosinophilia) • Chemistry panel: depending on underlying condition (↑ alkaline phosphatase) • Cytology: neutrophils and bacteria • Skin scrapings: ectoparasites • Culture: bacteria isolation and identification • Skin biopsy: to confirm folliculitis	• Culture: bacteria isolation and identification • Skin biopsy: non-follicular subcorneal pustules
	Imaging	• Not applicable	• Not applicable	• Not applicable
	Procedures	• Skin scraping and biopsy • Intradermal skin tests • Hypoallergenic test diet or novel elimination diet trial	• Skin scraping and biopsy • Intradermal skin tests • Hypoallergenic test diet or novel elimination diet trial	• Not applicable

(Continued)

Table 5.4 / **Pyoderma (Continued)**

Disease		Pyoderma		
		Deep	Superficial (superficial bacterial folliculitis or superficial pustular dermatitis)	Surface: acute moist dermatitis (hot spots), skinfold dermatitis (intertrigo)
Treatment	General	• Symptomatic • Fluid therapy (severe cases) • Whirlpool baths	• Symptomatic	• Symptomatic • Wound management • Surgery: fold correction
	Medication	• Antibiotics: variable • Medicated shampoos: benzoyl peroxide, chlorhexidine • Dilute bleach rinses (up to ¼ cup per gallon; must be made fresh daily)	• Antibiotics: variable • Medicated shampoos: antibacterial • Dilute bleach rinses (up to ¼ cup per gallon; must be made fresh daily) • Management of pruritus: Corticosteroids, oclacitinib, canine immunobiologic • Topical: products with corticosteroids, antihistamines, or anesthetics (pramoxine)	• Antibiotics (oral and/or topical): variable • Corticosteroids (topical): nystatin cream and Neo-Predef® powder
	Nursing care	• Clip hair coat on long-coated breeds	• Treated as outpatient	• Treated as outpatient
Follow-up	Patient care	• Bathe twice daily for 1–2 weeks then once to twice weekly. • Whirlpool baths • Provide a high-quality diet • Supplementation of essential fatty acids • Padded bedding to ease pressure point pyoderma	• Bathe two to three times weekly for 2–3 weeks, ± dilute bleach rinses • Prevent self-trauma • Provide a high-quality diet • Supplement with essential fatty acids	• Maintain a clean and dry wound • Prevent self-trauma: restraint, collars, etc.
	Prevention/ avoidance	• Determine the underlying cause • Bathe regularly with appropriate shampoo	• Determine the underlying cause • Bath with appropriate shampoo, especially after swimming	• Determine the underlying cause • Clean and dry the skin folds routinely with astringents.
	Complications	• Bacteremia or septicemia • Scarring	• Deep pyoderma • Recurrence	• Superficial or deep pyoderma
	Prognosis	• Excellent if underlying cause is determined	• Excellent	• Excellent
Notes		• German shepherds • Antibiotic therapy may be required for several months	• If persistent pruritus, ectoparasitism or allergy may be present as underlying etiology	• Cocker Spaniel, Springer Spaniel, Saint Bernard, Irish Setter, Shar-Pei, Basset Hound, Bulldog, Boston Terrier, Pug • Corrective surgery may be performed on chronically infected skin folds

DEMODECTIC MANGE

Demodectic mange is in inflammatory parasitic disease characterized by unusually high numbers of *Demodex* mites. In dogs, *D. canis* is the most common; others include *D. injai* and *D. cornei*. Infection can be adult onset or juvenile onset. It is non-contagious. In cats, the disease is characterized by the presence of, typically, *D. gatoi* and *D. cati*. *D. gatoi* is contagious.

Table 5.5 / **Demodectic mange**

Disease		Demodectic mange	
		Canine	Feline
Presentation	Clinical signs	• Erythema, alopecia, comedones, papules, pustules, lichenification, hyperpigmentation, seborrhea, otitis, pruritus is variable • Lesions localized or generalized	• Alopecia, erythema, papules, scale, crusts, hyperpigmentation, otitis, pruritus is variable but can be intense • Can be localized or generalized
Diagnosis	General	• History • Clinical signs	• History • Clinical signs
	Laboratory	• Not applicable	• Not applicable
	Imaging	• Not applicable	• Not applicable
	Procedures	• Skin scraping and/or hair plucks • Cytology: bacterial or fungal secondary infection • Biopsy	• Skin scraping and/or hair plucks • Cytology: bacterial or fungal secondary infection • Biopsy

(Continued)

Table 5.5 / Demodectic mange (Continued)

Disease		Demodectic mange	
		Canine	Feline
Treatment	General	• Symptomatic • Skin treatment • Systemic treatment	• Symptomatic • Skin treatment • Systemic treatment

	Medication	• Topical:
		  • Localized: ear mite treatment, rotenone ointment
		  • Generalized: amitraz (Mitaban® is the only licensed product in the United States to treat demodectic mange), fluralaner (off-label), lime sulfur (off-label), sarolaner (off-label)
		• Generalized oral: (all off-label use) ivermectin, doramectin, moxidectin, milbemycin oxime, fluralaner, afoxolaner, lotilaner, sarolaner
		• Immunosuppressants should be used with caution (corticosteroids) or not at all (oclacitinib)
		• Medicated shampoo: benzoyl peroxide as an adjunct treatment
		• Antibiotics/antifungals to treat concurrent secondary infections
			• Topical:
			  • Localized: ear mite treatment
			  • Generalized: amitraz, (off-label) fluralaner (off-label), sarolaner (off- label), lime sulfur (off-label). Extreme care should be taken to avoid ingestion of lime sulfur and amitraz
			• Generalized subcutaneous: (all off-label use) ivermectin, doramectin
			• Immunosuppressants should be used with caution (corticosteroids) or not at all (modified cyclosporine)
			• Medicated shampoo: benzoyl peroxide as an adjunct treatment
			• Antibiotics/antifungals to treat concurrent secondary infections

	Nursing care	• Treated as outpatient	• Treated as outpatient
Follow-up	Patient care	• Prevent self-trauma • Frequent shampooing to treat/prevent secondary infections • Continue treatment 4 weeks post-negative skin scrapings (total of two negative scrapings)	• Prevent self-trauma • Shampooing to treat/prevent secondary infections if the cat allows • Continue treatment 4 weeks post-negative skin scrapings (total of two negative scrapings)
	Prevention/ avoidance	• Relapses are possible requiring periodic or lifelong treatment	• Relapses are possible requiring periodic or lifelong treatment
	Complications	• Deep pyoderma	• Deep pyoderma
	Prognosis	• Good to fair	• Good to fair
Notes		• English Bulldogs, Shar-Pei, American Staffordshire Terrier, Staffordshire Bull Terrier, West Highland White Terrier, Scottish Terrier, Boston Terrier, Weimaraner, Airedale Terrier, Alaskan Malamute, Shih Tzu, Great Dane, And Afghan Hound • Underlying causes should be investigated (autoimmune, neoplasia, endocrine) • Neutering affected animals with juvenile onset is recommended	• Siamese, Burmese • Underlying causes should be investigated (autoimmune, neoplasia, endocrine)

SCABIES (SARCOPTIC, NOTOEDRIC MANGE)

Sarcoptic mange is a canine parasitic skin disease caused by a superficial burrowing skin mite, *Sarcoptes scabei* var. *canis*. It is contagious and zoonotic.

Notoedric mange is a feline parasitic skin disease characterized by presence of a superficial burrowing sarcoptic skin mite, *Notoedres cati*. It is contagious and zoonotic.

Table 5.6 / Scabies (sarcoptic mange, notoedric mange)

Disease		Sarcoptic mange	Notoedric mange
		Canine	Feline
Presentation	Clinical signs	• Erythema, alopecia, papules, pustules, crusts, excoriations, lichenification, intense pruritus, peripheral lymphadenopathy • Typically affects the hocks, elbows, and pinnal margins but can spread to the entire body with chronicity	• Alopecia, erythema papules, scale, crusts, lichenification, hyperpigmentation, intense pruritus, peripheral lymphadenopathy • Lesions first appear on pinnal margins, spread toward the head, face, and neck, and can spread to the legs and perineum
Diagnosis	General	• History • Clinical signs	• History • Clinical signs
	Laboratory	• ELISA detects circulating IgG antibodies against Sarcoptes antigens, can have false negatives in puppies and immunosuppressed dogs or false positives in dogs successfully treated	• Not applicable
	Imaging	• Not applicable	• Not applicable
	Procedures	• Superficial skin scraping and/or hair and crust plucks. Mites are difficult to find. Lack of presence is non-diagnostic • Cytology: bacterial or fungal secondary infection, eosinophils usually present • Pinnal–pedal reflex • Biopsy	• Superficial skin scraping and/or hair and crust plucks. Mites are typically present in high numbers • Cytology: bacterial or fungal secondary infection, eosinophils usually present • Biopsy

(Continued)

Table 5.6 / Scabies (sarcoptic mange, notoedric mange) (Continued)

Disease		Sarcoptic mange	Notoedric mange
		Canine	Feline
Treatment	General	• Symptomatic • Skin treatment • Systemic treatment	• Symptomatic • Skin treatment • Systemic treatment
	Medication	• Topical: selamectin (only licensed product in the United States to treat sarcoptic mange), fluralaner (off-label), lime sulfur (off-label), moxidectin (off-label), fipronil spray (off-label), ivermectin (PO or SQ), doramectin (PO or SQ), milbemycin oxime (PO), fluralaner (PO), afoxolaner (PO), lotilaner (PO), sarolaner (PO); all off- label • Corticosteroids to minimize pruritus • Medicated shampoo: antibacterial and/or antifungal to help treat/prevent secondary infection. Warm water may worsen pruritus • Antibiotics/antifungals to treat concurrent secondary infections	• Topical: moxidectin/imidacloprid, selamectin, fluralaner, selamectin/sarolaner, lime sulfur, doramectin, moxidectin, fipronil spray, amitraz Extreme care should be taken to avoid ingestion of lime sulfur and amitraz. In general, cats can be extremely sensitive to amitraz (All are off-label use) • Ivermectin (PO or SQ), doramectin (SQ); all off-label use • Corticosteroids to minimize pruritus • Medicated shampoo: if tolerated, antibacterial and/or antifungal to help treat/prevent secondary infection. • Antibiotics/antifungals to treat concurrent secondary infections
	Nursing care	• **Treated as outpatient**	• Treated as outpatient
Follow-up	Patient care	• Prevent self-trauma • Frequent shampooing or topicals to treat/prevent secondary infections	• Prevent self-trauma • Shampooing or topicals to treat/prevent secondary infection if the cat allows
	Prevention/avoidance	• Relapses are possible requiring periodic or lifelong treatment. • Treatment of all animals in contact with one another is necessary if isolation is not possible.	• Not applicable
	Complications	• Deep pyoderma • Zoonosis	• Deep pyoderma • Zoonosis
	Prognosis	• Good	• Good
Notes		• Owing to the contagious and zoonotic nature, exposure can come from direct contact with other dogs, visiting a kennel or grooming facility, and/or wildlife • Avermectins should be used with caution in animals with the multiple drug resistant gene ABCB1 (formerly MDR1) • Mites can live in the environment for up to 21 days so treatment using a parasiticide may be beneficial • Worsening of pruritus can be seen as treatment begins	• *Notoedres* is highly contagious by direct contact but survives off the host for only a few days. • Pyrethrin/permethrin substances are toxic to cats

Chapter 6

Internal Medicine

H. Edward Durham Jr, CVT, RVT, LATG, VTS (Cardiology); Paula Plummer, LVT, VTS (ECC), (SAIM); Eleonora Mitelberg, LVT, VTS (SAIM); Kathleen Dunbar, BA, RVT, VTS (Clinical Practice C/F); Liza W. Rudolph, BAS, RVT, VTS (Clinical Practice- C/F), (SAIM); Wendy Davies, BS, CVT, CCRVN, VTS (Physical Rehabilitation); Stephanie Gilliam, RVTg, MS, CCRP, VTS (Neurology); Jenny Cassibry Fisher, RVT, VTS (Oncology); Tina De Victoria, BS, CVT, VTS (Clinical Practice C/F)

Veterinary Technician and Nurse's Daily Reference Guide: Canine and Feline, Fourth Edition. Edited by Mandy Fults and Kenichiro Yagi.

Companion website: www.wiley.com/go/fults/veterinary

Abbreviations

2AVB, second-degree atrioventricular block
2ME-TAT, 2-mercapto-ethanol tube agglutination test
3AVB, complete atrioventricular block
5-FU, fluorouracil
ACE, angiotensin-converting enzyme
AChR, acetylcholine receptors
ACT, activated clotting time
ACTH, adrenocorticotropic hormone
ACVIM, American College of Veterinary Internal Medicine
ADH, antidiuretic hormone
AGID, agar gel immunodiffusion
AHS, American Heart Society
ALP, alkaline phosphatase
ALT, alanine aminotransferase
ANA, antinuclear antibody
ANNPE, acute non-compressive nucleus pulposus extrusion
APC, atrial premature contraction
aPTT, activated partial thromboplastin time
ASD, atrial septal defect
AST, aspartate aminotransferase
ATE, aortic thromboembolism
AV, atrioventricular
BUN, blood urea nitrogen
Ca+, calcium ion
CBC, complete blood count
CGE, canine granulocytic ehrlichiosis
CHF, congestive heart failure
CK, creatine kinase
CME, canine monocytic ehrlichiosis
CN, cranial nerve
CNS, central nervous system
CORA, center of rotation of angulation
CRI, constant rate infusion
CRT, capillary refill time
CSF, cerebrospinal fluid
CSM, cervical spondylomyelopathy
CSTD, closed-system transfer device
CT, computed tomography
DCM, dilated cardiomyopathy
DIC, disseminated intravascular coagulation
DJD, degenerative joint disease
DMSO, dimethyl sulfoxide
DSS, dioctyl sodium sulfosuccinate
ECG, electrocardiogram
ELISA, enzyme-linked immunoassay
EMG, electromyography
EPI, exocrine pancreatic insufficiency
FBD, feline bronchopulmonary disease
FCE, fibrocartilaginous embolism
FCoV, feline coronavirus
FCV, feline calicivirus
FDP, fibrin degradation product
FeLV, feline leukemia virus
FHV-1, feline herpesvirus type 1
FIP, feline infectious peritonitis
FIV, feline immunodeficiency virus
FLUTD, feline lower urinary tract disease
FNA, fine-needle aspiration
fPLI, feline pancreatic lipase immunoreactivity
GGT, gamma glutamyl transpeptidase
GME, granulomatous meningoencephalomyelitis
HAC, hyperadrenocorticism;
IBD, inflammatory bowel disease
IGF, insulin-like growth factor
IgG, immunoglobulin G
IgM, immunoglobulin M
IFA, immunofluorescent assay
IM, intramuscular
IMHA, immune-mediated hemolytic anemia
IMPA, immune-mediated polyarthritis
IMT, immune-mediated thrombocytopenia
IN, intranasal
IV, intravenous
IVDD, intervertebral disc disease
L-MTP-PE, liposome-encapsulated muramyl tripeptide phosphatidylethanolamine
LA, left atrium
LMN, lower motor neuron
LV, left ventricle
MCV, mean corpuscular volume
MCHC, mean corpuscular hemoglobin concentration
MRI, magnetic resonance imaging
MUO, meningoencephalomyelitis of unknown origin
MV, mitral valve
MVD, myxomatous valvular degeneration
NIOSH, National Institute for Occupational Safety and Health
NLE, necrotizing leukoencephalitis
NME, necrotizing meningoencephalitis
NT-proBNP, N-terminal pro B-type natriuretic peptide
NSAIDs, non-steroidal anti-inflammatory drugs
PABA, para-aminobenzoic acid
PaO2, partial pressure of oxygen
PCE, pericardial effusion
PCR, polymerase chain reaction
PCV, packed cell volume
PDA, patent ductus arteriosus
PDT, photodynamic therapy
PFK, phosphofructokinase
PK, pyruvate kinase
PLE, protein-losing enteropathy
PLI, pancreatic lipase immunoreactivity
PLN, protein-losing nephropathy
PMMA, polymethyl methacrylate
PO, orally
PTE, pulmonary thromboembolism
PTH, parathyroid hormone
PTHrP, parathyroid hormone-related protein
PTT, partial thromboplastin time
PUFA, polyunsaturated fatty acid
RA, right atrium
RAT, reflexes, atrophy, tone
RBC, red blood cells
RSAT, rapid slide agglutination test
RV, right ventricle
SAS, subaortic stenosis
SDMA, symmetric dimethylarginine
SIRS, systemic inflammatory response syndrome
SLE, systemic lupus erythematosus
SOD-1, superoxide dismutase 1
SpO2, peripheral capillary oxygen saturation
SQ, subcutaneously
T3, triiodothyronine
T4, tetraiodothyronine
TAT, tube agglutination test
TLI, trypsin-like immunoreactivity
TSH, thyroid-stimulating hormone
TV, tricuspid valve
UMN, upper motor neuron
USG, urine specific gravity
USMI, urethral sphincter mechanism incompetence
UTI, urinary tract infection
VPC, ventricular premature contraction
VSD, ventricular septal defect
WCC, white cell count

CARDIOLOGY

The following information concerning specific disease conditions should be understood to include clinical signs, findings, and therapies for patients which present with undiagnosed congestive heart failure caused by the disease state being discussed. A separate table has been listed to include patients with congestive heart failure from all causes.

Congestive Heart Failure

Heart failure is the inability of the heart to maintain normal cardiac output in the presence of normal or enhanced preload. The inability to maintain cardiac output stimulates maladaptive mechanisms which contribute to hypotension, fluid retention and tissue congestion which cause clinical signs. Mechanisms of heart failure include myocardial systolic dysfunction (e.g. dilated cardiomyopathy), myocardial diastolic dysfunction (e.g. hypertrophic cardiomyopathy), volume overload (e.g. mitral valve regurgitation, or congenital shunt), pressure overload (e.g. subaortic stenosis), rhythm disturbances (e.g. third-degree (complete) atrioventricular block or supraventricular tachycardia), high-output states (e.g. hyperthyroidism) and toxicities (e.g. doxorubicin). The term "left-sided" heart failure represents increased pressure in the left atrium and left ventricle, leading to pulmonary edema, pleural effusion and/or pericardial effusion in cats, and only pulmonary edema in dogs. The term "right-sided" heart failure refers to increased pressure in the right atrium and right ventricle, leading to asities, and organomegaly, and pleural effusion. Congestive heart failure (CHF) can also be biventricular, which will exhibit signs from both left and right sides.

ACVIM Heart Disease Classification System (Paraphrased)[1]

Stage A:	Patients at risk of heart, with no structural changes identifiable
Stage B1:	Patients with identifiable heart disease (e.g. murmur) but have never developed CHF, nor have echocardiographic or radiographic evidence of chamber enlargement
Stage B2:	Patients with identifiable heart disease (e.g. murmur) but have never developed CHF, but do have identifiable cardiac remodeling exhibited by chamber enlargement
Stage C:	Patients with identifiable heart disease that are in or have been in CHF and have their clinical signs managed adequately
Stage D:	patients with CHF but refractory to medical management

Table 6.1 / Congestive heart failure

Disease		Congestive heart failure	
		Left-sided	Right-sided

Presentation	Presenting clinical signs	• Progression: sudden onset or gradual, especially if therapy previously initiated
		• Anorexia, cough; especially nocturnal, exercise intolerance, dyspnea, lethargy, syncope, orthopnea, tachypnea, wheeze
		• Cats: two presentations
		  • Pulmonary distress: anorexia, collapse, depression, dyspnea, hypothermia, open-mouth breathing, inactivity, restlessness, reluctance to move, tachypnea
		  • Aortic thromboembolism: ± all the above + hind-limb paralysis, pain vocalization
			• Progression: generally gradual onset but may be sudden dependent on cause (e.g. pericardial effusion)
			• Anorexia, abdominal distension, cachexia, dyspnea, orthopnea, pallor, tachypnea, syncope

	Physical examination	• Arrhythmias → pulse deficit, rales or crackles, cyanosis, ↑ CRT, femoral pulses weak, murmur + left hemithorax, ± right hemithorax, pallor, tachycardia, weak pulses • Cats: all the above plus: atrial gallop, abdominal distension, muffled heart sounds, ± systolic murmur, fluid line • ATE: ± all the above + limb paralysis, cyanotic nailbeds, ± generalized hypothermia, hypothermia in affected limb, pain, pale mucous membranes, no CRT, pulse absent, vocalization	• Ascites→ fluid wave, arrhythmia → pulse deficit, femoral pulses weak, fluid line,, jugular vein distention, ± jugular pulses, organomegaly, ± muffled heart sounds, ± murmur right, left, or bilateral

(Continued)

Table 6.1 / **Congestive heart failure (Continued)**

Disease		Congestive heart failure	
		Left-sided	Right-sided
Diagnosis	General	• History, clinical signs, physical examination • Cardiac/pulmonary auscultation	• History, clinical signs, physical examination • Cardiac/pulmonary auscultation
	Laboratory	• CBC: non-specific • Chemistry panel: often non-specific, ↑ ALT, AST, ALP, BUN, creatinine and rarely potassium, ↓ sodium, protein possible • Heartworm tests: rule out microfilaria and adult antigen as necessary • NT-proBNP: may be useful in discriminating dogs with CHF from those with murmurs and primary respiratory disease presenting in respiratory distress.[2] NT-proBNP marked ↑ with CHF • Cardiac troponin-I ↑ with myocardial damage	• CBC: heartworm non-specific generally, *D. immitis* = regenerative anemia, eosinophilia, basophilia, thrombocytopenia all possible but inconsistent • Chemistry panel: often non-specific; ↑ ALT, AST, ALP, GGT, BUN, creatinine, and ↓ sodium, protein possible • Urinalysis: non-specific, heartworm caval syndrome → hemoglobinurea • Heartworm tests: rule out microfilaria and adult antigen as necessary • Cardiac troponin ↑ with myocardial damage • NT-proBNP ↑
	Imaging	• Radiographs, thoracic: ↑ cardiac size, especially LA and LV, pulmonary vein dilation, pulmonary edema or perihilar edema • Cats: all the above + pleural effusion, pericardial effusion • Echocardiogram: diagnose cause (acquired vs. congenital) and progression of disease, ↑ LA size, assess systolic function, diagnose pericardial or pleural effusion, neoplasia, or heartworm disease. See specific etiology for more detail	• Radiographs, thoracic: ↑ cardiac size, globoid cardiac silhouette with PCE, ↑ vena cava and ± pulmonary arteries, pleural effusion, ± pulmonary edema • Echocardiogram: diagnose cause (acquired vs. congenital) and progression of disease, assess LA/LV involvement, RA ± enlarged, LA tear, pleural effusion, PCE, tamponade, neoplasia, or heartworm • Ultrasonography: ascites, enlarged liver, dilated hepatic veins
	Procedures	• ECG: may be normal, or ↑ P wave amplitude and duration, ±↑ R wave amplitude, APC, VPC, sinus tachycardia, atrial fibrillation, sustained or paroxysmal ventricular tachycardia • Blood pressure: hypotension	• ECG: may be normal, ↑ P wave amplitude, ± mean electrical axis right shift, AVP, VPC, sinus tachycardia, atrial fibrillation, sustained or paroxysmal ventricular tachycardia • Blood pressure: hypotension

(*Continued*)

Table 6.1 / Congestive heart failure (Continued)

Disease		Congestive heart failure	
		Left-sided	Right-sided
Treatment	General	• Acute: improve oxygenation, reduce edema, improve cardiac output; medications: diuretic (furosemide), oxygen, ± venodilator ointment, ± sedation, ± positive inotrope prn • Chronic: diuretics, ACE inhibitors, inodilator, aldosterone antagonist • Cats: Thoracocentesis as soon as possible as indicated • Pericardiocentesis-only if tamponade present • ATE: opioid analgesia together with CHF and anticoagulant therapy • Surgery: pacemakers for symptomatic bradycardia; none for acquired myocardial heart disease. Cardiopulmonary bypass surgical options in certain congenital disease, and valve replacement in unique patients with acquired valve disease. Interventional radiology with embolization device or valvuloplasty for congenital heart disease	• Acute: improve oxygenation, reduce edema, improve cardiac output, abdominocentesis, diuretic, oxygen, ± venodilator ointment, ± inodilator, ± positive inotrope • Acute PCE: pericardiocentesis, *no diuretic*, IV fluids, antiarrhythmics as necessary, treat concurrent disease appropriately • Chronic: treat underlying cause if possible (neoplasia, pericardiectomy) diuretics, ACE inhibitors, inodilator, aldosterone antagonist, abdominocentesis as necessary • Surgery: pacemakers for symptomatic bradycardia; none for acquired myocardial heart disease. Cardiopulmonary bypass surgical options in certain congenital disease, and valve replacement in unique patients with acquired valve disease. Interventional radiology with embolization device or valvuloplasty for congenital heart disease
	Medication	• ACE inhibitor: benazepril, captopril, enalapril, lisinopril • Aldosterone antagonist: spironolactone • Arterial dilators: acute – hydralazine or nitroprusside (emergency) • Ca^{+} channel blocker: diltiazem, *use with caution* for arrhythmias • Diuretics: acute – furosemide; chronic – furosemide, torsemide • Inodilator: pimobendan • Platelet aggregation inhibitor: clopidogrel bisulfate • Phosphodiesterase inhibitors: pimobendan, sildenafil • Positive inotropes: digoxin, dobutamine, or dopamine • Sedation: acepromazine maleate, benzodiazepines, opioids • Supplements: taurine, potassium, magnesium, L-carnitine or coenzyme Q10 • Venodilators: nitroglycerin ointment • Warfarin	• ACE inhibitor: benazepril, captopril, enalapril, lisinopril • Aldosterone antagonist: spironolactone • Ca^{+} channel blocker: diltiazem, *use with caution* for arrhythmias • Diuretics: acute – furosemide; chronic – furosemide, torsemide • Inodilator: pimobendan • Phosphodiesterase inhibitors: pimobendan, sildenafil • Positive inotropes: digoxin, dobutamine, or dopamine • Sedation: acepromazine maleate, benzodiazepines, opioids • Supplements: fish oil, taurine, potassium, magnesium, L-carnitine, • Venodilators: nitroglycerin ointment
	Nursing care	• Restrict stress: handling only for extremely necessary procedures • Cats: failed attempts at thoracocentesis are often safer than radiographs with suspected pleural effusion • Body cavity centesis as necessary	

(*Continued*)

Table 6.1 / **Congestive heart failure (Continued)**

Disease		Congestive heart failure	
		Left-sided	Right-sided
Follow-up	Patient care	• Instruct client in counting respiratory rates to monitor for tachypnea at home. Respiratory rate > 40 at rest = emergency • Restrict activity and ↓ anxiety • Oxygen therapy until respiratory rate < 30 on room air • Monitor BUN and creatinine when using diuretics and ACE inhibitors • Monitor ECG, radiograph, echocardiogram, serum chemistries concentrations regularly • Encourage eating	
	Prevention/avoidance	• Regular screening of at risk patients • Early use of inodilator therapy (see dilated cardiomyopathy and endocardiosis) • Early use of antiplatelet drugs in cats with ↑ LA size for ATE • Minimize stress and regulate exercise according to disease condition • Avoid high altitudes for patients with heart disease but not CHF	
	Complications	• Aortic thromboembolism (feline) • Arrhythmias • Azotemia • Cachexia • Electrolyte imbalances • Hypotension • Digoxin toxicity (if used) • Renal failure • Sudden death • Syncope • Worsening clinical signs leading to euthanasia	
	Prognosis	• Dependent on underlying disease • Not curable unless underlying condition can be corrected (some congenital heart disease, thyroid conditions, arrhythmias, nutritionally responsive)	• Dependent on underlying disease • Not curable unless underlying condition can be corrected (heartworm disease, arrhythmias, thyroid conditions, pericardial effusion)
Notes		• Caution: fluid therapy must be monitored closely for overload and worsening disease. • Instruct client in counting respiratory rates to monitor for tachypnea at home. Respiratory rate > 40 breaths/minute at rest = emergency	

Cardiomyopathy

Hypertrophic (Diastolic Dysfunction)

Idiopathic hypertrophic cardiomyopathy is a disease that occurs independently of other cardiac diseases. It is common in felines, rare in canines. It is characterized by concentric hypertrophy of the ventricle. Predominantly effects the left ventricle. This leads to decreased ventricular compliance and ventricular diastolic dysfunction, volume overload and congestive heart failure.

Restrictive (Diastolic Dysfunction)

Restrictive cardiomyopathy is a group of myocardial diseases that result in impaired ventricular filling. The exact etiology is unknown, and it results in related delayed myocardial relaxation and/or endocardial fibrosis leading to decreased compliance. This leads to ventricular diastolic dysfunction and biventricular CHF.

Table 6.2 / Cardiomyopathy, hypertrophic

Disease		Cardiomyopathy, hypertrophic (diastolic dysfunction)	Cardiomyopathy, restrictive (diastolic dysfunction)
Presentation	Presenting clinical signs	• Asymptomatic • Pulmonary compromise • Aortic thromboembolism • Signs of CHF, anorexia, collapse, depression, dyspnea, tachypnea, hypothermia, open-mouth breathing, inactivity, reluctance to move, • ATE: all the above + hind-limb paralysis, hypothermia, vocalization, pain • Sudden death	
	Physical examination	• Arrhythmia, atrial gallop, ± systolic murmur, tachycardia, finding of CHF and or paresis if ATE present	• Arrhythmia, atrial gallop, ascites, cyanosis, jugular distention, jugular pulse, ± systolic murmur, tachycardia, findings of CHF and or paresis if ATE present

(*Continued*)

Table 6.2 / **Cardiomyopathy, hypertrophic (Continued)**

Disease		Cardiomyopathy, hypertrophic (diastolic dysfunction)	Cardiomyopathy, restrictive (diastolic dysfunction)
Diagnosis	General	• History/clinical signs • Cardiac auscultation • Pulmonary auscultation	• History/clinical signs • Cardiac auscultation • Pulmonary auscultation
	Laboratory	• Chemistry panel: ↑ CK, AST, ALT, and azotemia • Thyroid panel (T4, Free T4, T3): Rule out hyperthyroidism; ↑ in 2nd-degree cases due to 1st-degree hyperthyroidism • NT-proBNP: ↑ • Coagulation: typically within normal limits	• Chemistry panel: ↑ CK, AST, ALT, creatinine, potassium and azotemia • Plasma taurine levels • NT-proBNP: ↑ • Coagulation: typically within normal limits
	Imaging	• Radiographs: thoracic ↑ cardiac size, valentine-shaped heart, elongated, LA enlargement, signs of CHF ± pleural effusion • Abdominal: ascites, organomegaly, negative flow during arteriogram if ATE • Echocardiogram: hypertrophy of the intraventricular septum, LV posterior wall, papillary muscles, left and ± right atrial enlargement, spontaneous echo-contrast and hyperdynamic contractility • MRI: uncommon, identifies mild disease and assessing response to therapy • Angiocardiography: arterial thrombosis – negative flow during arteriogram	• Radiographs: thoracic ↑ cardiac size, valentine-shaped heart, elongated, LA enlargement, signs of CHF ± pleural effusion, ± caudal vena cava enlargement • Abdominal: ascites, organomegaly, negative flow during arteriogram if ATE • Echocardiogram: bilateral atrial dilation, LV or RV, myocardial fibrosis, myocardial hypertrophy in septum or LV, valvular regurgitation, altered or prominent papillary muscles, ± normal systolic function • Angiocardiography: arterial thrombosis – negative flow during arteriogram
	Procedures	• ECG: sinus rhythm, sinus tachycardia, APC, VPC, ↑ P wave duration, ↑ R wave amplitudes, ↑ QRS width, uncommon atrial fibrillation • Blood pressure: rule out hypertension as cause of LV hypertrophy, hypotension	• ECG: sinus rhythm, sinus tachycardia, APC VPC, ↑ amplitude and duration of P waves, ↑ R wave amplitudes, ↑ QRS width, uncommon atrial fibrillation • Blood pressure: hypotension

(*Continued*)

Table 6.2 / Cardiomyopathy, hypertrophic (Continued)

Disease		Cardiomyopathy, hypertrophic (diastolic dysfunction)	Cardiomyopathy, restrictive (diastolic dysfunction)
Treatment	General	• Minimize stress • Symptomatic (Table 6.1) • Asymptomatic – none, ± β-blockers, or Ca+ channel blocker	• Minimize stress • Symptomatic (Table 6.1) • Asymptomatic – none, ± β-blockers, or Ca+ channel blocker
	Medication	• β-blockers: propranolol or atenolol • ACE inhibitor: benazepril, captopril, enalapril, lisinopril • Aldosterone antagonist: spironolactone • Antiarrhythmic: lidocaine • Aspirin • Bronchodilator: aminophylline, theophylline • Ca+ channel blocker: diltiazem • Diuretics: furosemide • Inodilator: pimobendan • Platelet aggregation inhibitor: clopidogrel bisulfate • Vasodilator: nitroglycerin ointment, captopril	• β-Blockers: propranolol or atenolol • ACE inhibitor: benazepril, captopril, enalapril, lisinopril • Aldosterone antagonist: spironolactone • Antiarrhythmic: lidocaine • Aspirin • Bronchodilator: aminophylline, theophylline • Ca+ channel blocker: diltiazem • Diuretics: furosemide • Inodilator: pimobendan • Platelet aggregation inhibitor: clopidogrel bisulfate • Positive inotropes: dobutamine, dopamine • Vasodilator: nitroglycerin ointment
	Nursing care	• Heat support • Low-stress environment • Restricted activity	• Heat support • Low-stress environment • Restricted activity
Follow-up	Patient care	• Observe closely for return of clinical signs. • Monitor blood values dependent on the medical treatment chosen (e.g. azotemia). • Repeat echocardiogram after 3–6 months of initiating treatment • Sodium-reduced diet • Warfarin use; monitor prothrombin time • Monitor physical condition, radiographs, ECG, blood pressure, and renal profile at regular intervals initially • Reevaluate patients every 2–4 months	• Observe closely for return of clinical signs. • Monitor blood values dependent on the medical treatment chosen (e.g. azotemia) • Repeat echocardiogram after 3–6 months of initiating treatment • Sodium-reduced diet • Monitor respiratory rate; ↑ rate may indicate worsening condition • Monitor physical condition, radiographs, ECG, blood pressure, and renal profile at regular intervals initially. • Reevaluate patients every 2–4 months
	Prevention/avoidance	• Idiopathic – no specific prevention • Selected breeding away from genetic carrier lines • DNA testing available for Maine Coon and Ragdoll breeds	• Idiopathic – no specific prevention

(*Continued*)

Table 6.2 / **Cardiomyopathy, hypertrophic (Continued)**

Disease		Cardiomyopathy, hypertrophic (diastolic dysfunction)	Cardiomyopathy, restrictive (diastolic dysfunction)
	Complications	• Congestive heart failure • Cardiac arrhythmias • DIC • Mitral valve regurgitation • Sudden death • Thromboembolism	• Congestive heart failure • Cardiac arrhythmias • DIC • Mitral valve regurgitation • Sudden death • Thromboembolism
	Prognosis	• Fair to good with some forms if diagnosed and treated early • Poor with CHF	• Poor: 3–12 months following diagnosis
Notes		• Caution: *any* fluid therapy (including saline used to flush catheter) must be monitored closely for fluid overload and worsening disease • Pain and crying may indicate thromboembolism to posterior aortic branches • Avoid β-blockers in patients with emboli	• Caution: *any* fluid therapy (including saline used to flush catheter) must be monitored closely for fluid overload and worsening disease • Pimobendan is not approved for clinical use in cats, but has been used extra label safely[3–5] • Pain and crying may indicate thromboembolism to posterior aortic branches
Client education		• Instruct client in counting respiratory rates to monitor for tachypnea at home. Respiratory rate > 40 breaths/minute at rest = emergency	• Instruct client in counting respiratory rates to monitor for tachypnea at home. Respiratory rate > 40 breaths/minute at rest = emergency

Dilated (Systolic Dysfunction)

Dilated cardiomyopathy (DCM) is a disease of the ventricular muscle. Advanced cases of disease show dilation of all chambers, eccentric hypertrophy, and poor contractility. Causes are typically idiopathic but have been linked in some cases to nutritional deficiencies, volume overload, viral, protozoan, chemotherapy, and immune-mediated mechanisms. Large breeds of dogs are more represented than small breeds. This disease leads to low cardiac output and/or CHF.

DCM is uncommonly seen in cats. Advanced cases of disease show dilation of all chambers, with or without eccentric hypertrophy, and poor contractility. It is most commonly caused by taurine deficiency and may be reversible. It may also be idiopathic. DCM may be noted at the end stage of another feline myocardial disease. This disease leads to low cardiac output and/or CHF.

Table 6.3 / Cardiomyopathy, dilated

Disease		Cardiomyopathy, dilated	
		Canine (systolic dysfunction)	Feline (systolic dysfunction)
Presentation	Presenting clinical signs	• Signs of CHF generally left sided or biventricular, including: abdominal distention, anorexia, ± ascites, cachexia, collapse, cough, dyspnea, exercise intolerance, lethargy, syncope, tachypnea	• Signs of CHF, anorexia, collapse, depression, dyspnea, tachypnea, hypothermia, open-mouth breathing, inactivity, reluctance to move, • ATE: all the above + hind-limb paralysis, hypothermia, vocalization, pain • Sudden death
	Physical examination	• Finding of left-sided CHF arrhythmias → pulse deficits, ↑ CRT, crackles, elicited cough, cyanosis, ± gallop, organomegaly, ± jugular distension and jugular pulse, soft heart sounds, left systolic murmur, sinus tachycardia with or without ectopy, chaotic tachycardia-presumed atrial fibrillation, weak femoral pulse, wheezes	• Arrhythmia, atrial gallop, ascites, cyanosis, jugular distention, jugular pulse, ±systolic murmur, tachycardia, ocular fundus lesion (↓ taurine), findings of CHF and or paresis if ATE present
Diagnosis	General	• History/clinical signs • Cardiac auscultation • Pulmonary auscultation	• History/clinical signs • Cardiac auscultation • Pulmonary auscultation
	Laboratory	• Chemistry panel: ↑ BUN, creatinine, ALT and ↓ sodium, chloride, potassium, protein • Plasma taurine and L-carnitine: ↓ • (see notes) • NT-proBNP ↑ • Cardiac troponin ↑	• CBC: stress leukogram • Chemistry panel: ↑ creatine kinase, AST, ALT, BUN, creatinine, glucose, and ↓ potassium • Urinalysis: ↑ myoglobin • Plasma taurine < 40 nmol/l (see notes) • Pleural effusion analysis: total protein < 4.9 g/dl and nucleated cell count < 2500/ml are supportive of CHF diagnosis
	Imaging	• Radiographs, thoracic: LA, LV ↑ size, ± caudal vena cava ↑, pulmonary venous ↑, pulmonary edema • Radiographs abdominal: organomegaly, ascites • Echocardiogram: LV, LA dilation often severe, ± biventricular involvement = dilation of the RA and RV, eccentric hypertrophy, reduced to markedly reduced systolic function, ± mitral, tricuspid, aortic valve regurgitation	• Radiographs, thoracic: ↑ cardiac size, rounding of cardiac apex, caudal vena cava, sign of left sided CHF, pulmonary veins enlarged, pleural effusion, pulmonary edema • Radiographs abdominal: organomegaly, ascites • Echocardiogram: dilation of LA and LV, ↓ LV contractility, valvular regurgitation, low aortic outflow velocity or LV muscle thinning • Ultrasonography, abdominal: arterial thromboembolism • Angiocardiography: arterial thromboembolism
	Procedures	• ECG: sinus rhythm, sinus tachycardia, atrial fibrillation, APC, VPC, low voltages (v), ↑ P wave size and duration, ↑ QRS duration	• ECG: APC, VPC, ↑ amplitude and duration of P waves, ↑ QRS duration, sinus rhythm, sinus tachycardia, rarely atrial fibrillation

(*Continued*)

Table 6.3 / **Cardiomyopathy, dilated (Continued)**

Disease		Cardiomyopathy, dilated	
		Canine (systolic dysfunction)	Feline (systolic dysfunction)
Treatment	General	• Symptomatic (Table 6.1)	• Symptomatic (Table 6.1) • Thoracocentesis • Pericardiocentesis ±
	Medication	• β-blockers (caution!): sotalol, carvedilol • ACE inhibitors: benazepril, captopril, enalapril, lisinopril • Aldosterone-antagonist: spironolactone • Antiarrhythmic: lidocaine, procainamide, mexiletine • Bronchodilators: aminophylline • Diuretics: furosemide, torsemide • Inodilator: pimobendan • Positive inotropes: digoxin and dobutamine • Sedation: acepromazine maleate, benzodiazepines, opioids • Taurine or L-carnitine supplementation • Vasodilators: hydralazine, nitroprusside (emergency) • Venodilator: nitroglycerin ointment	• ACE inhibitor: benazepril, captopril, enalapril, lisinopril • Aspirin • Bronchodilator: aminophylline • Diuretics: furosemide • Inodilator: pimobendan • Platelet aggregation inhibitor: clopidogrel bisulfate • Positive inotropes: dobutamine, dopamine • Sedation: acepromazine maleate, benzodiazepines, opioids • Taurine supplementation • Vasodilators: hydralazine, nitroprusside (emergency) • Venodilator: nitroglycerin ointment
	Nursing care	• Low-stress environment • Acute: CHF therapy ± CRI-positive inotropes • Chronic CHF therapy	• Low-stress environment • Acute: CHF therapy ± CRI-positive inotropes • Chronic CHF therapy

(Continued)

Table 6.3 / Cardiomyopathy, dilated (Continued)

Disease		Cardiomyopathy, dilated	
		Canine (systolic dysfunction)	Feline (systolic dysfunction)
Follow-up	Patient care	• Monitor physical condition, radiographs, Doppler echocardiogram, ECG, blood pressure, renal profile and electrolytes as necessary • Sodium-reduced diet • Check thoracic radiographs and blood pressure after 1 week of initiating treatment	• Monitor taurine • Monitor physical condition, radiographs, Doppler echocardiogram, ECG, BP, renal profile and electrolytes as necessary • Check thoracic radiographs and blood pressure after 1 week of initiating treatment
		• Activity: asymptomatic-normal self-regulated. Symptomatic – reduced exercise based on disease severity • Radiograph as necessary	• Repeat echocardiogram after 3–6 months of initiating treatment • Intermittent thoracocentesis may be required • Sodium-restricted diet
	Prevention/avoidance	• Occult: inodilator pimobendan started in the preclinical phase improves clinical outcomes[6] • Increased incidence linked to boutique, exotic, and grain-free diets, even in breeds not predisposed to DCM[7] • DNA testing: available for Doberman PDK4 (NCSU DCM1) and NCSU DCM2, Boxer cardiomyopathy, and ventricular arrhythmia in Rhodesian Ridgebacks. Selected breeding away from genetic carrier lines	• Feed a high-quality diet with adequate taurine supplementation
	Complications	• Sudden death • Hypothyroidism	• Hyperthyroidism • Thromboembolism
	Prognosis	• Poor to grave: 6–24 months following diagnosis	• Good with taurine supplementation after survival of first 2 weeks • Poor for idiopathic causes
Notes		• Caution: fluid therapy, including saline flush must be monitored closely for volume overload and worsening disease. • Monitoring resting respiratory rates can alert to potential decompensation. • Instruct client how to perform respiratory rates at home > 40 = emergency • Large breed dogs, especially Great Danes, Irish Wolfhound, Saint Bernard, Doberman Pinschers, Springer Spaniel, and Cocker Spaniel • Blood taurine levels are ideally run on both whole blood and plasma. If only one if available whole blood is preferred. Samples should immediately be put into an ice bath post collection. Separating plasma in a refrigerated centrifuge is ideal. • Instruct client in counting respiratory rates to monitor for tachypnea at home. Respiratory rate > 40 breaths/minute at rest = emergency	• Caution: fluid therapy, including saline flush must be monitored closely for volume overload and worsening disease • Monitoring resting respiratory rates can alert to potential decompensation. • Instruct client how to perform respiratory rates at home > 40 = emergency • Burmese, Abyssinian, and Siamese • Pimobendan is not approved for clinical use in cats, but has been used extra label safely[3–5] • Blood taurine levels are ideally run on both whole blood and plasma. If only one if available whole blood is preferred. Samples should immediately be put into an ice bath post collection. Separating plasma in a refrigerated centrifuge is ideal • Instruct client in counting respiratory rates to monitor for tachypnea at home. Respiratory rate > 40 breaths/minute at rest = emergency

Congenital Heart Diseases

All congenital heart diseases in veterinary medicine comprise fewer than 1% of all veterinary patients. Congenital heart disease is the most common heart condition in animals less than one year of age. Congenital heart diseases are embryological malformations of the heart and great vessels. Table 6.4 covers only the four most common congenital cardiac defects; patent ductus arteriosus (PDA), ventricular septal defect (VSD), subaortic stenosis (SAS), and pulmonic stenosis. While other congenital defects exist, they represent less than 1% of the 1% and are rarely seen in practice. Many will be listed in the definitions for reference purposes only. Information covering presentation to notes is strictly for the four conditions listed here.

Obstructions

The most common obstructions are from dysplastic heart valves. Dysplasia of a valve may cause incompetence, stenosis, or both. Pulmonic stenosis, subaortic stenosis, mitral valve dysplasia, and tricuspid valve dysplasia are examples. Pulmonic stenosis is most often seen in small-breed dogs, yet can be seen in large-breed dogs, especially Boxers, and Labrador Retrievers. Subaortic stenosis is most often present in large-breed dogs, especially Golden Retrievers, Newfoundlands, and Boxers. The lesion is a narrowing leading to the aortic valve, not the valve itself. Valvular aortic stenosis is uncommon in dogs. Tricuspid dysplasia is over-represented in Labrador Retrievers. Mitral dysplasia is most often seen in Bull Terriers, but can be identified in any breed. Other examples of congenital obstructions include cor triatriatum dexter and sinister, and coarctation of the aorta.

Shunts

Congenital defects that allow blood from one chamber or vessels to abnormally pass into another are termed shunts. Mixing of oxygenated blood into deoxygenated a blood pool is a "left-to-right" shunt (more common that right-to-left shunts) and deoxygenated blood with oxygenated blood is referred to as a "right-to-left" shunt. Examples of a left-to-right shunt include PDA, VSD, and atrial septal defect (ASD). Examples of right-to-left shunting defects include tetralogy of Fallot, patent foramen ovale, "reversed PDA, and VSD with pulmonary hypertension (Eisenmenger syndrome). Typical left-to-right shunting PDA and VSD both may lead to left-sided CHF from volume overload as extra volume circulates through the lungs back to the left atrium. VSD is the most common congenital heart defect in cats.

Table 6.4 / Obstructions and shunts

Disease		Obstructions	Congenital heart disease-shunts
Presentation	Presenting clinical signs	• Dependent on defect and severity. May be normal with murmur. Tricuspid valve dysplasia may be silent. Exercise intolerance, lethargy, failure to thrive, signs of either right or left sided CHF (arrhythmias → pulse deficit, crackles, cyanosis, ↑ CRT, femoral pulses weak, murmur + left, ± right, pallor, tachycardia, weak pulses), syncope	• Dependent on chronicity and shunt volume • PDA/VSD: asymptomatic presentation not uncommon. Murmur often identified at the first vaccination. Exercise intolerance, lethargy, failure to thrive, signs of left-sided CHF, syncope
	Physical examination	• May be within normal limits except for: • SAS – grade 2–6 left basilar systolic murmur, loud murmur may be heard radiating to the right hemithorax, and/or up carotid arteries. ±arrhythmias, ± weak pulses, severe cases →signs of left-sided CHF • Pulmonary stenosis – grade 2–6 left basilar systolic murmur, ± arrhythmias, jugular distension, jugular pulses, positive hepatojugular reflux, severe cases → right-sided CHF	• May be within normal limits except for: • PDA – grade 3–6 extreme left basilar (axillary) continuous murmur, secondary 2–5 left apical systolic murmur, hyperkinetic pulses • VSD – grade 4–6 right basilar systolic murmur, ± signs of left-sided CHF • PDA, VSD chronic cases: ± signs of left-sided CHF, atrial fibrillation

(Continued)

Table 6.4 / Obstructions and shunts (Continued)

Disease		Obstructions	Congenital heart disease-shunts
Diagnosis	General	• History/clinical signs • Physical examination • Cardiac auscultation	• History/clinical signs • Physical examination • Cardiac auscultation
	Laboratory	• CBC: PS rarely polycythemia if patent foramen ovale with significant shunt is present • Chemistry panel: SAS – non-specific, ± azotemia; PS ± ↑ hepatic enzymes, and ↓ albumin, globulin, azotemia	• CBC: non-specific except any right to left shunt can lead to polycythemia
	Imaging	• Radiographs, thoracic • SAS: may be normal with mild obstruction. ± LV and LA enlargement, loss of cranial waist on lateral, ± bulge at 1 : 00 on VD view. Severe cases – signs of left-sided CHF • Pulmonary stenosis: may be normal with mild obstruction. ± RV and RA enlargement, loss of cranial waist on lateral, reverse "D" RV shape, prominent bulge at 2–3 : 00 on VD, ± under size pulmonary arteries (under circulated) • Radiographs, abdominal: PS only – ± asities, organomegaly, ↑ caudal vena cava • ECG • SAS: ± LV concentric hypertrophy, ± LA dilation, normal systolic function unless advanced, MV regurgitation, increased Doppler velocity across aortic valve, severity assigned by Doppler derived pressure gradients • Pulmonary stenosis: RV dilation and hypertrophy, RA dilation, tricuspid valve regurgitation, ± patent foramen ovale, PA dilation, ± fused PV leaflets • ECG • SAS: Normal, sinus rhythm, sinus tachycardia, ± ↑ P wave duration, ± QRS ↑ duration, VPC, sustain or paroxysmal ventricular tachycardia • PS: sinus rhythm, sinus tachycardia, MEA right axis shift, ± ↑ P wave amplitude, ± ↑ QRS duration ± VPC, rare atrial arrhythmias	• Radiographs, thoracic • PDA: ↑ LA and LV size, pulmonary arterial over-circulation, "triple bump" sign on VD from 12 : 00 to 3 : 00, signs of left-sided CHF if present • VSD: May be normal, dependent on volume of shunt, ↑ LA and LV size, pulmonary arterial over-circulation, signs of left sided CHF if present • ECG • PDA: LA, LV dilation, normal or enhanced systolic function unless advanced, MV regurgitation by Doppler, ± pulmonary vein enlargement, ± ↑ mild increase in trans-aortic valve velocity, continuous Doppler retrograde color flow in the main pulmonary artery, often PV regurgitation, ± ductus visualization • VSD: cardiac remodeling dependent on volume of shunt and chronicity at presentation. Cardiac dimension and systolic function may be normal in the cases of minute to small defects. Doppler color imaging of flow crossing from LV to RV in systole near the aortic valve. This may be seen in short and long axis views. Larger defects lead to LA, LV dilation, MV regurgitation by Doppler, ± pulmonary vein enlargement, ± ↑ mild increase in trans-aortic valve velocity, eventually systolic dysfunction. Very large defects may impair the integrity of the aortic valve causing regurgitation hastening the advancement toward CHF. Signs of right-sided CHF uncommonly develop unless pulmonary hypertension should occur • ECG • PDA: Normal, sinus rhythm, sinus tachycardia, ↑ QRS amplitude, ± ↑ P wave duration, advanced disease→ atrial fibrillation, APC, VPC • VSD: sinus rhythm, sinus tachycardia, ± ↑ P wave duration, ± ↑ QRS amplitude, advanced disease→ atrial fibrillation, APC, VPC
	Procedures	• Blood pressure: ± hypotension	• Blood pressure: ± hypotension

(*Continued*)

Table 6.4 / **Obstructions and shunts (Continued)**

Disease		Obstructions	Congenital heart disease-shunts
Treatment	General	• Symptomatic (Table 6.1) • SAS: β-blockers, antiarrhythmics as necessary, antibiotics for any medical procedure (see notes) • Surgery: none superior to medical therapy at this time • Pulmonary stenosis: β-blockers • Surgery/interventional radiology: balloon valvuloplasty, patch graft/valvulotomy procedure, conduit graft procedure	• Symptomatic (Table 6.1) • PDA: medical management of CHF • Surgery – recommended therapy, open thoracic surgical ligation or transcatheter occlusion device • VSD: Medical management of CHF • Surgery: cardiopulmonary bypass open heart closure, transcatheter occlusion devices of minimal use in veterinary medicine
	Medication	• ACE inhibitor: benazepril, captopril, enalapril, lisinopril • Aldosterone antagonist: spironolactone • Antiarrhythmic: lidocaine or procainamide, sotalol • β-blockers: atenolol, carvedilol, propranolol, sotalol • Ca^{+} channel blocker: diltiazem • Diuretics: furosemide, torsemide • Inodilator: pimobendan • Phosphodiesterase inhibitors: pimobendan, sildenafil • Vasodilators: hydralazine, nitroprusside (emergency)	• ACE inhibitor: benazepril, captopril, enalapril, lisinopril • Aldosterone antagonist: spironolactone • Antiarrhythmic: lidocaine or procainamide • Arterial dilators: hydralazine or nitroprusside (emergency) • Ca^{+} channel blocker: diltiazem prn arrhythmias. *Use with caution* • Diuretics: furosemide, torsemide • Inodilator: pimobendan • Positive inotropes: digoxin • Phosphodiesterase inhibitors: pimobendan, sildenafil
	Nursing care	• Care for CHF as necessary • Intensive care following interventional or surgical procedure	• Care for CHF as necessary • Intensive care following interventional or surgical procedure
Follow-up	Patient care	• Puppies will generally self-regulate activity • Following interventional procedures activity is restricted during recovery and rehabilitation	• Monitor for clinical signs of CHF • PDA: Approximately two thirds of dogs with PDA will develop CHF by 1 year is not closed. • VSD: non-repaired – (annually during asymptomatic period); monitor radiographs and echocardiograms at regular intervals • Restrict activity if CHF • Sodium-reduced diet as necessary
	Prevention/avoidance	• Selected breeding away from genetic carrier lines • DNA testing: research continuing for SAS in Newfoundland dogs	• Selective breeding – do not breed affected dogs
	Complications	• CHF • Arrhythmias • SAS: sudden death	• CHF • Arrhythmias • Death
	Prognosis	• Good to guarded, depending on the degree of obstruction and response to therapy	• PDA: excellent with early closure; patient can live a normal life; guarded without surgery • VSD: outcome is vary with shunt volume – small shunt = good prognosis, large shunt = poor prognosis

(*Continued*)

Table 6.4 / Obstructions and shunts (Continued)

Disease	Obstructions	Congenital heart disease-shunts
	• Innocent murmurs in puppies, and kittens common. Distinguish from pathological congenital murmurs; murmur grade 3 or less, heard best that the left-heart base, gone by 16 weeks of age; murmur gets softer over the vaccination schedule. Murmurs not meeting those criteria should have a cardiology evaluation	
Notes	• Instruct client in counting respiratory rates to monitor for tachypnea at home. Respiratory rate > 40 breaths/minute at rest = emergency • SAS: dogs with moderate to severe SAS are likely to develop clinical signs, and severe cases may exhibit sudden death. Dogs with mild SAS may not develop clinical signs. Any degree of SAS obstruction predisposes the patient to bacterial endocarditis following any medical procedure, or serious infection. Dog with diagnosed SAS and those breeds at risk of SAS with left basilar murmurs should be given antibiotics before and after any planed procedure, e.g. dentistry, spay or neuter unless SAS has been excluded by echocardiography • Pulmonary stenosis: Onset of clinical signs is variable compared with degree of obstruction. Boxers and Bulldogs may develop an anomalous coronary artery that causes pulmonary stenosis. These cases need open thoracic surgery to repair	• Instruct client in counting respiratory rates to monitor for tachypnea at home. Respiratory rate > 40 breaths/minute at rest = emergency • PDA: standard of care is closure of the PDA at the earliest reasonable opportunity. • VSD: standard for care for most small animals is medical management of CHF when it occurs

Endocardiosis

Endocardiosis (chronic myxomatous valvular degeneration, MVD) is the most common cardiovascular disease in dogs. The disease is non-inflammatory degeneration in a structure of the valve apparatus (leaflets, papillary muscles, chordae tendinous) causing regurgitation and progressive cardiac remodeling and eventually CHF. The mitral valve is most often affected, with the tricuspid valve second in incidence; the semilunar valves may also be affected. Any or all valves may be affected at once. Rupture of a chordae tendineae leads to sudden onset of CHF. Chronic MVD does not predispose the patient to bacterial endocarditis. It is most common in small-breed dogs, but may be seem in elderly large-breed dogs. It is uncommon in cats.

Heartworm Disease

Heartworm disease is most commonly diagnosed in dogs, although cats may be affected. It is an infection of the nematode *Dirofilaria immitis*, which is transmitted by many species of mosquitoes There is wide distribution of the parasite in the United States. Adult parasites live in the pulmonary artery and its branches. Large populations can extend into the right ventricle, right atrium and both parts of the vena cava. Caval syndrome is seen in patients with heavy parasite loads, which reduce venous return, interfere with the operation of the tricuspid valve, and generates a shock response. Heartworm infection is the leading cause of pulmonary hypertension in dogs. Inflammatory response of patient more causative of clinical signs than parasite load. Cats typically have low parasite loads (fewer than eight) but a single worm can cause clinical signs of anaphylaxis.

Table 6.5 / Cardiovascular: endocardiosis and heartworm disease

Disease		Endocardiosis	Heartworm disease
Presentation	Presenting clinical signs	• Asymptomatic, or signs of CHF (usually left sided; right sided may also occur alone or concurrently), dyspnea, exercise intolerance, lethargy, syncope, tachypnea, cough, wheezing, ± anorexia	• Cachexia, cough, dyspnea, exercise intolerance, hemoptysis, dyspnea, sign of right-sided CHF, syncope, vomiting, wheezes • Cats: asymptomatic, cough, dyspnea, episodic vomiting, sudden death
	Physical examination	• Maybe normal with only a systolic murmur or click. Murmur grade not well correlated with severity of disease. Sinus rhythm or sinus arrhythmia in asymptomatic dogs. Or findings of left-sided CHF, arrhythmias → pulse deficits, ↑ CRT, crackles, elicited cough, cyanosis, ± jugular distension and jugular pulse, left, right or bilateral systolic murmur, sinus tachycardia with or without ectopy, chaotic tachycardia-presumed atrial fibrillation, ± weak femoral pulse, wheezes	• May be normal or findings of right-sided CHF, APC, VPC, cyanosis, crackles, wheezes, harsh lung sounds, fluid line, gallop, murmur, split S2 sound, jugular distension, ± jugular pulses, organomegaly, tachycardia • Severe: DIC, epistaxis, pulmonary thromboembolism, hemoglobinuria • Cats: may be normal, or dyspnea, muffled lung sounds, tachycardia, fluid line, ± gallop, ± murmur

(*Continued*)

Table 6.5 / Cardiovascular: endocardiosis and heartworm disease (Continued)

Disease		Endocardiosis	Heartworm disease
Diagnosis	General	• History/clinical signs • Cardiac auscultation • Pulmonary auscultation	• History/clinical signs • Cardiac auscultation • Pulmonary auscultation
	Laboratory	• CBC: stress leukogram • Chemistry panel: ↑ BUN, creatinine, phosphorus, ALT, AST, ALP, ↓ albumin • Urinalysis: ↑ protein, albumin, granular cast, WCC, occult blood • NT-proBNP: may be useful in discriminating dogs with CHF from those with murmurs and primary respiratory disease presenting in respiratory distress.[2] NT-proBNP marked ↑ with CHF • Cardiac troponin: ↑ with advanced disease	• CBC: regenerative anemia, eosinophilia, basophilia, thrombocytopenia all possible but inconsistent • Chemistry panel: ↑ hepatic enzymes, bile acids and ↓ albumin, globulin, azotemia • Urinalysis: ↑ protein, globulin, albumin, granular casts, hemoglobinuria • ELISA: adult female worm antigens • Cats: false negative not uncommon due to unisex infection • Direct blood smear, Knott test or Millipore filter test: microfilaria – must differentiate from *Acanthocheilonema* (formerly *Dipetalonema) reconditum* • Cats: false (negative) possible due to short microfilarial stage • Immunodiagnostic screens: microfilaria antigen • Serology: + *Dirofilaria*
	Imaging	• Radiographs, thoracic: may be normal in early stages, disease progression gradually ↑ LA, LV size, elevation mainstem bronchi, pulmonary edema esp. in perihilar, and dorsocaudal regions, TV involvement shows signs of right sided CHF • Echocardiogram: findings dependent on stage of disease. Earliest stage may only show MV/TV regurgitation with normal cardiac size and function. Progressive ↑ of LA, then LV. Likewise with RA, and RV in disease. Advanced disease-systolic dysfunction, dilated pulmonary veins, marked atrial enlargement, valve prolapse, flail leaflet, Doppler MV/TV regurgitation, ± aortic and pulmonary valve regurgitation, ± pericardial effusion (LA rent or tear), rarely ruptured chordae tendineae	• Radiographs, thoracic: dilated, truncated or tortuous pulmonary arteries, ↑ RA and RV, pneumonitis, localized or generalized interstitial or alveolar infiltrates, ± pleural effusion, ± caudal vena cava ↑ • Cats: broncho-interstitial infiltrates, pulmonary artery changes less prominent than dogs, RV/RA ↑ also less prominent, ± lung consolidation • Echocardiogram: RA, RV, pulmonary artery ↑, TV and PV regurgitation, positive iditol dehydrogenase parasite (specific not sensitive, slightly better in cats), Doppler-derived evidence of pulmonary hypertension • Severe: intraventricular septal flattening, LV pseudohypertrophy, TV entanglement, • Ultrasounds: hepatic congestion, enlarged vena cava, ± heartworms in vena cava with caval syndrome
	Procedures	• ECG: normal or ↑ P wave amplitude and/or duration, APC, ± ↑ QRS amplitude, sinus rhythm, sinus arrhythmia, sinus tachycardia, supraventricular tachycardia (sustained or paroxysmal) atrial fibrillation, VPC • Blood pressure: hypotension	• ECG: Normal, or APC, VPC, mean electrical axis shift to right, ↑ P amplitude, tachycardia • Angiography: demonstrate thromboembolism

(*Continued*)

Table 6.5 / **Cardiovascular: endocardiosis and heartworm disease (Continued)**

Disease		Endocardiosis	Heartworm disease
Treatment	General	• Symptomatic (Table 6.1) • Oxygen therapy as necessary • Low stress environment	• Symptomatic (Table 6.1) • Stabilize CHF before therapy • Platelet count prior to melarsomine therapy • Surgery: caval syndrome only – worm removal via jugular vein
	Medication	• ACE inhibitor: benazepril, captopril, enalapril, lisinopril • Adrenergic blocking agent: prazosin • Aldosterone blocker: spironolactone • Antiarrhythmics: lidocaine, procainamide, mexiletine, sotalol if ventricular arrhythmia present • Vasodilators: hydralazine, nitroprusside (emergency) • Aldosterone antagonist: spironolactone • Ca^{+} channel blocker: diltiazem • Diuretics: furosemide, torsemide • Inodilator: pimobendan • Positive inotropes: digoxin, dobutamine • Venodilator: nitroglycerin ointment	• Adulticide: melarsomine, or rarely thiacetarsamide sodium • All drugs listed in Table 6.1 • Antibiotics: doxycycline • Anticoagulant: heparin, aspirin (low dose) • Corticosteroids: prednisone or prednisolone (cats) • Microfilaricide: macrocyclic lactones: milbemycin oxime, moxidectin, ivermectin, selamectin, abamectin, doramectin, and eprinomectin • 2018 AHS "recommends use of doxycycline and a macrocyclic lactone prior to the 3-dose regimen of melarsomine (one injection 2.5 mg/kg followed by at least 1 month later followed by 2 injections at the same dosage 24 hours apart) for the treatment of both asymptomatic and symptomatic dogs. Any method utilizing macrocyclic lactone as a slow-kill adulticide is not recommended"[8] • Cats: 2018 AHS: "Adulticide (melarsomine) use is not recommended for use in cats due to insufficient experience and preliminary data which suggest that melarsomine is toxic to cats at doses as low as 3.5 mg/kg. Ivermectin administered at 24 µg/kg monthly given for 2 years has been reported to reduce worm burdens by 65% as compared with untreated cats. Because most cats have small worm burdens, it is not worm mass alone that is problematic but the 'anaphylactic' type reaction that results when the worms die. To date, there are no studies that indicate any form of medical adulticidal therapy increases the survival rate of cats harboring adult heartworms"[9]
	Nursing care	• CHF nursing care • Low-stress environment • Oxygen as necessary	• Read melarsomine manufacturer instructions carefully and follow exactly • Feed patient ½ hour prior to injection to observe for anorexia • Monitor for jaundice, fever, depression, dyspnea, or other signs of thromboembolism • Closely monitor after administering injection for signs of toxicity (inflammation at injection site, vomiting, anorexia, lethargy, icterus and ↑ BUN, ALT, or bilirubin
	Surgery	• Cardiopulmonary bypass surgical valve replacement available in select patients	• Not applicable

(Continued)

Table 6.5 / Cardiovascular: endocardiosis and heartworm disease (Continued)

Disease		Endocardiosis	Heartworm disease
Follow-up	Patient care	• Asymptomatic normal activity • Monitor physical condition, ECG, and radiography 1 week after initiating therapy. • Monitor therapy through radiographs every 6–12 months, or as clinical signs dictate • Activity: asymptomatic-normal self-regulated. Symptomatic – reduced exercise based on disease severity. • Normal or sodium-reduced diet	• Monitor for jaundice, fever, depression, dyspnea, or other signs of thromboembolism. • Cage confinement for 3–4 weeks followed by 2–3 weeks of strict confinement for severe cases • Instruct client in counting respiratory rates to monitor for tachypnea at home. RR > 40 RR at rest = Emergency • Radiograph prn
	Prevention/avoidance	• ACVIM class B2: inodilator pimobendan started in the preclinical phase improves clinical outcomes[10,11]	• Prophylactic therapy: milbemycin oxide, ivermectin, moxidectin, selamectin • Heartworm surveillance testing: 6–12 months of initiating preventative and then at annual intervals
	Complications	• Atrial fibrillation • CHF left and/or right sided • LA rent or tear • Tachyarrhythmia • Tamponade • Sudden death • Dependent of severity of disease	• Acute pulmonary thromboembolism • Caval syndrome • DIC • CHF • Reinfestation if prophylaxis is not started • Thrombocytopenia • Sudden death
	Prognosis		• Good when subclinical or mild disease • Fair with moderate to severe disease • Guarded if untreated, very high worm burden, of CHF present • Grave if caval syndrome present
Notes		• Instruct client in counting respiratory rates to monitor for tachypnea at home. Respiratory rate> 40 beaths/minute at rest = emergency • Client monitoring of exercise, diet, appetite, and heart rate is helpful to early detection of developing clinical signs • Poodle, Yorkshire terrier, Cavalier King Charles Spaniel, Schnauzer, Cocker Spaniel	• Caution: IM injection can cause pain and sterile abscesses with melarsomine; apply pressure at injection site during and after needle withdrawal. Cough, gagging, vomiting, anorexia, fever all reported complications with melarsomine therapy • Transplacental microfilaria infestation is possible • Necropsy may be necessary for a definitive diagnosis in cats with sudden death

Hypertension

Hypertension is an increase in pulmonary or systemic arterial blood pressure. Pulmonary hypertension may be either a primary or secondary condition. Pulmonary hypertension may be caused by disease of the circulatory (e.g. secondary to left-sided CHF) or respiratory (e.g. interstitial pulmonary fibrosis) systems. Systemic hypertension is typically secondary in dogs and cats, but may be primary in geriatric cats. Systemic disease linked to causing systemic hypertension are renal disease, hyperadrenocorticism in dogs, and hyperthyroidism in cats. Systemic hypertension is diagnosed with non-invasive blood pressure measurement repeated over several measurements ideally over several days. Pulmonary arterial hypertension is diagnosed by cardiac catheterization or estimated with a Doppler echocardiogram.

Table 6.6 / Hypertension

Disease		Hypertension	
		Pulmonary	Systemic
Presentation	Presenting	• Cough • Exercise intolerance • Syncope	• Sudden blindness, especially in cats • "Silent" disease • Target organs damaged: brain, eyes, heart, kidneys
	Clinical signs	• Signs of right heart failure including abdominal distention, anorexia, coughing, dyspnea, exercise intolerance, hemoptysis, lethargy, syncope, tachypnea	• Most commonly blindness (acute), • Rarely signs of cerebral vascular accident (circling, depression, dilated pupils, head tilt, nystagmus, paralysis, seizures) epistaxis, • occasionally CHF in cats, not reported in dogs • polyuria/polydipsia
	Physical examination	• Sign of right heart failure, atrial gallop, crackles, hypoxemia, right systolic murmur, ± left diastolic murmur, ± split S2 sound	• Intraocular hemorrhage, gallop sound, ± murmur, ± papilledema, retinal detachment

(Continued)

Table 6.6 / Hypertension (Continued)

Disease		Hypertension	
		Pulmonary	Systemic
Diagnosis	General	• History/clinical signs	• History/clinical signs
	Laboratory	• CBC: non-specific or possible ↑ packed cell volume • ELISA: adult female heartworm antigens • Modified knots: microfilaria	• CBC: typically normal • Chemistry panel: BUN, creatinine, ALP, ALT, glucose, and ↓ potassium. Information on effect and potential cause. • Urinalysis: ↑ protein, blood, glucose, and ↓ specific gravity • Dependent on underlying condition: thyroid disorders, nephrology disorders, hyperadrenocorticism
	Imaging	• Radiographs thoracic: dilated caudal vena cava, pulmonary artery dilation or tortuous vessels, neoplasia, bronchial collapse, pleural effusion, right ventricle and atrial enlargement, tracheal narrowing • Radiographs, abdominal: ascites, hepatomegaly or abnormal kidney size or shape • Echocardiogram: ± RV and RA dilation, RV hypertrophy related to degree of pressure elevation, intraventricular septum flattened, ± paradoxical septal motion, LV pseudohypertrophy, main pulmonary artery dilation, tricuspid valve regurgitation Doppler-derived velocities used to calculate peak pulmonary artery systolic pressure, pulmonary vein insufficiency, ± pleural or pericardial effusion, rule in heartworm disease (specific but not sensitive for heartworm) • Dependent on underlying condition: CT, MRI, transtracheal wash, bronchoalveolar lavage, lung aspirate or biopsy	• Radiographs, thoracic: ↑ cardiac size, prominent and or undulant aorta in cats • Radiographs, abdominal: hepatomegaly or abnormal kidneys • Echocardiogram: LV hypertrophy, ↑ LA size if MV regurgitation present • Cats: diastolic dysfunction • Ultrasound: adrenal enlargement, evaluation of liver, kidneys and bladder, pheochromocytoma • Dependent on underlying condition: CT, MRI, thyroid scintigraphy
	• Procedures	• Arterial blood gases • ECG: sinus rhythm, sinus tachycardia, tall P waves, widening of QRS complex, ST segment alterations, deep S waves, rare slowed AV node conduction • Interventional radiology: invasive pulmonary artery catheterization for measurement	• Blood pressure measurement • Invasive arterial catheter-considered "gold-standard", systolic, diastolic and mean blood pressure and heart rate • Non-invasive BP measurement: Doppler method → systolic pressure and heart rate, oscillometric → systolic, diastolic, mean blood pressure and heart rate • ECG: sinus rhythm, generally within normal

(*Continued*)

Table 6.6 / **Hypertension (Continued)**

Disease		Hypertension	
		Pulmonary	Systemic
Treatment	General	• Symptomatic (Table 6.1) • Supportive • Oxygen therapy • Phosphodiesterase-5 inhibitors as pulmonary arterial dilator • Surgery: dependent on underlying condition (e.g. caval syndrome)	• Treat underlying condition if possible • Treated as outpatient with medication • Surgery: dependent on underlying condition (e.g. pheochromocytoma)
	Medication	• ACE inhibitor: benazepril, captopril, enalapril, lisinopril • Anticoagulant: aspirin, clopidogrel, heparin, warfarin • Bronchodilators: terbutaline, theophylline • Ca^{+} channel blocker: diltiazem or amlodipine (cats) • Diuretics: furosemide, torsemide • Inodilator: pimobendan • Phosphodiesterase inhibitor: pimobendan, sildenafil, tadalafil • Vasodilators: hydralazine, nitroprusside (emergency)	• α_1 adrenergic blocker: phenoxybenzamine • β-adrenergic blocker: propranolol, atenolol • ACE inhibitor: benazepril, captopril, enalapril, lisinopril • Aldosterone antagonist: spironolactone • Ca^{+} channel blocker: diltiazem or amlodipine (cats) • Diuretics: furosemide, torsemide, hydrochlorothiazide • Vasodilators: hydralazine, nitroprusside (emergency)
	Nursing care	• Treat as outpatient if possible to ↓ overall stress • Monitor hydration and body temperature • Restrict activity, especially if related to heartworm disease	• Treat as outpatient if possible to ↓ overall stress
Follow-up	Patient care	• Avoid high-salt diet • Restrict activity, especially if related to heartworm disease • Monitor for worsening clinical signs • Monitor Doppler echocardiogram for response to treatment • Monitor blood pressure for hypotension. • Monitor CBC/chemistry panel to monitor potential adverse effects (e.g. azotemia) from therapy • Radiograph as necessary	• Avoid high-salt diet • Monitor for signs of hypotension • Monitor blood pressure every 1–2 weeks then every 1–3 months • Monitor CBC/chemistry panel to monitor potential adverse effects (e.g. azotemia) from therapy
	Prevention/avoidance	• Maintain proper weight control. • Measure blood pressure in all patients with renal failure	• Measure blood pressure in all patients with renal failure, sudden blindness, and patients with cardiac hypertrophy by echocardiography • Maintain proper weight control
	Complications	• Right-sided heart failure • Arrhythmias • Syncope	• Renal failure • LV hypertrophy • Glomerulonephropathy • Retinopathy/blindness • Central nervous system signs
	Prognosis	• Guarded, based on underlying condition	• Good if underlying cause can be determined and treated

(*Continued*)

Table 6.6 / Hypertension (Continued)

Disease	Hypertension	
	Pulmonary	Systemic
Notes	• Avoid respiratory distress (high altitudes, cigarette smoke, cold or hot air, or excessive heat)	• Systemic hypertension (see notes)
	• Assure proper equipment usage and technique when performing non-invasive blood pressure measurements • Educate clients on monitoring signs of hypertension (retinal hemorrhage or detachment, renal, cardiac, or neurological signs) • Recommended hypertension values by American College of Veterinary Internal Medicine based on risk of target organ damage for dogs and cats. All values are systolic blood pressure only • Normotensive, blood pressure < 140 mmHg: minimal risk of target organ damage • Prehypertensive, blood pressure 140–159 mmHg: low risk of target organ damage • Hypertensive, blood pressure 160–179 mmHg: moderate risk of target organ damage • Severely hypertensive, systolic blood pressure ≥ 180 mmHg: high risk of target organ damage[12] • An average of 5–7 readings after discarding the first should be taken. Some patients will demonstrate a progressively lowering blood pressure over the course of the readings. In this case, repeat the recording as necessary until the blood pressure plateaus. An average of 5–7 consistent readings are recorded[12] • Maintain low stress before and during the blood pressure measurement • Arrhythmias will complicate the measurement	

Myocarditis

Myocarditis is an inflammation of the heart muscle. Causes may be infectious or non-infectious. Infectious causes include viral (e.g. acute parvovirus myocarditis), protozoan (e.g. *Trypanosoma cruzi*, *T. babesei*, toxoplasmosis), bacterial (e.g. *Bartonella vinsonii*, or related to endocarditis). Non-infectious causes include ischemic injury, trauma, or toxicity. Primary infection is rare; typically, other systemic diseases present first.

Pleural Effusion

Pleural effusion is an accumulation of fluid in the pleural cavity. It may be seen unilaterally or bilaterally. This is an abnormal process that has many causes, typically indicating a more severe underlying condition.

Table 6.7 / **Myocarditis and pleural effusion**

Disease		Myocarditis	Pleural effusion
Presentation	Presenting clinical signs	• Anorexia, signs of CHF, ± fever, sudden death, syncope, vomiting, weakness	• Anorexia, depression, dyspnea, exercise intolerance, pallor, pleuritis, open-mouth breathing, preference for sternal recumbency, tachypnea
	Physical examination	• Findings of CHF left or right sided, ± gallop, ± murmur, ± tachycardia	• Ascites, cyanosis, pyrexia, muffled heart and lung sounds, tachycardia
Diagnosis	General	• History/clinical signs (e.g. parvovirus, Chagas disease – geographic link) • Cardiac auscultation	• History/clinical signs • Cardiac auscultation • Pulmonary auscultation • Thoracic palpation and percussion
	Laboratory	• CBC: related to underlying cause • Chemistry panel: ↑ creatine kinase, LDH, AST vary depending on organ involvement • Blood culture: bacteria • Fluid analysis: identify infectious organism • Serology, *Parvovirus*, *Bartonella* toxoplasmosis • IFA test: trypanosomiasis cruzi • Cardiac troponin ↑ • NT-proBNP ↑	• CBC: leukocytosis and anemia • Chemistry panel: ↑ globulin and ↓ albumin: <1 g/dl • Serology: FeLV, FIP, FIV, or heartworm • Fluid analysis: color, clarity, viscosity, specific gravity, total protein, nucleated cell count, neutrophils, macrophages, mesothelial cells, lymphocytes, eosinophils, or neoplastic cells
	Imaging	• Radiographs, thoracic: ↑ cardiac silhouette, or rounded heart shape pulmonary edema, ↑ pulmonary vein, ± pleural effusion • Echocardiogram: ± pericardial effusion, thickened pericardium, abnormal echogenicity of myocardium, ↓ systolic function, ± ↓ regional wall motion	• Radiographs, thoracic: ↑ cardiac size, tumor, lung lobe torsion, diaphragmatic hernia, widening of mediastinum, rounded lung • lobe edges, obscured cardiac borders and diaphragm, ascites, and pleural fissure lines • Echocardiogram: thoracic evaluation (cardiac disease, neoplasia, diaphragmatic hernia) • Contrast study: tumor, diaphragmatic hernia, and cardiac disease
	Procedures	• ECG: infectious – AV node conduction defects, QRS,T voltage abnormalities, non-specific ST segment changes, ± tachyarrhythmias • ECG: traumatic – accelerated idioventricular rhythm, VPC ventricular tachycardia. Generally appear at 24–48 hours post-trauma and dissipate over 1–2 weeks • 24 hour ambulatory ECG (Holter) monitor: to assess arrhythmic frequency and severity	• ECG: amplitudes all depressed

(*Continued*)

Table 6.7 / Myocarditis and pleural effusion (Continued)

Disease		Myocarditis	Pleural effusion
Treatment	General	• Symptomatic (Table 6.1) • Primary therapy directed at cause if possible, and relief of symptoms • Possible pericardiocentesis → pericardiocentesis if tamponade present	• Symptomatic • Fluid therapy • Thoracocentesis • Chest tube placement • Surgery: thoracotomy
	Medication	• Treat underlying condition accordingly • ACE inhibitor: benazepril, captopril, enalapril, lisinopril • Aldosterone antagonist: spironolactone • Arterial dilators: acute: hydralazine or nitroprusside (emergency) • Ca^{+} channel blocker: diltiazem, *use with caution* for arrhythmias • Diuretics: acute – furosemide; chronic – furosemide, torsemide • Inodilator: pimobendan • Phosphodiesterase inhibitors: pimobendan, sildenafil • Positive inotropes: digoxin, dobutamine, or dopamine • Sedation: acepromazine maleate, benzodiazepines, opioids • Supplements: taurine, potassium, magnesium, L-carnitine or coenzyme Q10 • Venodilators: nitroglycerin ointment	• Antibiotics: dependent on type of bacteria isolated • Analgesics: bupivacaine, non-steroidal anti-inflammatory drugs, morphine, meperidine • Diuretics: furosemide
	Nursing care	• Restrict activity • Active warming as necessary	• Monitor temperature, respiratory rate and effort, and pulse. • Nutritional support • Chest tube management
Follow-up	Patient care	• Sodium-restricted diet • Monitor ECG and auscultation • Radiograph as necessary	• Monitor radiographs.
	Prevention/avoidance	• Vaccinate • Monitor echocardiogram with patients using doxorubicin • Avoid endemic areas (e.g. Gulf Coast – Chagas)	• Not applicable
	Complications	• Chronically impaired myocardial function • Congestive heart failure • Arrhythmias, especially ventricular	• Pulmonary edema • Death
	Prognosis	• Variable-dependent on extent and causative agent of disease	• Guarded to poor

Symptomatic Bradycardia Arrhythmia

Certain arrhythmias may cause sustained bradycardia resulting in clinical symptoms. The arrhythmias of complete atrioventricular block (3AVB), high-grade second-degree AV block, sinus arrest, and atrial standstill are the most common. Complete and second-degree AV block induce bradycardia by blocking the atrial impulse from entering the ventricle, thereby stopping a ventricular contraction. Second-degree AV block does not always cause bradycardia, but may do so. Sinus arrest and atrial standstill are pathologies of the atria; where the sinoatrial node does not discharge, or the depolarization is not conduction through the atrial tissue, respectively.

Table 6.8 / Symptomatic bradycardia arrhythmia

Disease	Symptomatic bradycardia arrhythmia	
Presentation	Presenting clinical signs	• Syncope • Exercise intolerance/lethargy • Signs of CHF • Sudden death
	Exam findings	• Bradycardia • ± murmur • Findings of CHF • ± hyperkinetic pulses • ± periods of asystole during auscultation

(*Continued*)

Table 6.8 / **Symptomatic bradycardia arrhythmia (Continued)**

Disease	Symptomatic bradycardia arrhythmia	
Diagnosis	General	• History/clinical signs • Cardiac auscultation
	Laboratory	• CBC: non-specific • Chemistry panel: often non-specific, ↑ ALT, AST, ALP, BUN, creatinine and rarely potassium, ↓ sodium, protein possible • Urinalysis: screen for protein losing nephropathy
	Imaging	• Radiographs thoracic: may be normal, or ↑ cardiac size, especially LA and LV, pulmonary vein dilation, pulmonary edema or perihilar edema. Atrial dilation may be marked in cases of atrial standstill
		• Abdominal ultrasound: rule out concurrent neoplasia before pacemaker implantation
		• ECG: dependent on arrhythmia. May appear normal, except when arrhythmia present. Often ↑ LA, LV, and possible RA, systolic function generally preserved unless advance disease present, concurrent heart disease may be identified, Doppler evidence of diastolic mitral valve regurgitation with 3AVB, rule out neoplasia, atrial standstill marked atrial dilation
	Procedures	• ECG • 3AVB – P waves occurring at a rate normal of 10–20% faster than normal with ventricular escape complexes around 30–60 beats/minute, and no association of the P waves to the QRS complexes • 2AVB: may appear normal with viable numbers of blocked P waves, leading to an overall bradycardia; ventricular or APC may be noted • Sinus arrest: appears normal with periods of asystole 6–20 seconds' duration. Cessation of asystole may be by VPC, junctional escape complex or sinus complex. Asystole lead to clinical signs • Atrial standstill: no P wave activity, ventricular escapes complexes around 30–60 beats/minute, ± ↑ P duration and amplitude • Atropine response test to separate high vagal tone from pathology as a cause of arrhythmia especially 2AVB and sinus arrest • Blood pressure: hypotension

(Continued)

Table 6.8 / **Symptomatic bradycardia arrhythmia (Continued)**

Disease	Symptomatic bradycardia arrhythmia	
Treatment	General	• Symptomatic: permanent pacemaker implantation
		• Treat CHF as necessary
	Medication	• ACE inhibitor: benazepril, captopril, enalapril, lisinopril • Aldosterone-antagonist: spironolactone • Antimuscarinic/anticholinergic: atropine, propantheline • β-agonists: albuterol, isoproterenol, terbutaline • Methylxanthine: theophylline • Diuretics: furosemide • Inodilator: pimobendan • Vasodilator: nitroglycerin ointment
	Nursing care	• Care of CHF • Post-pacemaker implantation intensive care: sedation, analgesia, CHF as necessary
Follow-up	Patient care	• Monitor heart rate at home • Restrict activity for 2–4 weeks • Monitor for signs of CHF as necessary • Treat concurrent disease accordingly • Pacemaker follow-up visit 10–14 days, 3 months then every 6 months as necessary • Radiograph every 6 months, echocardiogram annually • Program/check battery in pacemaker every 6 month
	Prevention/avoidance	• No specific
	Complications	• CHF • Sudden death
	Prognosis	• Good with pacemaker therapy, guarded to poor without. Advanced cases of cardiac remodeling may be irreversible
Notes	• Patients with symptomatic bradycardia, and no concurrent disease can return to mostly normal life following the recovery period after pace-maker implantation	

ENDOCRINOLOGY

Acromegaly

Acromegaly is a rare condition caused by the overproduction of the growth hormone somatotropin or hypothalamic neoplasia in the feline patient. When acquired as an adult, it will cause overgrowth of the bone, internal organs and soft tissue causing abnormalities is the appearance of the feline patient with the complicating factor of uncontrolled diabetes mellitus.

Diabetes Insipidus

Diabetes insipidus is a disorder of water metabolism due to a deficiency of antidiuretic hormone (ADH) caused by either a lack of release of ADH or renal tubular insensitivity to ADH.

Table 6.9 / Acromegaly and Diabetes Insipidus

Disease		Acromegaly (feline)	Diabetes insipidus
Presentation	Presenting clinical signs	• Polyuria/polydipsia • Weight loss or weight gain • Polyphagia • Unkept hair/coat	• Blindness, disorientation, incontinence, nocturia, polyuria/polydipsia, seizures, weight loss • Central – head trauma, neoplasia, anatomical malformation, inflammation, parasites or acquired. • Nephrogenic – severe polyuria/polydipsia between 8 and 12 weeks of age • Considered primary or secondary and if congenital[13]
	Exam findings	• Renomegaly • Hepatomegaly • Plantigrade stance suggestive of diabetic neuropathy • Abnormal appearance of the body (large head, paws or body, prognathia inferior) • Heart murmur • Gallop sound • Neurological findings such as ataxia, behavior changes, depression, circling, stupor, seizures • Lameness	• Dehydration • Hyposthenuria (urine specific gravity of less than or equal to 1.006)

(Continued)

Table 6.9 / **Acromegaly and Diabetes Insipidus (Continued)**

Disease		Acromegaly (feline)	Diabetes insipidus
Diagnosis	General	• History/clinical signs • Insulin resistance	• Clinical signs
	Laboratory	• Increased IGF-1 (see notes) • Increased growth hormone • CBC, chemistry and urinalysis will not show abnormalities specific to acromegaly but will confirm diabetes mellitus, hyperglycemia, glucosuria	• Chemistry panel: ↑ sodium • Urinalysis: ↑ protein (v), ↓ specific gravity: < 1.010 • Modified water deprivation test: urinalysis specific gravity of < 1.025 ug/dl • ADH response test: failure to concentrate urine after exogenous ADH administration
	Imaging	• MRI of the brain to identify pituitary mass • Radiographs to identify organomegaly • Echocardiogram • Abdominal ultrasound to identify to identify comorbidities	• Nuclear imaging and CT: identify pituitary or hypothalamic lesion
	Procedures	• Radiation therapy or surgery if indicated	
Treatment	General	• Symptomatic • Supportive • Surgical excision of the pituitary mass • Radiation therapy of the pituitary gland (most common therapy)	• Symptomatic • Fluid therapy • Monitor fluid in/out every 1–2 hours
	Medication	• Somatostatin analogues (not shown to benefit)[14] • Control of concurrent medical conditions (see Table 6.)	• ADH supplement: vasopressin, pitressin tannate • Treatments can be cost prohibitive
	Nursing care	• Free access to water • Low-stress environment, implement environmental enrichment techniques for feline patients (feline pheromones, hiding, quiet, low traffic areas)	• Free access to water • Urinary catheter care if necessary • Empty urinary catheter collection system every 1–2 hours • Disinfect urinary catheter as indicated

(Continued)

Table 6.9 / Acromegaly and Diabetes Insipidus (Continued)

Disease		Acromegaly (feline)	Diabetes insipidus
Follow-up	Patient care	• Control of clinical signs at home • Good quality of life • Home glucose monitoring	• Free access to water • Keep patient clean and dry • Sodium-restricted diet
	Prevention/avoidance	• None	• Avoid circumstances that might markedly increase water loss
	Complications	• Insulin resistance • Diabetic ketoacidosis • Diabetic neuropathy • Hypovolemic shock • Death	• Primary disease
	Prognosis	• Poor to guarded if untreated • Good with surgical or radiation therapy	• Very good prognosis with lack of release of ADH • Guarded prognosis with renal insensitivity to ADH

Notes		• Causes for a false negative IGF-1
		  • The patient is in early stages of acromegaly
		  • The high end of the reference range of the test is set too high to detect early or mild cases
		  • Uncontrolled concurrent medical conditions
		  • Starvation
		  • Lack of insulin (patient may need to be treated with insulin for a longer period)
		  • Diabetes mellitus is poorly controlled
		• Causes for a false positive IGF-1
		  • Vigorous or long-term insulin therapy
		  • Improper preparation methods used by the laboratory[14]
			• Water deprivation test is contraindicated in dehydrated animals

Diabetes Mellitus

Diabetes mellitus is a chronic disorder of carbohydrate metabolism characterized by persistent, fasted hyperglycemia and glucosuria resulting from inadequate (relative or absolute) production or use of insulin. type I is insulin dependent (low to absent secretory ability), and is more common in dogs. Type II is non-insulin dependent (inadequate or delayed insulin secretion or peripheral tissue insensitivity to insulin), and is more common in cats.

Table 6.10 / Diabetes mellitus

Disease	Diabetes mellitus	
Presentation	Presenting clinical signs	• Polyuria/polydipsia, polyphagia, and weight loss • Later stages: anorexia, lethargy, oily hair coat, dorsal muscle wasting, depression, and vomiting
	Exam findings	• Hepatomegaly, cataracts (canine), plantigrade stance (feline), muscle wasting, under conditioned, dull or unkempt hair/coat
Diagnosis	General	• History/clinical signs
	Laboratory	• CBC: eosinophilia and lymphocytosis, ↑ packed cell volume/total protein, mild non-regenerative anemia, Heinz bodies • Chemistry panel: ↑ glucose (> 200 mg/dl in dogs: > 250 mg/dl in cats), cholesterol, sodium, phosphate, ALP, ALT, AST and ↓ potassium, CO_2, metabolic acidosis • Urinalysis: ↑ glucose, ± ketones, and ↓ specific gravity
	Imaging	• Radiographs, thoracic: microcardia and hypoperfusion of lungs • Radiographs, abdominal: calculi, cystitis, pancreatitis • Ultrasound: pancreatic and liver pathology. Note: imaging modality only indicated to determine any comorbidities in patient with diabetes mellitus
	Procedures	• Liver biopsy (e.g. jaundiced patients) • Central line (e.g. sampling catheter) when hospitalized and serial sampling is required
Treatment	General	• Supportive • Fluid therapy only when indicated
	Medication	• Insulin: protamine zinc insulin, neutral protamine Hagedorn, glargine, detemir, Vetsulin® (Table 6.11) • See regular insulin CRI protocol to be used with diabetic ketoacidosis patients (Table 6.12)
	Nursing care	• Free access to water • Try to mimic the same feeding and insulin administration schedule used at home • Low-stress environment, implement environmental enrichment techniques for feline patients (feline pheromones, hiding, quiet, low traffic areas)

(Continued)

Table 6.10 / **Diabetes mellitus (Continued)**

Disease	Diabetes mellitus	
Follow-up	Patient care	• Maintain a regimented feeding and medication schedule • Monitor for signs of iatrogenic hypoglycemia, polyuria/polydipsia, appetite, and body weight • Provide a consistent amount of exercise every day to prevent fluctuations in insulin requirements • Proper nutrition will help keep the patient's insulin regulated. If the patient will not eat on their own, a feeding tube should be placed • Monitor serial blood glucose (initially every few weeks and then, once regulated, every few months) • Monitoring serum fructosamine can be used as an aide but should not replace blood glucose curves when monitoring treatment protocols • Screen for predisposing disease if resistant (> 2 u/kg/dose)
	Prevention/ avoidance	• Prevent or correct obesity • Identify, correct, and properly treat any comorbidities • Eliminate any patient risk factors • Ovariohysterectomy is recommended, due to interference with progesterone • Avoid unnecessary use of corticosteroids or megestrol acetate
	Complications	• Anemia and hemoglobinemia with severe hypophosphatemia

		• Diabetic complications:
		  • Insulin resistance (feline)
		  • Somogyi effect
		  • Diabetic ketoacidosis
		  • Diabetic neuropathy (feline)
		  • Secondary infections
		  • Hypoglycemia
		  • Hypertrophic hyperosmolar syndrome
		  • Cataracts (canine)

		• Risk factors for complications include:
		  • Insulin resistance
		  • Pancreatitis
		  • Acromegaly
		  • Hyperadrenocorticism/hypoadrenocorticism
		  • Hypothyroidism/hyperthyroidism
		  • Renal disease
		  • Secondary infections
		  • Inflammation
		  • Glucocorticoid usage
		  • Obesity

	Prognosis	• 75–90% of newly diagnosed cats may go into remission with aggressive treatment of long-acting insulin and close monitoring. A long-term diabetic may have only a 30% chance of remission, with the remaining patients having permanent disease. Remission in the feline patient can take up to 6 months to 1 year to achieve. They should be normoglycemic for at least 4 weeks to be in remission • Dogs have permanent disease; insulin treatment is necessary for life • Normal life span is expected with treatment

(*Continued*)

Table 6.10 / Diabetes mellitus (Continued)

Disease	Diabetes mellitus
Notes	• The use of oral hypoglycemics in the feline patient are not proven to be effective in the feline patient[15] • Meals should coincide with the administration of insulin • Feline nutrition – high protein (> 40% metabolizable energy), low carbohydrate (< 15% metabolizable energy) and ideal body condition score will help achieve remission[16] • Canine nutrition – high fiber with complex carbohydrates to minimize post-prandial fluctuation • Feed canned or dry commercial diabetic diet • Patients scheduled for surgery: nil by mouth after 12 a.m.; give one-half of the normal dose of insulin on the morning of the surgery; monitor blood glucose levels and administer regular insulin if needed; following the surgery, maintain the patient on a 5% dextrose IV drip until food intake has resumed • Proper client education on topics such as insulin administration, nutrition, home monitoring, insulin care, and clinical signs will greatly help owners and potentially prevent complications • Uncontrolled daily management is most often the cause of patient instability Factors to consider with complications include: • Inactive insulin (expired) • Improper handling of insulin • Improper insulin dosing • Improper frequency of insulin administration

Insulin Types

Insulin availability is continuously changing. There is no predictor for which insulin will work for which patient; however, dogs are typically started on neutral protamine Hagedorn, while cats are typically started on glargine. Considering clinical signs and laboratory work, insulin type, amount, and frequency are adjusted.

Glipizide is an oral antidiabetic alternative for cats with uncomplicated diabetes mellitus. The starting dose is 2.5 mg/kg twice daily, but full effects may take four to eight weeks to be seen.

Table 6.11 / Insulin types

Type	Long acting	Intermediate acting				Short (rapid) acting
Drug	Detemir	Glargine	Protamine zinc	Porcine Insulin Zinc Suspension	Neutral protamine Hagedorn	Regular
Product	Levemir®	Lantus®	PROZINC	Vetsulin®	Humulin-N® Novolin® N	Humulin-R®, Novolin® R
Units/ml	100	100	40	40 or VetPen®	100	100
Use	Canine	Canine and feline	Feline	Canine and feline	Canine and feline	Canine and feline
Route	SQ	SQ	SQ	SQ	SQ	IV, IM, SQ (with adequate hydration)
Rate of onset	1–2 hours	1–4 hours	1–4 hours	0.5–2 hours	0.5–2 hours	IV: immediate IM/SQ: 10–30 minutes
Peak	4–10 hours	2–8 hours	4–8 hours	Canine: 1–10 hours Feline: 2–6 hours	Canine: 2–10 hours Feline: 2–8 hours	IV: 0.5–2 hours IM: 1–4 hours SQ: 1–5 hours
Duration	10–15 hours	10–16 hours	Canine: 6–28 hours Feline: 6–24 hours	Canine: 14–24 hours Feline: 8–12 hours	Canine: 6–18 hours Feline: 4–12 hours	IV: 1–4 hours IM: 3–8 hours SQ: 4–10 hours
Starting dose	Canine: 0.1 u/kg twice a day Feline: 0.25 u/kg twice a day	Canine: 0.3 u/kg twice a day Feline: 0.25 u/kg twice a day	0.25–0.5 u/kg twice a day	Canine: 0.5 u/kg once a day (twice a day if once-daily dose not regulate) Feline: 1–2 u/kg twice a day	0.5 u/kg twice a day	0.2 u/kg twice a day, subsequent dosing at 0.1–0.2 u/kg every 3–6 hours

Constant Rate Regular Insulin Infusion Protocol

Table 6.12 / Constant rate regular insulin infusion protocol

Blood glucose (mg/dl)	Insulin rate (ml/hour)	Fluid/dextrose concentration
> 400	10	0.9% sodium chloride
250–399	10	0.9% sodium chloride
200249	10	0.9% sodium chloride + 2.5% dextrose
150–199	5	0.9% sodium chloride + 2.5% dextrose
100–149	5	0.9% sodium chloride + 5% dextrose
< 100	Stop	0.9% sodium chloride + 5% dextrose
< 60	Stop	Give 1–2 ml/kg bolus of 25% dextrose, recheck blood glucose at end of bolus; continue 0.9% sodium chloride + 5% dextrose

1. Regular insulin is administered as a constant rate infusion (CRI) at a dose of 2.2 u/kg/day for the canine patient. The insulin CRI should be started after vascular volume is restored in the patient.
2. Mix the daily dose of regular insulin into a 250 ml bag of 0.9% saline. The insulin CRI must be in a separate bag of fluids. Mixing the insulin with the replacement fluids will lead to inadequate rehydration of the patient or improper glucose control.
3. Infusion rate of the Insulin CRI *must* be given with an infusion pump to ensure accuracy.
4. Once the saline/insulin solution is made, 50 ml should be run through the intravenous tubing as insulin is adsorbed to the plastic tubing to allow saturation.
5. Insulin dose is adjusted according to the above scale. Additional fluids should be piggybacked or administered in a separate catheter.
6. Blood glucose should be decreased no more than 75–100 mg/dl/hour. If the glucose is dropped too quickly it can result in cerebral edema and a coma.
7. Measure blood glucose every two hours. Increase to every 30 minutes to hourly blood glucose measurements if the blood glucose drops rapidly.
8. Dextrose should be added when the blood glucose reaches 250 mg/dl, and can be adjusted to keep the blood glucose in the range of 150–250 mg/dl.
9. Monitor electrolytes every 6–24 hours for changes in sodium, magnesium and correction of acidosis, depending on the patient's individual needs.
10. Once the patient is rehydrated, electrolytes are staying within normal ranges, ketosis has resolved and appetite returns, then maintenance insulin is initiated.

Hyperadrenocorticism

Hyperadrenocorticism is most commonly found in middle to old aged canines and is considered rare in cats. It is caused by the excessive secretion of cortisol by the adrenal glands. The excess glucocorticoid comes from excessive secretion of adrenocorticotropic hormone from a pituitary adenoma, or from an adrenocortical tumor. Excessive administration of corticosteroids can also result in iatrogenic hyperadrenocorticism, a separate syndrome.

Hyperparathyroidism

Hyperparathyroidism results from excessive secretion of the parathyroid hormone (PTH). This can be caused by an adenoma, carcinoma, or hyperplasia of the parathyroid gland.

Table 6.13 / Hyperadrenocorticism and hyperparathyroidism

Disease		Hyperadrenocorticism (canine Cushing syndrome)	Hyperparathyroidism
Presentation	Clinical signs	• Behavior changes, bilaterally symmetric alopecia, circling, dull hair coat, dyspnea, excessive panting, infertility, pendulous, distended or pot-bellied abdomen, polyphagia, polyuria/polydipsia, recurrent skin infections, seizures	• Anorexia, ataxia, constipation, depression, facial pruritis, lethargy, muscle tremors, polyuria/polydipsia, seizures, shivering, stiff gait, twitching, vomiting, weakness
	Exam findings	• Muscle and testicular atrophy, thin skin with hyperpigmentation and ↑ fragility (especially in felines), symmetrical alopecia	• Cataracts, tachycardia
Diagnosis	General	• History • Clinical signs	• Clinical signs
	Laboratory	• CBC: steroid leukogram and mild erythrocytosis • Chemistry panel: ↑ ALP, cholesterol, ALT, CO_2, glucose • Urinalysis: ↑ protein, blood, bacteria, WCC, cortisol : creatinine ratio (> 35) and ↓ specific gravity: < 1.020 • ACTH stimulation test: to diagnose type, > 20 µg/dl with endogenous HAC, blunted or no response with iatrogenic HAC • Low-dose dexamethasone suppression test: to confirm diagnosis, >1 µg/dl during 8-hour test • High-dose dexamethasone suppression test: to differentiate type, <1.5 µg/dl with pituitary-dependent HAC and > 1.5 µg/dl with adrenocortical neoplasia • Endogenous plasma ACTH concentration: to differentiate type, > 40 pg/ml with pituitary-dependent HAC and < 20 pg/ml with adrenocortical tumors	• Chemistry panel: ↑ calcium, ALT, ALP, and ↓ phosphorus • Urinalysis: ↓ specific gravity serum ionized calcium: ↑ values • Serum parathyroid hormone concentration: ↑ values
	Imaging	• Radiographs, thoracic: mineralization of bronchial walls • Radiographs, abdominal: adrenal tumors and hepatomegaly • Ultrasound: ↑ liver and adrenal glands • CT: visualization of pituitary tumors or adrenal tumor (radiographs and ultrasounds can be used but are not as accurate)	• Radiographs, skeletal: generalized osteopenia, ↑ bone resorption (alveolar bone of the jaw) and cyst-like areas in the bone • Ultrasound: visualization of the parathyroid gland, urolithiasis, and renal abnormalities • CT: enlarged parathyroid gland(s)
	Procedures	• Blood pressure	• ECG: premature ventricular complexes

(Continued)

Table 6.13 / **Hyperadrenocorticism and hyperparathyroidism (Continued)**

Disease		Hyperadrenocorticism (canine Cushing syndrome)	Hyperparathyroidism
Treatment	General	• Symptomatic • Radiation therapy: pituitary macroadenoma or microcarcinoma[17] • Surgery: removal of adrenal tumor, removal of pituitary (hypophysectomy)	• Symptomatic • Fluid therapy • Surgery: removal of the parathyroid gland adenoma with postoperative radiation therapy (patient dependent)
	Medication	• Trilostane • Mitotane	• Corticosteroids • Diuretics: furosemide • Calcium supplements: calcium, calcitriol (postoperatively for transient iatrogenic hypocalcemia)
	Nursing care	• Treated as outpatient	• Standard postoperative care
Follow-up	Patient care	• Monitor for recurrence of previous clinical signs • Perform an ACTH response test 5–10 days initiation of medication (except L-deprenyl) or after dose change then every 3–6 months once regulated • Monitor for inappetence, severe decreased water consumption, attitude change, activity, vomiting, or diarrhea relating to the medication	• Monitor serum calcium once or twice daily for 1-week postoperatively • Diet of ↑ phosphorus and ↓ calcium
	Prevention/avoidance	• Not applicable	• Not applicable
	Complications	• Thromboembolism • Congestive heart failure • Hypertension • Recurrence of clinical signs • Progression of central nervous system signs • Infection: skin and urinary • Diabetes mellitus	• Hypocalcemia (iatrogenic) • Renal failure
	Prognosis	• Good to guarded due to the number of complications associated with this disease	• Excellent with proper treatment • Poor with associated renal disease
Notes		• Easy cutaneous bruising (canine); venipuncture should be performed with extra care • Screening tests are originally performed to diagnose HAC followed by tests to differentiate between adrenocortical tumor and pituitary-dependent hyperadrenocorticism • Cortisol : creatinine ratio commonly has false positive; confirm with ACTH stimulation test • Most commonly seen in Poodles, Dachshunds, Boston Terriers, and Boxers	• This is the only condition that causes an ↑ phosphorus and ↓ calcium • Keeshond, German Shepherds, Norwegian Elkhounds, and Siamese cats

Hyperthyroidism

Hyperthyroidism is a multisystemic metabolic disorder most commonly seen in middle-aged to geriatric felines. It is caused by an excessive amount of circulating thyroid hormone. The disease causes an increased basal metabolic rate that, in turn, causes the disease's clinical signs.

Hypoadrenocorticism

Hypoadrenocorticism is a disease of the adrenal gland resulting in a deficiency of glucocorticoid or mineralocorticoid secretion from the adrenal cortex. The cause is often thought to be immune mediated or sometimes due to infection, hemorrhagic infarctions, metastatic neoplasia, trauma, and amyloidosis. It is mostly seen in young to middle-aged female dogs.

Table 6.14 / Hyperthyroidism and hypoadrenocorticism

Disease		Hyperthyroidism (feline)	Hypoadrenocorticism (Addison's disease)
Presentation	Clinical signs	• ↑ Appetite, weight loss, muscle wasting, increased vocalization, behavioral changes, diarrhea, dyspnea, excessive shedding and matting, heat intolerance, hyperexcitability, hyperventilation, panting, polyuria/polydipsia, restlessness, tachypnea, unkept hair/coat, vomiting, weakness	• Intermittent anorexia, collapse, depression, diarrhea, lethargy, melena, muscle weakness, polyuria, polyuria/polydipsia, shivering, vomiting, weight loss
	Exam findings	• Arrhythmia, enlargement of one or both thyroid glands (e.g. thyroid slip), gallop sound on cardiac auscultation, hypertension, lymphadenopathy, pallor, retinal detachment, systolic murmur, tachycardia	• Arrhythmias, dehydration, progressing to bradycardia, shock, weak pulses when patient is experiencing an Addisonian crisis (see notes)

(Continued)

Table 6.14 / **Hyperthyroidism and hypoadrenocorticism (Continued)**

Disease		Hyperthyroidism (feline)	Hypoadrenocorticism (Addison's disease)
Diagnosis	General	• History/clinical signs • Palpation of thyroid gland(s) • Cardiac exam • Renal exam	• History/clinical signs
	Laboratory	• CBC: erythrocytosis (variable), mature leukocytosis, eosinopenia, monocytosis, ↑ PCV, MCV, Heinz bodies (variable) • Chemistry panel: ↑ ALT, AST, ALP, BUN, creatinine, glucose, phosphorus, bilirubin, lactate • Basal serum total thyroid hormone concentration > 4 μg/dl	• CBC: normocytic, normochromic nonregenerative anemia, eosinophilia, lymphocytosis • Chemistry panel: ↑ ALT, AST, ALP, calcium, potassium, creatinine, BUN and ↓ phosphorus, sodium, chloride, CO_2, cholesterol, glucose • Urinalysis: ↑ ketones, glucose, ↓ specific gravity: < 1.030 • ACTH stimulation test: primary hypoadrenocorticism is < 1 μg/dl • Plasma concentration of ACTH: primary is > 500 pg/ml and 2nd-degree is < 20 pg/ml • Plasma aldosterone: ↓ value • Sodium: potassium ratio: < 27 : 1
	Imaging	• Radiographs, thoracic: cardiomegaly, pulmonary edema, valentine-shaped heart, metastasis due to thyroid carcinoma • Ultrasound, abdominal: abnormal renal findings suggestive of underlying renal disease • Echocardiography: atrial and LV dilation, hypercontractility, evidence of hypertrophic cardiomyopathy • Thyroid gland nuclear scintigraphy: diagnosis and location of abnormal tissue	• Radiographs, thoracic: hypoperfused lung fields, microcardia and narrowed posterior vena cava, hypoperfusion of caudal vena cava, or descending aorta • Radiographs, abdominal: cystic or renal calculi, cholecystitis, and pancreatitis • Ultrasound, abdominal: small adrenal glands
	Procedures	• ECG: atrial fibrillation, APC, VPC, tachycardia • Blood pressure: hypertension	• ECG: peaking of T waves, prolonged P-R waves until P wave ultimately disappears, QRS complex widens and R-R intervals become irregular
Treatment	General	• Symptomatic • Radioiodine therapy • Surgery: thyroidectomy	• Supportive • Fluid therapy (acute cases)
	Medication	• β-adrenergic blocking drugs when indicated • Antiarrhythmics: propranolol when indicated • Antithyroid: methimazole • Diet: Hills Prescription Diet™ y/d™ thyroid care	• Corticosteroids: prednisolone sodium succinate, dexamethasone, prednisone • Mineralocorticoids: desoxycorticosterone pivalate, fludrocortisones, hydrocortisone hemisuccinate, hydrocortisone phosphate • Calcium gluconate • Sodium bicarbonate
	Nursing care	• Treated as outpatient	• Monitor blood pressure, urine output, ECG, electrolytes, acid–base status (acute cases) • Treated as outpatient

(Continued)

Table 6.14 / Hyperthyroidism and hypoadrenocorticism (Continued)

Disease		Hyperthyroidism (feline)	Hypoadrenocorticism (Addison's disease)
Follow-up	Patient care	• Monitor CBC, BUN, creatinine, and serum T4 every 2–4 weeks during first 3 months of methimazole treatment to allow adjustment of medication, monitor for methimazole adverse effects and unmasking of renal disease, then every 6 months once regulated	• Monitor electrolytes weekly until stabilized
		• Thyroidectomy as treatment option: monitor serum total T4 postoperatively at 1 week, 1 month and then every 3–6 months (patient dependent). Monitor ionized calcium levels for 1-week postoperatively to monitor for iatrogenic hypoparathyroidism • I-131 as a treatment option: monitor T4 in the second week and then every 3–6 months after radioiodine therapy • Highly digestible diet with quality protein	• Monitor electrolytes, BUN, and creatinine monthly for 3–6 months, then every 3–12 months • Perform ACTH stimulation test to monitor adequacy of mineralocorticoid therapy once weekly until stabilized, then every 3–6 months
	Prevention/avoidance	• Not applicable	• Not applicable
	Complications	• Congestive heart failure • Death • Dehydration • Diarrhea • Hypothyroidism (iatrogenic) • Renal damage • Retinal detachment • Hypoparathyroidism (surgery) • Laryngeal paralysis (surgery)	• Polyuria/polydipsia from medication
	Prognosis	• Excellent with treatment • Poor with thyroid carcinoma	• Good to excellent with proper diagnosis and treatment • Poor prognosis with tumors as the cause of disease
Notes		• Clinical signs are expected to completely resolve with proper treatment • Radioiodine therapy is the gold standard of treatment to cure the disease • Renal disease may become apparent once euthyroid is established	• Most commonly seen in female dogs < 7 years old[18] • Glucocorticoids (e.g. prednisolone) need to be ↑ during times of stress such as travel, hospitalization, and surgery • Addisonian crisis (true emergency) • Clinical signs – hypovolemia, dehydration, hypotension • Bloodwork abnormalities-potassium, glucose, acid–base • Treatment – (aggressive) correct hypovolemia, correct acid–base and electrolyte derangements (dextrose, calcium gluconate, regular insulin), corticosteroids • Treatment is lifelong • Great Danes, Rottweilers, Portuguese Water Spaniel, West Highland White Terriers, Wheaten Terriers, and Standard Poodles

Hypoparathyroidism

Hypoparathyroidism is a deficiency in the secretion of the PTH. This condition is most commonly seen in dogs as naturally occurring and typically following thyroidectomy in cats.

Hypothyroidism

Hypothyroidism is the most commonly diagnosed endocrine disease in the dog. A condition that results from inadequate production and release of T4 (tetraiodothyronine); caused by either destruction of the thyroid gland or impaired secretion of thyroid-stimulating hormone by the pituitary gland.

Table 6.15 / Hypoparathyroidism and hypothyroidism

Disease		Hypoparathyroidism	Hypothyroidism (canine)
Presentation	Clinical signs	• Anorexia, ataxia, depression, diarrhea, listlessness, muscle spasms, nervousness, panting, rigid limb extension, seizures, stiff gait, tremors, twitching, vomiting, weight loss	• Abortion, anestrus, cold intolerance, exercise intolerance, infertility, lethargy, mental dullness, muscle weakness, weight gain
	Exam findings	• Cataracts, tachycardia, weak pulses	• Bradycardia, hyperpigmentation, impaired myocardial contractility, myxedema, neuropathies, pyodermas, testicular atrophy • Bilaterally symmetrical nonpruritic alopecia on ventral and lateral trunk, caudal thighs, dorsal tail, dorsal nose and ventral neck
Diagnosis	General	• Clinical signs	• Clinical signs
	Laboratory	• Chemistry panel: ↑ phosphorus and ↓ calcium • Serum parathyroid hormone concentration: ↓ value	• CBC: mild normocytic, normochromic, non-regenerative anemia • Chemistry panel: ↑ cholesterol, triglycerides, ALT, AST, ALP, creatine kinase, and ↓ calcium, sodium • Basal serum T4 levels: < 1.0 μg/dl • Serum thyroid-stimulating hormone concentration: ↑ value • Free T4 by equilibrium analysis: ↓ value
	Imaging	• Not applicable	• Ultrasound: changes in thyroid gland
	Procedures	• ECG: prolongation of QT and ST segments, deep wide T waves, and tachyarrhythmias	• Not applicable
Treatment	General	• Supportive • Fluid therapy	• Symptomatic
	Medication	• Calcium supplementation: calcium gluconate, calcium lactate, calcium carbonate • Vitamin D supplementation: vitamin D, calcitriol	• Sodium levothyroxine
	Nursing care	• Treated as outpatient	• Treated as outpatient

(Continued)

Table 6.15 / Hypoparathyroidism and hypothyroidism (Continued)

Disease		Hypoparathyroidism	Hypothyroidism (canine)
Follow-up	Patient care	• Check serum calcium weekly for 1 month, monthly for 6 months, then every 2–4 months once regulated • Diet of ↑ calcium and ↓ phosphorus	• Check serum T4 levels after 1 month of therapy followed by every 6–8 weeks for the first 6 months and then every 6–12 months as maintenance once regulated
	Prevention/avoidance	• Not applicable	• Not applicable
	Complications	• Hypercalcemia (iatrogenic) • Hypocalcemia • Renal disease	• Thyrotoxicosis from administration of high doses of L-thyroxine
	Prognosis	• Excellent with close monitoring of calcium levels	• Excellent with proper treatment • Poor if disease is due thyroid carcinoma
Notes		• Check albumin level as it is the most common cause for pseudohypocalcemia • Felines with transient hypoparathyroidism post-thyroidectomy typically regain normal function by 4–6 months • Educate clients on monitoring hypo- or hypercalcemia – Toy Poodle, Miniature Schnauzer, German Shepherd, Labrador Retriever and Scottish Terrier	• Failure of clinical signs to significantly improve within 3 months may be due to an incorrect diagnosis. • Improvement should be seen within 1–2 weeks after initiating treatment (e.g. mostly behavior and appetite) • Serum T4 levels should be checked 4–6 hours post-administration of L-thyroxine • Diagnosis and testing must be evaluated in conjunction with current medications as many alter results (e.g. non-steroidal anti-inflammatory drugs, phenobarbital, glucocorticoids, sulfonamides) • Treatment is lifelong • Golden Retriever, Doberman Pinscher, Irish Setter, Great Dane, Airedale Terrier, Old English Sheepdog, Miniature Schnauzer, Cocker Spaniel, Poodle and Boxer

GASTROINTESTINAL AND HEPATIC DISEASE

Anal Sac Disease

Anal sac disease is the most common disease of the anal area in small animals, especially dogs. It is the impaction, inflammation, infection, abscess and rupture of the anal glands (see also Skill Box 2.12, page 62).

Cholangitis and Cholangiohepatitis

Cholangitis is inflammation confined to the bile ducts; cholangiohepatitis is the inflammation of the bile ducts and adjacent hepatocytes. The inflammatory infiltrates are either suppurative, most commonly seen in younger cats, or non-suppurative, mostly seen in older cats.

Table 6.16 / Anal sac disease, cholangitis, and cholangiohepatitis

Disease		Anal sac disease	Cholangitis and cholangiohepatitis
Presentation	Clinical signs	• Behavior change, biting, chewing, discomfort in sitting, licking, malodorous, painful defecation, rubbing at perianal area, scooting, tail chasing, tenesmus	• Anorexia, depression, diarrhea, lethargy, vomiting, weight loss
	Exam findings	• Perianal discharge, swollen anal glands	• Abdominal pain, ascites, dehydration, generalized lymphadenopathy (rare), hepatomegaly (variable), pyrexia, jaundice
Diagnosis	General	• Clinical signs • Palpation of the anal glands	• History/clinical signs
	Laboratory	• Cytology, exudate/secretion: WCC and bacteria • Culture: bacteria isolation and identification	• CBC: mild nonregenerative anemia, neutrophilia with a left shift, poikilocytosis, Heinz body hemolysis • Chemistry panel: ↑ bilirubin, ammonia, cholesterol, ALT, AST, ALP, GGT, globulin; ↓ albumin, BUN • Urinalysis: ↓ bilirubin • Bile acid concentrations: ↑ values • Coagulation profile: prolonged • TLI and fPLI: ↑ values Biopsy: • Suppurative: ↑ neutrophils, intrahepatic • Non-suppurative: lymphocytic portal infiltrates • Culture, bile: bacteria isolation and identification
	Imaging	• Not applicable	• Radiographs, abdominal: hepatomegaly and cholelithiasis • Ultrasonography: cholelithiasis, cholecystitis, obstruction, pancreatic abnormalities and ↑ echogenicity of the liver
	Procedures	• Not applicable	• Cholecystocentesis • Fine-needle aspiration: liver or biliary structure • Laparoscopy: direct visualization and biopsy

(*Continued*)

Table 6.16 / **Anal sac disease, cholangitis, and cholangiohepatitis (Continued)**

	Disease	Anal sac disease	Cholangitis and cholangiohepatitis
Treatment	General	• Expression of glands • Duct cannulation, irrigation, and infusion of medication • Surgery: anal sacculectomy	• Supportive • Fluid therapy • Laparotomy to relieve obstruction
	Medication	• Antibiotics (systemic): chloramphenicol, penicillin, or aminoglycosides • Antibiotics (topical): Panalog®	• Antibiotics: ampicillin, amoxicillin cephalosporins, enrofloxacin, metronidazole, vancomycin • Corticosteroids (non-suppurative): prednisolone • Supplementation: vitamin E, water-soluble vitamins, S-adenosylmethionine, thiamine, milk thistle • Ursodeoxycholic acid: ursodiol (Actigall®) • Vitamin K1 therapy
	Nursing care	• Treated as outpatient • Standard postoperative care if surgery	• Nutritional support to prevent hepatic lipidosis
Follow-up	Patient care	• High-fiber diet • Exercise and weight control • Express anal glands every 3–14 days until material is normal	• Check liver enzymes and bilirubin every 7–14 days initially then quarterly
	Prevention/avoidance	• High-fiber diet • Routine expression	• Control inflammatory bowel disease
	Complications	• Fecal incontinence following anal sacculectomy • Rupture • Septicemia	• Death • Diabetes mellitus • Hepatic lipidosis • Pancreatitis and triad disease • Recurrence of non-suppurative forms
	Prognosis	• Excellent • Guarded to poor with fecal incontinence	• Good with early treatment of suppurative disease • Variable with non-suppurative

Notes		• Color and consistency of anal gland contents:
		  • Clear or pale yellow-brown, thin, and watery: normal
		  • Thick, pasty brown: impaction
		  • Creamy yellow or thin green: infection
		  • Yellow: inflammation
		  • Red-brown exudate: abscessed
			• Caution: drugs used must be selected with care not to further damage the liver through metabolism
			• Caution: corticosteroids should not be used in suppurative forms
			• Himalayan, Persian, and Siamese cats

Constipation and Megacolon

Constipation is a condition of prolonged fecal transit time, which contributes to increased water absorption leaving a hard, dry fecal mass. These fecal masses can cause irritation and inflammation of the intestinal mucosa and disrupt normal motility.

Megacolon is a persistent dilation of the colon along with hypomotility. Chronic constipation with unsuccessful medical treatment may lead to megacolon.

Table 6.17 / **Constipation and megacolon**

Disease		Constipation	Megacolon
Presentation	Clinical signs	• Anorexia, depression, hematochezia, mucus, tenesmus, lack of fecal output, unkempt hair/coat, vomiting, weakness	• Anorexia, depression, hematochezia, mucus, tenesmus, lack of fecal output, unkempt hair/coat, vomiting, weakness
	Exam findings	• Dehydration, distended and painful abdomen, hard and dry feces, enlarged prostate, narrowed pelvic canal, mass, stricture, foreign body material	• Dehydration, distended and painful abdomen, hard and dry feces, enlarged prostate, narrowed pelvic canal, mass, stricture, foreign body material
Diagnosis	General	• History/clinical signs • Abdominal palpation: enlarged colon with large fecal mass and a colon full of hypersegmented fecal balls • Digital rectal exam: fecal impaction and possible detection of underlying condition	• History/clinical signs • Abdominal palpation: enlarged colon with large fecal mass and a colon full of hypersegmented fecal balls • Digital rectal exam: fecal impaction and possible detection of underlying condition
	Laboratory	• CBC: stress leukogram and ↑ PCV/total protein • Chemistry panel: ↑ azotemia, calcium, ↓ chloride and potassium • T4 (felines): ↑ values	• CBC: stress leukogram and ↑ PCV/total protein • Chemistry panel: azotemia, electrolyte abnormalities (variable) • T4 (felines): ↑ values
	Imaging	• Radiographs, abdominal: enlarged colon with large fecal mass, colon full of hypersegmented fecal balls, possible detection of underlying) condition (e.g. pelvic fracture, spinal cord abnormalities, foreign body) • Contrast, barium enema contrast • Ultrasound: obstructive tumors or prostatic disease	• Radiographs, abdominal: enlarged colon with large fecal mass, possible detection of underlying) condition (e.g. pelvic fracture, spinal cord abnormalities, foreign body) • Ultrasound: obstructive tumors or prostatic disease
	Procedures	• Colonoscopy: obstructive mass, strictures, or lesions	• Colonoscopy: obstructive mass, strictures, or lesions

(Continued)

Table 6.17 / Constipation and megacolon (Continued)

Disease		Constipation	Megacolon
Treatment	General	• Supportive • Fluid therapy/rehydration • Anesthesia/analgesics required for manual evacuation of colon • Enema: avoid Fleet phosphate enema's in cats (toxic). Administer slowly, either warm water, saline, DSS, or mineral oil through a lubricated red rubber catheter • Surgery, following unsuccessful medical and dietary management: subtotal colectomy, pelvic osteotomy	• Supportive • Fluid therapy/rehydration • Anesthesia/analgesics required for manual evacuation of colon • Enema: avoid Fleet phosphate enema's in cats (oxic). Administer slowly, either warm water, saline, DSS, or mineral oil through a lubricated red rubber catheter • Surgery: subtotal/total colectomy, pelvic osteotomy

	Medication	• Antibiotics: broad-spectrum
		• Laxatives:
		  • Emollient: DSS
		  • Lubricant: mineral oil
		  • Osmotic: Miralax ®, lactulose
		• Prokinetics (avoid with obstruction): cisapride, nizatidine, neostigmine
			• Antibiotics: broad-spectrum
			• Laxatives:
			  • Emollient: DSS
			  • Lubricant: mineral oil
			  • Osmotic: Miralax, lactulose
			• Prokinetics (avoid with obstruction): cisapride, prucalopride, ranitidine, nizatidine, erythromycin

	Nursing care	• Encourage to defecate: clean litter pan or frequent walks	• Encourage to defecate: clean litter pan or frequent walks
Follow-up	Patient care	• Encourage activity and exercise after postoperative recovery • Dietary fiber • Probiotics/prebiotics • Low-residue diet	• Encourage activity and exercise after postoperative recovery • Dietary fiber • Probiotics/prebiotics • Low-residue diet
	Prevention/avoidance	• Same as above • Correction of narrowed pelvic canal (e.g. fracture repair)	• Same as above • Correction of narrowed pelvic canal (e.g. fracture repair)
	Complications	• Megacolon • Obstipation • Diarrhea with overuse of laxatives • Perforation of colon wall during manual evacuation • Peritonitis, diarrhea, or stricture formation post-surgery	• Reoccurrence • Perforation of colon wall during manual evacuation • Peritonitis, diarrhea, or stricture formation post-surgery
	Prognosis	• Fair with lifelong treatment	• Poor
Notes		• Typically seen in the transverse and descending colon • Verify adequate hydration before adding dietary fiber supplements • Diet with increased fiber content may exacerbate the condition; if so, feed a low-residue and low-fiber diet to decrease fecal amount	• Diet with increased fiber content may exacerbate the condition; if so, feed a low-residue and low-fiber diet to decrease fecal amount • Treatment is often lifelong

Diarrhea

Diarrhea can be acute or chronic (lasting longer than three to four weeks), and involves either the small bowel or the large bowel. The causes range from dietary indiscretion, toxins, drugs, intestinal parasites, infectious diseases, and systemic or metabolic disturbances.

Table 6.18 / Diarrhea

Disease		Diarrhea	
		Acute	Chronic
Presentation	Clinical signs	• Anorexia, lethargy, vomiting • Clinical signs of an underlying condition • Small-bowel diarrhea: watery, voluminous, and fetid • Large-bowel diarrhea: watery, mucoid, bloody feces with tenesmus, and ↑ sense of urgency	• Anorexia, lethargy, vomiting • Clinical signs of an underlying condition • Small-bowel diarrhea: watery, voluminous, and fetid • Large-bowel diarrhea: watery, mucoid, bloody feces with tenesmus, and ↑ sense of urgency
	Exam findings	• Abdominal pain, dehydration, ileus, pyrexia	• Abdominal pain, dehydration, ileus, pyrexia
Diagnosis	General	• History/clinical signs • Abdominal palpation: mass lesions, pain, mesenteric lymphadenopathy, thickened or fluid-distended bowel loops • Digital rectal palpation: masses, strictures, or anal diseases	• History/clinical signs • Abdominal palpation: mass lesions, pain, mesenteric lymphadenopathy, thickened or fluid-distended bowel loops • Digital rectal palpation: masses, strictures, or anal diseases
	Laboratory	• Chemistry panel: electrolyte abnormalities (variable) • Cytology, fecal: bacteria, fungi, protozoan, inflammatory cells • Culture, fecal: + *Tritrichomonas foetus* (feline) • ELISA: parvovirus, *Giardia*, rotavirus • Fecal flotation: parasites or bacteria • Fecal direct smear: cysts, larvae, and trophozoites • Folate and cobalamin: ↓↑ depending on different conditions • IFA Giardia/Cryptosporidium: positive • TLI and PLI: ↑ values (↓ with EPI)	• Dependent on suspected underlying condition (e.g. thyroid function, bile acids, urinalysis, hormonal assays, serology testing) • CBC: eosinophilia, macrocytosis, and anemia • Culture, fecal: bacteria isolation and identification • Cytology, fecal: infectious agents or inflammatory cells • Fecal flotation: parasites or bacteria • Folate and cobalamin: ↓↑ depending on different conditions • PCR, fecal: +, identifying active infections • TLI and PLI: ↑ values (↓ with EPI)
	Imaging	• Radiographs, abdominal: foreign bodies, obstruction, intussusceptions, and ileus • Contrast study: foreign body • Ultrasound, abdominal: foreign body	• Radiographs, abdominal: obstruction, mass, foreign body, organomegaly, abdominal disease • Contrast study: bowel wall thickening or irregularity, tumor, stricture, or foreign body • Ultrasound, abdominal: bowel wall thickening or irregularity, mass, foreign body, intussusception, ileus, or other disease process
	Procedures	• ± endoscopy: obtain biopsies	• Endoscopy: direct visualization and biopsy

(*Continued*)

Table 6.18 / **Diarrhea (Continued)**

Disease		Diarrhea	
		Acute	Chronic
Treatment	General	• Supportive • Fluid therapy • Surgery: laparotomy to remove obstruction	• Supportive • Fluid therapy • Surgery: laparotomy to remove obstruction or mass, or obtain full thickness biopsy
	Medication	• Antibiotics • Anthelmintics: fenbendazole and metronidazole • Local protectant: bismuth subsalicylate (canine) • Motility modifiers: opiates, loperamide, diphenoxylate • Probiotics	• Dependent on underlying condition • Anthelmintics: fenbendazole and metronidazole
	Nursing care	• Nil by mouth for at least 24 hours • Provide a clean litter box or frequent walks • Limit activity	• Provide a clean litter box or frequent walks
Follow-up	Patient care	• Recheck fecal analysis following treatment for parasites • Small, frequent meals • Bland or hypoallergenic diet	• Bland or hypoallergenic diet • Monitor fecal output: consistency, frequency, volume • Monitor body weight
	Prevention/avoidance	• Avoid indiscriminate eating (e.g. garbage, food other than high-quality diet) • Yearly fecal analysis • Vaccinate	• Avoid indiscriminate eating (e.g. garbage, food other than high-quality diet) • Yearly fecal analysis • Vaccinate
	Complications	• Intussusception	• Dehydration • Abdominal effusion with intestinal adenocarcinoma • Inflammatory bowel disease
	Prognosis	• Excellent in mild cases and with proper treatment of severe cases	• Poor with chronic diarrhea unresponsive to treatment
Notes		• Most acute diarrhea is self-limiting within 3–4 days • Do not administer bismuth subsalicylate to cats • Begin probiotics with certain medications to prevent diarrhea	

Exocrine Pancreatic Insufficiency

Exocrine pancreatic insufficiency is the insufficient secretion of digestive enzymes in the small intestines, with subsequent clinical signs of malabsorption. It can occur with the severe progressive loss of acinar tissue from atrophy, pancreatitis, or obstruction of the pancreatic duct. It is most commonly seen in middle-aged to older dogs or young German Shepherds.

Gastric Dilatation Volvulus

Gastric dilatation volvulus is the process by which the stomach becomes dilated with gas or fluid and rotates on its central axis. Gastric dilatation can also occur without torsion, but surgery is still indicated as there is an 80% recurrence rate.

Table 6.19 / Exocrine pancreatic insufficiency and gastric dilatation volvulus

Disease		Exocrine pancreatic insufficiency	Gastric dilatation volvulus (gastric torsion, bloat)
Presentation	Clinical signs	• Cachexia, coprophagia, diarrhea, dull hair/coat, excessive shedding, feces voluminous, flatulence, greasy oily hair around perineum, ↓ muscle mass, pica, ravenous appetite, unthrifty, vomiting, ↑ water intake	• Abdominal distention, belching, collapse, depression, excessive salivation, respiratory distress, retching, weakness
	Exam findings	• Borborygmus, dehydration	• ↑ Capillary refill time, cool extremities, pale mucous membrane, tachycardia, tachypnea, tympanic cranial abdomen
Diagnosis	General	• History/clinical signs	• History/clinical signs
	Laboratory	• CBC: mild lymphopenia and eosinophilia • Chemistry panel: ↑ ALT and ↓ cholesterol, lipids, polyunsaturated fatty acids • TLI assay: < 5 μg/dl (dogs) and < 31 μg/dl (feline) • TLI stimulation test: no response • Fecal elastase: < 10 μg/g • Fecal proteolytic activity: ↓ values • Oral bentiromide digestion test: minimal ↑ PABA • Folate: variable depending on different conditions • Cobalamin: ↓ value	• CBC: stress leukogram, packed cell volume/total protein (variable) • Chemistry panel: ↓ potassium, electrolyte abnormalities (v) • Urinalysis: ↑ specific gravity • Blood gas analysis: metabolic acidosis • Coagulation tests, prothrombin time, aPTT, FDP: ↑ time • Plasma lactate: < 6 mmol/l ↑ survival rate
	Imaging	• Not applicable	• Radiographs, abdominal: “double bubble” with air-filled pylorus
	Procedures	• Not applicable	• Abdominocentesis/cytology: gastric perforation and peritonitis

(Continued)

Table 6.19 / **Exocrine pancreatic insufficiency and gastric dilatation volvulus (Continued)**

Disease		Exocrine pancreatic insufficiency	Gastric dilatation volvulus (gastric torsion, bloat)
Treatment	General	• Symptomatic • Hyperglycemia treatment (severe cases)	• Symptomatic • Supportive • Fluid therapy • Oxygen therapy • Decompression with orogastric tube/trocarization/gastric lavage • Surgery: exploratory celiotomy with gastropexy
	Medication	• Antibiotics: tetracyclines, metronidazole, tylosin • H2-receptor blocker: famotidine, cimetidine, ranitidine • Pancreatic enzyme replacement (powder, fresh or frozen pancreas) added to each meal • Vitamin supplements: cobalamin, vitamin E, K1	• Alkalinizer: sodium bicarbonate • Analgesics: lidocaine, buprenorphine, hydromorphone, fentanyl • Antiarrhythmics: lidocaine, procainamide • Antibiotics: cefazolin, cefoxitin, enrofloxacin, metronidazole • Anticoagulant: heparin • Antiemetics: metoclopramide, dolasetron, ondansetron, maropitant • Corticosteroids: dexamethasone • H2 receptor: famotidine, ranitidine
	Nursing care	• Divide daily food intake into 2–3 meals • Diet should be low in fiber and highly digestible • Multivitamin, especially fat-soluble vitamins, cobalamin, and tocopherol	• Nil by mouth for 12–24 hours following surgery or as dictated by severity of disease • Fluid therapy • Oxygen therapy • Monitor: acid–base status, blood pressure, CBC, chemistry panel, central venous pressure, ECG, electrolytes, urine output
Follow-up	Patient care	• Monitor weight gain and fecal consistency • Monitor cobalamin concentrations until stable • Gradually ↓ enzyme replacement as animal returns to normal	• Gradually return to a normal diet • Restrict activity for 2 weeks postoperatively
	Prevention/avoidance	• Not applicable	• Feed smaller meals multiple times a day • Slow the rate of eating Avoid postprandial exercise
	Complications	• Small bowel bacterial overgrowth • Inadequate response to pancreatic enzyme replacement • Small intestine disease • Oral ulceration	• Gastric ulceration and peritonitis • Aspiration pneumonia • DIC • Cardiac arrhythmias
	Prognosis	• Good with dietary and enzyme management • Poor when associated with diabetes mellitus	• Guarded to grave without prompt surgical treatment • Good, patients recovering 7 days post-treatment

(*Continued*)

Table 6.19 / Exocrine pancreatic insufficiency and gastric dilatation volvulus (Continued)

Disease	Exocrine pancreatic insufficiency	Gastric dilatation volvulus (gastric torsion, bloat)
Notes	• Fecal elastase and proteolytic activity often have false positive and false negative results; results must be verified • Patients without improvements within 1 week should start antibiotics • Cobalamin must be given subcutaneously for absorption • Treatment is lifelong • German Shepherds, Rough-Coated Collies	• Feeding must begin as soon as possible to avoid enterocyte atrophy. • Clients of large- and giant-breed dogs should be aware of clinical signs • Large, deep-chested breeds: Irish Setters, Great Danes, Saint Bernards, Rottweilers, Alaskan Malamutes, Labrador Retrievers, German Shepherds

Hepatic Disease and Failure

"Hepatic failure" results from the sudden loss of over 75% of functioning hepatic mass, whereas "hepatic disease" is the accumulation of inflammatory cells in the liver over an extended period of time while maintaining adequate liver function. Causes include infectious agents, drugs, toxins, immune-mediated, traumatic injury, thermal injury, and hypoxia.

Table 6.20 / Hepatic disease and failure

Disease		Hepatic disease/failure (liver disease)
Presentation	Clinical signs	• Anorexia, circling, constipation, dementia, depression, diarrhea, disorientation, hematuria, hypersalivation, lethargy, weak, melena, nausea, polyuria/polydipsia, seizures, vomiting, weight loss, reluctant to walk due to superficial necrolytic dermatitis (hepatocutaneous syndrome) • Hepatic encephalopathy – head pressing, depression, ptyalism
	Exam findings	• Abdominal pain, ascites, ataxia, dementia, hemorrhages, hepatomegaly, pyrexia, jaundice, microhepatia, pallor, dehydration • Prolonged bleeding from venipuncture sites, epistaxis, melena on rectal exam • Neurological signs: dull mentation, blindness, obtunded, comatose, seizure activity – consistent with hepatic encephalopathy • Febrile due to infectious agents (bacteria, parasites, or viruses)

(Continued)

Table 6.20 / **Hepatic disease and failure (Continued)**

Disease		Hepatic disease/failure (liver disease)

Diagnosis	General	• Clinical signs:
		  • Vomiting, diarrhea, anorexia, lethargy, depression
		  • Acute hepatitis may have a very rapid onset
		• Abdominal palpation (abdominal pain): hepatomegaly and hepatodynia

	Laboratory	• CBC: normocytic, normochromic nonregenerative anemia, thrombocytopenia ± nucleated • WCC can be normal, increased due to inflammation/response to infection, or low if infection is overwhelming • RBC may be normal or nonregenerative (chronic disease) • Hematocrit/PCV can be normal, elevated due to dehydration, or low due to blood loss from hemorrhage (secondary to coagulations factors) • Mild thrombocytosis may be seen with chronic hemorrhage
		• Chemistry panel: ↑ ALT, AST, ALP, GGT, total bilirubin, globulin, ammonia, BUN (acute), glucose (chronic), cholesterol and ↓ albumin, BUN (chronic), glucose (acute), and cholesterol • Most consistent laboratory finding with acute hepatitis is an elevated ALT (continuing hepatocyte damage) • Elevated ALP and total bilirubin • Low BUN, ALB, cholesterol – poor function of protein synthesis, protein breakdown, and bile acid production • Hypoglycemia due to overwhelming infection/decreased hepatic function • If jaundice present, run a fasting blood ammonia level to rule out encephalopathy • If no jaundice present, run fasting and postprandial bile acids
		• Urinalysis: ↑ bilirubin, urobilinogen, ammonia, bilirubin crystals, ammonium biurate crystals and ↓ specific gravity • Isosthenuria and bilirubinuria • If bilirubin > 2 mg/dl and visible jaundice, may see bilirubin crystals on urinalysis (more significant in cats) • Coagulation profile, ACT, PTT, prothrombin time: prolonged • PTT prolonged due lack hepatic production of coagulation factors • Coagulation panel recommended prior invasive procedures • Bile acids concentrations: ↑ values (not recommended if visible icterus) • Fasting bile acids concentrations: > 30 μmol/l • Postprandial bile acids concentrations: > 30 μmol/l • Blood ammonia concentrations: ↑ values • Ammonia tolerance test: ↑ values • Cytology/biopsy liver

(*Continued*)

Table 6.20 / **Hepatic disease and failure (Continued)**

Disease		Hepatic disease/failure (liver disease)
	Imaging	• Radiographs, thoracic: metastasis to lung parenchyma • Radiographs, abdominal: ↑ or ↓ in liver size, changes in tissue characteristics and contours • Hepatomegaly may be demonstrated by extension of the liver past the caudal rib margin and with caudal deviation of the gastric axis • Microhepatica with cranial displacement of gastric axis and other abdominal organs • If patient has ascites, this can obscure the visual detail • Ultrasonography: masses, abscesses, cysts, obstructions, and lesions • Chronic hepatitis – tissue architecture loss and liver parenchyma may appear irregular and nodular • Liver capsule may lose its smooth appearance; may look undulant or "lumpy bumpy" • Gallbladder and biliary tree scanned for obstructions • Portal hypertension and ascites may be present-fluid may be hypocellular to acellular • Hemorrhage fluid will appear more cellular • Fluid can be obtained if present and submitted for a cytological analysis, protein content and cell count • "Swiss cheese" appearance to liver – hepatocutaneous syndrome

	Procedures	• Biopsy to determine the nature and severity of hepatic disease
		• Surgical exploratory vs. laparoscopic biopsies:
		  • Coagulation status must be assessed prior to biopsy
		  • Recommended samples to submit: histopathology, bacterial culture and sensitivity (liver and bile), copper quantification
		• Ultrasound biopsies are not routinely helpful due to limited amount of tissue obtained and risks of bleeding due to prolonged coagulation
		• Ultrasound-guided fine needle aspiration performed for cytological evaluation
		• Skin biopsies for hepatocutaneous syndrome
		• Considerations with anesthesia:
		  • Analgesic therapy using agents that require minimal hepatic metabolism
		  • While anesthetized, monitor blood glucose levels, blood pressure, body temperature
		  • Dextrose infusions, pressor support, and external warming may be needed
		  • Cerebral edema

Treatment	General	• Symptomatic
		• Signs typically vague and nonspecific:
		  • Polyuria/polydipsia, weight loss, vomiting, anorexia/hyporexia
		  • Neurological abnormalities – mental dullness, circling, head pressing (hepatic encephalopathy)
		• Supportive:
		  • Primary support
		  • Multidrug therapies
		• Fluid therapy:
		  • Crystalloid therapy – correction of dehydration and replacing ongoing fluid losses
		  • Colloid therapy – used for animals unable to maintain oncotic pressure due to hypoalbuminemia
		  • Plasma transfusion/cryoprecipitate – coagulation support
		  • Fluid additives – dextrose if hypoglycemic
		• Paracentesis with respiratory distress

(Continued)

Table 6.20 / **Hepatic disease and failure (Continued)**

Disease	Hepatic disease/failure (liver disease)

Medication	• Antibiotics – used in cases of bacterial hepatitis, pyoderma (HCS): penicillin, ampicillin, cephalosporins, metronidazole, aminoglycosides
	• Antiemetics: metoclopramide, ondansetron, chlorpromazine, and maropitant
	• Antioxidants: vitamin E, C, S-adenosyl-L-methionine, and N-acetylcysteine, milk thistle
	• Immunosuppressants indicated when an immune mediated hepatitis is diagnosed: azathioprine (use cautiously)
	• Colchicine – antifibrotic agent (helpful cases with hepatic fibrosis and cirrhosis) – efficacy is unknown
	• Corticosteroids: prednisolone
	• Gastrointestinal protectants: sucralfate
	• H2 blocker: famotidine, ranitidine, and cimetidine
	• Lactulose (oral/rectal) – hepatic encephalopathy
	• Liver protectants:
	  • milk thistle – antioxidant
	  • ursodeoxycholic acid – increases bile flow in cases with cholestasis
	• Osmotic diuretic: mannitol
	• Phenobarbital, diazepam, NSAIDs, acetaminophen, xylitol – toxic hepatopathy
	• Vitamin K therapy (oral/injectable) – used on animals who are coagulopathic
	• Penicillamine – chelating agent; useful in patients with severe metal (copper) accumulation
	• Zinc – induces intestinal metallothionein, which binds dietary copper to prevent its absorption. This therapy is reserved for maintenance treatment of patients completing chelator therapy or for treating asymptomatic patients. Monitor zinc levels to prevent zinc toxicity
	• Therapy beneficial for hepatocutaneous syndrome
	• Supplements:
	  • Omega-3 fatty acids (cutaneous lesions)
	  • Amino acid intravenous infusions
	• Intravenous fluid additives:
	  • B complex vitamins
	  • Potassium chloride
	  • Dextrose
	• Antioxidant agents:
	  • N-acetylcysteine
	  • S-adenosylmethionine
	  • Silymarin
	  • Vitamin E
	• Appetite stimulants
	  • Mirtazapine
	  • Cyproheptadine
	  • Entyce® (capromorelin oral solution)

(*Continued*)

Table 6.20 / Hepatic disease and failure (Continued)

Disease		Hepatic disease/failure (liver disease)

Follow-up	Nursing care	• Moderate activity restriction to aid in liver regeneration
		• Nutritional support:
		  • Animals with copper associated chronic hepatitis need to be fed a low copper diet.
		  • Protein restriction recommended for animals with hepatic encephalopathy (not advised for HCS)
		  • Feeding tubes considered for hyporexic/anorexic patients (common for hepatic lipidosis patients)
		  • Total or partial parenteral nutrition if animal does not tolerate enteral feedings
		• Monitor:
		  • Serial physical exams, appetite, abdominal pain, energy level, body weight, pulse, respiration, oxygenation parameters, mental status, blood pressure, and perfusion (pulse quality, temperature, urine output)
		  • Vigilant monitoring for signs of infection
		• Place head at 30-degree elevation if cerebral edema is suspected
		• Vitamin and mineral supplements

	Patient care	• Monitor CBC and serum biochemistry frequently depending on severity of presenting condition • Follow up biopsies at 6 and 12 months • Dietary modifications (e.g. ↓ copper)
	Prevention/avoidance	• Vaccinate against infectious agents • Screen susceptible breeds • Avoid hepatotoxic drugs and environmental toxins
	Complications	• Death • DIC and bleeding diathesis • Gastrointestinal ulceration • Liver failure and liver encephalopathy • Renal disease or failure • Sepsis
	Prognosis	• Dependent on the amount of viable liver mass left after treatment • ↑ Prognosis with determination of underlying cause

Notes		• Caution: drugs used must be selected with care to not further damage the liver through metabolism
		• Caution: avoid alkalinizing agents (e.g. lactate, sodium bicarbonate) with patients with hepatic encephalopathy
		• Toxic environmental hepatopathy:
		  • Aflatoxins (fungal toxin)
		  • Sago palm
		  • Several types of wild mushrooms

Hepatic Lipidosis

Hepatic lipidosis is seen almost exclusively in cats. It is the result of more than 50% of cells in the liver accumulating excessive triglycerides. This occurs when there is a difference in the rates of deposition and metabolism of fat. Hepatic lipidosis often occurs with prolonged anorexia and will result in death if left untreated. It occurs with severe energy (calorie) and/or protein restriction, or rapid weight loss in obese cats.

Inflammatory Bowel Disease

Inflammatory bowel disease (IBD) is a group of gastrointestinal diseases with infiltration of the mucosa and submucosa with inflammatory cells. It may involve the stomach, small and large intestines, or a combination. Lymphocytic plasmacytic is the most common type of IBD, and is found in both dogs and cats. It is a subtype of protein-losing enteropathy diseases.

Table 6.21 / Hepatic lipidosis and inflammatory bowel disease

Disease		Hepatic lipidosis (fatty liver disease)	Inflammatory bowel disease
Presentation	Clinical signs	• Constipation, depression, diarrhea, lethargy, prolonged anorexia, vomiting, weakness, weight loss	• Diarrhea, flatulence, hematochezia, intermittent vomiting, listless, mucus, poor hair/coat, steatorrhea, tenesmus, vomiting, weight loss
	Exam findings	• Dehydration, hepatomegaly, jaundice, muscle wasting, pallor	• Mesenteric lymphadenopathy, thickened bowel loops
Diagnosis	General	• History/clinical signs: obesity	• Clinical signs • Canine IBD Analysis Index
	Laboratory	• CBC: normocytic, normochromic nonregenerative anemia with poikilocytosis (if prolonged) and neutrophilia and lymphopenia (v) • Chemistry panel: ↑ALP, ALT, AST, GGT, ammonia, bilirubin, and ↓ potassium, phosphorous, albumin, BUN, and azotemia (v) • Urinalysis: ↑ lipids and bilirubin, ↓ specific gravity • Coagulation profile, ACT, PTT, prothrombin time: can be prolonged • Bile acid concentrations: ↑ values • B12 concentrations: ↓ values	• CBC: mild, nonregenerative anemia or mild leukocytosis without a left shift (feline), and neutrophilic leukocytosis with a left shift (canine) • Chemistry panel: ↑ ALT, ALP, T4 (feline), ↓ protein (canine) and albumin (feline) • Cobalamin and folate assays: ↓↑ depending on different conditions • Fecal flotation: parasites • FeLV/FIV: + results • Serum C-reactive protein: ↑ values • TLI and PLI: to rule out exocrine pancreatic insufficiency
	Imaging	• Radiographs, abdominal: hepatomegaly • Ultrasonography: hepatomegaly and hyperechoic liver	• Radiographs, abdominal: survey films to rule out other diseases • Barium contrast study: mucosal abnormalities and thickened bowel loops • Ultrasonography: measure stomach and intestinal wall thickness, mesenteric lymph node, and rule out other diseases
	Procedures	• Biopsy: hepatocellular vacuoles versus underlying disease causing • Ultrasound-guided fine-needle aspiration or Tru-Cut® biopsy • Cytology: highly vacuolated cytoplasm consistent with lipid accumulation (vacuolar hepatopathy). Pathologist will grade mild, moderate, or severe	• Endoscopy: intestinal biopsies • Hypoallergenic test diet or novel elimination diet trial

(*Continued*)

Table 6.21 / **Hepatic lipidosis and inflammatory bowel disease (Continued)**

Disease		Hepatic lipidosis (fatty liver disease)	Inflammatory bowel disease
Treatment	General	• Supportive • Fluid therapy	• Symptomatic • Fluid therapy if vomiting • Surgery: enterotomy biopsies
	Medication	• Antiemetic: metoclopramide, ondansetron, or maropitant • Antibiotics: ampicillin, amoxicillin, metronidazole • H2 blocker: famotidine • Lactulose if constipated • Vitamin K therapy • Vitamin supplementation: vitamin B12, vitamin E, phosphate, thiamine, taurine, arginine, ʟ-carnitine and L-citrulline	• 5-Aminosalicyclic drugs: sulfasalazine, olsalazine, and mesalamine • Antibiotics: metronidazole, oxytetracycline, tylosin • Antidiarrheal drugs: loperamide and diphenoxylate • Corticosteroids: prednisolone, budesonide • Chemotherapy: chlorambucil • Immunosuppression: azathioprine, cyclosporine A • Probiotics • Vitamin supplementation: folic acid, cobalamin, omega-3, vitamin B12, fat-soluble vitamins
	Nursing care	• Aggressive nutritional support via syringe (caution to prevent aspiration), nasogastric tube, esophagostomy tube or percutaneous endoscopic gastrostomy tube • Vitamin supplementation • Monitor phosphate levels every 3–6 hours until > 2 mg/dl	• Nutritional support if severely malnourished • Vitamin supplementation
Follow-up	Patient care	• Continuous feeding via tube by owners for 4–6 weeks or for 10 days post-vomiting, eating on their own, and normal biochemical values • Monitor electrolytes (potassium and phosphorus) • Monitor body weight and hydration	• Hypoallergenic dietary management • Periodic evaluations until patient stabilizes
	Prevention/avoidance	• Prevent anorexia (especially obese felines) • Monitor food intake in obese cats during times of stress or other disease processes • Weight loss should not exceed lb/month or 10% of body weight/month	• Not applicable
	Complications	• Vomiting • Tube dysfunction • Hepatic failure • Death	• Adverse drug reactions • Anemia • Malnutrition and dehydration • Protein-losing enteropathy • Small-intestinal bacterial overgrowth
	Prognosis	• Grave if left untreated • 85% of patients recover with proper treatment	• Good with continuous maintenance of remission and control of relapses • Course of disease tends to be progressive in prone breeds

(Continued)

Table 6.21 / Hepatic lipidosis and inflammatory bowel disease (Continued)

Disease	Hepatic lipidosis (fatty liver disease)	Inflammatory bowel disease
Notes	• Caution: avoid dextrose supplementation as it interferes with fat oxidation • Majority of felines are obese before this disease process starts • Vitamin K should be given IM at least 12 hours before biopsies or jugular catheter placement • Biopsy samples typically float when placed in formalin	• A hypoallergenic protein source refers to one the patient has not yet been exposed or a hydrolyzed diet. • The diet should also be void of artificial colorings, flavors, and preservatives. • Feed a novel protein source for six weeks while the gastrointestinal tract heals, then switch to another novel protein source • Basenjis, Soft-Coated Wheaten Terriers, and Shar-Peis

Megaesophagus

Megaesophagus (esophageal hypomotility) is a segmental or diffuse hypomotility and dilation of the esophagus. There are three main causes: congenital, acquired idiopathic, or secondary to another condition (e.g. myasthenia gravis, brainstem lesion, tetanus).

Table 6.22 / Megaesophagus

		Megaesophagus (esophageal hypomotility)
Presentation	Clinical signs	• Cough, dyspnea, emaciation, generalized muscle weakness or atrophy, halitosis, mucopurulent nasal discharge, regurgitation, salivation, weight loss
	Exam findings	• Pyrexia, neurological deficits, pulmonary crackles, raspy fluid sounds in the esophagus
Diagnosis	General	• History/clinical signs • Palpation of dilated esophagus
	Laboratory	• CBC: neutrophilia and left shift (variable depending in underlying condition) • Acetylcholine receptor antibody titer: screen for myasthenia gravis • Dependent on underlying condition, e.g. ACTH stimulation test, thyroid screen, lead and cholinesterase levels, edrophonium (Tensilon®) response test
	Imaging	• Radiographs, thoracic: distention of esophagus with air, fluid or food, aspiration pneumonia, tracheal displacement • Contrast study: ↓ movement and pooling of fluid
	Procedures	• Fluoroscopy: ↓ strength and coordination or peristaltic contractions • Endoscopy: dilated esophagus, foreign body, neoplasia, and esophagitis • Nuclear scintigraphy: dilated esophagus, foreign body, neoplasia, and esophagitis

(Continued)

Table 6.22 / **Megaesophagus (Continued)**

		Megaesophagus (esophageal hypomotility)
Treatment	General	• Symptomatic • Supportive
	Medication	• Antibiotics for aspiration pneumonia: variable • Antiemetics: metoclopramide • Antimucolytics: N-acetylcysteine • H2 blockers: sucralfate, ranitidine, cimetidine, and famotidine • Prokinetic agents: cisapride
	Nursing care	• Nutritional support to ensure passage of food past the dilated esophagus (trials with different food consistencies, elevate food 45–90 degrees off the floor, maintain upright position for 10–15 minutes) • ↑ Caloric density diet • Monitor thoracic radiographs with aspiration pneumonia until resolved
Follow-up	Patient care	• Offer small frequent meals with the patient in an upright position for 10–15 minutes following the meal • Monitor weight regularly
	Prevention/ avoidance	• Diligent feeding rituals will increase lifespan • Early detection of recurrent pneumonias
	Complications	• Weight loss • Aspiration pneumonia
	Prognosis	• Fair with diligent supportive care • Guarded
Notes		• Caution: take care to avoid aspiration of contrast material during contrast studies • Offer food in different consistencies to determine the least regurgitation (e.g. small meatballs, slurries to liquid gruel) • Treatment is typically lifelong

Pancreatitis

Pancreatitis is inflammation of the pancreas, which can be either acute or chronic. Unlike acute, chronic pancreatitis is often seen with morphological changes in the pancreas. It can be caused by obesity, ingestion of excessive fat, drugs (e.g. azathioprine), or multiple other disease processes.

Peritonitis

Peritonitis is a life-threatening condition that requires progressive medical management for resolution. It is an inflammatory process involving all or part of the peritoneal cavity.

Table 6.23 / **Pancreatitis and peritonitis**

Disease		Pancreatitis	Peritonitis
Presentation	Clinical signs	• Anorexia, depression, diarrhea, jaundice, panting, praying position, restlessness, tachypnea, trembling, vomiting, weakness	• Diarrhea, praying posture, reluctance to move, tachypnea, tucked-up abdomen, vomiting
	Exam findings	• Dehydration, pyrexia, cranial abdominal pain, and mass effect	• Abdominal pain, dehydration, pyrexia, shock, tachycardia
Diagnosis	General	• History/clinical signs • Abdominal palpation: enlarged and painful pancreas	• History/clinical signs • Abdominal palpation: pain or organomegaly
	Laboratory	• CBC: neutrophilia with or without a left shift, leukocytosis, thrombocytopenia, toxic neutrophils, anemia • Chemistry panel: ↑ amylase, lipase, ALP, ALT, bilirubin, BUN, creatinine, cholesterol, lipids, glucose, azotemia (acute), and ↓ albumin, calcium (variable) • PLI: ↑ value • TLI: ↑ value	• CBC: neutrophilia with or without a left shift, leukocytosis, ↑ PCV, and anemia • Chemistry panel: ↑ amylase, lipase, ALT, AST, bilirubin, azotemia, and ↓ protein, glucose, potassium, electrolyte imbalances • Chemistry, abdominal fluid: ↑ BUN, creatinine, amylase, bilirubin, ALP (dependent on underlying condition) • Cytology, abdominal: degenerate neutrophils and intracellular bacteria • ± culture: bacteria isolation and identification • Protein electrophoresis, abdominal fluid: feline infectious peritonitis
	Imaging	• Radiographs, thoracic: pulmonary edema or pleural effusion (rare) • Radiographs, abdominal: displacement of stomach and duodenum, ↑ density, ↓ contrast gastric distention, static gas pattern, thickened and corrugated walls of the duodenum • Ultrasound: irregular enlargement and abscesses of the pancreas, hyper- and hypoechoic changes, peripancreatic fluid accumulation • Contrast CT: identification and management	• Radiographs, abdominal: free fluid or air, ↓ detail, ileus, distention of loops of bowel with fluid or gas • Iodinated Contrast studies: gastrointestinal tract to locate perforation • Ultrasound: free fluid, abscesses, masses, and cause of peritonitis
	Procedures	• Central line	• Paracentesis • Abdominocentesis and diagnostic peritoneal lavage

(*Continued*)

Table 6.23 / **Pancreatitis and peritonitis (Continued)**

	Disease	Pancreatitis	Peritonitis
Treatment	General	• Symptomatic • Supportive • Fluid therapy • Surgery: laparotomy	• Supportive • Fluid therapy • Peritoneal lavage • Surgery: laparotomy, correct primary etiology, lavage and drain placement
	Medication	• Analgesics: buprenorphine, meperidine HCl and butorphanol • Antibiotics: ampicillin, penicillin, cephalosporins, trimethoprim sulfa, and enrofloxacin • Antiemetics: chlorpromazine, dolasetron, ondansetron, metoclopramide, maropitant • Corticosteroids (shock): prednisone • Glucagon • Plasma • Somatostatin • Vasopressin • Supplements: potassium	• Analgesics: variable • Antibiotics: penicillin, cephalosporins or aminoglycosides, ampicillin, enrofloxacin
	Nursing care	• Monitor hydration, body weight, PCV, total protein, BUN, and urine output • Monitor PLI to assess treatment • Nutritional support unless vomiting • Complete rest and confinement	• Standard postoperative care • Limit activity • Nutritional support, tube placement if needed
Follow-up	Patient care	• After vomiting has stopped, slowly reintroduce water followed by a gradual reintroduction of a low-fat diet	• Check CBC, chemistry profile, and urinalysis every 1–2 days even in patients who are responding • If drain placed, check fluid cytology daily
	Prevention/avoidance	• Avoid fatty foods and dietary indiscretion • Maintain optimum weight control • Avoid corticosteroid treatment	• Not applicable
	Complications	• ↓ Protein and oncotic pressure • Peritonitis • Renal failure, acute • Septic shock • Thromboembolic disease • Worsening pancreatitis	• Herniation of abdominal contents • Adhesions
	Prognosis	• Fatal without treatment • Poor with complications	• Poor even with adequate treatment

(Continued)

Table 6.23 / **Pancreatitis and peritonitis (Continued)**

Disease	Pancreatitis	Peritonitis
Notes	• Patients with recurrent pancreatitis may try a trial period of enzyme therapy	• Caution: do not use povidone-iodine solution for lavage as it may be absorbed and may produce toxic effects • Use a contrast medium with minimal abdominal effects in case of leakage (e.g. iohexol)

Protein-Losing Enteropathy

Protein-losing enteropathy is a disease of excessive loss of serum protein into the intestinal tract. It can be a primary disease of the gastrointestinal tract or the result of a generalized condition such as congestive heart failure, or metastatic neoplasia.

Vomiting

Vomiting is the forceful, reflex expulsion of gastric or proximal small bowel contents from the oral cavity. Its duration can be acute or chronic (lasting for more than 14 days).

Table 6.24 / **Protein-losing enteropathy and vomiting**

Disease		Protein-losing enteropathy	Vomiting
Presentation	Clinical signs	• Diarrhea, dyspnea	• Anorexia, depression, hypersalivation, nausea, repeated swallowing, and licking of lips • Others, depending on underlying disease
	Exam findings	• Ascites, edema, pleural effusion, thickened bowel loops	• Abdominal distention or pain
Diagnosis	General	• History/clinical signs • Abdominal palpation: thickened bowel loops	• History/clinical signs • Examination of vomitus
	Laboratory	• CBC: ± anemia, ± lymphopenia • Chemistry panel: ↓ albumin, globulin, calcium and cholesterol • Urinalysis: protein: creatinine ratio • Fecal α1-proteinase inhibitor concentration: ↑ values • Fecal examinations: rule out parasites and bacterial overgrowth • TLI and folate: results dependent on disease process • Cobalamin: ↓ values • Serum bile acids: assess hepatic function • T4: ↑ values (felines)	• Dependent on underlying condition • CBC: ↑ PCV, total protein
	Imaging	• Radiographs, thoracic: rule out cardiac disease or fungal disease • Radiographs, abdominal: rule out fungal disease, tumors or intestinal obstruction • Contrast: tumor or bowel disease • Echocardiogram: thoracic abnormalities or tumors • Ultrasound: abdominal abnormalities or tumors	• Radiographs, thoracic: heartworm disease • Radiographs, abdominal: foreign body, pancreatitis, or pyometra • Contrast: foreign body • Ultrasound: abdominal abnormalities or tumors
	Procedures	• Endoscopy: mucosal visualization and biopsy • Hypoallergenic test diet or novel elimination diet trial	• Endoscopy: stomach and proximal duodenal abnormalities

(*Continued*)

Table 6.24 / Protein-losing enteropathy and vomiting (Continued)

Disease		Protein-losing enteropathy	Vomiting
Treatment	General	• Symptomatic • Supportive • Blood or hetastarch transfusions • Abdominocentesis or pleurocentesis • Surgery: laparotomy for diagnostic full thickness biopsies	• Symptomatic • Fluid therapy • Surgery: exploratory laparotomy
	Medication	• Antibiotics: metronidazole, tylosin or sulfasalazine • Anticoagulant: aspirin, clopidogrel • Chemotherapy: chlorambucil • Corticosteroids: prednisone • Diuretics: furosemide • Immunosuppressant: azathioprine, cyclosporine	• Dependent on underlying condition • Antiemetic: metoclopramide, diphenhydramine, prochlorperazine, chlorpromazine, maropitant • Antisecretory: cimetidine, famotidine, ranitidine omeprazole • Gastrointestinal protectants: sucralfate
	Nursing care	• Treated as outpatient • Standard postoperative care	• Nil by mouth
Follow-up	Patient care	• Dietary modifications depending on underlying cause • Recheck body weight, CBC, liver enzymes, and protein concentrations every 7–14 days. • Monitor for recurrence of clinical signs	• After vomiting has stopped for 12–24 hours, slowly reintroduce water, followed by a gradual reintroduction of an easily digestible diet • Wean back to regular diet over 4–5 days.
	Prevention/avoidance	• Control inflammatory bowel disease.	• Avoid dietary indiscretion, table scraps, high-fat treats
	Complications	• Diarrhea, severe • Malnutrition, severe • Respiratory difficulty • Slow wound healing	• Dehydration • Electrolyte imbalances • Aspiration pneumonia
	Prognosis	• Guarded	• Excellent in mild cases and with proper treatment of severe cases

Notes		• ↑ Risk of morbidity postoperatively due to slow wound healing because of ↓ albumin; serosal patch graft may be necessary; respiratory difficulty
		• Treatment is based on underlying conditions and is often lifelong
			• Types of vomiting:
			  • Undigested or partially digested food > 12–16 hours: delayed gastric emptying
			  • Projectile vomiting: gastric or upper small bowel obstruction
			  • Praying mantis position: gastrointestinal pain
			• Physical appearance of vomit:
			  • Bile: gastroduodenal reflux
			  • Fresh blood: recent bleeding in proximal gastrointestinal tract
			  • Digested blood: ulcer disease
			  • Mucus: concurrent irritation of stomach and intestines

HEMATOLOGIC AND IMMUNOLOGIC DISORDERS

Anemia

Anemia is a decreased number of necessary red blood cells and is a primary bone marrow dysfunction. It is characterized by adequate or inadequate reticulocytosis. Anemia is caused by loss of red blood cells, hemolysis, or depression of production. It is divided into two types: regenerative (loss and hemolysis) and nonregenerative (depression of production). Regenerative anemia can be primary or secondary immune-mediated hemolytic anemia.[19,20]

Table 6.25 / Anemia

Disease		Anemia: Nonregenerative	Anemia: Regenerative
Presentation	Clinical signs	• Anorexia, collapse, depression, dyspnea, exercise intolerance, melena, tachypnea, weakness	
Presentation	Exam findings	• Ectoparasite infestation, icterus, lymphadenopathy, pallor, petechiae, pyrexia, retinal hemorrhages, soft systolic murmur, splenomegaly, tachycardia, gallop rhythm	
Diagnosis	General	• History/clinical signs	
Diagnosis	Laboratory	• CBC: ↑ MCV, ↓ PCV, MCHC, total protein, leukopenia, thrombocytopenia, alterations based on underlying condition • Chemistry panel: dependent on underlying condition (e.g. kidney or liver disease) • Urinalysis: ↑ blood, ± bilirubin • Coagulation testing: alterations (variable) • Fecal analysis: hookworms,[21] whipworms,[22] lungworms,[23,24] coccidia[25] • Fecal occult blood • testing + • Coombs' test and ANA serology: + results • Cytology, bone marrow: erythroid hypoplasia • ELISA: FeLV/FIV/*Dirofilaria* • Serology: *Ehrlichia*,[26] Anaplasma,[27] *Babesia*,[28] *Bartonella*,[29] *Borrelia*[30] • PCR: Mycoplasma hemofelis (cats)[31] • DNA testing: PK/PFK deficiency[32–34] • Iron/ferritin/transferrin: ↓ values[35] • Reticulocyte count: < 500 000/μl (feline) and <60 000/μl (canine)[19]	• CBC: ↑ ± MCHC, ↓ PCV, ± MCV, total protein, reticulocytosis, neutrophilia, thrombocytosis, nucleated RBC, basophilic stippling, spherocytes (canine, IMHA), RBC ghost cells[36,37] • Chemistry panel: ↑ hepatic enzymes • Coagulation testing: alterations (variable) • Cytology, bone marrow: erythroid hyperplasia • Coombs' test and ANA serology: + results • Direct immunofluorescence: + antibodies (IMHA) • Fecal analysis: hookworms,[21] whipworms,[22] lungworms,[23,24] coccidia[25] • DNA testing: PK/PFK deficiency[32–34] • Reticulocyte, corrected: > 1%[38,39] • Reticulocyte count: > 500 000/μl (feline) and > 60 000/μl (canine)[19] • Slide agglutination test: positive results indicate anemia is immune mediated • Rapid osmotic fragility testing: + (IMHA)[20,40]
Diagnosis	Imaging	• Radiographs, abdominal: splenomegaly/neoplasia • ECG: abnormal ST segment in *Ehrlichia* and *Babesia*[41] • Echocardiogram: heart alterations[42,43]	• Radiographs, thoracic: fluid • Radiographs, abdominal: fluid/metallic foreign body (i.e. zinc coin)[38] • Echocardiogram: heart alterations[42,43]
Diagnosis	Procedures	• Bone marrow biopsy: RBC hyperplasia (regenerative), architecture and cellularity • Abdominocentesis (if fluid wave): effusion • Blood pressure measurement: hypotension (variable)	

(Continued)

Table 6.25 / Anemia (Continued)

Disease		Anemia	
		Nonregenerative	Regenerative
Treatment	General	• Supportive • Blood transfusions • Auto-transfusions if redeemable blood loss • Fluid therapy • Oxygen therapy if SpO_2 < 95% or PaO_2 < 80 mmHg	• Supportive • Blood transfusions • Auto-transfusions if redeemable blood loss • Fluid therapy • Oxygen therapy if SpO_2 < 95% or PaO_2 < 80 mmHg
	Medication	• Corticosteroids:[19,44,45] prednisone, prednisolone, dexamethasone • Immunosuppressants:[19,44,45] cyclosporine, mycophenolate, azathioprine • Erythropoietic agent:[19,44,45] erythropoietin, darbepoetin • Supplements:[44,45] iron dextran or ferrous sulfate • Antiparasitics • Antibiotics (for ectoparasite-borne infections) • Anticoagulant: low-molecular-weight/unfractionated sodium heparin (inconclusive)[46–48]	• Antibiotics: tetracyclines • Corticosteroids:[20,38,39] prednisone, prednisolone, dexamethasone • Immunosuppressant:[20,38,39] mycophenolate, azathioprine, leflunomide azathioprine, chlorambucil • Supplements:[20,38,39] iron dextran or ferrous sulfate • Antiparasitics • Anticoagulant: low-molecular-weight/unfractionated sodium heparin (inconclusive)[46–48]
	Nursing care	• Monitor for adverse reactions to drugs and transfusions • Measure PCV/total protein every 8–12 hours initially, during a relapse, or if blood loss • During acute event, monitor mentation, respiratory rate, heart rate, pulses, capillary refill time, mucous membranes, and respiratory effort at frequent intervals • Provide heat support necessary • Restrict activity • Score body condition and provide nutritional support	

(*Continued*)

Table 6.25 / Anemia (Continued)

Disease		Anemia	
		Nonregenerative	Regenerative
Follow-up	Patient care	• If stable blood loss/hemolytic/IMHA anemia, measure PCV/total protein/CBC every 12–24 hours, then every 1–4 weeks until stable[39,44,45] • If pure red-cell aplasia, measure PCV/CBC every 3–4 days, then weekly until normal[38] • Perform CBC for any anemia monthly once regulated or when tapering meds[38,39,44,45] • Measure blood pressure (before venipuncture) at same time as CBC rechecks • Dogs receiving azathioprine should have hepatic values checked during the first four weeks of therapy[49]	
	Prevention/ avoidance	• Monitor CBCs of patients receiving chemotherapeutic agents[50]	
	Complications	• Transfusion reactions • Erythropoietin carries greater risk of pure red cell aplasia than darbepoetin[51–53] • Hemorrhage • Sepsis • Long-term immunosuppression increases risk of infections • Hyperadrenocorticism[54]	• Transfusion reactions • Cardiac arrhythmias • DIC • Embolisms • Hypoxia • Long-term immunosuppression increases risk of infections • Hyperadrenocorticism[54]
	Prognosis	• Guarded to poor unless underlying disease can be diagnosed and treated[44,45,55] • Recovery may take weeks to months.	• Poor to good prognosis with appropriate treatment • Guarded to poor prognosis with IMHA[56,57]
Notes		• Lack of regeneration does not eliminate IMHA; 30% of dogs have non-regenerative anemia upon presentation[39] • Evaluate blood smear before transfusions, as spherocytes can appear after transfusions	• IMHA: Cocker Spaniel, Shih Tzu, Lab, Irish Setter, English Springer Spaniel, Maltese, Poodle, Jack Russell Terrier, Dachshund, Beagle[39] • Microcytosis can occur in Shiba Inus and Akitas; do not confuse with spherocytes[58,59] • Evaluate blood smear before transfusions, as spherocytes can appear after transfusions

Disseminated Intravascular Coagulation

Disseminated intravascular coagulation is an exaggerated activation of normal hemostatic processes. It is never a primary condition. Fibrin is deposited, disrupting microvasculature and blood flow to vital organs. Risk factors are inflammation, infection, hypotension, neoplasia, and trauma.[60,61]

Table 6.26 / Disseminated intravascular coagulation

Disease		Disseminated Intravascular Coagulation (DIC)
Presentation	Clinical signs	• Clinical signs of underlying disease • Dyspnea, melena, petechiae, collapse, spontaneous hemorrhage from orifices (dogs more than cats)[46,62]
	Exam findings	• Pyrexia, subcutaneous hematoma and petechiae, ecchymosis, tachycardia, bradycardia (cats)[62]
Diagnosis	General	• History/clinical signs
	Laboratory	• CBC: stress or inflammatory leukogram, thrombocytopenia, schistocytes, keratocytes, acanthocytes, ↓ platelet count, fibrinogen levels, and presence of fibrin degradation products • Chemistry panel: ↑ renal and hepatic values, ↑ lactate[46,60,61,63] • Blood gas: abnormalities • Urinalysis: hematuria • FDP and D-dimers assay: + • Coagulation tests, prothrombin time, PTT, ACT: ↑ times • Adrenocortical tumor: ↓ (dogs) • Protein culture and sensitivity ↓ • Viscoelastic testing: determine stage of condition[64,65]
	Imaging	• Radiographs, thoracic/abdominal: underlying disease/thromboembolism/hemorrhage
	Procedures	• Scoring system designed (dogs): predict mortality/diagnose occult/chronic condition[63,66] • Blood pressure measurement: hypotension (variable)
Treatment	General	• Treat primary condition • Symptomatic • Aggressive fluid therapy • Blood transfusions • Oxygen therapy if $SpO_2 < 95\%$ or $PaO_2 < 80$ mmHg
	Medication	• Antibiotics (sepsis) • Anticoagulant: low molecular weight/unfractionated sodium heparin (inconclusive)[46–48,67] • Cryoprecipitate
	Nursing care	• Monitor CBC and coagulation panels daily until improvement is seen • Avoid intramuscular injections and neck leads • Strict confinement • Feed soft foods • Use peripheral blood vessels for blood draws and catheter placement

(*Continued*)

Table 6.26 / Disseminated intravascular coagulation (Continued)

Disease		Disseminated Intravascular Coagulation (DIC)
Follow-up	Patient care	• Monitor blood pressure • Monitor urine output (indicative of organ function)
	Prevention/avoidance	• Do not use heparin, hetastarch, and dextrans if severe thrombocytopenia or if coagulation times are prolonged[61] • Do not use jugular vessels • Avoid corticosteroids as they may inhibit fibrinolysis and encourage thrombosis[39,68]
	Complications	• Pulmonary thromboembolism • Thromboembolism • Hemorrhage
	Prognosis	• Depends on underlying condition[66] • Poor to grave in fulminant and hemorrhagic cases[46]
Notes		• Venipuncture sites can lead to excessive hematomas; place pressure wraps following procedure • Pay close attention to patients with DIC risk factors

Thrombocytopenia

Thrombocytopenia is a deficiency of circulating platelets. Primary immune-mediated thrombocytopenia is one of the most common types.[69] It destroys platelets with no cause. Secondary causes include drug therapy, infection, neoplasia and hereditary. The condition may occur as a single entity or with a combination of other immune-mediated diseases.[70,71]

Table 6.27 / **Thrombocytopenia**

Disease		Thrombocytopenia
Presentation	Clinical signs	• Anorexia, dyspnea, retinal and mucosal hemorrhages, epistaxis, hematochezia, melena, lethargy, obtundation, seizures, vomiting, weakness
	Exam findings	• Murmur, pallor, petechiae, ecchymosis, pyrexia, tachycardia
Diagnosis	General	• History/clinical signs • Patient response to treatment
	Laboratory	• CBC: thrombocytopenia < 50 000/µl, microthrombocytosis, neutrophilia or neutropenia, schistocytes, autoagglutination, anemia[70,71] • Chemistry panel: ↑ BUN, mild ↑ ALT and ALP (variable) and ↓ protein[70,71] • Urinalysis: ↑ protein and blood (rare) • Platelet count: thrombocytopenia, ↑ shift platelets, immature platelets • Cytology: bone marrow: ↑ or ↓ megakaryocytes[70,71] • Platelet-surface associated IgG (sensitive but not specific): +IMT[70] • Serology: Ehrlichia,[26] Rickettsia rickettsii,[72] Anaplasma,[27] and Leptospira[73] • Screening: FeLV/FIV • ANA titer: + results (variable) • Coagulation profiles: normal to ↓[70,71]
	Imaging	• Radiographs, thoracic: neoplasia • Radiographs, abdominal: neoplasia/splenomegaly
	Procedures	• Blood pressure measurement: hypotension (variable)
Treatment	General	• Supportive • Fluid therapy • Blood transfusion • Surgery: splenectomy
	Medication	• Corticosteroids: prednisone, prednisolone, dexamethasone • Immunosuppressants: vincristine, azathioprine, danazol, cyclosporine, mycophenolate mofetil, leflunomide • Human immunoglobulin
	Nursing care	• Strict confinement • Use peripheral blood vessels for blood draws and catheter placement • Feed liquid or soft food to limit damage to gingival surfaces

(Continued)

Table 6.27 / **Thrombocytopenia (Continued)**

Disease		Thrombocytopenia
Follow-up	Patient care	• Strict confinement until normal platelet counts return • Ensure patient avoids self-trauma • Score body condition and monitor for obesity[71] • Monitor platelet counts every 48 hours initially, then periodically following recovery[70,71]
	Prevention/avoidance	• Avoid cyclophosphamide for treatment as hemorrhagic cystitis can be fatal[71] • Avoid unnecessary vaccinations • Minimize stress • Avoid medications that are suspected of having caused initial IMT • Monitor CBC of patients receiving chemotherapeutic agents
	Complications	• Long-term immunosuppression increases risk of infections • Gastrointestinal ulceration • CNS hemorrhage • Hemorrhagic shock
	Prognosis	• Good once response to treatment is known; affected animals with melena or ↑ BUN associated with poorer outcome[74,75]
Notes		• Spontaneous bleeding can occur at thrombocytes <30 000/ul[70] • Avoid intramuscular injections, jugular venipuncture, and cystocentesis • Apply extended pressure followed by a pressure wrap after venous access • The shortest duration of treatment is 4–6 months[75] • This condition can coexist with IMHA (Evans syndrome) • IMT: Cocker Spaniels, Poodles, German Shepherds, and Old English Sheepdogs[71] • Inherited macrothrombocytopenia – benign: Cavalier King Charles Spaniels

Innate and Adaptive Immune System Dysregulation

The immune system identifies entities that are non-self and mounts a response against them. It does that via the innate and adaptive immune systems. Each system has two modes of supporting their functions: humoral and cellular immunity. Both systems work to maintain immune homeostasis. If either system dysregulates, or if inflammation is chronic, pathological immune conditions ensue. Although the innate and adaptive immunity perform very different tasks, they intersect and are not mutually exclusive.[76–78]

Table 6.28 / **Innate and Adaptive Immune System Dysregulation**[76–78]

Response	Innate	Adaptive
Type of defense	• Generic	• Specialized
Speed	• Fast (minutes to hours)	• Slow (days to weeks)
Recall	• No memory	• After exposure has memory
Humoral immunity players	• Complement system • Natural antibodies • Acute-phase proteins • Antimicrobial peptides • Soluble lectins	• Complement system • Immunoglobulins
Cellular immunity players	• Neutrophils • Macrophages • Mast cells • Lymphoid cells • Basophils • Eosinophils	• Dendritic cells • T lymphocytes • B lymphocytes
Effectiveness	• Does not improve	• Improves with exposure

Anaphylaxis

Anaphylaxis is an acute allergic reaction that occurs after exposure to inciting antigens (drug, vaccine, venom, and in rare cases, food). It is the product of widespread release of mast cell mediators, including histamine.[79,80]

Table 6.29 / **Anaphylaxis**

Disease		Anaphylaxis
Presentation	Clinical signs	• Severe pruritus, vomiting, diarrhea, defecation, hypersalivation, respiratory distress, depressed/excited, collapse
	Exam findings	• Hypotension, bronchospasm, urticaria, erythema, pharyngeal and laryngeal edema, dyspnea (usually cats)[61,79,80] tachycardia, pale mucous membranes, poor capillary refill time, coma, death

(Continued)

Table 6.29 / **Anaphylaxis (Continued)**

Disease		Anaphylaxis
Diagnosis	General	• History/clinical signs
	Laboratory	• CBC: usually unremarkable • Chemistry panel: ↑ ALT (dogs)[81] • Coagulation factors: abnormal (variable)
	Imaging	• Radiographs, thoracic: pulmonary disease if respiratory/cardiac signs[80] • Ultrasound, abdominal: thickened, striated gallbladder (dogs)[81]
	Procedures	• Blood pressure: hypotension
Treatment	General	• Establish patent airway: intubation/tracheostomy • Oxygen therapy if $SpO_2 < 95\%$ or $PaO_2 < 80$ mmHg • Obtain vascular access • Fluid therapy for hemodynamic support • Fresh frozen plasma: if coagulopathy

	Medication	• Acute/severe:
		  • Epinephrine: treat hypotension, bronchoconstriction and block mediators
		  • Aminophylline: for bronchospasm not responsive to epinephrine
		  • Vasopressor: dopamine or vasopressin for hypotension
		• Chronic/mild:
		  • Glucocorticoids: dexamethasone, prednisone
		  • Antihistamine: diphenhydramine, famotidine

	Nursing care	• If recumbent, encourage sternal recumbency to reduce risk of atelectasis and aspiration pneumonia
Follow-up	Patient care	• Severe cases require serial assessment of temperature, heart rate, respiratory rate and effort, blood pressure, capillary refill time, mucous membrane color
	Prevention/avoidance	• Give IV medications slowly to reduce anaphylaxis incidence • Pretreat patients with a history of vaccine reactions with antihistamines and/or glucocorticoids • If affected animal has a severe reaction, do not revaccinate • Epinephrine and aminophylline can cause arrhythmias when used together[80,82] • Epinephrine and aminophylline should not be administered in the same IV line, as they are incompatible[82]
	Complications	• Cardiac arrhythmia • Organ failure
	Prognosis	• Affected patients can die in 1 hour if left untreated or severe • Antigens administered parenterally have most severe clinical signs and poorer outcome[83]
Notes		• If sudden and unexplained cardiovascular and respiratory collapse, anaphylaxis should be considered[80] • In anaphylaxis, the target shock organs for dogs are the liver and gallbladder. In cats the target shock organ is the respiratory tract. Clinical signs will correlate with these target organs[83,84] • Urticaria: Boxers and Pitbulls more commonly affected[80]

Systemic Lupus Erythematosus

Systemic lupus erythematosus (SLE) is a multisystemic disease that affects two or more organ systems. Diagnosis is not based on a single test, but rather is established on two separate expressions of autoimmunity with a positive antinuclear antibody titer, or three expressions of autoimmunity without a positive antinuclear antibody titer.[85–87]

Table 6.30 / Systemic lupus erythematosus

Disease		Systemic lupus erythematosus
Presentation	Clinical signs	• Lethargy, reluctance to walk, inappetence, erythema, hair loss, skin scaling and crusting, depigmentation
	Exam findings	• Lameness, swollen/painful joints (particularly carpi, tarsi, elbows and stifles), pyrexia, lymphadenopathy, splenomegaly, cutaneous lesions, especially at mucocutaneous junction or skin exposed to ultraviolet light, mucosal ulcers
Diagnosis	General	• History/clinical signs • Symptoms frequently wax and wane
	Laboratory	• CBC: possible anemia, leukocytosis, or leukopenia • Chemistry panel: depends on site of inflammation • Urinalysis: ↑ protein • Urine protein/creatinine ratio: abnormal (variable) • Urine culture and sensitivity: + • Serum ANA titer: +[86–88] • Lupus erythematosus cell test (↑ false negatives): +[87,89] • Tickborne disease titer/FeLV/FIV (screening): + (variable)
	Imaging	• Radiographs, nonerosive joint swelling; pleural or pericardial effusion
	Procedures	• Arthrocentesis: neutrophilic inflammation[85,87] • Skin biopsies: inflammatory infiltrates • Immunoperoxidase and immunofluorescent staining of skin biopsies: immunoglobulin and complement deposits[90] • Renal histopathology: histological changes[85,86]
Treatment	General	• Avoid sunlight/use topical sunscreen if photosensitization occurs[85] • Rest and restrict activity if painful • Use a modified, high-quality protein diet
	Medication	• Glucocorticoids: prednisone, prednisolone • Immunosuppressants: mycophenolate mofetil, chlorambucil (cats)[85] • Enalapril if proteinuria • Supplements (especially if proteinuria): omega 3[85,86,91]
	Nursing care	• Measure and document pain score regularly

(*Continued*)

Table 6.30 / Systemic lupus erythematosus (Continued)		
Disease		**Systemic lupus erythematosus**
Follow-up	Patient care	• Monitor adverse effects of mycophenolate mofetil, as the drug can cause diarrhea[92] • Monitor blood pressure in proteinuric patients • Score all patients for body condition; implement weight gain/loss plan if necessary
	Prevention/avoidance	• Patients can be painful, so be cognizant when handling • Avoid stress to decrease symptom reoccurrence
	Complications	• Long-term immunosuppression increases risk of infections • Progressive kidney disease • Monitor CBC of patients receiving chemotherapeutic agents
	Prognosis	• No documented studies; anecdotally outcome is good[84,85] • If progressive kidney disease, prognosis is guarded[93]
Notes		• Clients should be reminded that symptoms can wax and wane; aggressive treatment not always necessary, as clinical signs are unpredictable • German Shepherds may be at increased risk[86]

Immune-Mediated Polyarthritis

Immune-mediated polyarthritis (IMPA) is the neutrophilic inflammation of two or more joints. This condition can be primary or secondary to an immunogenic stimulus (reactive). Primary IMPA is divided into non-erosive (SLE, breed-associated and idiopathic) or erosive (breed-associated or idiopathic). Polyarthropathy that develops secondary to drugs and vaccination is caused by the synovial deposition of immune complexes.[94,95]

Table 6.31 / **Immune-mediated polyarthritis**

Disease		Immune-mediated polyarthritis
Presentation	Clinical signs	• Inappetence, difficulty walking, weakness, inability to rise, stiffness, lameness, lethargy, weight loss, vomiting and diarrhea
	Exam findings	• Symmetrical joint swelling, pyrexia, peripheral lymphadenopathy
Diagnosis	General	• History/clinical signs
	Laboratory	• Complete blood count: anemia, leukocytosis • Chemistry panel: to assess organ function • Urinalysis: ↑ protein • Culture and sensitivity (synovial joint fluid): + • Echocardiogram: bacterial endocarditis • Serum antinuclear antibody titer: + (variable) • Rheumatoid factor titers: ↑ • Tickborne disease titer (screening): +
	Imaging	• Radiographs, extremities: distinguish erosive from non-erosive (erosive: subchondral bone destruction may not be visible right away;[96] non-erosive: no bony abnormalities) • Ultrasound, abdominal/thoracic: infection, neoplasia and gastrointestinal disease
	Procedures	• Arthrocentesis: of at least four joints,[94] especially tarsi and carpi: loses viscosity and strand formation and > 10% neutrophils[95] • Cerebrospinal fluid tap: meningitis (variable)
Treatment	General	• Avoid weight gain • Rest and restrict activity if painful • Treat obesity • If septic arthritis, perform joint lavage and drainage[95] • Arthrodesis for severe erosive cases[96,97]
	Medication	• Depends on etiology • Glucocorticoids: prednisone, prednisolone • Immunosuppressants: azathioprine (dogs), cyclophosphamide, gold salts, methotrexate, leflunomide[95] • Analgesics: non-steroidal anti-inflammatories for Shar Pei fever[95] • Supplements: omega 3,methylsulfonylmethane,vitamin E, selenium if Shar-Pei fever[95] • Antibiotics: if septic arthritis or secondary cause • Analgesics: gabapentin, tramadol, amantadine[94]
	Nursing care	• Measure and document pain score at regular intervals • Passive range of motion exercises if tolerable/non-infectious[98] • Class IV laser therapy, massage, and cold/heat therapy[99–102]

(*Continued*)

Table 6.31 / Immune-mediated polyarthritis (Continued)

Disease		Immune-mediated polyarthritis
Follow-up	Patient care	• Do regular CBC for patients receiving cyclophosphamide and azathioprine[50] • Dogs receiving azathioprine should have liver values checked during the first four weeks of therapy[49]
	Prevention/avoidance	• Patients can be painful, so be cognizant when handling • Avoid stress to decrease symptom reoccurrence
	Complications	• Long-term immunosuppression increases risk of infections • Hyperadrenocorticism[54]
	Prognosis	• Good to guarded for non-erosive types[94,95] • Guarded for erosive types • Most patients encounter joint deterioration eventually[97,103]
Notes		• Owners usually describe cats as lethargic; lameness can be missed unless cats are witnessed walking[95] • Relapses are possible, even with treatment • Mainly affects young animals[95]

Pemphigus Complex

Pemphigus complex is a collection of autoimmune skin diseases. Cats and dogs with this disease make autoantibodies against intracellular adhesive proteins located between keratinocytes. The loss of protein leads to the formation of vesicles within the skin. Currently, subsets are grouped based on the severity of vesicles. Superficial (pemphigus foliaceus, immunoglobulin A pemphigus) and deep (pemphigus vulgaris, pemphigus vegetans and paraneoplastic pemphigus) are accepted subsets.[103–105] In the future, these groups may be categorized based on the action of autoantibodies.[106]

Table 6.32 / **Pemphigus complex**

Disease		Pemphigus complex
Presentation	Clinical signs	• Crusting, scaling, and pustules on skin, footpads, nailbeds (often bilaterally symmetrical), hair loss, lameness if affected area is on extremity
	Exam findings	• Pyrexia, lymphadenopathy, pruritus, anorexia, limb edema, oral ulceration, hypersalivation, halitosis and weight loss if mouth is affected
Diagnosis	General	• History/clinical signs
	Laboratory	• Complete blood count: mild non regenerative anemia, leukocytosis • Chemistry panel: hypoalbuminemia • Skin scraping (ectoparasites): exclude • Culture and sensitivity (of affected area for secondary infections): + • Cytology of pustule contents or exudate: neutrophils, eosinophils, clusters of acantholytic keratinocytes[106]
	Imaging	• Radiographs, thoracic/abdominal: if neoplastic subset of complex, exclude metastasis • Ultrasound, thoracic/abdominal: if neoplastic subset of complex, exclude metastasis
	Procedures	• Skin biopsies (confirmatory): acantholysis with pustule formation • Immunohistochemical/immunofluorescent analysis of skin: "chicken-wire" pattern[78]
Treatment	General	• Apply Elizabethan collar if risk of further trauma • Studies from human medicine have found class IV laser therapy to be of benefit[108]
	Medication	• Depends on subset • Glucocorticoids: prednisone, prednisolone, dexamethasone, triamcinolone • Immunosuppressants: azathioprine (dogs), chlorambucil (cats), cyclosporine, tetracycline and niacinamide • Topical glucocorticoids or tacrolimus[105] • Antibiotics: for secondary infection • Analgesics (for severe, painful cases): gabapentin, opioids, tramadol
	Nursing care	• Measure and document pain score at regular intervals, as affected animals in some subsets can have high pain scores
Follow-up	Patient care	• Apply sunscreen when taking outside, as ultraviolet radiation exacerbates acantholysis[105,106]
	Prevention/avoidance	• If treating with laser therapy, use non-contact technique to decrease risk of future nosocomial infections
	Complications	• Long-term immunosuppression increases risk of infections • Cats receiving chlorambucil and dogs receiving azathioprine should have regular CBC checked[51] • Dogs receiving azathioprine should have liver values checked during the first four weeks of therapy[49]
	Prognosis	• Owners should be prepared for spontaneous relapses during the lifetime of their pet • Superficial/mild cases have a fair to good outcome; severe cases have a grave prognosis[109–112]
Notes		• Advise clients to wear gloves when applying topical medication • Obtain entire medication history, as some subsets are drug-induced

Systemic Inflammatory Response Syndrome

Systemic inflammatory response syndrome (SIRS) is a type of shock. It is an ubiquitous systemic inflammation caused by a primary infectious or non-infectious disease. The syndrome is marked by an imbalance of hypo- and hyperinflammatory mediators. As SIRS progresses, perfusion problems, microcirculation disturbances and organ injury unfold.[113] Criteria for SIRS are met when at least two abnormal clinical findings (body temperature, heart rate, respiratory rate, white cell count) are present.[113,114]

Table 6.33 / Systemic inflammatory response syndrome

Disease		Systemic inflammatory response syndrome (SIRS)
Presentation	Clinical signs	• Depends on underlying disease • Acute collapse, abdominal distention
	Exam findings	• Depends on underlying disease and the syndrome's phase upon presentation • Abdominal pain, abdominal distention, retching, vomiting, petechiae, ecchymosis, dull mentation • Dogs: initially pyrexia, injected mucus membranes, tachycardia, bounding pulses; later will be hypotension, pallor, and hypothermia[113] • Cats: pallor, tachypnea, bradycardia, poor pulse quality, hypotension, hypothermia[63,113,115]
Diagnosis	General	• History/clinical signs • Diagnosis cannot be made without meeting SIRS criteria[113]
	Laboratory	• CBC: leukocytosis with a left shift or leukopenia, thrombocytopenia • Chemistry panel: hypoalbuminemia, hyper/hypoglycemia, hyperbilirubinemia, ↑ BUN/creatinine,[117] ↑ hepatic enzymes[63,117,118] • Urinalysis: ↑ protein[117] • PPT and aPTT: prolonged • Lactate: ↑ • Adrenocortical tumor activity: ↓ • Protein C: ↓[119] • D-dimer concentration: ↑ • Blood gas: disturbances (variable)
	Imaging	• Radiographs, thoracic/abdominal: effusions/neoplasia • Ultrasound, thoracic/abdominal: effusions/neoplasia
	Procedures	• Blood pressure • Culture and sensitivity (blood, urine, wound exudate, peritoneal fluid, bronchoalveolar lavage fluid, synovial fluid): +[113]

(Continued)

Table 6.33 / **Systemic inflammatory response syndrome (Continued)**

Disease		Systemic inflammatory response syndrome (SIRS)
Treatment	General	• Isotonic/hypertonic fluid therapy: hemodynamic support • Dextrose and electrolyte supplementation if required • Oxygen therapy if $SpO_2 < 95\%$ or $PaO_2 < 80$ mmHg • Isolate injured organ, monitor and support function • Fresh whole blood or fresh frozen plasma for blood loss/coagulation factors • Colloids/albumin: possible adverse effects lack evidence in veterinary medicine; not recommended in human medicine[120–122]
	Medication	• Antibiotics: broad spectrum while cultures pending; empiric treatment for antibiotic resistant bacteria if iatrogenic is suspected[113]
	Nursing care	• Passive range-of-motion exercises if recumbent • Encourage sternal recumbency to reduce risk or atelectasis • Encourage short intervals of standing and walking when recovering • Implement parenteral or enteral nutrition • Monitor urine output (indicative of organ function)
Follow-up	Patient care	• Serial assessment of temperature, heart rate, respiratory rate and effort, and blood pressure • WCC and chemistry: monitor for progression, patterns and appearance of multiple-organ dysfunction syndrome
	Prevention/avoidance	• Do not use a "cookie-cutter" approach to fluid therapy; tailor needs to individual patient to avoid fluid insufficiency or overload • Certain antibiotics can lead to further organ injury (i.e. amikacin affects kidneys)[82] and should be avoided
	Complications	• Can lead to DIC very quickly • Non-infectious SIRS can develop into infection/sepsis because of nosocomial infections or risk of aspiration pneumonia in recumbent/ vomiting patients
	Prognosis	• High mortality if untreated or severe[115,118,123–125] • Outcome depends on primary cause and severity
Notes		• Sepsis is the most important exclusion for SIRS; no single test is available to differentiate sepsis from SIRS[113] • Early empiric antimicrobial therapy increases survival time[113]

INFECTIOUS DISEASES

Canine Transmissible Diseases

Infectious Canine Hepatitis

Canine adenovirus type-1 is the causative virus for infectious canine hepatitis, which affects the liver, eyes, and endothelium.

Canine Infectious Respiratory Disease

Canine infectious respiratory disease (CIRD; also known as "kennel cough" or infectious tracheobronchitis) is a contagious respiratory disease. It is caused by a variety of pathogens: viral (e.g. canine parainfluenza virus, canine ademovirus-2, canine herpesvirus-1, canine influenza virus) and bacterial (e.g. *Bordetella bronchiseptica, Mycoplasma cynos*). Infection results in coughing, nasal discharge, and dyspnea. CIRD is rarely a single pathogen and coinfections are common.

Table 6.34 / Infectious canine hepatitis and canine infectious respiratory disease

Disease		Infectious canine hepatitis (ICH)	Canine infectious respiratory disease (CIRD)
Presentation	Presenting clinical signs	• Depression, lethargy • Fever, laryngitis, coughing, vomiting, diarrhea, disorientation, seizures, stupor, coma	• Coughing (typically loud and persistent), nasal discharge, dyspnea, laryngitis, anorexia.
	Examination findings	• Tachycardia, tachypnea, abdominal pain, hepatomegaly, harsh lung sounds, anterior uveitis, corneal edema, fever, hepatic encephalopathy, tonsillitis/pharyngitis, hypoglycemia, pale mucous membranes, petechial/ecchymotic hemorrhages, epistaxis, nonsuppurative encephalitis, DIC	• Fever, increased bronchovesicular sounds, tracheal sensitivity
Diagnosis	General	• History/clinical signs	• History/clinical signs • History of frequenting locations where other canines congregate
	Laboratory	• CBC: leukopenia with lymphopenia and neutropenia, thrombocytopenia • Chemistry: ↑ AST, ALT, hypoglycemia, possible serum protein alternations • Urinalysis: proteinuria • Bile acids: mild to moderately high • Coagulation tests: prolonged prothrombin time, aPTT, hypofibrinogenemia • Complement fixation: serum • Fluorescent antibody: serum • Hemagglutination inhibition: serum • Histology: tissue • Immunohistochemistry: hepatic tissue • PCR: blood, urine, hepatic tissue • Viral inclusion: oropharyngeal swab, urine, feces • Viral neutralization: serum	• CBC: mild leukopenia, neutrophilic leukocytosis with a left shift or normal • ELISA: nasal swab, tissue • Culture: nasal swab, transendotracheal wash, bronchoalveolar lavage • Fluorescent antibody test: blood, buffy coat smear, conjunctival scraping, CSF, transendotracheal wash, bronchoalveolar lavage, tissue • Hemagglutination inhibition: serum, CSF, nasal swab, tissue • Histology: tissue • Immunohistochemistry: tissue • PCR: Serum, blood, urine, CSF, nasal, swab tissue • Viral inclusion: serum, transendotracheal wash, bronchoalveolar lavage, oropharyngeal swab, tissue • Viral neutralization: serum, CSF, tissue
	Imaging	• Abdominal radiographs: hepatomegaly • Ultrasound: hepatomegaly and abdominal effusion	• Thoracic radiographs: interstitial density, alveolar pattern, evidence of pneumonia (severe form)
	Procedures	• Not applicable	• Bronchoscopy, tracheal wash/bronchioalveolar lavage

(Continued)

Table 6.34 / Infectious canine hepatitis and canine infectious respiratory disease (Continued)

Disease		Infectious canine hepatitis (ICH)	Canine infectious respiratory disease (CIRD)
Treatment	General	• Symptomatic • Supportive • Fluid therapy • Transfusion	• Supportive
	Medication	• Antibiotics for secondary pneumonia or pyelonephritis	• Antibiotics – do not typically alter course if given by mouth; can nebulize • Bronchodilators • Antitussives
	Nursing care	• Frequent feedings to avoid hypoglycemia • Restricted activity/cage rest	• Encourage outpatient care for uncomplicated disease • Airway humidification • Strict confinement with low stress and few canines • Nutritional support • ↑ Fluid intake • Fresh air flow
Follow-up	Patient care	• Monitor blood chemistries • Monitor dehydration, acid–base balances, body weight, physical assessment, and electrolytes	• Adequate fluid intake • Airway humidification • Strict rest for 14–21 days
	Prevention/avoidance	• Vaccinate • Avoid urine: shedding time is 6 months or more	• Consider vaccination based on risk assessment • Prevent fomite spread with bleach diluted 1 : 32 • Isolate infected animals • Shed for up to 3 months, infectious risk is greatly ↓ after recovery of discharge and cough
	Complications	• Hepatic failure or chronic active hepatitis • Acute renal failure, glomerulonephritis • DIC	• Pneumonia
	Prognosis	• Guarded to good • Some have a complete recovery	• Complete recovery expected unless severe disease develops
Notes		• Transmitted through direct contact of body secretions/excretions and environmental fomites • Shed for 6–9 months following recovery • Highly resistant to inactivation and disinfection; susceptible to some quaternary ammonium compounds, bleach (1 : 32 dilution), and hydrogen peroxide products	• Highly contagious via aerosol spread and fomites • Disinfect with bleach, Rescue, Nolvasan, or Roccal wound cleanser • Incubation period: 3–10 days

Coronavirus

Coronavirus is a contagious viral disease affecting the gastrointestinal tract, resulting in sporadic outbreaks of vomiting and diarrhea; diarrhea is caused by the virus invading the enterocytes of the villous tips.

Distemper

Distemper is an acute to subacute infection, which is often fatal. It is a highly contagious viral disease with respiratory, gastrointestinal tract, and central nervous system manifestations.

Table 6.35 / Coronavirus and distemper

Disease		Coronavirus	Distemper virus
Presentation	Clinical signs	• Most infected canines are asymptomatic and fewer signs are exhibited in adult canines	• Mucosal phase: malaise, nasal discharge followed by pneumonia, vomiting, diarrhea, and fever
		• Anorexia, depression, diarrhea (yellow-green to orange, malodorous), and vomiting	• CNS phase: seizures, circling, pacing, ataxia, and paresis
	Examination findings	• Dehydration, mild respiratory effects	• Abdominal pustules, anterior uveitis, conjunctivitis, dental enamel hypoplasia, hyperkeratosis of foot pads, keratoconjunctivitis sicca, myoclonus, optic neuritis, retinal degeneration, and rhinitis
Diagnosis	General	• History/clinical signs	• History/clinical signs
	Laboratory	• Electron microscope • Fluorescent antibody tests	• CBC: lymphopenia, leukopenia, thrombocytopenia in early disease • Fluorescent antibody test: detection of virus in intact cells (e.g. conjunctival scrapings, buffy coat, urine sediment, CSF, transtracheal wash) • IgM: serum antibodies measured by ELISA • IgG: serial titers on two serum samples 2 weeks apart to detect ↑ titers • PCR: virus detection in respiratory secretions, CSF, feces, and urine
	Imaging	• Not applicable	• Thoracic: interstitial or alveolar pneumonia
	Procedures	• Not applicable	• Not applicable
Treatment	General	• Symptomatic • Supportive • Fluid therapy	• Supportive • Fluid therapy
	Medication	• Antidiarrheals	• Antibiotics • B vitamin supplementation • Anticonvulsant therapy • Antiemetics

(*Continued*)

Table 6.35 / **Coronavirus and distemper (Continued)**

Disease		Coronavirus	Distemper virus
Follow-up	Nursing care	• Not applicable	• Humidification of airways, nebulization, and coupage • Clean discharge from eyes and nose • Nutritional support • Adequate fluid intake or therapy • Isolation to avoid infecting other patients
	Patient care	• Not applicable	• Monitor dehydration and electrolytes. • Recheck thoracic radiographs if persistent cough occurs
	Prevention/avoidance	• Not typically vaccinated against this virus • Clean up feces: (will be shed in the feces for typically 6–9 days but can be for many months)	• Vaccinate • Avoid infected canines or wildlife. • Clean up feces: shedding time typically < 2–3 months
	Complications	• Persistent diarrhea for 10–12 days • Dehydration and electrolyte imbalances	• Occurrence of CNS signs (including seizures) may appear for up to 2–3 months after initial clinical signs
	Prognosis	• Complete recovery expected	• Ranges from slight to mortality • Mortality rate 50%
Notes		• Optional part of vaccine series • Consider vaccinating high-risk canines: field trial dogs and kenneled dogs • Transmitted by fecal–oral route	• Unvaccinated puppies 6–12 weeks of age are most at risk • Transmitted through body secretions, body excretions, and airborne • Easily destroyed by heat and most disinfectants; survives no more than a few days outside the host • Recovered canines are not carriers • Incubation period: 1–5 weeks

Leptospirosis

Leptospirosis is an acute and chronic multiorgan bacterial disease, particularly of the lungs, kidneys, and liver, which is zoonotic.

Borreliosis (Lyme Disease)

Borreliosis is caused by infection of the spirochete *Borrelia burgdorferi*, which causes inflammation of various tissues, including skin, joint capsules, lymph nodes, kidney, liver, and heart.

Table 6.36 / **Leptospirosis and Borreliosis (Lyme Disease)**

Disease		Leptospirosis	Borreliosis
Presentation	Presenting clinical signs	• Anorexia, lethargy, vomiting, dehydration, myalgia, and signs consistent with acute renal and/or hepatic disease	• Polyarthritis: lethargy, stiff gait, shifting leg lameness, joint swelling, dehydration • Nephropathy: vomiting, anorexia, polyuria/polydipsia, weight loss, peripheral edema, ascites
	Examination findings	• Fever, uveitis, conjunctivitis, renomegaly, hepatomegaly, renal discomfort/pain, oliguria/anuria, polyuria/polydipsia, icterus • Severe vasculitis, DIC, petechia/ecchymosis, increased lung sounds	• Fever, lymphadenopathy, lameness, swollen joints, and polyarthritis
Diagnosis	General	• History and clinical signs	• History (including travel) and clinical signs • Joint palpation: lameness, swelling, and pain
	Laboratory	• CBC: inflammatory leukogram ± left shift, thrombocytopenia • Chemistry: azotemia, hyperphosphatemia, increased ALT and ALP, bilirubinemia, hyponatremia, hypochloremia, hypokalemia • Urinalysis: glucosuria, proteinuria, granular casts, and isosthenuria • Fluorescent antibody: tissue or body fluids • Histology: kidney, placenta, urine, fetal fluid • Immunohistochemistry: tissue • Latex agglutination: serum • Microscopic agglutination test: serum • PCR: kidney, urine, blood	• Polyarthritis: routine labs may be normal • Nephropathy: azotemia, hyperphosphatemia, hypercholesterolemia, hypoalbuminemia, proteinuria, glucosuria, hematuria, and renal casts (cylindruria) • ELISA: serum • Fluorescent antibody: serum, tissue • Immunoblot: serum, tissue • PCR: blood
	Imaging	• Abdominal imaging: liver, spleen, and/or kidney enlargement • Abdominal ultrasound: hydronephrosis, medullary rim (hyperechoic) sign • Thoracic radiographs: interstitial, nodular, or patchy alveolar lung patterns in patients with respiratory involvement	• Polyarthritis: radiographs may revel joint effusion and characterize the arthritis • Nephropathy: abdominal ultrasound may help to rule in/out other causes of renal failure
	Procedures	• Not applicable	• Not applicable
Treatment	General	• Supportive • Fluid therapy • Transfusion therapy	• Supportive • Fluid therapy
	Medication	• Antibiotics, antiemetics, analgesics	• Antibiotics, antiemetics, analgesics
	Nursing care	• Restrict activity/cage rest • Nutritional support	• Restrict activity/cage rest • Pain management

(Continued)

Table 6.36 / **Leptospirosis and Borreliosis (Lyme Disease) (Continued)**

Disease		Leptospirosis	Borreliosis
Follow-up	Patient care	• Monitor blood chemistries and urinalysis	• Restricted activity • Nephropathy: monitor laboratory values
	Prevention/avoidance	• Avoid stagnant/slow-moving water sources where animals (particularly rodents) may have urinated • Consider vaccination based on risk assessment	• Appropriate environmental tick control measures • Periodically check canines for ticks • Consider vaccination based on risk assessment
	Complications	• DIC • Permanent renal and/or hepatic dysfunction • Can be lethal	• Seizures, behavior changes, and arrhythmias have been reported • Renal failure
	Prognosis	• Acute severe leptospirosis has a guarded prognosis	• Recovery expected but recurrence possible within weeks to months
Notes		• Zoonotic disease; proper personal protective equipment is necessary for hospitalized patients • Transmitted through direct contact (urine) and indirect contact (contaminated fomites) • Enters through skin or mucous membranes or by ingestion of contaminated water • Disinfect with Rescue, Nolvasan, bleach 1 : 10 dilution • Onset is a few days to 30 days, typically 3–14 days	• Vector-borne: *Ixodes* spp. tick • Infected animals pose little risk to humans as this is vector-borne disease

Brucellosis

Brucellosis is a zoonotic disease predominately caused by *Brucella canis*.

Ehrlichiosis

Ehrlichiosis is a rickettsial disease of dogs caused by *Ehrlichia* spp. Canine monocytic ehrlichiosis can result from multiple species, but *E. canis* is the most common pathogen. Canine granulocytic ehrlichiosis is associated with *E. ewingii*.

Table 6.37 / **Brucellosis and Ehrlichiosis**

Disease		Brucellosis	Ehrlichiosis
Presentation	Presenting clinical signs	• Variable; asymptomatic • Lethargy, hyporexia, weight loss • Male: epididymitis, scrotal edema, orchitis • Female: abortion, infertility and vaginal discharge for 1–6 weeks post-abortion • Less common: abnormal gait, ataxia, weakness	• Acute phase lasts 2–4 weeks, clinical signs resolve, and the dog enters a subclinical stage that may last months to years. • Acute CME: non-specific (fever, anorexia, lethargy, lymphadenomegaly), multisystemic (lameness, ataxia, seizures, hyperesthesia, bruising, changes in eye color • Chronic: non-specific and multisystemic, dyspnea, epistaxis, pallor, spontaneous bleeding, weakness, weight loss • Subclinical: no clinical signs • CGE: polyarthritis
	Examination findings	• Anterior uveitis, ascites, corneal edema, epididymitis, lymphadenopathy, paralysis, paresis, pyrexia, spinal hyperesthesia, splenomegaly	• Acute: lymphadenopathy, organomegaly, pyrexia, vestibular dysfunction • Chronic: arthritis, intermittent limb edema, neurological signs, organomegaly, pyrexia, uveitis
Diagnosis	General	• History/clinical signs	• History/clinical signs • Ocular exam: retinal detachment and hemorrhage
	Laboratory	• Chemistry panel: ↑ globulin and ↓ albumin • Urinalysis: ↑ protein, albumin • RSAT: serum • AGID: serum • TAT/2ME-TAT: serum • ELISA: serum • PCR: blood • Culture: blood, urine, semen, vaginal discharge, aborted fetuses, *B. canis* identification • Cytology, lymph node: nonspecific reactive hyperplasia • Cytology, semen: > 80% of sperm are morphologically abnormal, inflammatory cells • Fluid analysis, CSF: pleocytosis, ↑ protein	• CBC: acute – thrombocytopenia, anemia, leukopenia and chronic, nonregenerative anemia, thrombocytopenia, lymphocytosis, pancytopenia, leukopenia or leukocytosis. Subclinical – mild thrombocytopenia • Chemistry panel: acute – ↑ globulin, mild ↑ ALT, ALP, BUN, creatinine, and ↓ albumin; chronic – ↑ globulin, BUN, creatinine, and ↓ albumin • Urinalysis: acute – ↑ protein, ↓ specific gravity • Prolonged clotting times • Immunofluorescent assay: serum, titers > 1 : 10 (2–3 weeks after exposure, titers not available for all species) • ELISA: serum, blood • PCR: blood • Buffy coat smear: presence of *Ehrlichia* morulae • Cytology, bone marrow: plasmacytosis • Fluid analysis, CSF: mononuclear pleocytosis, ↑ protein
	Imaging	• Radiography, spine: diskospondylitis; if found, then check for brucellosis	• Not applicable
	Procedures	• Lymph node biopsy	• Bone marrow biopsy

(Continued)

Table 6.37 / **Brucellosis and Ehrlichiosis (Continued)**

Disease		Brucellosis	Ehrlichiosis
Treatment	General	• Supportive • Surgery: neuter	• Supportive • Blood transfusion • Fluid therapy
	Medication	• Antibiotics: often combination therapy; tetracyclines (e.g. minocycline, doxycycline), dihydrostreptomycin, enrofloxacin	• Antibiotics: doxycycline, minocycline, tetracycline, chloramphenicol • Corticosteroids (short term): prednisone, prednisolone
	Nursing care	• Treated as outpatient	• Restrict activity
Follow-up	Patient care	• Multiple courses of antibiotic treatment • Serologic titers monthly for 3 months, then at 6 months • Blood cultures monthly for 3 months • Restrict activity in working dogs	• Restrict activity • Continuing laboratory monitoring and rechecks as needed
	Prevention/avoidance	• Neuter infected animals • Quarantine and test all new dogs and breeding individuals	• Appropriate environmental tick control measures • Periodically check canines for ticks
	Complications	• Infertility • Sexual transmission	• Not applicable
	Prognosis	• Good with early treatment • Guarded with late detection	• Excellent • Poor if bone marrow is severely hypoplastic
Notes		• Transmitted through ingestion and oronasal contact and can be found in the lymphatic system, genital tract, eye, kidney, and intervertebral disks • Transmission typically follows breeding or abortion, or contact with semen, vaginal discharge, or urine by penetration of oronasal, conjunctival, or genital mucous membranes • Lasts for 6–64 months • Low risk of human infection with proper hygiene, mild and easily treated	• Transmission is most seen through the bite of the brown dog tick, *Rhipicephalus sanguineus*, or the lone star tick, *Amblyomma americanum* • *E. canis* can also be transmitted via blood transfusion • Incubation period is 7–21 days • German Shepherds may be overrepresented

Rocky Mountain Spotted Fever

Rocky mountain spotted fever is a tick-borne disease caused by *Rickettsia rickettsii.*

Salmon Poisoning Disease

Salmon poisoning disease is a multisystemic rickettsial disease caused by *Neorikettsia helminthoeca*, which is found in the Pacific Northwest. It attacks the tissue of the small intestinal epithelium and associated lymph system.

Table 6.38 / **Rocky Mountain spotted fever and salmon poisoning disease**

	Disease	Rocky Mountain spotted fever	Salmon poisoning
Presentation	Presenting clinical signs	• Non-specific • Abnormal gait, anorexia, ataxia, convulsions, depression, diarrhea, dyspnea, epistaxis, face and limb edema, lethargy, myalgia, weakness	• Diarrhea, hematochezia, melena, anorexia, lethargy, vomiting, weight loss, respiratory involvement, abdominal pain, weakness, polydipsia
	Physical exam findings	• Anterior uveitis, arthritis, ascites, conjunctivitis, lymphadenopathy, ocular pain, petechial hemorrhages, pyrexia, scleral injection, tachycardia, vasculitis, vestibular signs	• lethargy, acute pyrexia, ± development of hypothermia 7–10 days post-onset, tachycardia, dehydration, peripheral lymphadenopathy, respiratory involvement, neurologic
Diagnosis	General	• History/clinical signs	• History/clinical signs • Recent ingestion of raw or partially cooked fish containing *Nanophyetus Salmincola*
	Laboratory	• CBC: leukocytosis with a left shift, ±toxic neutrophils, monocytosis, mild anemia, thrombocytopenia • Chemistry panel: ↑ ALT, ALP, BUN, creatinine, cholesterol, albumin, and hyponatremia, hypochloremia, hypoproteinemia, metabolic acidosis • Urinalysis: ↑ protein, blood • Prolonged coagulation times • Direct immunofluorescence; skin biopsies: rickettsial antigens as early as 3–4 days post-infection • Micro-immunofluorescent assay: serum, titers > 1 : 128 • PCR: blood	• CBC: Non-specific, thrombocytopenia commonly reported • Chemistry panel: hypocalcemia and hypoalbuminemia most common finding. hypokalemia, hyponatremia, hypochloremia, hyperphosphatemia, azotemia, increased ALT and ALP • Urinalysis: proteinuria, hematuria, bilirubinemia • Direct fecal smear and sedimentation: operculated fluke eggs (*N. salminicola*) • Lymph-node aspirate: evaluate for rickettsial inclusion bodies • PCR: blood • Histopathology
	Imaging	• Not applicable	• Radiographs: unremarkable or focal areas of decreased detail and fluid-filled intestinal loops • Abdominal ultrasound: lymphadenomegaly, fluid-filled intestinal loops, ± organomegaly
	Procedures	• Skin biopsy	• Lymph node biopsy

(*Continued*)

Table 6.38 / Rocky Mountain spotted fever and salmon poisoning disease (Continued)

Disease		Rocky Mountain spotted fever	Salmon poisoning
Treatment	General	• Supportive • Blood transfusions • Fluid therapy	• Supportive • Fluid therapy
	Medication	• Antibiotics: tetracycline, doxycycline, chloramphenicol, enrofloxacin • Corticosteroids: prednisone	• Antibiotics: tetracycline, oxytetracycline, chloramphenicol • Anticestodal: praziquantel
	Nursing care	• Restrict activity.	• Restrict activity
Follow–up	Patient care	• Monitor platelet count every 3 days until normal • Micro-immunofluorescent assay titers 2–4 weeks after initial titer: 2–4-fold rise in titer • Restrict activity	• Monitor temperature, hydration, electrolytes, acid–base balances
	Prevention/avoidance	• Tick and rodent control • Using gloves or instruments, check daily for ticks, and remove the entire tick if found	• Prevent eating of raw fish • Thoroughly cook or freeze fish
	Complications	• Not applicable.	• Not applicable
	Prognosis	• Good if early diagnosis and treatment • Poor if in later stages with CNS disease	• Good with early diagnosis and treatment
Notes		• Caution: handling of an infected tick may result in transmission of the disease even without attachment • Transmitted by the American deer tick, wood tick, lone star tick, and transfusions • The tick must be attached for 5–20 hours to infect dogs. • Primary hosts – rodents and rabbits • Incubation time is 2 days to 2 weeks • High titers can be seen for 1 year following successful treatment	• Transmitted through eating raw salmon or related fish carrying encysted forms of the fluke *N. salminicola* • Incubation of 5–7 days • If untreated, death typically occurs within two weeks of the dog eating the infected fish

Canine Parvovirus

Canine Parvovirus is a highly contagious disease causing severe enteritis and affecting the lymphatic system. The disease typically affects puppies between weaning and six months of age.

Rabies

Rabies is a virus that can infect almost all warm-blooded animals and is considered untreatable. It infects the nervous system, causing death from paralysis.

Table 6.39 / **Canine parvovirus and rabies**

Disease		Canine parvovirus	Rabies
Presentation	Clinical signs	• Anorexia, depression, vomiting, lethargy • Diarrhea: profuse, liquid, hemorrhagic, and distinct metallic odor • Symptoms may vary in older canines	• Classically described as having three phases, but presentation can be quite variable and atypical signs are commonly observed • Prodromal phase (duration 2–3 days): fever, apprehension, nervousness, anxiety, solitude; behavior changes (e.g. friendly animals become shy or irritable and vice versa) • Furious/psychotic phase (duration 1–7 days): irritability, restlessness, excitable, photophobia, hyperesthesia, vocalizing, ataxia and seizures • Paralytic phase (duration 2–4 days, range 1–10 days): progressive paralysis, depression, coma, and, ultimately, death from respiratory paralysis
	Examination findings	• Extreme dehydration, fever, abdominal discomfort/pain, septic shock, hypothermia	• Prodromal phase: slow corneal and palpebral reflexes
Diagnosis	General	• History/clinical signs	• History/clinical signs • Atypical signs are possible, so rabies should be considered in any animal that suddenly develops significant behavioral changes, lower motor neuron paralysis, or both
	Laboratory	• CBC: severe leukopenia and lymphopenia, PCV variable • Chemistry panel: ↑ bilirubin, ALT, and AST, and ↓ potassium, sodium, and chloride, hypoglycemia • ELISA: serum, feces • Electron microscopy: feces, intestinal mucosa • Fluorescent antibody: feces, intestinal mucosa • Hemagglutination: feces, intestinal mucosa • Hemagglutination inhibition: feces, intestinal mucosa • PCR: blood, feces	• CSF: minimal ↑ protein and leukocytes • Fluorescent antibody: brain tissue • Histology: brain tissue • Immunohistochemistry: brain tissue
	Imaging	• Radiographs, abdominal: gas and fluid distention in gastrointestinal tract	• Not applicable
	Procedures	• Not applicable	• Not applicable

(*Continued*)

Table 6.39 / **Canine parvovirus and rabies (Continued)**

Disease		Canine parvovirus	Rabies
Treatment	General	• Symptomatic • Supportive • Fluid therapy: aggressive • Transfusion	• Supportive
	Medication	• Antibiotics • Antiemetics • Gastric protectants	• Not applicable
	Nursing care	• Limited fasting after vomiting • Early enteral nutrition leads to shorter hospitalization and recovery time • Quarantine protocol	• Strictly inpatient/quarantine • Runs and cages should be locked
Follow-up	Patient care	• Canines should remain isolated for 1 week after complete recovery	• None
	Prevention/avoidance	• Vaccinate up to at least 16 weeks; 18–20 weeks in high-risk situations	• Vaccinate • Strict quarantine for those suspected of having rabies according to local health department protocols • Euthanize all animals known to have rabies
	Complications	• Septicemia • Secondary bacterial pneumonia • Intussusception	• Not applicable
	Prognosis	• Survival of 3–4 days is usually followed by rapid recovery • Immunity by natural infection is at least 20 months, but is likely longer	• Almost 100% fatal
Notes		• Transmitted by direct contact (oronasal exposure or ingestion of feces) and indirect contact (contaminated fomites), flies have also been shown to play a role in the infection of dogs • Stable in the environment for months to years • Rottweilers, American Pit Bull Terriers, Doberman Pinschers, English Springer Spaniels, and German Shepherds may be at higher risk • Resistant virus; disinfect with 1 : 30 dilution of bleach and water, Rescue • Incubation period: 5–10 days	• Transmitted via direct contact with saliva (bite wound or open wounds/abrasions) • Inactivated by routine disinfectants • Head should be refrigerated, not frozen, and sent to a laboratory for brain tissue analysis

Feline Transmissible Diseases

Feline Calicivirus

Feline calicivirus is one of the major causes of feline upper respiratory disease. It is an acute, highly contagious viral disease causing oral ulceration, pneumonia, and occasionally arthritis.

Table 6.40 / Feline calicivirus

Disease		Feline calicivirus (FCV)
Presentation	Clinical signs	• Anorexia, depression, dyspnea, mild conjunctivitis, mild sneezing, oculonasal discharge • Strains of FCV can differ and a wide range of clinical signs are possible
	Examination findings	• Oral ulceration, facial and limb edema, fever, gingivitis, limping syndrome, interdigital paw ulcers
Diagnosis	General	• History/clinical signs
	Laboratory	• CBC: neutrophilia and lymphopenia • Chemistry panel: ↑ bilirubin, creatine kinase • Electron microscopy: oropharyngeal swab, intestinal and fecal swab • Fluorescent antibody: serum, oropharyngeal, intestinal, and fecal swabs • Viral inclusion: oropharyngeal, intestinal, and fecal swabs • Viral neutralization: serum
	Imaging	• Thoracic radiographs: generalized ↑ density of the lungs
	Procedures	• Not applicable
Treatment	General	• Supportive
	Medication	• Antibiotics • Pain medication, nonsteroidal anti-inflammatory medications
	Nursing care	• Oxygen supplementation if complicated pneumonia • Nutritional support

(Continued)

Table 6.40 / Feline calicivirus (Continued)

Disease		Feline calicivirus (FCV)
Follow-up	Patient care	• Keep eyes and nose clear of discharge • Support nutrition and fluid intake • Airway humidification • Provide soft foods if oral ulcers
	Prevention/avoidance	• Vaccinate • Prevent contact with FCV-infected cats
	Complications	• Interstitial pneumonia • Secondary bacterial infections
	Prognosis	• Excellent unless pneumonia develops • Recovered cats may shed the virus in their saliva for long periods
Notes		• Transmission is through direct contact (mucosal secretions) and indirect contact (contaminated fomites) • Disinfect with 1 : 32 dilution of bleach in water • Cats that recover may remain subclinical carriers for months to years, but a minority of patients it may be lifelong • Cats should be tested for FIV or FeLV to rule out underlying immunodeficiency syndromes • Coinfections are common, particularly FHV-1 • Incubation period: 1–5 days • Feline chronic gingivostomatitis has been associated with FCV infection

Feline Infectious Peritonitis

Feline infectious peritonitis (FIP) is a systemic viral disease with high mortality. The disease arises from a mutation of a benign virus, feline coronavirus), commonly found in the gastrointestinal tract of cats. There are two different forms: the wet/effusive form, and the dry/non-effusive, granulomatous form. FIP is essentially a pyogranulomatous vasculitis and its presentation is a reflection of the organ/tissues affected.

Table 6.41 / Feline infectious peritonitis

Disease		Feline infectious peritonitis (FIP)
Presentation	Clinical signs	• Wide variety of signs • Ataxia, behavioral changes, depression, diarrhea, failure to thrive, inactivity, paresis, poor condition, seizures, urinary incontinence, vomiting, weight loss
		• Non-effusive form: weight loss, hyporexia, lethargy • Effusive form: abdominal distention
	Examination findings	• Fever, icterus, pallor
		• Non-effusive form: ocular signs (iritis, changes in retinal vasculature, retinal pyogranuloma), neurological signs (altered mental status, ataxia, nystagmus, seizures) • Effusive form: dyspnea, tachypnea, muffled heart sounds, abdominal or pleural effusion
Diagnosis	General	• History and clinical signs; likely after other conditions have been ruled out
	Laboratory	• CBC: lymphopenia, non-regenerative anemia, thrombocytopenia • Chemistry panel: ↑ bilirubin, ALP, ALT, globulins and bile acids, BUN, creatinine • Urinalysis: ↑ bilirubin and protein • Rivalta test: effusion • ELISA: serum • Fluorescent antibody: serum, tissue • Protein electrophoresis: serum • Histology: tissue • Immunohistochemistry: tissue, CSF, lymphoid tissue, effusion fluid
	Imaging	• Thoracic radiographs: effusion • Abdominal radiographs: effusion, organomegaly, lymphadenopathy, and occasionally ileocolic mass
	Procedures	• Abdominocentesis or thoracocentesis: straw-colored fluid, viscous, clots, fibrinous and ↑ protein • Tumor biopsy: granulomatous inflammation
Treatment	General	• Fluid therapy • Supportive
	Medication	• Corticosteroids • Immunosuppressive drugs • Immunomodulators • Non-steroidal anti-inflammatory medications
	Nursing care	• Supportive • Nutritional support

(Continued)

Table 6.41 / **Feline infectious peritonitis (Continued)**

Disease		Feline infectious peritonitis (FIP)
Follow-up	Patient care	• Confine to prevent exposure to other cats
	Prevention/avoidance	• Prevent contact with FIP-positive cats; transmission is rare between cats • Intranasal vaccine, questionable efficacy • Routine disinfection
	Complications	• Gastrointestinal obstruction • Neurological disease (non-suppurative granulomatous meningitis) • Pleural effusion, peritoneal
	Prognosis	• Almost 100% mortality • Length of disease is a few days to months
Notes		• Cats < 2 years of age are at the greatest risk, followed by those > 10 years of age • FCoV is transmitted through direct contact (ingestion of feces) and indirect contact (contaminated fomites) • FIP develops from spontaneous mutations of FCoV within infected cats • Once clinical disease FIP develops, death is likely to occur in a few days to weeks • Survives in the environment for several weeks • Readily inactivated by commonly used disinfectants

Feline Panleukopenia

Feline panleukopenia is an acute, systemic and enteric viral disease caused by feline parvovirus. It has a sudden onset, is highly contagious, and has a high mortality rate.

Feline Immunodeficiency Virus

Feline immunodeficiency virus is an immunodeficiency syndrome characterized by chronic and recurrent infection, which gradually selects and destroys T lymphocytes. This process makes cats more prone to secondary syndromes. Affected cats can be asymptomatic for more than five years.

Table 6.42 / **Feline panleukopenia and feline immunodeficiency virus**

Disease		Feline panleukopenia	Feline immunodeficiency virus
Presentation	Presenting clinical signs	• Often subclinical • Abdominal pain (crouching position and head between front paws), anorexia, depression, diarrhea, vomiting, diarrhea, rough and dull hair coat	• Often described as progressing in three stages: • Transient/primary subclinical stage (fever, neutropenia, and lymphadenopathy) • Chronic asymptomatic stage, which may last years • Terminal phase: anorexia, cachexia, and other signs associated with secondary infections • Nonspecific; weight loss • Various signs may present due to opportunistic secondary infections
	Examination findings	• Fever which can progress to hypothermia and progressive dehydration • Dehydration, abdominal pain, thickened intestinal loops, mesenteric lymphadenomegaly, retinal lesions may be present	• Lymphadenopathy, fever, anterior uveitis, gingivitis, periodontitis, stomatitis, chronic upper respiratory viral disease, conjunctivitis, gingivitis, otitis, periodontitis, pneumonia, rhinitis, skin infections, stomatitis, tachycardia, urinary tract infections
Diagnosis	General	• History/clinical signs	• History/clinical signs of exposure
	Laboratory	• CBC: leukopenia, ± thrombocytopenia • Chemistry panel: can be non-specific; ↑ liver values, azotemia, and electrolyte imbalances • ELISA: feces, serum • Electron microscopy: feces, tissue • Fluorescent antibody: serum • Hemagglutination inhibition: serum • Histology: tissue • PCR: feces, tissue • Viral inclusion: feces, tissue • Viral neutralization: serum	• Various abnormalities have been observed due to concurrent disease • CBC (stage 3): anemia, lymphopenia, neutropenia • Chemistry panel: ↑ protein and globulins • Urinalysis: ↑ protein • ELISA: serum, whole blood • Immunoblot: serum, whole blood • Indirect fluorescent antibody: serum, whole blood • PCR: whole blood, bone marrow, lymphoid tissue
	Imaging	• MRI/CT – cerebellar/cortical defects in patients with neurological signs (infected in utero)	• Not applicable
	Procedures	• Not applicable	• Not applicable

(Continued)

Table 6.42 / Feline panleukopenia and feline immunodeficiency virus (Continued)

Disease		Feline panleukopenia	Feline immunodeficiency virus
Treatment	General	• Supportive • Fluid therapy • Blood transfusions	• Symptomatic • Fluid therapy • Dental care
	Medication	• Antibiotics • Antiemetics	• Antibiotics for secondary infection • Appetite stimulants • Corticosteroids • Immunostimulants • Treatment for secondary conditions
	Nursing care	• Heat support if hypothermic • Monitor hydration, electrolytes, and CBC	• Supportive
Follow-up	Patient care	• Heat support • Nutritional support	• Semi-annual wellness visits with a focus on preventive medicine (vaccination, laboratory monitoring, dental care, etc.)
	Prevention/avoidance	• Vaccinate • Prevent contact with infected cats • Clean up feces	• Neuter males and minimize roaming behaviors • Quarantine and test all incoming cats regardless of age • Retest high-risk cats regularly • Consider vaccination in cats based on risk assessment and permanent identification (microchip)
	Complications	• Hypothermia and shock • DIC • Liver/renal failure	• Stomatitis • Secondary infections • Neurological signs • Ocular disease • Neoplasia
	Prognosis	• Poor prognosis in terminal phase: ≤1-year survival	• > 50% remain asymptomatic within 2 years after diagnosis Poor prognosis in terminal phase: ≤ 1-year survival
Notes		• Transmitted by direct contact (ingestion of feces or transplacental transfer), indirect contact (contaminated fomites) • Disinfect with 1 : 32 dilution of bleach solution • Survives months to years in the environment • In utero or transmission from infected queen leads to cerebellar hypoplasia in kittens. • Incubation period: < 14 days • Recovered cats have lifetime immunity against feline parvovirus	• Transmitted by direct contact (inoculation of saliva through bite wounds and transplacental transfer); transmission through blood transfusion has been documented • Shed in the saliva • Most commonly seen in unneutered roaming males • A kitten may test + when < 6 months of age, due to maternal antibodies; retest at 8–12 months after all maternal antibodies are gone • Readily inactivated by commonly used disinfectants

Feline Leukemia Virus

Feline leukemia virus is a retrovirus causing bone marrow disorders, neoplasia, and immunosuppression. Cats may clear initial infection, but there is no cure for persistent infection, which ultimately leads to death.

Feline Rhinotracheitis

Feline rhinotracheitis is a highly contagious viral disease causing rhinitis, conjunctivitis, and ulcerative keratitis. It is caused by feline herpesvirus type 1, one of the major causes of feline upper respiratory disease.

Table 6.43 / Feline leukemia virus and feline viral rhinotracheitis

Disease		Feline leukemia virus (FeLV)	Feline viral rhinotracheitis (FVR)
Presentation	Presenting clinical signs	• Hyporexia/anorexia, weight loss, lethargy • Clinical signs are variable based on associated conditions	• Hyporexia/anorexia, sneezing, conjunctivitis, oculonasal discharge • Anorexia, cough, depression, hypersalivation, loss of voice, photophobia
	Physical examination findings	• Fever, pallor, dehydration, rhinitis, diarrhea, conjunctivitis, oral inflammation, lymphadenopathy, abscesses, stomatitis, uveitis	• Fever, conjunctivitis, uveitis, dermal/oral ulcerations, rhinitis; possibly ulcerative keratitis, corneal ulcers/sequestration
Diagnosis	General	• History/clinical signs	• History and clinical signs
	Laboratory	• CBC: lymphopenia, neutropenia, nonregenerative anemia, thrombocytopenia, granulocytopenia • ELISA: serum, whole blood • Fluorescent antibody: blood smear, buffy coat, bone marrow, tissue • PCR: lymphoid tissue, bone marrow • Rapid immunomigration: blood, serum • Viral inclusion: blood, serum	• CBC: transient leukopenia, leukocytosis • ELISA: serum, whole blood • Electron microscopy: serum, whole blood • Fluorescent antibody: serum, whole blood • Immunohistochemistry: tissue • PCR: conjunctival/pharyngeal swabs, tissue • Viral inclusion: tissue, respiratory wash, feces, oropharyngeal swabs, conjunctival smears, CSF, whole blood, body fluids • Viral neutralization; serum, whole blood
	Imaging	• Not applicable	• Radiographs, skull: chronic disease shows changes in the nasal cavities and frontal sinuses
	Procedures	• Not applicable	• Not applicable

(*Continued*)

Table 6.43 / Feline leukemia virus and feline viral rhinotracheitis (Continued)

Disease		Feline leukemia virus (FeLV)	Feline viral rhinotracheitis (FVR)
Treatment	General	• Supportive • Symptomatic	• Supportive • Fluid therapy
	Medication	• Antibiotics, (e.g. *Mycoplasma haemofelis* infection) • Immunomodulatory drugs	• Antibiotics (secondary infection) • Antibiotics (ophthalmic)
	Nursing care	• Blood transfusions many may be necessary. Using blood from FeLV vaccinated cats may reduce the level of FeLV antigenemia in some cats	• Nutritional support, feeding tube placement • Facial hygiene, eyes and nose clear of discharge • Airway humidification
Follow-up	Patient care	• Semiannual wellness visits with a focus on preventive medicine (vaccination, laboratory monitoring, dental care, etc.) • Symptomatic	• Confine indoors to decrease environmentally induced stress
	Prevention/avoidance	• Vaccinate outdoor cats and those living with an FeLV-positive cat • Quarantine and test all new cats to the household or local environment • Consider vaccination based on risk assessment	• Vaccinate • Prevent contact with FHV-infected cats • Virus shed intermittently
	Complications	• Bone marrow disorders (e.g. pure red cell aplasia) • Neoplasia (lymphoma) • Immune-mediated hemolytic anemia • Glomerulonephritis • Toxoplasmosis • M. haemofelis	• Pneumonia • Chronic rhinosinusitis • Persistent nasal discharge • Herpetic ulcerative keratitis • Permanent closure of nasolacrimal duct • Recrudescent disease usually occurs during times of stress or glucocorticoid administration
	Prognosis	• > 50% of cats die from related diseases in 2–3 years	• Good; recovery in 7–14 days
Notes		• All FeLV-positive cats must remain indoors to prevent further spread of the disease • Test each cat prior to first vaccine or if there has been a long period of time without vaccines • More false-positive results when using whole blood on the ELISA test • False negatives can be seen in cats infected within the last 1–3 months • Transmission is through direct contact (saliva and nasal secretions); transmission through blood transfusion and contaminated needles has been documented • Readily inactivated by commonly used disinfectants	• Transmission is through direct contact (oronasal or conjunctival secretions) and fomites • Most patients become lifelong latent carriers, with viral reactivation and shedding occurring during periods of stress • Readily inactivated by commonly used disinfectants • Cats should be tested for FIV and FeLV to rule out underlying immunodeficiency syndromes

Tetanus

Tetanus is a disease caused by *Clostridium tetani*, which is found in the soil and as part of the normal bacterial flora of the intestinal tract of mammals.

Toxoplasmosis

Toxoplasmosis, which is caused by the intracellular coccidian protozoan parasite, *Toxoplasma gondii*, can invade and multiply in any cell in the body and can infect almost all mammals.

Table 6.44 / Tetanus and toxoplasmosis

Disease		Tetanus	Toxoplasmosis Zoonotic
Presentation	Clinical signs	• Ataxia, convulsions, disoriented, dyspnea, ears erect, forehead wrinkled, hypersalivation, lips retracted, localized or generalized muscle rigidity, seizures, stiffness, tetanic spasms, trismus, walking difficulty, weakness	• Subclinical most of the time • Anorexia, ataxia, depression, diarrhea, dyspnea, exercise intolerance, lethargy, paralysis, paresis, seizures, stiff gait, tremors, vomiting, weakness, weight loss
	Exam findings	• Altered heart and respiratory rates, hyperventilation, laryngeal spasms, pyrexia, tachycardia	• Lethargy, anterior and posterior uveitis, blindness, icterus, musculoskeletal pain and stiffness, neurological abnormalities, pyrexia, cardiac arrhythmia
Diagnosis	General	• Clinical signs • Recent wound (especially with high levels of necrosis and anaerobic conditions)	• Clinical signs

	Laboratory	• CBC: initial leukopenia followed by leukocytosis
		• Chemistry panel: ↑ AST, creatine kinase
		• Urinalysis: ↑ myoglobin
		
		• Culture, **CSF**, blood: bacteria recognition and identification (meningitis)
			• CBC: nonregenerative anemia, neutrophilic leukocytosis, lymphocytosis, monocytosis, neutropenia, eosinophilia
			• Chemistry panel: ↑ protein, ↑ bilirubin, ALT, ALP, creatinine, amylase, lipase
			• Urinalysis: ↑ protein and bilirubin
			• PCR assays
			• Serology:
			  • ELISA antibody IgG and IgM
			  • Modified agglutination test
			  • Indirect fluorescent antibody test
			  • Cytologic evaluation of fluids (affusion, CSF) and tissue samples for *T. gondii* tachyzoites

	Imaging	• Not applicable	• Radiographs, thoracic: effusion, patchy alveolar and interstitial pulmonary infiltrates
	Procedures	• Not applicable	• ECG: arrhythmia, cardiac irregularity

(*Continued*)

Table 6.44 / **Tetanus and toxoplasmosis (Continued)**

Disease		Tetanus	Toxoplasmosis Zoonotic
Treatment	General	• Supportive • Fluid therapy • Wound management: debridement, H_2O_2 flushing, cleaning	• Supportive • Fluid therapy
	Medication	• Antibiotics: amoxicillin, metronidazole, tetracycline, clindamycin • Sedatives/analgesia: diazepam, chlorpromazine, phenobarbital, pentobarbital, propofol, butorphanol • Muscle relaxants: methocarbamol • Tetanus antitoxin	• Antibiotics: clindamycin, pyrimethamine, trimethoprim-sulfonamide • Ophthalmic drops: 1% prednisone
	Nursing care	• Keep the patient in a dark quiet area and do not disturb. • Provide soft bedding and rotate every 4 hours to prevent decubital sores and atelectasis • Consider an indwelling urinary catheter • Nutritional support • Monitor blood pressure and ECG	• Treat as outpatient • Confine patients with neurological signs or with severe disease.
Follow-up	Patient care	• Not applicable	• Continuing monitoring and rechecking • Provide a high-quality diet, biannual physical exams, annual blood work, vaccines, and prompt attention to illness
	Prevention/avoidance	• Prevent skin wounds: maintain clean and safe runs and yards • Give proper wound care management • Aseptic surgical technique	• Prevent ingestion of raw meat, bones, viscera, or unpasteurized milk • Prevent free roaming to hunt prey or access to the housing of food-producing animals
	Complications	• Respiratory dysfunction • Uncontrolled hyperthermia	• Not applicable
	Prognosis	• Good with early treatment • Extremely guarded when severely affected	• Guarded: can be become carriers and relapse clinically if immunocompromised
Notes		• Clinical signs show up 5 days to 3 weeks later and may take up to 4 weeks to resolve. • Animals can be pretested for anaphylactic reaction to the antitoxin by giving an intradermal injection first and monitoring for 30 minutes • Force feeding is not advised as it may cause a tetanic state and increases risk of aspiration • The use of "cold sterile" instruments for these patients is discouraged	• Caution: disease can be transmitted to an unborn fetus by an infected human mother • Transmitted by ingesting infected animal tissues, cat feces, and transplacental infection • Excrete eggs 3–10 days after infection for 1–2 weeks; can shed again if stressed (feline) • Oocysts must first sporulate to become infectious, > 24 hours. • Oocysts can last in the soil for > 1 year

MUSCULOSKELETAL DISEASES AND CONDITIONS

Arthritis

There are two types of clinically diagnosed arthritides: degenerative and acute inflammatory. Acute arthritis is a pathogenic organism within the closed space of a joint. Degenerative joint disease (DJD) or osteoarthritis is a progressive deterioration characterized by a loss of hyaline cartilage matrix and death of chondrocytes. There is no cure for DJD; treatment is based on alleviating clinical signs and slowing progression.

Table 6.45 / Arthritis

Disease		Arthritis	
		Acute	Degenerative joint disease (DJD)
Presentation	Clinical signs	• Joint swelling, lameness, pain, reluctance to jump or climb stairs, stiff gait	• Abnormal gait, ataxia, exercise intolerance, ↑ lameness following moderate to heavy exercise, stiff upon rising after recumbency, swelling, walking difficulty
	Exam findings	• Crepitus, laxity, pain, ↓ range of motion	• Crepitus, edema, laxity, muscle atrophy, pain
Diagnosis	General	• History/clinical signs • Joint palpation and manipulation	• History/clinical signs • Joint palpation
	Laboratory	• CBC: leukocytosis, neutrophilia • Urinalysis: ↑ protein • ANA test: + results • Tick-borne agent serology: + results • Synovial fluid analysis: ↑ WBCs and bacteria • Biopsy, synovial: neoplasia • Cytology, synovial: ↑ WBCs, turbidity, bacteria • Culture, synovial: bacteria, yeast, fungi, additional organisms • Mucin clot test: clot poor	• Synovial fluid analysis: ↑ mononuclear cells (e.g. lymphocytes), protein, and ↓ viscosity, cell count (compared to septic or inflammatory arthritis) • Culture: negative for bacteria • Mucin clot test: clot poor • Serum titers: + Borrelia, Ehrlichia, and Rickettsia • Coombs test, ANA serology, rheumatoid factor: + with immune mediated

	Imaging	• Radiograph, affected joint:
		  • Early disease: joint capsular distension, soft tissue thickening, joint effusion
		  • Late disease: bone lysis, erosion and destruction, irregular joint space
			• Radiograph, affected joint: osteophytes, subchondral sclerosis, narrowed joint space and remodeling of subchondral bone/epiphyses
			• Nuclear scintigraphy, bone: subtle changes

	Procedures	• Arthrocentesis: joint drainage and lavage • Arthroscopy: visual examination, lavage and biopsy	• Arthrocentesis

(Continued)

Table 6.45 / Arthritis (Continued)

Disease		Arthritis	
		Acute	Degenerative joint disease (DJD)
Treatment	General	• Supportive • Surgery: arthrotomy, reconstructive procedures, arthrodesis	• Supportive • Surgery: resection arthroplasty, joint replacement, arthrodesis
	Medication	• Antibiotics: variable • Chondroprotective agents: polysulfated glycosaminoglycan (Adequan®), glucosamine with chondroitin sulfate • Corticosteroids: prednisone or triamcinolone • Immunomodulators • Methyl sulfonyl methane • NSAIDs: aspirin, carprofen, deracoxib, etodolac, firocoxib, meloxicam, tepoxalin, Galliprant	• Chondroprotective agents: glucosamine with chondroitin sulfate • Corticosteroids: prednisone or triamcinolone • NSAIDs: aspirin, carprofen, deracoxib, etodolac, firocoxib, meloxicam, tepoxalin, Galliprant® • Supplements: omega-3 and -6
	Nursing care	• Standard postoperative care • Initial joint immobilization may provide comfort, but long-term use can cause worsening damage • Monitor synovial fluid cytology for response to treatment • Monitor joints for swelling and pain • Treated as outpatient	• Standard postoperative care • Monitor joints for swelling and pain • Treated as outpatient
Follow-up	Patient care	• Moderate activity but restricted to a level that minimizes discomfort • Strict confinement with acutely painful episodes • Obesity control • Physical therapy: hot/cold treatment, swimming, range of movement exercises, and massage	• Weight control • Encourage moderate and consistent exercise for muscle tone and strengthening (e.g. swimming – low impact). • Physical therapy: hot/cold treatment, swimming, range of movement exercises, and massage
	Prevention/avoidance	• Maintain appropriate weight control. • Early recognition to prevent proceeding to secondary condition	• Maintain proper weight control. • Early use of glucosamine with chondroitin sulfate to slow progression
	Complications	• Arthritis, erosive • Non-ambulatory • DJD • Osteomyelitis • Recurrence of infection	• Non-ambulatory
	Prognosis	• Good with septic form • Fair to guarded with immune-mediated form	• Progressive
Notes		• Antibiotics are given for 4–8 weeks	• When switching NSAIDs, provide a 3-day washout period

Cruciate Disease

Cruciate disease results in a partial or complete instability of the stifle joint. The tearing of the anterior cruciate ligament can be done acutely or as a degenerative process.

Hip Dysplasia

Hip dysplasia is the most common condition of the hip joint and cause of osteoarthritis. Hip dysplasia is a faulty development of the hip joint contributing to joint laxity and subluxation early in life. Joint instability occurs as muscle development and maturation lag behind the rate of skeletal growth.

See also Skill Box 2.7, page 53.

Table 6.46 / Cruciate disease and hip dysplasia

Disease		Cruciate disease (cranial cruciate rupture)	Hip dysplasia
Presentation	Clinical signs	• Abnormal gait, acute or intermittent lameness, ataxia, walking difficulty	• Abnormal gait, ataxia, exercise intolerance, hind limb lameness
	Exam findings	• Deformed stifle joint, edema, joint effusion, muscle atrophy of hind limb musculature, swelling	• Barden's sign, Barlow's sign, crepitus, joint laxity, muscle atrophy, Ortolani + test, pain, ↓ range of motion
Diagnosis	General	• History/clinical signs • Joint palpation: + anterior drawer sign, cranial tibial thrust	• History/clinical signs • Joint palpation
	Laboratory	• Synovial fluid analysis: rule out sepsis and immune-mediated disease	• Not applicable
	Imaging	• Radiograph, stifle joint: joint effusion with capsular distention, periarticular osteophytes, compression of infrapatellar fat pad and calcification of cruciate ligament • MRI or CT: confirmation and severity of disease	• Radiographs, skeletal: joint subluxation of femoral head, flattening of femoral head, shallow acetabulum, periarticular osteophytes, or widening of joint space between femoral head and cranial acetabulum
	Procedures	• Arthrocentesis • Arthroscopy: confirmation and severity of disease	• Not applicable

(Continued)

Table 6.46 / **Cruciate disease and hip dysplasia (Continued)**

Disease		Cruciate disease (cranial cruciate rupture)	Hip dysplasia
Treatment	General	• Symptomatic • Cage rest • Surgery: tibial plateau leveling osteotomy, "over-the-top" fascia lata graft, fibular head transposition imbrication procedure, extracapsular reinforcing procedures, CORA-based leveling osteotomy and tibial tuberosity advancement	• Surgery: triple pelvic osteotomy, femoral head and neck excision arthroplasty, pectineal myectomy, or total hip replacement
	Medication	• Chondroprotective drugs: polysulfated glycosaminoglycan (Adequan®), glucosamine with chondroitin sulfate • NSAIDs: aspirin, carprofen, deracoxib, etodolac, firocoxib, meloxicam, tepoxalin, Galliprant®	• Analgesics: variable • Chondroprotective agents: Adequan or glucosamine with chondroitin sulfate • Corticosteroids: prednisone, triamcinolone (short term use) • Prostaglandin E1 analog: misoprostol • NSAIDs: aspirin, piroxicam, carprofen, etodolac, Galliprant • phenylbutazone, meclofenamic acid
	Nursing care	• Placement of Robert Jones bandage • Pain management • Surgery, postoperatively: cryotherapy, laser therapy, range of movement exercises, electrical stimulation, controlled weight-bearing and balance exercises	• Postoperative radiographs to evaluate surgery • Physical rehabilitation and hydrotherapy • Restrict activity
Follow-up	Patient care	• Physical rehabilitation: range of movement exercises, massage, underwater treadmill, and ball, stairs, walking, and balance board exercises • Restricted activity: controlled weightbearing leashed walks and no use of stairs for 3 months postoperatively • Re-radiograph at 8 weeks • Full exercise by 6–9 months postoperatively or 3–4 months for patients with rehabilitation • Control obesity	• Restrict activity. • Physical rehabilitation and hydrotherapy • Monitor radiographs to assess degeneration
	Prevention/avoidance	• Selective breeding • Maintain proper weight control	• Selective breeding • Nutritional manipulation for large breed dogs during growth and development • Avoid excessive exercise • Maintain proper weight control

(*Continued*)

Table 6.46 / **Cruciate disease and hip dysplasia (Continued)**

Disease		Cruciate disease (cranial cruciate rupture)	Hip dysplasia
	Complications	• Osteoarthritis • Additional surgery due to meniscal damage	• Osteoarthritis • Non-ambulatory
	Prognosis	• Excellent with surgery, > 85% success rate • Fair without surgery, mostly dependent on dog size	• Good depending on severity of disease and treatment choice
Notes		• Joint is palpated for drawer motion, movement of tibia relative to femur during the tibial compression test, and thickening of joint capsule • 30–40% of canines rupture the opposite cranial cruciate ligament within 17 months • Dogs weighing < 15 kg typically have a 65% recovery rate with cage rest, while dogs > 15 kg often only have a 20% recovery rate • Rehabilitation often requires 2–4 months • Rottweilers and Labrador Retrievers	• Condition is progressive without surgical intervention • Care should be taken to rule out knee involvement before surgical intervention on the hips • Rehabilitation is the key to surgical and long-term success

Osteochondrosis

Osteochondrosis, or osteochondritis dessicans (OCD), is a defect in endochondral ossification leading to an excessive retention of cartilage. This defect may occur in the elbow, shoulder, and knee joints. Ununited anconeal process and fragmented coronoid process may also be seen along with osteochondrosis or separately. It is often seen in animals between 5 and 10 months of age.

Osteomyelitis

Osteomyelitis is an infection of the bone and its soft tissue elements and membranes. Infectious organisms often complicate an existing condition leading to a very difficult, sometimes impossible, infection to treat.

Table 6.47 / **Osteochondrosis and osteomyelitis**

Disease		Osteochondrosis	Osteomyelitis
Presentation	Clinical signs	• Abnormal gait, anorexia, cachexia, forelimb or hindlimb lameness, reluctance to exercise, walking difficulty	• Anorexia, cachexia, depression, exercise intolerance, lameness, lethargy, rising difficulty, weakness
	Exam findings	• Arthritis, crepitus, hyperextension pain, joint effusion, joint pain, muscle atrophy, swelling	• Edema, inflammation, intermittent draining tracts, pain, paralysis, paresis, pyrexia, swelling, tachycardia
Diagnosis	General	• History/clinical signs • Joint palpation	• History/clinical signs • Skeletal palpation • Neurological examination
	Laboratory	• Joint tap and fluid analysis: confirms involvement and mononucleated cells	• CBC: neutrophilic leukocytosis • Urinalysis: ± aspergillosis • Cytology: toxic neutrophils, phagocytized bacteria, or fungal organisms • Culture: bacteria isolation and identification and sensitivity
	Imaging	• Radiographs, skeletal: joint abnormalities, bone lengths, arthritis, sclerosis of underlying bone or bone flap/fragments (joint "mice") • CT/MRI: location and severity of lesion • Arthrogram: identifies cartilage flap or loose cartilage via contrast enhanced joint radiographs after intraarticular injections	• Radiographs, skeletal: soft tissue swelling, bone resorption, sclerosis, bone sequestra, fracture nonunion, cortical thinning, widening of fracture gap, reactive periosteal new bone, foreign bodies, or fungal lesions • Contrast: sinus location and severity, foreign bodies • Radionuclide imaging: detecting osteomyelitis
	Procedures	• Arthroscopy: confirming cartilage lesion	• Fluid aspirates or tissue biopsy
Treatment	General	• Symptomatic • Surgery: arthrotomy or arthroscopy	• Symptomatic • Wound management: debridement, drainage, and irrigation • Surgery: sequestrectomy, amputation, bone grafts, or biopsy
	Medication	• Analgesics • NSAIDs: aspirin, carprofen, deracoxib, etodolac, firocoxib, meloxicam, tepoxalin	• Analgesics • Antibiotics: variable • Antifungals: itraconazole
	Nursing care	• Cryotherapy postoperatively • Place modified Robert Jones bandage • Restricted activity	• Sterile dressing applied to surgical wounds left to close by secondary intention • Irrigate daily with sterile saline • Physical rehabilitation

(*Continued*)

Table 6.47 / **Osteochondrosis and osteomyelitis (Continued)**

Disease		Osteochondrosis	Osteomyelitis
Follow-up	Patient care	• Cryotherapy for 15–20 minutes three times daily for 3–5 days if no bandage placed • Physical rehabilitation: range of movement exercises • Restrict activity for 4 weeks then gradually increase to normal activity over the next 4 weeks • Re-radiograph 4–6 weeks postoperatively • Obesity management	• Monitor radiographs for fracture healing every 4–6 weeks • Repeated bone culture if persistent infection
	Prevention/avoidance	• Selective breeding • Maintain proper weight control • Nutritional manipulation for large-breed dogs during growth and development	• Proper wound and fracture management
	Complications	• Osteoarthritis • Disuse atrophy	• Recurrence and relapse • Limb deformity or impaired function • Neurological disease • Neoplasia
	Prognosis	• Good with early surgical repair (forelimb) • Guarded with stifle or tarsal osteochondrosis	• Good with acute disease • Poor with chronic disease
Notes		• Great Danes, Labrador Retrievers, Newfoundlands, Rottweilers, Bernese Mountain Dogs, English Setters, Old English Sheepdogs	• Saint Bernards, German Shepherds, Labrador Retrievers, Golden Retrievers, and Rottweilers

Panosteitis

Panosteitis is a very painful disease of young large-breed dogs that begins in the medullary bone marrow in the region of the nutrient foramen. Its cause is unknown. It gives intermittent lameness of one or multiple limbs. The disease is self-limiting, but its clinical signs will remain for months.

Patella Luxation

Medial patellar luxation is generally a concern of small-breed dogs. It is typically a congenital or developmental malformation of the stifle joint, which causes the patellar to displace from the femoral trochlea. Luxations are graded on a scale of I–IV, which allows guidance of treatment options.

Table 6.48 / **Panosteitis and patella luxation**

Disease		Panosteitis (enostosis)	Medial patellar luxation
Presentation	Clinical signs	• Anorexia, ataxia, cachexia, depression, forelimb and hind limb lameness, lethargy, shifting leg lameness, walking difficulty	• Abnormal gait, ataxia, intermittent lameness of hind limb, skipping, walking difficulty
	Exam findings	• Pain on palpation of diaphysis, pyrexia	• Arthritis, pain, stifle joint deformity
Diagnosis	General	• History/clinical signs • Bone palpation	• History/clinical signs • Patella palpation: laxity
	Laboratory	• CBC: eosinophilia (variable)	• Cytology, synovial fluid: ↑ mononuclear cells
	Imaging	• Radiograph, skeletal: ↑ density, progressive mottling and radiopacity within the medullary cavity, new bone formation, thickened bone cortices • Scintigrams, bone: bone lesions	• Radiographs, hind limb: bowing and/or torsion of tibia or femur, shape of femoral trochlea, and luxated patella
	Procedures	• Bone biopsy	• Arthrocentesis
Treatment	General	• Supportive	• Supportive • Symptomatic • Surgical: trochleoplasty, trochlear sulcoplasty, recession sulcoplasty, trochlear chondroplasty, chondroplasty, wedge recession, patelloplasty, tibial crest transposition, or tibial tuberosity translocation
	Medication	• Analgesics • Corticosteroids: prednisone • NSAIDs: aspirin, piroxicam, carprofen, etodolac, deracoxib, firocoxib, Galliprant	• Analgesics • Chondroprotective agents: polysulfated glycosaminoglycan (Adequan) or glucosamine with chondroitin sulfate • NSAIDs: aspirin, carprofen, deracoxib, etodolac, piroxicam, Galliprant
	Nursing care	• Treated as outpatient	• Cryotherapy immediately postoperatively then 15–20 minutes daily for 3–5 days if no bandage • Placement of Robert Jones bandage • Physical rehabilitation: range of movement exercises and swimming

(Continued)

Table 6.48 / Panosteitis and patella luxation (Continued)

Disease		Panosteitis (enostosis)	Medial patellar luxation
Follow-up	Patient care	• Restrict activity • Recheck lameness every 2–4 weeks for more serious orthopedic problems	• Restricted activity: leash walk for 4 weeks and prevent jumping • Full exercise by 6–9 months postoperatively • Correct obesity
	Prevention/avoidance	• Not applicable	• Selective breeding • Maintain proper weight control
	Complications	• Not applicable	• Recurrence following surgery • Degenerative joint disease
	Prognosis	• Excellent	• Excellent with surgery
Notes		• Clinical signs may persist for weeks to months and other juvenile orthopedic diseases may develop • Clinical signs may reoccur up to the age of 2 years • German Shepherd, Irish Setter, Saint Bernard, Doberman Pinscher, Airedale, Basset Hound, Miniature Schnauzer	• Miniature and Toy Poodles, Yorkshire Terriers, Pomeranians, Pekingese, Chihuahuas, Boston Terriers

NEUROLOGY

Neurological Examination

See also Skill Box 2.6: Neurological Examination, page 52.

Table 6.49 / Neurological examination

Mentation	• Alert • Lethargic-depressed • Stuporous: responds to painful stimuli • Comatose: no response to painful stimuli
Involuntary movements	• Tremors: intention or resting • Fasciculations • Myoclonus
Posture	• Head tilt • Torticollis: head turn • Wide-based stance • Scoliosis: lateral deviation • Lordosis: sway back • Kyphosis: hunched back • Falling • Decerebrate rigidity: extension of all limbs and trunk • Decerebellate rigidity: thoracic limbs rigid, pelvic limbs flexed • Schiff–Sherrington phenomenon: increased tone of thoracic limbs, flaccid paralysis of pelvic limbs

Gait	• Paresis: weakness
	• Plegia – paralysis:
	  • Mono-one limb
	  • Hemi – one side (e.g. right thoracic and pelvic)
	  • Para – pelvic limbs
	  • Tetra/quadra – all 4 limbs
	• Circling-wide vs. tight circles
	• Ataxia:
	  • Proprioceptive – crossing over of feet, uncoordinated movement of limbs
	  • Vestibular – tight circling, head tilt, falling, rolling
	  • Cerebellar – dysmetria (overflexion of joints or overreaching)

Table 6.49 / Neurological examination (Continued)

Postural reactions	• Proprioception (knuckling; Figure 6.1) • Hopping • Hemi standing/walking • Visual placing • Tactile placing • Extensor postural thrust • Wheelbarrowing
Cranial nerve exam	• Olfaction: CN I • Vision: CN II • Menace response: CN II, VII, forebrain and cerebellum • Pupillary light reflex: CN II, III • Pupil size: anisocoria (mydriasis or miosis) • Horner's signs: miosis, ptosis, elevated third eyelid, enophthalmos • Strabismus: CN III (ventrolateral), IV (outward rotation), VI (medial) • Physiologic nystagmus (doll's eye): CN III, IV, VI, VIII • Pathologic nystagmus: CN VIII, horizontal, rotary, vertical or pendular • Masticatory muscle mass: CN V • Palpebral: CN V, VII • Facial sensation: CN V, ophthalmic, maxillary and mandibular branch • Facial muscles: CN VII • Hearing: CN VIII • Gag reflex/swallowing/voice: CN IX, X, XII • Tongue: CN XII, paralysis, atrophy

Spinal reflexes	• Thoracic limbs:
	  • Triceps: radial n. C7–T2
	  • Biceps: musculocutaneous n. C6–8
	  • Extensor carpi radialis: radial n. C7–T2
	  • Withdrawal: radial, ulnar, median and musculocutaneous C6–T2
	• Pelvic limbs:
	  • Patellar: femoral n. L4–6
	  • Cranial tibial: fibular branch of sciatic n. L6–7
	  • Gastrocnemius: tibial branch of sciatic n. L7–S1
	  • Withdrawal: sciatic n. L6–S1
	• Perineal reflex: pudendal n. S1–S3
	• Cutaneous trunci: lateral thoracic n. C8–T1

(*Continued*)

Table 6.49 / Neurological examination (Continued)

Nociception	• Superficial pain perception • Deep pain perception • Order of functional loss: (i) proprioception, (ii) motor function, (iii) superficial pain, (iv) deep pain
Spinal hyperesthesia	• Cervical • Thoracic • Lumbar • Sacral

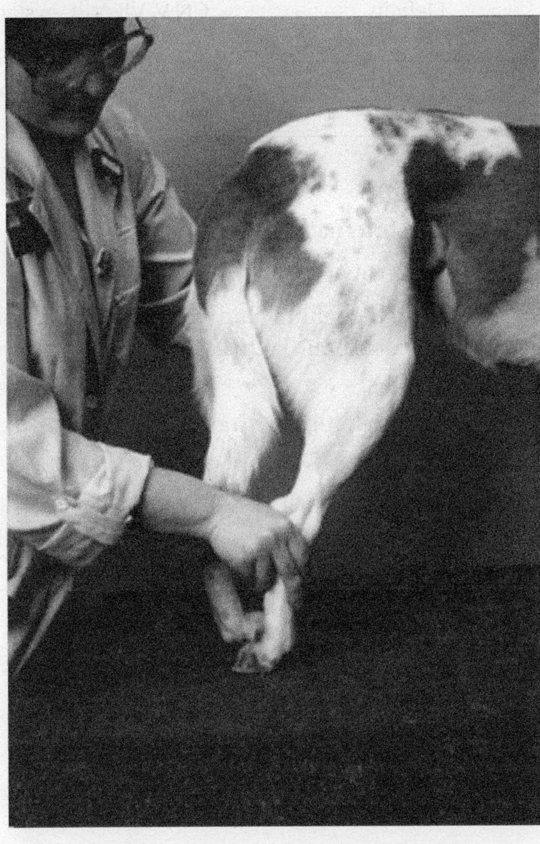

Figure 6.1 Proprioception (knuckling).

Lesion Localization

Table 6.50 / Lesion localization

Neuro RAT	Upper motor neuron	Lower motor neuron
Reflexes	Normal– increased	Decreased – absent
Atrophy	No neurogenic muscle atrophy	Neurogenic muscle atrophy
Tone	Normal – increased	Decreased – absent

Table 6.51 / Localization of lesions in the spinal cord

Spinal cord localization	Thoracic limbs	Pelvic limbs
C1–C5	UMN	LMN
C6–T2	LMN	UMN
T3–L3	Normal	UMN
L4–S3	Normal	LMN

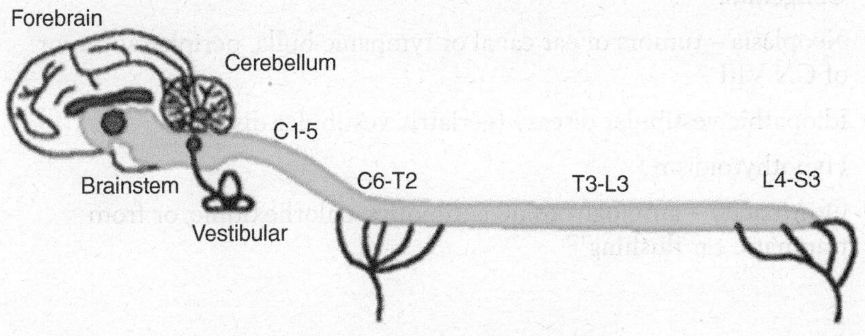

Figure 6.2 Lesion localization.

Table 6.52 / Localization of lesions in the brain

Lesion	Mentation	Posture/gait	Postural reactions	Cranial nerves
Forebrain	Behavior or mentation changes, seizures	• Normal, torticollis toward lesion; Hemi or tetraparesis	Deficits	CN I and II
Brainstem	Mentation changes – depressed, stuporous, comatose	• Normal, falling • Hemi or tetraparesis, ataxia	Deficits	CN III–XII
Peripheral vestibular	Normal	• Head tilt, circling, falling, rolling • Vestibular ataxia	Normal	CN VII, VIII, Horner syndrome, nystagmus
Central vestibular	Normal, depressed	• Head tilt, falling • Hemiparesis, vestibular ataxia	Deficits	CN V, VII, VIII, nystagmus
Cerebellum	Normal	• Normal, decerebellate, intention tremors • Cerebellar ataxia	Normal	Normal, may be decreased menace

Diseases Affecting the Brain

Vestibular Disease

The vestibular system is responsible for maintaining equilibrium and balance. Anatomically, it is divided into peripheral and central systems.

The peripheral system includes the vestibular division of vestibulocochlear nerve (CN VIII) and its receptors in the inner ear. Peripheral vestibular diseases are:

- Congenital
- Neoplasia – tumors of ear canal or tympanic bulla, peripheral tumor of CN VIII
- Idiopathic vestibular disease (geriatric vestibular disease)
- Hypothyroidism
- Ototoxicity – aminoglycoside antibiotics, chlorhexidine, or from traumatic ear flushing[126]
- Otitis media and otitis interna[127]
- Inflammatory polyps in cats.[127]

Central-nuclei located in cerebellum and rostral medulla oblongata with axons projecting to spinal cord, brain stem and cerebellum. Central vestibular diseases are:

- Infectious disease-bacterial, fungal, viral, protozoal, rickettsial and parasitic
- Meningoencephalitis of unknown origin
- Neoplasia – intracranial
- Cerebrovascular accident
- Metronidazole toxicity
- Thiamine deficiency
- Hypothyroidism

Epilepsy

Seizure is a clinical manifestation of abnormal electrical activity in the brain.[128,129] Epilepsy is a disease of the brain characterized by a predisposition to generate epileptic seizures. Practically defined as more than two unprovoked seizures over 24 hours apart.[130] Types of epilepsy are:

1. Idiopathic epilepsy – sub classified into three groups:
    a. Genetic – a causative gene has been identified.
    b. Suspected genetic – a genetic influence is supported.
    c. Unknown cause – the cause is not known; there is no evidence of structural epilepsy.
2. Structural epilepsy – epileptic seizures caused by intracranial pathology.[130]

Table 6.53 / Vestibular disease and epilepsy

Disease		Vestibular disease	Epilepsy
Presentation	Clinical signs	• Peripheral: • Asymmetric ataxia • Loss of balance • No weakness or proprioceptive deficits • Pathologic nystagmus can be horizontal or rotary and does not change direction with head position • Can affect facial nerve • Can cause Horner syndrome[131] • Central: • Altered consciousness • Paresis • Cranial nerve V–XII deficits • Proprioceptive deficits • Nystagmus can be horizontal, rotary or vertical and can change directions with head position131	Three stages of seizures: 1. Aura: period of time before seizure, usually seconds to minutes. Characterized by abnormal behaviors such as agitation, pacing or hiding. Caused by initial abnormal electrical activity in the brain[128] 2. Ictus: the actual seizure. Types of seizures: • Focal epileptic seizure – motor, autonomic and/or behavior signs that are regionalized. Any part of body can be involved depending on the area of the brain that is affected.[128] Signs indicate a specific region of the brain is affected. May be conscious or not during seizure. • Motor-ex: facial twitching, jerking head movements, rhythmic blinking.[130] • Autonomic – ex: hypersalivation or vomiting[130] • Behavioral – ex: anxiousness, restlessness, fear[130] • Generalized epileptic seizure – bilateral involvement; may be: • Tonic – muscle rigidity only • Tonic–clonic (most common) – muscle rigidity followed by rhythmic contraction of muscles (usually paddling of limbs and chewing with mouth); usually loses consciousness[128] • Atonic (rare) – sudden loss of muscle tone • Focal epileptic seizure evolving to generalized – starts in localized area of brain but spreads to involve both hemispheres[130] • Post-ictus – period immediately following ictus, lasting minutes to hours, behavioral changes, weakness, blindness, hungry, thirsty, depressed, pacing, or tired

(*Continued*)

Table 6.53 / Vestibular disease and epilepsy (Continued)

<table>
<tr><th>Disease</th><th></th><th>Vestibular disease</th><th>Epilepsy</th></tr>
<tr><td></td><td>Exam findings</td><td>• Peripheral:
  • Mentation: normal. May be disoriented
  • Posture/gait: head tilt (toward lesion),[131] vestibular ataxia
  • Proprioception: normal
  • Cranial nerves: pathologic nystagmus (horizontal or rotary – fast phase away from lesion)[129], positional strabismus
• Central:
  • Mentation – normal to comatose
  • Posture/gait – head tilt (to either side),[131] vestibular ataxia
  • Proprioception – deficits ipsilateral to lesion[131]
  • Cranial nerves: pathologic nystagmus (horizontal, rotary or vertical and may change direction with head position),[131] deficits of cranial nerves V–XII ipsilateral to lesion[131]</td><td>• Idiopathic epilepsy – physical and neurological exams are normal during interictal period
• Structural epilepsy – neurological exam findings dependent upon area of structural abnormality. May include cranial nerve deficits, proprioceptive deficits, behavioral/mentation changes and gait/posture abnormalities.
• If questioning whether deficits are due to postictal period, repeat exam in 24–48 hours[128,129]</td></tr>
<tr><td>Diagnosis</td><td>General</td><td>• History, signalment, clinical signs and neurological examination findings combined with laboratory tests and diagnostic imaging</td><td>• Idiopathic epilepsy diagnosis based on age of onset, lack of interictal abnormalities and exclusion of other causes[128]
• Structural epilepsy considered when seizures start before 1 or after 5 years of age, if patient has focal seizures, acute onset of multiple seizures, or if interictal abnormalities are detected[128]
• Historical findings
• Important history questions to ask owner:[129]
  • Age of the patient at first episode?
  • Time of day when episode occurred?
  • Any precipitating event (ex: exercise, sleep, etc.)?
  • Complete description of episode
  • Preictal, ictal and postictal
  • Muscle tone
  • Lateralized signs
  • Eye movements
  • Posture
  • Any autonomic signs (salivation, urination, defecation)?
  • Duration of episode?
  • Any behavior or other changes in between episodes?
  • Frequency of episodes?
  • Any family history of seizures?
  • Environment (indoor/outdoor, exposure to toxins)?
  • Any history of trauma?
  • Vaccination status
• Neurological exam: goal is to rule out signs of a structural brain lesion. If needed, repeat exam in 24–48 hours to rule out post-ictus as cause of exam findings[128,129]</td></tr>
</table>

(Continued)

Table 6.53 / **Vestibular disease and epilepsy (Continued)**

Disease		Vestibular disease	Epilepsy
	Laboratory	• CBC • Serum chemistry • Urinalysis	• CBC • Serum chemistry • Test for metabolic or endocrine disorders if indicated • Test for toxins if indicated
	Imaging	• Thoracic and abdominal radiographs and ultrasound – to look for metastatic lesions as well as evidence of infectious disease • CT – to evaluate external, middle or inner ear • MRI – to evaluate external, middle or inner ear as well as brain. Modality of choice for central disease	• Thoracic and abdominal radiographs and ultrasound – to look for metastatic lesions. • MRI – gold standard diagnostic imaging modality for brain.
	Procedures	• CSF – if safe and necessary based on imaging findings • Myringotomy – for otitis media interna; samples submitted for cytology and culture[131]	• CSF – if safe based on imaging findings

Treatment	General	• Treatment depends on the cause of vestibular signs
		• Idiopathic vestibular disease – supportive and symptomatic care
		• Metronidazole toxicity – discontinue metronidazole and supportive care. Diazepam
		• Inflammatory polyps – removal of polyp
		• Neoplasia – (treatment depends on type and location of neoplasia) surgery, radiation therapy
		• Otitis media/interna – if refractory to medical therapy or recurrent may require total ear canal ablation and bulla osteotomy[126]
			• Antiepileptic drug therapy initiated if:
			  • > 1 seizure/month
			  • History of cluster seizures or status epilepticus
			  • Seizure or postictal period considered severe
			  • Owner wants to treat despite frequency or severity
			• Client education is important:
			  • Goal is control, not cure
			  • Antiepileptic drug therapy is usually lifelong
			  • Do not miss doses of medications
			  • Patient will require visits to veterinarian every 6 months

Treatment	Medication	• Maropitant citrate: for nausea
		• Sedatives may be indicated if patient is severely disoriented
		• Hypothyroidism: thyroid hormone supplementation
		• Metronidazole toxicity: diazepam (0.5 mg/kg IV once, then 0.5 mg/kg PO q8h for 3 days) may speed recovery[132]
		• Neoplasia: palliative treatment with prednisone 0.5–1 mg/kg/day orally[131]
		• Otitis media/interna: 6–8 weeks of antibiotics dependent upon culture/sensitivity results[126]
			• Benzodiazepines (used for isolated or cluster seizures, and status epilepticus):
			  • Diazepam
			  • Dose: 0.5–1 mg/kg[133]
			  • Routes of administration: IV, IN, rectal
			  • Inactivated by light and adheres to plastic
			  • Midazolam
			  • Dose: 0.2–0.5 mg/kg[133]
			  • Routes of administration: IN, IM, IV, rectal
			  • Clorazepate
			  • Dose: 2–4 mg/kg orally every 12 hours for 3 days after initial seizure
			  • Used to prevent cluster seizures

(*Continued*)

Table 6.53 / **Vestibular disease and epilepsy (Continued)**

Disease	Vestibular disease	Epilepsy
		• Phenobarbital: • Dogs: 2.5–3 mg/kg every 12 hours • Cats: 1.5–2.5 mg/kg every 12 hours • Routes of administration: IV, IM or orally • Time to steady state concentration: 10–14 days • Route of elimination: hepatic • Adverse effects: sedation, ataxia, polyuria/polydipsia, hepatotoxicity, bone marrow suppression, hyperexitability[133] • Potassium bromide (KBr): • Dogs: 30 mg/kg every 24 hours • Cats: not recommended due to adverse respiratory problems • Routes of administration: oral • Time to steady state concentration: 100–200 days • Route of elimination: renal • Adverse effects: sedation, ataxia, vomiting, polyuria/polydipsia, polyphagia, pancreatitis[133] • Levetiracetam: • Dogs: 20 mg/kg every 8 hours (extended release form can be given every 12 hours) • Cats: 20 mg/kg every 8 hours • Routes of administration: oral, IV • Time to steady-state concentration: 1 day • Route of elimination: primarily renal, some enzymatic hydrolysis • Adverse effects: sedation, ataxia[133]Zonisamide: • Dogs: 5–10 mg/kg every 12 hours • Cats: 5 mg/kg every 12–24 hours • Routes of administration: oral • Time to steady state concentration:3–7 days • Route of elimination: hepatic • Adverse effects: sedation, ataxia, anorexia, vomiting, diarrhea[133]
Nursing care	• Dependent upon cause of vestibular signs	• Monitor for seizures and adverse effects of medications

(Continued)

Table 6.53 / **Vestibular disease and epilepsy (Continued)**

Disease		Vestibular disease	Epilepsy
Follow-up	Patient care	• Dependent upon cause of vestibular signs • Soft, padded cage if circling/rolling	• Monitor phenobarbital levels 2 weeks post-initiation or dose change and every 6 months thereafter • Therapeutic serum concentration: 15–35 μg/ml[134] • Monitor KBr levels 6–12 weeks post-initiation or dose change then every 12 months, or if toxicity is suspected • Therapeutic serum concentration: as combination therapy with phenobarbital – 810–2500 μg/ml, as monotherapy – up to 3000 μg/ml[134] • Monitor zonisamide levels 1–2 weeks post-initiation or dose change • Therapeutic serum concentration: 10–40 μg/ml[134] • Maintain a seizure log • Maintain a steady salt level in diet when giving KBr
	Prevention/avoidance	• Not applicable	• Castrate affected animals • Maintain antiepileptic medications
	Complications	• Otitis media/interna – rarely infection can spread causing central vestibular signs[127]	• Medication adverse effects • Status epilepticus – seizure lasting > 5 minutes or repeated seizures with failure to return to normal within 30 minutes
	Prognosis	• Dependent upon cause of vestibular signs • Idiopathic vestibular disease – good. Improvement seen within several days. Resolution of clinical signs within 3–4 weeks[126] • Metronidazole toxicity – good. Recovery within 1–11 days[131] • Neoplasia – dependent upon tumor type and location • Otitis media/interna – improvement usually seen within 1–2 weeks[126] • Cerebrovascular accident – prognosis usually good but is worse if predisposing condition is found[127] • Inflammatory polyps – excellent when polyp is removed[127]	• Idiopathic epilepsy – good with proper management • Structural epilepsy – dependent upon underlying cause
Notes		• Residual head tilt or facial paralysis is possible in patients treated for otitis media/interna	• Many seizures occur while sleeping or at rest, often at night or in early morning

Meningoencephalomyelitis of Unknown Origin

Meningoencephalomyelitis of unknown origin encompasses all non-infectious inflammatory central nervous system diseases, including:

- Granulomatous meningoencephalomyelitis
- Necrotizing meningoencephalitis (NME)
- Necrotizing leukoencephalitis (NLE).

NME and NLE have similar clinical signs, signalment and neuropathology, thus both are referred to as necrotizing encephalitis.

Table 6.54 / Meningoencephalomyelitis of unknown origin

Disease		Meningoencephalomyelitis of unknown origin (MUO)
Presentation	Clinical signs	• Clinical signs are reflective of area of CNS that is affected • GME – multifocal, focal or ocular forms. Clinical signs consistent with forebrain, brainstem or spinal cord lesions • Multifocal – acute, rapidly progressive. Commonly have forebrain and brainstem signs[135]Focal – slowly progressive. More commonly has forebrain signs alone[135] • Ocular – acute onset visual deficits due to optic neuritis. Uveitis also possible[136] • Necrotizing encephalitis – rapidly progressive. Forebrain and brainstem signs including seizures, mentation changes, vestibulocerebellar signs, visual deficits and death[137]
	Exam findings	• Signalment – can be any dog but small-breed females between age of 3–7 years most common[137] • NME – originally reported in Pugs but has been found in many breeds. • NLE – seen in Yorkshire Terriers[138] and French Bulldogs[139] • Neurological exam findings dependent upon area of CNS involved
Diagnosis	General	• Need to rule out infectious diseases based on geographic area • Neospora caninum, Cryptococcus spp., Ehrlichia spp., Anaplasma spp., Rickettsia rickettsia, *Coccidioides immitis*
	Laboratory	• CSF analysis – pleocytosis (> 50% mononuclear cells) and increased protein concentration[140]
	Imaging	• CT • GME – focal or multifocal, mass effect from edema and granuloma, ventricular asymmetry. Lesions may be difficult to see on CT[137] • Necrotizing encephalitis – multifocal hypoattenuation, no mass effect, no contrast enhancement[137] • MRI – gold standard imaging modality. Single, multiple or diffuse hyperintense intra-axial lesions on T2 weighted images[140]
	Procedures	• CSF tap • Brain biopsy – for definitive diagnosis. Using minimally invasive techniques such as CT- or MRI-guided stereotactic systems

(*Continued*)

Table 6.54 / Meningoencephalomyelitis of unknown origin (Continued)

Disease		Meningoencephalomyelitis of unknown origin (MUO)

Treatment	General	• Initial treatment may require stabilization consisting of:
		  • Oxygen for hypoxemia
		  • Fluid therapy for cerebral perfusion and hypotension
		  • Osmotic therapy (mannitol, hypertonic saline) for elevated intracranial pressure[137]
		• Goal of therapy is remission with minimal adverse effects

	Medication	• Immunosuppression • Corticosteroids (prednisone) – initially at anti-inflammatory dose (0.25–0.5 mg/kg orally every 24 hours) until results of infectious disease tests back, then increase to immunosuppressive dose (2–4 mg/kg orally every 24 hours) for 2–4 weeks, then gradually taper every 4 weeks when clinical signs are stable or improved[137] • Relapses are common. To maintain remission, many require other immunosuppressive drugs to avoid long-term corticosteroid therapy • Cytosine arabinoside – can give at 200 mg/m² as an IV infusion over 8 hours, or give 50 mg/m² SQ every 12 hours for 2 days. Repeat dose every 3 weeks for 4 cycles, then lengthen treatment interval by 1 week every 4 cycles with a maximum interval of 6–8 weeks[137] • Cyclosporine – 3–15 mg/kg orally every 12 hours[137] • Azathioprine – 2 mg/kg orally every 24 hours for two weeks, then decrease to 2 mg/kg every 48 hours. Goal is to alternate days with prednisone dose[137] • If patient is having seizures, they will also require antiepileptic medication
	Nursing care	• If elevated intracranial pressure – monitoring vitals, keep head elevated without compressing jugular veins. *No* jugular blood draws
Follow-up	Patient care	• Seizure monitoring • Monitoring for adverse effects of corticosteroids
	Prevention/avoidance	• Not applicable
	Complications	• Adverse effects of corticosteroid administration include polyuria, polydipsia, polyphagia, weakness, alopecia, thin skin, hypertension, hyperpigmentation, steroid hepatopathy and suppression of hypothalamic pituitary–adrenal axis[141]
	Prognosis	• Not well characterized • Dogs presenting with seizures have reduced survival time[142] • 15% of dogs with GME die before treatment is initiated[140] • Longer disease duration associated with longer survival time

Diseases Affecting the Spinal Cord

Intervertebral Disc Disease

Intervertebral disc disease is classified into two main types: Hansen types 1 and 2. A further type is acute non-compressive nucleus pulposus extrusion (ANNPE).

Hansen type I is chondroid metaplasia of the nucleus pulposus. The loss of glycosaminoglycans, increase in collagen and decrease in water results in decreased elasticity and ability to withstand pressure.[141] There is extrusion of nucleus pulposus into the spinal canal.

With Hansen type II there is fibrous metaplasia – fibrous collagenization of the nucleus pulposus with degeneration of annulus fibrosus.[142] There is protrusion of annulus fibrosus into the spinal canal.

In ANNPE, there is abrupt extrusion of non-degenerate nucleus pulposus into the spinal canal, which causes a spinal cord contusion but no compression.[143]

Fibrocartilaginous Embolism

In fibrocartilaginous embolism, fibrocartilaginous material, histochemically similar to the nucleus pulposus of an intervertebral disc, is found in the arterioles and veins of the meninges and the spinal cord, causing an ischemic necrotizing myelopathy. How this material makes its way into the circulation is unknown. The cause of the disease is also unknown.

Table 6.55 / Intervertebral disc disease and fibrocartilaginous embolism

Disease		Intervertebral disc disease (IVDD)	Fibrocartilaginous embolism (FCE)
Presentation	Clinical signs	• Hansen type I: • Chondrodystrophic breeds (e.g. Dachshund, Shih Tzu, Beagle) • Acute onset; progressive • Clinical signs vary from spinal hyperesthesia only to paresis or plegia • Clinical signs depend on site of disc extrusion and degree of compression/contusion. • Hansen type II: • Non-chondrodystrophic breeds (e.g. German Shepherd, Labrador Retriever) • Slowly progressive • Clinical signs vary from spinal hyperesthesia only to paresis or plegia • Clinical signs depend on site of disc protrusion and degree of compression • ANNPE: • Any breed can be affected but older large breeds are common[146] • Peracute onset. Often associated with running or trauma. Non-progressive after first 24 hours • Often severe neurological deficits and commonly lateralized signs[146] • May vocalize at onset of clinical signs but not severely painful thereafter[146]	• Common in non-chondrodystrophic breeds • Miniature Schnauzers, German Shepherds, Labrador Retrievers • Acute onset. Non-progressive. Maximum neurological deficits within 24 hours of onset[147] • Commonly present following episode of exercise • May be painful initially, but no spinal hyperesthesia noted after the first 24 hours • Clinical signs depend on location of infarct and severity of ischemia • Many times clinical signs are asymmetrical • Most common presentation is acute onset of asymmetric paraparesis

(*Continued*)

Table 6.55 / **Intervertebral disc disease and fibrocartilaginous embolism (Continued)**

Disease		Intervertebral disc disease (IVDD)	Fibrocartilaginous embolism (FCE)

	Exam findings	• Neurological exam findings dependent upon site of disc extrusion/protrusion and severity of contusion/compression. Signs progress in order of spinal hyperesthesia only to: (i) loss of general proprioception; (ii) loss of voluntary motor function; and (iii) loss of pain perception. Loss of bladder function usually occurs when patient becomes paraplegic[148]
		Clinical signs may be asymmetric:
		• Paresis (weakness), plegia (paralysis)
		• -Para – hind limbs; mono – one limb; hemi – both limbs of one side; tetra/quadra – all 4 limbs
		• -Proprioceptive ataxia – incoordination and loss of awareness of foot placement
		• Decreased – absent conscious proprioception
		• Spinal reflexes – may have upper motor neuron (UMN = normal-increased reflexes) or lower motor neuron (LMN = decreased-absent reflexes) signs depending on site of disc extrusion/protrusion
		  • C1-C5: UMN all 4 limbs
		  • C6-T2: LMN to thoracic limbs, UMN to pelvic limbs
		  • T3-L3: normal cranial to T3, UMN to pelvic limbs
		  • L4-S2: normal cranial to L4, LMN to pelvic limbs
		• Cutaneous trunci – may be absent caudal to the lesion
		• Pain perception – test for pain perception if patient is plegic
		• Spinal hyperesthesia
			• Neurological exam findings dependent upon site and severity of infarct
			• Cutaneous trunci may be absent caudal to the lesion
			• Pain perception – test for pain perception if patient is plegic
			• No spinal hyperesthesia

Diagnosis	General	• There are many other diseases that can mimic IVDD, so complete diagnostic evaluation is required for definitive diagnosis	• Antemortem diagnosis based on history, clinical signs and ruling out other causes
	Laboratory	• CBC/chemistry/urinalysis – minimum database • CSF analysis – may have pleocytosis and/or increased protein concentration[149]	• CBC/chemistry/urinalysis – minimum database • CSF analysis – not diagnostic for FCE but may rule out other causes

(Continued)

Table 6.55 / **Intervertebral disc disease and fibrocartilaginous embolism (Continued)**

Disease		Intervertebral disc disease (IVDD)	Fibrocartilaginous embolism (FCE)
	Imaging	• Radiographs – to rule out other differentials such as neoplasia, fractures or discospondylitis • May see narrowing of disc space or intervertebral foramen or mineralized disc material • Not able to distinguish exact location of disc extrusion on radiography • Myelography – injection of contrast medium into subarachnoid space. Thinning or deviation of the contrast column is suggestive of extradural compression. Axial deviation of contrast column required to determine lateralization[143] • CT – used with myelography or alone. Better for determining lateralization of lesion. Great for imaging bone, not modality of choice for soft tissue • MRI – gold standard modality for discs, spinal cord and associated structures	• Radiographs – within normal limits • Myelography – usually within normal limits • CT – within normal limits but may exclude other causes • MRI – gold standard modality. Focal, hyperintense, intramedullary lesions on T2 weighted images with varying degrees of contrast enhancement[150]
	Procedures	• CSF tap – if myelogram will be performed and CSF is needed, perform CSF tap first	• CSF tap
Treatment	General	• Conservative treatment – strict cage rest, pain medications and physical rehabilitation • Indicated if mild neurological deficits (i.e. patient is ambulatory), if owners have financial concerns or if patient has other medical conditions preventing surgery • Surgical treatment – decompressive procedures, such as hemilaminectomy, dorsal laminectomy and ventral slot • Indicated if refractory to conservative management, if progressive or if patient has severe neurological deficits (i.e. patient is non-ambulatory)	• Treatment is supportive care and physical rehabilitation
	Medication	• Prednisone – 0.25–0.5 mg/kg every 12 hours for 72 hours, then gradually taper[148] • NSAIDs – *not* combined with corticosteroids. Must have 72 hour "wash out" period in between if it has been on corticosteroids • Tramadol • Owners must understand that cage rest is the most important aspect of conservative management so dogs must stay confined even if pain is under control	• Corticosteroids controversial – goal is to reduce inflammation and edema, however, one study showed no positive effects with corticosteroid administration[151]
	Nursing care	• Careful handling of patients to protect the spine • Monitor for worsening neurological status • Monitor urine output – may require bladder catheterization or expression to void completely • Turn recumbent patients every 4 hours and keep well padded to prevent decubital ulcers and pulmonary edema	• Physical rehabilitation has been shown to have a positive effect on recovery[152] • Physical rehabilitation plan should be tailored to each patient. Recommend referral to a certified canine rehabilitation specialist

(*Continued*)

Table 6.55 / **Intervertebral disc disease and fibrocartilaginous embolism (Continued)**

Disease		Intervertebral disc disease (IVDD)	Fibrocartilaginous embolism (FCE)
Follow-up	Patient care	• Strict kennel rest for 6–8 weeks • Physical rehabilitation – recommend referring to a certified rehabilitation specialist for recommendations • Monitor for urinary tract infections • Use a harness instead of a collar for cervical disc disease	• Rest • Turn recumbent patients every 4 hours and keep well padded to prevent decubital ulcers and pulmonary edema • May require bladder catheterization or manual expression if unable to voluntarily urinate
	Prevention/avoidance	• Maintain ideal body condition	• Not applicable
	Complications	• Myelograms – up to 10% of patients have post-myelographic seizures[153]	• Not applicable
	Prognosis	• Pain perception is the most important prognostic indicator • If a patient has intact pain perception, usually has excellent prognosis with surgery • If patient does not have deep pain sensation but has surgery within 24 hours, prognosis ranges from 47 to 76%[148] • If patient does not have deep pain sensation for longer than 48 hours prognosis drops to less than 5%[148] • If deep pain sensation returns within two weeks post-op patient has good prognosis for functional recovery[148]	• If have LMN deficits or loss of deep pain perception prognosis is poor[147] • If UMN deficits have better prognosis • If patient has intact deep pain perception, prognosis is good • Animals with functional recovery within 2 weeks have better prognosis

Cervical Spondylomyelopathy (Wobbler Disease)

Cervical spondylomyelopathy (CSM) is referred to by 14 different names, the most common being cervical spondylomyelopathy, cervical spondylopathy, cervical vertebral malformation-malarticulation and cervical vertebral stenotic myelopathy. The disease is caused by dynamic and static compression of the spinal cord, nerve roots or both, which leads to a variable degrees of neurological deficits and cervical pain.

There are two types of CSM:

- Disc associated – mostly ventral compression caused by intervertebral disc degeneration and protrusion, which may be asymmetric or symmetric. There may also be dorsal compressions caused by vertebral canal stenosis or hypertrophy of ligamentum flavum. The most common sites affected are C5–6 and C6–7.[154] This type is osseus associated.
- Severe vertebral canal stenosis – compression caused by a combination of vertebral malformations and osteoarthritic changes.[155]

Degenerative Myelopathy

Degenerative myelopathy is an insidious, progressive loss of spinal cord function, involving primarily axonal degeneration. The disease starts at T3–L3 but progresses to affect lower motor neurons as well. The disease is histopathologically confirmed in many breeds, including the Pembroke Welsh Corgi, German Shepherd and Boxer.

Table 6.56 / Cervical spondylomyelopathy and degenerative myelopathy

Disease		Cervical spondylomyelopathy	Degenerative myelopathy
Presentation	Clinical signs	• Disc associated: middle-aged large-breed dogs; most common in Doberman Pinschers • Osseus associated: young adult giant-breed dogs; most common in Great Danes • Chronic progressive history	• Mean age of onset: 9 years in large breeds,[156] 11 years in Pembroke Welsh Corgis[157] • Progressive, asymmetric paraparesis and pelvic limb proprioceptive ataxia with no spinal hyperesthesia[158] • Progresses to cause LMN signs in the pelvic limbs and eventually the thoracic limbs
	Exam findings	• Proprioceptive ataxia in all 4 limbs. Pelvic limbs may be more severe than thoracic limbs • C1–5 lesion • "Floating" gait – long strided in all 4 limbs • Normal to increased spinal reflexes in all 4 limbs • C6–T2 lesion • "Two engine" gait – short and choppy in thoracic limbs, long strided in the pelvic limbs • Decreased to absent spinal reflexes in thoracic limbs, normal to increased in pelvic limbs • Para- or tetraparesis • Varies from mild paresis to non-ambulatory • Cervical spinal hyperesthesia	• Early disease: mild spastic paraparesis and proprioceptive ataxia of the pelvic limbs. May be asymmetric[158] • Spinal reflexes consistent with T3–L3 localization (normal-increased) • Late disease: progresses to LMN paraplegia (decreased-absent spinal reflexes, decreased muscle tone and muscle atrophy) and ascends to affect the thoracic limbs.[158] Will eventually cause a flaccid tetraplegia.
Diagnosis	General	• Not applicable	• Definitive diagnosis by postmortem histopathology only • Presumptive diagnosis based on history, clinical signs and diagnostics to rule out other causes • Other diseases that may mimic degenerative myelopathy: intervertebral disc disease, neoplasia and lumbosacral disease

	Laboratory	• Large breeds may have concurrent medical conditions precluding anesthesia and/or surgery so would require other tests in addition to minimum database such as:
		  • Thyroid function – for hypothyroidism
		  • Buccal mucosal bleeding time – for von Willebrand factor
		  • Electrocardiogram and echocardiogram – for dilated cardiomyopathy
			• SOD-1 mutation genetic test
			• Normal homozygotes are unlikely to develop degenerative myelopathy, will pass on protective allele to offspring
			• Heterozygotes are carriers, unlikely to develop degenerative myelopathy but can pass on mutant allele to half of their offspring
			• At-risk homozygotes are at risk of developing degenerative myelopathy, and will pass on one chromosome with mutant allele to offspring
			• CSF analysis – to rule out infectious disease

(Continued)

Table 6.56 / **Cervical spondylomyelopathy and degenerative myelopathy (Continued)**

Disease		Cervical spondylomyelopathy	Degenerative myelopathy
	Imaging	• Spinal radiographs – may see narrowing of disc space, changes to anatomy of vertebral bodies, osteoarthritic changes or vertebral canal stenosis[155] • Myelography – can define site and direction of compression. May also perform traction views to distinguish if lesion is static or dynamic[159] • CT – fast and can get transverse images. Usually used in combination with myelography. Better visualization of direction and severity of compression as well as better identification of most affected site[155] • MRI – gold standard modality. Main advantage is to visualize signal changes within the spinal cord. This allows better identification of affected site[155]	• Myelogram, CT or MRI – to rule out a compressive spinal cord disease. MRI is the gold standard
	Procedures	• Not applicable	• Electrodiagnostics – normal in early stages of disease, in later disease stage will see multifocal spontaneous activity on electromyography as well as decreased nerve conduction velocities[160] • Histopathology – axon and myelin degeneration of the spinal cord[158]
Treatment	General	• Conservative treatment • Exercise restriction – leash walk only, with harness instead of collar • Corticosteroids – anti-inflammatory dose of prednisone (0.5–1 mg/kg every 12–24 hours)[155] • Physical rehabilitation • Surgical treatment • 21 proposed surgical techniques • Direct decompressive techniques – used for static compressions. Dorsal laminectomy, ventral slot, hemilaminectomy • Indirect decompressive techniques – used for dynamic compressions. Distraction-stabilization – bone grafts, pins, screws, PMMA	• Physical rehabilitation may increase survival times[161] • Rehabilitation should begin at the first sign of disease • Controlled exercises – such as underwater treadmill, passive range of motion and other therapeutic exercises • Do not fatigue! • Rehabilitation plan should be designed by certified canine rehabilitation personnel
	Medication	• Prednisone 0.5–1 mg/kg every 12–24 hours	• None have been shown to slow disease progression
	Nursing care	• Care of non-ambulatory patient • Rotate sides every 4 hours and keep on dry, padded bedding	• Care of non-ambulatory patient in later disease stages

(Continued)

Table 6.56 / **Cervical spondylomyelopathy and degenerative myelopathy (Continued)**

Disease		Cervical spondylomyelopathy	Degenerative myelopathy
Follow-up	Patient care	• Physical rehabilitation – plan tailored to each individual patient. Recommend referral to a certified canine rehabilitation professional	• Assisted physical rehabilitation exercises • Bladder management in later disease stages may include manual expression or catheterization
	Prevention/avoidance	• Not applicable	• Not applicable
	Complications	• Surgical complications – postoperative worsening of neurologic status, implant failure, and death	• Decubital ulcers • Fecal and urine incontinence
	Prognosis	• Conservative treatment • Clinical signs either improved or stable in 81% of dogs managed medically[162] • Surgical treatment • About 80% of dogs improve after surgery[162] • Surgery leads to clinical improvement more consistently so should always be considered[155]	• Poor
Notes			• Wheelchair support may be desirable if the patient progresses to non-ambulatory

Discospondylitis

Discospondylitis is an infection of the intervertebral disc and adjacent vertebral bodies, usually by arterial spread from other infected areas of the body such as urinary tract, skin, mouth or heart.[163] The disease is usually bacterial but can be fungal or algal.

Steroid-Responsive Meningitis Arteritis

Steroid-responsive meningitis arteritis is immune mediated and is a combined meningitis and arteritis of leptomeningeal vessels.[164] It may occur together with immune-mediated polyarthritis.[165] There are two forms:

- Acute – the more common form, characterised by cervical rigidity, pain, pyrexia and polymorphonuclear pleocytosis of the cerebrospinal fluid.[164]
- Chronic – the less common form, which includes other neurological deficits and mononuclear pleocytosis of the cerebrospinal fluid.[164]

Table 6.57 / **Discospondylitis and steroid-responsive meningitis arteritis**

Disease		Discospondylitis	Steroid Responsive Meningitis Arteritis (SRMA)
Presentation	Clinical signs	• Most common in large breeds, middle-aged, males more than females[166] • Chronic, progressive • Spinal pain is the most common clinical sign. May also see fever, lethargy, anorexia, pelvic limb ataxia or paresis[148]	• May be seen in any breed but more common in Boxers, Beagles, Bernese Mountain Dogs, Weimaraners and Nova Scotia Duck Tolling Retrievers[164] • Typical age of onset 6–18 months[164] • Acute form: severe cervical hyperesthesia, depression, stiff gait and fever • Chronic form: relapse; variable degrees of paresis and ataxia, other cranial nerve deficits with severe disease[164]
	Exam findings	• Gait – may be stiff, paretic or ataxic • Spinal hyperesthesia • Signs of urinary tract infection or endocarditis • Systemic signs such as anorexia or pyrexia	• Severe cervical hyperesthesia, may have kyphosis and neck guarding • Fever • Lethargy • Paresis and ataxia – chronic form • Cranial nerve deficits – menace, anisocoria, strabismus – chronic form
Diagnosis	General	• Not applicable	• Not applicable
	Laboratory	• CBC – may have leukocytosis associated with endocarditis[148] • CSF – usually normal. May have elevated protein and mononuclear cells. • Blood cultures – positive results in about 45–75% of cases[148] • Urine culture – positive in about 25–50% of cases[148] • Staphylococcus pseudintermedius most common bacteria • Brucella – tube agglutination test. Confirm with IFA or PCR testing[148]	• Bloodwork – may have neutrophilia with left shift, increased erythrocyte sedimentation rate and elevated alpha2-globulin fraction[167] • CSF – increase in protein and neutrophils. Increased IgA concentrations
	Imaging	• Radiographs – usually diagnostic. Lysis of vertebral end plates and adjacent vertebral bodies. Collapse of intervertebral disc space[168] • Radiographic evidence of disease lags behind clinical signs by 2–3 weeks, so will need advanced imaging or repeat radiographs at later date if strongly suspected but not seen on radiographs[148] • CT – can identify osseous lesions sooner than radiography. Findings are similar to what is seen on radiographs[168] • MRI – modality of choice in humans. May identify sites not seen on radiographs[168]	• Not applicable
	Procedures	• Needle aspiration of lesion using fluoroscopy as a guide to obtain sample for culture	• Not applicable

(*Continued*)

Table 6.57 / Discospondylitis and steroid-responsive meningitis arteritis (Continued)

Disease		Discospondylitis	Steroid Responsive Meningitis Arteritis (SRMA)
Treatment	General	• Usually antibiotic therapy and pain medications alone. If severe spinal cord compression, or if not responding to therapy after 5 days will require surgery to decompress and stabilize[148]	• Not applicable
	Medication	• Antibiotics depending on culture/sensitivity results of blood/urine/infected tissue. Course of antibiotics should be at least 8 weeks[163] • Pain medications • NSAIDs for 3–5 days[163] • Avoid corticosteroids	• Prednisone 2–4 mg/kg every 24 hours • When clinical signs are controlled, dose is reduced by half. Dose is then gradually reduced over months until discontinued • Relapse is common is dose is too low or discontinued[148] • If not responding to prednisone alone, may require secondary immunosuppressant
	Nursing care	• Kennel rest for 6–8 weeks	• Avoid manipulation of the neck
Follow-up	Patient care	• Dogs with *Brucella canis* should be neutered	• CSF may be used to monitor response to therapy. When CSF values normalize, corticosteroid dose may be gradually reduced[164]
	Prevention/avoidance	• Not applicable	• Not applicable
	Complications	• Pathologic fracture or luxation • Owners should be made aware of zoonotic potential of *B. canis*	• Relapse if corticosteroid dose is too low or discontinued
	Prognosis	• If minimal neurologic deficits – good • If severe neurologic deficits – guarded • *B. canis* often responds to treatment but may reoccur and warrants periodic treatment[163] • Fungal infections commonly reoccur[163]	• Fair to good, especially in acute disease that is treated early[164]

Diseases Affecting the Peripheral Nervous System

Myasthenia Gravis

Myasthenia gravis is a disease of the neuromuscular junction.

Acquired myasthenia gravis is immune mediated. Autoantibodies against nicotinic acetylcholine receptors (AChR) of skeletal muscle result in decreased number of functional receptors. This reduces the probability that acetylcholine molecules will bind with the receptors and results in failure of neuromuscular transmission. The motor nerve ending repetitively fires, but the available receptors are soon bound with acetylcholine and further stimulation is prohibited. This results in fatigue and muscle weakness.[148]

Congenital myasthenia gravis is rare. In this form, there is a deficiency of AChR, but no autoimmunity.

Polyradiculoneuritis

Polyradiculoneuritis (also known as Coonhound paralysis) is the most common acute polyneuropathy in dogs.[169] It is seen mostly in dogs with raccoon exposure, but is also seen in those with no raccoon exposure. The disease is very similar to Guillain–Barré syndrome in humans, and is immune mediated. Segmental demyelination and axonal degeneration of ventral (motor) nerve roots and spinal nerves.

Table 6.58 / Myasthenia gravis and polyradiculoneuritis

Disease		Myasthenia gravis	Polyradiculoneuritis (Coonhound paralysis)

Presentation	Clinical signs	• Episodic muscle weakness that becomes worse with exercise and megaesophagus are most common signs in dogs[170]
		• 3 forms:
		  • Focal: megaesophagus with or without facial and pharyngeal weakness. May see ptosis, sialosis, regurgitation and dysphagia
		  • Generalized: tetraparesis with pelvic limbs worse, megaesophagus, facial and pharyngeal weakness
		  • Acute fulminating: acute, rapidly progressive. Severe muscle weakness, megaesophagus, regurgitation, respiratory distress
			• Clinical signs develop 7–14 days after raccoon exposure in some dogs[148]
			• Starts as paraparesis and hyporeflexia
			• Quickly progresses to tetraparesis within 24–48 hours
			• Decreased to absent spinal reflexes
			• Nociception (deep pain perception) remains intact
			• Decreased muscle tone
			• May have hyperesthesia in paws and along spine
			• Cranial nerves are usually normal
			• May develop respiratory paralysis

	Exam findings	• Gait becomes fatigued, develops short and choppy stride, and then lies down; strength returns after rest • Spinal and cranial nerves – may be normal but can be fatigued. The palpebral reflex is the most sensitive for this • Megaesophagus • Cats: megaesophagus not as common because they have more smooth muscle in the esophagus. Generalized weakness can manifest as flexion on the neck. Voice change, drop jaw, exercise intolerance, dysphagia and vomiting/regurgitation also common[171]	• Flaccid ascending paresis/paralysis • Decreased to absent spinal reflexes • Decreased to flaccid muscle tone

(*Continued*)

Table 6.58 / Myasthenia gravis and polyradiculoneuritis (Continued)

Disease		Myasthenia gravis	Polyradiculoneuritis (Coonhound paralysis)
Diagnosis	General	• Edrophonium chloride (Tensilon®) test: an ultra-short-acting anticholinesterase drug. It enables more acetylcholine molecules to be available in the neuromuscular junction to bind with the functional AChR. After inducing weakness, an injection of 0.1–0.2 mg/kg is given IV. If the patient's muscle strength improves shortly after giving it is considered positive. This only lasts for a few minutes. However, a negative test does not rule out myasthenia gravis and dogs with other neuromuscular diseases can have a partial response[148]	• Presumptive diagnosis based on rapidity of progression of signs and ruling out other differential diagnoses • Differentials include tick paralysis, botulism and myasthenia gravis
	Laboratory	• AChR serum autoantibodies for definitive diagnosis. Titer above 0.6 nmol/l in dogs and 0.3 nmol/l in cats is positive for myasthenia gravis[172] • Must be done before corticosteroids are administered as this can lower antibody concentrations	• CSF: increased protein with normal cell count[169]
	Imaging	• Thoracic radiographs to assess for megaesophagus, aspiration pneumonia and neoplasia	• Not applicable
	Procedures	• Electrophysiology • EMG: normal • Repetitive nerve stimulation: amplitudes will decrease by 10–20% in first 10 responses[148]	• Electrophysiology: evidence of denervation seen 5–7 days after exposure • EMG: increased insertion activity, fibrillation potentials and positive sharp waves. Evoked potentials slightly decreased but not by as much as with botulism or tick paralysis[148] • Nerve conduction velocities – decreased in later course of disease[148]

(Continued)

Table 6.58 / **Myasthenia gravis and polyradiculoneuritis (Continued)**

Disease		Myasthenia gravis	Polyradiculoneuritis (Coonhound paralysis)
Treatment	General	• Supportive care	• No specific treatment exists • Supportive care and physical rehabilitation
	Medication	• Anticholinesterase agents: prolong the action of ACh at the neuromuscular junction • Pyridostigmine bromide: 0.5–3 mg/kg orally 2–3 times a day • Neostigmine bromide: 0.4 mg/kg IM • Monitor AChr antibody titers until remission, then gradually decrease dose • Corticosteroids; prednisone starting at 0.2 mg/kg once a day (anti-inflammatory dose) and gradually increasing to 1–2 mg/kg twice a day (immunosuppressive dose) for 2–4 weeks[148] • May be contraindicated in patients at risk of or with aspiration pneumonia • When AChR antibody titer is normal can gradually decrease dose very slowly every 4 weeks[148] • Ultimate goal is alternate day therapy at lowest effective dose[148]	• Corticosteroids are not recommended
	Nursing care	• Megaesophagus: food and water elevated. May need to feed small amounts of soft food • Use of a Bailey chair to keep the dog in a vertical position in order to try to prevent aspiration pneumonia (Figure 6.3) • May require a gastrostomy tube	• Prevention of decubital ulcers, pneumonia, urinary tract infection • Keep on clean, padded bedding • Support respiratory function as needed • Patient may need help to completely empty the bladder by manual expression • Physical rehabilitation: plan should be made with goals of minimizing muscle atrophy/contracture and reestablishing neural pathways
Follow-up	Patient care	• Differentiation between vomiting and regurgitation in order to treat properly • Altered feeding as mentioned above	• Physical rehabilitation: may consist of passive range of motion, muscle massage, stretching, hydrotherapy, neuromuscular electric stimulation and other therapeutic exercises. Recommend referral to a certified canine rehabilitation professional for plan development
	Prevention/avoidance	• Spay female dogs and cats with myasthenia gravis as soon as possible because heat cycles and pregnancy can exacerbate the disease[172] • Do not over vaccinate, as vaccines may exacerbate active myasthenia gravis[172]	• Avoid exposure to raccoons

(*Continued*)

Table 6.58 / **Myasthenia gravis and polyradiculoneuritis (Continued)**

Disease	Myasthenia gravis	Polyradiculoneuritis (Coonhound paralysis)
Complications	• May require parenteral feeding • Aspiration pneumonia	• Aspiration pneumonia • Respiratory failure: may require ventilator support
Prognosis	• Cats with focal or generalized myasthenia gravis have better prognosis than dogs • Guarded prognosis in early stages • Mortality rate within 1 year of diagnosis is about 40%[173] • 87% of dogs in one study went into spontaneous remission without recurrence with supportive care or acetylcholinesterase drugs alone[174]	• Usually good • Recovery can take from 3 weeks to 4 months or longer • Improvement begins by 3 weeks with complete recovery generally at 6–8 weeks[148]

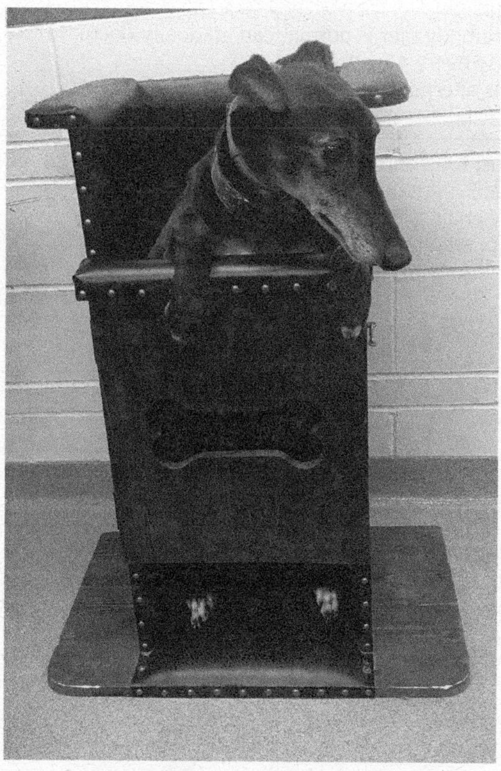

Figure 6.3 Bailey chair.

ONCOLOGY

Neoplasia

Neoplasia is the development of a new and abnormal formation of tissue, as a tumor or growth. It serves no useful function but grows at the expense of the healthy organism (benign or malignant). The common categories of cancer are leukemias, lymphomas, sarcomas, carcinomas, or a combination. Common tissue origins include round cell, epithelial cell and mesenchymal cell tumors. Benign behaving tumors tend to remain local without distant metastasis. Benign tumors can still be locally invasive and impair function. Malignant tumors retain the ability to not only be locally invasive but also spread to distant locations throughout the body. Lymphatic and vascular invasion can be direct indicators of metastasis potential. All cancer patients should be evaluated for definitive diagnosis and staging of disease.

Table 6.59 / Neoplasia

Disease		Neoplasia
Presentation	Clinical signs	• Presence of a tumor(s) effects attributable to adjacent organ/tissue injury (e.g. halitosis, swelling, pain) • Anorexia, depression, diarrhea, inappetence, lethargy, vomiting, weight loss • Impairment of normal function • Source of uncontrollable pain
	Exam findings	• Detection of tumor, variable (e.g. lymphadenopathy, organomegaly, hyperemic mucous membranes), additional disorders • Hematologic abnormalities
Diagnosis	General	• History/clinical signs • Physical exam: tumor and lymph node palpation • Lymph node and tumor measurement noted within medical record
	Laboratory	• CBC: variable (see specific tumor type), anemia: normocytic and normochromic • Paraneoplastic syndromes (hypercalcemia, anemia, etc.) • Chemistry panel: variable (see specific tumor type) • Urinalysis: variable (see specific tumor type) • Fine-needle aspirate, core biopsy or surgical biopsy of tumor or enlarged lymph node(s) • Cytology: cells fulfilling the criteria for malignancy • Histopathology: clean margins and tumor grade • Vascular or lymphatic invasion
	Imaging	• Radiographs, thoracic (ventrodorsal, left and right laterals): tumor identification, metastases, lymphadenopathy, pleural effusion • Radiographs, abdominal: tumor identification, metastases, lymphadenopathy, organomegaly • Ultrasound: tumor identification, lymphadenopathy, guided biopsy • MRI/CT: tumor identification, metastases, lymphadenopathy, tumor margins and tissue of origin
	Procedures	• Variable

(Continued)

Table 6.59 / Neoplasia (Continued)

Disease		Neoplasia
Treatment	General	• Symptomatic • Fluid therapy • Interventional radiology • Radiotherapy (local control) • Cryosurgery (local control • Photodynamic therapy • Surgery: excision with 2–3 cm clean margins (local control)
	Medication	• Variable: see specific tumor type • Chemotherapy agents (to aid in local control and prevent or slow metastasis) • Corticosteroids • Analgesics
	Nursing care	• Standard postoperative care following surgical excision • Supportive care for chemotherapy and radiation therapy adverse effects
Follow-up	Patient care	• Variable (see specific tumor type) • Monitor specific blood values • Monitor response to treatment (Skill Box 6.3), appetite, elimination, and energy level
	Prevention/avoidance	• Variable; cancer can be linked to many causes such as environmental factors (e.g. cigarette smoke, asbestos, herbicides), nutrition, castration, genetics
	Complications	• Variable (see specific tumor type) • Tumor related complications (obstruction, seizures, hemoabdomen) • Treatment-related complications (neutropenia, sepsis, skin toxicity)
	Prognosis	• Dependent on tumor type, size, location, time of discovery, and completeness of excision • Prognostic factors vary between tumor types

Histiocytoma

A histiocytoma is a benign skin tumor often found on the head, ear pinna, and limbs. Histiocytomas are most commonly seen in dogs less than two years of age. Most of these tumors will regress.

Mammary Gland Neoplasia

Mammary gland neoplasia is very prevalent among female, intact dogs and very rare in male dogs. The tumors show malignancy 50% of the time in canines. Mammary tumors in cats are malignant 80–90% of the time.

Mast Cell Tumor

Mast cell tumors are malignant tumors that arise from mast cells. They are a very unpredictable tumor in their appearance, growth rate, and response to treatment. These cells contain histamine and heparin, which can cause these tumors to bleed, grow and regress spontaneously.

Table 6.60 / **Histiocytoma, mammary gland neoplasia, and mast cell tumor**

Disease		Histiocytoma (button tumor)	Mammary gland neoplasia	Mast cell tumor
Presentation	Clinical signs	• Fast growing, firm, small, dome or button-shaped mass, solitary, nonpainful, ± ulcerated	• Firm nodular mass, ± ulceration • Nipples: red, swollen and exudate (e.g. tan, red) • Fever • Painful lesions	• Dogs: • Lymphadenopathy, erythema, and edema • Tumor: solitary skin or SQ mass, present for days to months, recent rapid growth • Cats: • Anorexia and vomiting • Tumor: found in SQ tissue or dermis, papular or nodular, solitary or multiple, hairy or alopecic and ulcerated
	Exam findings	• Not applicable	• Edematous hind limbs • Nodules or masses around nipple or within gland	• Lymphadenopathy, hepatomegaly, intestinal wall thickening, splenomegaly
Diagnosis	General	• Clinical signs	• Clinical signs • Mammary gland palpation • Inflammatory carcinoma • Worse prognosis • Cats or dogs	• History/clinical signs • Fine needle aspirate almost always diagnostic
	Laboratory	• Good with early treatment • Extremely guarded when severely affected	• Guarded: can be become carriers and relapse clinically if immunocompromised	• Good with early treatment • Extremely guarded when severely affected
	Imaging	• Not applicable	• Radiographs, thoracic: pleural effusion and lung metastases • Radiographs, abdominal: ascites and ↑ size of sublumbar lymph nodes • Ultrasound: ascites and size of sublumbar lymph nodes – measure when possible for monitoring	• Radiographs, abdominal: ↑ spleen, liver and lymph nodes • Radiographs, thoracic: metastases • Ultrasound, abdominal: visceral metastasis
	Procedures	• Not applicable	• Fine-needle aspirate for diagnosis	• Lymph node aspirates • Darier's sign: A tumor that has been manipulated will degranulate causing erythema and wheel formations

(Continued)

Table 6.60 / **Histiocytoma, mammary gland neoplasia, and mast cell tumor (Continued)**

Disease		Histiocytoma (button tumor)	Mammary gland neoplasia	Mast cell tumor
Treatment	General	• Spontaneous regression • Surgery: excision or cryosurgery	• Symptomatic • Surgery: mastectomy • Canines – conservative surgery may be indicated • Felines – more aggressive surgery linked to longer survival times	• Symptomatic • Chemotherapy • Radiotherapy • Cryosurgery (grade I, small, cutaneous) • Surgery: aggressive excision and splenectomy
	Medication	• Not applicable	• Chemotherapy: doxorubicin, cyclophosphamide, carboplatin, and mitoxantrone • NSAIDs • Corticosteroids	• Chemotherapy: vinblastine, doxorubicin, lomustine, torcerinib, masitinib, vincristine • Corticosteroids: prednisone • GI protectants: sucralfate • H1-blockers: diphenhydramine • H2-blockers: cimetidine, ranitidine
	Nursing care	• Standard postoperative care	• Standard postoperative care • Chemotherapy adverse effects if applicable	• Standard postoperative care • Chemotherapy adverse effects if applicable • Radiation therapy adverse effects if applicable
Follow-up	Patient care	• Monitor its growth and the presence of new tumors.	• Exam with special attention to mammary glands, incision line and lymph nodes, and thoracic radiographs every 2–3 months	• Monitor CBC and lymph node enlargement before each chemotherapy administration • Monitor for the presence of new tumors.
	Prevention/avoidance	• Not applicable	• Early hysterectomy: before 6 months • Some large-breed dogs spay before second heat cycle	• Not applicable
	Complications	• Not applicable	• Anemia • Ascites • DIC • Hypercalcemia • Osteoporosis • Pleural effusion • Metastasis	• Bleeding • Chemotherapy toxicity • Hemorrhagic gastroenteritis • Radiation reaction

(*Continued*)

Table 6.60 / Histiocytoma, mammary gland neoplasia, and mast cell tumor (Continued)

Disease	Histiocytoma (button tumor)	Mammary gland neoplasia	Mast cell tumor
Prognosis	• Excellent	• Dependent on size, time of detection, and the completeness of excision • Stage of disease (presence of metastasis) • Histologic grade of tumor • Metastatic sites include: brain bone, liver, spleen, lymph nodes	• Dependent on the area affected, time of detection, and the completeness of excision • Metastasis to regional lymph nodes, liver, spleen, bone marrow

Notes	• Boxers, Dachshunds, Cocker Spaniel, Great Danes, and Shetland Sheepdog	• Freely movable tumor implies benign and fixed to body wall or skin implies malignant.
		• Removal of all four glands of the affected chain is recommended.
		• Canine mammary tumor less than 2 cm more likely to be benign
		• Breed predisposition:
		  • Canines: Spaniels, Poodles
		  • Felines: Siamese, Persian
			• Animals with tumors on the extremities tend to live longer than animals with trunk tumors
			• Boxers, Boston Terriers, Bullmastiffs, Pugs, English Setters, and Siamese cats

Table 6.61 / Various neoplasias

Cancer type by body area	Clinical signs	Diagnosis	Treatment	Additional information
Carcinoma				
Adenocarcinoma				
Anal sac (mostly seen in geriatric female dogs with a very high rate of metastasis; can be unilateral or bilateral)	Dyschezia, tenesmus, polyuria/polydipsia, pruritus, ulceration, bleeding, weakness, paresis	• Chemistry panel: ↑ calcium, ↓ phosphorus • PTH: ± ↓ values • PTHrP: ↑ values • Radiographs, thoracic: metastasis (nodules) • Radiographs, abdominal: enlarged lymph nodes, fluid • Ultrasound, abdominal: enlarged lymph nodes, liver, or spleen nodules • Biopsy: confirmation • Biologic behavior/grade of tumor • Vascular or lymphatic invasion	• Chemotherapy: carboplatin, doxorubicin, melphalan • Calcitonin • Diuretics: furosemide • Fluid therapy • Radiotherapy • Surgery: tumor and lymph node excision/debulking • Bisphosphonates for increased calcium if applicable	• Follow-up: exam, radiographs, ultrasound and blood work every 3 months following surgery • Complications: fecal incontinence, metastasis, renal failure, reoccurrence, sepsis • Chemotherapy and radiation therapy management if applicable • Prognosis: poor

(Continued)

Table 6.61 / **Various neoplasias (Continued)**

Cancer type by body area	Clinical signs	Diagnosis	Treatment	Additional information
Nasal (most tumors begin as unilateral but progress to bilateral)	Epistaxis, epiphora, sneezing, nasal discharge, halitosis, and seizures; facial deformity: nasal bone swelling	• Radiographs, skull: tumor location, extent • Radiograph, thoracic: metastasis (nodules) • MRI/CT and rhinoscopy: tumor location, extent, and effect on surrounding structures and biopsy • Mycotic cultures: fungal rhinitis • Biopsy: confirmation • Regional lymph nodes aspirates	• Antiemetic: butorphanol • Chemotherapy: cisplatin (canine), cyclophosphamide, piroxicam, vincristine, doxorubicin • Radiotherapy • Surgery: tumor excision/debulking, hydropulsion	• Follow-up: survey radiographs, MRI/CT when clinical signs return • Complications: brain involvement across cribriform plate, 2nd-degree bacterial infections, hemorrhage, regrowth • Prognosis: fair with radiation or hydropulsion; poor with brain involvement
Pancreas (liver metastases are very common)	Ascites, icterus, maldigestion; palpable abdominal mass, pyrexia, vomiting, weakness	• CBC: mild anemia, neutrophilia • Chemistry panel: ↑ amylase, lipase • Radiograph, abdominal: metastasis, fluid, ascites • Ultrasound, abdominal: tumor, pancreatitis • Biopsy: confirmation	• Palliative • Surgery: tumor excision	• Follow-up: monitor quality of life • Complications: diabetes mellitus, EPI, intestinal or biliary obstruction, pancreatic abscess, pancreatitis, peritonitis • Prognosis: grave
Prostate (always malignant)	Cachexia, constipation, dyschezia, dyspnea, dysuria, exercise intolerance, rear-limb lameness, stranguria, tenesmus, hematuria, pyrexia	• CBC: inflammatory leukogram • Chemistry panel: ↑ ALP, azotemia • Urinalysis: pyuria, ↑ blood, malignant epithelial cells • Prostatic wash: malignant cells • Radiography, thoracic: metastasis • Radiograph, abdominal: lesions, prostate changes, lymphadenopathy • Ultrasound, abdominal: prostate changes (asymmetry) • Contrast cystography: distortion of prostatic urethra	• Analgesics • Chemotherapy: carboplatin, doxorubicin • Stool softeners • Radiotherapy • Surgery: prostate excision, castration	• Follow-up: monitor ability to urinate and defecate • Monitor pain levels • Complications: constipation, metastasis, urethral obstruction • Prognosis: guarded to poor

(*Continued*)

Table 6.61 / **Various neoplasias (Continued)**

Cancer type by body area	Clinical signs	Diagnosis	Treatment	Additional information
Salivary gland	Dysphagia, pain on opening mouth, swelling of upper neck, ear base, upper lip, maxilla, mucous membrane of lip	• Radiographs, thoracic: metastasis • MRI/CT: tumor location and extent • Biopsy: confirmation	• Radiotherapy (palliative or definitive intent) case dependent • Surgery: tumor excision • Chemotherapy may also be indicated if vascular/lymphatic invasion	• Follow-up: monitor for tumor growth every 3–6 months • Prognosis: fair
Thyroid (high rate of metastasis; biopsy and FNA can cause excessive bleeding; rare in felines. Biopsy often required for definitive diagnosis; can be unilateral or bilateral)	Dysphagia, dysphonia, dyspnea, polyuria/polysipsia, regurgitation; firm, nonpainful cervical mass, tachycardia (see Hypothyroidism; Table 6.15)	• CBC: nonregenerative anemia • Radiographs, cervical: displacement of normal structures • Ultrasound, thoracic: disease extent • CT: disease extent • Radioiodine study: thyroid hormone production • T4, T3, TSH concentrations • Thyroid gland scintigraphy: location	• β-blockers • Analgesics • Antiemetics • Chemotherapy: doxorubicin, carboplatin • Methimazole • Radioactive iodine (feline) • Radiotherapy • Surgery: tumor, gland, lymph node excision • Thyroxine (secondary hypothyroidism)	• Follow-up: exam tumor site and radiographs every 3 months; monitor calcium, thyroid concentration levels • Complications: anemia, DIC, hypoparathyroidism, hypothyroidism, laryngeal paralysis, respiratory distress • Prognosis dependent on size of tumor and lymph node involvement; larger fixed tumors have a poor prognosis
Squamous cell carcinoma				
Digit (often seen in large, black dogs; arises from subungual epithelium)	Chronic and progressive lameness, swelling, ulceration	• Radiographs, affected foot: lysis of the third phalanx • Radiographs, thoracic: metastasis • Ultrasound, abdominal: lymph node involvement • Biopsy: confirmation	• Analgesics: piroxicam • Chemotherapy: doxorubicin, mitoxantrone, bovine collagen matrix with 5-fluorouracil • Retinoids • Surgery: wide-margin amputation	• Follow-up: exam, radiographs, and ultrasound at 1 month, then every 3 months • Limit sun exposure; use sunscreen or tattoo low-pigmented areas of the paws • Prognosis: good

(*Continued*)

Table 6.61 / Various neoplasias (Continued)

Cancer type by body area	Clinical signs	Diagnosis	Treatment	Additional information
Ear (areas of low pigmentation and those subjected to solar radiation are more at risk)	Crusty eczematous lesions on edge of pinna, ulceration, discharge, pruritus	• Radiographs, skull: tumor extent • Radiographs, thoracic: metastasis; biopsy: confirmation	• Chemotherapy • Immune response modifier: imiquimod • Retinoid: acitretin • Cryosurgery • Electrochemotherapy • Hyperthermia • **PDT** • Radiotherapy • Surgery: amputation/pinnectomy ± ablation of ear canal • Vitamin E	• Follow-up: exam, radiographs, and lymph node evaluation at 1 month, then every 3 months • Limit sun exposure; use sunscreen or tattoo low-pigmented areas of the ears • Prognosis: good with complete excision
Gingiva	Bloody oral discharge, dysphagia, excessive salivation, halitosis, loose teeth, and facial deformity; loose teeth, plaque-like areas that bleed easily	• Radiographs, skull: bone involvement and lysis • Radiographs, thoracic: metastasis • CT: bone involvement and lysis, lymph node metastasis • Biopsy: confirmation	• Analgesics • Chemotherapy: cisplatin (canine), mitoxantrone, carboplatin • Cryosurgery • PDT • NSAIDs: piroxicam, ± meloxicam • Radiotherapy • Surgery: tumor excision/debulking	• Follow-up: exam, radiographs and lymph node evaluation at 1 month, then every 3 months • Feed soft foods or by enteral feeding tube • Complications: dysphagia, recurrence, malocclusion • Prognosis: poor due to local invasion (feline); the more rostral the tumor is located, the better the prognosis (canine)
Skin (areas of low pigmentation and those subjected to solar radiation are more at risk. Malignant tumor of squamous epithelium)	Crusty, pigmentation, ulceration; facial skin involvement (feline), nail bed involvement (canine)	• Radiographs, extremity: bone involvement • Radiographs, thoracic: metastasis • Ultrasound, abdominal: lymph node evaluation • Biopsy: confirmation	• Analgesics • Chemotherapy: carboplatin, mitoxantrone, bovine collagen matrix with 5-fluorouracil (canine) • Immune response modifier: imiquimod • Cryosurgery • Electrochemotherapy • Photodynamic therapy • Radiotherapy • Retinoids • Surgery: tumor excision/debulking	• Follow-up: reexam and radiographs every 3 months for 1 year then every 6 months for 1 year • Limit sun exposure; use sunscreen or tattoo low-pigmented areas of the skin • Prognosis: good with superficial lesions; guarded with nail-bed or digit involvement

(Continued)

Table 6.61 / **Various neoplasias (Continued)**

Cancer type by body area	Clinical signs	Diagnosis	Treatment	Additional information
Transitional cell carcinoma				
Bladder, urethra (high rate of metastasis; FNA may cause seeding of tumor cells along the needle tract. Metastatic sites include: bone, brain, liver, spleen, lymph node, lungs)	Dysuria, hematuria, pollakiuria, polyuria/polydipsia, recurrent stranguria, tenesmus, urinary incontinence	• Chemistry panel: azotemia if at trigone • Urinalysis: ↑ blood, malignant epithelial cells • Urine culture: urinary tract infection • Radiograph, thoracic: metastasis • Double-contrast cystography: irregularities or mass lesions • IV pyelography, voiding urethrogram or vaginogram • Ultrasound, abdominal: extent of disease, proximity to trigone • Biopsy through cystoscopy, laparotomy, catheterization, or ultrasound: confirmation	• Chemotherapy: doxorubicin, carboplatin, mitoxantrone • NSAIDs: piroxicam, meloxicam • Radiotherapy • Interventional radiology: stenting • Surgery: tumor excision, urethral stenting	• Follow-up: cystography or ultrasonography every 6–8 weeks • Thoracic radiographs every 2–3 months • Complications: transplantation of cells during surgery or biopsy, urinary incontinence, urethral or ureteral obstruction, renal failure, urinary tract infection • Prognosis: grave
Sarcoma				
Chondrosarcoma				
Bone (affects large-breed dogs)	Lameness, nasal discharge, visible mass, pain, swelling	• Radiograph, affected limb: lesion • Radiograph, thoracic: metastasis • CT: extent of disease • Nuclear bone scan: staging of disease • Biopsy: definitive diagnosis	• Analgesics • Chemotherapy: Cyclophosphamide, carboplatin, doxorubicin • Radiotherapy • Surgery: tumor excision, amputation	• Follow-up: thoracic radiographs monthly for 3 months, then every 3 months • Complications: brain involvement • Prognosis: poor to excellent, dependent on tumor grade
Nasal and paranasal sinus Affects large breed dogs	Epiphora, halitosis, nasal discharge, seizures, sneezing, epistaxis Facial deformity, pain	• Radiographs, skull: tumor, fluid, and destruction of caudal turbinates • Radiographs, thoracic: metastasis • MRI/CT: integrity of cribriform plate and orbital invasion • Rhinoscopy: tumor identification • Biopsy: definitive diagnosis	• Corticosteroids: prednisone radiotherapy • Surgery: tumor excision/debulking	• Follow-up: radiographs every 2–3 months • CT/MRI may be repeated when clinical signs return • Complications: brain involvement • Prognosis: fair; poor with brain involvement (cribriform plate destruction)

(Continued)

Table 6.61 / Various neoplasias (Continued)

Cancer type by body area	Clinical signs	Diagnosis	Treatment	Additional information
Fibrosarcoma				
Bone (primarily affect the axial skeleton)	Lameness, pain, swelling, pallor; pathologic long bone fracture	• Radiograph, affected limb: lesion • Radiograph, thoracic: metastasis • CT: extent of disease • Biopsy: definitive diagnosis	• Analgesics • Chemotherapy: carboplatin, doxorubicin • Radiotherapy • Surgery: tumor excision, amputation	• Follow-up: thoracic radiographs monthly for 3 months, then every 3 months • Complications: pathologic fractures • Prognosis: guarded
Gingiva	Bloody oral discharge, dysphagia, excessive salivation, halitosis Facial deformity, loose teeth	• Radiographs, skull: bone involvement • Radiographs, thoracic, metastasis • Biopsy: intraoral • CT: extent of disease	• Analgesics • Chemotherapy: doxorubicin, cisplatin • Cryosurgery • Radiotherapy • Surgery: tumor excision/ debulking	• Follow-up: feed soft foods • Exam, radiographs every 2–3 months • Complications: dysphagia • Prognosis: fair with early detection and aggressive treatment
Hemangiosarcoma				
Bone	Lameness, pain, swelling, pallor; pathologic long-bone fracture	• CBC: regenerative anemia, nucleated RBC, poikilocytosis, anisocytosis, thrombocytopenia, leukocytosis, ↓ protein • FDP, prothrombin time, PTT: ↑ values • Fibrinogen: ↓ values • Radiographs, bone: lysis • Radiographs, thoracic: metastasis • Ultrasound: metastasis • CT: extent of disease	• Analgesics • Chemotherapy: doxorubicin, cyclophosphamide, vincristine • Radiotherapy • Surgery: tumor excision, amputation	• Follow-up: exam, thoracic radiographs and ultrasound every 3 months for 1 year then every 6 months • Complications: pathologic fractures, rupturing tumors causing hemorrhage • Prognosis: unknown
Heart (pulmonary metastasis very common; right atrium common site)	Dyspnea, exercise intolerance, syncope, weight loss; abdominal and pleural effusion, arrhythmia, hepatomegaly, hind limb paresis, jugular distention, pulse deficits	• CBC: anemia, nucleated RBC, schistocytes, thrombocytopenia • Chemistry panel: azotemia • Ultrasound, thoracic: location of tumor • Biopsy, heart: definitive diagnosis	• Chemotherapy: doxorubicin, vincristine, cyclophosphamide • Pericardial and pleural centesis • Surgery: tumor excision/ debulking	• Follow-up: exam, thoracic radiographs and ultrasound monthly • Complications: centesis and surgery complications • Prognosis: guarded to poor

(Continued)

Table 6.61 / **Various neoplasias (Continued)**

Cancer type by body area	Clinical signs	Diagnosis	Treatment	Additional information
Spleen, liver (rapid growth and widespread metastatic vascular neoplasia; patients may also have right-atrium hemangiosarcoma)	Ataxia, dementia, intermittent collapse, lameness, paresis, seizures, weakness, enlarged abdomen, pale mucous membranes, peritoneal fluid, tachycardia	• CBC: regenerative anemia, polychromasia, reticulocytosis, nucleated RBC, anisocytosis, leukocytosis, neutrophilia, thrombocytopenia • Chemistry panel: ↑ liver enzymes • FDP, prothrombin time, PTT: ↑ values • Radiograph, abdominal: tumor detection, fluid • Radiograph, thoracic: metastasis • Ultrasound, abdominal: tumor location and metastasis • Ultrasound, heart: right atrial tumor • MRI/CT • Abdominocentesis	• Antihistamines: diphenhydramine • Biological response modifier L-MTP-PE • Blood transfusions • Chemotherapy: cyclophosphamide, doxorubicin, chlorambucil, methotrexate, piroxicam, vincristine • Fluid therapy • Surgery: splenectomy • Radiotherapy	• Follow-up: restrict activity; CBC and platelet count before each cycle of chemotherapy; thoracic and abdominal radiographs and abdominal ultrasound every 2 months • Complications: sepsis, skin sloughs, tumor rupture leading to hemorrhage, vomiting and diarrhea • Prognosis: poor
Lymphosarcoma/lymphoma				
Feline (most common sites are alimentary tract, anterior mediastinum, nasal, liver, spleen, and kidneys) • Lymphoblastic: large cell, more aggressive, solitary lesions possible • Lymphocytic: small cell, typically more diffuse disease; can be managed long term	Dependent on form (mediastinal, renal, alimentary, solitary, or multicentric); coughing, open-mouth breathing, regurgitation, vomiting, weight loss; renal failure signs, thickened intestines	• CBC: anemia, leukocytosis, and lymphoblastosis • Chemistry panel: ↑ creatinine, BUN, ALT, AST, calcium, and ↓ albumin • Urinalysis: ↑ bilirubin, protein, isosthenuria • Serology: + FeLV • Cobalamin and folate: ↓ values • Radiography, abdominal/thoracic • Ultrasound, abdominal • Endoscopy • Cytology: bone marrow, tumor, lymph nodes • Histopathology: clean margins and tumor grade • Fine needle aspirate of enlarged lymph nodes	• Chemotherapy: vincristine, vinblastine, cytosine, cyclophosphamide, chlorambucil, procarbazine, doxorubicin, actinomycin-D, lomustine, mechlorethamine • Corticosteroids: prednisolone • Surgery • Radiotherapy	• Follow-up: exam, CBC and platelet count before each weekly cycle of chemotherapy • Nutritional support • Complications: leukopenia, sepsis, and tumor lysis syndrome (rare) • Prognosis: variable depending on stage of the disease, patient's health and response to therapy, treatment chosen, and care given

(*Continued*)

Table 6.61 / **Various neoplasias (Continued)**

Cancer type by body area	Clinical signs	Diagnosis	Treatment	Additional information
Canine (seen most commonly in solid tissues: lymph nodes, bone marrow, and visceral organs; ↑ risk with exposure to the herbicide: 2,4-dichlorophenoxyacetic acid; 80% of canine patients present with multicentric or peripheral lymph node enlargement; stages 1–5, substages A, B)	Coughing, drooling, dysphagia, dyspnea, exercise intolerance; anterior uveitis, ascites, lymphadenopathy, lymphoid infiltrate, organomegaly	• CBC: anemia, lymphocytosis, lymphopenia, neutrophilia, monocytosis, circulating blasts, and thrombocytopenia • Chemistry panel: ↑ ALT, ALP, proteins, and calcium • PTHrP: ↑ values • Radiographs, abdominal/thoracic • Echo: cardiac contractility • Ultrasound, abdominal • Cytology: bone marrow, tumor, lymph nodes – FNA • Histopathology: clean margins and tumor grade • Immunochemical staining of lymphocytes – B or T cell • Prognostic factors include immunophenotype, stage, substage and response to therapy. • FNA of enlarged lymph nodes	• Chemotherapy: doxorubicin, vincristine, cyclophosphamide, l-asparaginase • Corticosteroids: prednisone • Fluid therapy • Radiotherapy • Bone marrow transplant • Retinoids • Surgery • Thoraco- and abdominocentesis	• Follow-up: restrict activity of patients with ↓ WCC or platelet count; monitor CBC and platelet count during chemotherapy. Echo and ECG: cardiotoxicity of doxorubicin • Nutritional support • Complications: alopecia, DIC, leukopenia and neutropenia, pancreatitis, sepsis, tissue sloughing, vomiting, diarrhea, tumor lysis syndrome (rare) • Prognosis: variable depending on stage of the disease, patient's health and response to therapy, treatment chosen, and care given; mean survival time of B cell with CHOP is 12–18 months
Osteosarcoma (most common bone tumor in dogs, typically affecting the appendicular skeleton of large to giant breeds)	Lameness, pain, swelling; pathologic long-bone fracture; most common locations – proximal humerus and distal radius	• Radiograph, affected bone: bone lysis, proliferation in the metaphyseal region of long bones, soft tissue swelling • Radiograph, thoracic: metastasis • 90% of patients have pulmonary metastasis at the time of diagnosis • Nuclear bone scans: bony or soft tissue metastatic disease • Bone aspirate or biopsy • Use radiographs or ultrasound for lesion isolation	• Analgesics: piroxicam, fentanyl, morphine, pamidronate • Biological response modifiers: L-MTP-PE • Bisphosphonate • Chemotherapy: carboplatin, doxorubicin • Radiotherapy • Surgery: amputation, limb spare	• Follow-up: restrict activity. • Monitor radiographs every 2–3 months; monitor CBC and platelet count 7–10 days after chemotherapy; carboplatin may have double or triple nadir • Complications: metastasis (90% of cases at examination) and hypertrophic osteopathy • Prognosis: guarded once metastases is present

(*Continued*)

Table 6.61 / Various neoplasias (Continued)

Cancer type by body area	Clinical signs	Diagnosis	Treatment	Additional information
Injection site sarcoma (typically, fibrosarcoma, but may be many other types of sarcoma; reported with multiple types of injections including vaccines)	Firm, painless, SQ swelling located at a previous vaccination site or injection site; these sarcomas tend to be extremely locally invasive with deep "tendrils" within multiple tissue layers	• Radiograph, tumor site: bone lysis or extension of the tumor along other tissue planes • Radiograph, thoracic: metastasis • Contrast CT: extent of disease and for surgical planning • Requires extensive surgical margins • Biopsy: confirm diagnosis • Histopathology: clean margins and tumor grade	• Analgesics • Chemotherapy: doxorubicin, cyclophosphamide, carboplatin, ifosfamide • Radiotherapy – pre- or post-surgical • Surgery	• Follow-up: • Evaluate monthly for 3 months, then every 3 months • Monitor CBC and platelet count before each chemo treatment • Complications: recurrence, new lesions • Prognosis: poor

Chemotherapy

The administration of chemotherapeutic drugs is one of the treatment options for cancer (e.g. metastatic carcinoma, sarcomas, and hematologic malignancies). Cancer drugs selectively attack cells that are actively dividing and at times select for certain stages of division. The inability of cancer drugs to select for only cancer cells limits the duration and quantity of use. Healthy cells most commonly attacked are from blood, mucosa, crypt cells of the gastrointestinal tract, epidermis, gametes, and fetal tissue.

With the administration of chemotherapy, the first concern is for the safety of the staff, patient, and owner. Proper training is essential to deal with the potentially hazardous nature of these drugs. Routes of exposure include absorption, inhalation, and ingestion. Each clinic should have documented preparation, storage, disposal, and spill protocols for the various agents.

Together with safety concerning the administration of chemotherapy, care must be taken from the arrival of the medication at the hospital. Chemotherapy drugs should be unpacked, clearly labeled, and stored in a designated section of the clinic. Gloves should be worn when unpacking in case of breakage during transport, breakage during unpacking, or contamination from possible drug residue on the drug container. Spill kits should be readily available.

Skill Box 6.1 / Chemotherapy Administration

Step 1. Drug calculation

- Review the patient's record and recheck the chemotherapy protocol and drug calculations.
- Five right rules of chemotherapy (drug, route, dose, interval, patient).
- Verify the drug calculations with a second person.

Note: Chemotherapy drugs differ as to their body weight calculations (e.g. kilograms, pounds, or square meters). Be sure to verify the correct form. Also, most drugs are based on lean body weight, not actual body weight.

Step 2. Personnel supplies

- Prepare yourself and your assistant with safety gear regardless of administration technique:
  - Latex gloves: high-risk gloves or two pairs of regular gloves
  - ASTM International approved
  - Two pairs for handling NIOSH group one hazardous drugs (*Tip*: with the two-pair system, wear one pair under the cuff of gown and one pair over the cuff of the gown)
  - Goggles, full face shield or protective eyewear
  - Mask: dust or mist respirator or a mask with a filter
  - Note: Surgical masks do not have a filter and are not sufficient.
  - Gown: disposable with long sleeves, closed front, impervious and cuffs

Step 3. Administration supplies

Oral:

- Chemotherapy agent
- Hemostat or pill gun
- Spill kit

Subcutaneous/intramuscular:

- Drop cloth with plastic backing
- Chemotherapy agent
- Gauze sponges
- Closed system transfer device
- Spill kit

Intravenous:

- Same as SQ/IM together with:
  - Catheter
  - Clippers
  - Scrub preparation materials
  - Tape
  - Spill kit

Step 4. Drug preparation

1. Prepare in a type-2B biological safety cabinet or a well-ventilated area.
2. Use a closed-system transfer device (CSTD; e.g. Phaseal™, Equashield®) following manufacturer's guidelines to add diluent or to draw up the drug. If a CSTD is not available, the following steps should be followed with the knowledge that risk of exposure to personnel and patient is high:
   a. Remove plastic cover of vial and wipe the top with an alcohol swab.
   b. Insert the hydrophobic filter (e.g. chemo-pin) into the vial to normalize pressure and to avoid aerosolization.
   c. Attach the syringe to the filter while holding the vial upright.
   d. If adding a diluent, add slowly and then mix the contents of the vial completely with the Luer-Lok™ syringe left in place.
   e. Turn vial upside down and aspirate the drug into the syringe slowly to avoid excess air bubbles.
   f. Push any excess air back into the syringe before separating from the vial.
   g. Wrap gauze around the connection between the syringe and the vial and gently pull apart.
   h. Place a covered needle onto the syringe.
      – Do not inject air into the vial; maintaining a negative pressure within the vial reduces the risk of aerosolization.
      – When not using a hydrophobic filter, all the above steps are accomplished with a needle attached to the end of a Luer-Lok syringe.
      – Do not fill a syringe more than two thirds full to prevent the plunger from detaching from the end of the syringe.
      – If an agent is to be administered via a fluid bag, fill the administration set with plain diluent before adding the chemotherapy agent to reduce the risk of contamination when attaching the line to the patient.
      – If prepared drugs need to be moved throughout the hospital, they should be transported in a sealed plastic bag or container.

Step 5. Patient preparation

1. A plastic-lined absorbent pad is placed under the patient's leg with all the catheter and administration supplies on top.
2. Select vein: peripheral veins are recommended because they provide better visualization of any drug that becomes extravascular.
3. Aseptically clip and prepare the site.

(*Continued*)

Skill Box 6.1 / Chemotherapy Administration (Continued)

4. Place a catheter: butterfly, over-the-needle, or through-the-needle intracatheter. The use of a smaller size catheter allows for reduced patient pain and scarring, both important for future administration.
5. Assure patency of the catheter by flushing at least 12 ml non-heparinized 0.9% sodium chloride. Once a vein has been unsuccessfully punctured, a new vein should be used. If this is not possible, it is recommended that time be allowed for the proper clotting to occur before a proximal site is used. Heparinized saline should not be used as it may cause the drug to form a precipitate.

Step 6. Drug administration

1. With an alcohol-soaked gauze around the end of the catheter, insert the needle into the catheter and administer the drug at the correct rate but at an even pace to avoid leakage around venipuncture site.
2. Flush the catheter with 3–5 ml non-heparinized 0.9% sodium chloride after administration to avoid irritation to the vein.
3. Monitor for allergic reactions for up to 1 hour after administration of certain drugs (e.g. L-asparaginase).
4. Apply a pressure wrap after removing the catheter and maintain pressure for several minutes. Place an alcohol-soaked gauze sponge over the injection site whenever inserting or removing the needle or catheter to avoid aerosolization of the drug. Do not aspirate the drug back into the catheter after administration to avoid dilution and residual drug in the catheter injection port.

Step 7. Disposal

1. Place all items in a zipped bag to prevent aerosolization.
2. Dispose of the waste into an appropriate chemotherapy container.
3. Clean the preparation and administration surfaces thoroughly with bleach or soap and water and disposable towels. Before removing gloves, place capped syringes and any other used products that may aerosolize into your hands, pull gloves off over the materials, and then dispose of them in a chemotherapy approved container. A surface wipe test can be done for drug detection and removal (e.g. Chemoglo™).

Step 8. Post-administration patient care

1. Wear a double layer of gloves when handling waste from the patient for the first 72 hours.
2. Wipe down cages; avoid the use of a hose or spray to reduce aerosolization of excreted drugs.
3. Closely monitor response to the drug (e.g. attitude, appetite, eliminations, and general behavior).

Note: Chemotherapy administration should take place in a well-ventilated, low-traffic area of the hospital.

Skill Box 6.2 / Extravasation Injury

Extravasation injury is the accidental infusion of a drug outside of the vein into the perivascular tissues. These injuries can result in tissue necrosis of the area and possible loss of the limb. The cause can be an improperly placed intravenous catheter, patient movement, or fragile veins. Due to this high risk, only a catheter with perfect placement on the first attempt should be used for chemotherapy administration. Once a vein has been unsuccessfully punctured, a new vein should be used. If this is not possible, proper clotting should occur before a proximal site is used. Peripheral veins should be saved for chemotherapy treatment with the jugular veins used for blood collection. The vein used should be recorded at each treatment and rotated.

The patient should be continuously monitored during chemotherapy administration for adverse clinical signs. Signs of extravasation injury are pain, redness, swelling, or resistance to infusion of medication.

Chemotherapy drug	Treatment for extravasation injury
Cisplatin	• Stop administration immediately. • Do not remove needle and withdraw as much of the drug as possible (canine 10 ml blood; feline 5 ml blood). • Instill 1 ml of isotonic sodium thiosulfate for every milliliter extravasated.
Doxorubicin	• Stop administration immediately. • Do not remove needle and withdraw as much of the drug as possible (canine 10 ml blood; feline 5 ml blood). • Drug administration • Instill dexrazoxane IV for 10 times the milligram amount extravasated; repeat at 24 and 48 hours. • Paint twice the size of the affected area with a saturated pad of dimethyl sulfoxide 99%. Allow to air dry and repeat every 6 hours for 14 days; do not cover with bandaging. • Apply cold packs for 15 minutes every 2 hours to site for 72 hours, then every 6–8 hours for 10–14 days.
Vincristine vinblastine	• Stop administration immediately. • Do not remove needle and withdraw as much of the drug as possible (canine 10 ml blood; feline 5 ml blood). • Instill 3–5 ml of 0.9% saline. • Instill 2 ml of hyaluronidase (150 u/ml) diluted in 6 ml of 0.9% saline into 5–6 sites weekly until tissues are healed. • Apply warm packs for 15 minutes every 6–8 hours for 24–48 hours.

Chemotherapy Toxicity

Chemotherapy is the process of administering drugs to attack actively growing and dividing tumor cells. Unfortunately, these agents are not selective for tumor cells and will attack other cells (e.g., bone marrow cells, gastrointestinal cells). With the administration of any chemotherapy agents the patient must be monitored for adverse reactions and toxicities. Toxicities may not appear for several days following administration or until an accumulation of toxic levels have been obtained within the body. Most protocols are generally designed to result in less than 5% hospitalization rate (e.g. sepsis) for chemotherapy toxicity and less than 1% direct mortality rate from any particular toxicity.

Table 6.62 / Chemotherapy toxicity

System	Complication	Treatment	Comments
Hematologic	• Neutropenia • Anemia, thrombocytopenia (rare)	• Neutropenia: • < 2000/µl • ↓ dose by 10–25% • < 1500/µl • ↓ dose by 10–25% • Drug administration (e.g. trimethoprim-sulfa, fluoroquinolones) • Monitor temperature • Neutropenia and fever: • Hospitalization, IV fluids, antibiotics, bloodwork, blood culture, urinalysis and culture, thoracic radiographs, ± colony stimulating factors • Thrombocytopenia: • Delay administration when platelet counts are < 50,000–100,000/µl	• CBC and platelet count are required 12–24 hours before administration of chemotherapy agents known to cause myelosuppressive (e.g., cyclophosphamide, lomustine, vincristine, vinblastine, carboplatin, doxorubicin) • Severely neutropenic patients may not be able to show signs of infection or fever • Nadir is typically seen 5–10 days after administration • Some drugs many have double and triple nadirs (lomustine, carboplatin) • Delay of chemotherapy for 1 week typically allows for bone marrow recovery
Cardiac	• Arrhythmias • Acute, rare, transient • Cardiomyopathy • Chronic, cumulative • Most seen with doxorubicin in dogs *not* cats	Prevention: • Drug administration with iron-chelating cardioprotective agents (e.g. dexrazoxane) • Drug infusion over 15 minutes or a constant rate infusion over several hours • ECG monitoring Treatment: • Discontinue drug use if rhythm abnormalities are seen • Drug administration (e.g. antiarrhythmics)	• Mostly seen with canine doxorubicin administration • Limit total cumulative dose to < 180 mg/m² as a guideline for doxorubicin • Cardiotoxicity is typically irreversible and fatal
Dermatologic	• Alopecia, delayed hair regrowth, hyperpigmentation, hair color alterations	• No treatment necessary	• Mostly seen in non-shedding breeds (e.g. Poodles, Terriers, Old English Sheepdogs) • Regrowth seen soon after discontinuing chemotherapy • Change in color or textures may be initially seen, but often resolve with time

(Continued)

Table 6.62 / Chemotherapy toxicity (Continued)

System	Complication	Treatment	Comments	Hematologic
	• Local tissue necrosis • Secondary to extravasation injuries	Prevention: • Knowledge of the drugs and their toxicities • Meticulous catheter placement and monitoring Treatment: • Discontinue infusion • Do not remove needle, withdraw as much of the drug as possible • Follow extravasation guidelines and antidote therapy • Wound and surgical treatment, antibiotics, analgesics with tissue necrosis and sloughing		• Mostly seen with vincristine, doxorubicin and cisplatin • Clinical signs may appear from 1 to 7 days, sloughs at 7–10 days, and treat as open wounds • Bandages and E-collars can be used to avoid additional self-trauma • Potential limb amputation if severe necrosis

Gastrointestinal	• Nausea, inappetence, vomiting, diarrhea, enterocolitis	• Symptomatic therapy (e.g. highly palatable food, appetite stimulants, antiemetics, motility modifiers)
		• Severe:
		  • IV fluids
		  • Nutritional support
		  • Antibiotic therapy
		  • Preemptive antiemetics (e.g. ondansetron)
				• Mostly mild and self-limiting, except cisplatin, which can be severely emetogenic
				• Typically occur 5–7 days post-administration

Hypersensitivity	• Urticaria, erythema, restlessness, head shaking, vomiting, diarrhea, hypotension, pallor • Cardiovascular collapse (canine, rare), anaphylaxis • Respiratory distress (feline)	Prevention: • Drug administration (e.g. diphenhydramine, dexamethasone) Treatment: • Slowing or discontinuing drug infusion in hypersensitive patients • IV fluids • Drug administration (e.g. dexamethasone, diphenhydramine, epinephrine) preemptively or during symptoms • Monitor laboratory work, ECG, and radiographs		• Mostly seen with doxorubicin and L-asparaginase administration • The dose, rate, route, and frequency of administration can be altered to ↓ incidence of hypersensitivity
Neurological	• Cerebellar ataxia • Peripheral neuropathy (e.g. constipation, hyporeflexia, weakness, motor dysfunction)	Peripheral neuropathy: • Bulk laxatives • Remain within guidelines of dosages (e.g. 5-FU < 20 mg/kg PO)		• Mostly seen with 5-FU (cerebellar ataxia) and vincristine (peripheral neuropathy)
Urologic	• Nephrotoxicity • Dehydration, fever, tachycardia, weakness, hematuria, polyuria/polydipsia, disorientation	• IV fluid diuresis (pre and post) • Correct electrolyte abnormalities • Monitor serum creatinine, urine output, and specific gravity		• Mostly seen with cisplatin (canine) and doxorubicin (feline). • Use caution in felines with existing renal disease • Avoid use in canines with existing renal insufficiency

(Continued)

Table 6.62 / **Chemotherapy toxicity (Continued)**

System	Complication	Treatment	Comments
Hematologic			
	• Hemorrhagic cystitis • Stranguria, pollakiuria, hematuria	• Prevention: • Altering dosing frequency or drug choice • Administer in the morning to allow more time to empty bladder • Drug administration (e.g. furosemide, mesna) • IV diuresis around time of injection • Provide access to fresh water and frequent trips outside • Treatment: drug administration (e.g. analgesics, antibiotics, DMSO, 1% formalin)	• Mostly seen with canine cyclophosphamide and ifosfamide administration • Do not repeat if cystitis occurs • Mild cases are often self-limiting
Acute tumor lysis syndrome	• Vomiting, seizures, acute collapse, and shock • Results from massive cell death in response to treatment, causing intra-cellular contents released within the blood stream • Lymphoma/leukemias most common	• Fluid therapy • Lab work monitoring • ECG (e.g. bradycardia and wave alterations) • Drug administration (e.g. sodium bicarbonate, dextrose, insulin, calcium gluconate)	• Rare condition, but typically seen 48 hours after initial chemotherapy • Multiple electrolyte imbalances (e.g. hyperkalemia, hyperphosphatemia, hypocalcemia). • Extensive treatment for lymphoma or leukemia with rapid tumor breakdown and subsequent release of excess phosphorus and potassium.

Oncology Resources

ACVIM, ECVN, and ECEIM, Consensus Statements. https://onlinelibrary.wiley.com/page/journal/19391676/homepage/free_reviews_and_consensus_statements.htm (accessed 14 July 2021).

American Association of Feline Practitioners. 2020 AAFP Feline Retrovirus Management. https://catvets.com/guidelines/practice-guidelines/retrovirus-management-guidelines (accessed 14 July 2021).

American Veterinary Medical Association. Occupational hazards: Protect yourself and your staff when handling hazardous drugs. https://www.avma.org/blog/occupational-hazards-protect-yourself-and-your-staff-when-handling-hazardous-drugs (accessed 14 July 2021).

Hazardous Drug Consensus Group. Consensus Statement on the Handling of Hazardous Drugs Per USP Chapter 800, March 2017. https://pdf4pro.com/view/consensus-statement-on-the-handling-of-hazardous-drugs-3c3dc0.html ().

National Institute for Occupational Safety and Health. NIOSH List of Antineoplastic and Other Hazardous Drugs in Healthcare Settings, 2016. DHHS (NIOSH) Publication Number 2016-161 (Supersedes 2014-138). https://www.cdc.gov/niosh/docs/2016-161/default.html (accessed 14 July 2021).

United States Pharmacopeial Convention. Compounding standards. https://www.usp.org/compounding (accessed 14 July 2021).

RESPIRATORY DISEASES

Asthma and Bronchitis

Asthma and bronchitis are secondary to inflammation and airway disorders causing bronchoconstrictive episodes. The distress is often seen on expiration or as coughing fits. The causes may be allergic, bacterial, infection, pulmonary parasites, heartworm disease, or inhaled irritants.

Brachycephalic Airway Syndrome

Brachycephalic breeds have a congenital condition of obstructive airways where the soft palate overlaps the tip of the epiglottis, although the condition can also be acquired. Common contributing causes are stenotic nares and elongated soft palate; secondary everted laryngeal saccules are a sequela.

Table 6.63 / Asthma, bronchitis and brachycephalic airway syndrome

Disease		Asthma, bronchitis	Brachycephalic airway syndrome
Presentation	Clinical signs	• Open-mouth breathing, coughing, wheezing, gagging, sneezing (variable), dyspnea, vomiting, lethargy, inappetence	• Coughing, gagging, panting, open-mouth breathing, dyspnea, tachypnea change in voice, exercise intolerance
	Exam findings	• Tracheal sensitivity, tachypnea, cyanosis, respiratory crackles, tachy- or bradycardia	• Stertor, stridor, ↑ respiratory effort, enlarged tonsils
Diagnosis	General	• History/clinical signs	• History/clinical signs • Airway examination • Common breeds: English Bulldogs, Pugs, Boston Terriers, Shih Zeus, Persian cats • Congenital abnormalities: stenotic nares, elongation, thickening of soft palate, redundant pharyngeal tissue, tracheal hypoplasia • Acquired abnormalities: secondary to chronic congenital abnormalities. Everted laryngeal saccules, enlarged pharyngeal mucosa and soft palate tissue, laryngeal edema, laryngeal collapse
	Laboratory	• CBC: neutrophilia, monocytosis (variable) and eosinophilia (variable) • Fecal analysis: parasites (e.g., *Capillaria*, *Paragonimus*) • Baermann technique: parasites (e.g., *Aelurostrongylus*) • Heartworm tests: antigen and antibody	• Blood gas analysis
	Imaging	• Radiographs, thoracic: pulmonary hyperinflation, aerophagia, flattened diaphragm, peribronchial or interstitial infiltration, atelectasis of the middle lung, lung collapse or pronounced bronchial pattern • Echocardiography: heartworm disease or pulmonary hypertension	• Radiographs, cervical/pharyngeal: thickened and lengthened soft palate and tracheal stenosis • Tracheal hypoplasia can be seen • Radiographs, thoracic: tracheal stenosis or aspiration pneumonia • Fluoroscopy: degree of obstruction

(*Continued*)

Table 6.63 / **Asthma, bronchitis and brachycephalic airway syndrome (Continued)**

Disease		Asthma, bronchitis	Brachycephalic airway syndrome
	Procedures	• ECG: heart disease screen • Bronchoscopy: tumors and airway pathology • Cytology, tracheal or bronchial wash: eosinophils, activated macrophages, nonregenerative neutrophils, bacteria, parasites	• Pulse oximetry • Laryngoscopy/pharyngoscopy: laryngeal and pharyngeal abnormalities • Sedation or light anesthesia: significant respiratory effort is required to diagnose laryngeal paralysis • Tracheoscopy: location and severity of stenotic tracheal lesions and pharyngeal abnormalities
Treatment	General	• Symptomatic • Oxygen therapy	• Surgery: nasal wedge resection, laryngeal sacculectomy, or staphylectomy
Treatment	Medication	• Anthelmintics: based on diagnosis or clinical signs and geographic location • Antibiotics: chloramphenicol, amoxicillin/clavulanic acid (Clavamox®), trimethoprim-sulfa, tetracycline, or quinolones • Bronchodilators: aminophylline, theophylline, terbutaline albuterol, or ipratropium bromide • Corticosteroids (systemic): prednisolone, dexamethasone • Corticosteroids (inhalers): fluticasone • Cyproheptadine • Sympathomimetic: epinephrine, isoproterenol, terbutaline, albuterol	• No specific medications • Sedatives to ↓ anxiety • Recommended treatment is surgical to correct stenotic nares, everted laryngeal saccules, and elongated soft palate • Extreme dyspnea presentation: IV catheter, anesthesia, endotracheal intubation
Treatment	Nursing care	• Handle gently to avoid added stress	• Intensive monitoring postoperatively (e.g. vital signs) for signs of airway collapse • Monitor temperature due to dyspneic animals in distress overheating • Monitor for gastric distention due to dyspneic patients tendency to swallow excess air

(Continued)

Table 6.63 / **Asthma, bronchitis and brachycephalic airway syndrome (Continued)**

Disease		Asthma, bronchitis	Brachycephalic airway syndrome
Follow-up	Patient care	• Monitor clinical signs	• Monitor for several days postoperatively for signs of aspiration while eating. • Do not encourage exercise and limit exercise in ↑ environmental temperatures
	Prevention/avoidance	• Early detection of recurrent infections • Eliminate any contributing environmental factors (e.g. cigarette smoke, air fresheners, hair sprays, dirty furnace filters, or certain cat litters)	• Maintain appropriate weight control • Selective breeding
	Complications	• Progression of disease • Bronchiectasis • Long-term use of corticosteroids (e.g. diabetes mellitus, immunosuppression)	• Death from hypoxia during or following an anesthetic procedure • Incisional hemorrhage leading to laryngeal occlusion • Excessive resection and subsequent nasal aspiration of food • Hyperthermia
	Prognosis	• Guarded • Excellent with determination of environmental allergen	• Fair • Guarded if severely affected
Notes		• Most cases are chronic and progressive • Avoid use of β-2 antagonists (e.g. propranolol)	• Caution: endotracheal tubes should be left in place as long as possible following an anesthetic procedure to prevent tracheal occlusion (see Table 20.14: Postanesthetic monitoring, page 902).
Client education		• Continue medication despite the disappearance of clinical signs • Lifelong medication and environmental changes may be necessary	• Dogs should not be exercised extensively or in hot weather • Surgery can improve the condition but will not completely correct the airway

Laryngeal Paralysis and Laryngitis

Laryngeal paralysis is unilateral or bilateral paralysis of the muscles moving the arytenoid cartilages. It can be congenital or acquired, but is more commonly acquired, and is seen in large to medium older retrievers.

Laryngitis is inflammation, swelling and irritation of the larynx.

Table 6.64 / Laryngeal paralysis and laryngitis

Disease	Laryngeal paralysis	Laryngitis
Presentation	• Inspiratory noise(stridor) and exercise intolerance • Acquired can be due to excessive panting	• Dogs: mild, self-limiting cough • Cats: systemic illness (anorexia, ptyalism, fever, dyspnea)
Diagnostic testing	• Laryngeal exam under heavy sedation/light anesthesia • Avoid drugs that depress respiratory effort • Thoracic radiographs to rule out pneumonia, pulmonary edema, megaesophagus, and masses	• Laryngeal exam under sedation • Biopsy to rule out neoplasia • Radiographs to rule out pneumonia • Cats: may see leukocytosis
Treatment	• If severe respiratory distress, sedation, endotracheal intubation recommended • IV fluids to correct hyperthermia • Unilateral arytenoid lateralization surgery	• Antitussive medications • Tracheostomy tube if upper airway obstruction
Nutrition	• Prevent obesity • Feed small meatballs slowly post-surgery	• Prevent obesity • Feed small meatballs slowly post-surgery

Mediastinitis, Pneumomediastinum, and Mediastinal Masses

Mediastinitis is inflammation of the mediastinum (area between lungs). Pneumomediastinum is the accumulation of air in mediastinum. Most cases are self-limiting and mild.

Mediastinal masses form the most common mediastinal disease. Neoplasia is the most common, consisting of lymphoma, thymoma, thyroid carcinoma, parathyroid carcinoma, and chemodectoma. Non-neoplastic masses include abscesses, granulomas, hematomas, and cysts.

Table 6.65 / **Mediastinitis, pneumomediastinum, and mediastinal masses**

Disease	Mediastinitis	Pneumomediastinum	Mediastinal masses
Presentation	• Gagging, ptyalism, dysphagia, vomiting, lethargy, respiratory distress, swelling of head, neck or front legs, weight loss, fever • Full or partial blockage in esophagus/trachea • Infection due to trauma	• Pneumothorax, pneumoperitoneum, and pneumopericardium • Trauma to esophagus, trachea, pharynx, or pulmonary injury • Respiratory distress, dyspnea, subcutaneous emphysema, tissue trauma, muffled heart sounds • Less common causes: pneumonia, pulmonary abscess, neoplasia, chronic granulomatous infection, or pulmonary parasitic infection • Iatrogenic causes: tracheal wash, tracheostomy, e-tube placement, over-inflammation of e-tube cuff	• Inspiratory distress • Coughing, regurgitation, pleural effusion, palpable tissue mass, respiratory distress, facial edema
Diagnostics	• Ultrasound • Echocardiogram • CBC/chemistry • Blood gas • Thoracic and abdominal radiographs • Fluoroscopy swallow study • Endoscopy	• Thoracic radiographs • Ultrasound • CT • Thoracocentesis	• Thoracic radiographs • Thoracocentesis • Cytology • Ultrasound • FNA • CT • Fluoroscopy swallow study • Endoscopy • Biopsy
Treatment	• Severe case: hospitalization with IV fluids, antibiotics, and chest tube • Abscess: surgery recommendation • Foreign body: removal via endoscopy or surgery • Medical management ranges from 2 weeks to 6 months (depending on type infection)	• Chest tube • Medical management-most common • Surgical management	• Varied (neoplastic vs. non neoplastic) • Medical vs. surgical • Chemotherapy • Radiation therapy

Bronchitis

In dogs, bronchitis is usually a progressive condition leading to permanent damage. Less frequently, it can be acute with reversible damage. The causes include viral, bacterial, mycoplasma, infection, pulmonary parasites, heartworm disease, allergic, inhaled irritants, or foreign bodies.

Feline Lower Airway Disease

Feline lower airway disease encompasses a variety of lower airway conditions, predominantly asthma and bronchitis, which causes airflow limitation by a combination of factors, including airway inflammation, accumulation of mucus in the airway, and smooth muscle contraction.

Table 6.66 / **Bronchitis**

Disease		Bronchitis (canine)	Feline lower airway disease (asthma, chronic bronchitis)
Presentation	Clinical signs	• Cachexia, coughing, dyspnea, gagging, open-mouth breathing, shortness of breath, tachypnea, wheezing, exercise intolerance	• Wheezing, coughing, respiratory distress, , open mouth breathing, lethargic
	Exam findings	• Arrhythmias, cyanosis, dehydration, pyrexia, murmur, pulmonary crackles, syncope, tachycardia, tracheal sensitivity	• Open mouth breathing, cyanotic mucous membranes, orthopneic posture, auscultation (may have wheezing or crackles, increased lung sounds)
Diagnosis	General	• History/clinical signs • Airway examination • Cardiac auscultation	• History/clinical signs • Airway examination • Cardiac auscultation

	Laboratory	• Blood gas analysis
		• CBC: neutrophilia or monocytosis, eosinophilia and ↑ PCV
		• Chemistry panel: ↑ ALT and ALP
		• Urinalysis: ↑ specific gravity
		• Fecal analysis: parasites
		• Heartworm tests: microfilaria and adult antigen
		• Cytology, transtracheal or bronchial wash: bacterial clusters, eosinophils, macrophages, neutrophils
		• Bacterial and fungal culture, transtracheal or bronchial wash: isolation and identification
			• CBC: eosinophilia (> 1500 cells/µl)
			• FIV/FeLV test (if +, may affect prognosis)
			• Heartworm test
			• Baermann fecal test: lungworm evaluation
			• Lower airway cytology:
			  • Evaluate for *Mycoplasma* spp., *Aelurostrongylus* larvae, neoplastic cells
			  • Allergic asthma ≤ 17% eosinophils
			  • Chronic bronchitis: non-degenerate neutrophils
			  • Asthmatic bronchitis: mixed eosinophils and neutrophils

	Imaging	• Radiographs, thoracic: normal in acute disease or ↑ cardiac size (variable), ↑ interstitial density, aerophagia, peribronchial infiltrates, lung lobe atelectatic, flattening diaphragm, dilated airways, hyperinflation, or bronchial pattern • Echocardiogram: right heart enlargement, pulmonary hypertension, and rule out of congestive heart failure	• Thoracic radiographs – to bronchointerstitial pattern, hyperinflation (flattened diaphragm, expanded lung field), hyperlucent lungs, collapsed right middle lung lobe, aerophagia
	Procedures	• Bronchoscopy: sputum sample, tumor, inflammation, foreign bodies and parasites • ECG: sinus arrhythmia, peaked P waves and a wandering atrial pacemaker	• Bronchoscopy – airway injury, inflammation, narrowing, mucous plugs, airway collapse

(Continued)

Table 6.66 / **Bronchitis (Continued)**

Disease		Bronchitis (canine)	Feline lower airway disease (asthma, chronic bronchitis)
Treatment	General	• Supportive • Oxygen therapy	• Supportive • Oxygen therapy
	Medication	• Antibiotics: chloramphenicol, amoxicillin/clavulanic acid (Clavamox®), trimethoprim-sulfa, cephalothin, enrofloxacin, or quinolones • Antitussives: hydrocodone or butorphanol • Bronchodilators: aminophylline, theophylline, or terbutaline • Corticosteroids: prednisone, dexamethasone • Corticosteroids (inhalers): fluticasone • Sympathomimetic: epinephrine, isoproterenol, terbutaline, albuterol • Tranquilizers	• Glucocoticoids • Bronchodilator (if bronchoconstriction is suspected): theophylline, terbutaline, albuterol • Sedation to decrease stress (butorphanol) • Antibiotic therapy: *Mycoplasma*-positive cats • Inhalation therapy: fluticasone propionate (glucocorticoid) • Salbutamol (bronchodilator, short-term use only) • Cyproheptadine (anti-serotonin/antihistamine) • Febendazole for *Aelurostrongylus abstrusus* (lungworm)
	Nursing care	• Nebulization • Chest-wall coupage	• Oxygen • Reduce environmental stressors
Follow-up	Patient care	• Weight loss	• Weight loss
	Prevention/avoidance	• Maintain appropriate weight control • Use a harness instead of a collar • Eliminate any contributing environmental factors (e.g. cigarette smoke and dirty furnace filters) • Humidifier followed by light exercise to encourage expelling of sputum • Maintain oral health • Heartworm prevention	• Eliminate any environmental factors (e.g. cigarette smoke, dusty litter, and dirty air filters) • Weight management
	Complications	• Pneumonia • Bacterial infection • Bronchiectasis • Syncope • Pulmonary hypertension	• Pneumonia • Spontaneous pneumothorax (secondary to asthma) • Bacterial infection • Bronchiectasis • ?? Pulmonary hypertension
	Prognosis	• Good • Poor with irreversible changes from chronic bronchitis	• Good with prompt treatment • Variable, depending on severity
Notes		• Caution: equipment used (e.g. nebulizer) needs to be thoroughly cleaned to prevent bacterial contamination	
Client education		• Harnesses should be used in place of collar • Weight loss may improve symptoms • Exercise assists in clearing airways; limit if this results in coughing • Dental care reduces secondary bacterial infections	

Other Pulmonary Diseases and Conditions

Other pulmonary diseases and conditions are described in Tables 6.67 and 6.68.

Table 6.67 / Other pulmonary diseases

Disease	Description
Pulmonary edema	• Accumulation of fluid in the pulmonary interstitium and alveoli • Heart failure • Fluid overload • Increased vascular hydrostatic pressure • Hypoalbuminemia, vasculitis, decreased lymphatic drainage • Treatment includes diuretics and oxygen
Pulmonary contusions	• Hemorrhage into pulmonary interstitium and alveoli caused by blunt trauma to the thorax • common in animals hit by cars • radiographic changes appear within 24 hours of trauma • traumatic myocarditis warrants continuous ECG monitoring • hypoventilation • Treatment includes pain management, oxygen, ventilation support
Eosinophilic bronchopneumopathy and eosinophilic granulomatosis	• Idiopathic inflammatory disorder • Pulmonary infiltrates with eosinophils • Commonly seen in middle aged large-breed dogs • Progressive exercise intolerance • Cough (often productive) • Nasal discharge • Thoracic radiographs: varying lung patterns and combination of unstructured interstitial, bronchial and alveolar changes • Heartworm disease, lungworm infection, pulmonary migration of other parasites, fungal, neoplasia • Treatment: corticosteroids • Environmental control
Lung lobe torsion	• Lung lobe rotates around axis of the lobar bronchus, closing off the bronchus and blocking venous drainage • Can be secondary to pleural effusion, trauma, or consolidation or atelectasis of the lung lobe • Seen more in dogs than cats • Radiograph findings – pleural effusion, lung lobe consolidation, abnormal positioning of bronchus • Diagnostics: bronchoscopy • Pleural fluid cytology: chyle, modified transudate, exudate or hemorrhage • Treatment: oxygen, thoracocentesis in prep for lung lobectomy

(Continued)

Table 6.67 / Other pulmonary diseases (Continued)

Disease	Description
Idiopathic pulmonary fibrosis	• Definition: progressive interstitial lung disease of dogs (cats rare) • End result of pulmonary inflammation or secondary to inhaled toxins (drugs, neoplasia) • Common in West Highland White Terriers (middle aged or older) • Clinical signs include exercise intolerance, dyspnea, and nonproductive cough. Tachypnea and inspiratory crackles on physical exam • Thoracic radiographs show diffuse interstitial patterns; may see right-heart enlargement if pulmonary hypertension present • Lung biopsy • Corticosteroids • Other immunosuppressive drugs (azathioprine) • Pulmonary vasodilators • Bronchodilators • Weight management • Environmental control
Pulmonary thromboembolism	• Obstruction of a pulmonary vessel or vessels by a thrombus that forms in a vessel or by an embolus that forms elsewhere and travels to the lung • Secondary condition • Seen in patients with heartworm infection, IMHA, PLE and/or PLN, hyperadrenocorticism, cardiac disease, sepsis, and trauma • Clinical signs: tachypnea and respiratory distress • Thoracic radiographs: variable but can look normal • Plasma D-dimer • Scintigraphy, angiography, CT, MRI • Treatment: oxygen, anticoagulants, thrombolytic treatment (tPA or streptokinase)
Acute respiratory distress syndrome (ARDS)	• Rapidly progressive acute respiratory failure due to acute lung injury • Secondary condition • Sepsis (most common), aspiration/bacterial pneumonia, drug or transfusion reaction, severe inflammatory disease, trauma • Clinical signs: acute respiratory distress, crackles, wheezes • Thoracic radiographs 0 bilateral alveolar or mixed pulmonary changes • Echocardiogram • Treatment: oxygen and treating underlying disease • Mechanical ventilation, diuretics • High mortality
Smoke inhalation	• Definition: airway and lung injury due to heat, toxic gases, and particles inhaled • Tissue injury, edema, and tissue hypoxia • Inflammation, increased respiratory secretions, and decrease oxygen uptake due to carbon monoxide toxicity • Treatment: oxygen, IV fluids for rehydration, nebulization, bronchodilators, corticosteroids, antibiotics for secondary infections
Pulmonary neoplasia	• Metastatic neoplasia most common • Neoplastic lesions can be difficult to distinguish between inflammatory/infectious lesions on thoracic radiographs • Diagnostics: lung aspiration, transtracheal wash, bronchoalveolar lavage • Treatment: depends on type of neoplasia (chemotherapy, surgery, radiation)

Table 6.68 / **Other pulmonary conditions**

Condition	Definition	Clinical signs	Diagnostics	Treatment

Pleural effusion	• Abnormal accumulation of fluid in the pleural space
	• Transudate, modified transudate, exudate, hemorrhagic, chylous
		• Tachypnea, shallow breathing, dyspnea, orthopnea, cyanosis, cough
		• Fever, anorexia, weight loss, heart murmur, arrhythmias, jugular pulses, ascites
			• Thoracic radiographs
			• Transudates:
			  • increased capillary hydrostatic pressure (congestive heart failure, pericardial effusion/cardiac tamponade, PTE, heartworm disease, decreased vascular oncotic pressure, or hypoproteinemia)
			  • appears clear, protein concentration < 2.5 g/dl, cell count < 1500 ul
			• Modified transudates:
			  • increased vascular permeability or vasculitis (infection/inflammation), increased lymphatic permeability (neoplasia), increased hydrostatic pressure (lung lobe torsion)
			  • appearance hazy, protein concentration 2.5–4.5 g/dl, cell count 1000–3000 ul
			• Exudates – high protein and cell count:
			  • increased vascular or lymphatic permeability or reduced lymphatic drainage (FIP, neoplasia, chronic diaphragmatic hernia)
			  • appears turbid to opaque, protein concentration >3 g/dl, cell count > 3000 ul
				• Removal of sufficient volume of pleural fluids to relieve respiratory distress (thoracentesis or chest tube placement)
				• Treatment of underlying cause (diuretics, colloids)

Pneumothorax	• Presence of free air in the pleural space • Can be secondary to trauma • Spontaneous pneumothorax not associated with trauma • Iatrogenic can be a result of injury following an aspiration procedure	• Tachypnea, shallow breathing, dyspnea, orthopnea, cyanosis. Cough. fever, anorexia, weight loss, heart murmur, arrhythmias, jugular pulses, ascites	• Thoracic radiographs: air in the pleural space	• Cage rest for subclinical to mild presentation • Thoracocentesis recommended when there is difficulty breathing. • Chest tube placement if thoracocentesis required often

(*Continued*)

Table 6.68 / Other pulmonary conditions (Continued)

Condition	Definition	Clinical signs	Diagnostics	Treatment
Hemothorax	• Accumulation of blood in the pleural space • Can be secondary to trauma, ulcerated thoracic/lung mass(s), lung lobe torsion, PTE, or system coagulation disorders)	• Tachypnea, shallow breathing, dyspnea, orthopnea, cyanosis, cough • External wounds may be present	• Thoracic radiographs	• Removal of a sufficient volume of pleural blood to relieve respiratory distress • Treating underlying cause • Blood transfusion if patient anemic
Chylothorax	• Accumulation of lipid rich chyle in the pleural space • Idiopathic vs. secondary to injury or obstruction • Hazy to milky appearance	• Tachypnea, shallow breathing, dyspnea, orthopnea, cyanosis, cough • External wounds may be present	• Chyle fluid has higher triglyceride concentration than serum	• Thoracocentesis to relieve respiratory distress. Caution removing large volumes • Low fat diet recommended
Pyothorax	• Accumulation of purulent pleural fluid • Thoracic wall injury, migrating foreign body, pulmonary infection	• External wounds may be present • Febrile frequently	• Aerobic and anaerobic cultures • Cytology	• Thoracocentesis • Chest tubes • Lavage via chest tube • Antimicrobial therapy • Surgical exploration to rule out foreign body
Ciliary dyskinesia	• Function of cilia impaired • Failure of the mucociliary clearance mechanism • Hereditary vs. acquired	• Chronic or recurring respiratory infections	• Thoracic radiographs – bronchiectasis, situs inversus, or dextrocardia • Electron microscopic examination of ciliated cells (samples from respiratory epithelium or sperm)	• Control of secondary infection and accumulation of secretions • Antibiotics, nebulization • Prevention, avoidance: smoke, aerosol sprays, and other irritant particles; antitussives; obesity

Pneumonia

Pneumonia is an inflammatory response of the terminal airways and pulmonary interstitium. It is most commonly caused by bacteria but can also be caused by aspiration of ingesta, fungi, allergic, foreign body, viral, neoplasia, lung parasites, or contusions. It has a high rate of mortality and morbidity, especially in hospitalized animals.

Table 6.69 / Pneumonia

Disease		Pneumonia
Presentation	Clinical signs	• Cachexia, dyspnea, mucopurulent nasal discharge, productive cough, tachypnea, wheezes, generalized weakness
	Exam findings	• Crackles, cyanosis, dehydration, pyrexia, loud or asymmetric bronchial sounds, tachycardia
Diagnosis	General	• History/clinical signs • Pulmonary auscultation
	Laboratory	• CBC: neutrophilic leukocytosis with or without a left shift and monocytosis • Cytology, tracheal wash: ↑ neutrophils and bacteria • Culture, tracheal wash: bacteria isolation and identification • PCR, viral: +
	Imaging	• Radiographs, thoracic: ↑ lung density, lung consolidation, pulmonary artery enlargement or interstitial pattern with air bronchograms • Contrast study: swallowing disorders, megaesophagus
	Procedures	• Bronchoscopy: foreign body or neutrophilic inflammation • Bronchial alveolar lavage • Transtracheal wash • Tracheal wash • Lung aspirate

(Continued)

Table 6.69 / **Pneumonia (Continued)**

	Disease	Pneumonia
Treatment	General	• Supportive • Fluid therapy • Oxygen therapy • Surgery: lung lobectomy (rare)
	Medication	• Antibiotics: (broad spectrum) dependent on type of bacteria isolated and one with good penetration into lung tissue (e.g. enrofloxacin) • Combination of an aminopenicillin or first generation cephalosporin and fluoroquinolone or an aminoglycoside • Antibiotics typically recommended 1–2 weeks past resolution of clinical and radiographic evidence of disease. • Antifungal: amphotericin, flucytosine, ketoconazole, fluconazole, itraconazole, posaconazole • Bronchodilators: theophylline or terbutaline uncommonly used • Mucolytic: N-acetylcysteine uncommonly used
	Nursing care	• Nebulization with bland aerosols followed by chest wall coupage and tracheal manipulation • Monitor respiratory rate and effort and perform frequent thoracic auscultation • Restrict activity • Alter the patient's position at least every 2 hours • Nutritional support
Follow-up	Patient care	• Airway humidification • Mild exercise • Radiograph at 48–72 hours, then after 2–6 weeks
	Prevention/avoidance	• Vaccinate
	Complications	• Chronic bronchitis • Secondary infection/sepsis
	Prognosis	• Good with early and aggressive treatment • Guarded with severe hypoxemia and sepsis

Rhinitis and Sinusitis

Infection of the nasal sinuses is a common veterinary problem. Acute rhinitis is self-limiting and chronic sinusitis may require constant treatment. The causes are bacterial, viral, fungi, foreign body, dental disease, infectious agents, or neoplasia.

Tracheal Collapse

A collapsing trachea is a trachea with a range of dynamic variations resulting in collapse somewhere along its length. It may also involve the mainstem bronchi causing them to collapse also. It can be an acquired weakness or congenital defect. It is most commonly seen in older toy breed dogs.

Table 6.70 / Rhinitis, sinusitis, and tracheal collapse

Disease		Rhinitis/sinusitis	Tracheal collapse
Presentation	Clinical signs	• Cough, gagging, mucopurulent nasal discharge, ocular discharge, open-mouth breathing, retching, sneezing	• Cachexia, change in voice, dyspnea, gagging, heat intolerance, intermittent "honking" cough, syncope
	Exam findings	• Bony swelling, pyrexia, lymphadenopathy, oral ulceration, ocular or neurological changes	• Cyanosis, enlarged tonsils, stertor, stridor
Diagnosis	General	• History/clinical signs • Nasal examination	• History/clinical signs • Airway examination
	Laboratory	• CBC: depending on underlying condition (anemia, leukocytosis, neutrophilia, eosinophilia) • Serology: FeLV and FIV • Cytology and culture: bacteria recognition and identification • Fungal culture: isolation and identification	• CBC: inflammatory leukogram • Chemistry panel: ↑ liver enzymes • Bile acids concentrations: ↑ values
	Imaging	• Radiographs, skull: ↑ fluid and bony changes (e.g. loss of bone detail and deviated septum) • Radiographs, thoracic: variable (neoplasia, lower airway disease, or fungal disease) • Radiographs, dental: periodontal disease • CT/MRI, skull	• Radiographs, thoracic: narrowing or ballooning of tracheal diameter and ↑ right-sided cardiac size • Radiographs, cervical/pharyngeal: narrowing or ballooning of tracheal diameter
	Procedures	• Rhinoscopy: foreign body and bony changes • Biopsy: inflammatory, bacteria, or fungi	• Bronchoscopy: severity (grading of I–IV) and small airway disease • Fluoroscopy: narrowing of tracheal diameter may be dynamic

(Continued)

Table 6.70 / **Rhinitis, sinusitis, and tracheal collapse (Continued)**

Disease		Rhinitis/sinusitis	Tracheal collapse
Treatment	General	• Supportive • Fluid therapy • Radiotherapy • Surgery: nasal exploratory, rhinotomy, or turbinectomy	• Symptomatic • Oxygen therapy • Surgery: application of intraluminal or extraluminal prostheses
	Medication	• Dependent on underlying cause • Antibiotics: cephalexin, trimethoprim-sulfa, chloramphenicol, and doxycycline • Antihistamines • Corticosteroids (systemic): prednisone • Corticosteroids (inhalers): fluticasone • Fungicides: enilconazole, itraconazole, thiabendazole, or ketoconazole • NSAIDs: piroxicam, carprofen, deracoxib • Supplements: l-lysine	• Antibiotics: doxycycline • Antitussives: butorphanol, hydrocodone • Bronchodilators: aminophylline, theophylline, terbutaline, guaifenesin • Corticosteroids: prednisone
	Nursing care	• Airway humidification • Nutritional support	• Intensive monitoring during and postoperatively for signs of hypoxia
Follow-up	Patient care	• Monitor for relapse of clinical signs.	• Limit activity • Weight loss • Chest harness
	Prevention/avoidance	• Vaccinate • Maintain good oral hygiene • Prevent exposure to bird feces (aspergillosis and cryptococcosis)	• Maintain proper weight control • Avoid respiratory distress (extreme temperature or humidity changes, cigarette smoke, pollen, dust, or other allergens)
	Complications	• Brain infection and neurological signs • Epistaxis	• Death from hypoxia (rare)
	Prognosis	• Fair to good	• Good with uncomplicated surgery • Guarded with symptomatic treatment
Notes		• Serous nasal discharge is indicative of acute or allergic disease. • Mucopurulent discharge suggests bacterial or fungal infection (infection may be only secondary to underlying neoplasia)	• Obtain both inspiratory and expiratory radiographs: Tracheal collapse may be seen at any point during breathing • Grade 1: reduction of tracheal lumen by 25%; grade II: 50%; grade III: 75%; grade IV: > 90% • Condition is irreversible; treatment is based on preventing cough triggers

URINARY AND RENAL DISORDERS

Cystic Calculi

Any macroscopic concretions found within the urinary bladder are called cystic calculi or uroliths. They can be found anywhere along the urinary tract but are most commonly seen in the urinary bladder.

Feline Lower Urinary Tract Disease

Feline lower urinary tract disease (FLUTD) is the inflammation of the lower urinary tract including the bladder and urethra. It is typically idiopathic. The inflammation can be caused by anxiety, a combination of early stressors, concurrent medical conditions and waxing/waning clinical signs that coincide with environmental stresses.[175] It can also occur secondary to bacterial infection, crystalluria or iatrogenic (e.g. urinary catheterization).

Pyelonephritis

Pyelonephritis is inflammation of the renal parenchyma, collecting diverticula, ureters and its pelves. It is typically used to refer to a kidney infection. It is most commonly due to bacterial invasion.

Table 6.71 / Cystic calculi, feline lower urinary tract disease, and pyelonephritis

Disease		Cystic calculi	Feline lower urinary tract disease	Pyelonephritis
Presentation	Clinical signs	• Dysuria, hematuria, malodorous, stranguria, pollakiuria, periuria	• Anuria, dysuria, hematuria, licking at perineal area, periuria, pollakiuria, polyuria	• Anorexia, arched back, cachexia, depression, dysuria, hematuria, lethargy, malodorous or discolored urine, pollakiuria, polyuria/polydipsia, stranguria, vomiting
	Exam findings	• Abdominal pain, dehydration	• Thickened, firm contracted bladder wall	• Abdominal and lumbar pain, dehydration, pyrexia, tachycardia
	General	• History/clinical signs: recurrent bacterial UTI • Bladder palpation (variable)	• History/clinical signs • Abdominal palpation: bladder • Perineal examination	• History/clinical signs • Abdominal palpation: kidney

(Continued)

Table 6.71 / **Cystic calculi, feline lower urinary tract disease, and pyelonephritis (Continued)**

Disease		Cystic calculi	Feline lower urinary tract disease	Pyelonephritis
Diagnosis	Laboratory	• Chemistry panel: dependent on type of calculi, ↑ potassium, BUN, calcium, creatinine and metabolic acidosis • Urinalysis: ↑ bacteria, crystals, change in pH (depending on type of calculi) • Urine culture: bacteria isolation and identification • Bile acids or ammonia concentration: ↑ with ammonium urate calculi and portosystemic shunts • PTH: rule out hyperparathyroidism • Stone analysis and bacterial culture: needed for long-term treatment	• Urinalysis: ↑ blood, neutrophils, protein, bacteria, crystals • Urine culture: bacteria isolation and identification	• CBC: neutrophilic leukocytosis with or without a left shift (variable) and nonregenerative anemia • Chemistry panel: ↑ BUN, creatinine, phosphorus, and azotemia, ↑ SDMA • Urinalysis: ↑ bacteria, neutrophils, blood, protein, leukocyte casts, crystals, ↓ specific gravity • Cytology, renal pelvis: bacteria and neutrophils • Urine culture: bacteria isolation and identification
	Imaging	• Radiographs, abdominal: radiopaque calculi (calcium oxalate, calcium phosphate, cystine, struvite) • Contrast: radiolucent calculi and vesicourachal diverticula (urate, xanthine, small radiopaque calculi) • Ultrasound, abdominal: calculi	• Radiographs, abdominal: anatomic abnormalities, calculi, urethral plugs, tumors, or urachal diverticula • Radiographs, contrast: urethral strictures, tumors, radiolucent calculi, or vesicourachal diverticula • Ultrasound, abdominal: anatomic abnormalities, calculi, tumors, or urachal diverticula	• Radiographs, abdominal: ↓ size of kidneys and contours (variable), nephroliths • Ultrasound, abdominal: dilation of renal pelvis and proximal ureter, kidney size, and nephroliths
	Procedures	• Not applicable	• Not applicable	• Pyelocentesis: urine culture and renal biopsy • Blood pressure: • Primary: narrowing of vasculature delivering blood to the kidneys • Secondary: increased blood pressure in response to electrolyte derangement, hypertension, hypotension (shock)

(*Continued*)

Table 6.71 / **Cystic calculi, feline lower urinary tract disease, and pyelonephritis (Continued)**

Disease		Cystic calculi	Feline lower urinary tract disease	Pyelonephritis
Treatment	General	• Symptomatic • Fluid therapy • Medical dissolution (struvite, urate, and cystine only) • Urohydropulsion • Surgery: shockwave lithotripsy, laparoscopic cystotomy, cystotomy, ureterotomy	• Symptomatic • MEMO (Multimodal Environmental Modifications)[175]	• Symptomatic • Surgery: nephrotomy, nephrectomy, shockwave lithotripsy
	Medication	• Allopurinol (ammonium urate) • Antibiotics: variable • MPG or D-penicillamine (cystine) • Urine alkalinizer: potassium citrate, sodium bicarbonate	• β-adrenergic blocker: phenoxybenzamine • Analgesics: buprenorphine, gabapentin • Antibiotics: variable • Glycosaminoglycan (variable): glucosamine, pentosan polysulfate sodium • Tranquilizers: diazepam • Tricyclic antidepressant: amitriptyline • Urine acidifier: DL-methionine, ammonium chloride	• Antibiotics: variable • Opioids: buprenorphine, fentanyl
	Nursing care	• Access to clean litter box or frequent walks • Monitor for anuria	• Access to clean litter box or frequent walks • Monitor for anuria • Treated as outpatient	• Access to clean litter box or frequent walks • Treated as outpatient

(*Continued*)

Table 6.71 / Cystic calculi, feline lower urinary tract disease, and pyelonephritis (Continued)

Disease		Cystic calculi	Feline lower urinary tract disease	Pyelonephritis
Follow-up	Patient care	• Monitor urine pH and specific gravity • Strict diet restrictions depending on type of calculus • Monitor dissolution monthly by radiographs, urinalysis, urine culture, and ultrasound • Monitor radiographs every 3–4 months on patients with surgical removal for reoccurrence	• Culture urine 1 week after beginning treatment and 1 week following completion of treatment • ↑ Water consumption by feeding canned food mixed with water, adding potassium or sodium chloride to the food or subcutaneous fluids • Monitor males for urethral obstruction	• Culture urine 3–5 days and 1 month after beginning treatment. • Perform a urinalysis and urine culture 7 and 28 days after completing treatment • ↑ Water consumption by feeding canned food mixed with water, adding sodium chloride to the food or subcutaneous fluids
	Prevention/avoidance	• Strict diet restrictions depending on the type of calculi • Monitor urine pH	• Acidifying or low-magnesium diet • Avoid stress • Encourage water consumption • Maintain a clean litter box • Avoid unnecessary use of urinary catheters	• Correct ectopic ureters • Encourage water consumption
	Complications	• Reoccurrence • Urethral obstruction/bladder rupture • Secondary bacterial UTI	• Urethral obstruction (feline, male) • Recurrence	• Chronic renal failure • Reoccurrence • Nephrolithiasis • Septicemia or septic shock • Metastatic infection
	Prognosis	• Excellent with treatment	• Excellent with treatment	• Fair to good: may have irreversible kidney damage
Notes		• Calculi and urine pH • Struvite: alkaline urine • Ammonium urate and silica: neutral to acid urine • Cystine: acid urine • Calcium oxalate: any urine pH • Radiolucent: cystine and ammonium urate • Radiopaque: calcium oxalate and struvite • Struvite more likely in females, also account for 41% of analyzed stones • Presence of crystals does not indicate the presence of stones[176]	• Stress is often a contributing factor; evaluate environmental stressors and offer solutions • Treatment efficacy can be evaluated by a negative urine culture 2–3 days after starting treatment	• Pyelonephritis should not be ruled out with a negative culture

Renal Failure

Acute kidney injury develops into a rapid decline in renal function. It is the accumulation of uremic toxins due to prerenal and renal causes of filtration failure, dysregulation of fluids, electrolytes and acid–base balances, as well as post-renal causes such as obstruction. Unlike chronic renal failure, this condition may be reversible if diagnosed quickly and treated aggressively.

Chronic renal failure is the progressive decline in the function of the kidneys leading to their shutdown over months to years. The damage is irreversible. The causes may be familial, medications, toxins, neoplasia, ischemia or infectious disease.

Table 6.72 / Renal failure

Disease		Renal failure	
		Acute	Chronic
Presentation	Clinical signs	• Anorexia, anuria, ataxia, bruising, diarrhea, dyspnea, lethargy, depression, oliguria, polyuria, seizures, tachypnea, vomiting	• Anorexia, blindness, coma, constipation, diarrhea, lethargy, nocturia, polyuria/polydipsia, seizures, vomiting, dehydration weakness, exercise intolerance
	Exam findings	• Bradycardia, cardiac abnormalities, dehydration, enlarged painful kidneys, halitosis, hypothermia, nonpalpable urinary bladder or large turgid bladder, oral ulcerations, pyrexia	• Ascites, dehydration, halitosis, oral ulcerations, small, firm nodular kidneys, subcutaneous edema
Diagnosis	General	• History/clinical signs • Abdominal palpation: kidney and bladder	• History/clinical signs • Abdominal palpation: kidney
	Laboratory	• CBC: leukocytosis with or without a left shift (variable), lymphopenia, monocytosis, ↑ PCV and nonregenerative anemia (variable) • Chemistry panel: ↑ BUN, creatinine, ↑ SDMA, phosphorus, phosphate, glucose, potassium, ALP, albumin, lipase, calcium (acute renal failure), and ↓ protein, calcium (ethylene glycol), and azotemia • Urinalysis: ↑ bacteria, crystals, neutrophils, albumin, glucose, cellular and granular casts, ↓ specific gravity (≤ 1.020 g/dl) • Protein: creatinine ratio: > 1 (3–5 severe) • Urine culture: bacteria isolation and identification • Blood gas: metabolic acidosis • Serology: leptospirosis or ehrlichiosis • PCR: Heterobilharzia • Ethylene glycol concentration: + results • Biopsy: confirmation, cause, and severity of disease	• CBC: nonregenerative anemia • Chemistry panel: metabolic acidosis, ↑ BUN, creatinine, SDMA, amylase, lipase, phosphate, and ↓ potassium, ±calcium, ↑↓ protein • Urinalysis: ↑ protein (v), ↓ specific gravity (< 1.030 canines and < 1.035 felines) • Protein: creatinine ratio: to determine severity of proteinuria and glomerular disease • Assay, microalbuminuria: +albumin • Culture, urine: bacteria isolation and identification • Biopsy, renal: confirmation, cause, and severity of disease

(Continued)

Table 6.72 / Renal failure (Continued)

Disease		Renal failure	
		Acute	Chronic
	Imaging	• Radiographs, abdominal: renal size and shape, renal uroliths, peritonitis • Ultrasound, abdominal: renal uroliths and parenchymal and anatomical abnormalities • CT, contrast: urethral obstruction or structural rupture	• Radiographs, abdominal: renal size and shape and renal uroliths • Radiographs, contract: obstruction or structural rupture • Ultrasound, abdominal: renal size and shape, renal uroliths, and polycystic kidneys
	Procedures	• Endoscopy: gastric ulcers • Blood pressure: hypertension • Percutaneous renal biopsy: cause and severity of disease	• Blood pressure: hypertension • Biopsy, renal
Treatment	General	• Symptomatic • Supportive • Fluid therapy, ± potassium • Hemodialysis • Peritoneal dialysis • Blood transfusions • Poison antidotes (e.g. ethylene glycol) • Surgery: renal transplantation, ureterotomy, ureteral stents, or resection	• Symptomatic • Supportive • Fluid therapy • Hemodialysis • Peritoneal dialysis • Blood transfusions • Surgery: renal transplantation
Treatment	Medication	• Alkalinizer: sodium bicarbonate • Antibiotics: variable • Antiemetics: maropitant, ondansetron, dolasetron, metoclopramide • Ca+ channel blocker: diltiazem • Calcium supplement: calcium gluconate • Diuretics: 10–20% mannitol, 10% dextrose, furosemide • H2-receptor antagonist: famotidine, cimetidine, ranitidine • Phosphate binders: aluminum hydroxide, calcium carbonate, calcium acetate, Epakitin® • Potassium supplement: potassium chloride, potassium gluconate • Proton pump inhibitors: pantoprazole, omeprazole[82]	• ACE inhibitors: enalapril, benazepril, amlodipine • Alkalinizer: sodium bicarbonate • Androgens: stanozolol, nandrolone decanoate • Antiemetics: maropitant, ondansetron, dolasetron, metoclopramide • Erythropoietics: erythropoietin, darbepoetin • H2-receptor antagonist: cimetidine, famotidine, ranitidine • Phosphate binders: aluminum hydroxide, calcium carbonate, calcium acetate, Epakitin • Potassium supplement: potassium chloride, potassium gluconate • Vitamin D: calcitriol
Treatment	Nursing care	• Monitor vomiting and provide nutritional support. • Monitor urine output, 1–3 ml/minute initially • Monitor hydration, temperature, and body weight, four times a day • Monitor PCV and blood values	• Nutritional support • Monitor urine output, 1–3 ml/minute initially • Monitor hydration, temperature, and body weight, four times a day • Monitor PCV and blood values

(*Continued*)

Table 6.72 / **Renal failure (Continued)**

Disease		Renal failure	
		Acute	Chronic
Follow-up	Patient care	• Monitor blood values until normal • Nutritional support • Renal diet: ↑ omega-3, caloric density, fiber, ↓ high-quality protein, phosphorus, sodium • Fresh water at all times to increase water consumption • Subcutaneous fluids for diuresis and hydration	• Nutritional support • Renal diet: ↑ omega-3, caloric density, fiber, ↓ high-quality protein, phosphorus, sodium • Fresh water at all times to increase water consumption • Subcutaneous fluids for diuresis and hydration • Monitor weekly initially then monitor hydration, weight, and blood values every 1–4 months depending on the severity of chronic renal failure
	Prevention/avoidance	• Anticipate acute renal failure in susceptible animals and conduct preventative fluids and medication • Avoid use of nephrotoxic drugs • Restrict exposure to antifreeze • Maintain adequate blood pressure during • anesthesia, especially in prolonged procedures and in older animals	• Anticipate acute renal failure in susceptible animals and conduct preventative fluids and medication • Avoid use of nephrotoxic drugs • Maintain adequate blood pressure during anesthesia • Selective breeding
	Complications	• Cardiac arrhythmias, congestive heart failure, pulmonary edema, uremic pneumonitis, or cardiopulmonary arrest • Gastrointestinal bleed • Pneumonitis (leptospirosis) • Hypovolemia, sepsis, and death • Seizures or coma • Death	• Anemia • Dehydration and constipation • Gastroenteritis • Hypertension • PLN • Uremic stomatitis • Urinary tract infection • Weight loss
	Prognosis	• Guarded to poor, but depends on severity and cause of injury	• Guarded to poor, long term due to progression of disease

Notes		• Modify all medications that require renal metabolism or elimination
		• Urine output:
		  • Anuria: ≤ 0.1 ml/kg/hour
		  • Oliguria: ≤ 0.25 ml/kg/hour (< 1 ml/kg/hour with fluid therapy)
		  • Non-oliguria: ≥ 2 ml/kg/hour
			• Isosthenuria seen before azotemia
			• Approximately 75% of the kidney must be nonfunctional before an elevation in serum BUN and creatinine is seen and 40% of the kidney must be nonfunctional before an elevation in SDMA in seen[177]
			• Monitor calcium and phosphorus levels when administering calcitriol

Common Causes of Acute Kidney Injury and Chronic Kidney Disease[177,178]

- Medications — Non-steroidal anti-inflammatory drugs, aminoglycosides, amphotericin B, cisplatin, cyclosporine
- Toxins — Ethylene glycol, rodenticide (vitamin D), raisins/grapes, lilies
- Bacterial infection — Leptospirosis, pyelonephritis, Rocky Mountain spotted fever, borreliosis, ehrlichiosis, babesiosis
- Ischemia — Anesthetic hypotension

Classification of Azotemia

- Prerenal azotemia – insufficient blood flow or increase in sources of nitrogenous waste: dehydration, hypotension (anesthetic), hypoadrenocorticism, trauma, shock, high-protein diet.
- Renal azotemia – injury to any part of the kidney: decreased perfusion, injury caused by medications, toxins, bacterial infection or ischemia.
- Postrenal azotemia – inability to excrete urine: obstruction, rupture.

Classification of Urine Specific Gravity

- **Normal**
  - **Canine > 1.030**
  - **Feline > 1.035**
- Isosthenuria 1.008–1.012
- Hyposthenuria < 1.008
  - While this low specific gravity may seem like a poor prognosticator, it indicates more renal function than isosthenuria because it requires more function to dilute urine to this level.
  - Dogs and cats can have an isosthenuric or hyposthenuric urine specific gravity (USG) normally, so without the proper symptoms (polyuria/polydipsia), their USG should not be overanalyzed.

Staging of Chronic Kidney Disease

Table 6.73 / Urine protein : creatinine ratio.[179,180]

Species	Non-proteinuric	Borderline	Proteinuric
Canine	< 0.2	0.2–0.5	> 0.5
Feline	< 0.2	0.2–0.4	> 0.4

Systolic Blood Pressure

Normotensive	< 140 mmHg
Prehypertensive	140–159 mmHg
Hypertensive	160–179 mmHg
Severely hypertensive	>180 mmHg

Urinary Tract Obstruction and Infection (Cystitis, Urethrocystitis)

Any obstruction will restrict the flow of urine along the pathway from the kidneys to the external urethral orifice. The obstruction can be from blood clots, urethral plugs, uroliths, tumors, or sloughed tissue fragments.

Urinary tract infection is usually a bacteria-induced inflammation of the lower urinary tract including the bladder and urethra. The cause is an ascending bacterial infection from the urethral orifice or is hematogenous.

Table 6.74 / Urinary tract obstruction and infection (cystitis, urethrocystitis)

Disease		Urinary tract obstruction	Urinary tract infection (cystitis, urethrocystitis)
Presentation	Clinical signs	• Anorexia, crouching, depression, dysuria, hematuria, lethargy, pollakiuria, ↑ size and velocity of urine stream, stranguria, vomiting, vocalizing	• Dysuria, hematuria, malodorous, periuria, pollakiuria, stranguria, urinary incontinence
	Exam findings	• Abdominal pain, bradycardia, dehydration, distended urinary bladder, hypothermia, renomegaly, protruding penis	• Thickened, firm contracted bladder wall
Diagnosis	General	• History/clinical signs • Abdominal palpation: kidneys and bladder • Digital rectal examination: stone or tumor	• History/clinical signs: recent catheterization or urinary tract surgery, chronic immunosuppressant administration, endocrinopathy (diabetes mellitus, HAC) • Abdominal palpation: kidneys and bladder • Digital rectal examination: prostate in males
	Laboratory	• CBC: ± stress leukogram • Chemistry panel: azotemia, metabolic acidosis, ↑ phosphorus, potassium, SDMA and ↓ calcium • Urinalysis: ↑ blood, protein, ± crystals • Blood gases: metabolic acidosis • Cytology, urinary tract: neoplasia, prostatic disease • Stone analysis and bacterial culture	• Urinalysis: ↑ blood, neutrophils, protein, bacteria, specific gravity • Urine culture: bacteria isolation and identification • Prostatic fluid analysis: bacteria and neutrophils

(*Continued*)

Table 6.74 / **Urinary tract obstruction and infection (cystitis, urethrocystitis) (Continued)**

Disease		Urinary tract obstruction	Urinary tract infection (cystitis, urethrocystitis)
	Imaging	• Radiographs, abdominal: anatomic abnormalities, extended bladder, calculi, urethral plugs, tumors, or urachal diverticula • Radiographs, contrast: urethral strictures, lesions, tumors, radiolucent uroliths, vesicourachal diverticula • Ultrasound, abdominal: anatomic abnormalities, extended bladder, calculi, tumors, or urachal diverticula	• Radiographs, abdominal: anatomic abnormalities, calculi, tumors, or urachal diverticula • Radiographs, contrast: radiolucent calculi • Ultrasound, abdominal: anatomic abnormalities, calculi, tumors, or urachal diverticula
	Procedures	• Cystocentesis: bladder decompression • Cystoscopy • ECG: bradycardia, atrial standstill	• Not applicable
Treatment	General	• Urinary catheter and decompression • Fluid therapy • Manage electrolyte abnormalities • Monitor • Fluids ins and outs • Hydration status • Vitals, particularly heart rate • Bladder size and patency of urinary catheter and collection • Surgery: urethrotomy, urethrostomy, lithotripsy	• Symptomatic
Treatment	Medication	• Antibiotics: variable • Calcium supplement: calcium gluconate • Potassium lowering drugs: sodium bicarbonate, insulin/glucose • Urethral relaxant: prazosin, phenoxybenzamine, bethanechol • Opioids: buprenorphine • Supplements: Cosequin® joint health supplement	• Antibiotics: variable • Probiotics
Treatment	Nursing care	• Monitor bladder size and urine output	• Treated as outpatient

(Continued)

Table 6.74 / Urinary tract obstruction and infection (cystitis, urethrocystitis) (Continued)

Disease		Urinary tract obstruction	Urinary tract infection (cystitis, urethrocystitis)
Follow-up	Patient care	• Monitor urine output and hydration status	• Culture urine 1 week after beginning treatment and 1 week following completion of treatment • Allow frequent access to litter box or outdoors
	Prevention/avoidance	• Dependent on the cause of obstruction	• Avoid glucocorticoid use • Avoid urethral catheterization and cystoscopy
	Complications	• Re-obstruction • Urinary tract infection • Urinary bladder rupture • Urethral trauma/stricture during catheterization • Shock • Death	• Pyelonephritis • Cystic calculi • Recurrence
	Prognosis	• Good with early detection and correction	• Excellent with uncomplicated bacterial UTI

Notes		• Caution: choose anesthetics carefully because of patient's compromised state (avoid IM ketamine due to its excretion in kidney)
		• Fluid therapy should not be started until obstruction has been relieved
		• Many different techniques are available for contrast radiographs, positive – contrast cystography, double-contrast cystography, excretory urography, retrograde positive urethrography
		• Post-obstruction care, monitoring and client education
			• Significant bacteria count:
			  • Cystocentesis: ≥ 1000 (cats and dogs)
			  • Catheter: ≥ 10 000 (dogs), ≥ 1000 (cats)
			  • Voided: ≥ 100 000 (dogs), ≥ 10 000 (cats)

Protein-Losing Nephropathy

Protein-losing nephropathy includes disorders that cause the loss of proteins due to disruption of the normal filtration barrier of the kidney. Conditions include glomerulonephritis (antibody/antigen complexes deposited in glomeruli causing inflammation and cell death) and amyloidosis (protein amyloid A is deposited in the kidneys in response to inflammation).[176]

Table 6.75 / Protein-losing nephropathy

Disease		Protein-losing nephropathy (glomerulonephritis and amyloidosis)
Presentation	Clinical signs	• Lethargy, vomiting, anorexia, weight loss, polyuria/polydipsia
	Examination findings	• unremarkable in early stages, but more advanced PLN can cause muscle wasting, pitting edema and ascites[181–183]
Diagnosis	General	• History/clinical signs • Abdominal palpation: kidney
	Laboratory	• Chemistry panel: azotemia, ↑ SDMA, hypoalbuminemia, hyperphosphatemia, metabolic acidosis • Hematology: anemia • Urinalysis: proteinuria
	Imaging	• Radiographs, abdominal: renal size and shape, and thoracic: possible neoplastic disease • Ultrasonography: increased cortical echogenicity[176]
	Procedures	• Renal biopsy to confirm and/or differentiate between glomerulonephritis and amyloidosis[183] • Blood pressure: systemic hypertension
Treatment	General	• Symptomatic, antihypertensives, dietary protein restriction, antithrombotic therapy
	Medication	• ACE inhibitors: enalapril, benazepril • Angiotensin II receptor blockers: telmisartan[82] • Antihypertensives: amlodipine • Immunosuppressive drugs: prednisone, mycophenolate • Anti-thrombotics: aspirin, clopidogrel • n-6 PUFA – direct supplementation or through diet • Amyloid A blocker: colchicine, DMSO[181]
	Nursing care	• monitor for peripheral edema, pale mucous membranes, blindness and weight loss
Follow-up	Patient care	• monitor UPC, azotemia and blood pressure
	Prevention/avoidance	• Proper flea and tick prevention, as some flea/tick-borne infectious diseases can be associated with GN
	Complications	• weight loss, hypertension/blindness, thromboembolic disease, nephrotic syndrome (proteinuria, hypoalbuminemia, ascites or edema and hypercholesterolemia)[183]
	Prognosis	• depends on the severity of azotemia and proteinuria. • In many cases, glomerulonephritis is progressive and the prognosis is poor
Notes		• PLN is rare in cats

Classification of Proteinuria

- Prerenal proteinuria – glomerulus receiving increased amounts of protein:
  - Physiologic prerenal proteinuria: caused by renal vasoconstriction, ischemia, congestion – strenuous exercise, fever, seizure, hyperthermia, inflammation
  - Pathologic prerenal proteinuria: small proteins too small to be filtered are excreted due to disease (hemoglobinuria, myoglobinuria, immunoglobulin light chains) – IMHA, rhabdomyolysis, dysproteinemias[176]
- Renal proteinuria:
  - Glomerular: injury to or dysfunction of the glomerulus – glomerulonephritis, amyloidosis[182]
  - Tubular: disease to the renal tubules that alters their ability to resorb proteins – CKD, Fanconi syndrome[176,182]
- Postrenal proteinuria: lower urinary tract inflammation or hemorrhage: UTI, urolithiasis, neoplasia, vaginitis

Table 6.76 / International Renal Interest Society Staging of Chronic Kidney Disease (modified 2019)[177,178]

Stage	1	2	3	4
Description	No azotemia	Mild azotemia	Moderate azotemia	Severe azotemia
Creatinine (mg/dl)				
Canine	< 1.4	1.4–2	2.1–5	> 5
Feline	< 1.6	1.6–2.8	2.9–5	> 5

Prostate Disease

Diseases of the prostate can include benign prostatic hyperplasia (BPH), prostatitis, prostatic infections and neoplasia of the prostate. BPH is an enlargement of the prostate over time in intact dogs due to the presence of testosterone. Fifty percent of intact dogs over five years of age exhibit some degree of BPH.[176,184]

Table 6.77 / Prostate disease

Disease		Prostate disease
Presentation	Clinical signs	• Hematuria, tenesmus, anorexia or fever possible with infection
	Examination findings	• Enlarged prostate on rectal examination • In prostatitis or prostate infections, exam may also include fever and lethargy, possibly painful prostate
Diagnosis	General	• History/clinical signs • Rectal examination: prostate • Histopathologic evaluation • Ultrasonographic evaluation • Urinalysis, semen evaluation
	Laboratory	• Urinalysis and urine culture: red blood cells, culture negative in BPH, bacteria seen with prostatitis • Prostatic fluid analysis and culture: red blood cells, epithelial cells, hematospermia, bacteria[184]
	Imaging	• Radiography • Ultrasound: enlargement and heterogeneity (small anechoic cysts)
	Procedures	• Biopsy of the prostate
Treatment	General	• castration • medical management if wanting to maintain breeding ability
	Medication	• 5-α-reductase inhibitor: finasteride[82,184] • Progestin: megestrol, medroxyprogesterone[82,184]
	Nursing care	• Monitor for dysuria, anuria, tenesmus or abdominal pain
Follow-up	Patient care	• Monitor for pain on prostatic exam • Monitor size via ultrasound and rectal exam • Monitor for worsening or changing of clinical signs, as prostatitis can occur in patients with BPH
	Prevention/avoidance	• Castration at a young age
	Complications	• Constipation • Perineal hernia
	Prognosis	• Prognosis with castration is very good with the prostate decreasing in size almost completely within 3 months[184] • Medical management has a good prognosis, but may not shrink the prostate as efficiently
Notes		• Scottish Terriers have a much larger prostate than other dogs of similar age and size[184]

Urinary Incontinence

Urinary incontinence is defined as an unconscious release of urine. This can be caused by a variety of conditions, including ectopic ureters, reflex dyssynergia and urethral sphincter mechanism incompetence (USMI). USMI is the most common cause of incontinence in adult female dogs.[176,185]

Table 6.78 / Urinary incontinence

Disease		Urinary incontinence
Presentation	Clinical signs	• Release of urine unconsciously
	Examination findings	• Often normal. May include urine staining, perivulvar dermatitis, erythematous vulva
Diagnosis	General	• history/clinical signs
	Laboratory	• Urinalysis: concentrated urine, otherwise normal • Chemistry, CBC and thyroid testing should be completed to help rule out other causes of disease or concurrent conditions exacerbating the incontinence

	Imaging	• To rule out other causes of urinary disease:
		  • Abdominal ultrasound
		  • Radiographs

	Procedures	• Cystoscopy to evaluate for and diagnose ectopic ureters • Surgical correction or laser ablation of ectopic ureters[186] • Cystoscopic injections of collagen to help narrow the urethra (urethral bulking)[176,185–187] • Cystometrogram with urethral pressure profile[186]
Treatment	General	• Increase muscle tone of the urethra
	Medication	• Sympathomimetics (USMI): phenylpropanolamine HCl, ephedrine sulfate • Estrogens (USMI): diethylstilbestrol, estradiol cypionate • Parasympathomimetic (reflex dyssynergia): bethanechol
	Nursing care	• Monitor for worsening of incontinence or changing clinical signs as conditions that cause polyuria/polydipsia will make incontinence worse

(Continued)

Table 6.78 / Urinary incontinence (Continued)

Disease		Urinary incontinence
Follow-up	Patient care	• Monitor for urine scalding and dermatitis • Frequent walks, particularly before times of rest or sleep
	Prevention/avoidance	• Many of these conditions are congenital or idiopathic with no known cause
	Complications	• Urine scalding • Dermatitis • USMI can occur in conjunction with ectopic ureters, therefore surgery or ablation alone may not be curative
	Prognosis	• Good with medical management • Phenylpropanolamine is effective in 85–90% of female dogs[187] • Surgery and laser ablation are effective for ectopic ureters

REFERENCES

1. Atkins, C., Bonagura, J., Ettinger, S. *et al.* (2009). Guidelines for the diagnosis and treatment of canine chronic valvular heart disease. *J Vet Intern Med* 23: 1142–1150.
2. Fine, D.M., DeClue, A.E., Reinero, C.R. (2008). Evaluation of circulating amino terminal-pro-B-type natriuretic peptide concentration in dogs with respiratory distress attributable to congestive heart failure or primary pulmonary disease. *J Am Vet Med Assoc* 232: 1674–1679.
3. Macgregor, J.M., Rush, J.E., Laste, N.J. *et al.* (2011). Use of pimobendan in 170 cats (2006–2010). *J Vet Cardiol* 13: 251–260.
4. Gordon, S.G., Saunders, A.B., Roland, R.M. *et al.* (2012). Effect of oral administration of pimobendan in cats with heart failure. *J Am Vet Med Assoc* 241: 89–94.
5. Reina-Doreste, Y., Stern, J.A., Keene, B.W. *et al.* (2014). Case–control study of the effects of pimobendan on survival time in cats with hypertrophic cardiomyopathy and congestive heart failure. *J Am Vet Med Assoc* 245: 534–539.
6. Summerfield, N.J., Boswood, A., O'Grady, M.R. *et al.* (2012). Efficacy of pimobendan in the prevention of congestive heart failure or sudden death in Doberman Pinschers with preclinical dilated cardiomyopathy (the PROTECT study) *J Vet Intern Med* 26: 1337–1349.
7. Freeman, L.M., Stern, J.A., Fries, R. *et al.* (2018). Diet-associated dilated cardiomyopathy in dogs: what do we know? *J Am Vet Med Assoc* 253: 1390–1394.
8. American Heartworm Society. (2018). *Current Canine Guidelines for the Prevention, Diagnosis, and Management of Heartworm*(Dirofilaria immitis) *Infection in Dogs.* Wilmington, DE: AHS; 2018.
9. American Heartworm Society. (2014). *Current Feline Guidelines for the Prevention, Diagnosis, and Management of Heartworm* (Dirofilaria immitis) *Infection in Cats.* Wilmington, DE: AHS; 2014.
10. Boswood, A., Häggstrom, J., Gordon, S.G. *et al.* (2016). Effect of pimobendan in dogs with preclinical myxomatous mitral valve disease and cardiomegaly: the EPIC study-a randomized clinical trial. *J Vet Intern Med* 30: 1765–1779.
11. Häggström, J., Boswood, A., O'Grady, M. *et al.* (2008). Effect of pimobendan or benazepril hydrochloride on survival times in dogs with congestive heart failure caused by naturally occurring myxomatous mitral valve disease: the QUEST study. *J Vet Intern Med* 22: 1124–1135.
12. Acierno, M.J., Brown, S., Coleman, A.E.*et al.* (2018). ACVIM consensus statement: guidelines for the identification, evaluation, and management of systemic hypertension in dogs and cats. *J Vet Intern Med* 32: 1803–1822.
13. Reusch, C. (2015). Water metabolism and diabetes insipidus. In: *Canine and Feline Endocrinology*, 4e (ed. E. Feldman, R. Nelson, C. Reusch *et al.*), 1–36. St. Louis, MO: Elsevier-Saunders.
14. Reusch, C. (2015). Disorders of growth hormone. In: Canine and Feline Endocrinology, 4e (ed. E. Feldman, R. Nelson, C. Reusch *et al.*), 37–77. St. Louis, MO: Elsevier-Saunders.
15. Sparkes, A., Cannon, M., Church, D. et al. (2015). ISFM consensus guidelines on the Practical Management of Diabetes Mellitus in cats. *J Feline Med Surg* 17: 235–250.
16. Zoran, D. and Rand, J. (2013). Feline diabetes, the role of diet in the prevention and management of feline diabetes. In: Veterinary Clinics of North America: Small Animal Practice (ed. J. Rand), 233–244. Philadelphia, PA: Elsevier.

17. Ramsey, I. and Reto, N. (2014). Canine hyperadrenocorticism therapy. In: *Kirk's Current Veterinary Therapy XV*. (ed. J. Bonagura and D. Twedt), 225–229. St. Louis, MO: Elsevier-Saunders.
18. Klein, S. and Peterson, M. (2010). Canine hypoadrenocorticism: part II. *Can Vet J* 51: 179–184.
19. Hohenhaus, A.E. and Winzelberg, S.E. (2017). Nonregenerative anemia. In: Textbook of Veterinary Internal Medicine (ed. S.J. Ettinger, E.C. Feldman and E. Côté), 2100–2112. St. Louis, MO: Elsevier.
20. Piek, C. (2017). Immune-mediated hemolytic anemias and other regenerative anemias. In: *Textbook of Veterinary Internal Medicine* (ed. S.J. Ettinger and E.C. Feldman), 2078–2099. St. Louis, MO: Elsevier.
21. Dracz, R.M., Mozzer, L.R., Fujiwara, R.T. *et al.* (2014). Parasitological and hematological aspects of co-infection with *Angiostrongylus vasorum* and *Ancylostoma caninum* in dogs. *Vet Parasitol* 200: 111–116.
22. Smith-Carr, S. (2015). Whipworm infection. In: *Clinical Veterinary Advisor* (ed. E. Côté), 1083–1084. St. Louis, MO: Elsevier.
23. Schnyder, M., Di Cesare, A., Basso, W. *et al.* (2014). Clinical, laboratory and pathological findings in cats experimentally infected with *Aelurostrongylus abstrusus*. *Parasitol Res* 113: 1425–1433.
24. Crisi, P.E., Aste, G., Traversa, D. *et al.* (2017). Single and mixed feline lungworm infections: clinical, radiographic and therapeutic features of 26 cases (2013–2015). *J Feline Med Surg* 19: 1017–1029.
25. Scott, K.D. (2015). Coccidiosis, intestinal. In: *Clinical Veterinary Advisor* (ed. E. Côté), 206–207. St. Louis, MO: Elsevier.
26. Parashar, R., Sudan, V., Jaiswal, A.K. *et al.* (2016). Evaluation of clinical, biochemical and haematological markers in natural infection of canine monocytic ehrlichiosis. *J Parasit Dis* 40: 1351–1354.
27. Chirek, A., Silaghi, C., Pfister, K. *et al.* (2018). Granulocytic anaplasmosis in 63 dogs: clinical signs, laboratory results, therapy and course of disease. *J Small Anim Pract* 59: 112–120.
28. Solano-Gallego, L., Sainz, A., Roura, X. *et al.* (2016). A review of canine babesiosis: the European perspective. *Parasit Vectors* 9: 336.
29. Goodman, R.A. and Breitschwerdt, E.B. (2005). Clinicopathologic findings in dogs seroreactive to Bartonella henselae antigens. *Am J Vet Res* 66: 2060–2064.
30. Littman, M.P., Goldstein, R.E., Labato, M.A. *et al.* (2006). ACVIM small animal consensus statement on Lyme disease in dogs: diagnosis, treatment, and prevention. *J Vet Intern Med* 20: 422–434.
31. Dowers, K.L., Tasker, S., Radecki, S.V. *et al.* (2009). Use of pradofloxacin to treat experimentally induced *Mycoplasma hemofelis* infection in cats, *Am J Vet Res* 70: 105–111.
32. Owen, J.L. and Harvey, J.W. (2012). Hemolytic anemia in dogs and cats due to erythrocyte enzyme deficiencies. *Vet Clin North Am Small Anim Pract* 42: 73–84.
33. Gultekin, G.I., Raj, K., Foureman, P. *et al.* (2012). Erythrocytic pyruvate kinase mutations causing hemolytic anemia, osteosclerosis, and secondary hemochromatosis in dogs. *J Vet Intern Med* 26: 935–944.
34. Harvey, J.W. (1996). Congenital erythrocyte enzyme deficiencies. *Vet Clin North Am Small Anim Pract* 26: 1003–1011.
35. Henderson, A.K. (2015). Anemia due to blood loss. In: *Clinical Veterinary Advisor* (ed. E. Côté), 63–64. St. Louis, MO: Elsevier.
36. Swann, J.W., Szladovits, B. and Glanemann, B. (2016). Demographic characteristics, survival and prognostic factors for mortality in cats with primary immune-mediated hemolytic anemia. *J Vet Intern Med* 30: 147–156.
37. Berentsen, S. and Sundic, T. (2015). Red blood cell destruction in autoimmune hemolytic anemia: role of complement and potential new targets for therapy. *Biomed Res Int* 2015: 363278.
38. Henderson, A.K. (2015). Anemia, hemolytic. In: *Clinical Veterinary Advisor* (ed. E. Côté), 65–66. St. Louis, MO: Elsevier.
39. O'Toole, T. (2015). Anemia, immune-mediated hemolytic. In: *Clinical Veterinary Advisor* (ed. E. Côté), 66–69. St. Louis, MO: Elsevier.
40. Paes, G., Paepe, D., Meyer, E *et al.* (2013). The use of the rapid osmotic fragility test as an additional test to diagnose canine immune-mediated haemolytic anaemia. *Acta Vet Scand* 55: 74.
41. Bhat, R.A., Dhaliwal, P.S., Saini, N. *et al.* (2017). Electrocardiographic evaluation in anemic dogs with blood parasitosis. *J Anim Res* 7: 205–207.
42. Wilson, H.E., Jasani, S., Wagner, T.B. *et al.* (2010). Signs of left heart volume overload in severely anaemic cats. *J Feline Med Surg* 12: 904–909.
43. Spotswood, T.C., Kirberger, R.M., Koma, L.M. *et al.* (2006). Changes in echocardiographic variables of left ventricle size and function in a model of canine normovolemic anemic. *Vet Radiol Ultrasound* 47: 358–365.
44. Barber, L.G. (2015). Anemia, aplastic. In: *Clinical Veterinary Advisor* (ed. E. Côté), 62–63. St. Louis, MO: Elsevier.
45. Barber, L.G. (2015). Anemia, nonregenerative and pure red cell aplasia. In: *Clinical Veterinary Advisor* (ed. E. Côté), 69–70. St. Louis, MO: Elsevier.
46. Estrin, M.A., Wehausen, C.E. Jessen, C.R. *et al.* (2006). Disseminated intravascular coagulation in cats. *J Vet Intern Med* 20: 1334–1339.
47. Levi, M., Toh, C.H. and Thachil, J. (2009). Guidelines for the diagnosis and management of disseminated intravascular coagulation. *Br J Haematol* 145: 24–33.
48. Ralph, A.C. and Brainard, B.M. (2012). Update on disseminated intravascular coagulation: when to consider it, when to expect it, when to treat it. *Top Companion Anim Med* 27: 65–72.
49. Wallisch, K. and Tepanier, L.A. (2015). Incidence, timing, and risk factors of azathioprine hepatotoxicosis in dogs. *J Vet Intern Med* 29: 513–518.
50. Miller, E. (1997). The use of cytotoxic agents in the treatment of immune-mediated diseases of dogs and cats. Semin. *Vet Med Surg (Small Anim)* 12: 157–160.

51. Randolph, J.E., Scarlett, J., Stokol. T, MacLeod JN. *et al.* (2004). Clinical efficacy and safety of recombinant canine erythropoietin in dogs with anemia of chronic renal failure and dogs with recombinant human erythropoietin-induced red call aplasia. *J Vet Intern Med* 18: 81–91.
52. Fiocchi, E.H., Cowgill, L.D., Brown, D.C. *et al.* (2017). The use of darbepoetin to stimulate erythropoiesis in the treatment of anemia of chronic kidney disease in dogs. *J Vet Intern Med* 31: 476–485.
53. Chaloub, S., Langston, C.E. and Farrelly, J. (2012). The use of darbepoetin to stimulate erythropoiesis in anemia of chronic kidney disease in cats: 25 cases. *J Vet Intern Med* 26: 363–369.
54. Huang, H.P., Yang, H.L., Liang, S.L. *et al.* (1999). Iatrogenic hyperadrenocorticism in 28 dogs. *J Am Anim Hosp Assoc* 35: 200–207.
55. Black, V., Adamantos, S., Barfield, D. *et al.* (2016). Feline non-regenerative immune-mediated anaemia: features and outcome in 15 cases. *J Feline Med Surg* 18: 597–602.
56. Grundy, S.A. and Barton, C. (2001). Influence of drug treatment on survival of dogs with immune-mediated hemolytic anemia: 88 cases (1989–1999). *J Am Vet Med Assoc* 218: 543–546.
57. Weinkle, T.K., Center, S.A., Randolph, J.F. *et al.* (2005). Evaluation of prognostic factors, survival rates, and treatment protocols for immune-mediated hemolytic anemia in dogs: 151 cases (1993–2002). *J Am Vet Med Assoc* 226: 1869–1880.
58. Degan, M. (1987). Pseudohyperkalemia in akitas. *J Am Vet Med Assoc* 190: 541–543.
59. Gookin, J.L., Bunch, S.E., Rush, L.J. et al. (1998). Evaluation of microcytosis in 18 shibas. *J Am Vet Med Assoc* ;212: 1258–1259.
60. Blois, S. (2017). Hyper-and hypocoagulable states. In: *Textbook of Veterinary Internal Medicine* (ed. S.J. Ettinger and E.C. Feldman), 2062–2077. St. Louis, MO: Elsevier.
61. Bach, J.F. (2015). Disseminated intravascular coagulation. In: *Clinical Veterinary Advisor* (ed. E. Côté), 286–287. St. Louis, MO: Elsevier.
62. Murphy, K. and Hibbert, A. (2013). The flat cat: 1. A logical and practical approach to management of this challenging presentation. *J Feline Med Surg* 15(3):175–88.
63. Goggs, R., Mastrococco, A. and Brooks, M.B. (2018). Retrospective evaluation of 4 methods for outcome prediction in overt disseminated intravascular coagulation in dogs (2009–2014): 804 cases. *J Vet Emerg Crit Care (San Antonio)* 28: 541–550.
64. Wiinberg, B., Jensen, A.L., Johansson, P.I. *et al.* (2008). Thromboelastographic evaluation of hemostatic function in dogs with disseminated intravascular coagulation. *J Vet Intern Med* 22: 357–365.
65. Vilar-Saavedra, P. and Hosoya, K. (2011). Thromboelastographic profile for a dog with hypocoagulable and hyperfibinolytic phase of disseminated intravascular coagulopathy. *J Small Anim Pract* 52: 656–659.
66. Wiinberg, B., Jensen, A.L., Johansson, P.I. *et al.* (2010). Development of a model based scoring system for diagnosis of canine disseminated intravascular coagulation with independent assessment of sensitivity and specificity. *Vet J* 185: 292–298.
67. Brainard, B.M., Buriko, Y., Good, J. *et al.* (2019). Consensus on the rational use of antithrombotics in veterinary critical care (curative): domain 5 – discontinuation of anticoagulant therapy in small animals. *J Vet Emerg Crit Care (San Antonio)* 29: 88–97.
68. Rose, L.J., Dunn, M.E., Allegret, V. *et al.* (2011). Effect of prednisone administration on coagulation variables in healthy beagle dogs. *Vet Clin Pathol* 40: 426–434.
69. Botsch, V., Kuchenhoff, H., Hartmann, K. *et al.* (2009). Retrospective study of 871 dogs with thrombocytopenia. *Vet Rec* 164: 647–651.
70. Callan, M.B. and Catalfamo, J.L. (2017). Immune-mediated thrombocytopenia, von Willebrand disease and other platelet disorders. In: *Textbook of Veterinary Internal Medicine* (ed. S.J. Ettinger, E.C. Feldman EC and E. Côté), 2120–2136. St. Louis, MO: Elsevier.
71. Stone, M. (2015). Thrombocytopenia, immune-mediated. In: *Clinical Veterinary Advisor* (ed. E. Côté), 995–997. St. Louis, MO: Elsevier.
72. Littman, M. (2015). Rocky mountain spotted fever. In: *Clinical Veterinary Advisor* (ed. E. Côté), 913–914. St. Louis, MO: Elsevier.
73. Barthelemy, A., Magnin, M., Pouzot-Nevoret, C. *et al.* (2017). Hemorrhagic, hemostatic, and thromboelastometric disorders in 35 dogs with a clinical diagnosis of leptospirosis: a prospective study. *J Vet Intern Med* 31: 69–80.
74. Simpson, K., Chapman, P. and Klag, A. (2018). Long-term outcome of primary immune-mediated thrombocytopenia in dogs. *J Small Anim Pract* 59: 674–680.
75. O'Marra, S.K., Delaforcade, A.M. and Shaw, S.P. (2011). Treatment and predictors of outcome in dogs with immune-mediated thrombocytopenia. *J Am Vet Med Assoc* 238: 346–352.
76. Gasteiger, G., D'Osualdo, A., Schubert, D. *et al.* (2017). Cellular innate immunity: an old game with new players. *J Innate Immun* 9:111–125.
77. Liu, J. and Cao, X. (2016). Cellular and molecular regulation of innate inflammatory responses. *Cell Mol Immunol* 13: 711–721.
78. Tizard, I. (2018). *Veterinary Immunology*, 10e. St. Louis, MO: Elsevier.
79. Waddell, L.S. (2017). Anaphylaxis. In: *Textbook of Veterinary Internal Medicine* (ed. S.J. Ettinger, E.C. Feldman and E. Côté), 1532–1538. St. Louis, MO: Elsevier.
80. Buckley, G.J. (2015). Anaphylaxis. In: *Clinical Veterinary Advisor* (ed. E. Côté), 58–60. St. Louis, MO: Elsevier.
81. Quantz, J.E., Miles, M.S., Reed, A.L. *et al.* (2009). Elevation of alanine transaminase and gallbladder wall abnormalities as biomarkers of anaphylaxis in canine hypersensitivity patients *J Vet Emerg Crit Care (San Antonio)* 19: 536–544.

82. Plumb, D.C. (2018). *Plumb's Veterinary Drug Handbook*, 9e. Ames, IA: Wiley Blackwell.
83. Schmuel, D.L. and Cortes, Y. (2013). Anaphylaxis in dogs and cats. *J Vet Emerg Crit Care (San Antonio)* 23: 377–394.
84. Litster, A. and Atwell, R. (2006). Physiological and haematological findings and clinical observations in a model of acute systematic anaphylaxis in Dirofilaria immitis-sensitized cats. *Aust Vet J* 84: 151–157.
85. Stone, M. (2017). Systemic lupus erythematosus. In: *Textbook of Veterinary Internal Medicine* (ed. S.J. Ettinger, E.C. Feldman and E. Côté), 2176–2186. St. Louis, MO: Elsevier.
86. Stone, M. (2015). Systemic lupus erythematosus. In: *Clinical Veterinary Advisor* (ed. E. Côté), 979–980. St. Louis, MO: Elsevier.
87. Smee, N.M., Harkin, K.R. and Wilkerson, M.J. (2007). Management of serum antinuclear antibody titer in dogs with and without systemic lupus erythematosus: 120 cases (1997–2005). *J Am Vet Med Assoc* 230: 1180–1183.
88. Bennett, D. and Kirkham, D. (1987). The laboratory identification of serum antinuclear antibody in the dog. *J Comp Pathol* 97: 523–539.
89. Kass, P.H., Farver, T.B., Strombeck, D.R. *et al.* (1985). Application of the log-linear and logistic regression in the prediction of systemic lupus erythematosus in the dog. *Am J Vet Res* 46: 2340–2345.
90. Chabanne, L.S. (2010). Systemic lupus erythematosus. In: *Schalm's Veterinary Hematology*, 6e (ed. D.J. Weiss and K.J. Wardrop), 383–392. Ames, IA: Wiley Blackwell.
91. Navarini, L., Bisogno, T., Margiotta, D.P.E. *et al.* (2018). Role of the specialized proresolving mediatory resolving D1 in systemic lupus erythematosus: preliminary results. *J Immunol Res* 2018: 5264195.
92. Ackermann, A.L., May, E.R. and Frank, L.A. (2017). Use of mycophenolate mofetil to treat immune-mediated skin disease in 14 dogs – a retrospective evaluation. *Vet Dermatol* 28: 195-e44.
93. Chabanne, L., Fournel, C., Rigal, D. *et al.* (1999). Canine systemic lupus erythematosus. Part II. Diagnosis and treatment. *Comp Contin Educ* 21: 402–408.
94. Stone, M. (2017). Immune-mediated polyarthritis and other polyarthritides. In: *Textbook of Veterinary Internal Medicine* (ed. S.J. Ettinger, E.C. Feldman and E. Côté), 2151–2160. St. Louis, Missouri, USA: Elsevier;. p..
95. Mahony O. (2015). Polyarthritis. In: *Clinical Veterinary Advisor* (ed. E. Côté), 821–823. St. Louis, MO: Elsevier.
96. Magen, L., Shaughnessy, M.L., Sample, S.J. *et al.* (2016). Clinical features and pathological joint changes in dogs with erosive immune-mediated polyarthritis: 13 cases (2004–2012). *J Am Vet Med Assoc* 249: 1156–1164.
97. Ralphs, S.C., Beale, B.S., Whitney, W.O. *et al.* (2000). Idiopathic erosive polyarthritis in six dogs (description of the disease and treatment with bilateral pancarpal arthrodesis). *Vet Comp Orthop Traumatol* 13: 191–196
98. Crook, T., McGowan, C. and Pead, M. (2007). Effect of passive stretching on the range of motion of osteoarthritic joints in 10 Labrador retrievers. *Vet Rec* 160: 545–547.
99. Dos Anjos, L.M.J., Salvador, P.A., de Souza da Fonseca, A. *et al.* (2019). Modulation of immune response to induced-arthritis by low-level laser therapy. *Biophototonics* 12(2): e201800120.
100. Sharp, B. (2012). Feline physiotherapy and rehabilitation: 1. Principles and potential. *J Feline Med Surg* 14: 622–632.
101. Formenton, M.R., Pereira, M.A.A. and Fantoni, D.T. (2017). Small animal massage therapy: a brief review and relevant observations. *Top Companion Anim Med* 32: 139–145.
102. Corti, L. (2014). Nonpharmaceutical approaches to pain management. *Top Companion Anim Med* 29: 24–28.
103. Carr, A.P. and Michels, G. (1997). Identifying noninfectious erosive arthritis in dogs and cats. *Vet Med* 92: 804–810.
104. Olivry, T. (2006). A review of autoimmune skin diseases in domestic animals I: superficial pemphigus. *Vet Dermatol* 17: 291–305.
105. Bizikova, P. (2017). Immune-mediated dermatologic disorders. In: *Textbook of Veterinary Internal Medicine* (ed. S.J. Ettinger, E.C. Feldman and E. Côté), 2161–2175. St. Louis, MO: Elsevier.
106. De Jaham, C. (2015). Pemphigus complex. In: *Clinical Veterinary Advisor* (ed. E. Côté), 786–788. St. Louis, MO: Elsevier.
107. Olivry, T. (2018). Auto-immune skin diseases in animals: time to reclassify and review after 40 years. *BMC Vet Res* 14: 157.
108. Yousef, M., Mansouri, P., Partovikia, M. *et al.* (2017). The effect of low level laser therapy on pemphigus vulgaris lesions: a pilot study. *J Lasers Med Sci* 8: 177–180.
109. Bizikova, P. and Burrows, A. (2019). Feline pemphigus foliaceus: original case series and comprehensive literature review. *BMC Vet Res* 15: 22.
110. Preziosi, D.E. (2019). Feline pemphigus foliaceus. *Vet Clin North Am Small Anim Pract* 49: 95–104.
111. Mueller, R.S., Krebs, I., Power, H.T. *et al.* (2006). Pemphigus foliaceus in 91 dogs. *J Am Anim Hosp Assoc* 42: 189–196.
112. Goodale, E. (2019). Pemphigus foliaceous. *Can Vet J* 60: 311–313.
113. DeClue, A.E. (2017). Sepsis and the systemic inflammatory response syndrome. In: *Textbook of Veterinary Internal Medicine* (ed. S.J. Ettinger, E.C. Feldman and E. Côté), 1492–1504. St. Louis, MO: Elsevier.
114. Okano, S., Yoshida, M., Fukushima, U. *et al.* (2002). Usefulness of systemic inflammatory response syndrome criteria as an index for prognosis judgment. *Vet Rec* 150: 245–246.
115. Brady, C.A., Otto, C.M., Van Winkle, T.J. *et al.* (2000). Severe sepsis in cats: 29 cats (1986–1998). *J Am Vet Med Assoc* 217: 531–535.

116. Schaefer, H., Kohn, B., Schweigert, F.J. *et al.* (2011). Quantitative and qualitative urine protein excretion in dogs with severe inflammatory response syndrome. *J Vet Intern Med* 25: 1292–1297.
117. Giunti, M., Troia, R., Bergamini, P.F. *et al.* (2015). Prospective evaluation of the acute patient physiologic and laboratory evaluation score and an extended clinicopathological profile in dogs with systemic inflammatory response syndrome. *J Vet Emerg Crit Care (San Antonio)* 25: 226–233.
118. DeClue, A.E., Delgado, C., Chang, C. *et al.* (2011). Clinical and immunologic assessment of sepsis and the systemic inflammatory response syndrome in cats. *J Am Vet Med Assoc* 238: 890–897.
119. Gommeren, K., Desmas, I., Garcia, A. *et al.* (2018). Inflammatory cytokine and C-reactive protein concentrations in dogs with systemic inflammatory response syndrome. *J Vet Emerg Crit Care (San Antonio)* 28: 9–19.
120. Wong, C. and Koenig, A. (2017). The colloid controversy: are colloids bad and what are the options? *Vet Clin North Am Small Anim Pract* 47: 411–421.
121. Frazee, E.N., Leedahi, D.D. and Kashani, K.B. (2015). Key controversies in colloid and crystalloid utilization. *Hosp Pharm* 50: 446–453.
122. Dastan, F., Jamaati, H., Emami, H. *et al.* (2018). Reducing inappropriate utilization of albumin: the value of pharmacist-led intervention model. *Iran J Pharm Res* 17: 1125–1129.
123. Covey, H.L, Connolly, D.J. (2018). Pericardial effusion associated with systemic inflammatory disease in seven dogs (January 2006–January 2012). *J Vet Cardiol* 20: 123–128.
124. Kenney, E.M., Rozanski, E.A., Rush, J.E. *et al.* (2010). Association between outcome and organ system dysfunction in dogs with sepsis: 114 cases (2003–2007). *J Am Vet Med Assoc* 236: 83–87.
125. Babyak, J.M. and Sharp, C.R. (2016). Epidemiology of systemic inflammatory response syndrome and sepsis in cats hospitalized in a veterinary teaching hospital. *J Am Vet Med Assoc* 249: 65–71.
126. Kent, M., Platt, S.R. and Schatzberg, S.J. (2010).The neurology of balance: function and dysfunction of the vestibular system in dogs and cats. *Vet J* 185: 247–258.
127. Lowrie, M. (2012). Vestibular disease: diseases causing vestibular signs. *Compend Contin Educ Vet* 34(7): E1.
128. Thomas, W.B. (2000). Idiopathic epilepsy in dogs. *Vet Clin North Am Small Anim Pract* 30: 183–206.
129. Melan, T. and Carrera-Justiz, S. (2018). A review: emergency management of dogs with suspected epileptic seizures. *Topics Comp Ann Med* 33: 17–20.
130. Berendt, M., Farquhar, R.G., Mandigers, P.J. *et al.* (2015). International veterinary epilepsy task force consensus report on epilepsy definition, classification and terminology in companion animals. *BMC Vet Res* 11: 182.
131. Rossmeisl, J.H. (2010). Vestibular disease in dogs and cats. *Vet Clin Small Anim* 40: 81–100.
132. Evans, J., Levesque, D., Kowles, K. *et al.* (2003). Diazepam as a treatment for metronidazole toxicosis in dogs: a retrospective study of 21 cases. *J Vet Intern Med* 17(3):304–310,.
133. Munana, K.R. (2013). Update seizure management in small animal practice. *Vet Clin Small Anim* 43: 1127–1147.
134. Podell M, Volk HA, Berendt M, et al. (2016). 2015 ACVIM small animal consensus statement of seizure management in dogs. *J Vet Intern Med* 30: 477–490.
135. Sorjonen, D.C. (1990). Clinical and histopathological features of granulomatous meningoencephalomyelitis in dogs. *J Am Anim Hosp Assoc* 26: 141–147.
136. Smith, R. (1995). A case of ocular granulomatous meningoencephalomyelitis in a German Shepherd dog presenting as bilateral uveitis. *Aust Vet Pract* 25: 76–78.
137. Coates, J.R. and Jeffery, N.D. (2014).Perspectives on meningoencephalomyelitis of unknown origin. *Vet Clin Small Anim* 44: 1157–1185.
138. Ducote, J.M., Johnson, K.E., Dewey, C.W. *et al.* (1999). Computed tomography of necrotizing meningoencephalitis in 3 Yorkshire terriers. *Vet Radiol Ultrasound* 40: 617–621.
139. Timmann, D., Konar, M., Howard, J. *et al.* (2007). Necrotising encephalitis in a French Bulldog. *J Small Anim Pract* 48: 339–342.
140. Granger, N., Smith, P.M. and Jeffery, N.D. (2010). Clinical findings and treatment of non-infectious meningoencephalomyelitis in dogs: a systematic review of 457 published cases from 1962 to 2008. *Vet J* 184: 290–297.
141. Miller, E. (1992). Immunosuppressive therapy in the treatment of immune-mediated disease. *J Vet Intern Med* 6: 206–213.
142. Bateman, S.W. and Parent, J.M. (1999). Clinical findings, treatment and outcome of dogs with status epilepticus or cluster seizures: 156 cases (1990–1995). *J Am Vet Med Assoc* 215: 1463–1468.
143. Brisson, B.A. (2010). Intervertebral disc disease in dogs. *Vet Clin Small Anim* 40: 829–858.
144. Hansen, H.J. (1952). A pathologic-anatomical study on disc degeneration in dog, with special reference to the so-called enchondrosis intervertebralis. *Acta Orthop Scand Suppl* 11: 1–117.
145. Decker, S.D. and Fenn J. (2018). Acute herniation of nondegenerate nucleus pulposus. Acute noncompressive nucleus pulposus extrusion and compressive hydrated nucleus pulposus extrusion. *Vet Clin Small Anim* 48: 95–109.
146. Fenn, J., Drees, R., Volk, H.A. *et al.* (2016). Comparison of clinical signs and outcomes between dogs with presumptive ischemic myelopathy and dogs with acute noncompressive nucleus pulposus extrusion. *J Am Vet Med Assoc* 249: 767–775.
147. Cauzinille, L. (2000). Fibrocartilaginous embolism in dogs. *Vet Clin Small Anim* 30: 155–167.

148. Lorenz, M.D., Coates, J.R. and Kent, M. (2011). *Handbook of Veterinary Neurology*, 5e. St Louis, MO: Elsevier Saunders.
149. Windsor, R.C., Vernau, K.M., Sturges, B.K. *et al.* (2008). Lumbar cerebrospinal fluid in dogs with type I intervertebral disc herniation. *J Vet Intern Med* 22: 954–960,.
150. De Risio, L., Adams, V., Dennis, R. *et al.* (2007). Magnetic resonance imaging findings and clinical associations in 52 dogs with suspected ischemic myelopathy. *J Vet Intern Med* 21: 1290–1298.
151. De Risio, L., Adams, V., Dennis, R. *et al.* (2008). Association of clinical and magnetic resonance imaging findings with outcome in dogs suspected to have ischemic myelopathy: 50 cases (2000–2006). *J Am Vet Med Assoc* 233: 129–135.
152. Gandini, G., Cizinauskas, S., Lang, J. *et al.* (2003). Fibrocartilaginous embolism in 75 dogs: clinical findings and factors influencing the recovery rate. *J Small Anim Pract* 44: 75–80.
153. Lewis, D.D. and Hosgood, G. (1992). Complications associated with the use of iohexol for myelography of the cervical vertebral column in dogs: 66 cases (1988–1990). *J Am Vet Med Assoc* 200: 1381–1384.
154. Burbidge, H.M., Pfeiffer, D.U. and Blair, H.T. (1994). Canine wobbler syndrome: a study of the Doberman pinscher in New Zealand. *N Z Vet J* 42: 221–228.
155. da Costa, R.C. (2010). Cervical spondylomyelopathy (wobbler syndrome) in dogs. *Vet Clin Small Anim* 40: 881–913.
156. Averill, D.R. (1973). Degenerative myelopathy in the aging German shepherd dog: clinical and pathologic findings. *J Am Vet Med Assoc* 162: 1045–1051.
157. Coates, J.R., March, P.A., Oglesbee, M. *et al.* (2007).Clinical characterization of a familial degenerative myelopathy in Pembroke Welsh Corgi dogs. *J Vet Intern Med* 21: 1323–1331.
158. Coates, J.R. and Wininger, F.A. (2010). Canine degenerative myelopathy. *Vet Clin Small Anim* 40: 929–950.
159. Seim, H.B. and Withrow, S.J. (1982). Pathophysiology and diagnosis of caudal cervical spondylo-myelopathy with emphasis on the Doberman Pinscher. *J Am Anim Hosp Assoc* 18: 241–251.
160. Awano, T., Johnson, G.S., Wade, C.M. *et al.* (2009). Genome-wide association analysis reveals a SOD1 mutation in canine degenerative myelopathy that resembles amyotrophic lateral sclerosis. *Proc Natl Acad Sci U S A* 106: 2794–2799.
161. Kathmann, I., Cizinauskas, S., Doherr, M.G. *et al.* (2006). Daily controlled physiotherapy increases survival time in dogs with suspected degenerative myelopathy. *J Vet Intern Med* 20: 927–932.
162. da Costa, R.C., Parent, J.M., Holmberg, D.L. *et al.* (2008). Outcome of medical and surgical treatment in dogs with cervical spondylomyelopathy: 104 cases. *J Am Vet Med Assoc* 233: 1284–1290.
163. Thomas, W.B. (2000). Diskospondylitis and other vertebral infections. *Vet Clin Small Anim* 30: 169–181.
164. Tipold, A. and Schatzberg, S.J. (2010). An update on steroid responsive meningitis-arteritis. *J Small Anim Pract* 51: 150–154.
165. Webb, A.A., Taylor, S.M. and Muir, G.D. (2002). Steroid-responsive meningitis-arteritis in dogs with noninfectious, nonerosive, idiopathic, immune-mediated polyarthritis. *J Vet Intern Med* 16: 269–273.
166. Kornegay, J.N. and Barber, D.L. (1980). Diskospondylitis in dogs. *J Am Vet Med Assoc* 177: 337–341.
167. Tipold, A. and Jaggy, A. (1994). Steroid-responsive meningitis-arteritis in dogs: long-term study of 32 cases. *J Small Anim Pract* 35: 311–316.
168. Ruoff, C.M., Kerwin, S.C. and Taylor, A.R. (2018).Diagnostic imaging of discospondylitis. *Vet Clin Small Anim* 48: 85–94.
169. Cuddon, P.A. (2002). Acquired canine peripheral neuropathies. *Vet Clin North Am Small Anim Pract* 32: 207–249.
170. Shelton, G.D., Schule, A. and Kass, P.H. (1997). Risk factors for acquired myasthenia gravis in dogs: 1154 cases (1991–1995). *J Am Vet Med Assoc* 211: 1428–1431.
171. Ducote, J.M., Dewey, C.W. and Coates, J.R. (1999). Clinical forms of myasthenia gravis in cats. *Compend Contin Educ Pract Vet* 21: 440–448.
172. Shelton, G.D. (2002). Myasthenia gravis and disorders of neuromuscular transmission. *Vet Clin North Am Small Anim Pract* 32: 189–206.
173. Dewey, C.W., Bailey, C.S., Shelton, G.D. *et al.* (1997). Clinical forms of acquired myasthenia gravis in dogs: 25 cases (1988–1995). *J Vet Intern Med* 11: 50–57.
174. Shelton, G.D. and Lindstrom, J.M. (2001). Spontaneous remission in canine myasthenia gravis: implications for assessing human MG therapies. *Neurology* 57: 2139–2141.
175. Buffington, C.A.T. (2018). Pandora syndrome in cats: diagnosis and treatment. *Today's Vet Pract* 30–39. https://todaysveterinarypractice.com/pandora-syndrome-in-cats (accessed 22 July 2021).
176. Merrill, L. (2012). Urinary and renal diseases. In: *Small Animal Internal Medicine for Veterinary Technicians and Nurses*. (ed. A. Aguirre and T. Darling), 289–347. Ames, IA: Wiley Blackwell.
177. Bilbrough, G., Evert, B., Hathaway, K. *et al.* (2018). IDEXX Catalyst SDMA Test for in-house measurement of SDMA concentration in serum from dogs and cats. https://www.idexx.com/files/catalyst-sdma-white-paper.pdf (accessed 22 July 2021).

178. Foy, D. (2014). Acute renal failure (acute kidney injury). Paper presented at the AAHA Conference, 20 March 2014, Music City Center, Nashville, TN.
179. International Renal Interest Society. (2019). IRIS Staging of CKD (modified 2019). http://www.iris-kidney.com/guidelines/staging.html (accessed 22 July 2021).
180. Robertson, J. (2017). A practical approach to using the IRIS CKD guidelines and the IDEXX SDMA test in everyday practice. 2017 Hill's Global Symposium, 6 May 2017, Washington, DC. https://files.brief.vet/migration/article/37636/robertson-proceedings_hgs2017_final_0-37636-article.pdf (accessed 22 July 2021).
181. Acierno, M. Protein-losing nephropathy. Paper presented at the Pacific Veterinary Conference, July 2017, Long Beach, CA.
182. Quimby, J. How to approach proteinuria. Paper presented at the Southwest Veterinary Symposium 2017, September 2017, San Antonio, TX.
183. Littman, M.P. (2011). Protein-losing nephropathy in small animals. *Vet Clin Small Anim* 41: 31–62.
184. Bowles, D. (2010). Prostatic disease in the dog (proceedings). *DVM360*. https://www.dvm360.com/view/prostatic-disease-dog-proceedings (accessed 3 September 2021).
185. Bartges, J. (2018). Management of urinary incontinence. Paper presented at the British Small Animal Veterinary Congress, April 2018, Birmingham, UK.
186. Adams, L.G. (2011). Diagnosis and treatment of refractory urinary incontinence. British Small Animal Veterinary Congress, 2011. April 2011, Birmingham, UK.
187. Bartges, J. (2018). Oops, I did it again: urinary incontinence. Paper presented at the Southwest Veterinary Symposium, Sept 2018, San Antonio Texas.

Chapter 7

Nutritional Diseases and Conditions

Kara M. Burns, MS, MEd, LVT, VTS (Nutrition)

Veterinary Technician and Nurse's Daily Reference Guide: Canine and Feline, Fourth Edition. Edited by Mandy Fults and Kenichiro Yagi.

Companion website: www.wiley.com/go/fults/veterinary

Abbreviations

CHF, congestive heart failure
CKD, chronic kidney disease
DER, daily energy requirement
DHA, docosahexaenoic acid
DMB, dry matter basis
EPA, eicosapentaenoic acid
FIC, feline idiopathic cystitis
FLUTD, feline lower urinary tract disease
kcal, kilocalorie
kg, kilograms
kJ, kilojoules
mg, milligrams
mOsm, milliosmoles
ppm, parts per million
RER, resting energy requirement
TNF-α, tumor necrosis factor alpha

Nutrition is one area of veterinary medicine that affects each pet that comes into the veterinary hospital. Of the three components that affect the life of an animal – genetics, environment, and nutrition – nutrition is the single factor that veterinary healthcare team members can impact. Proper nutrition and feeding management are the cornerstones to health and healing. Every patient, healthy or ill, that enters the veterinary hospital should have an evaluation of their nutritional status. This assessment is now known as the fifth vital assessment. Healthcare team members should make a nutritional recommendation based on this evaluation and should effectively communicate this recommendation to their clients.

Clients are wanting information on the proper nutrition for their pets. This nutrition discussion is best had with the veterinary healthcare team. There are numerous myths and misperceptions surrounding pet nutrition, which in some cases can be detrimental to the health and wellbeing of the pet. The healthcare team member must therefore initiate the discussion through proper nutritional history.

GASTROINTESTINAL DISEASE

Gastrointestinal problems are one of the most common reasons pet owners bring their pet to the hospital.[1] The main challenge to the veterinary healthcare team presented with a pet that has gastrointestinal dysfunction is to determine whether this is an emergency or potentially serious problem or a chronic or intermittent problem. The gastrointestinal tract is known for its resilience, and the veterinary healthcare team has seen countless pets with clinical signs of acute vomiting and/or diarrhea resolve uneventfully, sometimes without any supportive care. However, this cannot be held to all acute gastrointestinal events, as some may be life-threatening disorders, which if not identified and treated, could lead to poor patient management and/or death of the pet.

Vomiting and/or diarrhea are the hallmark symptoms of gastrointestinal disorders, and it is these obvious symptoms that result in pet owners bringing the pet to the hospital.

Following a diagnosis by the veterinarian, the vomiting and/or diarrhea will need to be managed. The healthcare team should be cognizant of key nutritional factors and their impact when managing a patient nutritionally. Nutritional management of patients suffering with vomiting and/or diarrhea should consider the following nutritional factors.

Water

Water is extremely important when working with patients with acute gastrointestinal distress, due to the potential for life-threatening dehydration from excess fluid loss and inability of the patient to replace the lost fluid. Patients with persistent nausea and vomiting should be supported with subcutaneous or intravenous rather than oral fluids.[1,2]

Electrolytes

Gastric and intestinal secretions differ from extracellular fluids in electrolyte composition, so their loss can result in systemic electrolyte abnormalities. Serum electrolyte concentrations are useful in tailoring appropriate fluid therapy and nutritional management of these patients. Mild hypokalemia, hypochloremia, and either hypernatremia or hyponatremia are the electrolyte abnormalities most commonly associated with acute vomiting and diarrhea. Initially, electrolyte disorders should be addressed and corrected with appropriate parenteral fluid and electrolyte therapy. Patients experiencing vomiting and/or diarrhea should begin nutritional therapy ideally containing levels of potassium, chloride, and sodium above the minimum allowances for normal dogs and cats. Recommended levels of these nutrients are 0.8–1.1% potassium (dry matter), 0.5–1.3% dry matter chloride and 0.3–0.5% dry matter sodium).

Protein

Nutritional therapy for gastrointestinal patients should not provide excess protein (no more than 30% for dogs and 40% for cats). Products of protein digestion (peptides, amino acids and amines) increase gastrin and gastric acid secretion. Hydrolyzed or novel protein foods have been recommended as dietary antigens are suspected to play a role in the etiopathogenesis.

Ideal elimination foods should: (i) avoid protein excess (16–26% for dogs; 30–40% for cats); (ii) have high protein digestibility (≥ 87%); and (iii) contain a limited number of novel protein sources to which the patient has never been exposed. Additionally, a food containing a protein hydrolysate may be used in nutritional management of the patient.[1,3]

Fat

Solids and liquids higher in fat empty more slowly from the stomach than comparable foods with less fat. Fat in the duodenum stimulates the release of cholecystokinin, which delays gastric emptying. Foods with less than 15% dry matter fat for dogs and less than 25% dry matter fat for cats are appropriate for dietary management.

Fiber

Foods containing gel-forming soluble fibers should be avoided as these fibers increase the viscosity of ingesta and slow gastric emptying. These fibers include pectins and gums. Overall, the crude fiber content should not exceed more than 5% dry matter.

Food Form and Temperature

Moist foods are the best form, since they reduce gastric retention time. For the same reason, the veterinary healthcare team should educate clients to warm foods to between room and body temperature (70–100°F; 21–38°C).

Vitamins and Trace Minerals

Iron, copper, and B vitamins may benefit patients with gastroduodenal ulceration and gastrointestinal blood loss. Hematinics should be used in patients with nonregenerative, microcytic/hypochromic anemias attributable to iron deficiency.

Acid Load

Alkalemia should be expected if vomiting patients lose hydrogen and chloride ions in excess of sodium and bicarbonate. Hypochloremia perpetuates the alkalosis by increasing renal bicarbonate reabsorption. Acidemia may occur in vomiting patients if the vomited gastric fluid is relatively low in hydrogen and chloride ion content (e.g. during fasting) or if concurrent loss of intestinal sodium and bicarbonate occurs.[1] It is best to correct severe acid–base disorders with parenteral fluid and electrolyte therapy. Foods for patients with acute vomiting and diarrhea should avoid excess dietary acid load. Foods that normally produce alkaline urine are less likely to be associated with acidosis.

OBESITY

Obesity is defined as an increase in fat tissue mass sufficient to contribute to disease. Dogs and cats weighing 10–19% more than the optimal weight for their breed are considered overweight; those weighing 20% or more above the optimum weight are considered obese.[4–6] Obesity has been associated with a number of disease conditions, as well as with a reduced lifespan. Excessive caloric intake, combined with decreased physical activity and genetic susceptibility are associated with most cases of obesity and the primary treatment for obesity is reduced caloric intake and increased physical activity. Obesity is one of the leading preventable causes of illness/death and with the dramatic rise in pet obesity over the past several decades, weight management, and obesity prevention should be among the top health issues that healthcare team members discuss with every client.

Obesity is a difficult disease to talk with owners about, as most pet owners do not recognize (or want to admit) that their pet is overweight. A successful weight management program includes consistent and accurate weight measurement/patient monitoring, effective and educational client communication, identification of compliance gaps, and use of tools to reinforce compliance, client and patient support and program restructure as needed.

Setting a weight-loss goal and calculating the appropriate energy intake starts with determination of the pet's ideal body weight. Ideal body weight is a starting goal that is adjusted for appropriate body condition as the pet loses weight. The healthcare team must determine the number of daily calories that will result in weight loss while subsequently providing adequate protein, vitamins and minerals to meet the pet's daily energy requirement (DER). The DER reflects the pet's activity level and is a calculation based on the pet's resting energy requirement (RER).[5–7] The most accurate formula to determine the RER for a cat or a dog is:

$$\text{RER kcal/day} = 70(\text{ideal body weight inkg})\ 0.75$$

or

$$\text{RER kcal/day} = (\text{kg} \times \text{kg} \times \text{kg}, \sqrt{}, \sqrt{}) \times 70$$

After RER is determined, DER may be calculated by multiplying RER by "standard" factors related to energy needs. The calculations used to determine energy needs for obese prone pets or for pets needing to lose weight are:[5–7]

- Obese prone dogs — DER = 1.4 × RER
- Weight loss/dogs — DER = 1.0 × RER
- Obese prone cats — DER = 1.0 × RER
- Weight loss/cats — DER = 0.8 × RER

Key Nutrients in Weight Management

- Energy density – foods for weight loss and prevention of weight regain should contain ≤ 3.4 kcal (≤ 14.2 kJ) metabolizable energy/g.
- Fat – foods for weight loss should contain ≤ 9% (dogs) and ≤ 10% cats.
- Fiber – foods for weight loss should contain 12–25%.
- Protein – foods for weight loss should contain ≥ 25%.
- Carbohydrate – foods for weight loss should contain ≤ 40%.
- L-carnitine – foods for weight loss should contain ≥ 300 ppm.
- Antioxidants – foods for weight loss should contain:
  - Vitamin E ≥ 400 iu vitamin E/kg
  - Vitamin C ≥ 100 mg vitamin C/kg
  - Selenium 0.5–1.3 mg selenium/kg.
- Sodium – foods for weight loss should contain between 0.2% and 0.4%.

FELINE LOWER URINARY TRACT DISEASE

Feline lower urinary tract disease (FLUTD) is a term used to describe any condition affecting the urinary bladder or urethra of cats and is a common reason for hospital visits and veterinary evaluation of our feline patients. Regardless of underlying cause, FLUTD is characterized by the following signs: dysuria, pollakiuria, stranguria, hematuria, and/or periuria (urination in inappropriate places). Lower urinary tract signs may result from disorders affecting the urinary bladder and/or urethra of cats and include feline idiopathic cystitis (FIC), urolithiasis, urethral plugs, neoplasia, anatomical abnormalities, and bacterial urinary tract infection.[8,9]

Key Nutrients in Managing Feline Lower Urinary Tract Disease

The goals of managing cats with FIC are to decrease severity of clinical signs and increase the interval between episodes of lower urinary tract disease.

Feeding moist food (> 60% moisture) has been associated with a decreased recurrence of clinical signs in cats with FIC. Beneficial effects have been observed in cats with FIC when urine specific gravity values decrease from 1.050 to values between 1.032 and 1.041. Additional methods for increasing water intake (e.g. adding broth to foods, placing ice cubes in the cat's water, and providing water fountains) also may be helpful for some cats.[10,11]

Omega-3 fatty acids are known to have potent anti-inflammatory effects and are recommended for managing FLUTD. Additionally, vitamin E and beta carotene are helpful for counteracting oxidative stress and reducing free radical damage, conditions that often accompany inflammation.

Treatment options for cats with struvite uroliths include physical removal of uroliths or dissolution via nutritional management. On average, approximately 30 days are required for dissolution of sterile struvite uroliths using these foods. Urine pH should remain less than 6.1, and if canned food is fed exclusively, the urine specific gravity should be less than 1.040. Nutritional management should be continued four weeks beyond radiographic resolution of the urolith.

After dissolution or removal of struvite uroliths or urethral plugs, nutritional management is indicated to prevent recurrence. The cat should be transitioned gradually to a struvite-prevention food that results in production of moderately acidic urine pH (e.g. 6.2–6.4).

Calcium oxalate crystals cannot be dissolved, therefore treatment should consist of urolith removal, followed by methods to prevent recurrence.

It is possible for one food, in the proper formulation, to manage both struvite uroliths and calcium oxalate uroliths. Nutritional management of struvite and calcium oxalate uroliths involves controlling mineral constituents in the urine, increasing urinary inhibitors of the uroliths, and controlling urine pH. This goal can be achieved by limiting the constituents in the food, reducing their absorption in the gastrointestinal tract, and/or reducing their excretion from the kidneys.

Controlling levels of magnesium, calcium, phosphorous, and oxalate will help to reduce the building blocks of crystals and uroliths. Adding citrate to the food will help inhibit crystals and uroliths. Vitamin B6 levels should be enhanced because a deficiency of this vitamin has been associated with increased urinary oxalate excretion. Nutritional management that includes antioxidants, specifically vitamin E and beta carotene, helps counteract oxidative stress and create an unfavorable environment for uroliths. Omega-3 fatty acids, specifically eicosapentaenoic acid (EPA) and docosahexaenoic acid (DHA), help to break the cycle of inflammation associated with uroliths and FIC.

CHRONIC KIDNEY DISEASE

Chronic kidney disease (CKD) affects over one million pets every year. Known as the "silent killer," CKD is the second most common cause of death in cats and the third most common cause of death in dogs.[12] This disease process results in a loss of functional renal tissue/kidney damage that has existed for at least three months. It is a progressive process with a reduction in glomerular filtration rate by more than 50%, persisting for at least three months.[13]

When addressing CKD, the goals of dietary management are to maximize the quality and quantity of life of the pet by ensuring adequate intake of energy, limiting the extent or uremia, and slowing the rate of progression of the disease.[13–15] Nutritional therapy is aimed at:

1. Reducing the workload of the kidney and improving kidney function.
2. Slowing continuing damage to the kidney.
3. Reducing the accumulation of toxic waste and signs of illness.
4. Providing highly palatable and optimally balanced nutrition.

Water

Kidney disease causes a progressive decline in urine concentrating ability, and maximal urine osmolality approaches that of plasma (300 mOsm/kg). Patients with CKD should have unlimited access to fresh water for free-choice consumption. If readily consumed by the patient, moist foods are preferred, because their consumption generally results in increased total water intake compared with dry food consumption.[14]

Energy

Endogenous protein catabolism resulting in malnutrition and exacerbation of azotemia will occur in the CKD patient unless sufficient amounts of energy are provided. Thus, prevention of malnutrition through adequate energy and nutrient intake is critical in the management of kidney disease. Carbohydrate and fat provide the non-protein sources of energy in the diet, with fat providing approximately twice the energy per gram compared with carbohydrates. Thus, fat increases the energy density of the diet, which allows the patient to obtain its nutritional requirements from a smaller volume of food. Providing a smaller volume of food will help to minimize gastric distention; consequently, reducing the incidence of nausea and vomiting.[16]

Protein

Avoiding excessive dietary protein intake is indicated to control clinical signs of uremia in dogs and cats with CKD. The extrarenal clinical and metabolic disturbances associated with uremia are typically direct results of the accumulated waste products derived from protein catabolism. Limiting accumulation of nitrogenous waste products and achieving nitrogen balance through the proportional decrease of protein intake as renal function declines, is the goal of managing cats and dogs with chronic renal disease. Studies show controlled protein food increases length and quality of life for dogs and cats with renal failure.[17,18] Protein levels in foods intended for most patients with CKD is 14–20% dry matter basis (DMB) for dogs and 28–35% DMB for cats. As CKD advances, foods with less protein may be needed to control signs of uremia. Protein should be highly digestible and of high biologic value.

Phosphorus

Decreasing the intake of dietary phosphorus in dogs and cats with CKD has been shown to be beneficial in limiting phosphorus retention, hyperphosphatemia, and secondary renal hyperparathyroidism. Limiting dietary phosphorus intake has also been shown to considerably prolong survival times compared with patients that were fed a higher phosphorus maintenance food.[17,18]

Alkalinizers and Buffers

Alkalinizers and buffers aid in counteracting the CKD patient's predisposition to metabolic acidosis, which is commonly seen in patients with kidney failure. They also help to decrease muscle wasting associated with acidosis. Plasma bicarbonate, venous blood pH and total CO_2 are commonly decreased in cats and dogs with uremia or end-stage chronic renal disease. It is recommended to feed a diet formulated to assist the kidney disease patient with alkalinizing the blood and urine, which in turn assists in minimizing acid load.[13]

Sodium and Chloride

Controlled amounts of sodium and chloride help control clinical signs associated with sodium and fluid retention (ascites/edema) and minimizes systemic and renal hypertension (primary). Recommendations for dietary sodium intake for CKD patients are 0.3% DMB or less for dogs and 0.4% DMB or less for cats. The minimum recommended allowances for chloride for dogs and cats are 1.5 times the recommended sodium levels.[14]

Potassium

Hypokalemia is frequently a complication of CKD. Inadequate potassium intake, acidifying diets, or increased urinary losses are all potential reasons for hypokalemia in CKD patients, as are vomiting and inappetence. Properly maintaining potassium in the body also helps preserve quality of life. The recommendation of amounts of potassium in foods for dogs with CKD is 0.4–0.8% DMB and for cats 0.7–1.2% DMB. Oral supplementation may be indicated in cats with CKD and hypokalemia.

Omega-3 Fatty Acids

The specific dietary fatty acid content of a food may play a role in the progression of CKD by affecting:

- Renal hemodynamics
- Platelet aggregation
- Lipid peroxidation

- Systemic blood pressure
- Proliferation of glomerular mesangial cells
- Plasma lipid concentration.

Omega-3 fatty acids (e.g. EPA and DHA) in foods compete with arachidonic acid to alter eicosanoid production. These alterations are renoprotective. It is suggested that the range for total omega-3 fatty acid content in foods for canine and feline CKD patients is 0.4–2.5% DMB. Current recommendation for the omega-6 to omega-3 fatty acid ratio is 1: 1 – 7: 1.[13,14]

B Vitamins

B vitamins help to compensate for urinary losses due to kidney disease. B-vitamin deficiency can be caused by decreased appetite, vomiting, diarrhea, and polyuria. Anorexia associated with renal failure may be exacerbated by thiamin and niacin deficiency.

Soluble Fiber

Growth of bacteria is dependent upon a source of nitrogen. Even though dietary protein provides some nitrogen, blood urea is the largest and most available source of nitrogen for bacterial protein synthesis in the colon. Soluble fiber encourages growth of beneficial bacterial in the colon. Urea is the major end product of protein catabolism in mammals. When blood urea diffuses into the large bowel it is broken down by bacterial ureases and used for protein synthesis and is then excreted in the feces.

CANCER

Nutritional management of dogs and cats with cancer is part of a multimodal approach to managing cancer patients. The provision of appropriate nutrition may improve quality of life, enhance the effectiveness of treatment, and increase survival time. Alterations in carbohydrate, protein, and fat metabolism precede obvious clinical disease and cachexia in dogs with cancer and may persist in animals with clinical remission of, or apparent recovery from, cancer. Pathophysiologic and therapeutic principles for cats with cancer should follow those of people and dogs with cancer.[19]

Soluble Carbohydrates and Fiber

Ingredients containing carbohydrates, such as starch, are used in commercial pet food because they are efficient energy sources and have properties that aid in manufacturing and cooking processes. However, soluble carbohydrates may be poorly used by animals with cancer and can contribute to increased lactate production. Therefore, soluble carbohydrates should make up 25% or less of a food's dry matter content.

Soluble (fermentable) and insoluble (poorly fermentable) fiber sources are important to help maintain intestinal health, especially in animals undergoing chemotherapy, radiation therapy, or surgery. Increased dietary fiber may help prevent and resolve abnormal stool quality (soft stools, diarrhea) encountered when changing from a high-carbohydrate commercial dry food to a high-fat commercial or homemade food. A crude fiber level greater than 2.5% dry matter is recommended.

Protein

Because patients with cancer experience altered protein metabolism, resulting in loss of lean muscle mass (cachexia), dietary protein should be highly digestible and exceed the level normally used for maintenance of adult animals. The protein level should be 30–45% dry matter in foods for dogs with cancer and 40–50% dry matter in foods for cats with cancer.[19]

Arginine

Arginine is an essential amino acid which may have specific therapeutic value in pets with cancer. A positive correlation between plasma arginine concentrations and survival in dogs with lymphoma receiving chemotherapy suggests that it is appropriate to provide more than 2.5% arginine on a dry matter basis.[19,20] Arginine has also been shown to improve immune function in cancer patients, promote wound healing, and inhibit tumorigenesis.

Glutamine

Glutamine is an essential precursor for nucleotide biosynthesis; as well as an important oxidative fuel for enterocytes. Glutamine has recently been recognized as a conditionally essential amino acid in certain physiologic states, including stress. Cancer would be considered to elicit a stressful physiologic response. Glutamine has several important biochemical roles and is a preferred source of energy for cells with rapid turnover, such as lymphocytes, enterocytes, and cancer cells. Glutamine has been shown to stabilize weight loss, improve protein metabolism, improve immune response, and improve gut barrier function in rodent cancer models and in human clinical trials.[19] Glutamine is best supplied by high-quality, high-protein pet foods.

Fat and Omega-3 Fatty Acids

Omega-3 fatty acids may have a preventive and therapeutic role in cancer therapy. There is epidemiologic evidence supporting the use of omega-3 fatty acids in human patients with cancer. Omega-3 fatty acids increase the immunologic response against tumor cells, increase tumor susceptibility to oxidative stress, and decrease TNF-α production. In patients with cancer, a high level of omega-3 fatty acids has many clinical benefits, including reduced tumorigenesis, tumor growth, and metastasis as well as anticatabolic effects.[21,22]

In clinical trials of dogs with spontaneous cancer, high dietary levels of omega-3 fatty acids (specifically EPA and DHA) and arginine were shown to benefit dogs with lymphoma, nasal carcinoma, hemangiosarcoma, and osteosarcoma.[20,23] Omega-3 fatty acids in conjunction with arginine were shown to influence clinical signs, increase survival time, provide longer remission time, and improve quality of life.[23]

CARDIAC DISEASE

In dogs and cats, cardiovascular disease is a common disorder with an estimated 11% of canines and 20% of felines affected.[24,25] Chronic valvular disease has been found to be the most common acquired heart disease in dogs, with an overall incidence greater than 40%.[26]

Sodium and Chloride

Sodium, chloride, and water retention are linked with congestive heart failure (CHF). Subsequently, the healthcare team should focus on these nutrients in patients with cardiovascular disease. A few hours after the ingestion of high levels of sodium, healthy dogs and cats easily excrete any excess in their urine. However, patients in early cardiac disease may lose this ability to excrete excess sodium. As heart disease worsens and CHF arises, the ability to excrete excess sodium is worsened. Chloride may act as a direct renal vasoconstrictor. When managing patients with cardiovascular disease, it is suggested that the sodium levels in foods be limited to 0.08–0.25% dry matter for dogs and 0.07–0.3% dry matter for cats. Recommended chloride levels are typically 1.5 times sodium levels.

It is important to remember that avoiding excess sodium chloride in cat foods is harder than in dog foods. This is because ingredients used to meet the higher protein requirement of cats likewise contain sodium and chloride; subsequently, the sodium chloride content of cat food may be increased.

Taurine

Taurine is an important amino acid in dogs and cats with myocardial failure. Taurine may function in inactivation of free radicals, osmoregulation, and calcium modulation. Taurine is also known for its direct effects on contractile proteins. Dilated cardiomyopathy and heart failure may result from an inciting or contributing factor combined with taurine deficiency. Taurine is an essential amino acid in cats, therefore a minimum recommended allowance for taurine is necessary in cat foods. Taurine content of foods for cats with cardiovascular disease should contain at least 0.3% dry matter. Levels of taurine typically recommended for supplementation of feline cardiovascular patients (250–500 mg taurine/day) provide approximately twice that much.

Taurine is not an essential amino acid for dogs. Nevertheless, an association between dilated cardiomyopathy and plasma taurine deficiency and low myocardial taurine concentrations, has been observed. Even in canine dilated cardiomyopathy, dogs with normal plasma and whole blood taurine levels, additional taurine may be warranted. Therefore foods for management of cardiovascular disease contain in dogs should contain added taurine. The level of taurine in foods for canine patients can be lower than for cats since dogs can synthesize taurine. The recommendation for taurine in foods for canine cardiovascular disease patients is at least 0.1% dry matter. This is somewhat lower than would be supplied by the typical recommendation for taurine supplementation of foods for dogs with dilated cardiomyopathy (500–1000 mg taurine/day).

L-Carnitine

Deficiency of L-carnitine in dogs has been linked to dilated cardiomyopathy in dogs. Cardiac muscle function benefits from carnitine because carnitine is a critical component of the mitochondrial membrane enzymes responsible for transporting activated fatty acids in the form of acyl-carnitine esters. These are transported across the mitochondrial membranes to the matrix. From here b-oxidation and high-energy phosphate generation occur. Free L-carnitine serves as a mitochondrial detoxifying agent.[27]

Currently, the recommendation for carnitine supplementation in dogs with dilated cardiomyopathy is 50–100 mg L-carnitine/kg body weight three times daily. It is widely accepted that even if the cause of cardiomyopathy in a heart disease patient is not carnitine deficiency, supplementing dogs with carnitine does not appear to do any harm and may in fact be beneficial. Foods for heart disease patients should provide at least 0.02% dry matter carnitine.

Phosphorus

Patients with cardiac disease are often suffering from concurrent disease conditions. It is understood that phosphorus is a nutrient of concern in patients with concurrent CKD and that kidney disease is one of the more prevalent diseases seen concurrently with cardiac disease. Therefore nutritional management should avoid excess phosphorus in patients with concurrent CKD. The recommended amount of phosphorous in nutritional management of cardiac disease is 0.2–0.7% dry matter in dogs and 0.3–0.7% dry matter in cats.

Potassium and Magnesium

Another concern in cardiac disease patients is the metabolism of potassium and magnesium. Hypokalemia, hyperkalemia, and hypomagnesemia all have the potential for complications when medication therapy is introduced in patients with cardiovascular disease. Potassium or magnesium homeostasis abnormalities can cause cardiac dysrhythmias, decrease myocardial contractility, produce profound muscle weakness, and potentiate adverse effects from cardiac glycosides and other cardiac drugs.

The amounts of potassium and magnesium recommended for adult maintenance in dogs and cats (0.4% and 0.52% dry matter potassium, respectively, and 0.06% and 0.04% dry matter magnesium) should be the minimum amounts included in nutritional management of CHF. If abnormalities in these electrolytes occur, the healthcare team should consider supplementation or switching to a different food.

Protein

Cardiac cachexia is a principal concern in patients with cardiac disease. The metabolic changes associated with cachexia and their effect on overall nutrient requirements are only recently being investigated. Many patients with cachexia present with concomitant disease (i.e. CKD), which also significantly affects nutrient requirements. Profound anorexia enhances protein–energy malnutrition in patients with cachexia. Subsequently, patients with cachexia or exhibiting signs potentially leading to cachexia should be encouraged to eat a complete and balanced food that contains adequate calories and adequate high-quality, highly digestible protein.

Omega-3 Fatty Acids

In cardiac cachexia, tumor necrosis factor and interleukin-1 cytokines have been implicated as pathogenic mediators. Fish oil (known to be high in omega-3, n-3, fatty acids) has been shown to alter cytokine production. Early investigations involving fish oil suggest that fish oil-mediated alterations in cytokine production may help dogs with CHF. Consequently, it is believed that heart failure patients with cachexia may benefit from the alterations of cytokine production through omega-3 fatty acid supplementation.

It is believed that omega-3 fatty acids electrically stabilize heart cells through modulation of the fast voltage-dependent Na(+) currents and the L-type Ca(2+) channels which results in the heart cells becoming resistant to dysrhythmias. Clinical studies of fish oil as a source of long-chain omega-3 fatty acids have confirmed the reduction in frequency of ventricular arrhythmia in Boxer dogs.

Omega-3 fatty acids have been shown to significantly affect survival times in dogs diagnosed with dilated cardiomyopathy or chronic valvular disease. The omega-3 fatty acids effect may be attributable to: anti-inflammatory effects, cachexia prevention, improved appetite, or anti-arrhythmic effects. The veterinary healthcare team should also be aware of further effects of omega-3 fatty acids on the patient. The healthcare team must be mindful of the fact that omega-3 fatty acids have the potential to alter immune function. This alteration in immune function may contribute to the cardiovascular effects of omega-3 fatty acids. Omega-3 fatty acids also reduce platelet aggregation resulting from the production of thromboxane B5. The reduction in platelet aggregation might be of benefit in cats with cardiac disease and at risk for thrombus formation. However, this effect is also important to be mindful of when using omega-3 fatty acids in animals with coagulopathies.[28]

At this point in time, no optimal dose of omega-3 fatty acids has been established for humans, cats, or dogs. The current recommendation from nutritionists studying fatty acids and cardiac disease is a dose of 40 mg/kg EPA and 25 mg/kg DHA for both dogs and cats.[28]

EPA and DHA can be provided through the diet or as a dietary supplement. There are a few therapeutic pet foods with high levels of EPA and DHA, but the majority of foods manufactured today do not achieve the recommended level of EPA and DHA. The current recommended dose is 40 mg/kg EPA plus 25 mg/kg DHA. A manufactured food would thus need to contain 80–150 mg/100 kcal EPA + DHA.[28]

Water

With all patients, veterinary technicians must remember to talk with clients about the importance of water for pets. Veterinary technicians need to remind clients that pets should be offered water free choice and it should be clean and fresh. Healthcare teams must also keep in mind that water quality varies considerably, even within the same community. We must be cognizant of the fact that water can be a significant source of sodium, chloride, and other minerals. Veterinary healthcare teams should be familiar with the mineral levels in their local water supply. Water samples can be submitted to state or other government laboratories for analysis. Also municipal water companies can be contacted to ask about mineral levels in local water supplies. Distilled water or water with less than 150 ppm sodium is recommended for patients with advanced heart disease and failure.

REFERENCES

1. Wortinger, A., Burns, K.M. (2015). Nutritional management of gastrointestinal disease. In: *Nutrition and Disease Management for Veterinary Technicians and Nurses*, 2e, 169–174. Ames, IA: Wiley-Blackwell.
2. Davenport, D.J., Jergens, A.E., Remillard, R.J. (2010). Inflammatory bowel disease. In: *Small Animal Clinical Nutrition*, 5e. (ed. M.S. Hand, C.D. Thatcher, R.J. Remillard *et al.*), 1065–1076. Topeka, KS: Mark Morris Institute.
3. Guilford, W.G., Jones, B.R., Markwell, P.J. *et al.* (2001). Food sensitivity in cats with chronic idiopathic intestinal problems. *J Vet Int Med* 15: 7–13.
4. Burns, K.M., Towell, T.L. (2011).Owner education and adherence. In: *Practical Weight Management in Dogs and Cats*. (ed. T.L. Towell), 3–21. Ames, IA: Wiley Blackwell.
5. Burns, K.M. (2006). Managing overweight or obese pets. *Vet Tech* June; 385–389.
6. Burns, K.M. (2013). Why is rocky so stocky? Obesity is a disease! *NAVTA J* Convention Issue; 16–19.
7. Toll, P.W., Yamka, R.N., Schoenherr, W.D., Hand, M.S. (2010). Obesity. In: *Small Animal Clinical Nutrition*, 5e (ed. M.S. Hand, C.D. Thatcher, R.J. Remillard *et al.*), 501–542. Topeka, KS: Mark Morris Institute.
8. Wortinger, A., Burns, K.M. (2015). Feline lower urinary tract disease. In: *Nutrition and Disease Management for Veterinary Technicians and Nurses*, 2e, 186–191. Ames, IA: Wiley-Blackwell.
9. Burns, K.M. (2014). FLUTD – using nutrition to go with the flow. *NAVTA J* Convention Issue; 7–12.
10. Markwell, P.J., Buffington, C.A., Chew, D.J. *et al.* (1999). Clinical evaluation of commercially available urinary acidification diets in the management of idiopathic cystitis in cats. *J Am Vet Med Assoc* 214: 361.
11. Burns, K.M., Forrester, S.D. (2007). Feline lower urinary tract disease. *NAVTA J* July/August.
12. Chew, D.J., DiBartola, S.P., Schenk, P.A. (2011). Chronic renal failure. In: *Canine and Feline Nephrology and Urology*, 2e. St. Louis, MO: Elsevier.
13. Ograin, V., Burns, K.M. (2017). Kidney disease and nutrition: yes they will eat! *NAVTA J* Convention Issue; 16–21.
14. Forrester, S.D., Adams, L.G., Allen, T.A. (2010). Chronic kidney disease. In: *Small Animal Clinical Nutrition*, 5e (ed. M.S. Hand, C.D. Thatcher, R.J. Remillard *et al.*), 765–809. Topeka, KS: Mark Morris Institute.
15. Polzin, D.J. (2007). 11 guidelines for conservatively treating chronic kidney disease. *Vet Med* 102: 788–799.
16. Elliott, D.A. (2012). Nutritional management of kidney disease. In: *Applied Veterinary Clinical Nutrition* (ed. A.J. Fascetti and S.J. Delaney) 251–268. Ames, IA: Wiley-Blackwell.
17. Ross, S., Osborne, C., Kirk, C. *et al.* (2006). Clinical evaluation of dietary modification for treatment of spontaneous chronic kidney disease in cats. *J Am Vet Med Assoc* 229: 949–957.
18. Jacob, F., Polzin, D.J., Osborne, C.A. *et al.* (2002). Clinical evaluation of dietary modification for treatment of spontaneous chronic renal failure in dogs. *J Am Vet Med Assoc* 220: 1163–1170.
19. Saker, K.E., Selting, K.A. (2010). Cancer. In: *Small Animal Clinical Nutrition*, 5e (ed. M.S. Hand, C.D. Thatcher, R.J. Remillard *et al.*), 587–607. Topeka, KS: Mark Morris Institute.
20. Forrester, S.D., Roudebush, P., Davenport, D.J. (2010). Supportive care of the cancer patient: nutritional management of the cancer patient. In: *Cancer*

Management in Small Animal Practice (ed. C.J. Henry and M.L. Higginbotham), 167–187. Maryland Heights, MO: Saunders Elsevier.

21. Bougnoux, P. (1999). Omega-3 polyunsaturated fatty acids and cancer. *Curr Opin Clin Nutr Metab Care* 2: 121–126.
22. Ross, J.A., Moses, A.G.W., Fearon, K.C.H. (1999). The anti-catabolic effects of omega-3 fatty acids. *Curr Opin Clin Nutr Metab Care* 2: 219–226.
23. Roudebush, P., Davenport, D.J., Novotny, B.J. (2004). The use of nutraceuticals in cancer therapy. *Vet Clin North Am Small Anim Pract* 34: 249–269.
24. Buchanan, J.W. (1999). Prevalence of cardiovascular disorders. In: *Textbook of Canine and Feline Cardiology*, 2e (ed. P.R. Fox, D. Sisson and N.S. Moise) 457–470. Philadelphia, PA: Saunders.
25. Paige, C.F., Abbott, J.A., Elvinger, F., Pyle, R.L. (2009). Prevalence of cardiomyopathy in apparently healthy cats. *J Am Vet Med Assoc*, 234: 1398–1403.
26. Rush, J.E. (2009). Chronic valvular disease in dogs. In: *Kirk's Current Therapy XIV: Small Animal Practice* (ed. J.D. Bongura and D.C. Twedt). St. Louis, MO: Saunders Elsevier.
27. Roudebush, P., Keene, B.W. (2010). Cardiovascular disease. In: *Small Animal Clinical Nutrition*, 5e. (ed. M.S. Hand, C.D. Thatcher, R.J. Remillard *et al.*), 733–763. Topeka, KS: Mark Morris Institute.
28. Freeman, L.M. (2010). Beneficial effects of omega-3 fatty acids in cardiovascular disease. *J Small Anim Pract* 51: 462–470.

Chapter 8

Ophthalmologic Diseases and Conditions

Natalie Herring, LVT, VTS (Ophthalmology)

Veterinary Technician and Nurse's Daily Reference Guide: Canine and Feline, Fourth Edition. Edited by Mandy Fults and Kenichiro Yagi.

Companion website: www.wiley.com/go/fults/veterinary

Abbreviations

CBC, complete blood count
FeLV, feline leukemia virus
FIV, feline immunodeficiency virus
KCS, keratoconjunctivitis sicca
NeoPolyDex, neomycin, polymyxin B sulfates, and dexamethasone
NSAIDs, non-steroidal anti-inflammatory drugs

ANTERIOR UVEITIS

Anterior uveitis is inflammation of the iris and ciliary body. Corneal ulceration, trauma, autoimmune, lens-induced, or infections can cause anterior uveitis.

CATARACTS

Cataracts are pathological changes in the eye that leads to opacity in the lens or lens capsule. The changes are in the lens protein composition or disruption of lens fiber arrangement. The general causes are hereditary, inflammatory, metabolic, traumatic, nutritional, and toxic.

Table 8.1 / Anterior uveitis and cataracts

Disease		Anterior uveitis	Cataracts
Presentation	Clinical signs	• Blepharospasm, blindness, elevation of nictitating membrane, epiphora, inappetence, lethargy, miosis, photophobia, redness, tearing	• Blindness, visual impairment
	Exam findings	• Aqueous flare, conjunctival hyperemia, hypopyon, hyphema, hypotony, corneal edema, fibrinous exudate	• Aqueous flare, any opacity in the lens, synechia, lens-induced uveitis
Diagnosis	General	• Clinical signs • Ophthalmic exam • Physical exam	• History/clinical signs • Ophthalmic exam
	Laboratory	• Chemistry panel: ↑ globulin • CBC • Cytology, ocular: causative agent • Serology: fungal, tick-borne, protozoal, bacterial, viral	• CBC/chemistry serology (dependent on other clinical signs): systemic mycoses, rickettsial disease, brucellosis, *Toxoplasma*, FeLV, FIV
	Imaging	• Radiographs, thoracic and abdominal: tumors, fungal disease • Ultrasound, abdominal: tumors • Ultrasound, ocular: foreign body, penetrating wounds, neoplasm, or retinal detachment	• Ultrasound, ocular: retinal detachment and lens capsule rupture

(*Continued*)

Table 8.1 / Anterior uveitis and cataracts (Continued)

Disease		Anterior uveitis	Cataracts
	Procedures	• Tonometry: ↓ pressure with uveitis or ↑ pressure with primary or secondary glaucoma • Ocular centesis: + causative agents • Systemic blood pressure	• Electroretinogram: degree of retinal atrophy • Gonioscopy: evaluation of the irideocorneal angle • Biomicroscopy or optical coherence tomography: examination of the anterior segment • Tonometry: ↓ pressure with uveitis or ↑ pressure with primary or secondary glaucoma
Treatment	General	• Symptomatic	• Supportive • Surgery: phacoemulsification, extracapsular extraction, intracapsular extraction, ± implantation of an intraocular lens
	Medication	• Antibiotics: variable • Corticosteroids (systemic): prednisone • Corticosteroids (topical) (no corneal ulcer): 1% prednisolone acetate, NeoPolyDex • Mydriatic/cycloplegic: topical atropine • NSAIDs (systemic): meloxicam, carprofen, • NSAIDs (topical): diclofenac, ketorolac	• Corticosteroids (topical): 1% prednisolone acetate, NeoPolyDex • Mydriatics: 1% tropicamide • NSAIDs (systemic): meloxicam, carprofen, • NSAIDs (topical): diclofenac, ketorolac • Mydriatic-cycloplegic: topical atropine
	Nursing care	• Treated as outpatient	• Treated as outpatient (non-surgical) • Surgical postoperatively (e.g. monitor inflammation, implant position, pressure, and retinal status) • Pain management
Follow-up	Patient care	• Reexamine 3–7 days after initiation of treatment then every 2–3 weeks dependent on the severity of the disease. • Monitor intraocular pressure and signs of secondary glaucoma	• Examine frequently for several months postoperatively, then every 6 months for life
	Prevention/ avoidance	• Proper treatment of underlying disease • Flea and tick preventative	• Prompt treatment of uveitis • Selective breeding and ocular screening • Well-balanced nutrition in hand-fed neonates • Glycemic control in diabetic animals

(*Continued*)

Table 8.1 / Anterior uveitis and cataracts (Continued)

Disease		Anterior uveitis	Cataracts
	Complications	• Blindness • Secondary glaucoma • Cataracts • Endophthalmitis or panophthalmitis • Iris atrophy • Lens luxation	• Anterior uveitis • Corneal endothelial damage • Glaucoma • Retinal detachment • Lens luxation
	Prognosis	• Depends on severity of disease upon presentation	• Dependent on stage and location of disease and age of animal • Good with surgery: 80–90% success rate
Notes		• Caution: corticosteroids are contraindicated in cases of primary conjunctivitis and corneal ulceration • Diagnostic testing is important as ocular clinical signs may indicate a systemic condition • Subconjunctival injections of triamcinolone acetonide may be necessary in severe cases	• Caution: Differentiate the type and stage of cataract from nuclear sclerosis, which is a decrease in the clarity of the nucleus of the lens and is a normal aging process • Special considerations must be taken with medications and procedures for patients with diabetes mellitus • Miniature Poodles, American Cocker Spaniel, Miniature Schnauzers, Golden Retrievers, Boston Terriers, Siberian Huskies, Persians, Birmans, Himalayans

CONJUNCTIVITIS

Conjunctivitis is a general term for inflammation of the ocular mucous membrane that covers the sclera and lines the inner surface of the eyelids. Its causes can be infectious, foreign body related, trauma related, tear film deficiency, chemical or environmental irritants, immune mediated, or due to other eye diseases.

ENTROPION

Entropion is the inward rolling of the eyelid margin causing contact of the eyelashes or eyelid hair with the eye.

Table 8.2 / **Conjunctivitis and entropion**

Disease		Conjunctivitis	Entropion
Presentation	Clinical signs	• Discharge, pain	• Blepharospasms, conjunctival hyperemia, epiphora, purulent discharge, visual impairment, excoriation of epidermal surface
	Exam findings	• Chemosis, hyperemia, tissue proliferation, discharge, and follicle formation	• Conjunctivitis, corneal rupture, corneal ulceration
Diagnosis	General	• History/clinical signs • Ophthalmic exam	• History/clinical signs • Ophthalmic exam
	Laboratory	• Serology: FeLV or FIV • Culture: bacteria or fungi isolation and identification • Cytology, conjunctival: inflammation, neoplasia, viral or chlamydial infection • Biopsy: neoplasia or preocular mucin deficiency	• Not applicable
	Imaging	• Not applicable	• Not applicable
	Procedures	• Schirmer tear test: ↓ tear production • Conjunctival scraping: FHV, chlamydia • Fluorescein stain: ulceration and nasolacrimal duct patency • Tonometry: ↑ pressure	• Fluorescein stain
Treatment	General	• Symptomatic • Surgery: keratectomy or removal of foreign body, hairs or mass	• Surgery, correction of anatomic entropion: temporary eversion of eyelid margins with sutures,
	Medication	• Amino acid: L-lysine (FHV-1) • Antibiotics (systemic): tetracycline, erythromycin, chloramphenicol, amoxicillin/clavulanic acid • Antibiotics (topical): triple antibiotic, oxytetracycline, erythromycin, tobramycin • Antiviral: idoxuridine, cidofovir famciclovir • Corticosteroids (systemic): megestrol acetate (caution with use!) • Corticosteroids (topical): NeoPolyDex, prednisolone acetate, megestrol acetate (no corneal ulcer) • Lacrimostimulants: cyclosporine, tacrolimus • Lacrimomimetics: hyaluronic acid, OTC artificial tears (no polyvinyl alcohol) • Systemic or topical NSAIDs	• Antibiotic (topical): variable • Lacrimomimetics: hyaluronic acid, OTC artificial tears (no polyvinyl alcohol)
	Nursing care	• Irrigate the eye with an eyewash solution to remove any exudates • Clip the hair surrounding the eye as needed • Apply an Elizabethan collar to prevent self-trauma	• Treated as outpatient

(Continued)

Table 8.2 / Conjunctivitis and entropion (Continued)

Disease		Conjunctivitis	Entropion
Follow-up	Patient care	• Maintain the eyes clear of exudates. • Examine 5–7 days after initiation of treatment and then as needed	• Apply an Elizabethan collar to prevent rubbing at eyes/sutures
	Prevention/avoidance	• Treat underlying condition if present • Isolate patients with infectious conjunctivitis • Minimize stress for patients with the herpetic conjunctivitis	• Selective breeding
	Complications	• Corneal • Symblepharon • KCS	• Conjunctivitis • Impaired vision • Corneal ulcer
	Prognosis	• Excellent with bacterial conjunctivitis • Fair with feline herpesvirus, immune-mediated diseases, or KCS	• Good
Notes		• Caution: corticosteroids are contraindicated in feline conjunctivitis and corneal ulcerations • Clean the eyes before instilling topical medications. • Determine the type of conjunctivitis to assist in treatment: bacterial, secondary, viral, allergic, follicular, eosinophilic	• Permanent corrective surgery is postponed until mature facial conformation, typically after 8 months of age (breed dependent) to increase surgical success • Temporary eyelid and/or brow tacking may be performed until mature facial conformation • Chow, Shar-Pei, Saint Bernard, hunting dogs, English Bulldogs, Rottweiler

CBC, complete blood count; FeLV, feline leukemia virus; FHV, feline herpesvirus; FIV, feline immunodeficiency virus; KCS, keratoconjunctivitis sicca; NeoPolyDex, neomycin, polymyxin B sulfates, and dexamethasone; NSAIDs, non-steroidal anti-inflammatory drugs; OTC, over the counter.

CILIA DISORDERS

Cilia disorders (distichiasis, trichiasis, and ectopic cilia) are the abnormal location or positioning of the eyelashes. Trichiasis is cilia arising from normal sites that are directed toward the eye. Distichiasis is the emergence of cilia from the meibomian glands and emergence from their ducts. Ectopic cilia are cilia that arise from the meibomian gland and erupt through the palpebral conjunctival surface.

GLAUCOMA

Glaucoma is an increase in intraocular pressure with subsequent damage to the optic nerve. It is categorized as primary (without preexisting ocular disease) or secondary (presence of other ocular abnormalities). Chronic glaucoma often results in blindness, retinal and optic nerve degeneration, and buphthalmos.

Table 8.3 / Cilia disorders and glaucoma

Disease		Cilia disorders	Glaucoma
Presentation	Clinical signs	• Blepharospasm, discharge, epiphora	• Blepharospasm, blindness, dilated pupil, epiphora, impaired vision, ↓ pupillary light response • Weak to absent menace response
	Exam findings	• Anisocoria, hyperemia, chemosis, pain, pigmentation, tissue proliferation, vascularization, corneal ulcerations can be present	• Buphthalmos, conjunctival hyperemia, corneal edema, luxated lens, retinal degeneration, exposure keratitis, lens changes, optic disc cupping
Diagnosis	General	• History/clinical signs • Ophthalmic exam	• History/clinical signs • Ophthalmic exam
	Laboratory	• Not applicable	• Dependent on underlying condition (secondary form)
	Imaging	• Not applicable	• Radiographs, skull: fungi or neoplastic lesions • Ultrasound, ocular: structural abnormalities
	Procedures	• Fluorescein stain	• Tonometry: ↑ pressure; > 25 mmHg (canine), > 27 mmHg (feline) • Fluorescein stain • Gonioscopy: evaluation of the irideocorneal angle
Treatment	General	• Surgery: cryoepilation, electroepilation (use caution), facial-fold resection, or medial canthal closure	• Supportive • Symptomatic • Surgery: transscleral cyclophotocoagulation, endocyclophotocoagulation, cyclophotoagglutination, intraocular prosthesis, enucleation, cyclodestruction
	Medication	• Antibiotics (topical): variable • Lacrimomimetics: Hyaluronic acid, OTC Artificial tears (no polyvinyl alcohol)	• Betablocker: timolol maleate 0.25–0.5% • Parasympathomimetic: demecarium bromide • Carbonic anhydrase inhibitors: methazolamide, dorzolamide, brinzolamide • Corticosteroids (topical/oral): dexamethasone, prednisolone • Diuretics: 20% mannitol or glycerin • Prostaglandins: latanoprost, travoprost, bimatoprost
	Nursing care	• Treated as outpatient	• Treated as outpatient

(Continued)

Table 8.3 / **Cilia disorders and glaucoma (Continued)**

Disease		Cilia disorders	Glaucoma
Follow-up	Patient care	• Elizabethan collar	• Warm, moist compresses twice daily for 5–7 days postoperatively • Monitor IOP closely • Treat the other eye with prophylactic antiglaucoma therapy (following initial diagnosis of primary glaucoma, onset in the opposite eye when left untreated is approximately 8 months. This timeframe is increased to approximately 30 months with prophylactic treatment)
	Prevention/ avoidance	• Clip hair on facial folds and around the eyes; it may make the hair more stiff and irritating to the patient	• Yearly ophthalmic exam in predisposed breeds • Examine unaffected eye 2–3 times a year when one eye already has glaucoma
	Complications	• Recurrence • Conjunctivitis • Keratitis	• Blindness • Chronic ocular pain • Corneal ulceration
	Prognosis	• Excellent with proper correction of affected areas • Fair to good with hair removal (can regrow)	• Fair with surgery • Poor with medical treatment alone
Notes			• Normal IOP is 15–25 mmHg • IOP readings can vary with tonometer used, time of day taken, and technique. It is important to consider the patient's overall ocular evaluation when determining the accuracy of the IOP readings • Determining the cause of glaucoma (primary vs. secondary) is important to the patient's long-term treatment and prognosis

IOP, intraocular pressure; OTC, over the counter.

KERATITIS

Keratitis is inflammation of the cornea. It can be caused by trauma, foreign bodies, bacterial infection, irritant, cilia disorders, keratoconjunctivitis sicca (KCS), feline herpesvirus, or corneal exposure. Keratitis can be classified into ulcerative and non-ulcerative. The non-ulcerative type is corneal inflammation that does not retain fluorescein stain. The ulcerative form is corneal ulceration/erosion.

Ulceration is the loss of epithelium. This can be caused by trauma, bacterial infection, *Pseudomonas*, feline herpesvirus, epithelial dystrophy, KCS, corneal dryness, neurotrophic keratitis, or complications from other diseases.

KERATOCONJUNCTIVITIS SICCA

KCS is a lack of normal tear production causing drying and inflammation of the cornea and conjunctiva. It is thought to be an immune-mediated disease against the lacrimal gland. It can also be caused by long-term use of sulfonamides, especially in susceptible or at-risk breeds.

Table 8.4 / **Keratitis and keratoconjunctivitis sicca**

Disease		Keratitis		Keratoconjunctivitis sicca (KCS)
		Non-ulcerative	Ulcerative	
Presentation	Clinical signs	• Blepharospasm, photophobia, squinting, rubbing at eyes, serous to mucopurulent discharge, tearing	• Blepharospasm, epiphora, photophobia, rubbing at eyes, serous to mucopurulent discharge	• Blepharospasms, reduced vision, eye rubbing, mucoid to mucopurulent discharge, periocular crust, photophobia, pruritus
	Exam findings	• Corneal edema, hyperemia, neovascularization, pigmentation	• Aqueous flare, corneal edema, corneal opacity, conjunctival hyperemia, hypotony, miosis, neovascularization, surface depression	• Chemosis, dull, opaque, or pigmentation of cornea, hyperemia, superficial vascularization, thickened conjunctiva, ulceration
Diagnosis	General	• History/clinical signs • Ophthalmic exam	• History/clinical signs • Ophthalmic exam	• History/clinical signs • Ophthalmic exam
	Laboratory	• Virus isolation: feline herpesvirus	• Virus isolation: feline herpesvirus • Culture: bacteria or fungi isolation and identification	• Thyroid panel
	Imaging	• Not applicable	• Not applicable	• Not applicable
	Procedures	• Corneal or conjunctival scraping • Schirmer tear test: ↓ production	• Fluorescein stain: • Schirmer tear test: > 15 mm/minute (proceed with caution: depth of ulcer should be noted prior to performing this test. Serum separator tube should be avoided in corneas with deep or infected corneal ulcers)	• Schirmer tear test: ↓ production, < 15 mm/minute • Fluorescein stain: retention of stain and identification of ulcers

(*Continued*)

Table 8.4 / Keratitis and keratoconjunctivitis sicca (Continued)

Disease		Keratitis		Keratoconjunctivitis sicca (KCS)
		Non-ulcerative	Ulcerative	
Treatment	General	• Symptomatic • Contact lenses	• Symptomatic • Debridement of ulcer edges (superficial) • Surgery: pedicle conjunctival flap, tissue adhesion, corneal transplant, corneoscleral transposition, keratectomy, linear keratotomy, contact lenses, and collagen shields	• Symptomatic • Surgery: transposition of the parotid salivary duct
	Medication	• Antibiotics (systemic): variable • Antibiotics (topical): variable • Antiviral: idoxuridine, cidofovir • Lacrimostimulant: cyclosporine, tacrolimus • Mydriatic/cycloplegic: atropine • Corticosteroids (topical): 0.1% dexamethasone, 1% prednisolone acetate • Mucolytics: acetylcysteine • NSAIDs: oral carprofen, meloxicam	• Antibiotics (systemic): variable • Antibiotics (topical): variable • Antiviral: Idoxuridine, cidofovir • Mydriatic/cycloplegic: atropine • NSAIDs	• Antibiotics (topical): variable • Lacrimomimetic artificial tears supplementation: hyaluronic acid, hydroxypropyl methylcellulose • Lacrimostimulant cyclosporine, tacrolimus
	Nursing care	• Treated as outpatient	• Restrict activity with deep ulcer to prevent rupture • Apply an Elizabethan collar to prevent self-trauma	• Clean eyes regularly to keep them clear of discharge

(Continued)

Table 8.4 / Keratitis and keratoconjunctivitis sicca (Continued)

Disease		Keratitis		Keratoconjunctivitis sicca (KCS)
		Non-ulcerative	Ulcerative	
Follow-up	Patient care	• Examine every 1–2 weeks to monitor progress until remission or ↓ clinical signs	• Monitor the healing process with fluorescein stain every 1–6 days depending on severity and until improvement is seen	• Monitor Schirmer tear test every 4–6 weeks until normal then periodically long-term • Clean eyes regularly to keep them clear of discharge
	Prevention/ avoidance	• Maintain health with FHV	• Lacrimomimetic administration (especially in brachycephalic breeds) long term • Continuous treatment with KCS	• Long-term treatment is necessary
	Complications	• Blindness • KCS • Keratitis, ulcerative • Ocular pain	• Descemetocele • Chronic ophthalmitis • Secondary glaucoma • Rupture of globe • Endophthalmitis • Blindness • Phthisis bulbi	• Keratitis, ulcerative • Corneal ulceration
	Prognosis	• Dependent on the severity of disease, may require lifelong treatment	• Fair to good: may take several weeks to heal	• Good with lifelong treatment
Notes		• Lifelong treatment is typical	• Caution: corticosteroids are contraindicated in cases of primary conjunctivitis and corneal ulceration • Descemetoceles are considered ocular emergencies	• Schirmer tear test: at least 15 mm/minute of wetting • Many with KCS have a secondary bacterial infection • Medical treatment (when effective) has the best level of patient comfort compared with surgery • Discontinue the use of sulfonamides • Cocker Spaniels, Bulldogs, West Highland Terriers, Lhaso Apsos, Miniature Schnauzers, Shih Tzus • Incidence is lower in felines

FHV, feline herpesvirus; NSAIDs, non-steroidal anti-inflammatory drugs.

LENS LUXATION

Lens luxation is the actual movement of the lens either anteriorly or posteriorly. It is often caused by glaucoma, uveitis, cataracts, trauma, or primary zonular degeneration.

PROLAPSED GLAND OF THE THIRD EYELID

Third eyelid gland prolapse (cherry eye) is caused by a weak attachment to the nictitating membrane gland allowing it to protrude or prolapse from the leading edge of the third eyelid.

Table 8.5 / Lens luxation and prolapsed gland of the third eyelid

Disease		Lens luxation	Prolapsed gland of the third eyelid (cherry eye)
Presentation	Clinical signs	• Blepharospasm, epiphora, redness, vision impairment	• Blepharospasms, discharge, epiphora, swelling at medial canthus, gland prolapse
	Exam findings	• Aphakic crescent, corneal edema, hyperemia, iridodonenesis, pain	• Conjunctivitis, hyperemia
	General	• Clinical signs • Ophthalmic exam	• History/clinical signs • Clinical signs
Diagnosis	Laboratory	• Not applicable	• Not applicable
	Imaging	• Radiographs, thoracic: metastasis from intraocular neoplasia • Ultrasound, ocular: structural abnormalities • Ultrasound, abdominal: metastasis from intraocular neoplasia • Electroretinography	• Not applicable
	Procedures	• Fluorescein stain • Tonometry: ↑ values	• Not applicable
Treatment	General	• Supportive (posterior luxation) • Surgery (anterior luxation): cyclocryosurgery, evisceration, intrascleral prosthesis, or enucleation	• Surgery: repositioning of the nictitating membrane gland and anchoring securely
	Medication	• Carbonic anhydrase inhibitors: methazolamide, Dorzolamide and brinzolamide • Corticosteroids (topical): 0.1% dexamethasone, 1% prednisolone acetate • Diuretics: mannitol • Miotics (topical): demecarium bromide, latanoprost, travoprost, bimatoprost (posterior luxation) • Mydriatics: 1% tropicamide • NSAIDS • Systemic steroids	• Antibiotics: variable • Corticosteroids (topical): 1% dexamethasone • NSAIDs
	Nursing care	• Treated as outpatient or inpatient	• Standard postoperative care

(Continued)

Table 8.5 / **Lens luxation and prolapsed gland of the third eyelid (Continued)**

Disease		Lens luxation	Prolapsed gland of the third eyelid (cherry eye)
Follow-up	Patient care	• Examine within 24 hours and then frequently after that until intraocular pressure stabilizes. • Examine every 3months	• Do not allow rubbing at eyes/sutures; use e-collar as needed.
	Prevention/ avoidance	• Selective breeding	• Selective breeding
	Complications	• Uveitis • Corneal edema • Dyscoria • Blindness • Synechia • Glaucoma • Retinal detachment • Vitreous entrapment in the incision	• Re-prolapse of the gland • Infection at surgery site • Corneal ulcer/erosion secondary to suture abrasion
	Prognosis	• Good with surgery (if caught early)	• Excellent with surgery
Notes		• Caution: anterior lens luxation should not be administered miotics • Anterior lens luxation should be seen and treated as soon as possible • Genetic testing is available to identify inherited ocular disease; recommended prior to breeding • Inherited in many terrier breeds. Prevalent in Poodles and many other breeds (not confirmed to be hereditary)	• Cocker Spaniels, Bulldogs, Pitbull Terriers, Beagles, Bloodhounds, Lhasa Apsos, Shih Tzus, Shar-Peis • When unilateral prolapse occurs prophylactic tacking of the opposite gland may be considered. • Tends to occur in younger patients • Removal of the gland should be avoided unless neoplasia is suspected (this is more commonly seen in older patients)

Chapter **9**

Reproductive Diseases and Conditions

Mandy Fults, MS, LVT, CVPP, VTS (Clinical Practice C/F)

Veterinary Technician and Nurse's Daily Reference Guide: Canine and Feline, Fourth Edition. Edited by Mandy Fults and Kenichiro Yagi.

Companion website: www.wiley.com/go/fults/veterinary

Abbreviations

2ME, 2-mercapto-ethanol
AGID, agar gel immunodiffusion
ALP, alkaline phosphatase
ALT, alanine aminotransferase
BPH, benign prostatic hyperplasia
bpm, beats per minute
CBC, complete blood count
ECG, electrocardiogram
ELISA, enzyme-linked immunoassay
FeLV, feline leukemia virus
FIP, feline infectious peritonitis
FIV, feline immunodeficiency virus
GnRH, gonadotropin hormone-releasing hormone
hCG, human chorionic gonadotropin
hpf, high power factor
OHE, ovariohysterectomy
PCV, packed cell volume
PGF2, prostaglandin F2
RBC, red blood cells
RSAT, rapid slide agglutination test
TAT, tube agglutination test
VPC, ventricular premature contractions

The Theriogenology Foundation defines theriogenology as:

> all aspects of veterinary reproductive medicine and surgery. This includes the basic sciences of anatomy, physiology, pathology and pharmacology, as well as all aspects of clinical practice related to male and female animal reproduction, obstetrics, and neonatology. The term Theriogenology is derived from the ancient Greek words *Therio* meaning beast or animal, 'gen' as in genesis meaning creation, generation, and 'ology' meaning study of. Theriogenology gathers mammals, both male and female, and reproduction, both physiology and pathology.[1]

ABORTION

An abortion is the termination of a pregnancy. It may be the result of difficulties with the mother, fetus, or placenta. Losses typically occur during the seventh week of gestation. Exposures to toxins or infections in the dam are well documented.

Table 9.1 / Reproductive diseases and conditions: abortion

Disease		Abortion
Presentation	Presenting clinical signs	• Anorexia, depression, lethargy, vomiting, and diarrhea • Early gestation: vaginal discharge, fetid and purulent • Late gestation: restlessness and abdominal contractions
	Exam findings	• Disappearance of previously documented (e.g. palpation, ultrasound, radiograph) fetuses

(*Continued*)

Table 9.1 / **Reproductive diseases and conditions: abortion (Continued)**

Disease		Abortion
Diagnosis	General	• History/clinical signs • Observe for any systemic signs of illness
	Laboratory	• Bacterial culture: bacteria isolation and identification • ELISA: FIV, FeLV, FIP • RSAT or AGID: *Babesia canis*, toxoplasmosis, *Neospora*, *Coxiella burnetii*, herpesvirus
	Imaging	• Radiographs, abdominal: retained fetuses • Ultrasound: uterine pathology and retained fetuses
	Procedures	• Vaginoscopy • Necropsy of dead fetuses
Treatment	General	• Symptomatic • Fluid therapy • Surgery: cesarean section
	Medication	• Antibiotics: variable • Prostaglandin
	Nursing care	• Post-parturition or postoperative nursing care
Follow-up	Patient care	• Physical exam 7–14 days after treatment
	Prevention/avoidance	• Ovariohysterectomy
	Complications	• Infertility • Peritonitis • Pyometra • Sepsis • Shock • Uterine rupture • Death
	Prognosis	• Excellent if treated early
Notes		• In the first trimester, it is very difficult to distinguish between abortion and infertility • Aborted fetuses or placenta may be infectious; isolate the animal from all other dogs, pups, and humans

DYSTOCIA

Dystocia results from abnormalities associated with parturition. They are due to either primary or secondary uterine inertia. Primary uterine inertia is the failure of uterine contractions sufficient to deliver. Secondary uterine inertia is fetal obstruction due to large pups, narrow birth canal, abnormal pup position, and so on.

ECLAMPSIA

Eclampsia can be a life-threatening condition often seen one to four weeks postpartum. It is due to extremely low serum ionized calcium levels.

Table 9.2 / **Dystocia and eclampsia**

Disease		Dystocia*	Eclampsia (Puerperal tetany)
Presentation	Clinical signs	• Abnormal vaginal discharge, active straining for > 45 minutes, crying and biting at vulvar area, intermittent weak contractions for > 2 hours, presence of fetal membrane in the vulva for > 15 minutes, resting phase for > 4–6 hours without straining	• Ataxia, convulsions, drooling, facial rubbing, muscle tremors, nervousness, pacing, panting, restlessness, salivation, seizures, stiff gait, tachypnea, tremors, whining
	Exam findings	• Vaginal stenosis, stress heart rate (heart rate < 196 and > 280 bpm) • Temperature dropped 2–3 degrees	• Dilated pupils, ↓ pupillary light response, pyrexia, tachycardia, tetany
Diagnosis	General	• History/clinical signs • Prolonged gestation: > 72 days from the first mating	• History/clinical signs
	Laboratory	• CBC: ↑ PCV/total protein; ↓ glucose and calcium • Progesterone concentration	• Chemistry panel: ↑ potassium; ↓ calcium (≤ 7 mg/dl), magnesium and glucose (rare)
	Imaging	• Radiographs, abdominal: pelvic conformation, number, position, and location of fetuses, fetal death (intrafetal gas patterns, fetal balling, collapsed spinal cord, overlapping of the skull bones) • Ultrasound: uterine pathology, placenta separation, and fetal distress (heart rate < 150 and > 280 bpm)	• Not applicable
	Procedures	• Abdominal palpation: confirm presence of fetuses • Vaginal exam	• ECG: prolonged QT interval, bradycardia, tachycardia or VPC

(*Continued*)

Table 9.2 / **Dystocia and eclampsia (Continued)**

	Disease	Dystocia*	Eclampsia (Puerperal tetany)
Treatment	General	• Symptomatic • Fluid therapy • Manual manipulation via vagina • Surgery: emergency cesarean section	• Symptomatic
	Medication	• Anesthesia: isoflurane or reversible induction agents • Ecbolic agents: oxytocin, calcium gluconate, ergonovine maleate or dextrose • Tranquilizer: acepromazine	• Supplementation: calcium gluconate, magnesium • Tranquilizers: diazepam
	Nursing care	• Post-parturition or standard postoperative care	• Calcium administration often leads to vomiting, which will subside • Cold water, alcohol baths, ice packs for hyperthermia • Hand-raise puppies until crisis is over and continue to supplement
Follow-up	Patient care	• Post-parturition care • Monitor growth and nursing habits of the neonates	• Monitor calcium levels • Supplement oral calcium throughout lactation
	Prevention/avoidance	• Ovariohysterectomy • Scheduled cesarean section	• Do not supplement with calcium during gestation • Ovariohysterectomy
	Complications	• Maternal or fetal death • ↑ risk in future pregnancies • Neonate stuck in birth canal	• Cerebral edema • Death
	Prognosis	• Excellent if discovered early • Poor to guarded if detected at 24–48 hours	• Good with immediate treatment • Poor with delayed treatment
Notes		• Rule out obstructive dystocia before administering ecbolic agents • Failure to manually deliver a fetus in the birth canal within 30 minutes requires a cesarean section • Welsh Corgis and brachycephalic breeds tend to have a congenitally small pelvis and the pups tend to have large heads and shoulders	• Response to treatment is rapid, therefore treat if the diagnosis is suspected while lab confirmation is pending • Probable reoccurrence with subsequent litters

* See Table 2.4: Normal parturition, page 40; Table 20.15: Case-based anesthesia, page 906.

MASTITIS

Mastitis is a bacterial infection of one or more of the lactating glands; seen in the postpartum dam and queen.

Table 9.3 / Mastitis

Disease		Mastitis
Presentation	Clinical signs	• Anorexia, cachexia, depression, lethargy, mammary gland abscess, neglected, bloated, crying, restless, failure to thrive neonates
	Exam findings	• Dehydration, pyrexia • Mammary gland(s): firm, swollen, warm, painful, purulent, or hemorrhagic discharge
Diagnosis	General	• History/clinical signs
	Laboratory	• CBC: leukocytosis with left shift or leukopenia with sepsis and ↑ PCV (variable) • Chemistry panel: ↑ total protein and BUN • Cytology and culture, milk: neutrophils, macrophages, RBC, bacteria isolation and identification
	Imaging	• Not applicable
	Procedures	• Not applicable
Treatment	General	• Supportive • Fluid therapy • Surgery: lance, debride, drain placement of infected glands
	Medication	• Antibiotics: variable, based on milk pH • Cabergoline
	Nursing care	• Hand-raise puppies or find a surrogate dam if glands are necrotic and need surgical care • Alternate cold and warm compress and manually milk glands several times a day
Follow-up	Patient care	• Same as above • Monitor the growth and feeding habits of the neonates
	Prevention/ avoidance	• Clean environment • Clip toenails of neonates • Shave hair around mammary glands

(*Continued*)

Table 9.3 / **Mastitis (Continued)**

Disease		Mastitis
	Complications	• Abscessed gland • Hand-raising of neonates
	Prognosis	• Good with prompt treatment
Notes		• Avoid antibiotics that may be passed in the milk and cause deleterious effects to the neonates • Green cabbage leaves can be applied and held to the affected glands to reduce engorgement. Overuse can cause the milk to dry up

PREGNANCY

Pregnancy is the condition of carrying a developing embryo in the uterus. Parturition consists of three stages. Stage one is characterized by restlessness, anxiety, nesting behavior, and shivering, and can last 6–12 hours. Stage two is the actual delivery of the fetus. There are visible contractions and the first fetus should be delivered within one to two hours from the onset of stage two. There may be a resting period for up to four hours after the delivery of a fetus. Stage three is the expulsion of the placenta typically following the delivery of each fetus.

PYOMETRA

Pyometra is a condition in which the uterus is filled with purulent exudate, involving both hormonal and bacterial factors, occurring during the luteal phase (the uterine environment in this phase is suitable for microbial growth). The condition typically affects middle-aged to older bitches and, rarely, queens. An open or closed cervix is possible and systemic illness can be mild to life threatening (endotoxemia and sepsis).[2]

Table 9.4 / **Pregnancy and pyometra**

Disease		Pregnancy	Pyometra
Presentation	Clinical signs	• Enlarged abdomen, mammary gland development and lactation, nesting instinct	• Anorexia, depression, lethargy, depression, diarrhea, vomiting • Open-cervix pyometra: mild systemic signs, polyuria/polydipsia, vaginal discharge (purulent, blood, mucus) • Closed-cervix pyometra: collapse, more severe systemic signs
	Exam findings	• Documented fetuses (e.g. palpation, ultrasound, radiograph)	• Mucopurulent to hemorrhagic vaginal discharge, abdominal distention and pain, enlarged uterus, pyrexic, tachycardia, weak pulse, depression

(*Continued*)

Table 9.4 / Pregnancy and pyometra (Continued)

Disease		Pregnancy	Pyometra
Diagnosis	General	• History/clinical signs • Abdominal palpation: 25–36 days after breeding in dogs and 21–28 days after breeding in cats	• History/clinical signs • Abdominal palpation: enlarged uterus in a closed-cervix pyometra • Vaginal discharge
	Laboratory	• Chemistry panel: ↑ relaxin and progesterone levels at 28 days of gestation	• CBC: neutrophilia with a left shift and mild nonregenerative anemia • Chemistry panel: ↑ globulin and total protein, ALT, ALP, azotemia and electrolyte imbalances • Urinalysis: ↑ protein and isosthenuric • Cytology and culture: bacteria isolation and identification • RSAT or AGID: *Brucella canis* • PGF2 metabolites: ↑ values
	Imaging	• Radiographs, abdominal: fetal skeletal calcification > 42 days of gestation • Ultrasound: after 16–20 days of gestation	• Radiographs, abdominal: enlarged or ruptured uterus and peritonitis • Ultrasonography: differentiate pyometra from pregnancy, intraluminal uterine contents, uterine wall thickened
	Procedures	• Not applicable	• Vaginoscopy: determine site of origin of purulent discharge
Treatment	General	• Treated as outpatient unless complications occur	• Surgery: OHE with abdominal lavage • Medical management
	Medication	• Not applicable	• Antibiotics: ampicillin, initial therapy (highly effective against *Escherichia coli*)[2] • Combination antimicrobial therapy, depending on disease severity and culture/sensitivity • PGF2α • Aglepristone (not available in United States)
	Nursing care	• Not applicable	• Standard postoperative care
Follow-up	Patient care	• Provide adequate nutrition throughout pregnancy. • Provide a quiet safe place for the dam/queen to deliver. • Monitor parturition to become aware of any complications.	• Re-examine medical managed pyometra cases one week after initiation of treatment • Monitor progesterone levels one week after discontinuing treatment. • Vaginal discharge may be seen for four weeks post treatment.
	Prevention/ avoidance	• OHE • Supervision	• OHE

(Continued)

Table 9.4 / Pregnancy and pyometra (Continued)

Disease		Pregnancy	Pyometra
	Complications	• Dystocia • Retained fetuses or placenta • Eclampsia • Mastitis	• Estrus sooner after treatment • PGF2α adverse effects • Recurrent pyometra with medical management • Sepsis and peritonitis • Uterine rupture
	Prognosis	• Excellent with proper prenatal care	• Good with OHE and no abdominal contamination • Guarded to good with medical management of open pyometra
Notes		• The length of gestation is 63 days from ovulation but may extend from 56 to 72 days. If the first day of diestrus can be determined, the gestation can be expected at 57–58 days • A transient temperature drop occurs within 24 hours of the onset of parturition • A normal fetal heart rate is twice that of the mother	• Do not perform cystocentesis when pyometra is suspected due to friable uterus and possible contamination of abdomen • Diluting PGF2α with 1 1 sterile saline and walking an animal for 30 minutes after giving the injection may ↓ adverse effects • Abdominal palpation must be performed gently on an enlarged uterus to prevent rupture

BRUCELLOSIS

Brucellosis is a zoonotic disease caused by *Brucella canis*. This bacterium is transmitted through ingestion or inhalation and can be found in the lymphatic system, genital tract, eye, kidney, and intervertebral disks.

BENIGN PROSTATIC HYPERPLASIA

Benign prostatic hyperplasia (BPH) is a condition affecting all intact male dogs, typically by four to eight years of age.[3,4] With the imbalance of the androgen estrogen ratio (higher concentration of estrogen), an increase in prostate androgen receptors occur to upregulate testosterone action. Conversion of testosterone into dihydrotestosterone occurs, leading to prostatic alterations.[5]

BPH is the most common prostatic disease in dogs.

Table 9.5 / Brucellosis and benign prostatic hyperplasia

Disease		Brucellosis	Benign prostatic hyperplasia
Presentation	Clinical signs	• Abnormal gait, anorexia, ataxia, exercise intolerance, weakness • Male: scrotal swelling or dermatitis, enlarged epididymis, testicular atrophy • Female: abortion, infertility and vaginal discharge for 1–6 weeks post-abortion	• Asymptomatic, hematuria, hematospermia, tenesmus
	Exam findings	• Anterior uveitis, ascites, corneal edema, epididymitis, lymphadenopathy, paralysis, paresis, pyrexia, spinal hyperesthesia, splenomegaly	• Non-painful and symmetrical enlargement of prostate on rectal exam

(Continued)

Table 9.5 / **Brucellosis and benign prostatic hyperplasia (Continued)**

Disease		Brucellosis	Benign prostatic hyperplasia
Diagnosis	General	• Clinical signs	• Not applicable

	Laboratory	• Chemistry panel: ↑ globulin and ↓ albumin
		• Urinalysis: ↑ protein, albumin
		• RSAT: accurate for negative dogs, detects infected dogs 3–4 weeks after infection
		• AGID: highly sensitive, detects infected dogs 4–12 weeks after infection
		• TAT/2ME-TAT: + titers, detects infected dogs 3–4 weeks after infection
		• Culture: *B. canis* identification
		• Cytology, lymph node: nonspecific reactive hyperplasia
		• Cytology, semen: > 80% of sperm are morphologically abnormal, inflammatory cells
		• Culture, blood, urine, semen, vaginal discharge, aborted fetuses: *Brucella* isolation and identification
			• Prostatic fluid evaluation- centrifuged at 1000 g for 10 minutes: the formed pellet can be used for:
			  • Aerobic culture
			  • Cytology ↑ RBC (> 20/hpf), ↑epithelial cells with mosaic appearance
			• Urinalysis: normal or ↑ RBC, ↑squamous epithelial cells
			• Urine culture: negative unless secondary prostatitis

	Imaging	• Radiography, spine: diskospondylitis; if found, then check for brucellosis	• Radiography: prostatomegaly • Ultrasonography: normal echogenicity or can be diffusely hyperechoic with small parenchymal cavities[6]
	Procedures	• Lymph node biopsy	• Not applicable
Treatment	General	• Supportive • Surgery: neuter	• Surgery: neuter; gland size reduction begins shortly after neutering, typically 50% reduced by 3 weeks[6]
	Medication	• Antibiotics: minocycline, doxycycline, tetracycline, enrofloxacin, dihydrostreptomycin	• Antiandrogens: finasteride, osaterone acetate • Progestins: medroxyprogesterone acetate, delmadinone acetate • Antiestrogen therapy: tamoxifen citrate, Anastrozole • GnRH agonists: deslorelin acetate
	Nursing care	• Treated as outpatient	• Treat as outpatient
Follow-Up	Patient care	• Multiple courses of antibiotic treatment • Serologic titers monthly for 3 months, then at 6 months • Blood cultures monthly for 3 months • Restrict activity in working dogs	• Medical management: monitor prostate size and clinical signs long term

(*Continued*)

Table 9.5 / Brucellosis and benign prostatic hyperplasia (Continued)

Disease		Brucellosis	Benign prostatic hyperplasia
	Prevention/ avoidance	• Neuter infected animals • Quarantine and test all new dogs and breeding individuals	• Preclinical screening test- Canine prostate-specific arginine esterase biomarker[3] • Neuter
	Complications	• Infertility • Sexual transmission	• Infertility (decreased semen quality)
	Prognosis	• Good with early treatment • Guarded with late detection	• Good with castration • Variable without treatment
Notes		• Transmission is following breeding or abortion, or following contact with semen, vaginal discharge, or urine by penetration of oronasal, conjunctival, or genital mucous membranes • Lasts for 6–64 months • Low risk of human infection with proper hygiene, mild and easily treated	

CRYPTORCHIDISM

Cryptorchidism is a condition in which one or both testes does not descend into the scrotum. The testes can be positioned anywhere caudal to the kidney up to the inguinal ring or subcutaneous, near the scrotum. Monorchidism and anorchidism are the unilateral or bilateral partial or complete absence of testicular tissue.

Table 9.6 / Cryptorchidism

Disease		Cryptorchidism
Presentation	Clinical signs	• None
Presentation	Exam findings	• Testicle(s) not palpable within the scrotum
Diagnosis	General	• Palpation • Canine: typically, testes can be palpated by 6–8 weeks of age, although can vary depending on breed • Tentative diagnosis if not descended by 8 weeks of age[9] • Diagnosis if not descended by 6 months of age[9] • Feline: definitive diagnosis of cryptorchidism should not be made in cats of < 7–8 months of age. The presence or absence of testes in a male without testes in the scrotum can be assessed by the presence of the penile spines, which totally disappear if the male has been castrated[7]

(Continued)

Table 9.6 / Cryptorchidism (Continued)

Disease		Cryptorchidism
	Laboratory	• hCG stimulation test • GnRH stimulation test • Anti-Müllerian hormone
	Imaging	• Ultrasound
Treatment	General	• Surgery: neuter
	Medication	• Not applicable
	Nursing care	• Not applicable
Follow-up	Patient care	• Not applicable
	Prevention/ avoidance	• Hereditary: patient not to be used for breeding • Gene linked to patellar luxation and hip dysplasia
	Prognosis	• Good with surgery before potential complications

	Complication	• Without surgery:
		  • Sertoli cell tumors are most commonly associated with retained testes in canines[8]
		  • Sterility[8]
		  • Testicular torsion[8]

Notes		• Prevalence of cryptorchidism in adult cats averages 1.7%[8] • Prevalence of cryptorchidism in dogs ranges from 0.8–9.8%[8] • Cryptorchidism is not completely understood. Continued research to understand the mechanism(s) involved with the development of cryptorchidism is under way[10]

REFERENCES

1. Theriogenology Foundation. What is theriogenology? https://www.theriofoundation.org/page/Theriodefinition (accessed 16 July 2021).
2. Hagman, R. Pyometra in small animals. *Vet Clin N Am Small Anim Pract* 2018; 8: 639–661.
3. Christensen, B. Canine prostate disease. *Vet Clin N Am Small Anim Pract* 2018; 48: 701–719.
4. Pinheiro, D., Machado, J., Viegas, C. *et al.* Evaluation of biomarker canine-prostate specific arginine esterase (CPSE) for the diagnosis of benign prostatic hyperplasia. *BMC Vet Res* 2017; 13:76.

5. Angrimani, D.S.R., Brito, M.M., Rui, B.R. *et al.* Reproductive and endocrinological effects of benign prostatic hyperplasia and finasteride therapy in dogs. *Sci Rep* 2020; 10: 14834.
6. Bowles, D. Prostatic disease in the dog (proceedings). *dvm360*, November 2010. https://www.dvm360.com/view/prostatic-disease-dog-proceedings (accessed 16 July 2021).
7. Verstegen-Onclin, K. Infectious and congenital diseases in cats. British Small Animal Veterinary Congress 2008. https://www.vin.com/doc/?id=3862916 (accessed 16 July 2021).
8. Felumlee, A.E., Reichle, J.K., Hecht, S. *et al.* Use of ultrasound to locate retained testes in dogs and cats. *Vet Radiol Ultrasound* 2012; 53: 581–585.
9. Romagnoli, S.E. Canine cryptorchidism. *Vet Clin N Am Small Anim Pract* 1991; 21: 533–544.
10. Khan, F.A., Gartley, C.J., Khanam, A. Canine cryptorchidism: an update. *Reprod Domest Anim* 2018; 53: 1263–1270.

Chapter **10**

Emergency Medicine

Megan Brashear, BS, RVT, VTS (ECC) and Tami Lind, BS, RVT, VTS (ECC)

Veterinary Technician and Nurse's Daily Reference Guide: Canine and Feline, Fourth Edition. Edited by Mandy Fults and Kenichiro Yagi.

Companion website: www.wiley.com/go/fults/veterinary

Abbreviations

ATE, arterial thromboembolism
CBC, complete blood count
CPR, cardiopulmonary resuscitation
CRT, capillary refill time
CSF, cerebrospinal fluid
CT, computed tomography
ECG, electrocardiogram
$ETCO_2$, end tidal CO_2
FAST, focused assessment with sonography in trauma
GDV, gastric dilation volvulus
IV, intravenous
IVDD, intervertebral disc disease
mEq, milliequivalent
MRI, magnetic resonance imaging
NaCl, sodium chloride
NSAIDs, non-steroidal anti-inflammatory drugs
PCV, packed cell volume
RAAS, renin–angiotensin–aldosterone system
SpO_2, peripheral capillary oxygen saturation

MEDICAL PREPAREDNESS

Emergencies can arrive at any hospital at any time. All team members must be trained and prepared to receive emergencies, including maintaining a designated area stocked and ready. Staff should be familiar with emergency triage, patient assessment, and monitoring. This chapter covers the basic supplies, patient support, and monitoring techniques necessary to handle common emergencies.

Please note that this chapter is not meant to be all inclusive; each clinic is urged to have regular emergency training and to maintain an emergency resource library.

Before an emergency arrives at the hospital, emergency supplies should be compiled and available either in a crash cart or at the emergency receiving station. Items listed are the most commonly used emergency supplies; clinics may need to alter this list based on preference, geographic location, and typical emergencies seen. The most important part of emergency preparedness is familiarity. Each staff member should know the location of the supplies and understand their use and operation.

Crash Cart

The items contained in the crash cart are limited to the first items used in an emergency. These items should be dedicated to emergencies only and not used for daily purposes. Staff should be designated to maintain and stock the crash cart on a regular basis. Resist the temptation to overstock the emergency area with supplies, as this will increase temptation to "steal" inventory from the area.

Supplies

Supplies can be organized by the ABCs – group all airway supplies together, circulation supplies together, drugs, and so on.

Table 10.1 / Supplies

	Equipment
Airway	• Endotracheal tubes of various sizes • Laryngoscope and small and large blade • Endotracheal ties or gauze • Cuff syringe • Sponge forceps and gauze squares to clear airway
Breathing	• Ambu-bag • Thoracocentesis kits (butterfly catheters, 1½″ needles, 3-way stopcock, extension sets)
Circulation	• IV catheters of various sizes • Injection caps • T-sets • 1-inch tape • Gauze squares • Flush syringes • Blood collection tubes • Fluid administration sets and extension sets • Drugs • Syringes of various sizes • Needles of various sizes • Emergency drug dose chart (RECOVER) • Epinephrine • Vasopressin • Atropine • Naloxone • Lidocaine • Calcium chloride or gluconate • 50% dextrose • 5 Fr and 8 Fr red rubber catheters for intratracheal infusion of medications • IV fluids (crystalloids and hypertonic saline)
Equipment	• Minor surgical instrument sterile pack (needle holders, scalpel handle, thumb forceps, hemostats) • Scalpel blades (multiple types) • Suture material (various sizes and materials) • Sterile gloves
Equipment nearby (not necessarily in/on the crash cart)	• Clippers • Oxygen supply/anesthesia machine and anesthetic tubing • Anesthetic masks for flow-by oxygen support • Multi-parameter anesthesia monitor (ECG, $ETCO_2$, SpO_2, blood pressure) ± defibrillator

Emergency Area

The emergency area of the hospital will contain items for patient support. These items have uses throughout the hospital but should be readily available for emergencies. They can be stocked in drawers or portable totes, or on carts to be moved to different areas:

- Bandaging material (tape of varying sizes, cast padding, roll gauze, self-adherent wrap)
- Heat support
- Doppler blood pressure monitor
- IV catheters – varied sizes
- Crystalloid fluids – various types
- Fluid drip sets and extension sets
- Pressure fluid infusion bag
- Thermometer
- Otoscope/ophthalmoscope
- Suction (bucket, suction tubing, ± portable suction machine).

CARDIOPULMONARY RESUSCITATION

Early recognition of cardiopulmonary arrest is the key to patient survival. Immediate initiation of cardiopulmonary resuscitation (CPR) is also known to increase patient survival. There are many causes of cardiopulmonary arrest, including hypoxia, trauma, anesthetic complications, organ failure, or environmental factors. Prevention of an impending arrest is easier than treating a patient during/after CPR. The facility should be always ready for a CPR event. A crash cart should always be stocked, and an oxygen source, a solid surface free of clutter, a multiparameter monitoring unit, an IV fluid pump, and a suction unit should always be available.

There are three phases of CPR: basic life support, advanced life support, and post-arrest care.

Basic Life Support

Basic life support includes:

1. Recognition of a cardiopulmonary arrest event.
2. Compressions/circulation.
3. Airway management/breathing (ventilation).

Compressions should start immediately. They can be performed in left or right lateral recumbency at a rate of 100–120 compressions per minute. The rate does not change based on the size of the patient. Hands should be placed at the highest point of the chest and compressions should be delivered with enough force to depress the chest by one third depth. In deep-chested patients, the hands should be placed at the fourth–fifth rib space. For cats and small dogs, compressions can be done directly over the heart. Compressions should be performed in two-minute cycles before a change in compressor.

Ventilation is managed by placing an endotracheal tube into a patient's airway at the same time that compressions are occurring. A laryngoscope should be used to visualize the airway. 100% oxygen delivered via a bag valve mask (Ambu bag) or anesthesia machine should be used once the patient is properly intubated. A technician should give one breath every six seconds, (10 breaths/minute), with a tidal volume of 10 ml/kg. End tidal CO_2 ($ETCO_2$) measurement can be used to confirm endotracheal tube placement and to provide the compressor information on compression success and efficacy. An $ETCO_2$ reading above 15 mmHg has been associated with a higher chance of achieving return of spontaneous circulation). Once basic life support is achieved, advanced life support is then started.

Advanced Life Support

Advanced life support includes:

1. Vascular access.
2. Drug administration.
3. Defibrillation.
4. Advanced monitoring.

Vascular access can be achieved in many ways. A peripheral venous catheter can be placed and is the most common. However, during cardiopulmonary arrest, this can be difficult to achieve because of decreased blood flow. Other ways to achieve vascular access are:

- Jugular vein catheter
- Intraosseous catheter.

Drugs can be administered via the intratracheal route if venous access is not achieved. Consult the drug charts shown in Figures 10.1, 10.2 and 10.3 for appropriate drugs and dosages during CPR events.

Defibrillation is the recommended therapy for ventricular fibrillation and pulseless ventricular tachycardia. There are two types of defibrillators – a monophasic and biphasic. It is recommended that you familiarize yourself with the type of defibrillator your practice owns.

Post-Cardiac Arrest Care

Post-arrest starts when a patient has a spontaneous heartbeat. These patients must be monitored extremely closely by the technician. Every organ system must be evaluated constantly. Some 2–10% of patients survive to discharge after cardiac arrest.

More RECOVER information is provided in Figures 10.1–10.3, and on the RECOVER website (recoverinitiative.org).

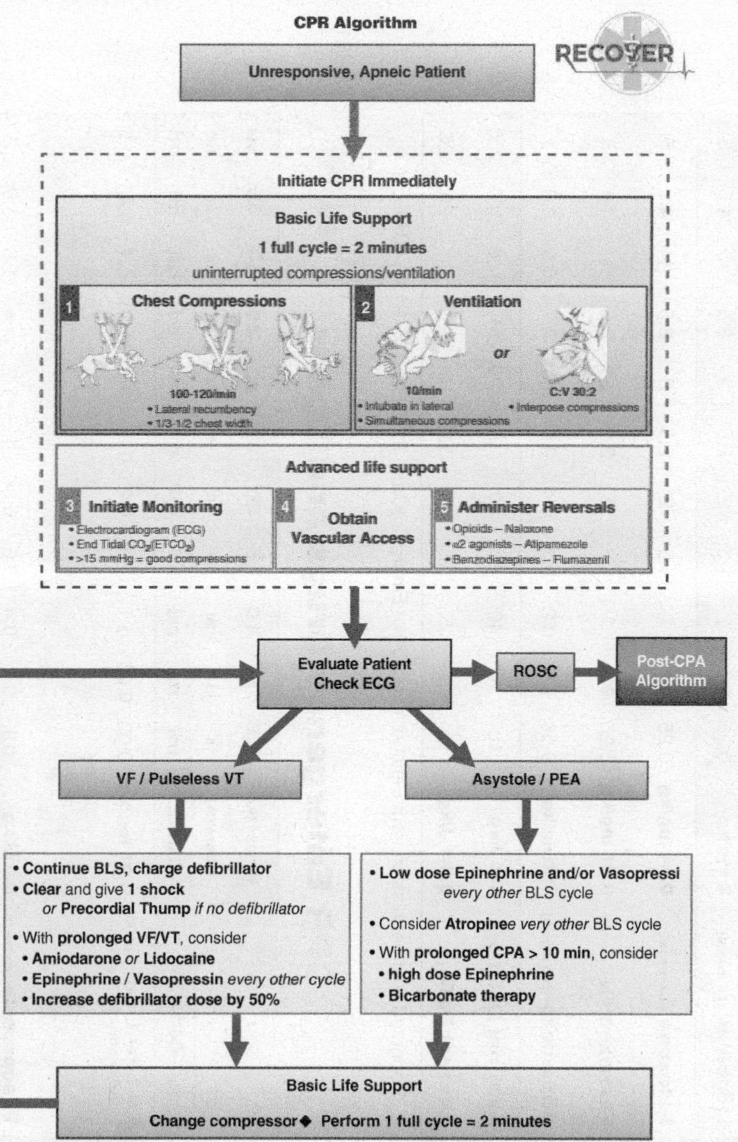

Figure 10.1 RECOVER cardiopulmonary resuscitation algorithm.

CPR Emergency Drugs and Doses

RECOVER

	DRUG	DOSE	2.5 kg (5 lb) ml	5 kg (10 lb) ml	10 kg (20 lb) ml	15 kg (30 lb) ml	20 kg (40 lb) ml	25 kg (50 lb) ml	30 kg (60 lb) ml	35 kg (70 lb) ml	40 kg (80 lb) ml	45 kg (90 lb) ml	50 kg (100 lb) ml
Arrest	Epi Low (1:1000; 1mg/ml) every other BLS cycle x3	0.01 mg/kg	0.03	0.05	0.1	0.15	0.2	0.25	0.3	0.35	0.4	0.45	0.5
Arrest	Epi High (1:1000; 1 mg/ml) for prolonged CPR	0.1 mg/kg	0.25	0.5	1	1.5	2	2.5	3	3.5	4	4.5	5
Arrest	Vasopressin (20 U/ml)	0.8 U/kg	0.1	0.2	0.4	0.6	0.8	1	1.2	1.4	1.6	1.8	2
Arrest	Atropine (0.54 mg/ml)	0.04 mg/kg	0.2	0.4	0.8	1.1	1.5	1.9	2.2	2.6	3	3.3	3.7
Anti-Arrhythmic	Amiodarone (50 mg/ml)	5 mg/kg	0.25	0.5	1	1.5	2	2.5	3	3.5	4	4.5	5
Anti-Arrhythmic	Lidocaine (20 mg/ml)	2 mg/kg	0.25	0.5	1	1.5	2	2.5	3	3.5	4	4.5	5
Reversal	Naloxone (0.4 mg/ml)	0.04 mg/kg	0.25	0.5	1	1.5	2	2.5	3	3.5	4	4.5	5
Reversal	Flumazenil (0.1 mg/ml)	0.01 mg/kg	0.25	0.5	1	1.5	2	2.5	3	3.5	4	4.5	5
Reversal	Atipamezole (5 mg/ml)	100 μg/kg	0.06	0.1	0.2	0.3	0.4	0.5	0.6	0.7	0.8	0.9	1
Defib Monophasic	External Defib (J)	4-6 J/kg	10	20	40	60	80	100	120	140	160	180	200
Defib Monophasic	Internal Defib (J)	0.5-1 J/kg	2	3	5	8	10	15	15	20	20	20	25

Reprinted with permission from Fletcher et al., *J Vet EmergCritCare*, 22(S1): S102-S131, 2012

CPR Emergency Drugs and Doses

RECOVER

	DRUG	DOSE	2.5 kg (5 lb) ml	5 kg (10 lb) ml	10 kg (20 lb) ml	15 kg (30 lb) ml	20 kg (40 lb) ml	25 kg (50 lb) ml	30 kg (60 lb) ml	35 kg (70 lb) ml	40 kg (80 lb) ml	45 kg (90 lb) ml	50 kg (100 lb) ml
Arrest	Epi Low (1:1000; 1mg/ml) every other BLS cycle x3	0.01 mg/kg	0.03	0.05	0.1	0.15	0.2	0.25	0.3	0.35	0.4	0.45	0.5
Arrest	Epi High (1:1000; 1 mg/ml) for prolonged CPR	0.1 mg/kg	0.25	0.5	1	1.5	2	2.5	3	3.5	4	4.5	5
Arrest	Vasopressin (20 U/ml)	0.8 U/kg	0.1	0.2	0.4	0.6	0.8	1	1.2	1.4	1.6	1.8	2
Arrest	Atropine (0.54 mg/ml)	0.04 mg/kg	0.2	0.4	0.8	1.1	1.5	1.9	2.2	2.6	3	3.3	3.7
Anti-Arrhythmic	Amiodarone (50 mg/ml)	5 mg/kg	0.25	0.5	1	1.5	2	2.5	3	3.5	4	4.5	5
Anti-Arrhythmic	Lidocaine (20 mg/ml)	2 mg/kg	0.25	0.5	1	1.5	2	2.5	3	3.5	4	4.5	5
Reversal	Naloxone (0.4 mg/ml)	0.04 mg/kg	0.25	0.5	1	1.5	2	2.5	3	3.5	4	4.5	5
Reversal	Flumazenil (0.1 mg/ml)	0.01 mg/kg	0.25	0.5	1	1.5	2	2.5	3	3.5	4	4.5	5
Reversal	Atipamezole (5 mg/ml)	100 μg/kg	0.06	0.1	0.2	0.3	0.4	0.5	0.6	0.7	0.8	0.9	1
Defib Monophasic	External Defib (J)	2-4 J/kg	5	10	20	30	40	50	60	70	80	90	100
Defib Monophasic	Internal Defib (J)	0.2-0.4 J/kg	1	2	2	3	4	5	6	7	8	9	10

Reprinted with permission from Fletcher et al., *J Vet EmergCritCare*, 22(S1): S102-S131, 2012

Figure 10.2 RECOVER cardiopulmonary resuscitation emergency drugs and doses.

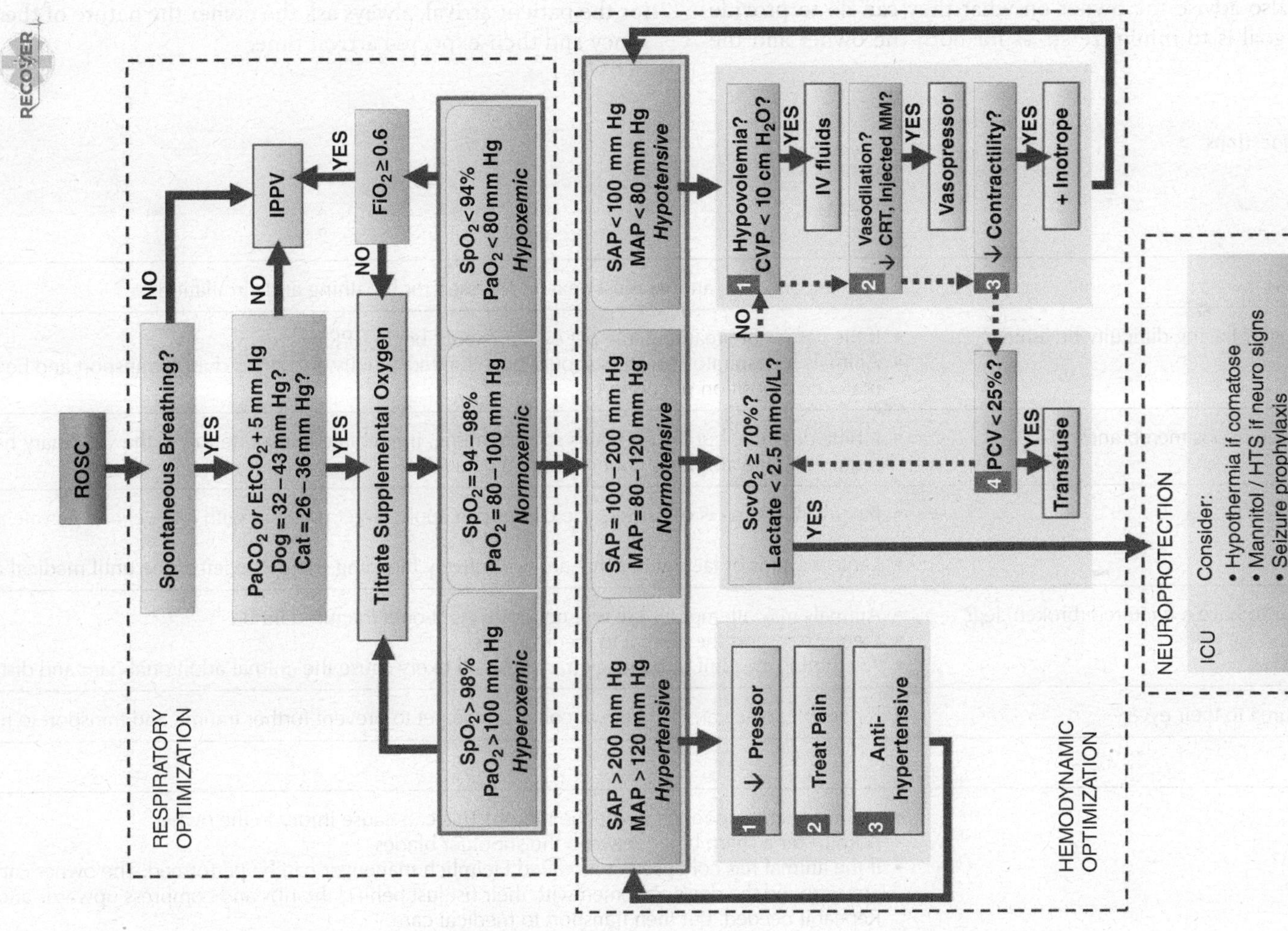

Figure 10.3 **RECOVER post-cardiac arrest algorithm.**

TELEPHONE TRIAGE

When a client calls with an emergent situation, they should be asked specific questions that will assist in the team preparing for their arrival (Table 10.2). These questions can also advise the owner on what they can do to provide immediate care. The goal is to minimize stress for both the owner and the patient. Stressed pet owners may not be able to retain information well, and the same questions may need to be asked or answered multiple times. Regardless of the nature of the situation, if the owner perceives it to be an emergency it must be handled as such. To assist the medical staff in preparing for the patient arrival, always ask the owner the nature of the injury or emergency and their expected arrival time.

Table 10.2 / **Owner questions**

Question	Comments
Trauma	
Is your pet unconscious?	• Any unconscious animal must next be assessed for breathing and circulation
Is your animal breathing or having difficulty breathing?	• If the pet is not breathing, the pet owner should begin CPR • Animals in respiratory distress should have limited activity and stress during transport and be able to maintain a position of comfort
What color are the pet's mucous membranes?	• If blue or white, but the animal is still breathing, immediate transportation to the veterinary hospital is required. If the animal is not breathing, begin CPR
Is the pet bleeding?	• If active bleeding is occurring, the owner can apply direct pressure with a towel and elevate above the heart (if able) • Large wounds or lacerations that are not actively bleeding should be left alone until medical assessment
Does the animal appear to have a fractured (broken) leg?	• Animals may attempt to, but will not put weight on a fractured limb • Gently transport the animal to medical care • Attempting to splint or bandage fractures will likely cause the animal additional pain and distress
Did the pet sustain trauma to their eye/s?	• If possible, place an Elizabethan collar on the pet to prevent further trauma and transport to medical care
Acute conditions	
Is the pet choking?	• *Do not* attempt to reach inside the mouth! This can cause injury to the owner • Administer a sharp blow between the shoulder blades • If the animal has collapsed, a modified Heimlich maneuver can be performed. The owner can place their arms around the dog's abdomen with their fist just behind the ribs and compress upwards and inwards. Repeat if needed, but then transport to medical care
Is the pet coughing or have increased respiratory effort?	• Keep the pet calm and transport to medical care

(*Continued*)

Table 10.2 / Owner questions (Continued)

Question	Comments
Does the pet have a distended abdomen?	• Do not apply pressure to the abdomen • Transport the pet to medical care as soon as possible
Is the pet vomiting?	• A single episode of vomiting warrants watching the pet closely, but may not require medical intervention • A pet with multiple episodes of vomiting should have food and water access removed and receive medical attention • If a dog is retching and/or attempting to vomit without producing vomit it should receive medical attention as soon as possible
Is the pet having diarrhea?	• A single episode of diarrhea warrants watching the pet closely, but may not require medical intervention • A pet with multiple episodes of diarrhea should receive medical attention; the owner should bring a sample if possible • If there is blood in the diarrhea the pet should receive medical attention • A pet experiencing vomiting and diarrhea should receive medical attention
Is the pet having a seizure?	• If possible, move furniture away from pet to prevent injury; do not intervene as that risks injury to the owner • If the seizure lasts longer than 3 minutes wrap the pet in a towel/blanket to pick up and transport to medical care immediately • If the seizure ceases on its own, use caution approaching the pet, as some can act aggressively immediately after a seizure, and transport to medical care
Did the pet ingest something toxic?	• Remove the pet from the toxin • If any symptoms are present, the pet should be immediately transported for medical care • If possible, the owner should bring any packaging • If no symptoms are present, the owner can contact Animal Poison Control for further instructions
Does the pet have hives?	• Hives ± facial swelling should receive medical attention • If vomiting and/or diarrhea is also occurring, the pet should receive immediate medical attention
Does the owner suspect the pet is suffering from heatstroke or the pet has a rectal temperature > 106°F (> 41°C)?	• Bring the pet inside or in the shade and soak them with cold water then immediately transport to medical care • If the elevated temperature is not due to environmental exposure (rather due to infection), do not soak the pet with water but immediately transport to medical care
Is the pet in labor?	• Active labor (witnessed abdominal contractions/pushing) that extends 30 minutes or longer without producing a puppy or kitten warrants medical attention • A puppy or kitten stuck in the birth canal for longer than 30 minutes warrants medical attention • Dogs and cats may go hours between each delivery; if no active labor is witnessed the bitch/queen should be left to rest

TRIAGE

When an animal presents to the veterinary hospital with an emergent condition, the best outcome requires team preparedness, teamwork, appropriate triage, and a quick response to abnormalities. Triage is the process of organizing patients and symptoms in the order of most to least critical. It generally occurs in the lobby of the hospital, but is also a continuing process with any hospitalized patient. Emergency triage is a quick assessment of the three major body systems:

- Respiratory – observe the animal for any increase in respiratory rate and effort. Listen for wheezes, stertor, stridor, or any wet breathing sounds.
- Cardiovascular – palpate a femoral pulse if possible to ascertain pulse quality and pulse rate. Examine the mucous membranes and capillary refill time.
- Neurological – examine the level of consciousness and the animal's awareness and response to their surroundings. Stress can change this so be sure to ask the owner how the pet was behaving at home prior to coming to the hospital.

If the animal has gross abnormalities with any of the three major body systems, it should be brought immediately to the treatment area for a complete physical exam and any necessary immediate treatment.

Primary Survey

When performing a physical exam on any emergent patient, begin with a primary exam (Table 10.3). The primary exam is a brief physical exam meant to identify life-threatening conditions. Begin by briefly observing the animal and noting their presenting complaint. Next address any arterial bleeding. Then auscultate the heart and lung sounds proving supplemental oxygen if necessary. Assess pulses and pulse quality comparing them with the heart rate. Assess the mucous membrane color and capillary refill time as well as the patient's body temperature. The final part of the primary exam is to evaluate the central nervous system by noting pupil position, pupillary light response, and reflexes.

Table 10.3 / Primary survey

System	Clinical signs	Physical exam	Causes	Immediate action
Respiratory	Panting, uncomfortable (constant changing positions), paradoxical respirations, open-mouth breathing, coughing, increased or decreased respiratory rate, extended head and neck with abducted elbows	No passage of air, loud inspiratory or expiratory sounds, paradoxical breathing, increased respiratory effort, pale/blue/muddy mucous membrane color	Pleural space disease, respiratory system trauma; cardiac disease; neurologic disease; pneumonia	Supplemental oxygen, sedation/pain management; specific treatment following diagnosis
Cardiovascular	External hemorrhage, panting, weakness and collapse, abdominal distention, cough exacerbated by activity or exercise	Change in mucous membrane color and moisture, prolonged CRT, bounding or weak pulses, variable heart rate and rhythm, hyper- or hypothermia, cold extremities, crackles in lung fields, pulse deficits	Trauma; structural cardiac disease; myocardial infection	Hemostasis, supplemental oxygen, sedation; specific treatment following diagnosis
Central nervous system	Altered level of consciousness, abnormal head position, seizures, changes in ambulation (front limb rigidity, Schiff–Sherrington posture, generalized weakness/paralysis)	Abnormal pupillary response/size/position, strabismus, nystagmus, absent or altered motor reflexes, amplified pain response, hyperthermia, hypertonia, hyperreflexia	Head trauma, intoxication, spinal cord injury, seizures, bacterial/parasitic infections, vestibular syndrome, IVDD	Supplemental oxygen, anticonvulsant therapy as needed; pain management; specific treatment following diagnosis
Body condition	Lacerations, fractures, eye injuries, abdominal distention, burns	Changes in conformation/limb angles, amplified pain response, soft tissue wounds, bleeding	Trauma	Supplemental oxygen therapy, analgesics, basic wound care, specific treatment following diagnosis

Hemostasis

If arterial bleeding is present, it must be controlled before additional treatments are pursued. If the bleeding artery can be identified it should be clamped and ligated when possible.

- Direct digital pressure:
  - Apply direct digital pressure over the injury.
  - If the injury is to an extremity or the tail, encircle the area proximal to the injury and apply pressure.
- Pressure wraps:
  - Can be applied to wounds for short periods of time (< 10 minutes).
  - If the bandage soaks through, apply more bandage material on top of the soiled material – do not remove it.
- Tourniquets are generally not recommended, but if they are used, they should not be applied for longer than 10 minutes.

Secondary Survey

After the primary survey, the patient is resuscitated and treated for any life-threatening problems. Once stable, a repeat of the primary survey, examination of a thorough past and current medical history, and laboratory database is performed. This is followed by a reassessment of the original treatments:

- Past medical history:
  - Chronic medical conditions, drug therapies, allergies, vaccination history, surgical history, previous blood transfusions.

- Current medical history:
  - Presenting complaint, when animal was last normal, recent medical history, chronology and progression of clinical signs, potential toxin ingestion, physical trauma, signs of collapse or weakness, travel history, access to other animals, affinity to eat abnormal things.
- Physical examination:
  - Repeat the primary survey to evaluate any changes and assess the current treatment plan followed by a complete examination of the organ systems not immediately involved:
    - Thoracic (imaging, thoracocentesis).
    - Abdominal (imaging, abdominocentesis).
    - Rectal
    - Urinary
    - Wound care
    - Fracture stabilization.
- Stat lab database:
  - Can consist of some or all of the following depending on patient status: packed cell volume/total protein; chemistry panel and electrolytes, complete blood count, blood gases, cytology, urinalysis, coagulation tests.

SHOCK

Shock in small animals is the result of inadequate cellular energy production due to decreased oxygen delivery or consumption. Simply put, cellular oxygen demand is not met by the body's oxygen supply to the cells. Shock can be the result of numerous disease processes and must be recognized and treated immediately. The goal, regardless of cause, is to optimize oxygen delivery to tissues. In many cases this is achieved by increasing preload thereby increasing cardiac output by administering intravenous fluids. It is important to rule out cardiac disease (and thereby cardiogenic shock) prior to fluid administration.

Shock can be divided into three categories which occur as the body attempts to compensate for decreased perfusion (Table 10.4). It is important for the veterinary technician and nursing team to recognize these changes and respond with appropriate treatment and monitoring.

Table 10.4 / Categories of shock

Shock type	Description	Clinical signs
Compensated	Subtle changes occur to maintain adequate perfusion (splenic contraction, peripheral vasoconstriction due to RAAS activation)	• Tachycardia; bounding pulses; CRT 1 second
Early decompensated	More dramatic clinical signs as the body begins to peripherally vasoconstrict to maintain perfusion to vital organs	• Canine: tachycardia (significant); bounding or weak/thready pulses; pale mucous membranes, prolonged CRT; hypothermia/cold extremities; dull mentation; weakness • Feline: bradycardia; hypothermia; hypotension, pale mucous membranes
Late decompensated	Terminal stage; tissue hypoxia leads to cellular death	• bradycardia, obtunded mentation, pale/cyanotic mucous membranes, weak/absent pulses

Shock treatment must begin as soon as clinical signs are noted and focus on immediate needs determined during the primary survey:

- Respiratory: provide oxygen support in the form of flow by or nasal prongs.
- Cardiovascular: an abdominal focused assessment with sonography in trauma (FAST) can diagnose pericardial effusion; ECG can diagnose deadly cardiac arrhythmias.
- Neurological: mentation changes due to intoxication, head trauma.
- Body condition: apply pressure to bleeding wounds.
- Always collect full vital signs (body temperature, heart rate, pulse quality, respiratory rate and effort, mucous membrane color, capillary refill time, blood pressure, mentation) on any emergency patient.

Patients can present on emergency suffering from different types of shock. While appropriate shock treatment is important, so is determining the origin of shock. Any initial treatment plan must focus on correcting the inciting disease process.

Veterinary technicians must monitor these patients closely to note the success of treatment. Frequent and continued monitoring of patient heart rate, respiratory rate and effort, mucous membrane color, capillary refill time, and blood pressure is required until the patient is stable (vital signs consistently normal). Once the patient has responded to therapy and is less critical, additional diagnostics such as radiographs, ultrasounds, and complete blood work can be performed and evaluated.

Table 10.5 / **Types of shock**

Shock type	Description	Causes	Treatment
Hypovolemic	Fluid loss leading to decreased perfusion (oxygen delivery) to cells	Vomiting, diarrhea, decreased food/water intake, blood loss	IV catheter placement; IV fluid therapy (balanced crystalloid); pain management as needed
Cardiogenic	Decrease in forward blood flow from the heart leading to decreased perfusion (oxygen delivery) to cells	Primary cardiac disease or malformation, cardiac injury, cardiac infection, pericardial disease	oxygen therapy, mild sedation as needed; cardiac medications as needed to treat pulmonary edema, tachycardia, bradycardia; abdominal FAST to diagnose and treat pericardial effusion
Obstructive	Mechanical obstruction to blood flow resulting in decreased perfusion (oxygen delivery) to cells	Distended stomach (GDV, food bloat, gas bloat); arterial thromboembolism (ATE; "saddle thrombus" in cats)	IV catheter placement; IV crystalloid fluids (all but ATE); pain management as needed
Distributive	A lack of systemic vascular resistance results in decreased perfusion (oxygen delivery) to cells	sepsis, SIRS, anaphylaxis	IV catheter placement; IV crystalloid fluids; drugs to increase vascular resistance

TRAUMA EMERGENCIES

Traumatic emergencies happen any time a patient is in contact with an outside force that can cause injury. Some examples of these emergencies are patients that have been hit by a car, animal attacks, gunshot wounds, fire burns, and electrocution.

To successfully treat trauma, ensure that the hospital is equipped with a crash cart/triage area, oxygen supplementation, and well-trained technicians who know how to respond to an emergency. It is important for the technician to triage the patient appropriately and treat life-threatening problems first (primary survey).

- Airway: ensure that the patient has a patent airway; trauma can lead to blood obstructing the airway and/or injury to the neck and trachea.
- Breathing: ensure that the patient can move air – trauma to the thorax and lungs can greatly impair breathing; supply supplemental oxygen.
- Bleeding: check for catastrophic arterial bleeding and apply pressure to bleeding wounds.
- Circulation: assess pulse quality and heart rate; trauma patients are at great risk for hypovolemic shock.
- Consciousness: quickly assess level of consciousness; determine whether patient is in shock or has head trauma and neurological deficits.

For more information about traumatic emergencies, refer to the specific organ system emergencies in the remainder of this chapter.

RESPIRATORY EMERGENCIES

Table 10.6 / Respiratory emergencies

Emergency	Clinical signs	Clinical concerns	Diagnostics	Treatment
Airway obstruction (includes brachycephalic airway syndrome, laryngeal paralysis, physical airway obstruction)	Brachycephalic breed disposition, large-breed dog disposition, respiratory distress, cyanosis, stridor, stertor, no air movement, collapse	Hypoxia, hyperthermia, anxiety, death	Patient history, physical exam, pulse oximetry, arterial blood gas	Supplemental oxygen therapy, sedation/general anesthesia, removal of obstruction, intubation, ± definitive surgical correction
Upper airway trauma	Respiratory distress, cyanosis, hemorrhage	Hypoxemia, hyperthermia, hypertension, anxiety, pain, sudden death	History, physical exam, pulse oximetry, arterial blood gas	Oxygen therapy, sedation, pain medication, IV catheter, ± intubation, ± surgical correction
Pleural space disease (can include pyothorax, hemothorax, chylothorax, and pneumothorax)	Respiratory distress, cyanosis, lethargy, anorexia, decreased lung sounds	Hypoxia, hypotension, pain, death	Patient history, thoracocentesis, pulse oximetry, radiographs, arterial blood gas	Thoracocentesis, supplemental oxygen therapy, treatment dependent on diagnosis
Pulmonary edema	Respiratory distress, cyanosis, nasal discharge, coughing	Hypoxia, anxiety, pain, death	Patient physical exam, radiographs	Supplemental oxygen therapy, intubation, sedation, furosemide
Thoracic trauma	Respiratory distress, hemorrhage, cyanosis, recumbent, hypothermic	Pain, hypotension, hypovolemia, hypoxia, tachycardia, shock, death	Patient physical exam, radiographs, thoracic FAST, arterial blood gas	Control hemorrhage, oxygen therapy, IV catheter, pain medication, fluids, intubation, ± blood products, ± surgery
Pneumonia	Tachypnea, coughing, fever, cyanosis, respiratory distress	Hypoxia, sudden death	Radiographs, CBC, pulse oximetry, arterial blood gas	Supplemental oxygen therapy, antibiotics, IV catheter placement, IV crystalloid fluid therapy
Neurologic disease affecting ventilation	Respiratory distress, apnea, paralysis, anxiety	Inability to expand chest, hypoxia, hypercapnia, hypertension	Neurologic exam, radiographs, arterial blood gas, ± MRI, ± CSF tap	Supplemental oxygen therapy, intubation, manual ventilation, pain management, other treatments depending on underlying cause

CARDIOVASCULAR EMERGENCIES

Table 10.7 / Cardiovascular emergencies

Emergency	Clinical signs	Clinical concerns	Diagnostics	Treatment
Arterial or venous injury	External or internal bleeding, weakness, pain, distended abdomen, pale mucous membranes, tachycardia	Hypovolemic shock, anemia, poor perfusion leading to tissue death and limb loss, infection	Patient physical exam, abdominal and thoracic FAST, direct pressure to bleeding wounds, IV catheter placement, IV crystalloid fluid therapy, pain management, wound care	Direct pressure to bleeding wounds, IV catheter placement, IV crystalloid fluid therapy, pain management, wound care
Cardiac arrhythmias	Weakness; cough; exercise intolerance; weak pulses; asynchronous pulses; respiratory distress; syncope	Cardiogenic shock; sudden death	ECG; echocardiogram	IV catheter placement; specific treatment following diagnosis
Congestive heart failure	Weakness; cough; ± distended abdomen; ± cardiac arrhythmia; hypotension; hypothermia; respiratory distress; pulmonary edema	Cardiogenic shock; sudden death	Thoracic radiographs; ECG; echocardiogram; CBC; blood chemistry profile	Supplemental oxygen therapy; ± anxiolytic medication; diuretic; ± positive inotrope; specific treatment due to underlying cardiac disease
Cardiovascular system trauma	Cardiac arrhythmia following thoracic trauma; respiratory distress; hypotension; pericardial effusion	Cardiogenic shock; arrhythmias; hemothorax; sudden death	ECG; thoracic FAST; thoracic radiographs	Oxygen therapy; ± antiarrhythmic; treatment will depend on diagnosis
Feline aortic thromboembolism	Pain; respiratory distress; acute paralysis; ± underlying cardiac disease	Severe pain; sudden death	Physical exam; cold affected extremities; lack of pulse in affected extremities	IV catheter placement; pain management; treatment for underlying cardiac disease; anti-platelet medication; oxygen therapy
Pericardial effusion	Tachycardia; weak pulses; weakness; lethargy; hypotension; collapse; cardiac arrhythmia; respiratory distress	Cardiogenic shock; sudden death	Thoracic FAST	Treatment: IV catheter placement; IV crystalloid therapy; mild sedation; ECG monitoring; pericardiocentesis

NEUROLOGICAL EMERGENCIES

The neurological system controls other body functions such as the respiratory and cardiac system. It is important to evaluate the entire patient when presenting with a neurologic emergency.

Table 10.8 / Neurological emergencies

Emergency	Clinical signs	Clinical concerns	Diagnostics	Treatment
Seizures	Altered mentation, repetitive limb, eye, muscle movements, inability to stand, disorientation, hypersalivation	Hyperthermia, hypoxia, hypertension or hypotension, miosis, decreased platelet/ lymphocyte ratio, sudden death	Neurologic exam, CBC, Chemistry, blood glucose, ± MRI, ± CSF tap	• Direct pressure to bleeding wounds, IV catheter placement, IV crystalloid fluid therapy, pain management, wound care • Status epilepticus: general anesthesia may be required if traditional drug therapies are not effective
Traumatic brain injury	Facial or head wounds, anisocoria, obtunded mentation, respiratory distress	Hyper/hypotension, hypoxia, hypo/hyperglycemia, anemia, tachycardia, seizures, sudden death	Radiographs, pulse oximetry, blood glucose, venous or arterial blood gas, blood pressure	IV catheter placement, supplemental oxygen therapy, IV crystalloid fluid therapy, pain management, hypertonic fluid administration, mannitol
Vestibular disease	Altered mentation, nystagmus, Horner syndrome, head tilt, ataxia, depression, anorexia, paresis	Hypo/hypertension, anxiety, nausea	Patient history, otologic exam, CBC, blood chemistry panel, blood glucose, thyroid panel, urinalysis, blood pressure, ± MRI or CT	Anti-nausea medication, antiemetic, anti-anxiety medications, antibiotics for otitis media/interna
Spinal cord injury	Ataxic, paresis, tetraparesis	Hypoxia, hypotension, hypoperfusion, spinal fracture	Patient history, radiographs, CBC, blood chemistry panel, ± MRI, ± CSF tap	Pain management, cage restriction, ± surgery, physical rehabilitation

Other neurological conditions:

- Myasthenia gravis
- Tick paralysis
- Botulism
- Electrolyte imbalances
- Neoplasia
- Parasitic infections.

OPHTHALMIC EMERGENCIES

Ophthalmic emergencies can occur due to trauma, congenital malformation, chronic systemic disease, and cancer.

Table 10.9 / Ophthalmic emergencies

Emergency	Clinical signs	Clinical concerns	Diagnostics	Treatment
Traumatic proptosis	Unilateral or bilateral globe proptosis	Blindness, pain, potential head trauma	Patient physical exam	Pain management, apply water-based lubricant to proptosed globe(s), E-collar on patient, prepare for surgical replacement or enucleation
Corneal ulcer	Pain, blepharospasm, photophobia, increased tear production, mucoid ocular discharge, rubbing at eye, observable corneal defect	Infection, loss of sight, eventual loss of eye	Diagnostics: patient history, ocular exam, fluorescein stain	Ocular antibiotic therapy, pain management, E-collar placed on patient
Descemetocele (deep corneal ulcer so that only the Descemet's membrane remains to maintain the integrity of the eyeball)	Pain, blepharospasm, photophobia, increased tear production, mucoid ocular discharge, rubbing at eye, observable corneal defect	Pain, globe rupture, blindness	Ocular exam, Schirmer tear test, fluorescein stain	Potential surgical conjunctival graft, ocular antibiotics, systemic antibiotics, pain management, E-collar placed on patient, decreased handling as patient stress can lead to globe rupture
Acute blindness	Anxiety, pain (depending on reason), hypertension (depending on disease process), acute blindness	Dependent on underlying disease causing blindness: can be systemic disease, pain, coagulopathy, organ dysfunction/failure, death	Blood pressure, CBC, complete chemistry panel, clotting panel, ocular exam, neurologic exam, intraocular pressure exam, CT/MRI	Will be dependent on underlying disease process and results of diagnostics
Glaucoma	Acute blepharospasm, corneal edema, mydriasis, exophthalmos	Pain, blindness, if untreated will lead to necessary enucleation	Intraocular pressure measurement, ocular exam	IV catheter placement, mannitol administration, topical antiglaucoma medications
Acute uveitis	Blepharospasm, excessive watering of the eyes, corneal edema, aqueous flare	Blindness, underlying disease process	Ocular exam, fluorescein stain, CBC, complete chemistry profile, urinalysis, tick titers (searching for underlying disease)	Topical ocular corticosteroids (if no ulcer diagnosed), treatment will be dependent on underlying disease process

GASTROINTESTINAL EMERGENCIES

Table 10.10 / Gastrointestinal emergencies

Emergency	Clinical signs	Clinical concerns	Diagnostics	Treatment
Gastric obstruction	Vomiting, diarrhea, anorexia, lethargy	Abdominal pain, dehydration, hypovolemic shock	Abdominal radiographs, abdominal ultrasound	IV catheter placement, IV crystalloid fluid therapy, pain management, gastroprotectants, ± surgery/endoscopy, ± antibiotics
Gastric dilation volvulus	Distended abdomen, non-productive retching, weakness, hypotension, weak to absent pulses, injected mucous membranes, respiratory distress, collapse	Pain, obstructive shock, gastric necrosis, gastric rupture, hemoabdomen, splenic necrosis, sudden death	Abdominal radiographs	IV catheter, IV crystalloid fluid therapy, pain management, gastric decompression, surgery
Acute hemorrhagic diarrhea syndrome	Hemorrhagic diarrhea, vomiting, anorexia, lethargy, collapse	Hypovolemic shock, pain, sepsis	CBC, blood chemistry profile, abdominal radiographs, abdominal FAST	IV catheter placement, IV crystalloid fluid therapy, nutritional support, antiemetic, gastroprotectants, ± antibiotics
Canine parvovirus	Vomiting, diarrhea, lethargy, anorexia, abdominal pain, hypotension	Hypovolemic shock, dehydration, tachycardia, hypotension, prolonged CRT	Parvovirus test, CBC, blood chemistry panel, abdominal radiographs	IV catheter placement, IV crystalloid fluid therapy, antibiotics, antiemetic, nutritional support, pain management
Pancreatitis	Vomiting, diarrhea, lethargy, abdominal pain, icterus	Hypovolemic shock, dehydration, pain	CBC, blood chemistry panel, abdominal ultrasound	IV catheter placement, IV crystalloid fluid bolus, nutritional support, antiemetics, gastroprotectants, pain management

KIDNEY AND URINARY EMERGENCIES

Table 10.11 / Kidney and urinary emergencies

Emergency	Clinical signs	Clinical concerns	Diagnostics	Treatment
Uroabdomen (can be the result of blunt force abdominal trauma, urethral rupture, ureteral rupture, or bladder rupture due to obstruction or cancer)	Pain, vomiting, anorexia, lethargy, anuria (will depend on cause for uroabdomen and length of time since uroabdomen occurred)	Azotemia, hyperkalemia, cardiac arrhythmias, pain, hypovolemic shock, collapse, death	Blood chemistry profile, ECG, abdominal FAST, contrast cystogram	IV catheter placement, IV crystalloid fluid therapy, treatment for hyperkalemia (if present), pain management, urinary catheter placement, ± peritoneal catheter placement, ± exploratory laparotomy
Urinary tract infections	Pollakiuria, stranguria, inappropriate urination	Pain, pyelonephritis, prostatitis, progression to systemic infection, sepsis	CBC, complete blood chemistry, urinalysis, urine culture, abdominal ultrasound	Antibiotic therapy guided by urine culture results
Urethral obstruction (can occur due to physical obstruction such as a urolith or urinary crystal plug, as the result of urethral stricture, or the result of urethral spasm and inflammation)	Abdominal pain, vomiting, anorexia, stranguria producing only drops of urine, anuria, palpable turgid bladder	Pain, azotemia, hyperkalemia, bladder rupture, death	Physical exam, patient history, CBC, blood chemistry profile, urinalysis, ECG	Pain management, IV catheter placement, IV crystalloid fluid therapy, ± decompressive cystocentesis, treatment for hyperkalemia, ± general anesthesia to pass urinary catheter to relieve obstruction
Ureteral obstruction	Vomiting, anorexia, abdominal/ kidney pain, azotemia, hyperkalemia	Pain, azotemia, hyperkalemia, uroabdomen, death	CBC, blood chemistry profile, urinalysis, abdominal ultrasound, abdominal radiographs	IV catheter placement, IV crystalloid therapy, pain management, ± laser lithotripsy, ± surgical correction, diet change for stone dissolution
Acute kidney injury (can occur due to abdominal trauma, toxin ingestion, prolonged hypotension, urinary obstruction)	Can vary depending on cause of kidney injury; can include pain, azotemia, hyperphosphatemia, hyperkalemia, dehydration	Cardiac arrhythmias, pain, hypotension, hypovolemic shock, fluid overload	Patient history, CBC, blood chemistry profile, urinalysis, abdominal ultrasound	IV catheter placement, IV crystalloid fluid therapy, correction of electrolyte disturbances, blood pressure management
Acute on chronic kidney disease occurs when a patient with chronic kidney disease has an acute crisis	Anorexia, vomiting, weakness, lethargy, hypothermia, dehydration, oral ulcers	Hypovolemic shock, gastric ulcers, electrolyte abnormalities, cardiac arrhythmias, azotemia, anemia, pain, hypertension	CBC, blood chemistry panel, venous blood gas, urinalysis, abdominal ultrasound	IV catheter placement, IV crystalloid fluid therapy, electrolyte management, pain management, RBC transfusion as indicated, hypertension treatment as indicated, patient warming, nutritional therapy
Toxins (ingestion of kidney toxins including ethylene glycol; grapes, raisins, currants; NSAIDs; vitamin D3)	Can vary depending on toxin; include abdominal pain, ataxia, vomiting, hypersalivation, polydipsia, polyuria	Acute kidney injury, hypovolemic shock, electrolyte abnormalities, cardiac arrhythmias, death	Patient history, CBC, blood chemistry panel, urinalysis	± decontamination, IV catheter placement, IV crystalloid fluid therapy, ECG monitoring, hemodialysis

REPRODUCTIVE AND GENITAL EMERGENCIES

Reproductive and genital emergencies can affect both male and female patients. A technician should always ask if a patient is intact or not. It is important to get a breeding history if known.

Table 10.12 / **Reproductive and genital emergencies**

Emergency	Clinical signs	Clinical concerns	Diagnostics	Treatment
Dystocia	Bitch/queen in active labor unable to pass a puppy/kitten for 30 minutes, abnormal vaginal discharge, resting for more than 4 hours between births, weak contractions, muscle tremors, weakness, collapse	Hypertension, pain, fetal death, queen/bitch death	Radiographs, abdominal FAST, blood glucose, CBC, blood chemistry panel, electrolytes	IV catheter placement, ± IV crystalloid fluid therapy, oxytocin, calcium gluconate, ± surgery
Pyometra: closed and open	Lethargy, anorexia, vomiting, polydipsia, polyuria, fever, vaginal discharge (if open pyometra)	Hypovolemic shock, sepsis, death	Radiographs, abdominal FAST, CBC, blood chemistry panel	IV catheter placement, IV crystalloid fluid therapy, pain management, antibiotics, surgery
Uterine torsion	Distended abdomen, abdominal pain, anorexia	Hypo/ hypertension, pain, hypovolemic shock	Abdominal radiographs, abdominal ultrasound, CBC, blood chemistry profile	Pain management, IV catheter, IV crystalloid fluids, ovariohysterectomy
Uterine prolapse	Uterus visible outside of the vagina, pain, anxiety	Pain, hypertension, hypotension, sepsis	Patient history, physical exam	IV catheter placement, pain management, E-collar on patient, IV crystalloid fluid therapy, abdominal radiographs, manually reduce prolapse, ± surgery
Hypocalcemia (eclampsia)	Generalized muscle tremors, seizures, facial rubbing, panting, polyuria, polydipsia, hyperthermia	Hyperthermia, seizures	Blood chemistry panel, patient history	IV catheter placement, IV calcium gluconate • Special considerations: when giving calcium gluconate intravenously, administer slowly and monitor patient ECG for bradycardia and sudden death
Paraphimosis	Penis unable to retract back into the prepuce	Entrapment or strangulation of the penis, penile necrosis, pain	Patient history, physical exam	Pain management, manual retraction of penis; manual retraction of penis can be achieved by using lubricant and placing penis back into prepuce. Dextrose solution, granulated sugar, or ice can be used to decrease swelling
Prostatic disease (benign prostatic hypertrophy, neoplasia, prostatitis)	Lethargy, fever, abdominal pain, inability to urinate	Pain, hypertension, hyperkalemia	Abdominal radiographs, abdominal ultrasound, rectal exam, urinalysis, cbc	IV catheter placement, pain management, urinary catheter placement, antibiotic therapy, ± surgery

NEONATAL AND PEDIATRIC EMERGENCIES

Table 10.13 / Neonate and pediatric emergencies

Emergency	Clinical signs	Clinical concerns	Diagnostics	Treatment
Fading Puppy/ Kitten syndrome	Lethargy, inappetence, diarrhea, weight loss	Dehydration, hypothermia, malnutrition	CBC, blood chemistry panel	IV catheter placement, IV crystalloid fluid therapy, nutritional support, antibiotics
Hypoglycemia	Lethargy, anorexia, collapse	Hypoglycemia, bradycardia, hypothermia	Blood glucose, CBC, blood chemistry panel	IV catheter placement, IV crystalloid fluid therapy, IV/IO dextrose, nutritional support
Canine parvovirus	Vomiting, diarrhea, lethargy, anorexia, abdominal pain, hypotension	Hypovolemic shock, dehydration, hypoglycemia, sepsis, death	Parvovirus test, CBC, blood chemistry panel, abdominal radiographs	IV catheter placement, IV crystalloid fluid therapy, antibiotics, antiemetic, gastroprotectants, nutritional support, pain management
Neonatal isoerythrolysis	Lethargy, icterus, anorexia, tachycardia, tachypnea, pale mucous membranes	Anemia, dehydration, death	Blood type queen, blood type kitten, CBC, blood chemistry panel	IV catheter placement, blood transfusion
Septicemia in Neonates	Lethargy, anorexia, ecchymosis, fever	Hypotension, dehydration, hypoglycemia, death	CBC, blood chemistry panel	IV catheter placement, IV crystalloid fluid therapy, antibiotics, pain management, nutritional support
Parasites	Lethargy, anorexia, vomiting, diarrhea	Hypovolemia, hypotension, death	Fecal exam, CBC, blood chemistry panel	Anti-parasitics, IV catheter placement, IV crystalloid fluid therapy
Aspiration pneumonia	Tachypnea, cough, fever, cyanosis	Hypoxia, sudden death	Thoracic radiographs, CBC, blood chemistry panel	Supplemental oxygen therapy, antibiotics, IV catheter placement, IV crystalloid fluid therapy

HEMATOLOGIC EMERGENCIES

Hematologic emergences include autoimmune diseases leading to anemia, inability for blood to clot, and hemorrhage.

Table 10.14 / Hematologic emergencies

Emergency	Clinical signs	Clinical concerns	Diagnostics	Treatment
Parasitic anemia (can be caused by flea infestation; tickborne diseases; RBC parasites)	Weakness, tachycardia, tachypnea, pale mucous membranes, prolonged CRT, weak pulses, dull mentation	Hypovolemic shock, sudden death	CBC, blood smear evaluation, flea comb	Supplemental oxygen therapy, IV catheter placement, IV crystalloid fluid therapy, blood transfusion as indicated, anti-parasitics
Immune-mediated hemolytic anemia (caused by patient's immune system lysing red blood cells)	Weakness, tachycardia, tachypnea, pale mucous membranes, prolonged CRT, weak pulses, dull mentation, icterus	Hypovolemic shock, sudden death	CBC, blood smear evaluation, slide agglutination test	Supplemental oxygen therapy, IV catheter placement, IV crystalloid fluid therapy, RBC transfusion as indicated, immunosuppressive drug therapy
Immune-mediated thrombocytopenia (caused by patient's immune system attacking platelets)	Petechia, ecchymosis, epistaxis, inappropriate bleeding into body cavities (e.g. hemoabdomen, hemothorax, pericardial effusion), vomiting, lethargy, weakness	Anemia, hypovolemic shock, sudden death	CBC, blood smear evaluation, platelet count, clotting profile	Supplemental oxygen therapy as needed, IV catheter placement, IV crystalloid therapy as needed, blood transfusion as needed, immunosuppressive drug therapy
Hemorrhage (trauma)	Massive bleeding due to trauma, tachycardia, tachypnea, pale mucous membranes, prolonged CRT, weak pulses, distended abdomen, respiratory distress	Hypovolemic shock, anemia, sudden death	PCV/total solids (frequent monitoring), physical exam, abdominal and thoracic FAST	Direct pressure to bleeding, IV catheter placement, IV crystalloid fluid therapy, pain management, blood transfusion as indicated
Hemorrhage (coagulopathy; can be congenital or acquired; emergency treatment is similar regardless of cause)	Petechia, ecchymosis, inappropriate spontaneous bleeding, inability to stop bleeding from minor injury, hematemesis, hemoptysis, hematochezia, weakness, tachycardia, weak pulses, tachypnea, pale mucous membranes, prolonged CRT	Hypovolemic shock, respiratory distress, anemia, sudden death	CBC, blood smear evaluation, clotting profile, abdominal and thoracic FAST	Oxygen supplementation as indicated, IV catheter placement, IV crystalloid fluid therapy, blood transfusion as indicated

METABOLIC AND ENDOCRINE EMERGENCIES

Metabolic and endocrine emergencies include emergency presentation of diabetes, electrolyte disturbances, adrenal disorders, and acid base abnormalities.

Table 10.15 / Metabolic and endocrine emergencies

Emergency	Clinical signs	Clinical concerns	Diagnostics	Treatment
Hypoglycemia (can be due to insulin overdose, chronic seizure activity, toxin ingestion, and cancer)	Weakness, ataxia, confused mentation, collapse, seizure	Sudden death	Glucometer blood glucose, blood chemistry	IV catheter placement, IV glucose therapy
Diabetes mellitus	Polydipsia, polyuria, polyphagia, abdominal distention	Development of diabetic ketoacidosis, dehydration	CBC, blood chemistry, fructosamine levels, glucometer glucose reading	Insulin therapy, IV catheter as indicated, IV crystalloid fluid therapy as indicated
Diabetic ketoacidosis	Dehydration, weakness, dull mentation, tachypnea, tachycardia, vomiting	Hypovolemic shock, severe hyperglycemia, ketosis, electrolyte imbalance	Glucometer blood glucose, CBC, blood chemistry panel, venous blood gas, urinalysis	IV catheter placement, IV crystalloid fluid therapy, potassium supplementation, insulin therapy, antibiotic therapy as indicated
Hypercalcemia (can be due to cancer, toxin ingestion, hyperparathyroidism, hypoadrenocorticism, kidney disease)	Polyuria, polydipsia, anorexia, lethargy, weakness, seizures	Cardiac arrhythmias, kidney failure	Blood chemistry panel, ECG, abdominal ultrasound	IV catheter placement, IV fluid therapy (0.9% NaCl), furosemide, prednisone, calcitriol or pamidronate therapy as indicated
Hypocalcemia (can be due to recent parturition; kidney disease; hypoparathyroidism; toxin ingestion)	Generalized muscle tremors, seizures, facial rubbing, panting, polyuria, polydipsia, hyperthermia	Hyperthermia, seizures	Blood chemistry panel, patient history	IV catheter placement, IV calcium gluconate • Special considerations: when administering calcium gluconate, administer slowly and monitor patient ECG for bradycardia and sudden death
Hypernatremia (can be due to kidney disease, ingestion of excessive sodium, lack of access to water)	Neurologic changes, muscle tremors, seizures, polydipsia, lethargy, ataxia, coma	Seizures, death	Blood chemistry panel	IV catheter placement, IV fluid therapy (type will depend on acute vs. chronic hypernatremia; careful decrease of serum sodium levels is required with chronic changes)

(*Continued*)

Table 10.15 / Metabolic and endocrine emergencies (Continued)

Emergency	Clinical signs	Clinical concerns	Diagnostics	Treatment
Hyponatremia (can be due to kidney disease, water loss from vomiting/diarrhea, excessive ingestion of fresh water)	Weakness, ataxia, dull mentation, vomiting, seizures, coma	Seizures, death	Blood chemistry panel	IV catheter placement, IV fluid therapy (type will depend on acute vs. chronic hyponatremia; careful increase of serum sodium levels is required with chronic changes)
Hyperkalemia can be due to urinary obstruction, kidney disease, hypoadrenocorticism	Mental depression, weakness, cardiac arrhythmias	Cardiac arrhythmias, sudden death	Blood chemistry panel, ECG	IV catheter placement, IV fluid therapy, IV terbutaline, IV insulin/dextrose, IV calcium gluconate if ECG changes evident, correction of urinary obstruction if present, peritoneal or hemodialysis
Hypokalemia can be due to kidney disease, toxin ingestion, gastrointestinal loss, nutritional deficit, insulin therapy	Skeletal muscle weakness (ventroflexion; plantigrade stance), respiratory weakness, cardiac arrhythmias	Respiratory distress, cardiac arrhythmias, sudden death	Blood chemistry panel, ECG	IV catheter placement, IV crystalloid fluid therapy, IV potassium (not to exceed 0.5 mEq/kg/hour)
Hypoadrenocorticism (Addison's disease) is caused by decreased secretion of glucocorticoids and mineralocorticoids by the adrenal glands	Waxing and waning gastrointestinal signs (vomiting/diarrhea), lethargy, anorexia, polydipsia, polyuria, weakness, collapse	Hypovolemic shock, cardiac arrhythmias, electrolyte disturbances, death	CBC, blood chemistry profile, abdominal ultrasound, basal serum cortisol level, ACTH stimulation test	IV catheter placement, IV crystalloid fluid therapy, IV dextrose if indicated; treatment for hyperkalemia if indicated
Acid–base disturbances (can be due to metabolic diseases or respiratory diseases)				Acid–base status is generally corrected as the underlying disease process is corrected

ENVIRONMENTAL EMERGENCIES

Table 10.16 / Environmental emergencies

Emergency	Clinical signs	Clinical concerns	Diagnostics	Treatment
Bone fractures	Lameness, unwilling to bear weight, swelling, pain	Pain, infection, blood loss	Patient history, physical exam, radiographs	Bandaging, splinting, surgery
Bite wounds	Swelling, hemorrhage, lacerations, puncture wounds	Pain, infection, can penetrate thorax, abdomen, eyeballs	Patient physical exam, radiographs	Basic wound care, ± wound closure, ± bandage, ± antibiotics
Electrocution	Thermal burns of mouth and tongue, respiratory distress, muscle tremors/weakness	Tachypnea, pulmonary edema, cardiac arrhythmias, pain, altered mentation	Patient history, thoracic radiographs, thoracic and abdominal FAST	Supplemental oxygen administration, IV catheter placement, ± IV crystalloid fluid administration, oral care
High-rise syndrome	Injuries to the face, head, thorax, and limbs, respiratory distress, hemorrhage	Respiratory distress, pneumothorax, head trauma, hypovolemic shock, pain, fractured limbs, hemoabdomen	Survey radiographs, patient physical exam	Pain management, supplemental oxygen administration, IV catheter placement; specific treatment will depend on injuries
Hyperthermia (environmental hyperthermia, heatstroke: different from a fever and treatment is different; rely on patient history to differentiate)	Elevated body temperature, respiratory distress, petechial, ecchymosis, diarrhea/melena, collapse, seizures, coma	Hypovolemic shock, distributive shock, hypoglycemia, coagulopathy, sepsis, multiple organ failure, seizures, death	Patient history, physical exam, CBC, blood chemistry panel, coagulation panel	IV catheter placement, active patient cooling, IV crystalloid therapy, specific therapy will depend on severity of disease
Hypothermia	Low body temperature, shivering, dull/obtunded mentation	Bradycardia, hypotension, death	Patient history, physical exam	Rewarming
Burns (causes: exposure to fire, heating blankets, heat lamps, chemicals, boiling/hot liquid)	Hair loss, swelling, redness or discolored skin, open wound	Pain, infection, hypovolemia	Patient history, physical exam, CBC, blood chemistry panel	Wound management, IV crystalloid fluid therapy, pain management, nutritional support

TOXICOLOGICAL EMERGENCIES

Toxin ingestion in common in small animals and can cause these patients to present to the hospital with a wide variety of symptoms and clinical signs. It is important to methodically question owners as to the possibility of drugs, cleaners, foods, plants, and poisons so that treatment can be focused and appropriate whenever possible. Regardless of cause, emergency treatment for seizures, dehydration, and shock should be administered immediately.

Table 10.17 / Toxicological emergencies

Toxin	Toxic dose	Clinical signs	Clinical concerns	Treatment
Chocolate	Milk chocolate: weight (lb) × 0.3 = oz needed for reaction Dark chocolate: weight (lb) × 0.12 = oz needed for reaction Baking chocolate: weight (lb) × 0.04 = oz needed for reaction	Vomiting, diarrhea, muscle tremors, hyperexcitability, tachycardia, seizures; coma	Cardiac arrhythmias, hypovolemic shock, cardiogenic shock, death	Decontamination (vomit induction), activated charcoal; ± IV fluid therapy, ECG; ± treatment to decrease heart rate
Ethylene glycol	Canine: 4–6 ml/kg Feline: 1.5 ml/kg	Ataxia, depression, vomiting; seizures	Acute kidney failure, death	IV catheter placement, IV crystalloid fluid therapy, 4-methylpryazole, IV ethanol; hemodialysis, continuous renal replacement therapy
Xylitol	> 0.1 g/kg = hypoglycemia > 0.5 g/kg = hepatotoxicity	Weakness, seizures, vomiting, petechia, ecchymosis, icterus	Hypoglycemia, acute liver necrosis and failure, coagulopathy, death	IV catheter placement, IV crystalloid fluid therapy, IV dextrose, liver support
Ibuprofen	Canine: 25–125 mg/kg gastrointestinal signs (vomiting, diarrhea, abdominal pain, anorexia) > 175 mg/kg gastrointestinal signs + acute kidney injury > 400 mg/kg gastrointestinal and kidney injury + ataxia, seizures, coma > 600 mg/kg death Cats: Any dose: gastrointestinal ulcerations > 20 mg/kg renal injury	Will vary with dose: lethargy, vomiting, diarrhea, anorexia, melena, azotemia, polyuria, polydipsia, hypertension, seizures, coma	Gastrointestinal ulceration, hypovolemic shock, acute kidney injury, neurologic deficits, death	Vomit induction, activated charcoal administration, IV catheter placement, IV crystalloid fluid treatment, drugs for gastroprotection
Acetaminophen	Dogs: > 50 mg/kg Cats: > 10 mg/kg	Vomiting, weakness, brown mucous membranes, respiratory distress, facial edema	Hepatic necrosis, respiratory distress, tissue hypoxia, anemia, death	Vomit induction, activated charcoal administration, supplemental oxygen therapy, IV catheter placement, IV crystalloid fluid therapy, N-acetylcysteine, liver protectant medications, ± blood transfusion

(Continued)

Table 10.17 / **Toxicological emergencies (Continued)**

Toxin	Toxic dose	Clinical signs	Clinical concerns	Treatment
Tremorogenic toxins (compost/ molds/pyrethrins/ metaldehyde)	Will vary dependent on species, size, and amount ingested	Ataxia, generalized muscle tremors, seizures, coma	Seizures, hyperthermia, death	Vomit induction, enema, activated charcoal, IV catheter placement, IV crystalloid fluid therapy, muscle relaxants, sedation, anti-seizure medications
Rodenticides: anticoagulant (warfarin/ brodifacoum/ difethialone/ bromadiolone)	Any when ingested	3–5 days post-exposure: inappropriate bleeding (epistaxis, hematemesis, hematochezia, melena, hemoabdomen, hemothorax, hyphemia, bleeding around gums, ecchymosis, petechia)	Anemia, hypovolemic shock, death	Vomit induction, activated charcoal, CBC, clotting profile, IV crystalloid therapy, plasma transfusion, ± blood transfusion, vitamin K
Cholecalciferol	> 0.5 mg/kg	12–36 hours post-exposure: vomiting, diarrhea, anorexia, depressed mentation, polyuria, polydipsia	Acute kidney failure, cardiac arrhythmias, death	Vomit induction, activated charcoal, IV catheter placement, 0.9% NaCl IV fluid administration, ± furosemide, ± prednisone
Bromethalin	> 1 mg/kg (cats more sensitive)	Hyperexcitability, muscle tremors, CNS depression, seizures, hyperthermia	Seizures, death	Vomit induction, activated charcoal, IV catheter placement, anti-seizure medications, ± mannitol
Lily (Easter, stargazer, Japanese, tiger)	Ingestion of any part of the plant is toxic to felines	Anorexia, lethargy, vomiting	Acute kidney failure, death	Vomit induction, IV catheter placement, IV crystalloid fluid therapy
Mushrooms	Will vary based on species and clinical effects	Varies widely: hallucinations, vomiting, diarrhea, acute liver failure	Liver failure, hypovolemic shock, hyperthermia, death	Vomit induction, activated charcoal, IV catheter placement, symptomatic

Decontamination

Vomit Induction should be considered if ingestion occurred within four hours of presentation and toxin is not corrosive, caustic, or poses a risk to obstruction if vomited. The patient must be mentally appropriate and able to protect their airway.

Activated charcoal may or may not contain sorbitol (cathartic); it will absorb most toxins. It is important to re-dose in the case of toxins that undergo enterohepatic recirculation.

If the patient has received improper topical flea/tick prevention, has been sprayed with a toxin, or has any substance on their skin that is toxic if groomed and ingested, the animal should be bathed with a degreasing product.

Gastric lavage can be performed if the patient has ingested a toxin with no antidote and patient cannot or will not vomit. Gastric lavage requires general anesthesia and is not without risk.

An enema can be performed multiple times to eliminate toxin from the gastrointestinal tract, especially if the patient is sedated and/or the toxin has moved from the stomach into the intestines.

Inducing Vomiting at Home

Inducing vomiting is a common treatment for foreign body or toxic ingestions. However, care must be taken before advising over the phone to induce vomiting at home as it can be dangerous to the pet. Alkalis, acids, corrosive agents, petroleum products, or hydrocarbons should not be expelled via induced vomiting. Animals with the preexisting conditions of megaesophagus, epilepsy, cardiac disease, or that have altered mental status due to the ingested toxin should not be induced to vomit.

The best way to induce vomiting in a dog at home is by using 3% hydrogen peroxide and administering it within three hours of toxin ingestion. Even if the treatment is successful, only 40–60% of the stomach contents will be expelled. It is important for owners to verify that they are using 3% hydrogen peroxide and not a strength any higher, as higher concentrations will cause oral, esophageal, and gastric ulceration. Even appropriate dosing of 3% hydrogen peroxide can cause oral and esophageal ulcers. A maximum of two doses can be administered at home. If unsuccessful, the dog should be transported to medical care. The use of hydrogen peroxide in cats is discouraged due to esophageal and gastric ulcers.

Hydrogen peroxide dose:

- 5 ml (1 tsp) per 5lb body weight (1 ml/lb) to a maximum dose of 45 ml (5 tbs).
- If no vomiting within 10 minutes, the dose can be repeated once.

Tips for at-home vomit induction:

- Verify that the strength of hydrogen peroxide is 3% and is not expired.
- Before administering, feed the dog a small meal.
- Administer the hydrogen peroxide and then walk the dog around the yard.

Chapter 11

Musculoskeletal Diseases and Conditions

Wendy Davies, BS, CVT, CCRVN, VTS (Physical Rehabilitation)

Veterinary Technician and Nurse's Daily Reference Guide: Canine and Feline, Fourth Edition. Edited by Mandy Fults and Kenichiro Yagi.

Companion website: www.wiley.com/go/fults/veterinary

Abbreviations

ANA, antinuclear antibody
CBC, complete blood count
CBLO, cora based leveling osteotomy
CT, computed tomography
DJD, degenerative joint disease
MRI, magnetic resonance imaging
NSAIDs, non-steroidal anti-inflammatory drugs
ROM, range of movement
OCD, osteochondritis dessicans
TPLO, tibial plateau leveling osteotomy
TPO, triple pelvic osteotomy
WCC, white cell count

ARTHRITIS

There are two types of clinically diagnosed arthritides: degenerative and acute inflammatory. Acute arthritis is a pathogenic organism within the closed space of a joint. Degenerative joint disease (DJD) is a progressive deterioration characterized by a loss of hyaline cartilage matrix and death of chondrocytes. There is no cure for DJD; treatment is based on alleviating clinical signs and slowing progression.

Table 11.1 / **Arthritis**

Disease		Arthritis	
		Acute	Degenerative Joint Disease
Presentation	Clinical signs	• Joint swelling, lameness, pain, reluctance to jump or climb stairs, stiff gait	• Abnormal gait, ataxia, exercise intolerance, ↑ lameness following moderate to heavy exercise, stiff upon rising after recumbency, swelling, walking difficulty
	Exam findings	• Crepitus, laxity, pain, ↓ range of motion	• Crepitus, edema, laxity, muscle atrophy, pain

(*Continued*)

Table 11.1 / Arthritis (Continued)

Disease		Arthritis	
		Acute	Degenerative Joint Disease
Diagnosis	General	• History/clinical signs • Joint palpation and manipulation	• History/clinical signs • Joint palpation
	Laboratory	• CBC: leukocytosis, neutrophilia • Urinalysis: ↑ protein • ANA test: + results • Tick-borne agent serology: + results • Synovial fluid analysis: ↑ WCC and bacteria • Biopsy, synovial: neoplasia • Cytology, synovial: ↑ WCC, turbidity, bacteria • Culture, synovial: bacteria, yeast, fungi, additional organisms • Mucin clot test: clot poor	• Synovial fluid analysis: ↑ mononuclear cells (e.g. lymphocytes), protein, and ↓ viscosity, cell count (compared with septic or inflammatory arthritides) • Culture: negative bacteria • Mucin clot test: clot poor • Serum titers: + *Borrelia*, *Ehrlichia*, and *Rickettsia* • Coombs test, ANA serology, rheumatoid factor: + with immune mediated

	Imaging	• Radiograph, affected joint:
		  • Early disease: joint capsular distension, soft tissue thickening, joint effusion
		  • Late disease: bone lysis, erosion and destruction, irregular joint space
			• Radiograph, affected joint: osteophytes, subchondral sclerosis, narrowed joint space and remodeling of subchondral bone/epiphyses
			• Nuclear scintigraphy, bone: subtle changes

	Procedures	• Arthrocentesis: joint drainage and lavage • Arthroscopy: visual examination, lavage, and biopsy	• Arthrocentesis
Treatment	General	• Supportive • Surgery: arthrotomy, reconstructive procedures, arthrodesis	• Supportive • Surgery: resection arthroplasty, joint replacement, arthrodesis
	Medication	• Antibiotics: variable • Chondroprotective agents: polysulfated glycosaminoglycan (Adequan®), glucosamine with chondroitin sulfate • Corticosteroids: prednisone or triamcinolone • Immunomodulators • Methyl sulfonyl methane • NSAIDs: aspirin, carprofen, deracoxib, etodolac, firocoxib, meloxicam, tepoxalin, grapiprant (Galliprant®)	• Chondroprotective agents: glucosamine with chondroitin sulfate • Corticosteroids: prednisone or triamcinolone • NSAIDs: aspirin, carprofen, deracoxib, etodolac, firocoxib, meloxicam, tepoxalin, grapiprant (Galliprant) • Supplements: omega-3 and -6
	Nursing care	• Standard postoperative care • Initial joint immobilization may provide comfort, but long-term use can cause worsening damage • Monitor synovial fluid cytology for response to treatment • Monitor joints for swelling and pain • Treated as outpatient	• Standard postoperative care • Monitor joints for swelling and pain • Treated as outpatient

(*Continued*)

Table 11.1 / Arthritis (Continued)

Disease		Arthritis	
		Acute	Degenerative Joint Disease
Follow-up	Patient care	• Moderate activity but restricted to a level that minimizes discomfort • Strict confinement with acutely painful episodes • Obesity control • Physical therapy: hot/cold treatment, swimming, ROM exercises, massage	• Weight control • Encourage moderate and consistent exercise for muscle tone and strengthening (e.g. swimming – low impact) • Physical therapy: hot/cold treatment, swimming, ROM exercises, massage
	Prevention/ Avoidance	• Maintain appropriate weight control • Early recognition to prevent proceeding to secondary condition	• Maintain proper weight control • Early use of glucosamine with chondroitin sulfate to slow progression
	Complications	• Arthritis, erosive • Non-ambulatory • DJD • Osteomyelitis • Recurrence of infection	• Non-ambulatory
	Prognosis	• Good with septic form • Fair to guarded with immune-mediated form	• Progressive
Notes		• Antibiotics are given for 4–8 weeks	• When switching NSAIDs, provide a 3-day washout period

CRUCIATE DISEASE

Cruciate disease (cranial cruciate rupture) results in a partial or complete instability of the stifle joint. The tearing of the anterior cruciate ligament can be done acutely or as a degenerative process.

HIP DYSPLASIA

Hip dysplasia is the most common condition of the hip joint and cause of osteoarthritis. Hip dysplasia is a faulty development of the hip joint contributing to joint laxity and subluxation early in life. Joint instability occurs as muscle development and maturation lag behind the rate of skeletal growth. See Skill Box 2.7: Orthopedic Examination, page 53.

Table 11.2 / **Cruciate disease and hip dysplasia**

Disease		Cruciate disease (cranial cruciate rupture)	Hip dysplasia
Presentation	Clinical signs	• Abnormal gait, acute or intermittent lameness, ataxia, walking difficulty	• Abnormal gait, ataxia, exercise intolerance, hind limb lameness
	Exam findings	• Deformed stifle joint, edema, joint effusion, muscle atrophy of hind limb musculature, swelling	• Barden's sign, Barlow's sign, crepitus, joint laxity, muscle atrophy, Ortolani + test, pain, ↓ range of motion
Diagnosis	General	• History/clinical signs • Joint palpation: + anterior drawer sign, cranial tibial thrust	• History/clinical signs • Joint palpation
	Laboratory	• Synovial fluid analysis: rule out sepsis and immune-mediated disease	• Not applicable
	Imaging	• Radiograph, stifle joint: joint effusion with capsular distention, periarticular osteophytes, compression of infrapatellar fat pad and calcification of cruciate ligament • MRI or CT: confirmation and severity of disease	• Radiographs, skeletal: joint subluxation of femoral head, flattening of femoral head, shallow acetabulum, periarticular osteophytes, or widening of joint space between femoral head and cranial acetabulum
	Procedures	• Arthrocentesis • Arthroscopy: confirmation and severity of disease	• Not applicable
Treatment	General	• Symptomatic • Cage rest • Surgery: TPLO, "over-the-top" fascia lata graft, fibular head transposition imbrication procedure, extracapsular reinforcing procedures, CBLO, tibial tuberosity advancement	• Surgery: TPO, femoral head and neck excision arthroplasty, pectineal myectomy, total hip replacement
	Medication	• Chondroprotective drugs: polysulfated glycosaminoglycan (Adequan®), glucosamine with chondroitin sulfate • NSAIDs: aspirin, carprofen, deracoxib, etodolac, firocoxib, meloxicam, tepoxalin, grapiprant (Galliprant®)	• Analgesics: variable • Chondroprotective agents: Adequan or glucosamine with chondroitin sulfate • Corticosteroids: prednisone, triamcinolone (short-term use) • Prostaglandin E1 analog: misoprostol • NSAIDs: aspirin, piroxicam, carprofen, etodolac, Galliprant, phenylbutazone, meclofenamic acid
	Nursing care	• Placement of Robert Jones bandage • Pain management • Post-surgery: cryotherapy, laser therapy, ROM exercises, electrical stimulation, controlled weight-bearing, and balance exercises	• Postoerativep radiographs to evaluate surgery • Physical rehabilitation and hydrotherapy • Restrict activity

(Continued)

Table 11.2 / **Cruciate disease and hip dysplasia (Continued)**

Disease		Cruciate disease (cranial cruciate rupture)	Hip dysplasia
Follow-up	Patient care	• Physical rehabilitation: ROM exercises, massage, underwater treadmill, and ball, stair, walking, and balance board exercises • Restricted activity: controlled weight bearing leashed walks and no use of stairs for 3 months postoperatively • Radiograph at 8 weeks • Full exercise by 6–9 months postoperatively, with no physical rehabilitation and 3–4 months with rehabilitation • Control obesity	• Restrict activity • Physical rehabilitation and hydrotherapy • Monitor radiographs to assess degeneration
	Prevention/ avoidance	• Selective breeding • Maintain proper weight control	• Selective breeding • Nutritional manipulation for large-breed dogs during growth and development • Avoid excessive exercise until skeletally mature • Maintain proper weight control
	Complications	• Osteoarthritis • Additional surgery due to meniscal damage	• Osteoarthritis • Non-ambulatory
	Prognosis	• Excellent with surgery, > 85% success rate • Fair without surgery, mostly dependent on dog size	• Good depending on severity of disease and treatment choice
Notes		• Joint is palpated for drawer motion, movement of tibia relative to femur during the tibial compression test, and thickening of joint capsule • 30–40% of canines rupture the opposite cranial cruciate ligament within 17 months • Dogs weighing < 15 kg typically have a 65% recovery rate with cage rest, while dogs > 15 kg often only have a 20% recovery rate • Rehabilitation often requires 2–4 months • Rottweilers and Labrador Retrievers	• Condition is progressive without surgical intervention. • Care should be taken to rule out knee involvement before surgical intervention on the hips • Rehabilitation is the key to surgical and long-term success

OSTEOCHONDROSIS

Osteochondrosis or osteochondritis dessicans (OCD) is a defect in endochondral ossification leading to an excessive retention of cartilage. This defect may occur in the elbow, shoulder, and knee joints. Ununited anconeal process and fragmented coronoid process may also be seen, in association with osteochondrosis or separately. It is often seen in animals between 5 and 10 months of age.

OSTEOMYELITIS

Osteomyelitis is an infection of the bone and its soft tissue elements and membranes. Infectious organisms often complicate an existing condition leading to a very difficult, sometimes impossible, infection to treat.

Table 11.3 / **Osteochondrosis and osteomyelitis**

Disease		Osteochondrosis or osteochondritis dessicans	Osteomyelitis
Presentation	Clinical signs	• Abnormal gait, anorexia, cachexia, forelimb, or hindlimb lameness, reluctance to exercise, walking difficulty	• Anorexia, cachexia, depression, exercise intolerance, lameness, lethargy, rising difficulty, weakness
	Exam findings	• Arthritis, crepitus, hyperextension pain, joint effusion, joint pain, muscle atrophy, swelling	• Edema, inflammation, intermittent draining tracts, pain, paralysis, paresis, pyrexia, swelling, tachycardia
Diagnosis	General	• History/clinical signs • Joint palpation	• History/clinical signs • Skeletal palpation • Neurological examination
	Laboratory	• Joint tap and fluid analysis: confirms involvement and mononucleated cells	• CBC: neutrophilic leukocytosis • Urinalysis: ± aspergillosis • Cytology: toxic neutrophils, phagocytized bacteria, or fungal organisms • Culture: bacteria isolation and identification and sensitivity
	Imaging	• Radiographs, skeletal: joint abnormalities, bone lengths, arthritis, sclerosis of underlying bone or bone flap/fragments (joint "mice") • CT/MRI: location and severity of lesion • Arthrogram: identifies cartilage flap or loose cartilage via contrast enhanced joint radiographs after intraarticular injections	• Radiographs, skeletal: soft tissue swelling, bone resorption, sclerosis, bone sequestra, fracture nonunion, cortical thinning, widening of fracture gap, reactive periosteal new bone, foreign bodies, or fungal lesions • Contrast: sinus location and severity, foreign bodies • Radionuclide imaging: detecting osteomyelitis
	Procedures	• Arthroscopy: confirming cartilage lesion	• Fluid aspirates or tissue biopsy

(*Continued*)

Table 11.3 / Osteochondrosis and osteomyelitis (Continued)

Disease		Osteochondrosis or osteochondritis dessicans	Osteomyelitis
Treatment	General	• Symptomatic • Surgery: arthrotomy or arthroscopy	• Symptomatic • Wound management: debridement, drainage, and irrigation • Surgery: sequestrectomy, amputation, bone grafts, or biopsy
	Medication	• Analgesics • NSAIDs: aspirin, carprofen, deracoxib, etodolac, firocoxib, meloxicam, tepoxalin	• Analgesics • Antibiotics: variable • Antifungals: itraconazole
	Nursing care	• Cryotherapy postoperatively • Place modified Robert Jones bandage • Restricted activity	• Sterile dressing applied to surgical wounds left to close by secondary intention • Irrigate daily with sterile saline • Physical rehabilitation
Follow-up	Patient care	• Cryotherapy for 15–20 minutes three times daily for 3–5 days if no bandage placed • Physical rehabilitation: ROM exercises • Restrict activity for 4 weeks then gradually increase to normal activity over the next 4 weeks • Re-radiograph 4–6 weeks postoperatively • Obesity management	• Monitor radiographs for fracture healing every 4–6 weeks • Repeated bone culture if persistent infection
	Prevention/ avoidance	• Selective breeding • Maintain proper weight control • Nutritional manipulation for large breed dogs during growth and development	• Proper wound and fracture management
	Complications	• Osteoarthritis • Disuse atrophy	• Recurrence and relapse • Limb deformity or impaired function • Neurological disease • Neoplasia
	Prognosis	• Good with early surgical repair (forelimb) • Guarded with stifle or tarsal osteochondrosis	• Good with acute disease • Poor with chronic disease
Notes		• Great Danes, Labrador Retrievers, Newfoundlands, Rottweilers, Bernese Mountain Dogs, English Setters, Old English Sheepdogs	• Saint Bernards, German Shepherds, Labrador Retrievers, Golden Retrievers, Rottweilers

PANOSTEITIS

Panosteitis (enostosis) is a very painful disease of young large-breed dogs that begins in the medullary bone marrow in the region of the nutrient foramen. Its cause is unknown. It gives intermittent lameness of one or multiple limbs. The disease is self-limiting, but its clinical signs will remain for months.

MEDIAL PATELLAR LUXATION

Medial patellar luxation is generally a concern in small-breed dogs. It is typically a congenital or developmental malformation of the stifle joint that causes the patella to displace from the femoral trochlea. Luxation is graded on a scale of I–IV, which allows guidance of treatment options.

Table 11.4 / Panosteitis and medial patellar luxation

Disease		Panosteitis (Enostosis)	Patellar luxation, medial
Presentation	Clinical signs	• Anorexia, ataxia, cachexia, depression, forelimb and hind limb lameness, lethargy, shifting leg lameness, walking difficulty	• Abnormal gait, ataxia, intermittent lameness of hind limb, skipping, walking difficulty
	Exam findings	• Pain on palpation of diaphysis, pyrexia	• Arthritis, pain, stifle joint deformity
Diagnosis	General	• History/clinical signs • Bone palpation	• History/clinical signs • Patella palpation: laxity
	Laboratory	• CBC: eosinophilia (variable)	• Cytology, synovial fluid: ↑ mononuclear cells
	Imaging	• Radiograph, skeletal: ↑ density, progressive mottling and radiopacity within the medullary cavity, new bone formation, thickened bone cortices • Scintigrams, bone: bone lesions	• Radiographs, hind limb: bowing and/or torsion of tibia or femur, shape of femoral trochlea, luxated patella
	Procedures	• Bone biopsy	• Arthrocentesis

(*Continued*)

Table 11.4 / Panosteitis and medial patellar luxation (Continued)

Disease		Panosteitis (Enostosis)	Patellar luxation, medial
Treatment	General	• Supportive	• Supportive • Symptomatic • Surgical: trochleoplasty, trochlear sulcoplasty, recession sulcoplasty, trochlear chondroplasty, chondroplasty, wedge recession, patelloplasty, tibial crest transposition, or tibial tuberosity translocation
	Medication	• Analgesics • Corticosteroids: prednisone • NSAIDs: aspirin, piroxicam, carprofen, etodolac, deracoxib, firocoxib, grapiprant (Galliprant®)	• Analgesics • Chondroprotective agents: polysulfated glycosaminoglycan (Adequan®) or glucosamine with chondroitin sulfate • NSAIDs: aspirin, carprofen, deracoxib, etodolac, piroxicam, Galliprant
	Nursing care	• Treated as outpatient	• Cryotherapy immediately postoperatively then 15–20 minutes daily for 3–5 days if no bandage • Placement of Robert Jones bandage • Physical rehabilitation: ROM exercises and swimming
Follow-up	Patient care	• Restrict activity • Recheck lameness every 2–4 weeks for more serious orthopedic problems	• Restricted activity: leash walk for 4 weeks and prevent jumping • Full exercise by 6–9 months postoperatively • Correct obesity
	Prevention/ avoidance	• Not applicable	• Selective breeding • Maintain proper weight control
	Complications	• Not applicable	• Recurrence following surgery • DJD
	Prognosis	• Excellent	• Excellent with surgery
Notes		• Clinical signs may persist for weeks to months and other juvenile orthopedic diseases may develop • Clinical signs may reoccur up to the age of 2 years • German Shepherd, Irish Setter, Saint Bernard, Doberman Pinscher, Airedale, Basset Hound, Miniature Schnauzer	• Miniature and Toy Poodles, Yorkshire Terriers, Pomeranians, Pekingese, Chihuahuas, Boston Terriers

Section Five

Patient Care Skills

Chapter 12

Animal Behavior

Monique Feyrecilde, BA, LVT, VTS (Behavior)

Veterinary Technician and Nurse's Daily Reference Guide: Canine and Feline, Fourth Edition. Edited by Mandy Fults and Kenichiro Yagi.

Companion website: www.wiley.com/go/fults/veterinary

Abbreviations

BAER, brainstem auditory evoked response

Veterinary medicine relies on healthy intact human–animal bonds to exist. The veterinary team can and should be stewards of the human–animal bond in client families. A strong foundation in animal behavior improves our stewardship abilities, maintaining a better quality of life for families, improving on-the-job safety and job satisfaction for veterinary professionals.

INTRODUCTION TO BEHAVIOR

Behaviors are happening all the time! Humans and all other animals do "what works". Determining the animal's point of view for "what works" allows us to interact in a sensible and effective way with patients and the clients who love them. The veterinary team needs a basic understanding of why animals do the things they do, what may guide an animal's behavioral choices, and how our own actions and behavior can guide patients to cooperate with us.

THE TECHNICIAN'S ROLE

Technicians are sentinels for animal welfare and care. We can help with prevention and early detection of unwanted behaviors and certain disorders, and participate in treatment as a crucial member of the care team. Veterinarians are responsible for medical assessments of patients, diagnosing or ruling out behavioral disorders, prescribing medications and treatment protocols, prognostic predictions, and modifications to the treatment plan. Veterinary technicians can and should participate as much as possible to best leverage the time of the veterinarian and improve the quality of care provided.

Technicians may not perform diagnosis.[1] For example, determining whether a dog suffers from a separation or hyper-attachment disorder or whether a cat has a pain-related toileting disorder is the role of the veterinarian. These are medical diagnoses and outside the scope of practice for technicians. Technicians can provide a huge volume of support throughout the diagnostic and treatment process for the veterinarian, the patient, and the patient's family. Example tasks appropriate for the veterinary technician include:[1]

- Screening all patients for unwanted or abnormal behaviors during every wellness and illness visit.
- Teaching prevention classes for pets and clients.
- Providing preventive behavioral health education and demonstrating prevention protocols.
- Triaging incoming behavioral concerns and scheduling appropriately.
- Collecting a detailed history.
- Identifying risk factors for disorders and unwanted behaviors.
- Collecting laboratory samples with or without sample analysis.
- Educating the client about the veterinarian's diagnosis and treatment plan.
- Educating clients about pharmacology, and the expected and adverse effects of prescriptions
- Demonstrating behavior modification and training protocols.
- Observing and coaching the client to ensure effective implementation of behavior modification.
- Acting as a liaison between client, veterinarian, and any other professionals.
- Assisting in evaluating the qualifications and credentials of the referral pool (trainers, etc.).
- Providing emotional support to clients throughout the treatment period.

Understanding normal and abnormal behavior and how we can (intentionally or by accident) modify animal behaviors is crucial for veterinary technicians. Every interaction we have with a patient teaches that patient something about the veterinary setting, our team, and the treatment experience. What message would we like to send to our patients? How is this message sent? What can we do to improve the messaging we provide to pets? How does controlling what pets learn about the veterinary environment change our working conditions?

Patients who are fearful will often act in self-defense. Defensive behavior in animals generally looks like attempts to escape followed by defensive aggression. Preventing and reducing animal fear will directly reduce the number of escape behaviors and aggressive behaviors seen in the veterinary hospital.[2]

The most common unwanted behaviors described by pet owners include house soiling, destructive behavior, and aggression.[3] Technicians are crucial in preventing unwanted behaviors and being part of the team to reverse the behaviors should they occur.

In this chapter, we discuss normal and abnormal behaviors, animal development, the essentials of learning theory, and animal handling for veterinary procedures. A good basic foundation should assist the veterinary technician to incorporate awareness about behavior during every patient interaction, provide client education for preventive care, assist in interventional and diagnostic care, and improve the safety of the veterinary team within the hospital environment.

GENETICS AND BEHAVIOR

Every individual animal will have a given genetic potential for physical characteristics and behavioral characteristics. Proper socialization and training can help any individual animal to reach its best possible behavioral genetic potential but not to surpass it. Incorrect socialization and training can hinder the individual from reaching its potential. A combination of nature and nurture are required for successful human–animal bonding.[4]

Separate breeds will have probable behavior patterns. A Labrador Retriever is likely to enjoy picking up and carrying items, while a Border Collie is likely to become excited when they see rapid movements. That said, individuals within any breed can vary widely, particularly along the shy–bold spectrum. Puppies and kittens who are reluctant to approach new people, new situations, novel objects and sounds, and so on are at high risk for developing fear-related unwanted behaviors in the future. Early detection and intervention can help families to achieve the best possible results for these shy individuals. The technician plays a crucial role in early detection of potential problems.

NORMAL AND ABNORMAL BEHAVIOR: PUPPIES AND KITTENS

Puppies and kittens are born with their eyes and ears closed; they require stimulation to eliminate, and cannot thermoregulate unassisted. Once their eyes and ears open, the first socialization period begins. The primary socialization window closes at around 7 weeks of age for kittens, and around 14–16 weeks of age for puppies. For kittens, this presents a unique challenge, since the primary socialization opportunity to humans is completed prior to the time of adoption. For puppies, the primary socialization period extends into the first weeks usually spent with a new family.[5,6]

What is socialization? Socialization is a period of mental flexibility when animals learn who their primary social partners are (same species, other species), how to navigate social interaction, what is pleasurable or dangerous in the environment, and how to respond to potential threats. While animals continue to learn this information throughout their lives, it is learned most easily during this crucial time.

Clients should be advised to protect puppies and kittens from frightening experiences during this time, while strategically setting up pleasurable exposures to as many features of their planned adult lives as possible. The socialization period is an opportunity to create important positive associations (garbage truck sound = chicken treats) which can last a lifetime. Socialization and early learning are like behavioral vaccinations, helping to prepare pets for family life and protect against common sources of fear and stress.

Kittens and puppies visiting the veterinary hospital around seven to eight weeks of age should be prosocial. These young animals should willingly explore the environment, approach people, and accept social contact. Kittens and puppies who are shy, fearful, "slow to warm up", or not prosocial during these first visits may need immediate effective intervention. Families should be referred to a veterinary behaviorist (DVM, DACVB), veterinary treating behavior patients, certified applied animal behaviorist, or when those professionals are unavailable, a positive reinforcement trainer. Because there is no formal licensure process for trainers, veterinary teams should confirm the level of education, experience, and training style of a specific professional before providing referrals.[7]

BEHAVIORAL "VACCINATION"

Priming the mind of a young animal to become an adored member of the family takes planning. Veterinary teams should plan to provide information about protecting patients from the most common unwanted behaviors described by families, and prepare patients for a life of positive experiences with husbandry, grooming, and veterinary care.

Box 12.1 shows an example checklist of topics to discuss with puppy and kitten owners during juvenile wellness visits to prevent common problems. Spreading the topics out over several visits will facilitate successful communication between clients and team members.

Some very simple suggestions to help puppies and kittens become easily handled adult patients include:

- Use desensitization and classical conditioning when performing examinations, injections, grooming, and other treatments.
- Feed a variety of treats in the hospital, and include feeding from a syringe to simulate receiving oral medications
- If a pet is showing signs of stress such as moving away, avoidance, body language associated with fear, vocalizing, and so on, stop treatment and make a new plan.

Box 12.1 / Example Checklists for Topics to Discuss with Puppy and Kitten Owners during Juvenile Wellness Visits

Example Puppy Visit Topic Checklist

- Choosing a puppy class
- Housetraining
- Crate training, travel training
- Appropriate play including bite inhibition during play
- Introductions between your puppy and other pets
- Family lifestyle meeting: socialization to people, places, surfaces, sounds, odors, experiences
- How to choose food and treats
- Making a vaccine schedule and understanding exposure risks
- Anti-pulling devices such as harnesses for walking
- Teething and chewing – selecting appropriate chew items
- Internal and external parasite control and zoonosis
- Learning to accept handling and restraint for grooming and health care
- Toothbrushing
- Nail trimming
- Ear cleaning
- Skin and coat care
- Breed-specific health concerns and behavior tendencies
- Neutering: what, why and when?

Example kitten visit topic checklist

- Housetraining, including common litter Issues
- The health benefits of keeping cats indoors
- Crate training to make trips outside the house easy
- Appropriate play including bite and claw inhibition during play
- Introductions between your kitten and other pets
- How to choose food and treats
- Making a vaccine schedule and understanding exposure risks
- Appropriate toy choices and avoiding foreign object ingestion
- Teething and clawing – selecting appropriate items and developing good scratching habits
- Internal and external parasite control and zoonosis
- Learning to accept handling and restraint for grooming and health care
- Toothbrushing
- Nail trimming
- Ear cleaning
- Skin and coat care
- Breed-specific problems and tendencies
- Neutering: what, why and when?

NORMAL AND ABNORMAL BEHAVIOR: PRESENTATIONS AND DISORDERS

Animals presented to the veterinary hospital for any reason should be screened during the history for changes in behavior and unwanted behaviors. Often, the first sign of a medical problem is a change in behavior. However, the dichotomy between medical and behavioral conditions is false: every pet is a whole animal. Conditions are not medical or behavioral: any condition which impacts information transmitted by the nervous system can and will change behavior. For example, stress and anxiety are known to increase skin permeability and susceptibility to allergens and irritants. Pruritus is linked to irritability in humans and animals. Stress is associated with colitis, high blood pressure, changes in white blood cell counts, cystitis, and more. Increased or decreased sensory aptitude, acuity, or perception (vision loss, hearing loss, sensation changes, etc.) can result in what look like "training problems".[8]

When a patient has a change in behavior or a possible behavioral diagnosis, a minimum database of physical examination, neurological examination, serum biochemistries, complete blood count, urinalysis, and fecal analysis should be performed. Additional testing such as dermatologic evaluation, imaging including radiographs, computed tomography, magnetic resonance imaging, and BAER (brainstem auditory evoked response) hearing tests may also be required to establish the database of relevant information for an individual patient. Any abnormalities should be treated, even if they are not associated with any change in behavior. Assuring patients are having their basic needs met (safety, nutrition, hydration, sleep, exercise, and good overall health) is always the first step.[9]

When a behavioral diagnosis and intervention plan is made, or when a prevention and training plan is needed, the veterinary team must understand the fundamentals of how and what animals learn and the principles guiding each animal's decision-making process to best assist the family in achieving success.

HOW ANIMALS LEARN

All animals, including humans, do what "works". All behavior has a function in the mind of the individual doing the behavior. The function may be normal, abnormal, productive or harmful: but it is present. Making the animal's version of what works match the human's version of what works will result in successful behavioral change from the human's perspective. We must keep in mind the animal is simply doing what they have been conditioned or trained to do. Conditioning and training come from people, other animals, the environment, general experiences, specific contexts, and more. Learning is happening all the time when we are conscious. Helping animals learn the things we want them to learn, and avoid learning the things we want to prevent is the key to healthy human–animal bonding.

Animals will not perform behaviors out of spite, specifically to anger humans, to punish humans, because they are "bad" or "mean". Behaviors are means to function. Table 12.1 has a quick reference for common training and behavior modification procedures and their likely outcomes.

Table 12.1 / **Summary of common training and behavior modification procedures**

Procedure	Summary/outcomes
Classical conditioning	Event A is associated with event B
	Event B leads to emotion, secretion, reflex
	Event A will cause the emotion, secretion, reflex even if event B does not occur
	• Example: feeling happy when you hear the ice cream truck song
Counterconditioning	Event A leads to unwanted emotion, secretion, reflex (e.g. fear)
	Event B leads to wanted emotion, secretion, reflex (e.g. pleasure)
	Event A and event B are linked to replace the unwanted response with the wanted response (e.g. replace fear with happy)
	• Example: salivating when seeing the ear cleanser bottle
Operant conditioning	Learner performs a behavior
	What happens next from the learner's perspective determines whether the learner repeats the behavior in the future
	• Example: dog sits; treat delivered; dog sits again in the future

(*Continued*)

Table 12.1 / Summary of common training and behavior modification procedures (Continued)	
Procedure	**Summary/outcomes**
Desensitization	Gradual repeated exposure to a controlled stimulus
	Learner stops responding to the stimulus
	• Example: injection training
Habituation	Repeated exposure to the same unmodulated stimulus
	Learner stops responding to the stimulus
	• Example: ignoring planes overhead when you live near the airport
Sensitization	Repeated exposure to the same unmodulated stimulus
	Learner responds more and more strongly to the stimulus
	• Example: hitting a sibling who steals your pencil for the 10th time

Classical Conditioning

Classical conditioning is associative learning where the pairing of two stimuli eventually results in a predictable response from the learner. At the beginning of the process, one stimulus is meaningless and one stimulus causes a result in the form of an emotion, a secretion, or a reflex. When the stimuli are paired in a predictable way, the first initially meaningless stimulus will begin to cause the result of the emotion, secretion, or reflex.[10] Take, for example, Pavlov's dogs. A bell rings (meaningless). Meat powder is presented (salivation occurs). After enough repetitions of the bell predicting meat powder and salivation resulting, the bell rings and the dogs salivate even when the meat powder is absent. The previously meaningless bell now results in saliva production.

Classical conditioning is powerful. The dog who runs away when he sees a bottle of ear cleanser and the cat who disappears into thin air at the sight of a pet carrier have been classically conditioned to fear these inanimate and previously meaningless objects. The cat who comes running eagerly when her pill bottle rattles and the dog who runs happily to the refrigerator when the client reaches for the dog's insulin are also classically conditioned. Classical conditioning is an extremely useful tool both within and outside the veterinary context. Table 12.2 shows a stepwise example of classically conditioning a cat to gag at the sight of a syringe.

Table 12.2 / Example of classically conditioning a gag response to the sight of a syringe

Before conditioning	During conditioning	Result of conditioning
1. Syringe appears → no response 2. Bitter liquid administered → cat gags and salivates	Syringe appears → bitter liquid administered → cat gags and salivates	Syringe appears → cat gags and salivates

Counterconditioning

Counterconditioning involves replacing an existing response to a stimulus with an alternate response.[11] Replacing responses is an incredibly useful tool to use when providing veterinary care and husbandry as well as a crucial part of most behavior modification plans.

Example

Nail clippers appear → pet is held down while struggling → fear response
Nail clippers appear → fear response
Nail clippers appear → treats appear → pleasure response
Nail clippers appear → pleasure response

Timing matters with respect to classical conditioning and counterconditioning, and different patients will respond according to their individual learning style, preference, and learning history. Backward conditioning (also called distraction), delay conditioning, simultaneous conditioning, and trace conditioning are the four timing options for classical conditioning and counterconditioning.

Figure 12.1 shows a visual representation of the timing for the four types of conditioning, using the example of attempting to condition a pet to like touch by using something else the pet likes: food. In most cases, a predictive relationship creates the strongest conditioned response. Predictive relationships are pairs of stimuli that happen in a way the learner can easily learn to predict. For this reason, backward conditioning runs the risk of teaching the pet to be fearful when food is offered. If the pet fears being touched and the presence of food predicts the touch, soon the pet may fear the presence of food. For example, feeding a fearful dog peanut butter and then attempting to clip his nails while he is distracted may work short-term, but it can also result in the dog avoiding peanut butter in the future. In most situations, the use of simultaneous, delay, and trace conditioning are more safe and effective than backward conditioning (distraction).

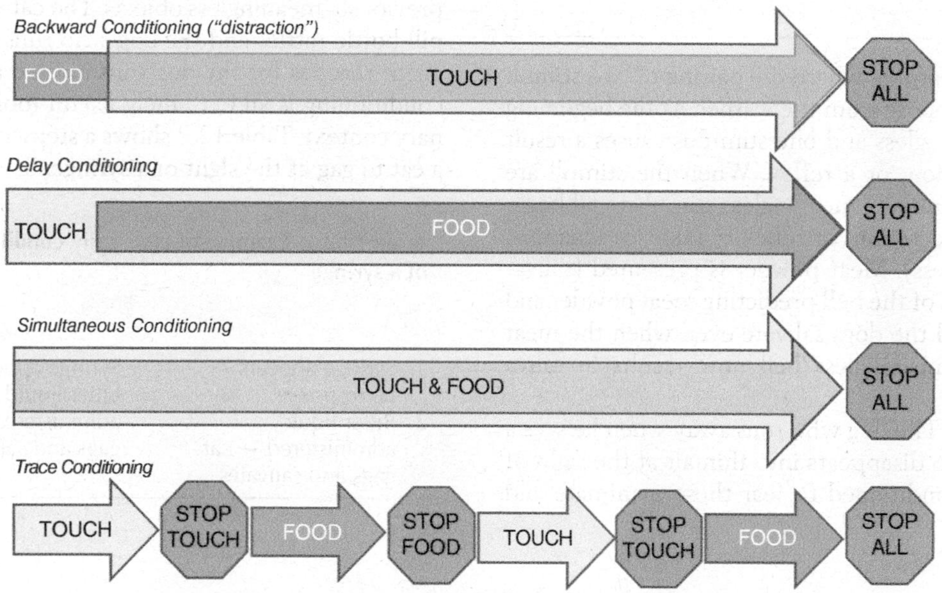

Figure 12.1 Timing application for four common conditioning practices.

Desensitization, Habituation, and Sensitization

Desensitization involves controlled gradual exposures to a stimulus, with the goal being for the learner to stop responding to the stimulus. The exposures must be well-planned and gradual so the learner is kept in a stress-free state. During desensitization procedures, the pet should choose to participate and should show no discernible response to the stimulus.[11]

To perform desensitization, a systematic approach is needed to control the trigger stimulus, often called an exposure hierarchy or exposure ladder. The ladder is a helpful visual representation, but it is crucial to remember the learner dictates the size and shape of the ladder, how many rungs there are, how far apart or close together the rungs sit, and how quickly the ladder might be climbed.

Controlling the intensity of a stimulus may mean how close or far the stimulus is from the learner, how big or small it is, how loud a sound is, how firm a touch is, the duration of time the stimulus is presented, which body part is touched (sensitive toes vs. less sensitive shoulders), the presence of equipment and products, and more. The starting point must always be non-stressful for the learner. For an example hierarchy of introducing ear cleansers, refer to Box 12.2. The procedure described in the box could require 30 seconds or 30 days, depending on the learner's history and feelings about ear care and the skill of the person implementing desensitization.

Box 12.2 / Example of Exposure Ladder for Desensitization to Basic Ear Cleansing

Following each approximation by delivering something the pet loves will combine desensitization and classical conditioning or counterconditioning, a common prevention plan and treatment plan for behavior modification.

Desensitization exposure ladder for ear cleansing

- Walk to cabinet where ear cleanser is stored
- Reach toward handle
- Open cabinet
- Touch ear cleanser bottle
  - Increase duration of touching bottle
- Lift ear cleanser bottle
- Remove from cabinet
- Ear cleanser bottle in learner's visual field 8 ft away
- Cotton ball in learner's visual field 8 ft away
- Bottle is moved closer in 6-inch increments
- Cotton ball is moved closer in 6-inch increments
- Bottle is opened so odor can escape
- Cotton ball approaches non-sensitive body part
- Non-sensitive body parts touched with cotton ball
  - Increase duration and pressure associated with touch
  - Glide touch toward ear
- Cotton ball (dry) approaches ear
- Cotton ball (dry) touches ear lightly for 1 second
  - Gradually increase duration and pressure of cotton ball (dry) contact
- Cotton ball (wet) approaches ear
- Cotton ball (wet) touches ear lightly for 1 second
  - Gradually increase duration and pressure of cotton ball (wet) contact
- After introduction of wet material, touch ear with two hands
- Massage of ear canal as appropriate for 1 second
  - Gradually increase duration and pressure of massage
- Cotton ball (dry) approaches cleaned ear
- Cotton ball (dry) touches cleaned ear lightly for 1 second
  - Gradually increase duration and pressure of cotton ball (dry) contact to wipe out ear

Because desensitization is a slow process and the goal is non-response, but the goal of most veterinary care training is a patient having a positive emotional response to handling, desensitization and classical conditioning or counterconditioning are generally used together. To combine desensitization and classical conditioning or classical counterconditioning, use the stimulus pairing procedure from the classical conditioning section. Each tiny approximation in the exposure ladder predicts something wonderful appearing or happening. Look again at Box 12.2, and imagine at the end of each line inserting the event "bites of steak appear!" Preparing the patient to accept treatments and husbandry events using desensitization and classical conditioning or counterconditioning is a powerful prevention and intervention tool to improve the behavioral wellbeing of pets and the safety of the veterinary team.

Habituation and sensitization involve exposing the learner to a stimulus that is not modulated.[11] Habituation results in the learner being indifferent to the stimulus, while sensitization means that the learner develops a much stronger response to the stimulus even though the stimulus itself is unchanged. An example of habituation would be living near the airport; one rapidly becomes oblivious to the sound of aircraft overhead because it is meaningless and does not impact the learner. An example of sensitization might include two siblings riding together in the back seat of the car. Sister pokes brother, brother whines. Sister pokes brother five more times, brother whines five times. The next time sister pokes brother, brother lashes out and hits sister. Sensitization means the stimulus (poke) is the same every time, but the response (whine vs. hit) gets more intense over time. Sensitization is a real risk with veterinary care and husbandry if we are not careful and control exposures to keep them within what the pet can comfortably tolerate.

Operant Conditioning

Operant conditioning is what many people commonly think of as "training". Operant conditioning is different from classical conditioning because it involves intentional behaviors which become stronger or weaker over time depending upon the consequence of the behavior (Figure 12.2). If a behavior is getting stronger over time (happening with greater frequency, intensity, or duration), reinforcement is occurring. If a behavior is getting weaker over time, punishment is likely occurring.[12] To determine whether reinforcement or punishment is happening, we must measure the behavior in question and assess whether the behavior is becoming stronger or weaker, then examine the consequence of the behavior to understand which quadrant(s) might be at work.

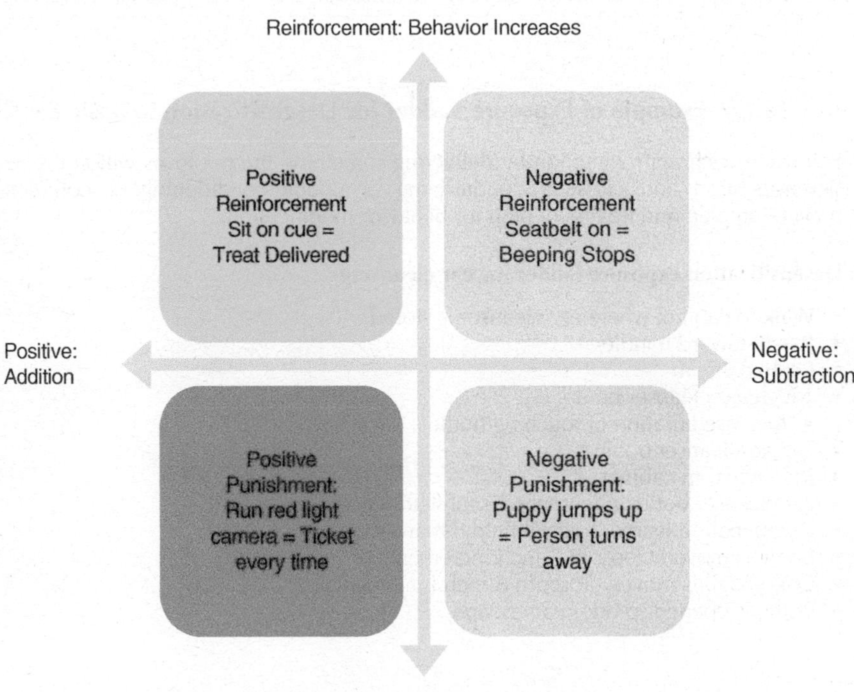

Figure 12.2 The quadrants of operant conditioning.

The term "consequence" often has a negative connotation, but consequences are simply what comes after a behavior. Consequences can be pleasant or unpleasant from the perspective of the learner. If a consequence is pleasant, behavior is likely to increase. If a consequence is unpleasant, behavior is likely to decrease. Remember, animals do what works.

In operant conditioning, there are two categories of reinforcement discussed: positive reinforcement and negative reinforcement. The same is true for punishment: positive punishment and negative punishment.

Positive simply means something is added to the situation from the perspective of the learner. Negative means something is subtracted. Successful training and learning are best done using reinforcement, especially positive reinforcement. The learner performs a behavior you wish to see repeated, add something the learner likes immediately. The learner is likely to do the behavior again in the future. For example, a cat scratches her claws on the scratching post and the owner immediately delivers a delicious treat.

When using operant conditioning, the three most common strategies are luring, capturing, and shaping. Luring means the animal follows something they want, and following results in the goal behavior occurring. Capturing means the trainer waits for the learner to do the behavior on their own, then marks the desired behavior and delivers a reward. Shaping means breaking the goal behavior down into small steps or approximations, then marking and rewarding each time the learner completes an approximation. Eventually the small baby steps or approximations will add up to a completed goal behavior.

The use of a marker can be very helpful in a wide variety of training contexts. Marker-based training means using a specific sound or signal to mark the right behavior before delivering a reward. Common markers include a clicker, a short word like "yes", a specific gesture such as pointing or thumbs up, a whistle, a flash of light, and many more. The type of marker used depends upon the preference of the learner, the preference of the trainer, and the practicality in a given situation.

Example: / Puppy Going to its Bed

Lure

Trainer holds out a delicious treat to get the puppy's interest. Once the puppy's nose is "magnetized" to the treat, the trainer moves the treat toward the bed. When the puppy has followed the treat to the bed, the trainer marks the behavior and delivers the treat.

Capture

The trainer sits where he can see both the puppy and the bed. While the puppy is exploring the area, the puppy wanders onto the bed. When the puppy accidentally moves onto the bed, the trainer marks the behavior and immediately delivers the treat.

Shape

The trainer sits where he can see both the puppy and the bed. While the puppy is exploring, the trainer watches carefully for any behavior which could lead to the goal of puppy on the bed and will mark *any* of these behaviors as they occur, giving a treat every time the marker (e.g. a click) is used. Possible approximations: Puppy glances at bed, looks at bed longer, turns toward bed, walks one step toward bed, walks several steps toward bed, sniffs bed, leans over bed, walks around bed, places any toe on the bed, places any paw on the bed, places more than one paw on the bed, places more than one paw on the bed for gradually longer duration, places all paws on the bed, places all paws on the bed for gradually longer durations.

Punishment Problems

The use of punishment is challenging. For punishment to be effective, it needs to be:

- Perfectly timed within one second of the undesired behavior.
- Consistent and constant. It must occur every time the undesired behavior does and when the punishment is ceased, the undesired behavior is likely to return. This is called suppression.
- Sufficiently unpleasant that the learner will actively work to avoid it.

Using punishment as a part of a training plan can lead to welfare concerns as well as decreasing the likelihood that the goal behavior will be learned.[13,14] The use of punishment shows the learner what not to do, but does not show the learner the goal behavior. The learner may avoid the "wrong" answers, but may not arrive on the goal behavior on his own. The learner may also become reluctant to try new behaviors, fearful of the trainer, fearful of the context of training, avoidant of training situations, and simply confused. Punishment, particularly positive punishment, can harm the human–animal bond because it damages trust between the pet and the human.

When pets are fearful, they have a limited number of ways to communicate their fear. Largely, this is by fleeing the situation (avoidance), fidgeting (displacement), and fighting (defensive aggression). The use of positive punishment such as prong collars, choke chains, shock collars, shocking mats, striking the animal, intentionally scaring the animal (booby traps, yelling), physically manipulating the animal ("alpha roll", "scruff and shake") can lead to the animal avoiding the situation or showing aggressive behaviors.

Aggression is communication. Aggressive behaviors are a means for an animal to show that it is uncomfortable and needs immediate change to feel safe or comfortable. When an animal resorts to aggression, many non-aggression body language cues have usually been displayed. For dogs, these include: lip licking when not hungry, yawning when not tired, sniffing uninteresting areas, ears held to the side/down/back, furrowed brows, wide eyes, turning to the side, turning away, moving away, lowering the tail, shaking off when not wet, panting with the lips held back, pupil dilation, changes in respiratory rate, trembling, staring, becoming stiff, piloerection, growling, showing teeth, and snapping without making contact. For cats, the signs are often similar: dilated pupils, ears held to the side/down/back, furrowed brows, whiskers flat, tail down or tucked to the side, turning away, moving away, concealing body parts (lying with feet or tail tight to or under the body), becoming tense or stiff, freezing, swishing or twitching the tail, whiskers forward, opening the mouth, vocalizing, hissing, biting near the threat without damage.

THE ABCS OF BEHAVIOR

In many situations, training and behavior modification can be simplified as remembering the ABCs. The ABC method is also referred to as the applied behavior analysis model, and works to determine the function of a behavior as well as the conditions surrounding the behavior. By understanding the conditions in which the behavior occurs and how the behavior is maintained, a plan for change or modification can be made.

A is for *antecedent*. Antecedents are what happens before a behavior. Antecedents can be contextual, location-based, visual, tactile, olfactory, auditory, taste, anything in the environment which is salient and predictive. Examples include the presence of a mat predicts the behavior of lying on the mat, the sound of rain predicts a change in behavior for a storm-phobic dog, the word "sit" predicts the cat or dog sitting.

B is for *behavior*. Behavior is anything a learner does, and particularly what the learner does following the presence of the antecedent.

C is for *consequence*. Consequences, as discussed earlier in this chapter, follow behavior and drive future behavioral decisions.

Careful observation surrounding the behavior of interest is a crucial skill to develop when working with patients in regular practice or in treating behavior disorders. Figure 12.3 shows Dr. Susan Friedman's guide for procedures to select when working to change behavior. To apply this algorithm to the ABCs, follow these steps:

1. Identify the *behavior* of interest.
2. Identify the *consequences* which are likely maintaining the behavior.
3. Identify the *antecedents* which predict the occurrence of the behavior.

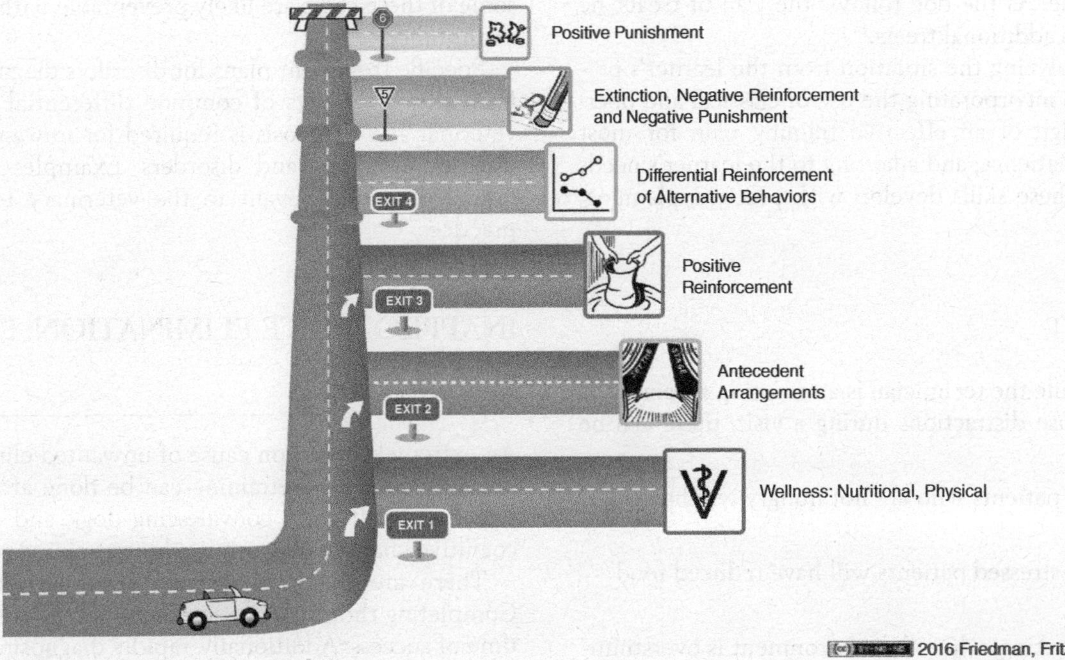

Figure 12.3 Recommended order for procedure selection in behavior modification and training. Source: courtesy of Susan G. Friedman.

Modifying the behavior may be extremely simple or very complex. For the purposes of this chapter's examples, we will keep the process simple.

Example: / A Dog Backs up Instead of Getting on the Scale.

1. B = Backing up.
2. C = Negative reinforcement – distance away from the frightening scale is increased.
3. A = Presence of the scale, the owner, and pressure from the owner pulling on the leash.

The simplest method of modifying this behavior is antecedent arrangement. Change the antecedents to see a different behavior. The desired behavior is the dog walking onto the scale.

1. B = Dog walks toward and then steps onto the scale.
2. C = Treats delivered for walking toward and onto the scale.
3. A = Presence of a non-slip soft mat on the scale and treats next to the scale. Owner is coached to stop applying leash pressure.

In this example, a non-slip soft mat is placed on the scale. Treats are strategically trailed onto the scale. As the dog follows the trail of treats, he walks onto the scale and receives additional treats.[14]

Taking a thorough history, analyzing the situation from the learner's perspective, applying the ABCs, and incorporating the use of classical and operant conditioning allow the design of an effective training plan for most situations. Creativity, ingenuity, patience, and adapting to the learner's needs are also necessary for success. These skills develop with practice, planning, patience, and time.

MY PATIENT WON'T EAT

When the patient will not eat while the technician is attempting a training or conditioning plan, or trying to use distractions during a visit, there can be several reasons:

- The patient may be satiated: patients who are not hungry will have reduced food acceptance.
- The patient may be stressed: stressed patients will have reduced food acceptance.
- The environment is too distracting: when the environment is overstimulating, pets will have decreased interest in food.
- The patient is not familiar with accepting treats: pets without a learning history around accepting treats may need to learn this skill.
- The behavior requested is too difficult: the conditioning plan may need to be broken down into smaller steps, or the skill being trained should be reviewed to verify the learner is ready to understand complex behaviors.

PREVENTION AND INTERVENTION FOR "THE BIG THREE"

The most common unwanted behaviors described by cat and dog owners who surrender their pets to shelters are inappropriate elimination, destructive behavior, and aggression. Each of these problems was owner-defined in the relevant studies, meaning that the definitions may be rather broad, but some of these cases are likely preventable with assistance from the veterinary community.

Specific treatment plans for disorders diagnosed are intentionally omitted from this text. Lists of common differential diagnoses are included, but a veterinarian's diagnosis is required for unwanted eliminations secondary to diseases processes and disorders. Examples provided in this chapter are intended to be relevant to the veterinary technician or nurse's scope of practice.

INAPPROPRIATE ELIMINATION: DOGS

Housetraining

An extremely common cause of unwanted elimination in dogs is incomplete housetraining. Housetraining can be done at any age: it is not restricted to puppies. Adult dogs, convalescing dogs, and dogs experiencing physical or cognitive changes may require housetraining plans.

There are many correct ways to housetrain a puppy or adult dog. Completing thorough housetraining on the first try can set dogs up for a lifetime of success. Additionally, rapidly diagnosing medical conditions linked to unwanted elimination is much easier if the dog has a strong established foundation of housetraining.

The following guidelines will help puppy and dog owners to successfully housetrain their pets. If following this plan diligently does not result in success, medical causes for housetraining challenges should be investigated by the veterinary team.

Guideline #1 : Have Realistic Time Expectations

Housetraining takes time. We consider a dog to be well housetrained when they have gone 12 weeks with no mistakes. For puppies, housetraining will take a minimum of two months and the puppy is unlikely to be reliable prior to six months of age. Setting the goal of housetraining taking time will decrease conflict between the client and the pet. It can also help to keep clients from feeling discouraged. Clients may balk initially, but remembering humans take two years or so to housetrain can be a helpful analogy to provide.

Guideline #2: Have a Supervision, Management, and Reinforcement Plan

Puppies and dogs who are in in training have three basic modes:

1. Be safely confined in a place where it is acceptable to eliminate.
2. Be on a leash or directly supervised within 6–10 feet of an observant owner.
3. Be safely confined in a place they will not soil (e.g. a properly sized crate or pen).

Puppies require practice learning to fully evacuate the bladder and colon. As puppies grow, they develop the ability to hold urine and feces and to void fully rather than in small amounts. Further, the great outdoors provides wonderful sights, smells, and general distractions to the task at hand. When taking puppies outdoors to eliminate, the puppy should be leashed and a timer set for about five minutes. Take the puppy to the desired elimination area and quietly wait. When elimination occurs, at the end of elimination celebrate with quiet, happy, verbal praise and a small delicious treat. After the puppy has eliminated, it can be allowed to play and explore the surroundings (assuming that the area is safe and fenced). Setting up this pattern teaches dogs to eliminate quickly when taken outdoors. Once the learner is beginning to understand the pattern, introducing a verbal or gestural cue to eliminate is helpful. Separate cues for urination and defecation can be used. Give the cue just prior to when the puppy is likely to eliminate, then have a quiet celebration afterward.

Learning to eliminate predictably, on cue, on leash, and in front of a person are useful life skills for travel, for healthcare (sample collection, monitoring quality and quantity of ins/outs), and to simplify dog ownership in general.

If the puppy is taken to the elimination area at a time elimination is likely and no elimination occurs, return the puppy to the safe confinement/no soil area for 10 minutes, then try again.

When taking puppies outdoors to eliminate, use a leash and spend five minutes per trip, even if the puppy has eliminated sooner. Most puppies need a few tries to fully empty themselves. When the puppy is successful, praise him in a quiet but happy voice and offer a delicious treat. If the yard is safe, the puppy can then be let off leash for a play and exploratory period. This way, puppies learn to eliminate immediately when they are taken out.

If you take the puppy out and know he needs to go, but he doesn't, take him back indoors and place him in his crate or pen for 10 minutes, then try again.

Mistakes happen. If the puppy is observed eliminating in an unapproved location, gently interrupt the process by clapping hands or saying something cheerful, then hurry the puppy to an approved area to finish. It will take time after an interruption for a puppy or dog to refocus on elimination, so allow several minutes for the task to be completed. Mistakes found after the fact should be cleaned up with a high-quality enzymatic cleanser. There is no value in showing mistakes to a puppy or dog, scolding the puppy or dog for the error, rubbing noses in eliminations, and so on. A mistake found after the fact is simply a sign that there was an error in the client's management and supervision plan. Further, the use of positive punishment during or after elimination may contribute to the puppy or dog being reluctant to eliminate in the presence of humans and can harm the human–animal bond. Fear of eliminating near a human can develop into covert elimination in other areas of the house, setbacks in housetraining due to fear of eliminating during planned elimination walks, and making sample collection impossible in the future.

Guideline #3: Housetraining is a Habit

Habits are formed by repetition. Creating the habit of eliminating in the approved location and on cue will occur through repeating the desired behavior numerous times. Clients should be coached to create the desired habit in their dog through repetition of right behavior and the use of management and positive reinforcement.

Guideline #4: Consistency Helps!

Providing meals, play time, and rest time on a coordinated and consistent schedule will help puppies and dogs to eliminate on a more consistent schedule as well. The ability to predict when the puppy is likely to eliminate (after meals, after sleep, after physical exertion, and after noteworthy water intake) allows the client to provide the best quality management, supervision, and training.

House Soiling in Housetrained Dogs

When a dog who has a history of good housetraining and begins eliminating in an unwanted way, or a puppy is challenging to housetrain, medical causes should be considered and ruled out before a strictly behavioral diagnosis is made.[9] Table 12.3 shows diagnoses commonly associated with a presenting complaint of unwanted eliminations for both dogs and cats. The elimination patterns in the table can occur simultaneously or separately, with only one sign present or several. Remember, some patients may also have concurrent diagnoses; for example, a dog may have primary hormone-related urinary incontinence and a urinary tract infection and renal disease. Additionally, crossover elimination is common in both dogs and cats, meaning that gastrointestinal disease can change urinary patterns, and diseases associated with urinary changes can impact defecation as well. These cases require a thorough and continuing workup if treating the first condition of concern does not result in a resolution of clinical signs.

Table 12.3 / Medical diagnoses commonly associated with unwanted elimination in dogs and cats*

Differential diagnoses	Possible elimination patterns observed
Urinary tract disease, e.g:	• Increased frequency • Urgency • Stranguria • Odor change, color change • Change in volume per elimination • Avoidance of usual substrate • Urine deposited in new or unusual locations • Soiling areas normally kept clean (e.g. crate, pen, bedding)
Bacterial infection	
Urolithiasis	
Prostate disease	
Urethritis	
Vaginitis	
Balanoposthitis	
Stress-related cystitis	
Any process associated with polyuria/polydipsia, e.g:	• Increased volume • Increased frequency of urination • Soiled bedding • Changes in location
Diabetes mellitus	
Renal insufficiency	
Adrenal disease	
Liver disease	
Ectopic ureter	
Neoplasia	
Toxicity	
Medication adverse effects	
Any process associated with changed stools, e.g:	• Increased frequency • Change in volume per elimination • Urgency • Tenesmus • Avoidance of usual substrate • Depositing feces in new or unusual locations • Soiling areas normally kept clean (e.g. crate, pen, bedding) • Changes in shape, odor, and/or color of feces
Dietary indiscretion, enteritis	
Stress-related colitis	
Infectious	
Adverse reaction to food	
Inflammatory bowel disease	
Neoplasia	
Malabsorption, any	
Adrenal disease	
Structural or obstructive gastrointestinal disease	
Heritable gastrointestinal disease	
Dietary indiscretion, enteritis	
Prostatic disease	

(Continued)

Table 12.3 / Medical diagnoses commonly associated with unwanted elimination in dogs and cats* (Continued)

Differential diagnoses	Possible elimination patterns observed
Any process associated with pain, e.g:	• Any changes can occur • Elimination in unusual or different locations • Eliminations near but not in the litter box/usual location • Changes in physical posture during elimination • Voiding pattern changes (frequency, volume per elimination)
Dental disease (70% of cats over age seven years)	
Osteoarthritis/DJD	
Intervertebral disc disease	
Trauma (any body part)	
Prostatic disease	

* These conditions require a veterinarian's diagnosis and treatment planning.

Behavioral causes of house soiling in dogs are less common than medical causes. The most common behavioral causes are listed in Table 12.4. Early detection is the key to rapidly restoring wellness and welfare for dogs with elimination concerns. Many clients will not volunteer information about changes in elimination patterns. Embarrassment, lack of knowledge, lack of supervision/observation, and not recognizing the importance of changes all contribute to underreporting by clients. Elimination concerns are at the top of the list for behavioral relinquishment and present a serious risk to the human–animal bond, so routine screening for elimination concerns should be performed at every visit. Each client should be asked about the quality and quantity of both urine and feces, if there are any unwanted eliminations, and if this is a change from the dog's previous condition.

Table 12.4 Behavioral diagnoses with an elimination component in dogs and cats.*

Differential diagnoses	Possible elimination patterns observed
Fears and phobias	• Eliminates when confined or alone • Eliminates in response to exposure to stimulus • Reluctance to eliminate when exposed to stimulus (e.g. will not eliminate outdoors on garbage truck day)
Separation distress	
Sound sensitivity/noise phobia	
Fear of any specific stimulus	
Generalized anxiety	
Substrate preference:	• Eliminates near but not in provided substrate • Reduced site selection behaviors • Does not dig/cover (cats) • Eliminates without touching substrate • Eliminates on similar substrates regularly (paper, clothing, towels, rugs)
Conditioned aversion (pain, infection)	
Conditioned preference for other	
Appeasement urination	• Urinates in socially overwhelming situations • Urination coincides with body language of appeasement
Excitement urination	• Urinates when overly excited or experiencing conflicting motivations • Urination coincides with body language of conflict (e.g. approach–retreat sequence) • Urination coincides with body language of high arousal
Stress-related elimination	• Any change in elimination habits
"Pandora's syndrome"	
(Feline interstitial/sterile cystitis)	
Cognitive dysfunction/changes	• Any change in elimination habits

* These conditions require a veterinarian's diagnosis and treatment planning.

Some urination is objectionable to clients but normal for animals, namely urine marking. Placing urine in socially important locations is a normal way for both male and female dogs and cats to communicate. Urine marking is a diagnosis of exclusion and history. Medical causes for increased frequency of urination should always be ruled out if urine marking is suspected. Dogs who are found to be engaging in urine marking should be housetrained using the protocol described earlier in this chapter.

Suggestions for decreasing unwanted urine marking in dogs include:

- Veterinarian has ruled out all medical and behavioral disorder diagnoses.
- Daily physical exercise and mental stimulation.
- Screen the pet for stress, reduce stressors as much as possible.
- If inter-dog competition or conflict is diagnosed within the household, treat accordingly.
- Opportunity is provided for urine marking in acceptable locations (e.g. on walks).
- Direct supervision and management to reduce opportunity to mark in unwanted areas.
- Positive reinforcement for all appropriate elimination.
- Placing urination on cue.
- Gentle interruption of precursors to mark (sniffing/flanking up to likely marking locations).
- Thorough cleaning of any urine contaminated areas.
- Judicious use of belly bands or diapers in select situations.*

* The use of belly bands or diapers will appeal to many clients but these strategies do not address the underlying concern and can have sequelae such as urinary tract infection, dermatologic problems, development of elimination disorders, and more. Veterinarians should be consulted prior to the use of these tools.

INAPPROPRIATE ELIMINATION: CATS

House soiling, or unwanted elimination, is the single most common unwanted behavior described by cat owners, and it poses a serious risk to the human–animal bond. Unwanted elimination is easiest to reverse when it is detected early and a comprehensive diagnostic and treatment plan is provided. The longer unwanted elimination has continued, the more guarded the prognosis becomes for the pet returning to the client's preferred elimination habits.

During every feline visit, the client should be questioned about any changes in the cat's elimination behavior, and if there is any elimination outside the litter box. Often, clients do not volunteer this information and must be asked. By establishing the habit of asking every cat owner during every visit, the technician takes the lead in early detection while simultaneously educating the client that changes in elimination should be promptly reported to the veterinary team. The technician or nurse should alert the veterinarian to any elimination concerns right away, regardless of the presenting complaint for the day's visit. Veterinarians should provide a complete medical workup for any cat showing signs of unwanted elimination. Underlying disease is a common cause of unwanted elimination in both cats and dogs. Once the unwanted elimination habit is established, it can present challenges to reverse and often a combination of treating both the physical illness and a comprehensive behavior modification plan will be required for successful resolution of unwanted elimination.

Housetraining for Cats

Prevention is crucial. Kitten and new cat owners should be counseled in providing what their cats need and prefer in an effort to prevent unwanted eliminations. Many cat owners may believe cats are "self-training" for litter use, and to a certain extent this may appear to be the case from the client's perspective. Clients need to understand how to arrange the environment and situation (antecedent arrangement) to promote litter box use over time.

Litter Box Etiquette

Much behavioral house soiling (toileting, substrate aversion) can be prevented by educating pet owners about litterbox etiquette. Many cat owners are unaware what cats need and want with respect to litterboxes. Most pet suppliers try to appeal to humans rather than cats, with the cats being the ultimate victims. Based on research, most cats prefer the following guidelines.[15]

Guideline #1: Size Matters!

Most cats prefer large, low, open, litter trays. Sweater boxes and storage containers make affordable, appropriate litter pans. Pet store litter trays are often too small. The cat should be able to enter the litter tray, turn around, dig, eliminate, cover, turn around, and exit the litter tray without touching the sides or top of the tray and without touching soiled litter. Figure 12.4 shows examples of litter trays constructed from storage boxes and sweater boxes commonly used for cats.

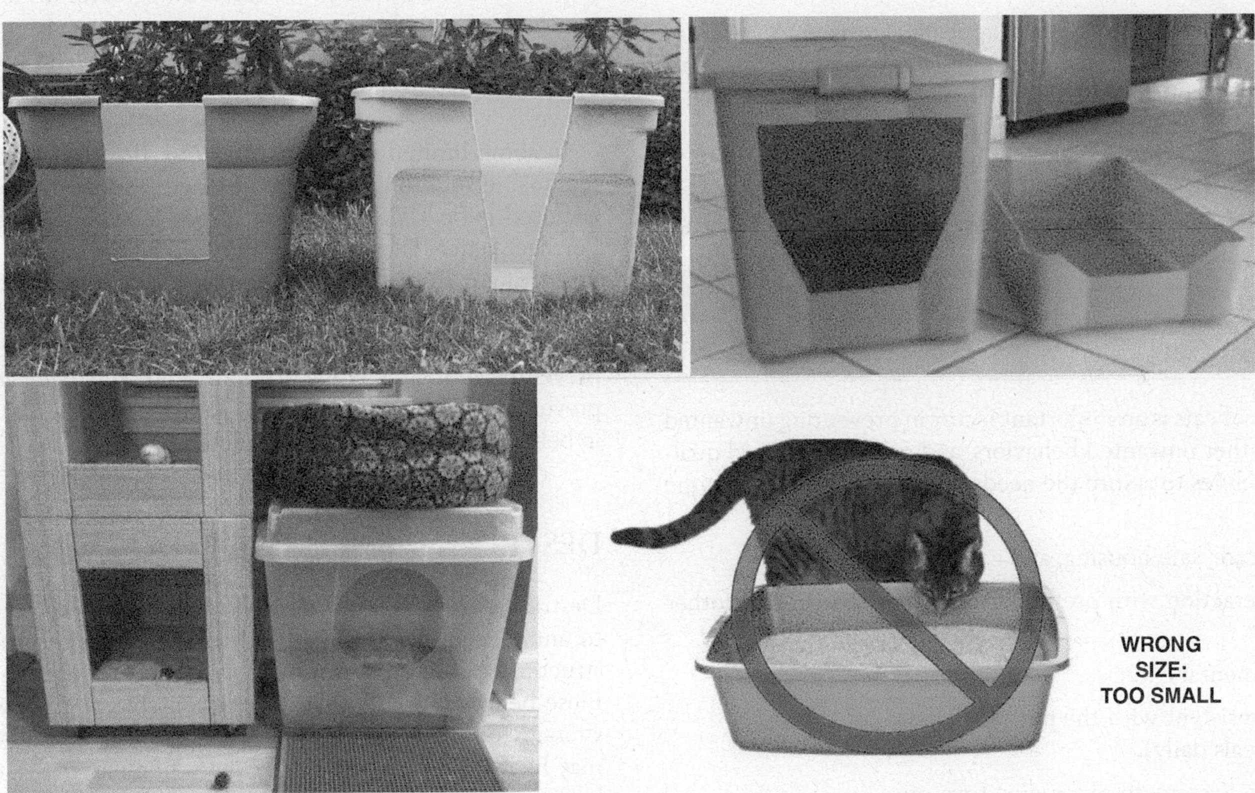

Figure 12.4 Three excellent examples of litter boxes, and one example showing a commercially available litter box that is too small for the cat.

Guideline #2: Substrate Matters

Kittens develop a substrate preference at a young age (prior to seven weeks), but this substrate preference can change over time and with experience. According to research, most cats prefer unscented fine grit clumping litter. If a kitten seems reluctant about a substrate, providing a "litter tray cafeteria" temporarily with several substrates available may allow the kitten to show the client which substrate is best for that individual.

Guideline #3: Litter Tray Hygiene

Litter trays should be kept clean to remain appealing to cats. An analogy which is helpful with some clients is the public restroom. Imagine you walk into a public restroom stall, push the door open, and find the toilet bowl is already soiled. What do you do next? Most humans will walk to the next stall and check that one, seeking a cleaner area to eliminate.

A good guideline is for litter to be scooped daily, dumped and replaced weekly, the litter trays scrubbed with soap and water monthly, and the litter trays replaced yearly.

Meeting the Needs of Cats

Meeting the basic needs of cats is an important factor in preventing unwanted elimination, as well as other unwanted behaviors, and providing a good quality of life .[16] A few guidelines to assure the needs of cats are being met in the home environment:

- Regular veterinary care, safe housing, and good nutrition.
- Adequate social interaction with preferred social partners (human/other species) daily.
- Daily physical and mental exercise.
- Feeding program consistent with the normal behavior of cats (numerous small meals daily).

Doc & Phoebe's Feeding System, food foraging toys, etc.

- Environment of plenty:
  - High perching areas
  - Enclosed hiding areas
- Multiple feeding stations and elimination stations, especially if a multi-cat household.
- Use of synthetic pheromone products may be helpful.

Urine Marking

As discussed in the canine section, depositing eliminations and secretions is normal behavior for animals, but the location selected can sometimes be unpalatable to humans. Prevention strategies for urine marking include meeting the basic needs of cats, working to create harmony in multi-cat households, and protecting cats from stress as much as possible. These strategies sound familiar because they are similar to the general strategies provided above.

In some limited situations, allowing the cat to have outdoor access is a reasonable solution. Cats provided with outdoor access should have a fully enclosed patio ("Catio"), or cat-proof fenced yard using a product such as PurrFect Fence. These options allow the cat to experience the outdoors while protecting it from fighting with other cats, automobile accidents, and often from predation or other injury.

Educating clients is the key to preventing problems when they can be prevented, and intervening promptly and effectively when the problem is not preventable. The technician's role in client education is a critical component in behavioral medicine and wellness.

DESTRUCTIVE BEHAVIOR: DOGS

Destructive behavior by dogs is described by many owners relinquishing dogs to animal shelters. Engaging in ripping, tearing, shredding, digging, deconstructing, and so on, is normal dog behavior. Dogs need an outlet to perform these behaviors in a way that is acceptable to the owner, and a prevention strategy for unwanted destructive behavior. While some destructive behavior may be associated with anxiety, fears, phobias, frustration disorders, or other behavioral diagnoses, a veterinarian's diagnosis is required in those cases.[17] A dog that is destructive when home alone may have separation anxiety, but this is not the only possible explanation and the veterinary team must remain mindful that a veterinarian's diagnosis may or may not be required when clients describe unwanted destructive behavior.

Technicians can coach pet owners on developing reasonable expectations for their dogs. Providing puppy and dog owners with education about preventing destructive behavior will protect the human–animal bond.

Guideline #1: Healthy Options

Dogs interact with their environments in a variety of ways, including chewing, shredding, and digging. Providing puppies and dogs with safe items to destroy can satisfy this urge without bringing the dog into conflict with the owner. Using toys, food toy puzzles, sand boxes for digging, shredding toys/cardboard items, refillable toys such as KONG products, and safe chews will guide dogs to make appropriate choices. For dental safety, chews should be firm enough the dog finds them satisfying, but soft enough to be flexed when held between two fists or indented when pressed firmly with the edge of a thumbnail.

Guideline #2: Management, Training, Supervision, and Guidance

Puppies and dogs need a well-managed environment and plenty of direct supervision while they are learning what owners want and expect. Setting an expectation for supervision helps dog owners understand they have an opportunity to give their dogs the skills needed to be successful family members. Additionally, supervision is needed to keep dogs safe from accidents and prevent ingestion of and interaction with dangerous items. Learning to be a canine good citizen takes time. Most dogs do not reach social maturity and adult decision-making capabilities until two to three years of age. Judicious use of safe confinement may help to prevent unwanted destructive behavior when dogs cannot be supervised.

Watch for what is right. Puppies and dogs are making many right choices every day. Playing with toys, lying on a dog bed, keeping their paws on the floor instead of the kitchen counter, running happily in the yard, checking in with the owners regularly, and so much more. Tell owners to constantly be on the lookout for opportunities to reward the behaviors they want.[18] Human nature is to ignore unconcerning behaviors and intervene when there is a problem. Intervening only when there is a problem can result in accidental reinforcement of unwanted behaviors from the puppy's point of view. For example, the puppy is playing with a toy and nothing happens. The puppy picks up a shoe and suddenly is being chased, cajoled, spoken to, and touched. Which behavior resulted in more attention? Picking up a shoe might be repeated in the future. Further, attending only unwanted behavior can also result in damage to the human–animal bond if punishment is used (see Punishment Problems).

When a puppy or dog begins to engage in an unwanted behavior, the client should gently interrupt and then redirect into a wanted activity. For example, if the puppy picks up a shoe to carry, he should be offered a toy instead and provided with positive reinforcement for engaging with the toy. Shoes should then be put out of reach. A dog who begins to dig in the yard should be gently interrupted and provided an alternate activity that the client finds acceptable, such as play with a toy or digging in a designated location and positive reinforcement given for the desired behavior. If evidence of undesired behavior is discovered after the fact, this is a signal to the client that an upgrade in management, training, supervision, or all three is appropriate.

Guideline #3: Meeting a Dog's Needs

Every dog needs sufficient mental and physical stimulation daily. Mental and physical exercise release endorphins resulting in feelings of wellbeing, promote relaxation, and improve the human–animal bond. Physical stimulation means the opportunity to reach its personal maximum speed at least one a day. Aerobic exercise needs will vary widely by individual dog, life stage, maturity, breed, and so on. For some dogs, a leash walk at the pace of a human will be enough, while others need running, biking, swimming, time with a "flirt pole", retrieving, or other higher-octane activity.

Mental stimulation is perhaps even more crucial than physical exercise. Keeping a dog's mind engaged will improve the human–animal bond, provide the dog with skills the owner finds valuable, and increase welfare. Examples of ways to provide mental stimulation include:

- Food foraging toys for meals (throw away that food bowl!).
- Games like hide and seek, retrieving.
- Quick training sessions (five minutes or shorter):
  - Manners
  - Life skills (recall, leash walking, doorbell manners, greetings, go to crate or bed)
  - Tricks.

- Sports for pets and people:
  - Nose work, agility, disc dog, dock dog, canine freestyle, and many more.
- Breed-specific skills/sports:
  - Stockdog, gundog, terrier/barn hunt, racing.

DESTRUCTIVE BEHAVIOR: CATS

When surveyed, clients describe destructive behavior by cats as predominantly clawing and scratching with some overlap of house soiling. Cats scratch items to mark their territory by leaving visual and odor markers, to maintain the feet and nails, and possibly because it feels pleasurable. Even cats who have had their claws amputated engage in this behavior. The need to scratch items is normal for all cats and every cat needs the opportunity to engage in this behavior. Just as each cat has an individual personality, most cats also have individual preferences for scratching.[16]

Technicians should seize the opportunity to educate clients about this crucial normal behavior. A few brief guidelines can set clients and cats up for a lifetime of success.

Guideline #1: Give Cats What They Want

Cats will have individual preferences about texture, location, and orientation of scratching surfaces. Most commercially available scratching items are made of cardboard, rope, or carpet. Many cats will like these, but others may prefer wood, fabric, or leather. Some cats will like horizontal, low scratchers while others like angled or vertical options placed higher up.

Provide cats with several substrate, location, and orientation options for scratching, and place them in socially important areas of the home. A scratching post in the back bedroom will be less appealing than the arm of the sofa in the living room: one function of scratching is communication. As the client learns the cat's preferences, clients can offer primarily what the cat prefers.

Guideline #2: Management, Supervision, and Training

Cats are smart and can be trained, but many clients may not realize this is true. As with puppies and dogs, kittens and cats should be encouraged and rewarded when they make right choices. Play with toys, laying on the cat tree or pet bed, scratching on desired items, staying on the kitchen floor instead of the counter, and so many more right choices present themselves daily. As with dogs, accidental reinforcement by only responding to unwanted behaviors can strengthen those behaviors while also endangering the human–animal bond. Coach clients to watch for wanted behaviors and reward the kitten or cat whenever wanted behaviors are observed.

Crate training is traditionally considered for dogs rather than cats, but the judicious use of safe confinement may help prevent unwanted destructive behavior for cats. A large dog crate or pen can be used for short periods and to encourage sleeping at night and activity during the day.

An effective product to promote training cats to scratch appropriately was released by Ceva Animal Health in 2018: Feliscratch. Application of the Feliscratch product has been clinically proven to prevent and reduce unwanted scratching behavior, and to promote ideal scratching behavior in cats and kittens.

Guideline #3: Meeting a Cat's Needs

Cats need physical and mental stimulation daily (refer to the list in the elimination section). The myth of cats sleeping all day and requiring little engagement or exercise is widespread. Combat this myth with high-quality client education from the start. The Ohio State University's Indoor Pet Initiative is an excellent resource for clients and professionals regarding meeting the needs of cats.[19]

AGGRESSION: DOGS AND CATS

In the National Council on Pet Population Study and Policy research, "aggression" is not carefully identified.[4] It is presumed to include lunging, growling, snapping, barking, biting, and other displays which could be interpreted as offensive or defensive on the part of the dog. Owners often identify aggression correctly, but many also misidentify normal behavior as abnormal aggression. In day practice, I often have owners tell me their puppies are "attacking" them. These puppies are engaging in normal play behaviors with insufficiently inhibited bites. Pet owners should be advised to avoid any type of play that elicits biting, cease play and all attention immediately after a bite, play using large soft toys rather than hands, and engage in a positive-reinforcement based bite-inhibition program.

Some aggressive behavior is attributable to medical diagnoses, so any dog described by the owner as aggressive should be worked up for possible medical causes before pursuing behavior modification.[9] Many dogs who give aggressive displays are motivated by fear; some are motivated by defensiveness, others may be engaging in resource guarding, territorial behavior, or numerous other explanations. The technician's role in this scenario is to detect the problem by asking the right history questions, get the veterinarian involved, and facilitate referral or treatment as needed.

Some types of aggression may be preventable, especially inappropriate play and aggression related to fear. To prevent fear, puppies and kittens should be regularly exposed, in a safe and non-threatening way, to a variety of stimuli for the purpose of socialization in the hopes of preventing future fears, phobias and fear-related aggressive displays. These stimuli include anything the dog or cat may need to tolerate or be accustomed to as an adult including a variety of people (adults, children, teens, both sexes, races, variable clothing, noise level, jerky movements, to name a few), locations, sensory experiences, handling needs, and situations. Make a list of topics in this category to discuss with puppy and kitten owners during their first few visits and demonstrate a little at each visit. Advise clients that animals need the opportunity to learn two things:

1. The stimulus is *not* dangerous and the owner will keep the animal safe.
2. The stimulus predicts *good* things!

Using the systems described earlier in this chapter of desensitization, classical conditioning, and operant conditioning, planned exposures can be done and the dog and cat taught life skills which will serve everyone well.

Inappropriate Play

Bite inhibition and learning appropriate play is part of the education every puppy and kitten owner should teach their new companion. A few tips for every client involving play:

- If play is too rough (teeth and claws, overstimulation), stop play as calmly as possible and take an immediate break.
- Watch for problem times of day when puppies or kittens are overstimulated or overtired and provide them with a quiet place to rest rather than engaging in rough play.
- Refrain from physical punishment and creating conflict between humans and pets.
- Use toys and never encourage animals to play or playfight with human hands or body parts.
- For puppies, use large toys and the human holds 10% while 90% is available to the dog.
- For kittens, use large toys for wrestling, and fishing-pole or other similar toys for chasing.
- Avoid chasing games with both dogs and cats.
- Any time the client is concerned, they should contact the veterinary office for advice or referral.

BEHAVIOR IN THE VETERINARY HOSPITAL

Every day, the veterinary team interacts with animals who are experiencing stress and distress. Whether the animal has a learned fear of the veterinary setting, encounters fear-related social signals from other animals, or is experiencing pain or illness, stress can complicate the behavior of companion animals.

Technicians should approach animals with compassion while maintaining human safety as the highest priority. Paying close attention to body language, responding early and often when animals are stressed, setting up the environment for success, and using gentle techniques which promote cooperation will help keep both humans and animals safe in the veterinary setting.

The Hospital Environment

The hospital environment contains many odors, pheromones, surfaces, sounds, sights, tactile experiences, social interactions, and potentially physically uncomfortable experiences – all of which can combine to increase stress in our patients. Imagine an animal's coping ability like a literal water reservoir. Each stressor removes a bit of water from the reservoir. Being loaded into a carrier, placed into the car, seeing another animal in the lobby, hearing a dog barking, hearing a cat hissing, walking across a slippery floor, being pulled into an exam room, and waiting to be seen are stressors which require emotional "juice" from the pet. Each stressor removes some of the pet's coping ability for the day. When the coping reservoir is dry, the animal is no longer capable of coping or cooperating and can respond with extreme avoidance or defensive aggression. Setting up the environment to maximize patient comfort can decrease underlying stress and allow the patient more emotional reserve to cope with treatments.

Ideas for making the environment more animal-friendly include:

- Reduce waiting time in the lobby: have clients call from the car and only invite them inside when a room is ready.
- When possible, have dogs and cats wait separately or where they cannot see one another.
- Customer service representatives should provide traffic control and coach clients to prevent social interactions between their pets and other clients or other animals.
- Communicate with team members when moving pets – do not allow social interactions between animals while handling or moving them through the hospital.
- Provide non-slip surfaces on the scale, the floor of the exam room, the examination table, treatment locations, and floor of housing units.
- Use synthetic pheromone products throughout the hospital.
- Play music evidenced to relax pets and people.
- Provide treats in the lobby, exam rooms, and all treatment areas.
- Store plenty of treats, administration tools, and toys in each exam room.
- Provide comfortable bedding.
- Use housing large enough for the pet to choose to rest in different locations.
- Allow hiding areas for cats in the exam room and all housing areas.
- Provide a water bowl and litter pan in the exam room.
- Provide high places for cats to explore.
- Choose furniture which is home-like, such as low ottomans or sofas where pets can join the client rather than hard or slippery individual chairs.

TALKING TO THE ANIMALS: BODY LANGUAGE OF DOGS AND CATS

Animals rely primarily on physical signaling to communicate their thoughts and emotions. While vocalization is part of how dogs and cats communicate, body postures and positions comprise the bulk of communication. When we are observing animals, we must observe the entire animal and the context rather than just individual body parts, but awareness of individual signs is also useful.

This guide uses three categories to assess animal comfort. These criteria are adapted from the scale provided in *Cooperative Veterinary Care*.[14] Monitor your patients for:

- Acceptance of food, treats, or tactile interactions.
- Chosen proximity to veterinary team members.
- Body language signs and signals.

In general, the higher the patient's acceptance of food/treats/touch, the closer proximity they choose to veterinary team members, and the fewer body language signs of stress observed, the more relaxed the patient is. Patients who are more relaxed and less stressed will be safer and easier to handle. The majority of aggressive displays shown by animals in all contexts are fear related, and this is especially true in the veterinary setting.

Body Language Cues

Body language cues have a function: the cues send a message about the desire for social contact, how safe or threatened an animal feels, and what the animal wishes to happen next.[5,6] The primary signals seen in veterinary environments are distance-decreasing signals, where animals desire social interaction, neutral signals or ambivalence, where the animal does not have a strong desire to interact nor a strong desire to move away, or stress and distance-increasing signals, where the animal is asking for increased personal space and decreased interactions.

When animals communicate with subtle signals and these signals are ignored, the animal may feel obligated to increase the intensity of the signals until the function or effect is achieved. By being sensitive to more subtle signals and responding in a way the pet understands, the veterinary team can de-escalate patient stress and decrease the instance of defensive aggression in the veterinary setting.

For a quick reference to body language signals, refer to Table 12.5. Figure 12.5 provides a guideline including illustrations for interpreting dog and cat body language called the spectrum of fear, anxiety, and stress.

Table 12.5 Quick reference for individual body signals and corresponding stress levels.

Individual physical characteristics	Relaxed	Mild stress	Moderate stress	Severe stress
Pupils	Normal for ambient light	Normal to mild dilation	Mild to moderate dilation	Fully dilated
Muscles	Soft	Soft	Some tension	Tense; some will be frozen
Haircoat	Flat	Flat	Flat	Some piloerection; cats may puff tail
Tail	Dog: midline or lower, soft Cat: midline or higher, crook tip	Midline or lower, soft	Dog: above or below midline, tense Cat: tucked, tense, tip may flick	Dog: high or tucked tight, tense Cat: tucked or lashing, tense
Gaze	Freely moves, chooses to look at and interact with people	Freely moves but looks away	Gaze will fix on threat or fix away from threat	Looking directly at or completely away from threat; direct staring
Mouth	Soft lips, closed mouth	Mouth may open, lips relaxed; dogs may pant lightly	Mouth tense, commissure of lips tight; dogs may pant with lips pulled back	Mouth tense, lips may be retracted to show teeth; dogs may pant heavily with lips pulled back, or close mouth with tight tense lips
Paws	All paws on the ground, freely moving	Dogs may lift a front paw, may place paws on humans	Cats: conceal one or several paws Dogs: lifting a front paw, pawing at humans	Cats: all paws tightly tucked, may strike with front paws Dogs: standing or crouching with weight forward or backward

THE SPECTRUM OF FEAR, ANXIETY & STRESS
RED: SEVERE SIGNS - FIGHT/AGGRESSION (FAS 5)
• Offensive aggression - pupils constricted or dilated. cat leaning forward. ears forward. moving forward. whiskers forward, tait is an inverted L (first inch of tail is horizontal with ground then the tail drops down), rump raised higher than front (on tip toes), staring, may be growling.
• Defensive aggression - ears back. pupils dilated. hunkered down. tail tight or tucked or tail thrashing, whiskers back, hissing, lips pulled back, staring. furrowed brow, could be swatting.
RED: SEVERE SIGNS - FIGHT/FREEZE/FRET (FAS 4)
• Flight - actively trying to escape, pupils dilated. ears back, whiskers back. tail down and bottle brushed, fleeing, turning to look at stimulus.
• Freeze/Fret - tonic immobility, dilated pupils. body flattened and tense, tail tucked, increased respiratory rate. ears back. staring. whiskers back.
YELLOW: MODERATE SIGNS (FAS 2-3)
• Ears further to the side, more pupil dilation but not completely dilated, increase in respiratory rate, brow furrowed. looking at stimulus instead of looking away, tail tight to body. possible tip of tail moving some, whiskers back. body crouched and leaning away.
GREEN: MILD/SUBTIE SIGNS (FAS 1)
• Avoids eye contact, turns head away without moving away, partially dilated pupils, head held just slightly down. slight brow furrowing. whiskers slightly back, ears partially to the side, body shifted slightly away. tail closer to body with possibly some slight flicking.
GREEN: PERKED/INTERESTED/ANXIOUS? (FAS 0-1)
• Looking directly but not intensely. tail up and winding, mouth closed with loose lips, ears perked forward. whiskers forward. slight pupil dilation.
GREEN: REIAXED (FAS 0)
A: Sleeping
B: Neutral - ears in neutral position. brow soft, eyes soft, mouth closed with relaxed lips. body loose, tail carriage U-shaped. pupils normal dilation.
C: Friendly greeting - tail up and winding, may elevate rear end slightly by standing on toes, ears neutral, forward. or slightly back. might have squinty eyes, brow relaxed, might cheek mark or rub on person or object.
(A)
(B)
(C)
ZZZ
FEAR FREE
www.fearfreepets.com
THE SPECTRUM OF FEAR, ANXIETY & STRESS
RED: SEVERE SIGNS - FIGHT/AGGRESSION (FAS 5)
• Offensive Aggression -lunging forward. ears forward, tail up. hair may be up on the shoulders. rump. and tail, showing only the front teeth, lip puckerlips pulled forward. tongue tight and thin. pupils poSSibly dilated or constricted.
• Defensive Aggression - hair may be up on the back and rump. dilated pupils, direct eye contact, showing all teeth including molars. body crouched and retreating, tail tucked ears back.
RED: SEVERE SIGNS - FIGHT/FREEZE/FRET (FAS 4)
• Flight - ears back. tail tucked, actively trying to escape - slinking away or running. mouth closed or excessive panting - tongue tight instead of loose out of mouth. showing whites of eyes, brow furrowed, pupils dilated.
• Freeze/Fret - tonic immobility, pupils dilated. increased respiratory rate. trembling, tense closed mouth, ears back, tail tucked, body hunched.
YELLOW: MODERATE SIGNS (FAS 3)
• Similar to FAS 2 but turning head away, may refuse treats for brief moments or take treats roughly, may be hesitant to interact but not completely avoiding interaction.
YELLOW: MODERATE SIGNS (FAS 2)
• Ears slightly back or to the side. tail down but not necessarily completely tucked, furrowed brow. slow movements or unable to settle, fidgeting, attention seeking to owner, panting with a tighter mouth, moderate pupil dilation.
GREEN: MILD/SUBTLE SIGNS (FAS 1)
• Tail up higher, looking directly, mouth closed, eyes more intense, more pupil dilation. brow tense, hair may bejust slightly up on the back and tail, may be expectant and excited or highly aroused.
GREEN: ALERT/EXCITED/ANXIOUS? (FAS 0-1)
• l ooking directly but not intensely, tall up slightly, mouth open slightly but lips loose, ears perked forward, slight pupil dilation.
GREEN: PERKED/INTERESTED/ ANXIOUS? (FAS 0-1)
• Looking directly but not intensely. tall up slightly, mouth open slightly but loose lips, ears perked forward, slight pupil dilation.
GREEN: REIAXED (FAS 0)
A: Sleeping.
B: Neutral- ears in neutral position, not perked forward, brow soft, eyes soft, mouth closed but lips relaxed, body loose, tail carriage neutral. pupils normal dilation.
C: Friendly greeting - slow back and forth tail and butt wag, ears just slightly back, relaxed brow and eyes, may have mouth slightly open with relaxed lips and loose tongue.
(A)
(B)
(C)
FEAR FREE
www.fearfreepets.com

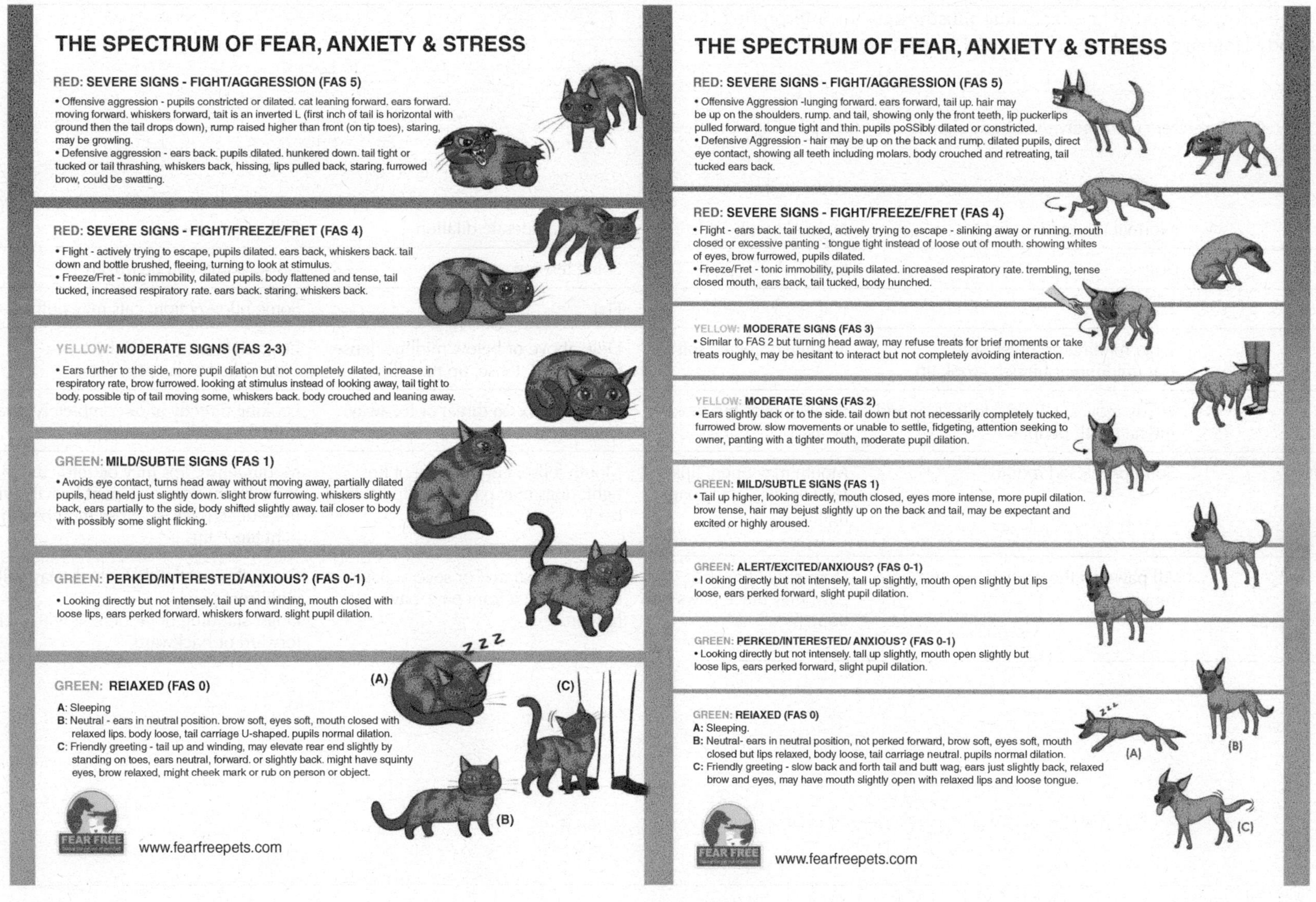

Figure 12.5 The spectrum of fear, anxiety and stress; body language signs associated with increased stress and decreased welfare. Source: courtesy of Fear Free.

Relaxed Body Language

Animals with relaxed body language are likely to seek social interaction and give distance-decreasing signals, indicating they are interested in being close to team members and involved. In some instances, animals may give distance-decreasing signals when they are feeling conflicted or ambivalent, so the animal's desire to come closer should be interpreted with respect to the overall body language displayed. Relaxed animals will willingly explore the environment and move around the examination room.

Relaxed dog body language includes soft muscles, a soft facial expression, normal pupil size, ears oriented forward or relaxing low for drop-ear breeds, whiskers held in a neutral position, tail held in the natural carriage or lower and softly wagging or hanging soft, mouth closed and soft or panting with a relaxed jaw and the tongue soft, sometimes with a curled tip.

Relaxed cat body language includes soft muscles, a soft facial expression, normal pupil size, ears erect and soft, relaxed brow, whiskers held neutral or slightly back, mouth closed, tail held up with a soft curve in the tip.

Mild Stress: Welfare and Safety Monitoring Indicated

Mildly stressed dogs will usually accept food/toy/tactile interactions and if they briefly disengage, they re-engage rapidly.

Dogs experiencing mild stress will show any or all of these signs, but infrequently: mild pupil dilation, mild muscle tension when touched, a soft facial expression with a more intent gaze, ears held slightly to the side or down, occasional lip licking, occasional yawning, looking away or moving away briefly but will return to the interaction, lifting a paw, tail held down or slightly higher than when relaxed.

Mildly stressed dogs may show stress signs when touched or handled, but will rapidly return to their baseline body language when touching is stopped.

Cats experiencing mild stress will show similar engagement and re-engagement to dogs. They may show any or all of these signs but infrequently: mild pupil dilation, looks away without moving away, ears slightly to the side, tail held tighter to the body, whiskers held closer to face, decreased desire to explore.

Mildly stressed animals can often be handled quickly and treatments performed, but they are at risk for increased stress levels over time, if serial treatments are needed, with hospitalization, and as they have repeated experiences with the veterinary hospital.

Moderate Stress: Welfare and Safety Likely Compromised

Moderate stress is a situation where team safety is easily compromised, and where animal welfare may also be compromised. When pets are experiencing moderate stress, the veterinarian should be consulted to triage wants compared with needs for the visit, and medication to reduce the stress associated with the visit and handling should be considered. While the veterinarian is responsible for determining which treatments and/or medications are appropriate to pursue, every member of the veterinary team is empowered to decide if they are comfortable handling a given animal, and if they believe handling that animal is in the animal's best interest.

Dogs experiencing moderate stress may show any of the signs listed under mild stress plus any or all of these signals: intermittently refusing food previously accepted, or taking food with a rough grab when previously gentle; looking away and moving away; choosing not to interact; furrowed brow; moderately dilated pupils; ears held back or down; lips held back; panting with tense lips held back and little tongue visible; tense muscles; inability to settle/sit still; seeking attention from the owner; generally fidgety. Signs of stress increase with handling.

Cats in moderate stress may show any of the signs listed under mild stress plus any or all of these signals: refusing food previously accepted; prefers not to interact; does not explore; tail held tight to the body; paws folded under the body when lying down; reluctant to leave carrier/prefers to hide; ears held to the side; looks away from and then at potential threats rather than only looking away; tail tip may twitch.

Severe Stress: Welfare and Safety Significantly Compromised

Severe stress should be relieved with medications and sedatives whenever possible, and a plan made for future visits to minimize continuing or repeated stressful events. Animals in extreme stress will generally either be "frozen", attempting to escape, or showing distance-increasing signals and/or defensive aggression. Severe stress significantly compromises the safety of veterinary team members, and has a significant impact on animal welfare. Severe fear-related distress can be both physically and emotionally harmful to animals. If a technician is handling an animal experiencing severe stress and the current treatment is not immediately life saving, treatment should be paused and a veterinarian involved to triage wants and needs and make a stress relief plan before resuming treatment.

Dogs in severe stress may show any of the above signs and/or the following: dilated pupils; ears held back; tail tucked; escape attempts; no interest in exploration or interaction; trembling; rapid panting with lips held tightly back; brow furrowed; whites of eyes visible (unless normal for that breed); cowering; staring; piloerection; showing teeth; growling; barking; snapping; biting.

Cats in severe stress may show any of the above signs and/or the following: dilated pupils; ears held flat; piloerection, especially of the tail; whiskers held completely flat or forward; escape attempts; body flattened; tail tucked tightly against the body or held out at the base then low; staring; hissing; growling; showing teeth; striking with paws and/or claws; biting.

HANDLING STRATEGIES: TIPS AND BASICS

Handling strategies have changed radically as we continue to better understand the motivations and needs of animals, as well as how to best assist them in feeling safe and comfortable during medical care. When handling animals, I encourage the concept of stabilization rather than older techniques referred to as restraint. Stabilization means supporting the animal at all times so that it feels secure and will not slip or fall, gently preventing unwanted movements, and communicating through touch both how to cooperate and what to expect next. Further, quality animal handling always involves good communication between team members, a contingency plan for how to safely change or stop the handling session should the animal's stress level escalate, and a hospital policy.

Multiple handling curricula are readily available for veterinary professionals and provide much-needed detail about appropriate handling techniques. *Low Stress Handling and Behavior Modification of Dogs and Cats* by Dr. Sophia Yin,[20] Low Stress Handling® University courses,[21] and the Fear Free® Professional Certification Program[22] all provide helpful detailed instruction in animal handling well beyond what can be discussed here. The language in this chapter reviews the Fear Free Certification Program's terminology.

Throughout a handling event, the veterinary team should monitor the patient for signs of increasing stress and always be ready to change the plan or triage some treatments to a later date. After creating an inviting environment as discussed earlier, we are ready to interact with patients. Some core guidelines for animal handling follow.

Before You Begin: Collecting Valuable Data

Before a pet's visit, the client should be questioned for possible warning signs about patient stress. Customer service team members can have a conversation about patient stress when scheduling an appointment, or a questionnaire can be easily emailed for the client to return when it is convenient. Incorporating the form into a mobile-friendly website is a good way to increase compliance. Figure 12.6 shows a sample online questionnaire designed by Fear Free.

PRE-VISIT QUESTIONNAIRE

FEAR FREE

Date: ______

Client Name: ______ Pet's Name: ______

As a Fear Free Certified Professional team, we want to make you pet's veterinary experience as enjoyable and as stress free as possible. As such, it's important for us to understand what your pet might find upsetting. The information will help us to adjust our care to better serve and comfort your pet. Please answer the following questions to the best of your ability so we can take into consideration both your & your pet's preferences.

Does your pet show any reluctance to getting in the carrier or car? Yes No

How and where does your pet travel in the car? (carrier, seatbelt, loose, etc.): ______

During travel to the veterinary hospital, does your pet do any of the following:

Eager & excited Reluctant Hide Drool Vomit Urine/BM

Subdued Bark/Meow Whine Pant Tremble Pace Other______

Does your pet prefer:

Female veterinary professional Male veterinary professional It doesn't matter

Check any situations listed below that your pet has shown avoidance or dislike of in the past. You can add additional comments at the end.

Getting in their carrier or the car
Entering the veterinary hospital
Other pets and/or people passing by while in reception/check-in
Waiting with other people and animals in the waiting area
Being approached by veterinary staff
Getting on the scale for a weight
Hearing the doorbell, overhead intercom, or phones ringing
Sounds coming from the back areas of the practice
Going into the exam room
Being put up on the table for examination
Having direct eye contact with the technician and/or veterinarian
Loud voices during examination
Having a rectal temperature taken
The use of instruments such as the stethoscope or otoscope (to look in the ears)
Being taken out of the exam room for procedures

How would you describe your pet around other animals and people?

Does your pet have any sensitive areas that s/he does not like to have touched by you or others?

Are there any procedures your pet has not liked having performed at the veterinary hospital in the past or that seemed difficult for you or the staff to do? (nail trims, weight, temperature, ear exam, blood draw) If so, how did you pet react?

What are your pet's favorite treats? (Please bring some to your next visit to our hospital):

Does your pet like to play with toys? If so what kinds?

Has your pet ever been prescribed any supplements or medications to help with a visit to the veterinary hospital? If so, what was it and what sort of results did you experience?

Anything else you would like us to know?

VETERINARY HEALTHCARE TEAM: Transfer all applicable information form questionnaire to the patient's Fear Free Emotional Medical Record.

Figure 12.6 Pre-visit questionnaire provided by Fear Free to assess patients and be better prepared prior to visits.

Guideline #1: Work Where the Pet is Comfortable

When possible and safe, work where a pet is most comfortable. This may be on the floor, the exam table, a bench or couch next to the client, in the bottom of a cat carrier, under a blanket or towel, or even referral for a house call.

Guideline #2: Use the Fear Free Touch Gradient Method

Animals have touch receptors all over their bodies, but they are not evenly distributed. Some areas of the body are naturally more sensitive than others based on distribution of nerve endings (Figure 12.7). Others may be more sensitive because of pain, individual conformation, individual preference, and learning history. For example, a dog with chronic otitis may flinch when a person reaches toward his ears even when an infection is not present due to learning history of ear touch predicting pain.

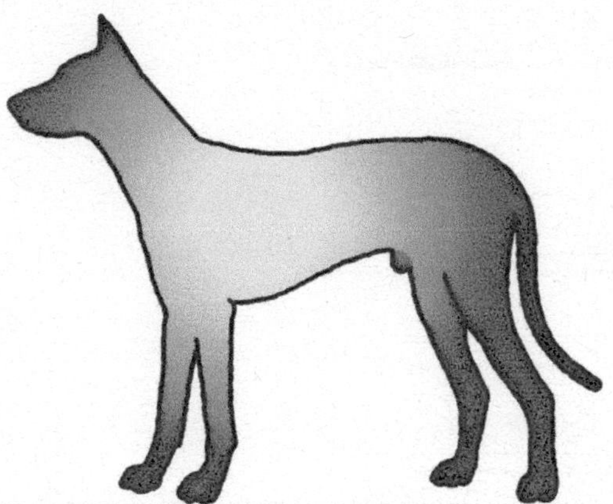

Figure 12.7 Body sensitivity. Source: Alicea Howell, Monique Feyrecilde, *Cooperative Veterinary Care*. **John Wiley & Sons, 2018.**

When touching animals, approach them from the side and begin touching in a non-sensitive body area – usually the sides of the trunk. Most dogs and cats find a hand over the head threatening, and many find touching of the hindquarters unpleasant or startling. Once you have established tactile contact with the pet, glide your hand or hands to each area of interest for examination or treatment. When possible, once tactile contact has begun, try to maintain some level of tactile contact until the handling session is complete. Many animals will startle each time touch is initiated, and reducing the number of times touch is started will reduce the number of startle responses.

Example : Paw Handling

- Begin touch at the shoulder, then glide to the elbow, forelimb, and paw.
- Only apply the amount of pressure needed to accomplish the current procedure.
- For hind limbs, begin touching on the side of the body, glide to the hip and then down the limb to the paw.

Guideline #3: Gentle Control and Stabilization

For many pets, "less is more" when it comes to stabilization. Use only the minimum amount of tactile contact and pressure to maintain the animal's position and keep the team safe. Be aware at all times of where the animal's head is, where it can move or is likely to move, and how you will respond when the pet moves. If the pet begins to show defensive aggression, quickly move away while maintaining team safety. This might mean holding the leash at an arm's length, allowing a cat to retreat into the carrier, or simply letting go and backing away from the pet. Care should be taken to make sure patients do not jump or fall off a table or out of an elevated cage – but human safety always comes first. In general, pausing treatments based on patient body language far before defensive aggression signs are shown will prevent team members from being placed in positions where safety is compromised. The days of simply physically overpowering an animal are behind us, much as they are in human pediatrics.[23]

If more than two people are required to hold a patient still for treatments, the handling strategy should be reviewed and changed. Forcefully placing animals on their sides or backs should be avoided. If a dog struggles for more than three seconds or three attempts, or a cat struggles for more than two seconds or two attempts, an alternate plan should be considered. Scruffing cats should also be avoided. These actions often prompt defensive aggression from patients, putting the veterinary team at risk of injury. Instead, the use of distractions, gentle handling, and medical stress reduction will be safer for everyone involved. Remember, every pleasant or unpleasant experience the animal has is recorded in its memory to draw upon when making decisions about how to behave in the veterinary setting in the future.

In many cases, the use of distractions is a desirable method of gentle control. Feeding treats during treatments using the desensitization and classical conditioning timing mentioned earlier in this chapter can be quite successful.

To use distractions, find a high value item the animal really enjoys (for a list of popular treat options for dogs and cats, see Box 12.3). While the animal is intrigued with the distraction, use touch gradient to initiate contact and perform brief treatments such as an ear swab, vaccination, or venipuncture. Distraction techniques are extremely useful for keeping relaxed and mildly stressed patients calm and content. However, in some patients, the use of distraction can lead to sensitization, as discussed earlier in this chapter.

Box 12.3 / Popular Treat Options for in-Hospital use for Dogs and Cats

Providing a variety of textures and tastes will improve the probability of treat acceptance.

Cats

- Kibble
- Canned cat food
- Canned cat food pureed
- Commercially produced cat treats, soft and crunchy
- Squeeze cheese/canned cheese
- Cream cheese packets
- Butter pats
- Bonito flakes/kitty caviar
- Flavored pastes commercially prepared (e.g. KONG)
- Freeze dried meats/organ meats/fish
- Baby food
- Liver paste/pate/braunschweiger
- Deli meat slices or cubes
- Canned whipped cream
- Anchovy paste
- Green olives (dice tiny)

Dogs

- Kibble
- Canned dog food
- Canned dog food pureed
- Commercially produced dog treats, soft and crunchy
- Squeeze cheese/canned cheese
- Cream cheese packets
- String cheese
- Flavored pastes commercially prepared (e.g. KONG)
- Nut butters (caution: some humans are allergic)
- Freeze dried meats/organ meats/fish
- Baby food
- Liver paste/pate/braunschweiger
- Deli meat slices or cubes
- Canned whipped cream
- Pretzel rods to administer soft foods
- Canned meats (SPAM, tuna, chicken, etc.)
- Pill Pockets/Pill Paste products
- Popcorn
- Goldfish crackers
- Cheerios or similar small cereals

To use desensitization and classical conditioning for an injection, this whole sequence may take only a few seconds in a comfortable animal:

1. Test to see whether the pet likes the treats, brushing, toy, or other reward being offered.
2. Touch a non-sensitive area → treat (toy, brushing, etc.).
3. Touch a non-sensitive area and glide to injection area → treat.
4. Glide to injection area and tent skin lightly → treat.
5. Glide to injection area, tent skin lightly and simulate injection with a pinch → treat.
6. If this is all well tolerated, glide to injection area, tent skin, inject while giving the treat.
7. Repeat step 2 twice to close the session.

Figure 12.8 shows several examples of patient positioning for common procedures.

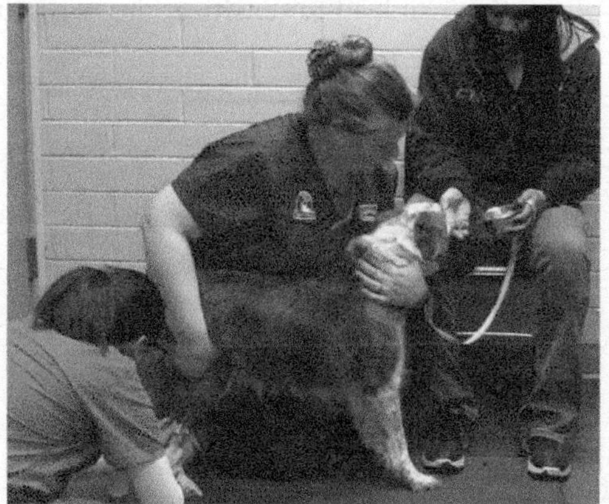
Standing lateral saphenous with stabilization, gentle control, and treats.

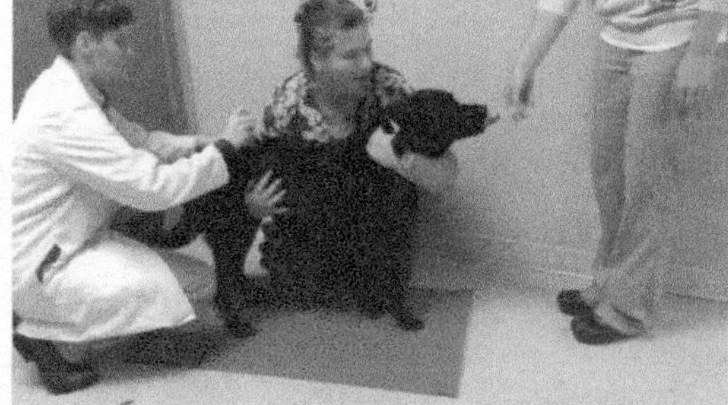
Intramuscular injection with stabilization, gentle control and treats.

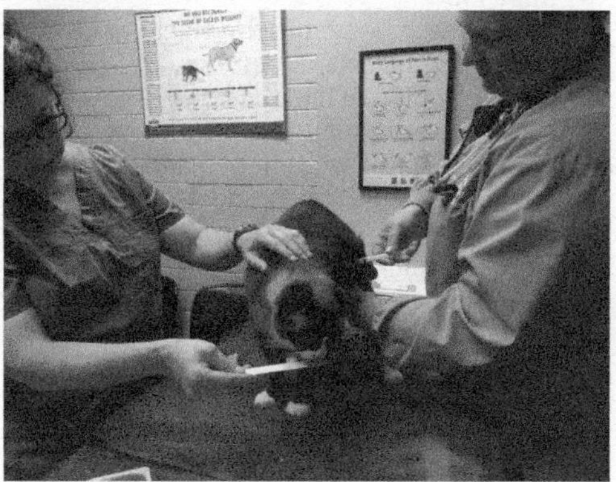
Standing cystocentesis, distraction method.

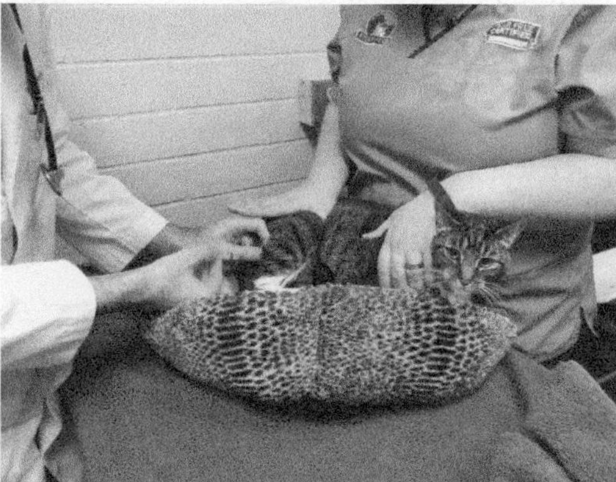
Distal vaccination in a soft bed with gentle control.

Figure 12.8 Common positioning for use of distractions, stabilization, and gentle control during basic procedures.

Guideline #4: Family Presence is Often Helpful

Family presence is calming for many pets. Hearing the owner's voice, seeing the owner, receiving treats and attention from the owner, and being able to seek comfort will all help patients relax in many situations. In human medicine, healing times are hastened, overall hospital stays are decreased in length, and patient perception of time spent in the hospital is more favorable if the family is encouraged to be present.

In rare instances, a veterinary team member may feel that the animal is being made more anxious by a client using a high-pitched voice, rapid stroking, or strong restraint. If this happens, the veterinary team can direct the client how to interact in a more helpful way. For example, "Ms. Taylor, can I hand you these 20 small treats? I would like you to drop one into this dish for Fifi to eat every 2 seconds. Before you drop each treat, tell Fifi you'll be dropping it by saying her name and then "treat". Many clients are anxious coming to the veterinary clinic, and they need to be able to trust the veterinary team. The veterinary team can and should direct the client how to remain safe but also be most helpful.

In more common instances, some veterinary team members may describe a patient as "better behaved without the owner present". Most patients who appear "better behaved" or "more cooperative" without the client are displaying the freezing behavior discussed earlier in this chapter in the section on severe stress. When the comfort of the client is removed, the patient's behavior becomes suppressed and fear inhibits them showing normal responses. Concerns about client safety in the presence of animals who are receiving treatment can be allayed by having clients stand within view but out of reach while a veterinary team member stabilizes the pet. It can be safe to have clients give treats during a variety of treatments, at the discretion and instruction of the veterinary team. When home treatments are prescribed, the client may be administering pills, injections, shampoos, salves, oral liquids, topical spot-on treatments, and any number of other medications. Instructing the client in proper administration keeping pet welfare and human safety in mind and then supervising while they practice is a necessary part of any treatment recommendation.

Practicing medicine with the client present can dramatically change the way the veterinary team helps both clients and patients. In the past, when strong physical restraint was normative, veterinary teams often separated the patient from the client so physical restraint could be applied in a large workspace where the client would not be present if the animal showed aggression. Keeping clients safe is crucially important, but handling animals with compassion and care is crucial as well. Further, it is difficult for clients to perceive the true value of treatments administered when it is all done out of view. A good rule of thumb is never to use a handling method or restraint hold on a patient that you would not use in front of that beloved pet's owner.

Guideline #5: Thick Towels, Blankets, Cones, and Basket Muzzles

Keep a stock of thick towels and blankets in the hospital for emergency use. Thick towels, blankets, and comforters can be used to safely lift and sedate many extremely fearful animals. By using a thick blanket or towel, the veterinary technician can protect his or her body and hands while safely and briefly securing the patient. When choosing a towel or blanket, choose material and fold it such that the thickness of the material is thicker than the length of the patient's canine teeth. If the patient bites the towel or blanket, this keeps hands safe. Refer to the low stress handling resources listed earlier in this chapter for detailed instructions on the use of towels and blankets.

For some pets, placing a cone collar designed to prevent self-trauma after surgery can help the pet relax and protect veterinary team members during brief procedures. Further, the use of basket muzzles, as shown in Figure 12.9, can help to keep team members safe and allow them to relax more when handling dogs that show defensive aggression. A towel rolled and placed around the neck of a dog or cat like a donut or scarf can often help the pet remain calm and provide safe control for sedation or a very brief procedure. Veterinary teams must remember that just because a patient is physically confined by a neck wrap, cone, or muzzle, we must also pay attention to the animal's body language. Safely "disarming" a pet using this equipment is not a permission slip to handle the animal with any less caution or consideration than we would use without that same equipment.

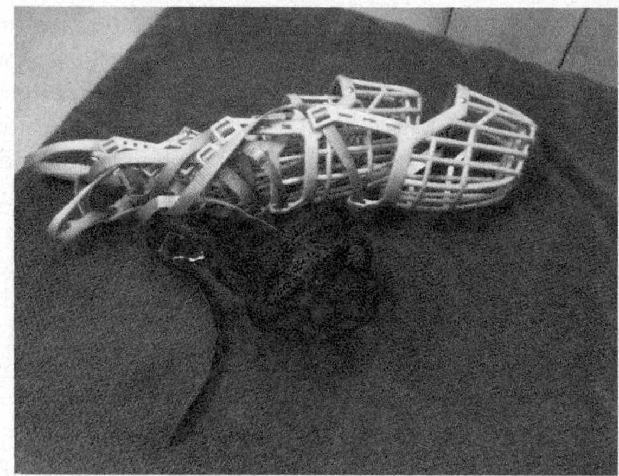

Figure 12.9 Assorted sizes of quick-snap basket muzzles.

Guideline #6: Rehearsing Conversations

Using the animal handling strategies outlined in this chapter will result in frequent use of stress-relieving medications and sedation. These medications are appropriate for many patients, and discussing their use should be a normal part of hospital culture. Having a strategy for discussing these medicines for clients prior to recommending them is important for gaining client compliance. Describing the medications as being used to decrease stress, decrease pain, and assure the pet does not form a negative memory of the experience will all help. Avoiding labels like "uncooperative", "fractious", "bad", or "mean", will improve internal hospital culture as well as facilitating compassionate client communication.

- Example:

  "Mrs. Smith, Fido has an infection of her left ear. It is red and inflamed, and we should flush it out thoroughly. Before treating this painful ear, the doctor would like to give her some medicine which will reduce pain, keep her calm, and make sure we can do a thorough job. With your permission, can we proceed?"

- Example:

  "Mr. Jones, I see Bowser is looking away, moving away, and panting when we touch his leg. These signs may mean he is painful and that touching his leg causes him stress. He will need an x-ray to help us make a diagnosis. Before the x-ray, the veterinarian will give him some medication to reduce any pain and stress as well as relax his muscles so the x-ray is high quality. May we proceed with that plan?"

- Example:

  "Ms. White, see how Muffin is pulling her legs tightly under her and flicking her tail tip? When she sees the syringe I would like to use to draw her blood, she tries to move away. The blood test is important but not time sensitive, and giving Muffin a pleasant experience is also important because stress can change the bloodwork results. I have some medicine the veterinarian would like to send home with you to give tonight and tomorrow morning. Then tomorrow when Muffin feels more relaxed, we can collect her blood and give her a better experience as well as getting more accurate test results."

Guideline #7: Write it Down!

Medical records are the perfect place to record a patient's body language, individual preferences (e.g. provider preference, location preference, favorite treats, individual sensitivities) and success strategies. By making specific notes about what works best for each patient, the veterinary team will streamline future handling events, improving both efficiency and profitability. Simple warnings or cautions do not provide instructions for how to proceed. Like animals, people learn best and achieve the most when we are instructed what to do rather than what not to do. Success Notes are key to making every visit better for the team, the patient, and the client over time.

MEDICAL TREATMENT OF FEAR

Administering medication is an excellent way to mitigate fear of the veterinary environment, procedures, and hospitalization. Every team member has an important role in noting signs of stress and fear in patients, and reporting these signs along with any physical findings as well as recording them in the chart. Patients who are hospitalized will often benefit from the addition of stress-relieving medications to their protocols. Pets who fear coming to the veterinary hospital or find specific treatments such as vaccinations and blood collection will be easier and safer to handle if their fear is reduced.

Many medications and combinations of medications can be given orally and by injection or even constant rate infusion to reduce fear. One caution: acepromazine should not be used as a sole agent. The sedative effects of acepromazine will slow the animal's ability to respond to stimuli, but research has demonstrated patients develop increasing severity of fear over repeated exposures when acepromazine has been administered.[24]

UNIQUE CHALLENGES: EMERGENCY/CRITICAL CARE PATIENTS

Many patients who are ill enough to require emergency and critical care will not accept food or are food-restricted for medical reasons. Food is not the only way to provide a low-stress handling event.

Use these tips to help reduce stress in the emergency care setting:

- Non-slip surfaces.
- Quiet work areas.
- Preventing social contact between patients.
- Using touch gradient for all physical contact.
- Provide non-medical touching before and after treatments for pets who like it.
- Use soft, comforting voices when talking to patients or to colleagues while in the patient areas.
- Work to keep patients in the wards quiet and comfortable to decrease everyone's stress.
- Allow family presence/family visitation to offer comfort.
- Work at the pet's pace – divide or combine treatments based on patient preference.
- Devise a hospital policy for reporting and recording emotional as well as physical changes in patients.
- Administer stress-reducing medications and comprehensive analgesia.
- Use a fresh needle for every injection (change after drawing up medications).
- Apply adhesive remover products prior to pulling off tape or other bandage materials.
- Use success notes for handling to help pets and people work together.

REFERENCES

1. Martin, K., Martin, D. (2015). The role of the veterinary technician in animal behavior. In: *Canine and Feline Behavior for Veterinary Technicians and Nurses* (ed. J. Shaw and D. Martin), 1–29. Ames, IA: Wiley.
2. Yin S. (2014). Calm pets, happy vets. Reducing stress and preventing and managing fear aggression in veterinary clinics. *Eur J Companion Anim Pract* 24: 28–36.
3. Salman, M.D., Hutchison, J., Ruch-Gallie, R. *et al.* (2000). Behavioral reasons for relinquishment of dogs and cats to 12 shelters. *J Appl Anim Welfare Sci* 3: 93–106.
4. Miklósi A. (2016). *Dog Behaviour, Evolution, and Cognition*. Oxford: Oxford University Press.
5. Leuscher, A. (2015). Canine behavior and development. In: *Canine and Feline Behavior for Veterinary Technicians and Nurses* (ed. J. Shaw and D. Martin), 30–50. Ames, IA: Wiley.
6. Martin, D. (2015). Feline behavior and development. In: *Canine and Feline Behavior for Veterinary Technicians and Nurses* (ed. J. Shaw and D. Martin), 51–69. Ames, IA: Wiley.
7. Becker, M., Radosta, L., Sung, W. *et al.* (2018). *From Fearful to Fear Free*. Deerfield Beech, FL: Health Communications.
8. Seibert, L. (2008). Diagnosis and management of patients presenting with behavior problems. *Vet Clin N Am Small Anim Pract* 38: 937–950.
9. Shaw, J. (2015). Specific behavior modification techniques and practical applications for behavior disorders. In: *Canine and Feline Behavior for Veterinary Technicians and Nurses* (ed. J. Shaw and D. Martin), 204–280. Ames, IA: Wiley.
10. Hout, M.V.D. and Merckelbach, H. (1991). Classical conditioning: still going strong. *Behav Psychother* 19: 59.
11. Price, V. (2015). Learning and behavior modification. In: *Canine and Feline Behavior for Veterinary Technicians and Nurses* (ed. J. Shaw and D. Martin), 113–144. Ames, IA: Wiley.
12. Burch, M.R. and Bailey, J.S. (1999). *How Dogs Learn*. Hoboken, NJ: Wiley.
13. Herron, M.E., Shofer, F.S. and Reisner, I.R. (2009). Survey of the use and outcome of confrontational and non-confrontational training methods in client-owned dogs showing undesired behaviors. *Appl Anim Behav Sci* 117: 47–54.
14. Howell, A. and Feyrecilde, M. (2018). *Cooperative Veterinary Care*. Hoboken, NJ: Wiley Blackwell.

15. Neilson, J.C. (2009). House soiling by cats. In: *BSAVA Manual of Canine and Feline Behavioural Medicine* (ed. D.F. Horwitz and D.S. Mills), 117–126. Gloucester: British Small Animal Veterinary Association.
16. Ellis, S.L.H., Rodan, I., Carney, H.C. *et al.* (2013). AAFP and ISFM feline environmental needs guidelines. *J Feline Med Surg* 15: 219–230.
17. Landsberg, G., Hunthausen, W. and Ackerman, L. (2013). Canine destructive behaviors. In: *Behavior Problems of the Dog and Cat*, 3e, 255–262. Edinburgh: Saunders Elsevier.
18. Sdao, K. (2012). *Plenty in Life Is Free: Reflections on dogs, training and finding grace*. Wenatchee, WA: Dogwise Publishing.
19. Ohio State University Indoor Pet Initiative. https://indoorpet.osu.edu/home (accessed 23 July 2021).
20. Yin, S. (2009). *Low Stress Handling and Behavior Modification of Dogs and Cats: Techniques for developing patients who love their visits*. Davis, CA: CattleDog Publishing.
21. Low Stress Handling University. CattleDog Publishing. https://lowstresshandling.com (accessed 23 July 2021).
22. Fear Free Professional Certification Program. https://fearfreepets.com (accessed 23 July 2021).
23. Loryman, B., Davies, F., Chavada, G. *et al.* (2006). Consigning "brutacaine" to history: a survey of pharmacological techniques to facilitate painful procedures in children in emergency departments in the UK. *Emerg Med J* 23: 838–840.
24. Overall, K.L. (1997). Pharmacologic treatments for behavior problems. *Vet Clin N Am Small Anim Pract* 27: 637–665.

Chapter 13

Physical Rehabilitation

Kristen L Hagler, BS(An.Phys), RVT, VTS (Physical Rehabilitation), CCRP, CVPP, COCM, CBW, VCC

Veterinary Technician and Nurse's Daily Reference Guide: Canine and Feline, Fourth Edition. Edited by Mandy Fults and Kenichiro Yagi.

Companion website: www.wiley.com/go/fults/veterinary

Abbreviations

ATP, adenosine triphosphate
FDA, US Food and Drugs Administration
NMES, neuromuscular electrical stimulation
PEMF, pulsed electromagnetic field
ROM, range of movement
TENS, transcutaneous electrical nerve stimulation

Physical rehabilitation is the treatment of injury or illness to decrease pain and restore function. It is used to address acute injuries, chronic injuries or diseases that have been affecting a patient for a long time and is often implemented, following musculoskeletal and neurological injuries or surgeries to strengthen muscle and increase flexibility and range of motion (ROM). This allows the patient to heal faster, return to function sooner, decrease pain levels and improve overall quality of life.

Patients are evaluated before beginning a physical rehabilitation treatment plan through physical exams, joint and muscle measurements, functional assessment measures and gait analysis. This baseline information allows for monitoring of patient responses to therapy. Routine evaluations to assess stability of any surgical repair (when present), the condition of tissues involved, pain assessment, and functional movement all help validate the patient's response to the therapeutic plans and make adjustments most appropriate for the condition being treated.

EXAMINATIONS

- Physical
- Body conditioning score
- Pain evaluation
- Neurological
- Orthopedic
- Gait analysis:
  - Evaluate the patient in at least two different gait speeds (e.g. walk, trot, running) and circumstances (e.g. walking toward, walking away, various surfaces, viewed from both sides, weight bearing)
- Postural and functional movement:
  - Evaluate the patient in a multitude of body postures (e.g. standing, sitting, lying down), on varied flooring textures (e.g. carpeting, slick, gravel) and environments (e.g. stairs, hills). Patients should be evaluated for posture and compensatory movements when performing a functional movement (e.g. difficulty rising from a lying down position or sitting asymmetrically with a pelvic limb)
- Radiographic

MEASUREMENTS

- Joint goniometry:
  - Measurements are taken to evaluate a joint's ROM using a goniometer (Figure 13.1).
  - Joint angles (e.g. hip, stifle, tarsus, shoulder, elbow, carpus) can be measured in either a standing or lateral recumbency position. Flexion and extension angles (Figures 13.2–13.13) are measured for each joint aforementioned and compared with established normal values (Table 13.1).[1] Varus and valgus measurements may be obtained for the carpus.
  - Comparison measurements are taken with opposite joints.
  - Measurements obtained may vary between breed and medical condition being evaluated.

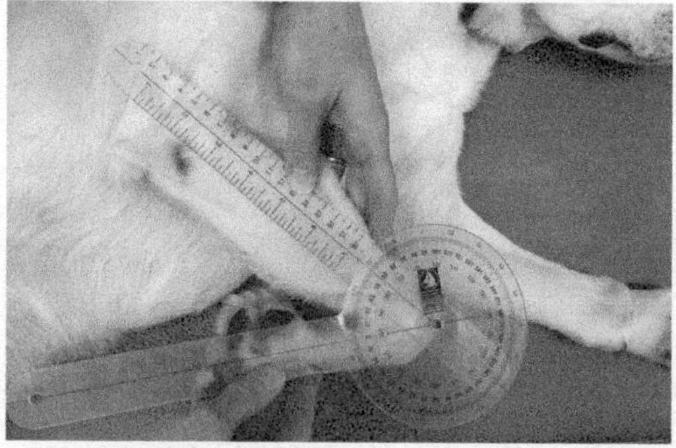

Figure 13.1 Goniometer. Source: image courtesy: Kristen L. Hagler © 2019 Golden Gait Canine.

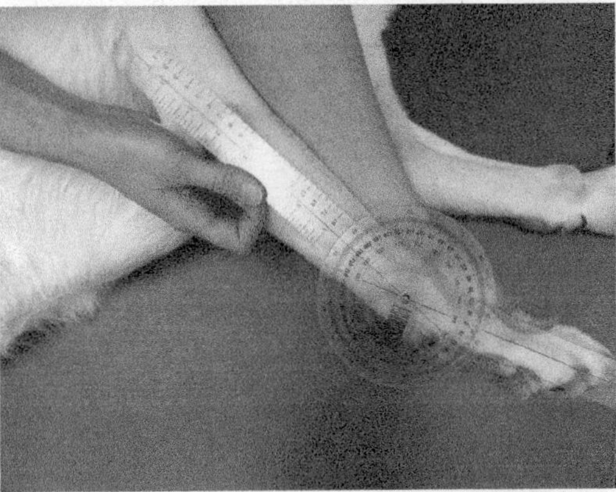

Figure 13.2 Goniometry carpal flexion. Source: image courtesy: Kristen L. Hagler, ©2019 Golden Gait Canine.

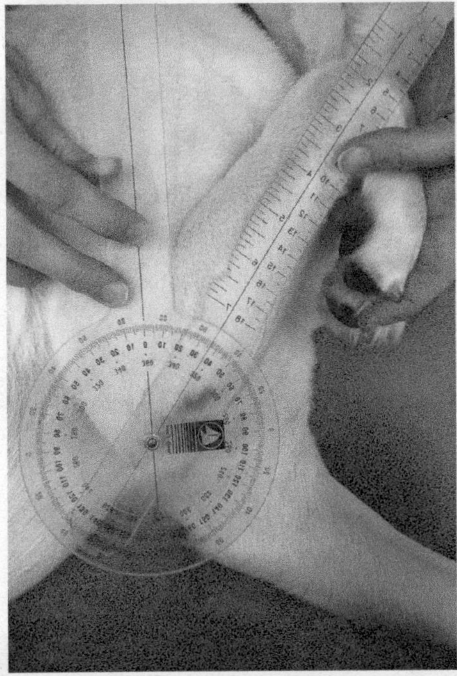

Figure 13.3 Goniometry carpal extension. Source: image courtesy: Kristen L. Hagler, © 2019 Golden Gait Canine.

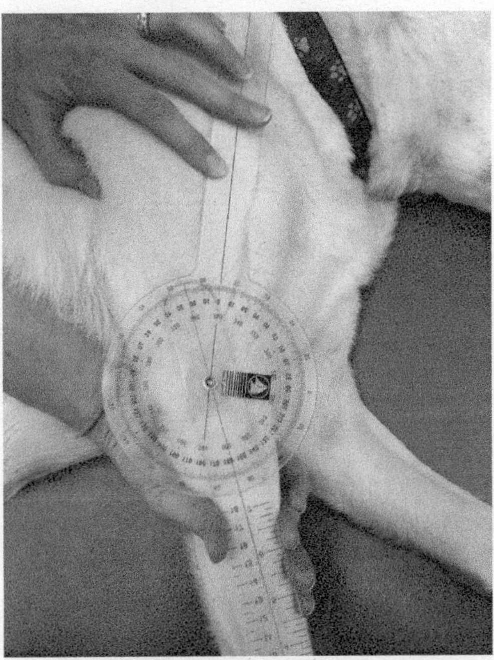

Figure 13.4 Goniometry elbow flexion. Source: image courtesy: Kristen L. Hagler, © 2019 Golden Gait Canine.

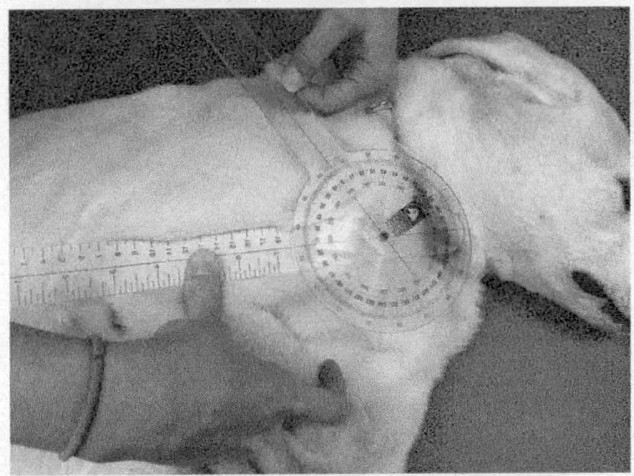

Figure 13.5 Goniometry elbow extension. Source: image courtesy: Kristen L. Hagler, © 2019 Golden Gait Canine.

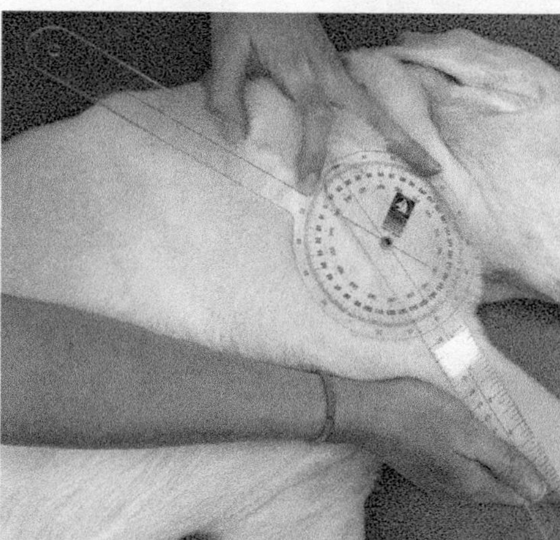

Figure 13.6 Goniometry shoulder flexion. Source: image courtesy: Kristen L. Hagler, © 2019 Golden Gait Canine.

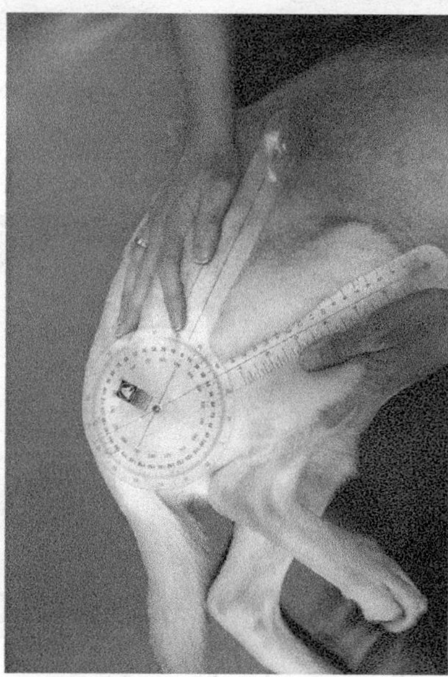

Figure 13.7 Goniometry shoulder extension. Source: image courtesy: Kristen L. Hagler, © 2019 Golden Gait Canine.

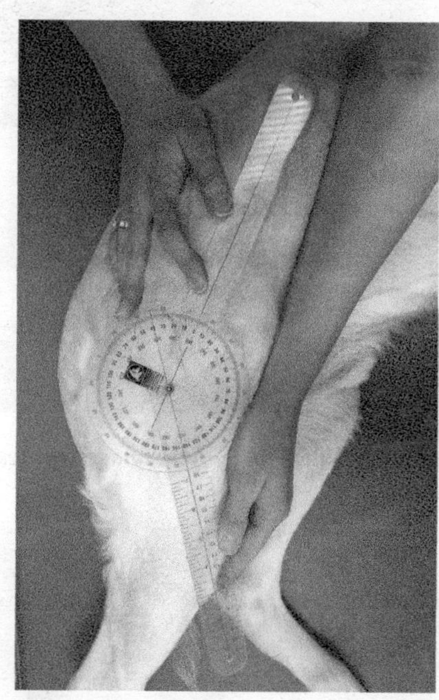

Figure 13.8 Goniometry hip flexion. Source: image courtesy: Kristen L. Hagler, © 2019 Golden Gait Canine.

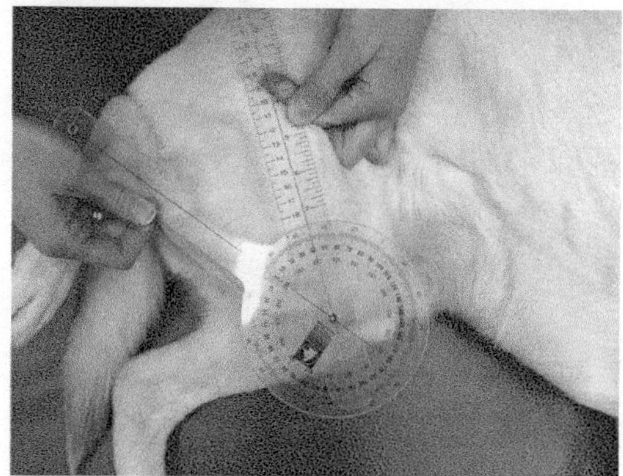

Figure 13.9 Goniometry hip extension. Source: image courtesy: Kristen L. Hagler, © 2019 Golden Gait Canine.

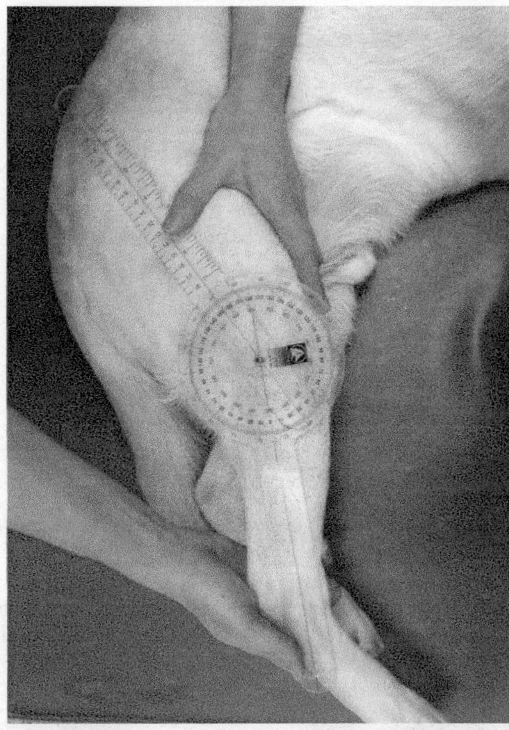

Figure 13.10 Goniometry stifle flexion. Source: image courtesy: Kristen L. Hagler, © 2019 Golden Gait Canine.

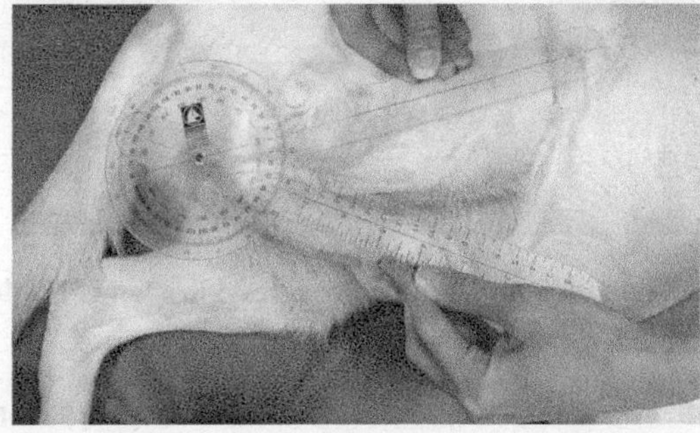

Figure 13.11 Goniometry stifle extension. Source: image courtesy: Kristen L. Hagler, © 2019 Golden Gait Canine.

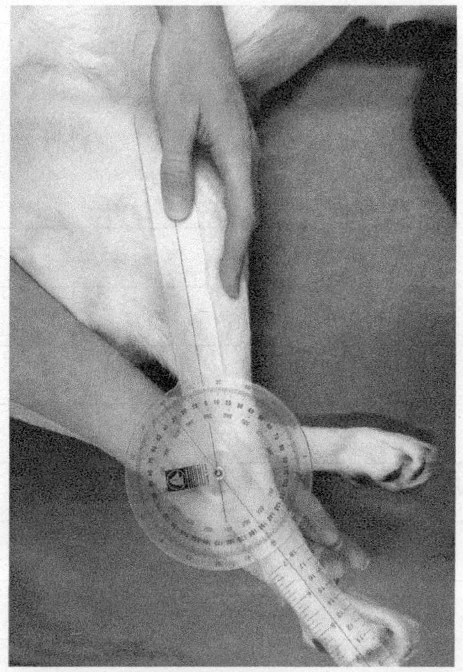

Figure 13.12 Goniometry hock flexion. Source: image courtesy: Kristen L. Hagler, © 2019 Golden Gait Canine.

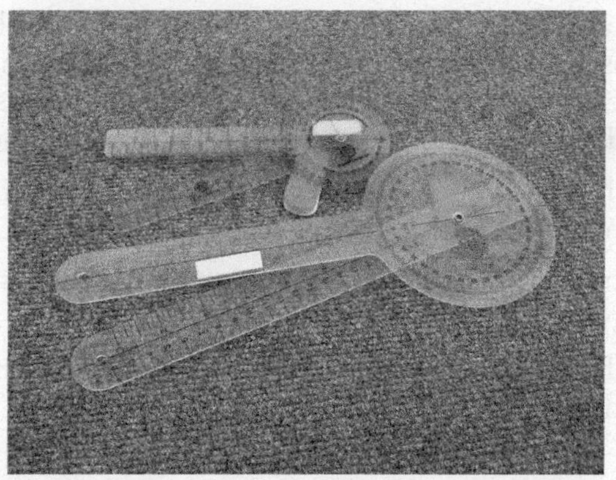

Figure 13.13 Goniometry hock extension. Source: image courtesy: Kristen L. Hagler, © 2019 Golden Gait Canine.

Table 13.1 / **Joint goniometric range of motion**[1]

Joint	Angle (degrees)	
	Flexion	Extension
Hip	50	162
Stifle	41	162
Hock	38	165
Shoulder	57	165
Elbow	36	166
Carpus	32	196
	Valgus	Varus
Carpus	12	7

- Muscle girth:
  - Relative measurements of the circumference of the hind limb and forelimb are obtained with the animal in a standing or lateral recumbency position using a spring tension tape measurer. The limb should remain relatively neutral with muscles relaxed and consistent tension is applied to each location to prevent errors in recording.
  - 70% thigh girth circumference evaluates the biceps femoris, semimembranosus, and semitendinosus musculatures.
  - Greater trochanter or upper thigh circumference assess gluteal musculatures (Figure 13.14).
  - 70% thigh girth circumference evaluates the biceps femoris, semimembranosus, and semitendinosus musculatures (Figure 13.15 and 13.16).
  - Antebrachial measurements assess extensor and flexor musculatures of the forelimb.
  - Distal humerus measurements assess triceps musculatures (Figure 13.17).

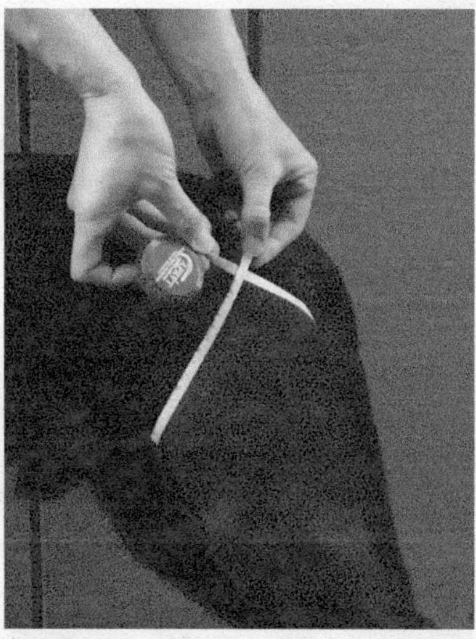

Figure 13.14 Muscle girth greater trochanter. Source: image courtesy: Kristen L. Hagler RVT, VTS (Physical Rehabilitation) © 2019 Golden Gait Canine.

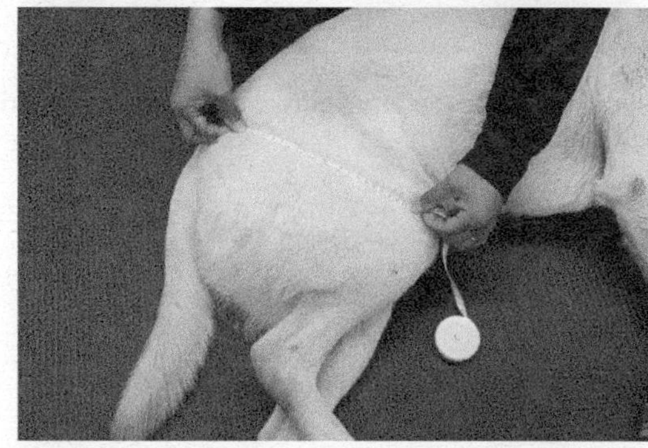

Figure 13.15 Thigh length. Source: image courtesy: Kristen L. Hagler, © 2019 Golden Gait Canine.

  - Antebrachial measurements assess extensor and flexor musculatures of the forelimb (Figure 13.18).
  - Deltoid musculatures using the acromion process as the anatomical landmark and the tension tape snugly fit in the axilla (Figure 13.19).

- Comparison measurements are taken with opposite limbs.
- Measurements obtained will vary between breed, body condition score, limb position, and measurement position.
- Evaluators must be able to reliably repeat measurements for proper medical record documentation. It is recommended to obtain the mean of three independent measurements to improve accuracy.

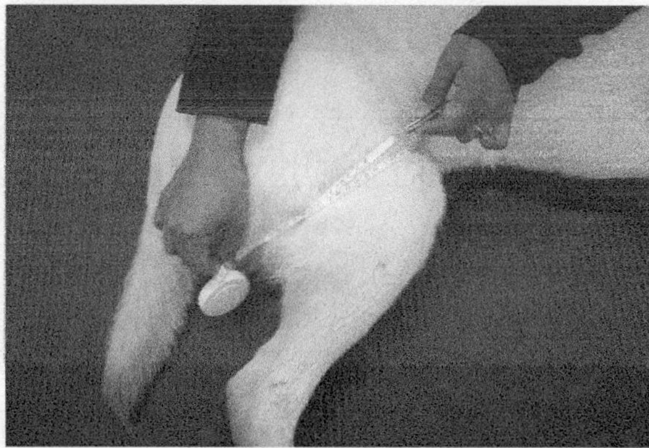

Figure 13.16 Thigh girth. Source: image courtesy: Kristen L. Hagler, © 2019 Golden Gait Canine.

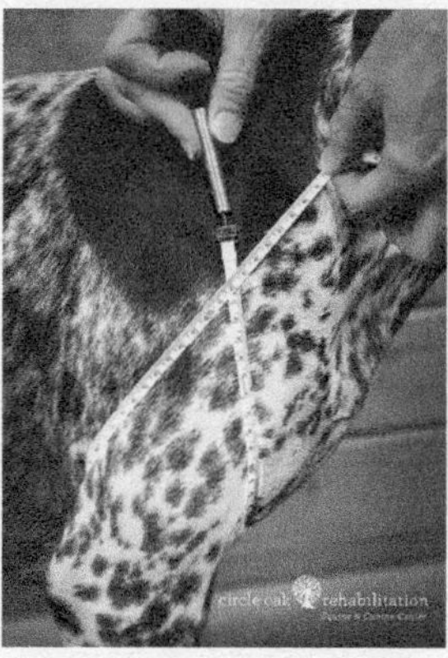

Figure 13.17 Muscle girth triceps. Source: image courtesy: Kristen L. Hagler, © 2019 Golden Gait Canine.

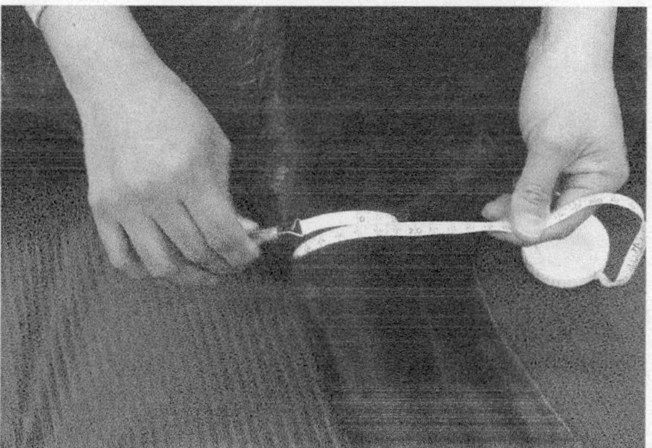

Figure 13.18 Muscle girth antebrachium. Source: image courtesy: Kristen L. Hagler, © 2019 Golden Gait Canine.

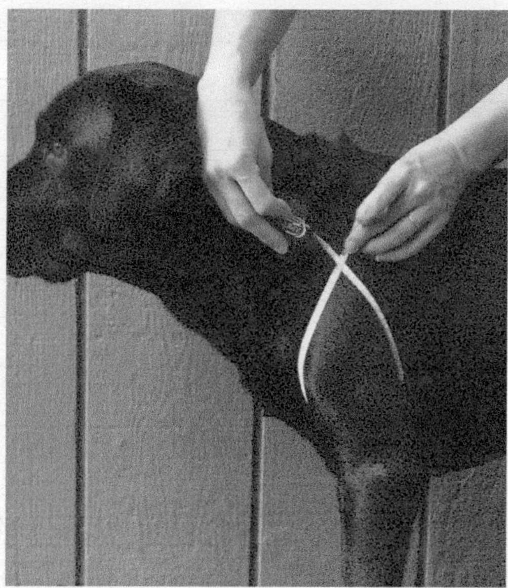

Figure 13.19 Shoulder musculatures. Source: image courtesy: Kristen L. Hagler, © 2019 Golden Gait Canine.

BENEFITS OF PHYSICAL REHABILITATION

Table 13.2 / Benefits of physical rehabilitation

Therapy	Assisted mobility devices	Hydrotherapy	Massage	Passive ROM	Active ROM	NMES	TENS	Laser therapy	Static magnets	PEMF	Cold	Heat	Therapeutic ultrasound
Improvement of function													
Balance	–	X	–	–	X	–	–	–	–	–	–	–	–
Blood flow	–	–	–	X	–	–	–	–	–	–	–	–	X
Cartilage regeneration	–	–	–	X	–	–	–	–	–	–	–	–	–
Circulation	–	X	X	–	–	X	–	–	–	–	–	X	–
Endurance	X	X	X	–	X	–	–	–	–	–	–	–	–
Enzyme activity	–	–	–	–	–	–	–	–	–	–	–	X	X
Flexibility	–	–	X	X	–	–	–	–	–	–	–	–	–
Mobility	X	X	–	X	–	–	–	–	–	–	–	–	–
Muscle relaxation	–	–	X	–	–	–	–	–	–	–	–	X	–
Oxygenation	–	–	–	–	–	–	–	–	–	–	–	X	–
Proprioception	–	–	–	–	X	–	–	–	–	–	–	–	–
ROM	–	X	X	X	X	X	–	–	–	–	–	X	X
Scar strength	–	–	–	X	–	–	–	–	–	–	–	–	–

(Continued)

Table 13.2 / **Benefits of Physical Rehabilitation (Continued)**

Therapy	Assisted mobility devices	Hydrotherapy	Massage	Passive ROM	Active ROM	NMES	TENS	Laser therapy	Static magnets	PEMF	Cold	Heat	Therapeutic ultrasound
Scar stretch	–	–	–	–	–	–	–	–	–	–	–	–	X
Strength	X	X	–	–	X	X	–	–	–	–	–	–	–
Vasoconstriction	–	–	–	–	–	–	–	–	–	–	X	–	–
Vasodilation	–	–	–	–	–	–	–	–	–	–	–	X	–
Wound healing	–	–	X	–	–	X	–	X	X	X	–	X	X
Decrease in symptoms													
Adhesions	–	–	X	X	–	–	–	–	–	–	–	–	–
Bleeding	–	–	–	–	–	–	–	–	–	–	X	–	–
Edema	–	–	X	–	–	X	–	–	–	–	X	–	–
Fibrosis	–	–	X	–	–	–	–	–	–	–	–	–	–
Joint stiffness	–	X	–	–	–	–	–	–	–	–	–	X	–
Metabolism	–	–	–	–	–	–	–	–	–	–	X	X	–
Muscle spasms	–	–	X	–	–	X	–	–	–	–	X	X	X
Pain	–	X	X	–	–	X	X	X	X	X	X	X	X

Skill Box 13.1 / Physical Rehabilitation Techniques

Effect	Technique	Uses	Comments
Assisted Mobility Devices			
• ↑ Mobility, endurance, strength, and independence	• Various carts and slings to assist with mobility	• Weak, painful, or paralyzed patients	• An adjustment period may be necessary for the patient to acclimate to the new device
• Prevent injury	• Various protective footwear	• Weakly ambulatory patients • Provide protection from excessive nail wear and wound development	• Protective footwear must be easily taken on/off, cleaned regularly and the patient should not be more hindered in ambulation when wearing the device
Hydrotherapy (Aquatic)			
• ↑ Flexibility, strength, mobility, circulation, endurance, balance, and ROM • ↓ Pain and joint stiffness • ↑ Muscle contraction and stretch • ↑ Metabolism and gastrointestinal motility • ↑Confidence • ↓ Fear, anxiety, stress • ↓ Edema	• Swimming • Underwater treadmill • Gait patterning • Exercises, massage, and stretching can be done before, during, or after water treatment. • Begun after all wounds have completely healed	• Osteoarthritis, postoperative orthopedic, gait retraining, neurological deficits, nerve damage, and athletic conditioning	• Action: provides resistance while limiting joint impact • Altering buoyancy, resistance, speed, and temperature allows creation of individual and progressive programs • Water temperature must be in a comfortable range to prevent hyper- or hypothermia • Underwater treadmill increases overall joint flexion • Swimming requires aerobic capacity and may benefit the forelimbs more than the hindlimbs • All patients must wear safety harnesses and personnel should wear personal protective equipment such as hip waders
Massage			
• ↑ Relaxation, circulation, flexibility, endurance, mobility, ROM, wound healing • ↓ Pain, edema, muscle spasms, fibrosis, adhesions	• In a quiet area, place the patient in a comfortable position and gently stroke the area. Begin massaging from the distal end moving proximal for approximately 30 minutes • *Effleurage:* apply broad, stroking motion to the long lines of the muscle fibers moving toward the heart. The hands always remain in contact with the skin. Use firm pressure when moving toward the heart and a lighter pressure when moving away from the heart. Affects connective tissue, blood flow, lymphatic flow, and promotes relaxation	• Orthopedic, neurological, or trauma patients • Postoperatively, muscle spasms, tissue tightness, chronic inflammation, or long-term medical conditions	• Action: ↑ circulation, release scar tissue, balance muscle function, relaxation • Contact is always maintained between the patient and the therapist's hands • Therapy time length is determined by patient willingness

(*Continued*)

Skill Box 13.1 / Physical Rehabilitation Techniques (Continued)

Effect	Technique	Uses	Comments
• Most studies done in humans with extrapolation to small animals	• *Pétrissage:* place hands in a C-shape; lift, roll, and knead together superficial and deeper soft tissues; ↑ blood flow and ↓ muscle stiffness • *Cross friction:* use a finger or thumb at a single point to rub the tissues against each other (rotary motion) while moving in a pattern • *Tapotement:* use a tapping or drumming motion of the fingers or hands to stimulate nerve endings or provide a sedative effect	• Relief of anxiety • Myofascial restrictions	• Contraindicated: acute inflammatory conditions, infections, unhealed incisions, unstable fractures, absent sensation, and bleeding disorders • Avoid: eyes, throat, kidneys, deep abdomen
Stretching (Passive ROM)			
• ↑ ROM, scar strength, flexibility, mobility, joint nutrition, cartilage regeneration, blood flow, endurance, and muscle relaxation • ↓Adhesions	• Begin with the most proximal joint and move distal. Place a hand above and below the joint to stabilize. Guide the limb through 10–20 alternating flexions and extensions at each joint, holding each end position for 10–30 seconds. Then cycle the entire limb through small circles ("bicycling") advancing to full comfortable ROM 10–20 times • All stretches should be pain free, and then gently moved slightly beyond while remaining comfortable for the patient • Performed on each joint separately postoperatively and in patients with ↓ mobility • Perform three times daily	• Orthopedic or neurological patients • Postoperatively (analgesia may be needed 30–60 minutes prior to stretching) • Chronic osteoarthritis	• Action: ↓ Dense connective tissues, enhances venous and lymphatic drainage • Contraindicated: joint instability • Avoid areas with damage to ligaments and tendons • Avoid hyperflexion of carpus and tarsus • Does not prevent muscle atrophy • Does not increase muscular strength
Therapeutic Exercise (Active ROM)			
• ↑ ROM, muscle mass and strength, endurance, balance, proprioception	• Therapeutic exercises are designed individually for each patient to provide variety for both patient and owner while ↑ the physical activity of the patient • Variety of therapeutic exercise prevents patient boredom and muscle accommodation • Exercise examples: standing, sit to stand, stand to down, balance board, controlled walks, cavaletti rails (Figure 13.9), walking, high-five or "wave", assisted balance on therapy balls, obstacle work, stair climbing, land treadmill, wheelbarrowing, dancing	• Orthopedic or neurological patients • Postoperatively, healing phase • Chronic osteoarthritis • Chronic compensatory issues	• Action: ↑ physical activity, increase balance, proprioception, flexibility and core strength • Contraindicated: dependent on patient's progress

ELECTRICAL STIMULATION THERAPY

Skill Box 13.2 / Electrical Stimulation Therapy

Effect	Technique	Uses	Comments
Neuromuscular			
↑ ROM, muscle strength and tone, wound healing, blood and lymph circulation, delivery of topical drugs (iontophoresis) ↓ Pain, muscle spasms, edema	• Clip the area and clean with alcohol. Locate the point where the motor nerve enters the muscle and place an electrode; place another at the distal end of the muscle. Using the lowest possible current, move the motor point electrode around until a good contraction is observed • Treatments are typically 15–20 minutes 1–2 times daily or every 2–3 day	• Orthopedic or neurological patients • Postoperatively, muscle atrophy prevention, reformation	• Action: muscle contraction through stimulation from an electrical current • Contraindicated: seizure disorders, thrombophlebitis, pregnant animals, and infection • Avoid exposure to: eyes, ears, cardiac pacemakers, heart, carotid sinus, areas of malignancy, ↓ sensation, and cervical ganglia
Transcutaneous Nerve			
↓ Pain	• Electrodes are placed directly on the skin at locations that are painful • Example: elbow joint arthritis, the electrode pads are placed at the medial and lateral joint regions so the electrical current crosses into the joint. Alternatively, the electrodes may be placed on the medial aspect of the joint so that the electrical current travels across the medial aspect of the joint • A TENS unit delivers an electrical current to stimulate faster sensory nerves to overload the interneurons inhibiting transmission of painful stimuli and creating analgesia	• Immediately postoperatively or prior to a painful part of therapy • Chronic joint or muscle pain	• Action: muscle stimulation from an electrical current • Results are of short duration • Avoid exposure to: eyes, ears, cardiac pacemakers, heart, carotid sinus, areas of malignancy, ↓ sensation, and cervical ganglia

LASER THERAPY

Skill Box 13.3 / Laser Therapy

Effect	Technique	Uses	Comments
• ↑ Wound healing • ↓ Pain and inflammation • ↑ Increase nerve regeneration • ↑ Cellular metabolism (ATP production, oxygenation)	• Low-energy lasers: power 3.5–500 mW. Considered class IIIb at tissue penetration depths up to 3 mm • High-power therapy lasers: power output greater than 500 mW. Includes class IV lasers, including surgical lasers (15–40 W). Therapeutic class IV lasers are classified as either heating or non-heating • The aperture tip of the laser is placed perpendicular to the target tissue 0–5 cm from the skin for direct application or a beam is used at a distance of 1–50 cm. Manufacturer guidelines must be followed for each individual laser class and aperture type • Long-coated breeds may need some light shaving to improve light penetration into the skin • Multiple treatments may be needed, with each lasting 3–10 minutes, depending on the size of the animal and the area being treated • Depth of photonic light penetration is dependent on wavelength. Longer wavelength penetrate deeper. Evidence supports 810–830 nm penetrating the skin most effectively, while 780–950 nm is better for deeper tissues • Personnel, and possibly the patient, are required to wear personal protective equipment such as safety eye lenses during treatments	Wound and ulcer healing, stomatitis, gingivitis, tendonitis, postoperative orthopedic and soft-tissue pain, neurological conditions or injury, osteoarthritis	• Action: use of monochromic and collimated light to alter cellular function and enhance healing nondestructively • Complications: retinal and thermal burns • Many parameters must be altered to achieve the desired treatment (e.g. wavelength, waveform, output power, power density) • Improvement is often seen starting from the second week of treatment. Some conditions may need continuing regular treatments • Contraindicated: long-acting steroid use or light sensitive drugs, over regions of hemorrhage, eyes, pacemakers, heart disease, carcinomas, pregnant uterus, epilepsy, tattoos, thyroid gland • Other terminology used: photobiomodulation, therapeutic laser, cold laser therapy • Veterinarians should prescribe the total energy provided to a location or "dose" for the specific condition • Therapeutic lasers are classified by the FDA based on power output and potential damage to the eye

MAGNETIC FIELD THERAPY

Skill Box 13.4 / Magnetic Field Therapy

Effect	Technique	Uses	Comments
Static Magnet			
• ↑ Wound healing • ↓ Pain	• A disturbed electrical field may lead to physical and emotional pain. Static or stationary magnets applied directly to the area of concern to provide continuous treatment. The magnet lines of force permeate the area of injury and stimulate healing. Magnetic fields can stimulate metabolism, enzyme action, and ↑ the amount of oxygen available to cells • Placement of magnets either in the cage (e.g. pad) or secured to the affected area on the animal for minutes, hours, or days • Magnets of different strengths (> 50 gauss) and sizes	Bone and wound healing, epilepsy, pain relief, slowing the growth rate of cancer and bacterial cells	• Because research regarding the use of magnets with animals is limited, testimony makes up the background for their use • The composition and size of the magnet affect its strength and intensity • The size and shape of a magnet are related to its depth of penetration • Magnet strength and size needed for each animal are highly variable and should begin with lower strengths and for short periods and then ↑ if well tolerated • Discontinue with worsening conditions (e.g.,↑ seizures and lethargy) • Do not use with pacemakers or partial cranial cruciate ruptures
Pulsed Electromagnetic Field			
• ↑ Wound healing and cell metabolism • ↓ Pain • ↓ Swelling • ↑ Bone healing	• PEMF is a pulsing current undergoing acceleration while moving through a coil of wire producing a magnetic field. Pulsed signal therapy is one type of PEMF typically used for the treatment of osteoarthritis with good to excellent results. It allows reconstruction of the disturbed electrical field, leading to ↑ production of proteoglycans and collagen • Coils are placed over the area to be treated for 30–60 minutes as frequently as daily • Battery-powered therapy devices consisting of several coils of wire, a control box with varying pulse settings, and a power source	Non-union fractures, acute and chronic injury (e.g. tendon, ligament), osteoarthritis, inflammatory joint disorders, poor lymphatic flow, traumatic brain injury, wound healing	• Action: Induce biological currents in the tissue • Numerous studies available validating its use • Technique: patient must remain still during treatment application time • Often implemented immediately after surgery or for management of chronic conditions • Discontinue with worsening conditions (e.g. ↑ seizures and lethargy) • An FDA approved therapy for safety and effectiveness

TEMPERATURE THERAPY

Skill Box 13.5 / Temperature Therapy

Effect	Technique	Uses	Comments
Cold (Cryotherapy)			
• ↑ Arteriolar vasoconstriction • ↓ Bleeding, metabolism, pain, muscle spasm, edema formation, and swelling	• Ice packs, moldable cold packs or towels soaked with cold water are laid over the affected area for 10–15 minutes and repeated every 2–3 hours • Observe the skin every few minutes for cyanotic changes resulting in frostbite • Place a wet towel between the cold pack and skin to ↑ conduction and monitor skin color at 10-minute intervals to avoid tissue damage (e.g. frostbite) • Bags with crushed ice provide the greatest deep tissue cooling • Additional methods: ice massage (rubbing ice over the affected area), cold baths, and whirlpools	Acute injury, postoperative orthopedic swelling and pain, muscle spasms, edema, musculoskeletal trauma (e.g. tendonitis, bursitis, sprains)	• Action: local arteriolar vasoconstriction and ↓ local tissue metabolism • Technique often implemented in the first 24–72 hours after injury or for chronic pain (e.g. osteoarthritis) • Contraindicated: areas of compromised circulation, ↓ or absent sensation, previous frostbite to that area, cold hypersensitivity, or hypothermia • Precautions: the very old, the very young, and areas with superficial nerves (e.g. peroneal and ulnar) • Tip: Moldable ice packs can be made by mixing one part isopropyl alcohol and three parts water and frozen in sealable bags
Heat (Thermotherapy)			
• ↑ Vasodilation, oxygenation, ROM, enzyme activity, muscle relaxation, circulation, wound healing • ↓ Pain, muscle spasms, metabolism, joint stiffness	• Moist hot packs (e.g. washcloths or towels soaked with water as hot as can be tolerated) or dry hot packs (e.g. hot water bottles, heating pads) are laid over the affected area for 15–45 minutes on and off cycles, reheating as necessary • Skin should be observed for red, mottled areas or white areas (e.g. thermal burns). • Plastic wrap can be placed over the wet towel to trap heat • Additional methods: warm baths and whirlpools (see Aquatic Therapy)	Areas of minimal soft tissue (e.g. joints) prior to stretching, pain relief, relaxation Muscle spasms, tissue tightness, adhesions (↓ scar tension), subacute and chronic traumatic and inflammatory conditions ↓ Ischemia via vasodilation	• Action: ↑ blood vessel diameter and ↓ smooth muscle tone • Superficial heat to no > 3 cm, typically 0–0.5 cm • Typically started 72 hours post-surgery or injury (the healing phase after most inflammation is gone) • Contraindicated: fever, acute inflammation, active bleeding, ↓ or absent sensation, neoplasms, active infection, areas of compromised circulation • Precautions: the very old, the very young

SOUNDWAVE THERAPY

Skill Box 13.6 / Soundwave Therapy

	Technique	Uses	Comments
Therapeutic Ultrasound			
• ↑ Stretching, blood flow, ROM, scar stretch, wound healing, enzyme activity, and delivery of topical drugs • ↓ Pain and muscle spasm (especially deep soft tissues, > 3 cm)	• An area twice the diameter of the probe head is clipped and ultrasound gel applied. Apply the ultrasound head and move in a pattern to cover the entire area. Continuously move the head to avoid thermal burns and observe the patient for discomfort • Stretching and exercises should be done during or immediately following the treatment for maximum benefit • Each treatment is about 5–10 minutes and begins daily, then ↓ as condition improves	Pain, muscle spasm, scar tissue contraction, wound healing (e.g. 2 weeks postoperatively, chronic), tendonitis, bursitis	• Action: use of sound waves through tissues to cause certain physiological effects (e.g. deep tissue heating up to 5 cm) • Contraindicated: eyes, testes, neoplasms, bony prominences, metal implants, infected wounds, pregnancy, thrombophlebitis, heart, cardiac pacemaker, and neck decompressive spinal surgeries
Extracorporeal Shockwave Therapy			
• ↑ Tissue repair and wound healing • ↓ Pain and stiffness • ↑ Bone osteogenesis • ↑ Antibacterial properties	• The areas to be treated are shaved and gently cleaned with alcohol. Chemical cleaners should be thoroughly removed to reduce intradermal introduction • Ultrasound transmission gel is applied to the treatment area • The Trode (sound wave applicator) is focused on the treatment area and moved in a scanning fashion, ensuring the treatment area is covered	Non-union fractures, management of chronic arthritis conditions, tendon and ligament repair, tendinopathies, chronic wounds including granulomas	• Action: high-energy focused sound waves generated by electrohydraulic spark, electromagnetic or piezoelectric (faster than 1500 m/s) • Treatment recommendations vary by condition; 2–3 treatments spaced 2–3 weeks apart are recommended • Dose or pulse recommendations are prescribed by the veterinarian and manufacturer • Patients must be sedated or anesthetized to reduce pain during administration • Contraindicated: unstable fractures, neoplasia
Extracorporeal Shockwave Therapy (Radial)			
• ↑ Tissue repair • ↓ Pain and stiffness	• Patients are not required to be shaved, but it is encouraged for long-coated dogs • Ultrasound transmission gel is applied to the treatment area • The electrode is used in a scanning method to cover the treatment area	Myofascial trigger points and superficial muscle pain	• Action: low-energy radial sound waves around 10 m/second

REFERENCE

1. Jaegger, G., Marcellin-Little, D.J. and Levine, D. (2002). Reliability of goniometry in Labrador retrievers, *Am J Vet Res* 63: 979–986.

Chapter 14

Patient Care Skills in Clinical Practice

Liza W. Rudolph, BAS, RVT, VTS (Clinical Practice- C/F), (SAIM)

Veterinary Technician and Nurse's Daily Reference Guide: Canine and Feline, Fourth Edition. Edited by Mandy Fults and Kenichiro Yagi.

Companion website: www.wiley.com/go/fults/veterinary

Abbreviations

ACD, acid citrate dextrose
ACVIM, American College of Veterinary Internal Medicine
ARDS, acute respiratory distress syndrome
ASA, American Association of Anesthesiologists
BP, blood pressure
bpm, beats per minute
CBC, complete blood count
CCL, cranial cruciate ligament
CHF, congestive heart failure
CNS, central nervous system
CO_2, carbon dioxide
COPD, chronic obstructive pulmonary disease
CPD, citrate phosphate dextrose
CPDA-1, citrate phosphate dextrose adenine
CRI, constant rate infusion
CRT, capillary refill time
CVP, central venous pressure
DEA, dog erythrocyte antigens
DKA, diabetic ketoacidosis
ECG, electrocardiogram
FDA, US Food and Drugs Administration
FeLV, feline leukemia virus
FIV, feline immunodeficiency virus
Fr, French
GDV, gastric dilation volvulus
GFR, glomerular filtration rate
H^+, hydrogen
HCO_3^-, bicarbonate
IV, intravenous
LA, left atrium
LDDST, low-dose dexamethasone suppression test
LL, left lateral
MAP, mean arterial pressure
NaCl, sodium chloride
NPH, neutral protamine Hagedorn
O_2, oxygen
OHE, ovariohysterectomy
$PaCO_2$, partial pressure of arterial carbon dioxide

PaO_2, partial pressure of arterial oxygen
pCO_2, partial pressure of carbon dioxide
PCV, packed cell volume
PICC, peripherally inserted central catheter
PTE, pulmonary thromboendarterectomy
$PvCO_2$, partial pressure of carbon dioxide in mixed venous blood
PvO_2, partial oxygen pressure in mixed venous blood
RA, right atrium
RBC, red blood cell
RL, right lateral
ROM, range of movement
SQ, subcutaneously
USG, urine specific gravity
UTI, urinary tract infection

PATIENT CARE

Caring for patients to help them achieve the most positive outcome is the veterinary technician's ultimate goal. Patient care encompasses not only monitoring and treating medical conditions but also tending to their physical and mental comfort. It is through continuous reassessment that changes and trends are seen and the appropriate actions are taken. Patient care is at the heart of our profession.

Established hospitalization levels serve as a guideline for inpatient care (Table 14.1). It is the goal that patients will move down to level 1 with eventual discharge. This movement can be rapid, over 12 hours with a young, healthy, dog spay, or may take days to weeks with a critically ill or injured pet. Each hospitalization level builds upon the one before it. For example, the monitoring parameters in level 2 will include all of level 1 together with some additional parameters. Three to five levels of hospitalization will fulfill the needs of most practices. The parameters monitored in each level will be specific and individualized for each patient, but these provide general guidelines.

As shifts and monitoring responsibilities change, it is critical that the veterinary technician become familiar with their patients to predict problems and recognize changing patterns. This begins with a review of all chart notes and laboratory work, together with discussing the patient with the veterinarian in charge and the veterinary technician who was previously providing care. An initial assessment should take place to evaluate all aspects of the patient and

Table 14.1 / Hospitalization level examples

Hospitalization level	Monitoring	Assessment	Actions
1.	• Observational hospitalization (blood glucose curve, LDDST, etc.) • Assess every 12 hours	• Temperature, pulse rate and quality, heart rate, weight, and hydration status • Mentation and pain level • Clean, dry, and comfortable • Elimination • Nutrition • Confirm adequate calorie intake • Medication administration	• Nutrition: free choice/portion controlled • Walk: no assistance required every 4–6 hours • Oral, topical, or ocular medications
2.	• Wounds, constipation, or urinary tract infection • Routine postoperative care ASA 1/II (OHE, neuter, CCL repair, etc.) • ± IV catheter (flush only) • Assess every 6 hours	• Level 1 monitoring • Auscultation • Wound/bandage care	• Nutrition: free choice/portion controlled ± restrictions • Walk: minimal assistance required every 4–6 hours • Wound checks and bandage replacement • Passive range of motion • Express bladder if necessary • Intermittent injectable medications • SQ fluid administration • E-collars

(Continued)

Table 14.1 / Hospitalization level examples (Continued)

Hospitalization level	Monitoring	Assessment	Actions
3.	• Non-critical patients (urethral obstructions, stable DKA, etc.) • Non-routine postoperative care ASA III/IV (splenectomy, GDV, etc.) • IV catheter with fluid therapy • Assess every 4 hours	• Level 1–2 monitoring • Vitals assessed every 4 hours • Laboratory monitoring • ECG (intermittent) • Blood pressure • Pulse oximetry	• Nutrition: restricted • Walk: non-ambulatory; assistance required • Recumbent patient care • Nutritional support via feeding tube • Nebulization/coupage • IV fluid therapy ± CRI

4.	• Critical care patients (uncontrolled seizure activity, unstable DKA, pneumonia, post-resuscitation, ventilator cases etc.)
	• Non-routine postoperative care ASA IV/V (thoracotomy)
	• Oxygen supplementation
	• Chemotherapy infusion
	• Assess every 1-2 hours
		• Level 1–3 monitoring
		• Monitor indwelling catheters and tubes
		• Neurological monitoring (mentation, PLR, menace response, etc.)
		• Appropriate cage padding
			• Nutrition: restricted, nil by mouth, parenteral
			• Recumbent patient care every 2–4 hours
			• IV fluid therapy, CRI (vasopressors, etc.)
			• Blood products
			• Monitor ins and outs:
			  • In: water consumption, fluid therapy, nutrition
			  • Out: urine, feces, vomiting, fluid lost from wounds
			• Tube care (tracheostomy, chest tube, etc.)
			• Preventative measures to prevent decubital sores

Notes	• Listed conditions in monitoring levels are basic guidelines, as each patient's condition will determine the frequency of monitoring. • See also Tables 2.1, 2.2, 2.3, 2.4, and 2.5; Skill Boxes 2.2, 2.3, 2.4, 2.5, 2.6, and 2.7; Chapter 18, Pain Management; Skill Boxes 14.11 and 14.18; Table 14.19.		

their care. The goal is to continually reassess the patient's status, response to treatment and the need for any alterations to the patient's management plan.

HOSPITALIZED PATIENT CARE

Providing nursing care to injured and sick animals is a core function of the veterinary technician. A strong foundation in veterinary nursing principles is essential for the veterinary technician to provide effective animal care. The basic tenets of animal welfare are upheld by veterinary technicians when providing nursing care. These were classified by the Farm Animal Welfare Council (now known as the Animal Welfare Committee) of the UK as the "five freedoms of animal welfare". These are:

1. Freedom from hunger and thirst: by ready access to fresh water and a diet to maintain full health and vigor.
2. Freedom from discomfort: by providing an appropriate environment, including shelter and a comfortable resting area.
3. Freedom from pain, injury, or disease: by prevention or rapid diagnosis and treatment.
4. Freedom to express normal behavior: by providing sufficient space, proper facilities, and company of the animal's own kind.
5. Freedom from fear and distress: by ensuring conditions and treatment that avoid mental suffering.

When caring for veterinary patients, the goal is to meet all basic patient needs. The five freedoms serve as important benchmarks for veterinary technicians to reach. In any patient intervention, veterinary technicians should constantly reflect upon the freedoms of their patients that they are impacting. Recognizing patient needs and providing an individualized patient care plan is ideal for every hospitalized patient.

THE VETERINARY NURSING PROCESS

The veterinary nursing process is a cyclical, structured method that encourages critical thinking and ensures that consistent quality care is provided to every patient. This is based on a structured systematic approach to nursing care called the nursing process, which was initially introduced to human nursing in 1958 and is considered a significant step forward for registered nurses ability to assess the individual needs of patients and provide appropriate nursing care, rather than making assumptions based on a diagnosis. Veterinary technicians work closely with attending veterinarians to ensure that changes in the patient's status are addressed promptly, on an as needed basis. The following four steps comprise the veterinary nursing process:

Step 1: Assessment

The veterinary technician gathers subjective and objective data to identify actual and potential health problems, followed by recording and communicating that information to the veterinary healthcare team. Subjective data collection is any information that is based on opinion, emotion, or interpretation (e.g. level of consciousness, general demeanor, or pain). Objective data are measurable and factual and are often collected through the application of a clinical skill (e.g. blood pressure measurement, heart rate, body temperature). It is important that when gathering information to prioritize the establishment of what is normal, particularly for that individual patient. In addition to collecting information and recording findings, having a verbal exchange of information or rounds when patient care transfers to another technician will facilitate communication between the veterinary healthcare team and promote continuity of care.

Information gathering may be accomplished in the following ways:

1. Gathering the initial medical history from the owner, or reviewing this information in the patient's chart if the initial history has been gathered by other veterinary health care team member(s).
2. Reviewing the medical record for past historical information.
3. Performing a physical examination.
4. Reviewing laboratory results and diagnostic, surgical, and medical reports.
5. Consulting with the attending veterinarian regarding any questions about the case not mentioned in the medical record.

Step 2: Planning

Based on the patient information gathered in the assessment phase of the nursing process, the veterinary technician analyzes the database and makes a clinical judgment regarding the physiologic and psychological needs of the patient. This judgment is called a technician evaluation and is based on the technician's independent critical thinking in identifying actual (current) problems, potential problems, and any additional factors such as the level of client knowledge and/or coping abilities that may or may not impair at-home care of the pet.

As an example, a patient with tachypnea, cyanosis, dyspnea, and a low pulse oximetry measurement (the data) would be given a technician evaluation of hypoxia. This assessment is separate from the medical diagnosis made by the veterinarian, which focuses on the cause of the problem, such as congestive heart failure (CHF). The technician is observing the patient's physiologic response to CHF and assigns technician evaluations independently based on the data gathered. Additionally, technician evaluations may include information on the owner's level of knowledge regarding care of the pet and the owner's ability to cope with the responsibility. Technician evaluations often refer to deficiencies in the five freedoms, compared with a systems approach that veterinarians use to diagnose a patient's medical condition.

Once a list of technician evaluations has been generated, each evaluation is prioritized in terms of importance to the life of the patient and interventions can be planned. For example, a patient with cyanosis and dyspnea has a body condition score of 5/5. The technician might document "hypoxia" and "overweight" as two separate technician evaluations. However, it is more important for the patient to breathe than it is to have an ideal body weight, so the technician evaluation of "hypoxia" takes precedence over the technician evaluation of "overweight" when the nursing plan is devised and implemented.

Step 3: Implementation

Once technician evaluations have been identified and prioritized, each should have a desired outcome associated with it. In our patient with hypoxia, for example, the desired outcome is adequate oxygenation and comfortable breathing, which would be evidenced by resolution of the dyspnea, tachypnea, the return of mucous membranes to a normal pink color, and a normal pulse oximetry measurement. Each technician evaluation is accompanied by one or more interventions, or actions, to help achieve the desired patient outcome. A technician intervention can be something seemingly simple, such as a nail trim, but when taken in the context of a feline patient who has forelimb paralysis and cannot use the scratching post to maintain healthy nails, a nail trim is an integral part of patient care because it prevents the nails from growing into the pads, causing an infection.

Step 4: Evaluation

The nursing care plan refers to the entire list of interventions specific to each technician evaluation for a particular patient. The care plan is continuously revised on the basis of patient response (positive or negative) to the interventions, and new technician evaluations are identified on the basis of changes in patient status. The evaluation step is most crucial as it focuses on a patient-centered approach and evaluates each patient's response to therapy, instead of a "one size fits all" approach. Taking the time to develop a nursing plan allows the veterinary healthcare team the opportunity to set specific parameters and goals. If these goals are not met it will prompt the veterinary heathcare team to review the current interventions, assess the patient, determine if goals were appropriate, and make any necessary adjustments. In some cases, additional data, such as laboratory and imaging studies, are required to fully assess the patient's response to nursing interventions and to the treatment prescribed by the attending veterinarian. In this way, the first phase of the veterinary technician practice model is repeated, underscoring its cyclical pattern.

ESTABLISHING NORMALCY

Patient comfort begins with understanding their normal routine. Animals are well adjusted to their daily routine at home and change can cause additional stress and anxiety that affects the recovery process. Providing care that incorporates some of those routines will help patients adjust to a hospital stay. Talking with the owner at admission and asking routine-directed questions will help with patient care:

- What diet does your pet typically eat and on what schedule?
- Are feeding dishes elevated?
- Do they avoid certain floor surfaces?
- How frequently do they go outside to eliminate?
- Where do they typically eliminate (e.g. pavement, grass)?
- What is their typical exercise each day?
- Do they prefer quiet and isolated spaces or to be with people?
- What type of surfaces or bedding due they typically rest on?

Table 14.2 / Hospitalized patient care

Patient care	Concern	Technique or treatment
Cage setup	• Slipping on cage or clinic surface • Forming decubital sores • Patient stress	• Provide a non-slip surface to stand on within and outside the cage (e.g. yoga mats, foam mats) • Provide boxes or cat beds for hiding places • Provide orthopedic mats and/or thick bedding to prevent pressure points and subsequent decubital sores • See also Table 14.6
Feeding	• Hyporexia/anorexia • Food aversion • Inability to access food	• Place bowls within easy reach • Offer palatable food, consider warming, add warm water or top dressing • Do not allow food to linger in cage • Measure/record food intake and weight patient at least daily to identify if feeding tube placement is required

(Continued)

Table 14.2 / **Hospitalized patient care (Continued)**

Patient care	Concern	Technique or treatment
Hygiene and grooming	• Patients unable to clean and groom themselves may get soiled (e.g. vomit, food, urine, fecal material)	• Brushing and combing daily to keep coat clean and provide an opportunity to observe for changes or abnormalities in the skin • Grooming stimulates the sebaceous glands and eliminates matting
Mental health	• ↑ Stress, anxiety, and boredom • Altered sleeping patterns/ 24-hour lighting • Elevated noise levels • Generalized lack of normalcy	• Enrichment activities • Puzzle feeders, pheromone sprays, and toys • Cats also benefit from a change in environment (e.g. empty exam room) and access to toys • Owner visits • Scheduling time for the owners to visit can often be very helpful to the patient • Assisting with attitude, feeding, medicating, progress, pain assessment • Some patients become more agitated and distraught with their owner present; these visits should be avoided until patients are stable • Providing time each day with low lights and noise and uninterrupted sleep • Caring attention (e.g. talking and gentle petting)
Physical therapy	• Reduced mobility • Post-surgery recovery • ↑ Edema and atelectasis • ↓ Circulation	• Certain movements can be beneficial to the patient (e.g. simple passive ROM exercises, cryotherapy, heat therapy) • See also Skill Box 13.1, Physical Rehabilitation, page 770.
Walks and exercise	• ↑ Elimination needs (e.g. high fluid rates, diabetes, UTI, and diarrhea) • Holding of eliminations • ↑ Stress, anxiety, and boredom	• Frequent trips outside; care must be taken to consider the patient's needs • Cardiac, respiratory, or anemia: slow walks to avoid exhaustion and collapse • Geriatric, trauma, fractures, wounds: slow, short walks on even ground • Neurological: assisted walks (e.g. slings, towels) • Head and neck conditions: use of harnesses • House-trained dogs often hold all eliminations until allowed outside • Even if patients do not eliminate on the walk, the fresh air and sun contribute to their mental health as well • Sunlight can be stimulating and helps with vitamin D production
Notes	• See also Tables 14.4, 14.5, and Table 14.6 for additional patient care information	

NEONATAL AND PEDIATRIC CARE

Providing the ideal conditions to a neonate is critical, as they rely solely on the care they receive to survive the first few months of life. The most important aspects of their care are nutrition, temperature, and elimination. Monitoring weight and temperature once or twice daily will allow quick recognition of changes.

Table 14.3 / Neonatal and pediatric care

Factor	Care	Technique	Notes
Housing	• A container providing a comfortable, warm, and safe place of confinement	• Container • Initially, the space should be limited to preserve heat and to prevent injury; larger spaces will be required as they grow • A box with tall sides to avoid escape, such as a cardboard pet carrier • A container that can be carried or easily moved is helpful • A small cat or dog kennel can be used but is often more difficult to keep clean once they begin eliminating on their own • Bedding • Line the bottom of the container with towels and place a diaper or moisture absorbent pad on top for easy cleaning	• Neonates like to nestle when sleeping; providing a stuffed animal or a rolled-up towel can be soothing • Avoid excessive bedding to prevent entanglement • Clean the box frequently to keep the neonates clean and dry
Temperature	• Neonates are unable to thermoregulate and therefore rely on the ambient temperature and the body temperatures of their littermates • Neonates are only able to maintain a temperature 12°F above ambient temperature.	• The environment should be draft free with an ambient temperature gradient across the container allowing the neonates to move away from the heat source • The temperature should be monitored and measured at the level of the neonates, never higher than 90°F • The ambient temperature should be 85–90°F for the first week, 80–85°F for weeks 2–4	• Extreme caution should be used with warming devices (e.g. low temperatures, padding, monitoring temperature) to avoid overheating and burns • Shivering reflex and peripheral vasoconstriction are not fully developed until at least 1 week of age, making hypothermia a significant concern
Diet	• Commercial replacement diets (e.g. Esbilac®, KMR®) that are formulated species specific are the best choice for diet replacement • Emergency formulas can be prepared but should only be used until a commercial diet is available	• Commercial diets: follow package directions for reconstituting • When commercial diets are not available, the following recipe can be used in the interim: ½ cup whole milk, ½ cup water, 1 tsp vegetable oil, 1 drop multivitamins, 2 egg yolks, 2 Tums® (antacid) crushed. Blend all ingredients in a blender; keep refrigerated and use within 48 hours	• Home-prepared diets may result in cataract formation, due to a deficiency in amino acids

(Continued)

Table 14.3 / Neonatal and pediatric care (Continued)

Factor	Care	Technique	Notes

Feeding	• Feeding a neonate is a time-consuming project, especially with larger litters.
	• A nipple bottle is most commonly used, but a feeding tube can be ideal in skilled hands for weak or premature neonates
		• Quantity
		• The diet should be gradually ↑ over 2–3 days to the recommended daily amount to avoid overfeeding and diarrhea:
		• 13–18 ml/100 g
		• Bottle feeding
		• Prepare the formula according to the manufacturer's directions and warm to 100°F in a bowl of hot water
		• Place the neonate in a comfortable dorsal position propped up on a rolled-up towel
		• Hold the bottle up in a position to closely mimic that of the mother while assuring that the nipple does not contain air
		• Following each feeding, burping may be necessary to expel excess air ingested
		• Tube feeding
			• Neonates are given 4–6 feedings daily for the first week, then 3–4 feedings/day until weaned
			• Neonates have a vigorous suckling response and can overfeed if not monitored (e.g. nose milk bubbles)
			• A satisfied neonate is quiet with a slightly enlarged abdomen
			• With all methods of feeding, care should be taken to avoid aspiration pneumonia, a complication seen with forced nursing, squeezing the bottle, nipple hole too large, improper feeding tube use and volume overload
			• Assess feeding plan based on overall appearance, hydration and activity level, and daily weight gain:
			  • Kittens: around 18–20 g/day
			  • Puppies: 1 g for every 2–5 g milk ingested

Weaning	• Weaning often begins at 3–4 weeks of age • Constant chewing on the nipple may be a sign that weaning should begin	• Offer gruel • Canned food with formula in a 1 : 2 ratio • Dry food softened with warm water can also be used • The food should be placed on a small plate that can be accessed for all sides and walked through • Putting gruel on the paws with a reluctant eater will cause them to lick and discover the new food • The amount of formula is slowly reduced	• Complete weaning is often by 7–8 weeks of age • Early weaning can cause health (malnutrition, stress-related diseases) and behavioral problems (timid, aggression) • Commercial food should be specifically made and tested for all life stages

Health	• Monitor daily:
	  • General appearance
	  • Activity level
	  • Hydration
	• Daily weight gain:
	  • Kittens: around 18–20 g/day
	  • Puppies: 1 g for every 2–5 g milk ingested
		• Monitor hydration, mucus membranes, eyes, and urine color
		• Weigh daily at the same time each day to assure accuracy
		• Urine specific gravity is not reliable until 8–10 weeks of age
		• Always wear exam glove when handling neonates
			• Crying for > 15 minutes is a sign of distress (e.g. hunger, cold, neglected, pain)
			• Neonates who did not nurse from the mother in the first 48 hours are lacking much needed antibodies; maintaining a strict cleaning protocol is crucial

(Continued)

Table 14.3 / **Neonatal and pediatric care (Continued)**

Factor	Care	Technique	Notes
Elimination	• Neonates are unable to voluntarily eliminate on their own • During the first 3 weeks, the neonate must be stimulated to urinate and defecate after each feeding	• Stimulation • Hold the neonate securely in one hand while supporting the spine • Placing them in a small towel or washcloth that is gently wrapped around their upper body will provide more security and comfort • While over a sink, gently massage the lower abdomen in a circular motion • The anal and genital areas may also be lightly rubbed with a warm, moist cotton ball • The genitals should be cleaned and dried after elimination to avoid skin irritation • Litter box • A small litter box can be introduced to kittens with a paper litter at 3–4 weeks of age • Pie pans or meat trays work well initially • Feces can be placed in the litter box as a guide, but the process is instinctive for most cats	• Feces should be soft but not green, yellow, or watery • Overfeeding is the most common cause of diarrhea; further dilute the formula by one third for 2 days if present • Urine and feces should be seen at almost every feeding during stimulation or in the box
Notes	• See also Table 2.3.		

REWARMING

Heat support is required for all animals unable to thermoregulate. Anesthetized, severely ill, and physically compromised patients are unable to regulate their body temperature and routinely require additional methods of heat support. Hypothermia is defined as less than 99°F and will significantly slow recovery. Severe hypothermia can cause cardiac arrhythmias, central nervous system deficits, and coagulation problems; prevention is better than management. Alternatively, monitoring the patient who is on heat support is also important to ensure that they do not become overheated or incidentally burned. Hospitalized or anesthetized patients are often unable to move away from an external heat source and have decreased peripheral blood supply, leading to sometimes severe thermal burns.

Shivering increases oxygen demand; additional oxygen should be provided if a patient is cold and shivering. Warming devices should be used immediately; otherwise, cooling will continue. The Bair Hugger™ temperature monitoring system, incubators, intravenous (IV) fluid warmers, and circulating warm air blankets are ideal. Warmed IV fluid bags, heating pads, and heating lamps are not recommended, as severe thermal burns can occur. There should be proper padding on all surfaces to control heat loss. It should be noted that rectal temperature is not core temperature, but allows trends to be assessed and should be measured regularly to ensure a return to normothermia. Esophageal temperature probes are reflective of core body temperature in anesthetized patients.

Basic heat support that does not require additional equipment includes keeping the patient dry, keeping patients away from air vents and air conditioners, maintaining warm room temperatures, and providing insulation materials against surgery tables and cages. Alongside providing heat support, it is also important to assure heat retention. Many quick methods have been devised, such as external covers, wrapping portions of the patient with bubble wrap or foil, placing the patient on foam padding, and placing baby socks on the paws.

Table 14.4 / **Rewarming**

Method	Use	Comments
Circulating heated water blankets	• A preheated circulating controlled warm water vinyl pad is placed under the patient	• Thermal burns may occur (rare) • Blankets or other protective coverings are placed on top of the pad to prevent inadvertent puncture • Provides a minimal amount of heat support
Heated air blankets (Bair Huggers)	• Blanket is placed over the patient • Place a cotton blanket over the blanket or gown for maximum effectiveness	• Do not use over transdermal medication as ↑ drug delivery and subsequent overdose may occur • Do not place blankets over the patient's head as corneal drying may occur • Use caution when using in surgery to avoid circulating contaminated air; do not turn on until the patient is fully prepped and draped • Best when placed near areas with a large blood supply (neck, abdomen, etc.)
Heated bags, heating pads/ lamps	• Expired IV fluid bags, rice, or oat bags • Wrap the bag in a blanket or towel and place to the side of the patient	• *Not* recommended, as severe thermal burns often occur • Bags/pads should never be placed on top, underneath, or next to a shaved area of skin • Remove the bag once it has cooled to prevent reverse heat exchange
Hot line IV fluid warmer	• Fluids are warmed within the administration set using metal warming channels or multilumen circulating warm water	• Additional methods can be used alone or along with fluid warmers: running the fluid administration set through a bowl of hot water, placing a circulating heated water blanket around the line, or coiling the line under the patient's heat source • Rewarming is determined by the rate of flow and the volume received; additional rewarming methods should be used
Lavage or rectal enema	• Administration of warmed fluids to the stomach, urinary bladder, pleura, peritoneum, or rectum	• Associated risks of vomiting and aspiration; should not be used as the first method of treatment
Warm blankets and towels	• Blankets and towels warmed by a clothes dryer	• Amount and length of heat are limited and best used for mildly hypothermic patients • The slowest rewarming method
Notes	• Note: Severely hypothermic patients should be handled gently, as excessive handling can cause ventricular fibrillation	

COOLING

Hyperthermia is the elevation of the body temperature past normal (> 103.5°F). This can be due to fever or inadequate heat dissipation.

Fevers change the temperature setpoint of the thermoregulatory center in response to pyrogens. Most pyrogens are pathogenic, such as bacteria or viruses, but nonpathogenic pyrogens such as pharmacological agents, tissue inflammation or necrosis may also induce fever. Patients with a fever, unlike those that are hyperthermic as a result of heat stroke, still have the ability to dissipate heat.

Heat stroke is the body's inability to dissipate excess heat due to external/environmental conditions such overexertion, being left in a hot car, or outside without shade or water. Brachycephalic patients and those with laryngeal paralysis or tracheal collapse have reduced ability to dissipate heat through their respiratory tract and therefore are at greater risk. Other conditions such as obesity and cardiovascular disease may compound the issue. Heat stroke patients, by definition, have a temperature of at least 104°F, but often present with temperatures much higher.

The goal is to rapidly cool the patient to 103.5–104°F. The cooling process should be discontinued once the patient reaches this temperature range as further cooling will result in rebound hypothermia. Temperatures should be taken every 5–10 minutes until consecutive temperatures maintain the same reading. The temperature should continue to be monitored every few hours for the next 24 hours.

Table 14.5 / Cooling

Method	Use	Comments
Cool water and fan	• Patient is soaked with cool to tepid water and a fan is placed nearby to dissipate heat	• Provides the best approach using both evaporation and convection and should be considered for the first method of treatment • Patients placed on a metal table will also benefit from conduction • Often the only treatment needed to reduce the temperature • Wet towels should not be placed on the patient as they may impede heat loss
Cold water and ice bath	• Patient is bathed in cold water and ice bath	• Used for extreme hyperthermia in humans, due to its rapid effects on temperature • Controversial as cold water/ice baths may cause cutaneous vasoconstriction and shivering
Enemas	• An enema is administered with cool to tepid water	• Subsequent rectal temperatures may be inaccurate
Ice packs	• Placed on the axillary and inguinal area	• Cooling by conduction, which is not the most effective; should not be used as the first method of treatment
Intranasal cooling	• Ice cubes are placed in an oxygen mask or cage while administering oxygen	• Provides cool, humidified oxygen therapy
IV fluids	• IV fluids are administered	• Do not cool fluids further as room temperature fluids are already around 30°F below the patient's temperature and will provide a cooling effect • Fluid therapy also provides ↑ blood volume and flow, allowing additional dispersion of heat
Lavage or rectal enemas	• Cool fluids are administered to the stomach, urinary bladder, peritoneum, or rectum	• Considered for large-breeds dogs needing further cooling; should not be used as the first method of treatment • Difficult to avoid rebound hypothermia

RECUMBENT PATIENT CARE

Decubital sores (pressure sores), urine and fecal scalding, and lung atelectasis can be the source of further patient complications and can lead to increased morbidity and mortality. Recumbent patients with neurological or orthopedic disease are at the greatest risk of acquiring these complications. Observant nursing care should prevent or identify these complications in their early stages.

Table 14.6 / Recumbent patient care

Condition	Cause	Prevention	Treatment	Comments
Decubital sores	• Excessive pressure, friction, or shearing forces over a bony prominence resulting in local or regional ischemia • Anatomical differences: thin breeds (↓ muscle or fat padding over bones), obese or large and giant breeds (excessive weight and pressure), thick hair coat (trapping of moisture and inability to monitor skin changes) • Underlying disease conditions (e.g. paralysis, inability or unwillingness to change position, malnutrition, impaired circulation, metabolic disease, or thick hair coat)	• Identifying at-risk patients • Monitor for early signs (e.g. erythema, edema, tenderness, exudate, or alopecia) • Adequate nutritional status • Beds (e.g. hammocks, air or water mattresses) • Bedding (e.g. orthopedic pads, thick blankets) • Keeping the patient's skin clean and dry • Repositioning every two to four hours • Passive exercise and massage to ↑ circulation	• Relieve pressure (e.g. "donuts," inflatable rings). • Clip and clean with an antiseptic. • Drug administration (e.g. systemic antibiotics) • Debridement, surgical and wound management (see also Skill Box 19.1: wound care, page 819)	• Patients should be lifted and turned as dragging or pulling across the floor can lead to disruption in skin integrity and the beginning of decubital sores • Greater trochanter is the most common site, but additional pressure points of forelimbs and hind limbs are also seen
Urine and fecal scalding	• Exposure to urine or feces for extended periods of time or with compromised skin integrity	• Clean bedding • Grates • Beds (e.g. nylon mesh hammock) • Protective topical ointments (e.g. petrolatum) applied to the perineal and inguinal areas • Bathing	• Clip and clean with an antiseptic • Drug administration (e.g. silver sulfadiazine, systemic antibiotics) • Debridement, surgical and wound management (see also Skill Box 19.1)	• Patients with urine-soaked fur are assumed to have urine-soaked skin • Can result in severe dermatitis and predispose to decubital ulcers
Lung atelectasis	• Extended periods of one-sided recumbency	• Repositioning every 2–4 hours	• Re-expansion (e.g. repositioning, removal of air or fluid from pleural space)	• Auscultation reveals localized areas of dullness

MEDICAL NURSING

Patient Monitoring

Monitoring of a hospitalized patient is one of the crucial responsibilities of a veterinary technician. This section includes some basic monitoring skills, blood pressure, blood gas analysis, central venous pressure (CVP), and cardiac values (ECG readings). See also Table 20.11: Anesthesia monitoring, page 889, and Table 20.14: Post-anesthetic monitoring, page 902.

Blood Pressure

Measuring accurate blood pressure on animals requires experience and attention to detail. Selection of the appropriate limb, proper cuff size, fit of the cuff, position of the animal so that no weight or pressure is on the measurement limb or cuff, a relaxed and still animal, and an experienced and very patient person all affect the results.

Measurement should be done in a quiet room after the patient has had 5–10 minutes to acclimate to their surroundings. Having the owner present may also decrease the patient's stress. The procedure should be done before other diagnostic procedures and with minimal handling. Consistency between visits with the same technician performing the procedure is beneficial to the overall accuracy of the results.

Research has shown that if an animal is upset or agitated due to handling or the measurement procedure itself, it will take 8–10 minutes after the animal is calmed and relaxed for the animal's blood pressure to return to normal. Measurements on an agitated animal are not indicative of their normal blood pressure.

Assessing pulse quality can be used when blood pressure monitoring equipment is not available. However, it does not provide the same information that monitoring equipment provides, and the results must be viewed in light of other physical monitoring parameters. The pressure felt is the difference between the systolic and diastolic pressure. Therefore, a patient with 100/60 mmHg would have a similar pulse pressure as a patient with 80/40 mmHg, but the mean arterial pressure (MAP) would be different. A reasonable assessment of adequate perfusion can be made with a palpable arterial pulse, together with adequate mucous membrane color, capillary refill time, and heart sound quality. MAP can be estimated by the feeling of the vessel. Vessels that are hard and stiff will have a higher MAP than a vessel that is soft and flaccid.

Pulse quality can be assessed at the femoral artery or the dorsal pedal artery on awake animals. Pulse pressure of the arteries can be visualized through the mesentery or the caudal aorta can be palpated during an anesthetic procedure. Pulse pressures are less reliable during anesthetic procedures due to the alterations caused by anesthetic agents.

Skill Box 14.1 / Blood Pressure Procedure

Method	Direct arterial pressure	Doppler ultrasound flow detectors	Oscillometric
Indications	• Monitoring during anesthesia, shock, fluid administration, and any other condition leading to secondary hyper- or hypotension	• Monitoring during anesthesia, shock, fluid administration, and any other condition leading to secondary hyper- or hypotension • Detection of flow in distal limbs (e.g. traumatic wounds, saddle thrombi) • Irregular pulse signals or rates may indicate cardiac arrhythmias	• Monitoring during anesthesia, shock, fluid administration, and any other condition leading to secondary hyper- or hypotension
Contraindications	• Using large vessels in patients with coagulopathies • Stressed, agitated, or active patients	• Stressed or agitated patients	• Stressed or agitated patients

(Continued)

Skill Box 14.1 / Blood Pressure Procedure (Continued)

Method	Direct arterial pressure	Doppler ultrasound flow detectors	Oscillometric
Setup	• Catheter (e.g. arterial, over-the-needle, through-the-needle) • Heparinized saline • Pressure transducer and monitor	• Equipment • Doppler unit • Probe • Appropriately sized cuff • Sphygmomanometer • ± Headphones • Ultrasonic gel	• Equipment • Oscillometric device • Appropriately sized cuff
Procedure	1. Catheter is placed in an artery (e.g. dorsal pedal, femoral, or auricular) and flushed with 1–1.5 ml heparinized saline 2. Catheter is thoroughly secured with tape to avoid dislodging or kinking and labeled to prevent inadvertent intra-arterial injections 3. Catheter is then connected to the pressure transducer by rigid tubing filled with heparinized saline 4. Refer to the manufacturer's guidelines for further setup and monitoring instructions 5. 5.Method for measuring CVP can also be used if a transducer system is not available	1. Place patient in a comfortable position (ideally lateral recumbent) 2. Select a cuff that has a width that is approximately 40% of the circumference of the patient's distal limb or tail. In cats, the measurement should be adjusted to 30–40% 3. Snugly place the cuff on any place where an artery is accessible, typically a limb distal to the elbow or hock or the base of the tail 4. Place the probe over the artery but distal to the cuff; turn on Doppler and listen for blood flow 5. Position the probe until a clear flow is heard. Headphones will improve the sound quality and will minimize stress to the patient. It may be desirable to clip the hair and tape the probe into place 6. Inflate the cuff and slowly release the trigger until the first flow sound is heard; this is the systolic pressure. The second sound heard is the diastolic, which often cannot be heard 7. The cuff should be inflated to approximately 40 mmHg above the systolic pressure to properly occlude the vessel and obtain an accurate value 8. Excessive inflation pressure should be avoided as it is unnecessary and uncomfortable to the patient	1. Place patient in a comfortable lateral recumbent position 2. Select a cuff that has a width that is approximately 40% of the circumference of the patient's distal limb or tail. In cats, the measurement should be adjusted to 30–40% 3. Snugly place the cuff on any place an artery is accessible, typically a limb distal to the elbow or hock or the base of the tail 4. Connect the cuff to the monitor and turn on 5. The cuff is slowly deflated by the machine and the microprocessor measures and records readings 6. The systolic, diastolic, mean arterial pressure, and heart rate will be displayed 7. Patients need to remain still during this process as these machines have decreased reliability when there is muscle movement (such as tremor/shaking)
Complications	• Exsanguination, thrombosis, infection, necrosis	• Poor contact between probe and artery • Relies on subjective interpretation of the operator; may be operator variations	• Patient movement, arrhythmias, bradycardia, and poor perfusion can lead to inaccurate results
Notes	• Blood pressure is significantly affected by body position. Sitting produces a significantly higher blood pressure reading, whereas lateral recumbency has been proven to have the least variable results.		

Table 14.7 **Blood pressure evaluation.**

Blood pressure	Normal	Abnormal
Canine	Systolic: 90–150 mmHg Diastolic: 60–85 mmHg Mean: 80–105 mmHg	Systolic: < 90 and > 150 mmHg Diastolic: >85 mmHg Mean: < 60 and > 105 mmHg
Feline	Systolic: 90–150 mmHg Diastolic: 80–90 mmHg Mean: 80–105 mmHg	Systolic: < 90 and > 150 mmHg Diastolic: > 90 mmHg Mean: < 60 and > 105 mmHg

The normal and abnormal values for blood pressure measurements are clearly defined in human medicine but have not yet been solidly established in veterinary medicine. Table 14.7 shows the ranges currently accepted.

MAP is the average pressure within an artery over a complete cycle of one heartbeat. Since two thirds of the cardiac cycle are spent near the diastolic pressure, MAP is not just an average of the systolic and diastolic. MAP can be calculated as:

$$\text{MAP} = \text{diastolic BP} + \tfrac{1}{3}(\text{systolic BP} \quad \text{diastolic BP}).$$

A MAP of about 60 mmHg is necessary to perfuse coronary arteries, brain, and kidneys.

Central Venous Pressure

CVP is a measurement of pressure within a central vein (usually the cranial vena cava) that provides an estimation of vascular volume and cardiac preload. Individual CVP readings are of limited value and trends are more relevant. Additionally, CVP must be interpreted in conjunction with other patient parameters and status. The pressure within the intrathoracic anterior vena cava is compared with a column of water in a manometer or pressure transducer and oscilloscope. Fluctuations are seen with changes in pressure. A raised CVP may indicate a backup of blood due to excessive volume (e.g. fluid overload), whereas a lower CVP can indicate a decrease in blood volume (e.g. dehydration) leading to hypovolemia.

Skill Box 14.2 / Central Venous Pressure

Method	**Central venous pressure**
Indications	Monitoring patients undergoing fluid therapy, particularly those at risk for volume overload and congestive heart failure
Contraindications	Burn, abrasion, pyoderma over site, severe coagulopathy, hypercoagulable, or thrombosis of chosen vein inhibiting jugular catheter placement
Setup	• Surgical site preparation materials • Three-way stopcock • IV jugular catheter • Bandaging materials • Heparinized saline • IV fluid setup
Procedure	• Place a jugular catheter and advance to the cranial vena cava (Skill Box 14.9) • Attach an extension set to the catheter, followed by a three-way stopcock • Attach the IV fluids to the open line of the stopcock • Attach the manometer to the upright opening of the stopcock • Place the patient in sternal recumbency and position the manometer at the level of the sternum • Turn off the fluids to the patient and fill the manometer with fluids • Open the extension set and allow the fluid level to equalize • The level at which the fluids stabilize is the central venous pressure reading. Alternatively, an electronic transducer system may be used with a compatible multiparameter monitor
Complications	• Blood clots or occlusions can $\uparrow$ values • If fluids are not running through the catheter, flush with heparinized saline every hour • Arrhythmias if catheter tip is placed inside the heart
Results	$\downarrow$ CVP: < 0 cm H_2O • May be indicative of hypovolemia $\uparrow$ CVP: > 10 cm H_2O • May be indicative of volume overload, right-sided heart failure, or an increase in intrathoracic pressure

Blood Gas Analysis

Blood gas analysis is used to monitor ventilation acid–base status, and oxygenation through the delicate balance between carbon dioxide (CO_2), bicarbonate (HCO_3^-), hydrogen (H^+), and oxygen (O_2). A change in CO_2 or HCO_3^- affects the body's pH, ultimately affecting its ability to carry out various enzyme activities. The lungs are primarily responsible for regulating CO_2 through respiration, while the kidneys regulate HCO_3^- through resorption and excretion in the proximal tubule. Since CO_2 and HCO_3^- are the main determinants of the acid–base status (pH) of a patient, a change in one factor can affect the other. It should be noted that only an arterial blood gas can provide information about oxygenation.

Skill Box 14.3 / Blood Gas Analysis

Method	Blood gas analysis
Indications	Patients with respiratory disease or metabolic disturbances (e.g. hypoadrenocorticism, diabetes mellitus, chronic renal failure)
Contraindications	Patients taking potassium bromide, severe coagulopathy, cellulitis, or open infection at collection site
Setup	• Blood gas syringe set or 25-gauge needle with 1-ml syringe • Heparin • ± Sterile red-top tube • Ice water bath (for temporary storage) • Blood gas analyzer

Procedure	• A syringe coated with heparin (1000 u/ml) is used to obtain a blood sample
	• A full 1 ml of blood should be obtained to avoid any dilution with heparin
	• All excess air is expelled from the syringe and the sample is analyzed immediately
	• If temporary storage is required, the sample can be stored at room temperature for $< 10–15$ minutes or $< 1–2$ hours in an ice bath once placed in a container with a tight-fitting cap (e.g. rubber stopper, red-top tube)
	• Arterial:
	  • Femoral, dorsal pedal, or lingual artery
	  • Hold off for 3–5 minutes and/or place a temporary pressure wrap to prevent hematoma formation
	• Venous:
	  • Jugular, cephalic, or saphenous vein

Complications	• Samples stored at room temperature for > 20 minutes: ↓ pH • Excessive heparin: ↓ HCO_3^-

(Continued)

Skill Box 14.3 / Blood Gas Analysis (Continued)

Method	Blood gas analysis	
Results:	**Canine:**	**Feline:**
Arterial normal	• pH: 7.35–7.45 • $PaCO_2$: 35–45 mmHg • PaO_2: 90–100 mmHg • HCO_3^-: 22–27 mEq/l • Base excess: −2 to +2	• pH: 7.24–7.45 • $PaCO_2$: 25–37 mmHg • PaO_2: 101–113 mmHg • HCO_3^-: 15–22 mEq/l • Base excess: −2 to +2.5
Venous normal	• pH: 7.32–7.5 • $PvCO_2$: 33–50 mmHg • PvO_2: 40–50 mmHg • HCO_3^-: 18–26 mEq/l • Base excess: −2 to +2	• pH: 7.28–7.41 • $PvCO_2$: 33–45 mmHg • PvO_2: 28–50 mmHg • HCO_3^-: 18–23 mEq/l • Base excess: −2 to +2.5
Abnormal	• Single or multiple alterations from normal • pH: <7.35, acidemia; > 7.45, alkalemia	
Critical values	• pH: < 7.2 or > 7.5 • $PaCO_2$: < 20 or > 55 mmHg • PaO_2: <60 mmHg (arterial sample) • HCO_3^-: < 13 or > 33 mEq/l • Base excess: > 8	
Notes	• Samples, particularly arterial, must be protected from air to avoid alterations • Refer to reference range for the blood gas analyzer in use • Base excess: represents the magnitude of acid–base abnormality contributed by metabolic components	

The results of the blood gas analysis are then evaluated to determine the status of the patient. This can often be a tricky process, but the basic interpretation is shown in Skill Box 14.4 is a five-step process.

Skill Box 14.4 / Arterial Blood Gas Interpretation

1. Evaluate the PaO_2 and determine whether the patient is hypoxemic (needs oxygen)
2. Evaluate the pH and determine whether the patient is normal, acidotic, or alkalotic:
   - pH = 7.4, normal
   - pH > 7.4, alkalosis
   - pH < 7.4, acidosis
3. Evaluate the $PaCO_2$ and determine whether it supports the pH findings:
   - Yes; moves in the same direction: condition is metabolic
   - No; moves in the opposite direction: condition is respiratory
4. Evaluate the HCO_3^- and determine whether it supports the pH findings:
   - Yes; moves in the same direction: condition is metabolic
   - No; moves in the opposite direction: condition is respiratory
5. Evaluate the parameter not responsible for abnormal conditions to assess for compensation

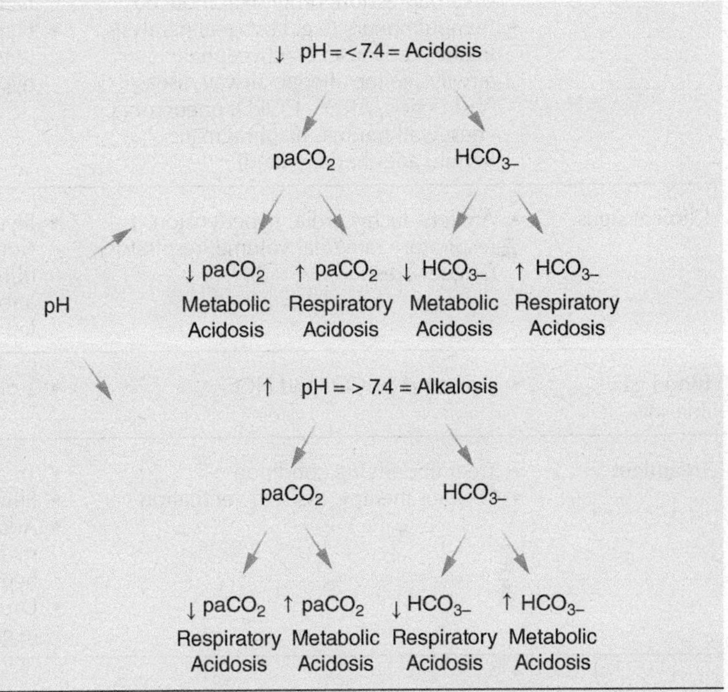

Source: adapted with permission from Nancy Shaffran.

Table 14.8 / Acid–base disturbances

	Respiratory acidosis	Metabolic acidosis	Respiratory alkalosis	Metabolic alkalosis
Cause	• Hypoventilation • Extrapulmonary (e.g. myasthenia gravis, tick paralysis, tetanus, hypokalemia, CNS depression, drug/toxin induced) • Intrapulmonary (e.g. laryngeal paralysis, tracheal collapse, brachycephalic airways, feline allergic airway disease, obstruction, ARDS, COPD, pneumonia, chest wall trauma, diaphragmatic hernia, anesthesia related)	• Intoxication (e.g. ethylene glycol, salicylate) • Ketoacidosis, uremic acidosis, lactic acidosis • Hypochloremia (e.g. diarrhea, renal failure, hypoadrenocorticism)	• Hyperventilation • Pulmonary (e.g. hypoxemia, ARDS, PTE, pulmonary edema, pneumonia) • Non-pulmonary (e.g. anxiety, fear, pain, anemia, septicemia, hyperthermia, CNS disease, corticosteroid administration, excessive assisted ventilation) • Secondary to metabolic acidosis	• Vomiting (often associated with an upper gastrointestinal obstruction) • Drug administration (e.g. furosemide, phosphate binders, sodium bicarbonate) • Hyperadrenocorticism
Clinical signs	• Anxiety, tachycardia, hypertension, ↓ respiratory rate/tidal volume, respiratory fatigue/arrest	• Hyperventilation, hypotension, tachycardia, ventricular fibrillation, tachypnea, anorexia, vomiting, and lethargy	• Variable signs associated with underlying condition	• Variable signs associated with underlying condition • ± ↑ Respiratory rate, effort and depth, vomiting, nausea, and muscle tremors
Blood gas analysis	• ↓ pH and ↑ pCO_2 and HCO_3^-	• ↓ pH, pCO_2, and HCO_3^-	• ↑ pH and ↓ pCO_2 and HCO_3^-	• ↑ pH, pCO_2, and HCO_3^-
Treatment	• Treat underlying condition • Oxygen therapy, assisted ventilation	• Treat underlying condition • Fluid therapy • Address electrolyte abnormalities (e.g. hypernatremia, hypokalemia, hypocalcemia) • Drug administration (e.g. sodium bicarbonate)	• Treat underlying condition • Fluid therapy	• Treat underlying condition • Fluid therapy • Address electrolyte abnormalities (e.g. hypokalemia, hypochloremia)

Electrocardiogram

An ECG is a graphical interpretation of the electrical activity of the cardiac muscle (Figure 14.1). Its use is required for accurate diagnosis of arrhythmias and conduction disorders. An ECG should be a regular part of any systemic disease workup as life-threatening arrhythmias (e.g. ventricular tachycardia, atrial tachycardia) are easily missed on auscultation. ECG is also used in the preoperative evaluation of geriatrics, during anesthetic procedures, and in assessing the effects of cardiac drugs. An ECG is also a necessary component of advanced life support during cardiopulmonary resuscitation.

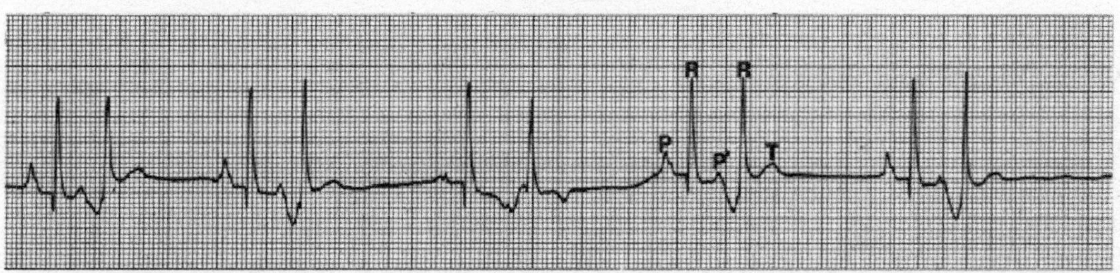

Figure 14.1 Normal canine electrocardiogram. Source: reprinted with permission from Larry Patrick Tilley (1992).

Skill Box 14.5 / Electrocardiogram Procedure

Method	Electrocardiogram
Indications	• To determine heart rate and rhythm • Cardiac arrhythmias and the status of the myocardium • Tachycardia, bradycardia, pulse deficits, irregular rhythm, murmurs, cardiomegaly, electrolyte disturbances, cardiopulmonary arrest • Exercise intolerance, panting, dyspnea, cyanosis, fainting, seizures, syncope, and shock,
Contraindications	**If animal is exhibiting severe dyspnea**
Setup	• Equipment • Limb leads (electrode cables) • Alligator clips/ electrode pads • Conducting solution (e.g. alcohol, gel) • Blanket or soft pad • Clippers • Recording/telemetry device

Procedure	• The procedure should take place in a calm and quiet environment
	• All devices that may cause electrical disturbances should be turned off (e.g. fluorescent bulbs, electrical equipment) and having a dedicated ECG outlet can help reduce interference
	• Using a nonconductive table (e.g. Formica or metal covered with an insulator such as blanket or pad), the patient should ideally be placed in right lateral recumbency. However, if the patient is in distress, other positions will provide information about the rate and rhythm, but will not provide information on cardiac enlargement patterns
	• The limbs should be extended and held parallel to each other and not touching. The forelimbs should be perpendicular to the long axis of the body
	• If using clips, moisten the areas of attachment with conductive gel, paste, creams, or alcohol
	• Apply the clips and reapply the conductive agent.
	  • RA/LA: proximal to the olecranon and on the caudal aspect (electrodes may need to be positioned halfway between the olecranon and carpus if cardiac interference is seen)
	  • RL/LL: patellar ligament on the anterior aspect
	  • ECG strips are recorded at 25 mm/second or 50 mm/second according to clinician preference and practice protocol

(*Continued*)

Skill Box 14.5 / Electrocardiogram Procedure (Continued)

Method	Electrocardiogram
Complications	• ↑ Stress can exacerbate already critical situations • Variations in the body conformation of many dog breeds may alter standard measurements • Drug administration (e.g. ketamine, valium) may alter results • See also Table 14.12

Tip: ECG activity may continue to appear normal even after all mechanical activity has ceased and the patient has no palpable pulse (e.g. deceased, electromechanical dissociation).
Tip: Some arrhythmias may manifest themselves when the patient is calm and resting, others when the patient is excited.
Tip: The teeth of the alligator clips may be bent out, flattened, or filed to improve patient comfort.
Tip: Conductive gel, paste, and creams are better at lowering the electrical resistance than alcohol and do not evaporate; however, alcohol-soaked pads may be used between the clip and skin.

Table 14.9 Electrocardiogram leads.

Lead	Measurement	Movement and electrode position	Use
Bipolar standard:	Between two limbs		
I		R arm (–) → L arm (+)	Abnormalities in P,QRS,T deflections and cardiac arrhythmias
II		R arm (–) → L leg (+)	Determining mean electrical axis
III		L arm (–) → L leg (+)	
Augmented unipolar limb:	From one limb to a point halfway in between the other two limbs		
aVR		L arm and leg (–) → R arm (+)	Determining mean electrical axis and heart position
aVL		R arm and L leg (–) → L arm (+)	Confirming information gained from other leads
aVF		L arm and R arm (–) → L leg (+)	

L, left; R, right.

Table 14.10 / **Electrocardiogram interpretation**

Cycle segment	Movement*	Image description	Normal ECG	Action

P wave	SA node → R Atrium → L Atrium → AV node	Positive wave
		Measurement:
		• Width:
		  • 0.04 second (two boxes)
		  • 0.05 second, giant breeds
		• Height:
		  • 0.4 mV (four boxes)
		  • 0.2 mV, feline
			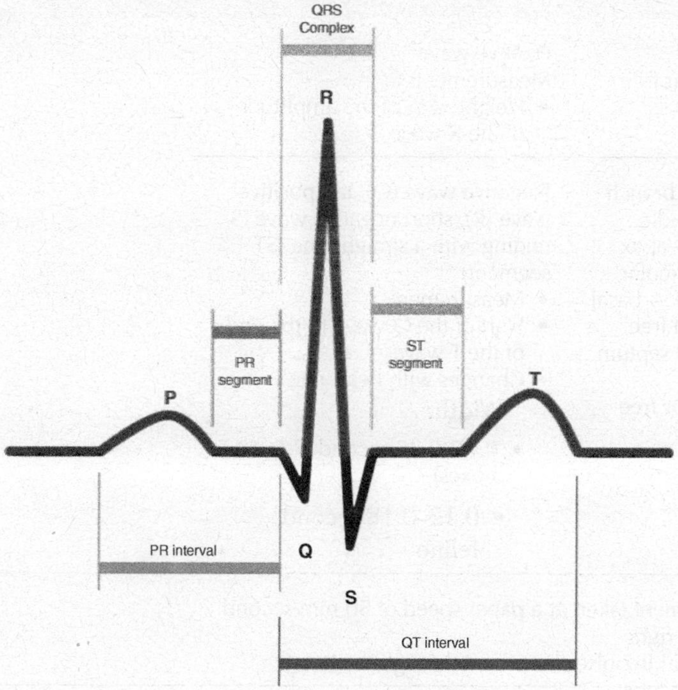 QRS Complex; R; PR segment; ST segment; P; T; PR interval; Q; S; QT interval	Depolarization of the R and L atrium triggering the atria to contract

PR Interval	SA node → AV Node → ventricle	P wave and ending straight line Measurement: • Start of the P wave to start of Q wave (R wave if no Q wave) • 0.06–0.13 second (3–6.5 boxes) • 0.05–0.09 second, feline		Time delay to allow filling of ventricles

QRS	R bundle branch and L bundle branch → apex and ventricular free walls → basal regions of free walls and septum	Negative wave (Q) followed by a tall positive wave (R) and ended with a short negative wave (S)
		Measurement:
		• Start of Q wave to the end of the S wave
		• Width:
		  • 0.05–0.06 second (2.5 boxes)
		  • 0.04 second, feline
		• Height:
		  • 2.5–3.0 mV (25–30 boxes)
		  • 0.9 mV, feline
				Depolarization of the ventricles triggering their contraction

ST interval	Basal regions of free walls and septum → apex and ventricular free walls	Straight line with no deviations Measurement: • End of the QRS complex to the start of the T wave • Width: 0.2 mV (two boxes) • Height: 0.15 mV (1.5 boxes)		Early phase of ventricular repolarization

(Continued)

Table 14.10 / Electrocardiogram interpretation (Continued)

Cycle segment	Movement*	Image description	Normal ECG	Action
T Wave	Apex and ventricular free walls	Positive wave Measurement: • Height: ≤ ¼ of the amplitude of the R wave		Repolarization of the ventricles
QT interval	R bundle branch and L bundle branch → apex and ventricular free walls → basal regions of free walls and septum → apex **ventricular free walls**	Negative wave (Q), tall positive wave (R), short negative wave (S) ending with a straight line (ST segment) • Measurement: • Start of the Q wave to the end of the T wave • Changes with heart rate Width: • 0.15–0.25 second (7.5–12.5 boxes) • 0.12–0.18 second, feline		Summation of depolarization and repolarization of the ventricles
Notes	Measurement taken at a paper speed of 50 mm/second L, left; R, right * Electrical impulse movement through the heart			

Skill Box 14.6 / Heart Rate Calculation

	ECG paper and grid lines	
Paper speed **Measurements**	25 mm/second Small box = 0.04 second Large box (five small boxes) = 0.20 second Set (15 large boxes) = 3 seconds	50 mm/second Small box = 0.02 second Large box (five small boxes) = 0.10 second Set (15 large boxes) = 1.5 seconds
Rhythm:		
Regular • Average heart rate • Instantaneous heart rate	Method 1: the number of complete complexes in one set × 20 = bpm	Method 1: the number of complete complexes in one set × 40 = bpm
	Method 2: 1500 ÷ the number of small boxes between two QRS complexes = bpm	Method 2: 3000 ÷ the number of small boxes between two QRS complexes = bpm
	Method 3: 300 ÷ the number of large boxes between two QRS complexes = bpm	Method 3: 600 ÷ the number of large boxes between two QRS complexes = bpm
	Method 4: heart rate calculator used according to provided directions	
Irregular • The fraction of the last cycle should be estimated in tenths	The number of cycles in two sets × 10 = bpm	Method 1: the number of cycles in two sets × 20 = bpm
		Method 2: the number of cycles in four sets × 10 = bpm Greater accuracy with slower rates

Table 14.11 / Common heart rhythm abnormalities

Rhythm pattern	Cause	Image	Associated conditions
Atrial fibrillation	• Rapid and disorganized depolarization pattern in the atria • ↓ Cardiac output	• P waves are absent and replaced by numerous fibrillatory *f* waves • QRS complexes may be normal or wide with varying amplitude 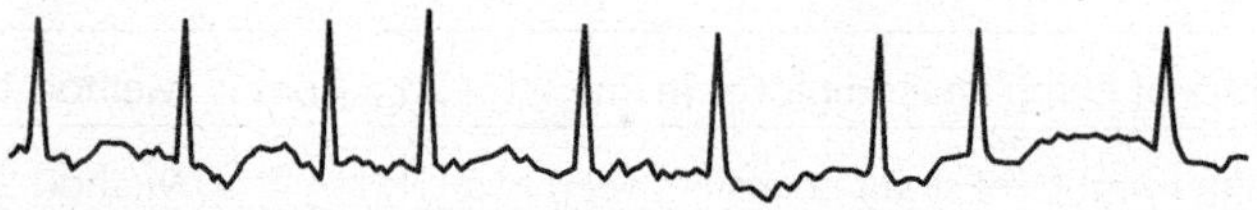	Atrial enlargement, congenital heart defects, drug reactions, anesthesia, heartworm disease, trauma, hypertrophic cardiomyopathy
Atrial premature contraction/ complexes (APC)	• Premature atrial beats originating outside the SA node	• Premature P wave • QRS complexes are normal unless the P wave is so premature they overlap with varying results • May occur as singles, couplets, or triplets (Figure 14.2) 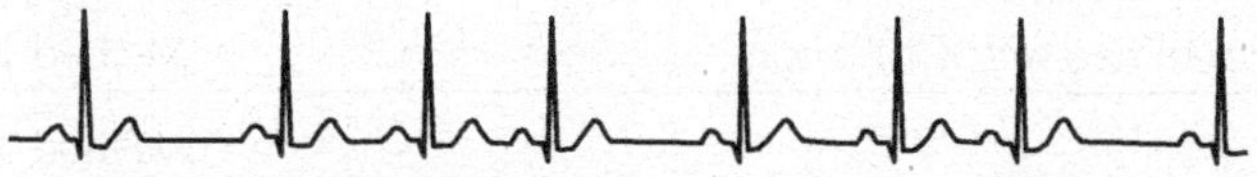	Congenital heart disease, cardiomyopathy, electrolyte imbalances, neoplasia, hyperthyroidism, drug reactions, toxemias, atrial myocarditis, normal variations in aged animals
Respiratory sinus arrhythmias	• Irregular sinus rhythm originating in the SA node • Respiratory rate ↑ during inspiration and ↓ during expiration	• Normal sinus rhythm • ↑ Number of cycles during inspiration and ↓ number of cycles during expiration 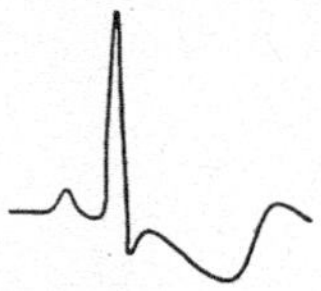	Normal finding (brachycephalic), vagal stimulation, chronic respiratory diseases
ST segment depression	• Net electrical event of myocardial cell repolarization	• Depression of the ST segment of the QRS complex 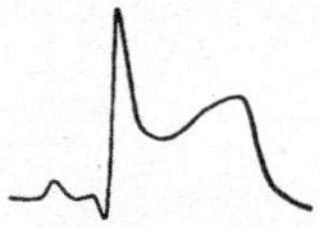	Normal finding, myocardial ischemia (inadequate circulation), hyper- or hypokalemia, cardiac trauma, acute myocardial infarction

(*Continued*)

Table 14.11 / **Common heart rhythm abnormalities (Continued)**

Rhythm pattern	Cause	Image	Associated conditions
ST segment elevation	• Net electrical event of myocardial cell repolarization	• Elevation of the ST segment of the QRS complex (Figure 14.3) 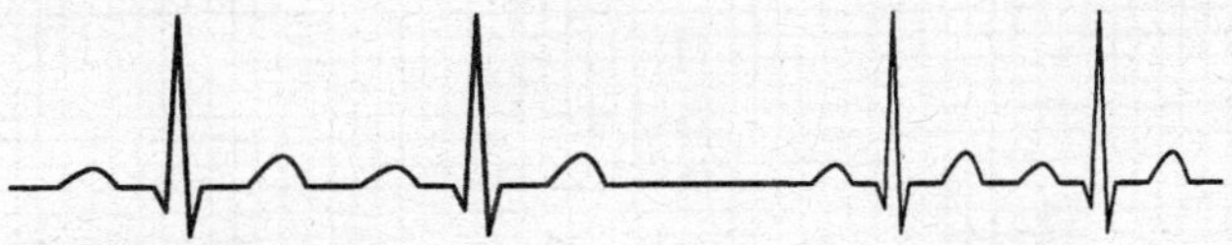	Normal finding, myocardial hypoxia (oxygen deficiency), myocardial infarction, pericarditis
Ventricular fibrillation	• Weak and uncoordinated ventricular contractions • ↓ to zero cardiac output	Completely irregular, chaotic, and deformed reflections of varying width, amplitude, and shape 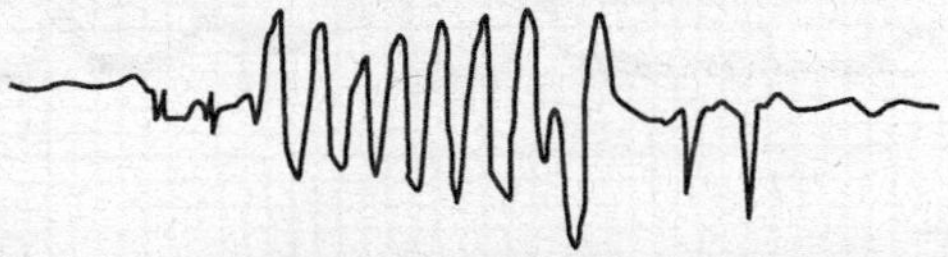	Shock, anoxia, trauma, electrolyte imbalances, drug reactions, aortic stenosis, cardiac surgery, electric shock, myocarditis, hypothermia
Ventricular premature contraction/ complexes (VPC)	• An impulse originating in the ventricles instead of the SA node	P wave is dissociated from the QRS complex Widened and bizarre QRS complex (Figure 14.4) 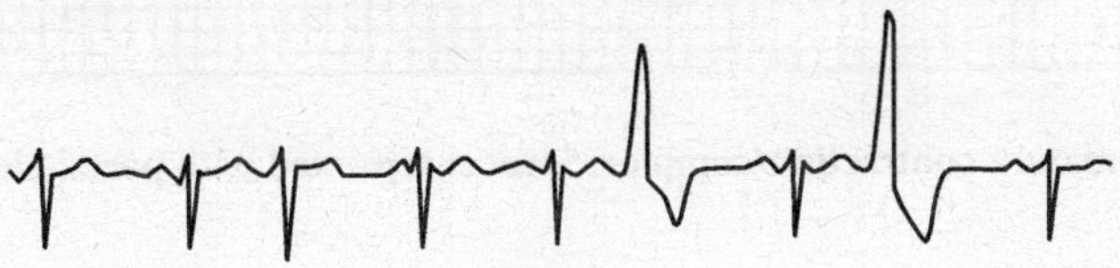	Cardiomyopathy, congenital defects, GDV, drug reactions, myocarditis, cardiac neoplasia, hyperthyroidism, chronic valvular disease

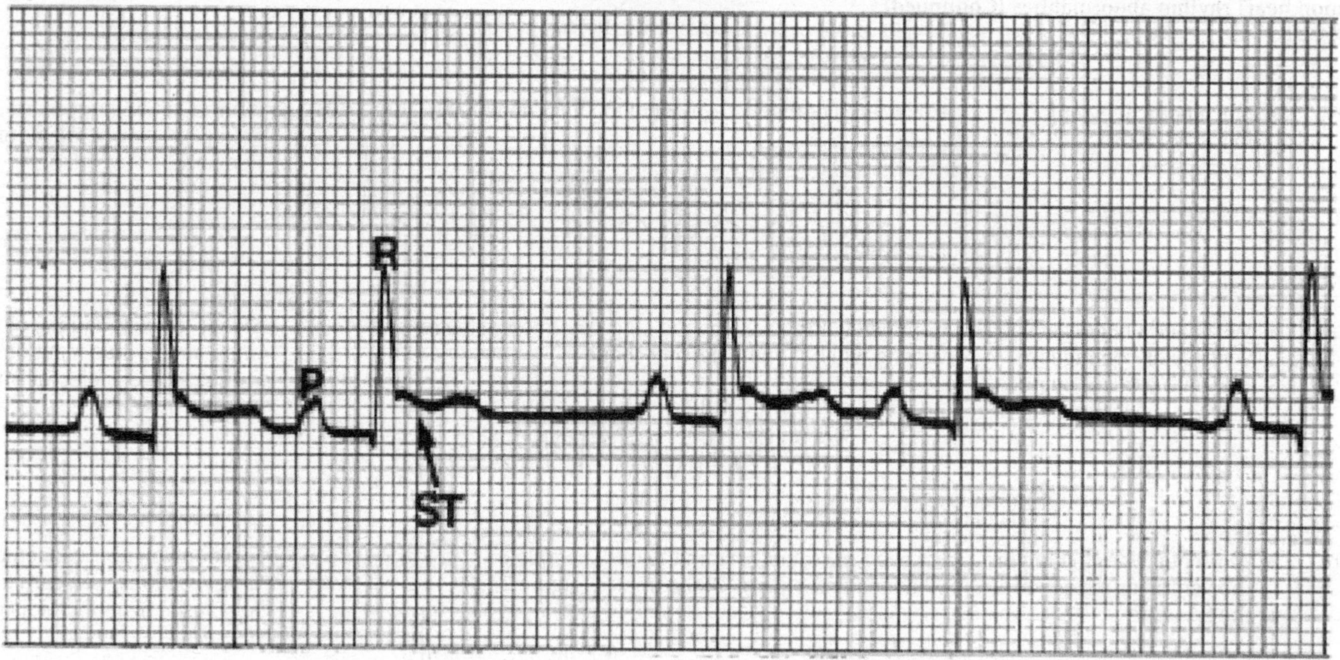

Figure 14.2 Atrial premature contraction/complex. Source: reprinted with permission from Larry Patrick Tilley (1992).

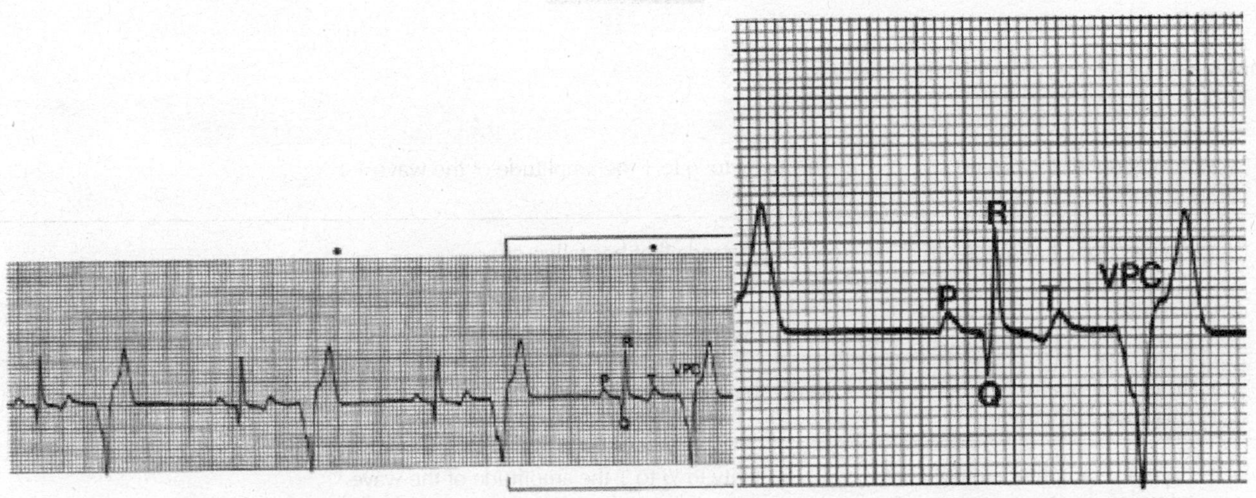

Figure 14.3 ST elevation. Source: reprinted with permission from Larry Patrick Tilley (1992).

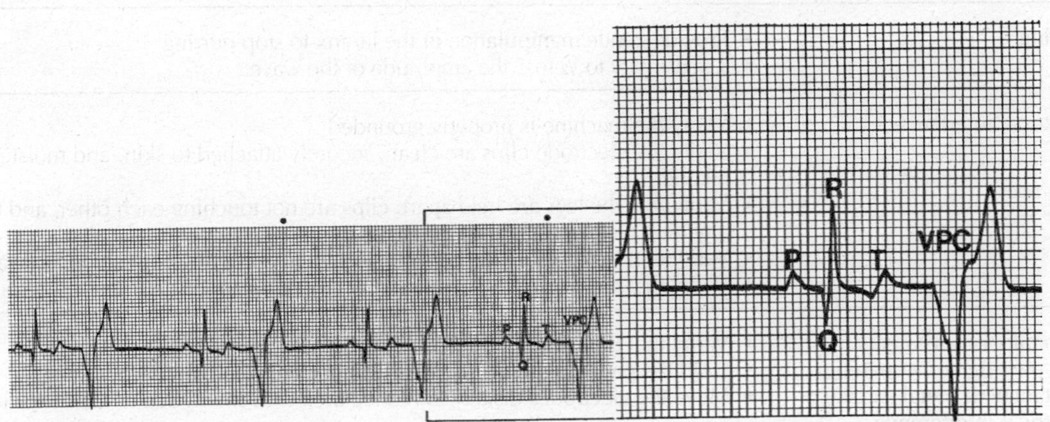

Figure 14.4 Ventricular premature contraction/complex. Source: reprinted with permission from Larry Patrick Tilley (1992).

Table 14.12 / Electrocardiogram problems and artifacts

Alteration	Problem	Solution
Baseline is not well defined	• Poorly defined baseline	↓ Sensitivity to ½ to ↓ the amplitude of the wave
Flat line	• An electrode has fallen off	Replace electrode that has fallen off: • Lead I works and leads II and III do not – replace L leg • Lead II works and leads I and III do not – replace L arm • Lead III works and leads I and II do not – replace R arm
Negative R wave	• True abnormality • Misplaced electrode	• Verify that the electrodes are placed in the correct position
QRS complex off the paper	• Excessive amplitude of QRS complex	• ↓ Sensitivity to ½ to ↓ the amplitude of the wave
Rapid and irregular vibrations of the baseline	• Muscle tremors	• Verify the patient is in a comfortable position and electrodes are comfortably placed
	• Body movements	• Place a hand over the chest wall with moderate pressure to ↓ body tremors
	• Purring	• Provide gentle manipulation of the larynx to stop purring • ↓ Sensitivity to ½ to ↓ the amplitude of the wave
Regular sequence of 60 sharp up and down waves	• Electrical interference	• Verify the machine is properly grounded • Verify the electrode clips are clean, securely attached to skin, and moistened (not saturated) with gel or alcohol • Verify that the legs are held apart, clips are not touching each other, and the patient is not touching anything metal (e.g. table) • Verify that the table is not touching electrical cords and is positioned away from electrical wiring • Verify that the cords are not tangled or coiled up on one another
Up and down movement of baseline	• Respiratory movements (e.g. panting and coughing) • Contact with metal surface or electrical interference • Crossed wires or legs	• Verify that the patient is in a comfortable and appropriate position • Hold the patient's mouth shut for short periods to obtain each tracing • Move the electrodes distally to reduce their movement due to the thoracic wall

VENIPUNCTURE

Venipuncture is the technique of puncturing a vein with a needle. While we typically think of venipuncture strictly in regard to blood sampling, the act of venipuncture is also performed to administer intravenous medications and in conjunction with intravenous catheter placement. Although a fairly straightforward skill, veterinary technicians must be cognizant to always actively engage in critical thinking even when attempting the most routine of tasks.

The most common venipuncture sites in small animals are the cephalic, lateral or medial saphenous, and jugular veins.

Blood Sampling

Venipuncture without the goal of indwelling intravenous catheterization placement can be performed with a needle or butterfly catheter and syringe or vacuum blood collection device with the appropriate blood tube(s). The factors that will influence the veterinary technician's choice include vessel size, amount of sample required, sample handling and processing considerations, and the individual's preference and skill level.

The steps for blood sampling are similar for all veins with only slight changes in position and technique.

Equipment

- Alcohol swab or equivalent
- Bandage material
- Blood collection tubes
- Clippers with #40 blade
- Gloves and surgical preparation materials (blood culture samples)
- Vacuum blood collection system *or*
- Needle
  - Needle choice is based on the comfort and size of the animal, and on vein health (small gauge), while maintaining the integrity of the cellular structure of the sample drawn (large gauge).
- Syringe
  - Syringe size should be related to the sample required, size of the vein, and the amount of back pressure it can apply; excessive back pressure can cause vein collapse, hemolysis, and altered laboratory values.
  - A large syringe may drain the vein faster than it can refill.
  - 20–22-gauge needles are often chosen for our patients, but 25-gauge may be appropriate for smaller patients and small sample sizes.

Site Preparation

The venipuncture site is prepped with 70% isopropyl alcohol, which will aid in removing superficial skin contaminants as well as improving vessel visualization. If the vessel is not readily apparent, clipping away a small amount of hair may improve visualization, increasing the likelihood of a successful and atraumatic venipuncture experience. Samples collected for blood culture are performed with a standard surgical preparation.

Vein Occlusion

The objective of digital occlusion of the vein is to confine its movement (e.g. rolling) between two points and to allow the vein to fill for easy palpation and sample collection.

Vein Palpation

Palpate for the vein by gently rubbing your fingertip horizontally across the furrow. An occluded vein will feel like a taut rope (e.g. pencil) and will slip on either side of your fingertip as you move across it. Small tapping motions can also be made in the area suspected of vein location as the occluded vein will bounce like an inflated balloon.

Venipuncture General Technique

Insert the needle at a 20–30-degree angle, with the bevel side up into the lumen of the vein. As a flash of blood is seen in the hub of the needle, slightly thread the needle further into the vein. Pull the plunger back slowly and steadily to fill the syringe with the blood sample. One key to success is keeping the needle and syringe in the same position throughout the procedure. If blood is not seen in the hub of the needle, slightly withdraw without removing the needle and reposition. Slow and thoughtful motions will help to decrease the pain of the procedure for the patient. Release pressure on the vein when the desired quantity is reached. Remove the needle and immediately apply digital pressure for at least 60 seconds. If needed, apply a pressure bandage and remove after 30–60 minutes.

Problem Solving

If blood stops flowing into the syringe prematurely, the vein may be drained and may need time to refill or the tip of the needle may be against the vessel wall. Begin by releasing back pressure on the syringe, waiting 1–2 seconds and then slowly applying a small amount of pressure. If drawing from an extremity, the paw can be pumped to increase flow. The backend of the syringe can also be slightly tilted up or the needle tip rotated to ensure that it is not against a vessel wall.

Skill Box 14.7 / Venous Blood Collection Techniques

Vein	Jugular			Cephalic	Saphenous
	Sternal	**Seated**	**Lateral**		
Location	Either side of the trachea in the jugular furrow		Right or left jugular furrow, depending on which side is facing up	Cranial portion of the front leg	Medial: inner thigh Lateral: outer leg between stifle and hock
Volume	Volume is determined by quantity needed, patient and vein size, and speed of collection, due to clotting Typical maximum amounts collected in healthy animals: Canine: 13–17 ml/kg Feline 10–12 ml/kg				
Quantity	10 ml			5–7 ml	1–3 ml
Restraint	Place the patient in sternal recumbency. With one hand, grasp the front legs and slightly hang them over the edge of a table while gently pulling forward to elongate the neck. The other hand should be placed over the head with the thumb and middle finger grasping under the mandible. Slightly lift the head and turn it to the opposite side of the intended venipuncture. Occluding of the vein will be done by the venipuncturist	Place the patient in a seated position. Stand with back against wall to prevent backward movement. Depending on the size and temperament of the patient, both hands may be used to hold and slightly lift and turn the head to the opposite side of the venipuncture. Occluding of the vein will be done by the venipuncturist	Stand behind the patient and place it in lateral recumbency. Use one hand to grasp the front legs and slightly pull them back and the other hand to grasp over the head. The thumb and the middle finger are placed on either side of the head below the mandible. The head is the lifted to raise the chin and expose the throat area. An additional restrainer may be necessary to manage the backend. Occluding of the vein will be done by the venipuncturist	Place the patient in sternal recumbency and stand behind the patient. Secure the head (see further), grab the leg with the other hand to occlude the vein. • Felines/small canines: Secure the head by placing one hand on the underside of the patient's muzzle and grabbing the ramus of the mandible on either side. • Canines: secure the head by placing the forearm under the patient's mandible and pulling toward yourself	• Canine: place the patient in lateral recumbency or in a standing position. Place one hand behind the stifle and the other hand across the patella. Push the hands together to occlude the vein while also keeping the leg straight • Felines and small canines: place the patient in lateral recumbency. Top hind leg is moved toward the body wall and then with the side of the hand, press straight down to occlude the saphenous vein

(*Continued*)

Skill Box 14.7 / Venous Blood Collection Techniques (Continued)

Vein	Jugular			Cephalic	Saphenous
	Sternal	Seated	Lateral		
Technique	• Occlude the vein in the jugular furrow at the thoracic inlet with the thumb of the non-syringe hand • The head should be slightly rotated away from the injection site for better visibility • The jugular vein typically lies in the cowlick of the fur running from the ramus of the mandible to the thoracic inlet • Palpate for the vein and insert the needle parallel to the skin in a cranial direction, aspirate for blood, and either inject contents of the syringe or withdraw blood • Avoid the carotid artery			• Once the vein is occluded by either a tourniquet or assistant, palpate for the vein • Lay your thumb alongside the vein to stabilize it and stretch the skin for better visibility • Insert the needle parallel to the skin in a cranial direction, aspirate for blood and withdraw blood • Avoid all nerves	
Notes	• Tip: When grasping the front legs, place your middle finger between the legs with the thumb and middle finger around the outside of the legs to ↑ increase the grip • The marginal ear vein is an additional option when small amounts of blood are needed. A common use is with monitoring glucose levels in diabetic cats. Collection can be done with a lancing device or a single needle; warming the pinna can ↑ volume obtained				

Skill Box 14.8 / Injections

Injection	Subcutaneous (SQ)	Intramuscular (IM)	Intravenous (IV)
Location	Anywhere the skin can provide a tent for injection	Lumbar region, semimembranous and semitendinosus muscles	Any accessible vein (e.g. cephalic, saphenous, pedal, lingual during anesthesia)
Volume	Fluid administration: 50–200 ml in one location depending on the size and species of the animal	< 3 ml per site	Large volumes can be administered

(Continued)

Skill Box 14.8 / **Injections (Continued)**

Injection	Subcutaneous (SQ)	Intramuscular (IM)	Intravenous (IV)
Technique	1. Gently pull an area of skin up to form a small "tent" 2. Insert the needle with the bevel side up at a 15-degree angle through the center of the tent. You should feel the needle pop through the skin 3. Aspirate for blood and then inject the contents intended	Rear leg: 1. Place the needle at least a thumb's width from the femur 2. Inject the needle in a slightly caudal direction, aspirate for blood, and inject the contents of the syringe 3. Avoid the sciatic nerve, femoral artery and vein, popliteal lymph node, and the femur Lumbar region: 1. Place your thumb on the wing of the ilium and your middle finger on a vertebra of the spine 2. Let your index finger fall naturally; where it lands is the location for the injection 3. Inject the needle straight into the muscle, aspirate for blood, and inject the contents of the syringe 4. Avoid all nerves and blood vessels	1. Once the vein is occluded by either a tourniquet or assistant, palpate for the vein 2. Lay your thumb alongside the vein to stabilize it 3. Insert the needle parallel to the skin in a cranial direction 4. Aspirate for blood to confirm the needle is well seated in the vein and either inject contents of syringe or withdraw blood 5. Avoid all nerves
Tips	• Use a fresh needle after the drug has been drawn to ensure a sharp needle • Gentle insertion of the needle typically results in much less of a reaction than thrusting • Pinching or flicking the injection site before administration desensitizes the area • Use distraction (e.g. treats, petting, talking to the patient) • Use topical anesthetic cream on prepared skin to desensitize the animal's reaction to insertion of the catheter. Place 1 g on shaved area, cover with dressing, and wait a minimum of 30 minutes for full effect (topical formulations containing lidocaine should be used with caution in cats)		

INTRAVENOUS CATHETER PLACEMENT

Catheters are used in veterinary medicine to gain access to the vascular system for administration of medications or fluids as well as to obtain blood samples.

Each patient should be assessed as an individual before intravenous catheterization. Veterinary technicians will need to determine insertion site and what kind of catheter to place (type, diameter, length). The following questions may be helpful when evaluating a patient for catheter selection:

- Who is my patient?
  - What is the signalment? How large/small is my patient? What is the conformation of the patient?
  - What are my best options for intravenous catheter insertion sites?
- What will I be using this IV catheter for?
  - Will I be infusing large volumes or repeated doses of medication? Will this pet need a constant rate infusion?
  - Will this patient be administered irritant drugs (i.e. chemotherapy)?
  - Will this patient require serial blood sampling that may necessitate the placement of a central line?
- How long do I expect this IV catheter to remain in place?
  - Is this a short-term placement for light intravenous sedation in an otherwise healthy patient?
  - Is this an unstable critical care case that is likely to be in the hospital for several days and a central line should be considered?

- Are there any medical or behavioral considerations?
  - Is this a stable patient? Would a large-bore catheter be ideal?
  - Is the patient scheduled for a procedure that may influence where an IV catheter may or may not be placed?
  - Is there a high likelihood of catheter contamination depending on the site chosen? Is the patient vomiting or hypersalivating? Is there diarrhea present or is the patient incontinent? Is there any evidence of skin infection or tissue damage?
  - Does the patient have any bleeding tendencies? Is there any concern about head trauma or increased intracranial pressure?
  - Are there painful areas that should be avoided?
  - Is the patient fearful, anxious, or stressed? Is the patient sensitive about having their feet touched? Are they head shy?

Skill Box 14.9 / Intravenous Catheter Placement: Peripheral and Jugular

Method	IV catheter	
	Peripheral	Jugular
Indications	IV access for fluids, medications, and anesthesia	IV access for fluids, medications, and anesthesia. Multilumen catheters are ideal for patients receiving incompatible medications, hypotonic solutions, parenteral nutrition or those requiring reliable/continuing blood sampling; patients with poor peripheral veins or circulation, CVP measurement, prolonged fluid therapy
Contraindications	Burn, abrasion, or pyoderma over site, thrombosis of chosen vein, infusion of hypertonic solutions (e.g. parenteral nutrition)	Burn, abrasion, or pyoderma over site, head trauma, severe coagulopathy, hypercoagulable, or thrombosis of chosen vein
Catheter sites	• Cephalic and saphenous veins, pedal vein	• External jugular vein • Saphenous vein – PICC
Setup	• Surgical site preparation materials • ½- and 1-inch tape • IV catheter • Saline flush • T-port primed with 0.9% saline	• Surgical site preparation materials, drape, surgical gloves • Sterile gauze: 3 × 3 • ½- and 1-inch tape • Central venous catheter kit • Saline flush • T-port(s) primed with 0.9% saline • Lidocaine 2%

(Continued)

Skill Box 14.9 / Intravenous Catheter Placement: Peripheral and Jugular (Continued)

Method	IV catheter	
	Peripheral	**Jugular**
Procedure	1. Clip a wide area of hair leaving a 2-inch border above and below the catheter insertion point 2. Wash hands and put on gloves 3. Perform a surgical scrub at the site 4. Attempt placement as distal as possible for the patient's conformation 5. Place the catheter in the vessel 6. When a "flashback" is seen, advance the unit slightly into the vein to ensure that the catheter is well seated into the vein 7. Advance the catheter off the stylet into the vein 8. Place an injection cap/T-port and secure the catheter according to technician preference and practice protocol	1. Set up all required materials 2. Identify the location of the jugular vein and carefully clip the area of the intended insertion site, avoiding clipper burn 3. Perform a surgical scrub at the site Peel-away sheath: 1. Wearing sterile gloves, tent the skin and insert the over-the-needle sheath into the vessel 2. When a "flashback" as seen, advance the unit slightly into the vein to ensure that it is well seated into the vein 3. Advance the over-the-needle sheath off the stylet into the vein; a slight back-and-forth rotation may help advancement 4. Remove the stylet and temporarily place a finger over the opening to prevent hemorrhage or air embolus 5. Insert the catheter into the sheath 6. Cap and aspirate until blood fills the port and flush the catheter with saline 7. Carefully pull apart the sheath and secure the catheter according to technician preference and practice protocol 8. Take radiographs to confirm proper placement Seldinger (guidewire): 1. Wearing sterile gloves, tent the skin and insert the over-the-needle sheath into the vessel 2. When a "flashback" is seen, advance the unit slightly into the vein to ensure that it is well seated into the vein 3. Advance the catheter off the stylet and place the guidewire into the vessel to the appropriate length 4. Keeping the guidewire in place, remove the catheter from the vessel 5. Place the dilator over the wire and advance 6. After dilation has been accomplished, remove the dilator and feed the catheter over the wire and into the vessel 7. Remove the guidewire 8. Cap the catheter and aspirate until blood fills the port and flush the catheter with saline. Repeat with all ports 9. Secure the catheter according to technician preference and practice protocol 10. Take radiographs to confirm proper placement
Complications	Phlebitis, non-patent, fever, and front limb edema	Phlebitis, non-patent, fever, facial and front limb edema
Removal	• Cut the tape with bandage scissors on the lateral aspect of the limb and slowly pull the catheter out • Place a cotton ball and vet-wrap adhesive bandage for 1–2 hours	• Cut the tape with bandage scissors on the lateral aspect of the limb and slowly pull the catheter out • Place a cotton ball and vet-wrap adhesive bandage for 1–2 hours for peripheral placement. For jugular placement, hold digital pressure on the site for 5 minutes, followed by a loose wrap
Tip	• The right external jugular maintains a straighter course and is preferred for jugular placement	

Skill Box 14.10 / Catheter Placement: Arterial and Intraosseous

Method	Catheter	
	Arterial	**Intraosseous**
Indications	Blood gas analysis, continuous blood pressure monitoring, and blood sampling	IV access for fluids, medications and transfusions
Contraindications	Drug or fluid administration, burn, abrasion, or pyoderma over site, thromboembolic disease, hypercoagulopathy, and ambulatory patients	Osteopenia, infected tissue over the site, adult and large-breed animals
Catheter sites	Dorsal pedal, femoral, and auricular arteries	Greater trochanter of the proximal femur, flat medial aspect of the proximal tibia (in obese animals), wing of ilium, greater tubercle of the humerus
Setup	• Surgical site preparation materials • ½- and 1-inch tape • IV catheter • Saline flush • T-port • 22-gauge needle	• Surgical site preparation materials • Sterile gauze: 3 × 3 • ½- and 1-inch tape • IV catheter • Saline flush • T-port primed with 0.9% saline • 22-gauge needle • Lidocaine 2% • No. 15 or no. 11 scalpel blade • 16-gauge bone marrow needle • Suture material • Triple antibiotic ointment
Procedure	1. Follow peripheral catheter protocol 2. Place a gauze square just below the insertion site to help maintain an aseptic area as well as absorb any blood 3. Using a smooth and steady technique, insert the catheter with bevel side facing up into the artery at a 30–45-degree angle. A flashback of blood is seen upon entering the artery 4. Palpate the pulse and then advance the catheter toward the strongest area of pulse; withdraw the needle stylet. Blood should be seen at the hub of the catheter 5. Cap the catheter with a T-port and flush with saline and secure with tape 6. Label the catheter as arterial	1. Set up all required materials 2. Clip the greater trochanter and perform a surgical scrub at the site 3. Inject bupivacaine or lidocaine SQ if the patient is responsive (0.1 ml at the catheter insertion site) 4. Place a sterile gauze square just below the insertion site to help maintain an aseptic area as well as absorb any blood 5. Incise the insertion site with a no. 15 or no. 11 scalpel blade 6. With the leg in adduction, place one hand along the side of the femur with the thumb pointing toward the greater trochanter 7. Pass the catheter through the insertion site, down the medial aspect of the greater trochanter, and into the trochanteric fossa 8. Push the catheter through the cortex by applying downward pressure and rotating a quarter turn with each rotation. A loss of resistance is felt when the catheter passes through the cortex. The catheter will bounce lightly down the bone 9. Verify placement by aspirating for bone marrow particulates and by rotating the femur; the catheter and femur should move as one 10. Suture to the skin and secure with bandaging 11. Remove cap and stylet and attach fluid set

(Continued)

Skill Box 14.10 / Catheter Placement: Arterial and Intraosseous (Continued)

Method	Catheter	
	Arterial	**Intraosseous**
Complications	Venous puncture, phlebitis, non-patent and fever	Osteomyelitis, fractures, growth plate damage and displacement, and sciatic nerve damage
Removal	• Cut tape with bandage scissors on the lateral aspect of the limb and slowly pull the catheter out • Place a pressure wrap for 10 minutes, followed by a cotton ball and vet-wrap adhesive bandage for 1–2 hours	• Cut tape with bandage scissors and slowly pull the catheter out
Tips	• Use topical anesthetic on prepared skin to desensitize the patient's reaction to insertion of the catheter. Place 1 g on the shaved area, cover with dressing, and wait a minimum of 30 minutes for full effect. Topical formulations containing lidocaine should be used with caution in cats • Intraosseous catheters can also be placed with hypodermic or spinal needles	

Skill Box 14.11 / Intravenous Catheter Monitoring and Maintenance.

Patient care:
- Strict aseptic technique is critical to patient care. The catheter site should be aseptically cleaned prior to initial placement and before securing into place.
- Monitor for signs of fever, lethargy, or changes in vital signs (which may represent sepsis).
- Monitor the paw for swelling and altered temperature.
- Swelling distal to the catheter often indicates restrictive bandaging and swelling proximal to the catheter is often due to extravasation.
- Remove bandage material and inspect the site at least every 24 hours to observe for phlebitis (e.g. hardening or ropiness of the vessel), swelling, redness, pain, hot to the touch, and displacement.
- In the event of phlebitis, remove the IV catheter immediately.

Catheter care:
- Flush catheter at least every six to eight hours with saline to assess patency and evaluate patient response.
- Replace bandaging whenever it becomes soiled or wet.
- Replace IV catheters if there is any sign of extravasation, infection, phlebitis, heat, pain/discomfort, fever, or redness; IO catheters are typically removed after 24–48 hours but can be maintained longer with diligent care.

Equipment care:
- Swab injection ports on catheter and fluid bags with an antimicrobial solution prior to each injection.
- Replace T-ports and administration sets with obvious wear or contamination, especially in critically ill and immunosuppressed patients.
- Observe strict aseptic technique when changing administration sets and fluid bags.

INSULIN THERAPY

Diabetes mellitus is a common endocrine condition resulting in chronic hyperglycemia. This is due to a loss or dysfunction of pancreatic beta cells. In both human and veterinary medicine, diabetes is generally divided into two broad categories called type 1 and type 2. Type 1 diabetes is the result of immune-mediated beta cell destruction, which usually leads to an absolute insulin deficiency necessitating insulin administration. This form is more prevalent in the dogs.

Type 2 diabetes is the most common form in the feline and is due to a combination of insulin resistance and beta cell dysfunction, which may be partially reversible if prompt glycemic control is achieved. Supplying exogenous insulin and monitoring diet and exercise are the mainstay of treatment for uncomplicated diabetes.

Although diabetes is a treatable condition, upon presentation these patients may require varying degrees of stabilization and will require long-term management. The two mainstays of diabetic treatment are insulin and diet. Successful management of the diabetic patient is individualized and requires an understanding of the pathophysiology itself, as well as the necessity of frequent reassessment, open client communication and education, and clearly defined goals for the pet's treatment plan. Further information on diabetes can be found in the American Animal Hospital Association *Diabetes Management Guidelines for Dogs and Cats.*[1]

Insulin availability is continuously changing. There is no predictor as to which insulin will work for which patient; however, dogs are typically started on lente or neutral protamine Hagedorn (NPH), whereas protamine zinc (PZI) or glargine is usually recommended for cats. Considering clinical signs and laboratory work, insulin type, amount, and frequency are adjusted.

Table 14.13 / **Insulin types**

Type	Long acting			Intermediate acting		Short (rapid) acting
	Detemir	Glargine	Protamine zinc (PZI)	NPH	Lente	Regular
Products	Levemir®, U-100	Lantus®, U-100	Prozinc®, U-40	Humulin®-N, Novolin®-N, U-100	Vetsulin®, U-40	Humulin-R, Novolin-R, U-100
Use	Canines and felines	Canines and felines	Canines and felines*	Canines and felines	Canines* and felines*	Canines and felines
Route	SQ	SQ	SQ	SQ	SQ	IV, IM, SQ (with adequate hydration)
Peak	Canine: limited data Feline: 12–14 hours	Canine: 6–10 hours Feline: 12–14 hours	Canine: 8–12 hours Feline: 5–7 hours	Canine: 0.5–8.5 hours Feline: 2–8 hours	Canine: 1–10 hours Feline: 2–8 hours	IV: 30 minutes–2 hours IM: 1–4 hours SQ: 1–5 hours
Duration	Feline: 12–24 hours	Canine: 12–20 hours Feline: 12–24 hours	Feline: 8–24 hours	Canine: 4–10 hours Feline: 4–12 hours	Canine: 10–24 hours Feline: 8–14 hours	IV: 1–4 hours IM: 3–8 hours SQ: 4–10 hours

(Continued)

Table 14.13 / **Insulin types (Continued)**

Type	Long acting			Intermediate acting		Short (rapid) acting
	Detemir	Glargine	Protamine zinc (PZI)	NPH	Lente	Regular
Starting Dose	Canine: 0.1 U/kg twice a day Feline: 0.5 U/kg twice a day if blood glucose > 360 mg/dl 0.25 u/kg twice a day if blood glucose < 360 mg/dl	Canine: 0.3 U/kg twice a day Feline: 0.5 U/kg twice a day if blood glucose > 360 mg/dl 0.25 u/kg twice a day if blood glucose < 360 mg/dl	Canine: 0.25–0.5 u/kg twice a day Feline: 1– 2 U/cat twice a day	0.25–0.5 u/kg twice a day	Canine: 0.25–0.5 u/kg twice a day Feline: 0.25–0.5 u/kg twice a day; not to exceed 3 u/cat	0.2 u/kg twice a day, subsequent dosing at 0.1–0.2 u/kg every 3–6 hours
Notes	• Vetsulin must be shaken prior to administration • Detemir is very potent in dogs and should be used with caution • Compounded PZI can be formulated to U-40 or U-100; always confirm the type of insulin and syringes that is being used • Glipizide is an oral antidiabetic that has an extremely inconsistent response in cats and is not recommended or considered appropriate as a first-line treatment. However, it may be considered in very select cases of non-compliance if there is no other alternative * FDA approved in this species					

Insulin Storage and Handling

Insulin should be stored and handled according to manufacturer drug label, but most insulin is stored in the refrigerator and is discarded when past its expiration date, opened for longer than four to six weeks, previously frozen, exposed to excess heat (typically > 80°F), or if discolored. Insulin should be protected from direct light.

Insulin Syringes

Insulin syringes are specific to insulin concentration and are labeled for either U-100 or U-40 insulin. Human insulin (e.g. glargine or insulin isophane, Humulin-N®) has a concentration of U-100, with each milliliter containing 100 units of insulin. Veterinary insulin (e.g. PZI) has a concentration of U-40, with each milliliter containing 40 units of insulin. Not being aware of this difference can overdose or underdose a patient. Syringes are also available in different sizes (e.g. 100, 50, and 30 units) to allow more accurate dosing. It is strongly recommended to use the correct size of syringe to avoid dosing mistakes; however, the following information is for the rare and single event when a U-40 syringe is unavailable.

Tuberculin Syringes

Multiply the required units of U-40 insulin by 0.025 (e.g. 10 units of U-40 insulin would be 0.25 ml of a TB syringe).

U-100 Syringes

Multiply the required units of U-40 insulin by 2.5 (e.g. 10 units of U-40 insulin would be 25 units of a U-100 syringe).

Note: The use of diluted insulin requires determining the correct syringe type due to the change in concentration and is generally not recommended.

Blood Glucose Curve

Blood glucose curves are done routinely on diabetic animals to evaluate how food and medications affect their body's ability to control glucose. The results of the curve help to determine the proper dose of insulin. The goal of insulin therapy is to maintain blood glucose levels below the renal threshold (180–220 mg/dl in dogs and 250–300 mg/dl in cats) while avoiding the occurrence of hypoglycemia (< 60 mg/dl).

Obtaining a single reading or a small number of readings may cause confusion with interpretation and so a 12-hour curve is recommended. The blood glucose curve is the only method of diabetic patient monitoring that provides information on insulin efficacy including the nadir (lowest reading) and the duration of action (results in the ideal range) of the insulin. It is thus the preferred diagnostic test on which to determine insulin dosing adjustments. In addition to test results, the veterinarian will take into consideration the overall status of the patient including fluctuations in weight and the presence of clinical signs when making recommendations.

If a diabetic management is proving difficult, client compliance should be reviewed. Information on all aspects of insulin handling, storage, and administration, syringe type and technique, and feeding schedule should be discussed to rule out owner related causes for poor regulation. Further investigation would include a review of all medications (including topical and ophthalmic) and diagnostics to rule out concurrent diseases that could contribute to insulin resistance.

Blood glucose curves can be performed in hospital or at home. Although in-home blood glucose monitoring is strongly recommended, it may not be the best decision for every pet and owner.

Table 14.14 / Blood glucose curves

Location	In-hospital	In-home
Advantages	• Sampling performed by a skilled veterinary technician may be more reliable and consistent • Having the patient in the hospital allows the veterinarian to evaluate the whole patient (physical exam, weight, status, clinical signs, and diagnostics) prior to making any insulin dosing recommendations • Possibly less disruptive to the pet and owner's human-animal bond to have veterinary staff perform testing	• Performing testing in the home reduces patient stress and is less disruptive to the pet's schedule, so the values are more representative of a typical day • Facilitates owner education by direct observation of the inverse relationship of glucose and insulin • Promotes a team-oriented approach to diabetic management • Owners feel more confident and in the event of a hypoglycemic episode, can quickly determine whether the pet needs emergency veterinary care • More cost effective than in-hospital testing
Disadvantages	• Patient stress due to transport, hospitalization, and handling can skew test results and lead to stress hyperglycemia • Unable to mimic daily routine during hospitalization • Not cost effective • Practice: in an effort to make curves more affordable, charges are often insufficient to cover the associated costs • Pet owner: cost of repeated testing may be problematic to owners with financial limitations	• Initially, owner-reported results may be less reliable, as it takes time and experience for owners to become technically proficient and find what works best for their pet • Patient cooperation may be problematic for some owners and assistance may be required • If an owner feels that their human–animal bond has been negatively affected, it may be necessary to discontinue in-home testing

In-Hospital Protocol

Patients should receive their morning meal and dose of insulin at home and should then be brought to the clinic within the hour. The patient's typical feeding routine should be followed throughout the day and their stress and appetite monitored. Blood glucose values are monitored upon arrival and then every two hours (three to four hours for long-acting insulin, e.g. glargine) as long as they maintain greater than 150 mg/dl. If they drop to less than 150 mg/dl, they should be monitored hourly and treated if necessary.

In-Home Protocol

Similar to in-hospital blood glucose curves, values are monitored every two hours or every three to four hours for patients receiving a long-acting insulin such as glargine. Blood samples may be obtained from the capillary bed of the ear margin and foot pads (canine and feline) and lip, elbow callus, and base of tail (canine). The day of the curve should be as routine and as representative of a typical day for that patient as possible. It may be elected to obtain a sample immediately prior to feeding and insulin administration to produce a more complete curve. If any measurements less than 150 mg/dl (clinician dependent), the owner should be directed to notify the veterinarian for instruction. Otherwise the results can be reported when the curve is complete.

Insulin Constant Rate Infusions

Patients in a ketoacidotic state often require hospitalization and receive a constant rate infusion of regular insulin after an initial period of fluid therapy to equilibrate fluid and electrolyte balance. The insulin constant rate infusion (CRI) can be set up by placing a calculated dose of regular insulin (2.2 units/kg) into a separate 0.9% saline fluid bag and piggybacked onto the main fluid line. Since insulin adheres to plastic, 50 ml insulin/fluid mixture must be flushed through the line and discarded before beginning treatment and the insulin bag should be discarded every 24 hours.

Table 14.15 Example insulin constant rate infusions.

Serum glucose level (mg/dl)	Insulin infusion rate (ml/hour)		Secondary fluid type
	Canine	Feline	
> 250	10	5	Crystalloid
200–250	7	3	Crystalloid + 2.5% dextrose
150–200	5	2	Crystalloid + 2.5% dextrose
100–150	5	2	Crystalloid + 2.5–5% dextrose
< 100	Discontinue	Discontinue	Crystalloid + 5% dextrose

The goal of treatment is to maintain the blood glucose level between 150 and 300 mg/dl until the patient is stable and eating. Patients are often rehydrated over a period of six to eight hours prior to beginning an insulin CRI. The insulin infusion is calculated at 2.2 units/kg and typically placed in a 250 ml/bag of 0.9% saline.

CLIENT EDUCATION

Insulin Administration

Prior to the administration of insulin, patients should be fed their standard measured meal to assure they have food available for the insulin to use and to prevent a hypoglycemic state (see also Skill Box 14.14). Insulin should be given at the same time each day.

Skill Box 14.12 / Client Education: Insulin Administration

Preparation:

- For most insulin do not shake the vial; gently roll it between the palm of your hands to mix.
- Vetsulin is required to be shaken and well mixed prior to administration. Always follow manufacturer's instructions.
- Use a new syringe for each injection.

Drawing up the medication:

1. Pull back the plunger of the syringe to position the top of the plunger (part closest to the needle) at the desired dose.
2. Insert the needle into the vial and inject the air into the vial to prevent a vacuum.
3. Slowly pull back on the plunger to the desired amount and withdraw the needle from the vial.
4. Check to make sure there are no bubbles in the syringe; if present, pull back on the plunger and tap the syringe to move the bubbles to the top. Then push the plunger until all the air is out of the syringe.
5. Verify the correct amount of insulin is within the syringe.

Administering the insulin:

1. Locate an injection site from midneck to the last rib and halfway down on either side. The site should be changed with each injection.
2. Place your index finger against the back of the animal and use your thumb and middle finger to pull up skin to form a "tent" under your index finger.
3. Insert the needle; bevel side up into the skin at a 45° angle.
4. Pull back on the plunger to verify no blood or air fills the syringe; if present, remove the needle and try again.
5. Depress the plunger to insert the insulin under the skin.
6. Remove the syringe and immediately recap it.
7. Properly dispose of the syringe and needle.

Notes:

- Insulin that is not mixed properly will not provide the correct concentration and may over- or underdose the patient.
- Insulin pens are also available for many types of insulin. They are more accurate and often less intimidating to pet owners. However, most insulin pens can only adjust the dose in increments of 1 unit and this may be problematic for small patients that require smaller dosing changes. Additionally, small animal patients require longer insulin pen needles (i.e. 10 mm, 12 mm) for correct administration.

Monitoring Insulin Response

When caring for a diabetic patient, it is critical to have both diligent home monitoring and careful veterinary management. To manage a diabetic patient, physical exams are typically scheduled every two to six months with additional information obtained by the interpretation of glucose levels (preferably a curve), urinalysis, and fructosamine levels. Any time there is a dose adjustment, a blood glucose curve should be performed in 7–14 days. The health of most diabetic patients lies in the hands of the owner; their attention to detail and keen observations are critical. At-home monitoring includes the parameters listed in Skill Box 14.16. Observations should be communicated to the veterinarian to be considered in the treatment plan.

Skill Box 14.13 / Client Education: Monitoring Insulin Response

- Monitor:
  - Appetite
  - Attitude
  - Body condition/weight
  - Polydipsia/polyuria
  - Exercise
- Urine glucose levels can be helpful, but only reflect the average blood glucose during the time that the bladder was filling; they have a fairly low accuracy in dogs. It is not recommended to make dosing decisions based exclusively on urine glucose strips.
- Fructosamine levels reflect glycemic control over the past one to two weeks and it is particularly helpful in determining stress hyperglycemia from diabetes mellitus. As fructosamine indicates average glycemic control, individual results can be misleading. Monitoring fructosamine trends are more valuable than single results in diabetic patients.
- A blood glucose curve is the only test that has the ability to assess insulin efficacy, peak, and duration of effect. It should be noted that blood glucose curves will not be identical from day to day and variation is to be expected – particularly if there is a disruption to the pet's normal day.
- At-home monitoring:
  - Test every two hours (every three to four hours with glargine) starting before the morning insulin for 12 hours (until the evening insulin).
  - A variety of glucometers are available for home monitoring, but those validated for veterinary species are recommended.
  - Blood samples may be obtained from the capillary bed of the ear margin and foot pads (canine and feline) and lip, elbow callus, and base of tail (canine).

Monitoring for Hypoglycemia

Hypoglycemia is an abnormally low blood glucose level. This is often seen when there is an excess of insulin circulating in the bloodstream. This can be caused by overdose of insulin, missing or delaying a meal, eating less than normal, vomiting, strenuous exercise, stress, and certain medications. With a blood glucose level less than 60 mg/dl, most animals will show signs stumbling or staggering, and the administration of a carbohydrate source will result in a quick recovery. Animals with a blood glucose level less than 20 mg/dl often lose consciousness and seizures may occur. A carbohydrate source (e.g. Karo syrup) should be rubbed on the gums immediately, followed by immediate medical attention. Patients that are having a seizure or that are obtunded or unconscious should never be prompted to drink. Any patient that may have a diminished swallow reflex could be at risk for aspiration.

Skill Box 14.14 / Client Education: Monitoring for Hypoglycemia

Signs to watch for:
- Depression, lethargy
- Deviations from normal behavior
- Drunken state (e.g. stumbling, staggering)
- Lack of appetite
- Panting
- Seizures, comas

Actions to take:
- Give a carbohydrate source orally or transmucosally (e.g. Karo syrup, maple syrup).
- Seek veterinary care immediately.
- Keep the animal warm.

Prevention:
- Nutrition
  - Consistent food and feeding times.
  - Avoid table scraps or variations of regular diet.
  - Feed multiple meals each day.
  - Provide fresh clean water at all times.
- Exercise:
  - Maintain a consistent exercise program.
- Medication:
  - Do not administer insulin to a patient that is not eating.
  - Do not alter medications.

Note: consult the veterinarian before making changes to nutrition, exercise, or medication.

FLUID THERAPY

Fluid administration is necessary during times of dehydration, shock, excessive blood loss, surgery, or a disease resulting in depletion of the patient's normal fluid, electrolyte or acid–base balances. Fluid replacement is based on an animal's hydration status, reason for fluid loss, and its physical condition. Performing the assessments in Skill Box 14.18 will help to determine dehydration and perfusion status and will assist the veterinarian in the calculation of fluid requirements for the animal.

Skill Box 14.15 / Hydration Assessment

Hydration	Assessment	Significance
Physical Examination	• Assess dehydration status: • Skin turgor: assess the amount of time it takes for the skin to return to the patient's body when gently pulled up and twisted at the back of the neck or along the spine. Use two to three assessment locations • Obesity can falsely ↓ turgor and emaciation can falsely ↑ turgor • Not reliable in neonates due to high water and fat content • Mucous membranes: assess for dryness of gums and cornea (moist, tacky, dry) • Panting can falsely dry the gums (canines) • Eye position: assess the degree of eye sinkage into the bony orbit • Assess perfusion status: • Capillary refill time: direct digital pressure is applied to the mucous membranes until blanched and then timed for blood (pink color) to return (normal: < 1–2 seconds) • Mucous membranes: pink • Mucous membranes can also be pale due to reasons other than perfusion • Extremities: normothermic • Cool extremities may indicate poor circulation and subsequent concentration of fluids to the vital organs • Heart rate and pulse (femoral and metatarsal): assess the heart rate and pulse (amplitude and duration) • Weight of the animal: patient's normal body weight and current weight should be noted: 1 lb body weight = 1 pint (480 ml) fluid	< 5%: normal hydration: • No obvious clinical sign • Skin turgor: < 2 seconds • 6–8%: mild dehydration: • Skin: inelastic and leathery • Twist: disappears immediately • Skin turgor: > 3 seconds • Eyes: duller than normal and sunken • Mucous membranes: tacky to dry 8–10%: moderate dehydration: • Skin: inelastic and leathery • Twist: disappears slowly • Skin turgor: > 3 seconds • Eyes: duller than normal and sunken • Mucous membranes: tacky to dry • Heart rate: ↑ 10–12%: severe dehydration: • Skin: no elasticity • Twist: remains indefinitely • Skin turgor: remains indefinitely • Eyes: dry, deeply sunken • Mucous membranes: dry, cyanotic, and possibly cold • CRT: prolonged or absent • Heart rate: ↑ • Pulse: weak 12–15%: patient is in shock and death is imminent

(Continued)

Skill Box 14.15 / Hydration Assessment (Continued)

Hydration	Assessment	Significance
Laboratory Assessment	**Packed cell volume:** • Canines 37–55% • Felines 30–45%	Dehydration at > 45%
	Total protein—serum: • Canines: 5.4–7.5 g/dl • Felines: 5.7–7.6 g/dl	Dehydration at > 8.0 g/dl
	Urine specific gravity: • Canines: > 1.035 • Felines > 1.040	Evaluates kidney function more than hydration status; only reflects dehydration if kidneys are healthy
Medical history	Patient's history	**Fluid loss:** • Amount of vomiting, diarrhea, salivation • Amount of fluid and food intake
	Review of patient's file	Previous physical problems (e.g. heart disease, kidney disease) will influence fluid therapy

Calculating Fluid Requirements

The rates shown in Skill Box 14.16 are for those patients without pulmonary, cardiac, or severe renal disease and therefore are able to handle rapid or high fluid rates.

Skill Box 14.16 / Calculating Fluid Requirements

Purpose	Basis of calculations	Rate

Rehydration	• Basic rehydration formula
	  • Calculates the fixed rate of replacement fluids to correct the deficit over 4–6 hours
		• % dehydrated × body weight (kg) × 1000 ml/kg = ml of fluid replacement
		  • Example: animal weighing 20 kg is 6% dehydrated. Fluid needed for basic rehydration is calculated as:
		  0.06 × 20 (kg) × 1000 (ml/kg) = 1200 ml

(*Continued*)

Skill Box 14.16 / Calculating Fluid Requirements (Continued)

Purpose	Basis of calculations	Rate
	• Maintenance calculation • Calculates the amount of fluid to replace losses resulting from urination, feces, and respiration • Panting and fever will ↑ amount of fluid loss (evaporative loss)	• Feline: 80 × body weight (kg)$^{0.75}$ • Canine: 132 × body weight (kg)$^{0.75}$ • Dependent on the cause of the loss and patient's condition
	• Continuing losses • Calculates the amount of fluid loss attributable to excessive vomiting, diarrhea, polyuria, and third spacing of body fluids	• 20 ml vomit = 20 ml fluids
Anesthetic protocol	• Provide maintenance rate plus any replacement at < 10 ml/kg/hour	• Initial rate: • Feline: 3 ml/kg/hour • Canine: 5 ml/kg/hour • Adjustments made based on patient status
Postoperative protocol	• Calculated to account for rehydration, maintenance, and continuing losses	• Evaluation of rehydration above
Pediatric protocol	• Calculated to account for the rapid water turnover of neonates as their body weight is 80% water	• Neonate: 60–180 ml/kg/day • >6 weeks of age: 120–180 ml/kg/day
Shock protocol	• Calculated to establish a circulating blood volume to allow adequate tissue perfusion	• Crystalloids: • Full shock dose listed below, but administered in 25% increments over 10–20 minutes. Subsequent boluses are based on patient status • Canine: 90 ml/kg/hour • Feline: 55 ml/kg/hour • Colloids: • Controversial and have fallen out of favor due to acute kidney injury, coagulopathy, etc. • Rates are for patients with adequate/normal cardiopulmonary function

Table 14.16 / Routes of fluid administration

Route	Indication	Complications	Notes
Oral	• Minimal fluid loss • Recent anorexia, neonates	Accidental tracheal intubation and aspiration (e.g. neonates), vomiting, regurgitation, aerophagia	• Contraindicated: vomiting, diarrhea, dysphagia, or in life-threatening situations (e.g. shock) • Administration by bottle, syringe, or enteral feeding tubes
Subcutaneous	• Mild to moderate dehydration • Maintenance	Injection site infection (rare); do not use > 2.5% dextrose, as sloughing and abscesses may occur	• Contraindicated: infected or devitalized skin, hypothermia, or severely dehydrated • Warmed to body temperature and allow flow by gravity • Use only isotonic fluids • Use several sites; no more than 10–20 ml/kg • Absorption is expected within 6–8 hours • Technique: see Skill Box 14.8
Intravenous	• Severe dehydration • Perioperative precaution • Vomiting	Phlebitis, septicemia, embolism, and volume overload	• Contraindicated: severe anemia • Warmed to body temperature • Requires rate calculation • Requires closer monitoring especially in cardiac insufficiency cases • Flush catheter with saline at least every 6–8 hours • Technique: see Skill Box 14.9
Intraperitoneal	• Mild to moderate dehydration • Large volumes • Poor venous access	Peritonitis, intra-abdominal abscess	• Contraindicated: ascites, peritonitis, sepsis, pancreatitis, or expected abdominal surgery • Warmed to body temperature isotonic fluids • Absorption can take up to 20 minutes • Used to treat severe hyper- or hypothermia • Technique: caudal abdomen is aseptically prepared. An 18–22-gauge needle is inserted on the ventral midline, caudal to the umbilicus. The syringe is aspirated; if no fluid is seen (e.g. blood), the fluids are attached and administered. If fluid is seen, the needle is removed and repositioned
Intraosseous	• Small animals (< 5 kg), neonates, or animals with poor venous access	Osteomyelitis, fractures, growth plate damage	• Flush catheter with saline at least every 6–8 hours if fluid therapy is discontinued • An IV catheter should be placed as soon as possible (24–72 hours) • All IV medications and fluids can be administered IO • Technique: see Skill Box 14.10

Fluid Selection

Selecting the type of fluid to administer can be as important as the selected route and rate. In selecting a fluid, it is important to know the electrolyte status of the patient and the underlying disease. Fluids are then chosen based on what best fits the patient's condition and need.

Crystalloids are the most commonly used extracellular replacement fluid as they rapidly correct volume deficits. They contain electrolyte and nonelectrolyte solutes and are able to enter all body fluid compartments. However, only 20–33% remains in the vascular space after 30 minutes and only 10–20% after one hour following IV administration.

Colloids have a large molecular weight and remain in the plasma compartment to expand volume. However, synthetic colloids have fallen out of favor in human and veterinary medicine owing to concerns about acute kidney injury, coagulopathies, allergic reactions, and increased mortality in patients that are septic and critically ill. Currently crystalloids and blood products are often preferred for initial stabilization and volume replacement.

Table 14.17 / Commonly used fluids

Fluid type		Indications	Route	Comments
Synthetic colloids	Dextran 70	• Volume expansion • Shock therapy	IV slowly	• Monitor cardiac function. • Allergic responses (rare) • Possible coagulopathies, ↑ blood glucose levels, altered total protein, and blood cross-matching results • Remains within the vascular space for 4–8 hours
	Vetstarch™	• Hypoproteinemia • Shock therapy	IV	• Monitor cardiac function. • Allergic responses (rare) • Possible coagulopathies • Remains within the vascular space for 12–48 hours • ↑ Osmotic and oncotic pressure of blood
Crystalloids	Dextrose 5% in water (D5W – isotonic)	• Free water deficits • Hypernatremia	IV	• High dosages or prolonged use may produce pulmonary edema and dilution of electrolytes • Can cause fluid overload • Isotonic initially; dextrose is metabolized, providing free water (making it hypotonic) • Caution: not used in patients with increased intracranial pressure or during resuscitation due to hyperglycemia
	Lactated Ringer's solution (isotonic)	• Replacement fluid • Maintenance fluid (short term) • Acidotic states • Shock therapy	IV, SQ	• Will not exacerbate lactic acidosis

(Continued)

Table 14.17 / Commonly used fluids (Continued)

Fluid type	Indications	Route	Comments
Normosol-R (isotonic)	• Replacement fluid • Maintenance fluid • Acidotic states • Shock therapy	IV, SQ	• May sting when given SQ
Plasma-Lyte A (isotonic)	• Replacement fluid • Maintenance fluids • Acidotic states • Shock therapy	IV, SQ	• May sting when given SQ
0.45% NaCl (hypotonic)	• Long-term fluid therapy • Free water deficits • Hypernatremia • Sodium restrictions	IV	• Used for patients with high risk of fluid retention (i.e. cardiac disease)
0.45% NaCl with 2.5% dextrose (hypotonic)	• Replacement fluid • Maintenance fluid	IV	• Used for patients with congestive heart failure, liver disease, DKA, edema, and ascites
0.9% NaCl (isotonic)	• Replacement fluid • ↑ Plasma volume • Hyponatremia, hypochloremia, hyperkalemia, hypercalcemia • Bathes tissue during surgical procedures • Shock therapy	IV, SQ, IP	• Caution in patient with heart failure, pulmonary edema, renal impairment • Monitor: electrolyte concentrations and pulmonary pressure • Long-term infusion may cause electrolyte imbalances • Incompatible with amphotericin B • Compatible with blood products
7.5% NaCl (hypertonic)	• Volume expansion • Shock therapy	IV	• Normal hydration required before use • Administered in small boluses (e.g. 3–5 ml/kg)

Table 14.18 / **Fluid additives**

Additive	Indications	Route	Comments
Calcium gluconate and calcium chloride	Correction of hypocalcemia Eclampsia	IV slowly	• Contraindicated: hypercalcemia and ventricular fibrillation • Rate is variable depending on condition and other laboratory values • Monitor hypercalcemia, hypotension, cardiac arrhythmias (when given in conjunction with potassium), cardiac arrest, venous irritation
Dextrose 50%	Hypoglycemia	IV	• Contraindicated: hyperglycemia • See Chapter 15: Medical Calculations, page 693.
Potassium chloride	Prevention or correction of hypokalemia	SQ, IM	• Contraindicated: hyperkalemia, acute dehydration, and severe hemolytic reactions • Rate of infusion is critical (must be diluted): IV – do not exceed 0.5 mEq/kg/hour • Monitor hyperkalemia, bradycardia, or arrhythmias • Compatible with all commonly used IV fluids
Sodium bicarbonate	Correction of metabolic acidosis, hypercalcemic and hyperkalemic crises	IV	• Caution: congestive heart failure or other edema-causing conditions • Rate is variable depending on condition and other laboratory values • Monitor blood gas measurements and acidosis status
Vitamin B complex	Anorexic patients and renal disease	SQ, IM, IV	• Protect fluid bag from light

Skill Box 14.17 / **Calculating Drip Rates**

Method	Example:
	1200 ml administered over 5 hours, using a 15 drops/ml administration set
Determine the total minutes of fluid administration: • Multiply the total time (hours) by 60 = total minutes	5 hours × 60 = 300 minutes
Determine the amount of fluids needed per minute: • Divide the total fluid amount (ml) by the time (minute) = ml/minute	1200 ml ÷ 300 minutes = 4 ml/minute
Calculate the rate (drops/minute) based on the administration set: • Multiply the ml/minute by the drops/ml	4 ml/minute × 15 drops/ml = 60 drops/minute
Calculate a delivery rate to be monitored: • Drops/second or drops/10 seconds • Multiply the drops/minute by the drops/second	60 drops/minute × 1 minute/60 seconds = 1 drop/second

Monitoring Fluid Therapy

Fluid therapy consists of monitoring multiple parameters and observing for trends that reflect the patient's hydration status. Proper functioning of equipment (e.g. catheter, administration set, fluid bag, pump) must also be monitored.

Table 14.19 / Monitoring fluid therapy

Assessment	Dehydration	Normal	Overhydration	Comments
Physical				
Blood pressure	Hypotension	See Table 14.7	Hypertension	• See Skill Box 14.1
Capillary refill time	↓ CRT	1–2 seconds	↑ CRT	• Assesses peripheral perfusion
Heart rate, pulse rate and effort	Tachycardia, weak pulses	Canine: 60–120 bpm Feline: 160–220 bpm	Tachycardia, gallop Strong or bounding pulses	• Assesses cardiovascular and intravascular fluid volume status
Mentation	Depressed, dull	Calm, relaxed	Agitated, restless	
Physical exam	Sunken eyes	See Table 2.2, page 33	Serous nasal discharge, ↑ jugular pulses, pitting edema, chemosis, and dyspnea	• Performed multiple times a day to evaluate hydration and to calculate continuing losses
Pulmonary auscultation	Not applicable	Heard equally on both sides; smooth, quiet sound	Cough, pulmonary edema, harsh lung sounds, crackles, and rales	• See Skill Box 2.2, page 45
Respiratory rate and effort	Variable	Canine: 10–40 breaths/minute Feline: 20–40 breaths/minute	Tachypnea, dyspnea, and pulmonary crackles	
Skin turgor	↓ Skin turgor	< 2 seconds	↑ Skin turgor	• See Skill Box 14.15
Urine output	< 1 ml/kg/hour	1–2 ml/kg/hour	> 2 ml/kg/hour is consistent with polyuria, but should be interpreted in conjunction with patient status	• Assess renal function and perfusion (GFR) • A hydrated patient, with normal kidney function, receiving fluid therapy will have a USG of 1.010–1.020 • Monitoring of trends is important

(Continued)

Table 14.19 / Monitoring fluid therapy (Continued)

Assessment	Dehydration	Normal	Overhydration	Comments
Weight	↓ Weight	Variable	↑ Weight	• Monitor weight 3–4 times a day with aggressive fluid administration and daily with maintenance rates • An ↑ of 1 kg equals 1 l fluid (0.1 kg = 100 ml) • Rapid weight gain indicates fluid accumulation (e.g. pulmonary edema); rapid weight loss indicates fluid loss > replacement • Body weight ↑ by percentage of dehydration indicates a need to change to a maintenance fluid rate
Laboratory				
Electrolytes	N/A	See Table 3.3 page 74	N/A	• Evaluated to determine need for replacement therapy
PCV	↑	Canine: 37–55% Feline: 30–45%	↓	• Assesses hydration status and hemodilution effect of rapid crystalloid infusion • Monitor once or twice daily • Severe dehydration may present with a variable PCV due to fluid shift within the body • Assess in conjunction with total protein
Temperature	Variable	100.5–102.5	Hypothermia, shivering	• A rise of 1.8 degrees may require a 10% ↑ in the maintenance fluid rate
Total protein	> 8.0 g/dl	Canine: 5.4–7.5 g/dl Feline: 5.7–7.6 g/dl	< 4.0 g/dl	• Assesses the relative serum oncotic pressure • A in oncotic pressure allows more fluid to flow into the interstitium causing edema (e.g. pulmonary, SQ)

BLOOD TRANSFUSIONS

The frequency of blood transfusions has increased with additional commercial and in-hospital donor programs available. Laboratory tests prior to the transfusion are critical to avoid severe and possibly life-threatening reactions.

Blood Types

Understanding blood types is important in performing a blood transfusion, to avoid transfusion reactions. Blood types are distinguished by different genetic markers on the surface of the red blood cell (RBC). These genetic markers are antigenic and can cause immune system reactions to unmatched transfused blood with the formation of antibodies (alloantibodies or isoantibodies). These antibodies are found in the plasma and can cause minor to severe transfusion reactions.

Dogs have seven recognized different blood types. The genetic markers on the RBC surface are known as dog erythrocyte antigens (DEA), and are designated as either positive or negative for a specific antigen (e.g. DEA 1+ or DEA 1−). DEA 1+ is found in over 55% of dogs and is currently the most clinically significant in dog transfusion reactions. Dogs do not have naturally occurring alloantibodies but can form them when receiving unmatched blood. Transfusing a DEA 1− dog (recipient) with DEA 1+ blood will cause the recipient to form alloantibodies. Less than ideal transfusions may lead to immediate, delayed, or potentially life-threatening reactions on following transfusions. There are also other known and unknown blood types (e.g. Dal, Kai 1, Kai 2) outside the DEA system, which can lead to transfusion reactions on the first and subsequent transfusions.

Cats have an AB system with three blood types (e.g. A, B, and AB). These blood types, as in dogs, are distinguished by specific antigens found on RBC membranes. All cats have naturally occurring antibodies, called alloantibodies, specifically directed against the antibody they lack (e.g. A or B). Therefore, a transfusion of mismatched blood types will lead to immediate and possibly life-threatening reactions. Even though the majority of cats have type A blood (95%), cats with blood type B have the strongest alloantibodies against type A blood and suffer the most severe and likely fatal reactions. Although uncommon, type B blood is typically found in certain breeds and concentrated in certain geographical locations. An additional blood group, called Mik, has been described in the literature. Cats can have alloantibodies against the Mik antigen leading to acute hemolytic reactions. Owing to the severity of transfusion reactions possible in cats, pre-transfusion blood typing and crossmatch are wise precautions.

Table 14.20 / **Feline blood types**

Feline blood types	Prevalence	Naturally occurring alloantibodies	Mismatched transfusion reactions
A	• Most prevalent worldwide • 95% of cats in United States	Weak "anti-B" antibodies at low titer	Administering type B blood: typically produces a mild and/or delayed hemolytic reaction
B	• 5% of cats • Possibly overrepresented in the Exotic Shorthair, Cornish and Devon Rex populations • Distribution geographically variable	Strong "anti-A" antibodies at a high titer	Administering type A blood: acute severe hemolytic reaction often leading to death
AB	• < 1% of cats • Possibly overrepresented in the Ragdoll population • Distribution geographically variable	Lack antibodies to type A or B blood; universal recipient	None based on blood type

Blood Collection and Administration

A strict collection protocol must be followed to assure safety of the donor and recipient. Potential donors go through a selection process including exams and laboratory work to determine their health. Once selected, dogs can safely donate up to 11–19 ml/kg and cats 10–15 ml/kg of blood monthly. Blood is collected into a closed system, which is also airtight and sterile. The most important step to blood collection is sterility to avoid non-immunogenic transfusion reactions. During collection, the donor's health status must be monitored (e.g. muscle mass, pulse rate and strength, respiratory rate) for any signs of compromise.

Skill Box 14.18 / Blood Collection

Donor requirements	Testing	Collection supplies	Procedure
Canine			

• No behavioral concerns
• No health concerns or current medications (aside from preventives)
• Current vaccinations
• Currently taking heartworm and ectoparasite preventative
• > 25 kg ideal
• 1–8 years of age
	• Complete physical exam
	• Blood typing
	• Minimum laboratory work:
	• CBC, blood chemistry, heartworm testing
	• Minimum infectious disease screening:
	• Anaplasma phagocytophilum/platys, Dirofilaria immitis, Ehrlichia canis, Babesia canis/gibsoni, Bartonella henselae/vinsonii, Ehrlichia canis/chaffeensis/ewingii, Leishmania donovani, Mycoplasma haemocanis
	• Additional testing may be necessary depending on breed and geographical area; refer to the ACVIM consensus statement on canine and feline blood donor screening[2]
		• Blood donor bag and tubing
		• Venipuncture needle
		• Anticoagulant:
		  • CPDA-1, CPD (shelf life 28–35 and 21 days, respectively); 14 ml/100 ml blood
		  • Sodium citrate: (shelf life 48 hours); 1 ml/7–8 ml blood
		• Guarded hemostat
		• Tube sealing:
		  • Aluminum sealing clips
		  • Electric sealer
		• Tubing sealer stripper or household pliers
			1. Clamp the tubing behind the needle
			2. Add anticoagulant to the blood donor bag adhering strictly to aseptic technique and ratio of anticoagulant to blood (1 : 9)
			3. Charge the tubing with anticoagulant as the blood must flow through the anticoagulant to the bag
			4. Prepare and perform sterile venipuncture
			5. Place the collection bag as far below the patient as the tubing will allow
			6. Frequently mix the bag and anticoagulant to prevent clotting during collection
			7. Collect the desired amount of blood then clamp the tubing next to the needle and remove from the donor
			8. Strip the tubing of blood, mix the bag and allow the tubing to refill with blood
			9. Seal the tubing, cut off excess and remove clamped hemostat

(*Continued*)

Skill Box 14.18 / Blood Collection (Continued)

Donor requirements	Testing	Collection supplies	Procedure
Feline			

• No behavioral concerns
• No health concerns or current medications (aside from preventives)
• Current vaccinations
• > 5 kg
• 1–7 years of age
• Indoor only
	• Complete physical exam
	• Blood typing
	• Minimum laboratory work: CBC, blood chemistry, heartworm testing, FeLV, FIV
	• Infectious disease screening: A. phagocytophilum, B. henselae, and M. haemofelis
	• Additional testing may be necessary depending on geographical area; refer to the ACVIM consensus statement on canine and feline blood donor screening[2]
		• Blood donor bag and tubing
		• 19-g butterfly catheter
		• 3-way stopcock
		• Anticoagulant:
		  • ACD, CPD (shelf life 28–35, 21 days, respectively); 1.4 ml/10 ml blood
		  • Sodium citrate (shelf life 48 hours); 1 ml/7–8 ml blood
		• Guarded hemostat
		• 12 ml syringe
		• 60 ml syringe:
		  • Tube sealing
		  • Aluminum sealing clips
		• Electric sealer
		• Tubing sealer stripper or household pliers
			1. Assemble the stopcock, donor bag, tubing, and syringe
			2. Place the stopcock in the off or closed position *Note:* At no time should the stopcock be positioned to allow outside air to enter the tubing leading to contamination
			3. Add anticoagulant to the injection port of the 60-ml syringe paying close attention to sterility
			4. Place the stopcock in the open position to charge the butterfly catheter tubing with anticoagulant as the blood must flow through the anticoagulant to the bag
			5. Remove the hemostat and connect the donor tubing to the catheter tubing
			6. Prepare and perform sterile venipuncture Note: sedation and IV fluids may be required for feline donors
			7. Gently and lightly aspirate blood into the syringe
			8. Collect the desired amount of blood, place the stopcock in the closed position, and remove the needle from the donor
			9. Gently invert the syringe several times to mix the anticoagulant with the blood
			10. Transfer the blood from the syringe into the blood donor bag
			11. Strip the tubing of blood, mix the bag, and allow the tubing to refill with blood
			12. Seal the tubing and cut off

Table 14.21 / Blood products

Blood product	Contents	Use/Action	Storage*	Preparation/Administration
Whole blood, stored	RBC, WBC, plasma proteins; 40% PCV	• Use • Anemia and hypoproteinemia • Large volume deficits • Pediatric patients • Action • ↑ Blood volume and oxygen-carrying capacity	• Storage: 4°C (39.2°F) • Shelf life: 48 hours with sodium citrate and 28 days with CPDA-1 • Bags should be stored separated and upright to allow air movement • Bags removed from storage are stable for 6 hours but can be returned to refrigeration for maximum 24 hours • Note: Whole fresh blood can be stored at room temperature for 6–8 hours without compromising platelets or clotting factors	Preparation: • A change in color (e.g. purple, brown, green) or texture (e.g. clots) may indicate contamination • Warm to < 35°C (98.6°F) Administration: • Volume: 6–12 ml/kg (2–3 ml whole blood/kg will raise the PCV 1%) • General: 10 ml/kg/hour until desired PCV is reached • Rate: initial rate of 0.1–1 ml/minute for 30 minutes, with a gradual ↑ to 4–6 ml/minute as patient allows • Caution: canine CHF: ≤ 5 ml/kg/day
Packed RBC	RBC, most supernatant plasma removed; 80% PCV	Use: • Anemia • Animals in fear of fluid overload (e.g. CHF) • ↓ Risk of exposure to plasma antigens Action: • ↑ Oxygen-carrying capacity	• Separated from unrefrigerated whole blood within eight hours of collection • Storage: 4°C (39.2°F) • Shelf life: 35 days with CPDA-1 and ACD and 21 days with CPD • Gently mix refrigerated bags twice weekly • Bags should be stored separated and upright to allow air movement • Bags removed from storage are stable for 6 hours but can be returned to refrigeration for a max of 24 hours	Preparation: • A change in color (e.g. purple, brown, green) or texture (e.g. clots) may indicate contamination • Warm to < 35°C (98.6°F) • Addition of 0.9% sterile saline may be needed to ↓ viscosity of pRBC Administration: • Volume: 10–20 ml/kg (1–1.5 ml of pRBC/kg will raise PCV 1%) • Rate: initial rate of 0.1–1 ml/minute for 30 minutes, with a gradual ↑ to 4–6 ml/minute as patient allows
Fresh frozen plasma	Plasma supernatant; hemostatic proteins, albumin, globulins, and coagulation factors	Use: • Coagulation factor deficits, DIC, severe liver disease, vitamin K deficiency, pancreatitis, severe parvovirus enteritis • Hypoproteinemia and hypoglobinemia • Prolonged PT/APTT • Control of active bleeding • Preoperative prophylaxis Action: • Full activity of all coagulation factors • Expand extracellular fluid volume	• Frozen within 8 hours of collection • Storage: –20°C (1°F) • Shelf life: 1 year, then can be relabeled as frozen plasma for an additional 4 years • Bags should be frozen lying flat and then stored separated and upright to allow air movement • Bags removed from storage are stable for 6 hours but can be returned to refrigeration for a maximum of 24 hours • Bags may be refrozen if thawed for <1 hour	Preparation: • Plasma bags are brittle and should be warmed in their transport box and then inspected for cracks prior to administration • Unopened bags can be refrozen with minimal loss of activity • Warm to < 35°C (98.6°F) Administration: • Volume: 6–12 ml/kg • Rate: initial rate of 1–2 ml/minute to a maximum rate of 3–6 ml/minute • Administer within 1–2 hours to allow therapeutic plasma levels to be obtained

(Continued)

Table 14.21 / **Blood products (Continued)**

Blood product	Contents	Use/Action	Storage*	Preparation/Administration
Frozen plasma	Plasma supernatant; hemostatic proteins, albumin, globulins, and coagulation factors (II, VII, IX, X)	Use: • Coagulation factor • Hypoproteinemia and hypoglobinemia Action: • Full activity of coagulation factors II, VII, IX, X • Low activity of coagulation factors V, VIII	• Frozen > 8 hours after collection • Storage: −20 °C (1°F) • Shelf life: 5 years • Bags should be frozen lying flat and then stored separated and upright to allow air movement • Bags removed from storage are stable for 6 hours but can be returned to refrigeration for a maximum of 24 hours (do not refreeze)	Preparation: • Plasma bags are brittle and should be warmed in their transport box and then inspected for cracks prior to administration • Unopened bags can be refrozen with minimal loss of activity • Warm to < 35°C (98.6°F) Administration: • Volume: 6–12 ml/kg • Rate: initial rate of 1–2 ml/minute to a maximum rate of 3–6 ml/minute • Administer within 1–2 hours to allow therapeutic plasma levels to be obtained
Cryoprecipitate	Heavy, cold-insoluble proteins; 50% yield of factor VIII; von Willebrand's factor, fibrinogen, fibronectin	Use: • Hemophilia A, von Willebrand's disease, fibrinogen deficiency or dysfunction • Topical hemostatic in surgery Action: • Coagulation factor replacement	• Storage: −20°C (1°F) • Shelf life: 1 year	Preparation: • Plasma bags are brittle and should be warmed in their transport box and then inspected for cracks prior to administration • Warm to < 35°C (98.6°F) • Thawed product may be refrozen within 2 hours without effect Administration: • Volume: 1–2 ml/kg (1 unit/10 kg) • Rate: slow IV bolus over 10–20 minutes
Oxyglobin (hemoglobin-based oxygen carrier)	Acellular oxygen-carrying replacement fluid Derived from bovine hemoglobin	• Use: • ↑ Intravascular volume • Alleviates the risk of RBC sensitization • ↑ Oxygen-carrying capacity Action: • Carries O_2 and CO_2 similar to hemoglobin • Expands extracellular fluid volume	• Storage: room temperature or refrigerated • Shelf life: 3 years	Preparation: • Warm to < 35°C (98.6°F). Administration: • Volume: 10–30 ml/kg • Rate: IV to a maximum rate of 10 ml/kg/hour • Used within 24 hours after removing the foil packaging • Indicated for canines only
Notes	• Self-defrosting freezers should not be used to store blood due to their temperature fluctuations and potential to dehydrate			

* Storage referring to blood collected in a closed collection system

Skill Box 14.19 / Blood Administration

Transfusion Protocol	Patient	Blood

Preparation	• Perform blood typing and a crossmatch before every transfusion.
	• Catheter: must be dedicated to transfusion use only
	• Technique:
	  • Place an IV catheter with strict aseptic technique
	  • To use an existing catheter, flush the catheter before and after the transfusion with 0.9% sterile saline
	• Note: flush an existing catheter with 0.9% NaCl for 10 minutes if there is previous exposure to calcium-containing products
		• Inspection:
		  • Verify the correct patient and blood type have been selected
		  • Each bag should be thoroughly inspected prior to administration for changes in the integrity of the bag and blood color and for the presence of hemolysis or clots
		• Temperatures > 37 °C (98.6°F) may lyse RBC (↓ oxygen-carrying capacity, inactivate proteins and clotting factors) and accelerate bacterial overgrowth
		• Techniques:
		  • Place the bag at room temperature for 30 minutes
		  • Place the blood bag (and transport box if included) into zipped bags (to avoid infusion port contamination and damage to brittle bags) and submerge bags into a container of cold to warm water for 15 minutes or until ≤ 37 °C (98.6°F)
		  • Run the IV tubing through warm water during the transfusion

Setup	• Place the patient in a clean comfortable cage with white bedding to observe for hemoglobinuria.
	• Place in an area of the hospital to allow continuous visual monitoring.
		• Filters
		  • A blood administration set with an inline 170–270-μm pore, non-latex filter should be used to remove clots and debris collected during storage
		  • Filters are functional for 2–4 units of blood or for a maximum use of 4 hours
		• No fluids (e.g. lactated Ringer's, 5% dextrose in water, hypotonic saline) or medications should be added to a blood bag except 0.9% sterile saline to avoid triggering coagulation (e.g. calcium in fluids)

Administration	• Monitoring
	• Obtain baseline vital signs before beginning the transfusion (e.g. urine color, PCV, temperature, pulse, and respiratory rate)
	• Obtain basic vital signs every 5 minutes for 15–30 minutes
	• Continue monitoring every 15 minutes for the duration of the transfusion
		• Routes: IV is the preferred route, but intraosseous catheters can be used in patients with difficult venous access with excellent results (e.g. femur, tibia, humerus)
		• Rate:
		  • Based on blood product, recipient size, and health status
		  • An initial slow rate of 0.1–1 ml/minute for 30 minutes, with a gradual ↑ to 4–6 ml/minute as patient allows
		  • Blood may be administered by gravity or through an infusion pump rated to deliver blood products to assure no harm to the cells
		  • Transfusions should be completed within 4 hours to ↓ bacterial overgrowth
		  • See Skill Box 14.17

Notes	• Blood samples from the donor and recipient can be stored for 1 week post-transfusion in the event of an adverse reaction • 10 ml/kg packed RBC or 20 ml/kg whole blood ↑ PCV by 10% if donor has a PCV of approximately 40%[3] • The unit can be aseptically divided and half stored in the refrigerator to extend administration over 8 hours	

Blood Transfusion Reactions

Despite careful attention to detail, transfusion reactions may still occur. Reactions are seen both acutely (within minutes to hours) or after a delay (days to years), and are divided into immunologic or nonimmunologic causes. Immunologic reactions are caused by an antigen–antibody response between the recipient and the donor blood product. Non-immunologic reactions are caused by problems with blood samples or administration techniques. Treatment for transfusion reactions are directed toward alleviating clinical signs and basic supportive care (e.g. fluid support, oxygen support, diuretics, antipyretics, steroids, antihistamines).

Table 14.22 / Blood transfusion reactions.

Reaction	Cause	Signs
Acute Immunologic: • Antibody–antigen reactions • Typically occurs within minutes of initiating transfusion • Transfusion must be stopped immediately and anaphylactic treatment started	RBC	Intravascular or extravascular hemolysis, fever, anaphylaxis, hypotension, tachy- or bradycardia, cyanosis, apnea, salivation, lacrimation, urination, defecation, emesis, collapse, acute renal failure, shock, and death
	Platelets, WBC	Fever and emesis
	Plasma proteins	Urticaria, facial edema, erythema, and pruritis
Acute non-immunologic	Contamination	Fever, sepsis, infection, hypotension, hemolysis, vomiting, DIC, renal failure, shock, emesis, and diarrhea Blood products: dark, discoloration of RBC, clumped cells, hemolysis, and air bubbles
	Improper collection	Hemolysis, emesis, edema, and dyspnea
	Volume overload	Dyspnea, emesis, retching, pulmonary edema, vocalization, tachycardia, coughing, tachypnea, and cyanosis
	Microaggregates	Thrombosis
	Citrate toxicity (hypocalcemia toxicity)	Tetany, tremors, cardiac arrhythmias, emesis, and ECG changes
Delayed immunologic: • Occurs over days	RBC	↓ PCV, fever, icterus, and shortened red cell survival Neonatal hemolysis
	Platelet	Thrombocytopenia and petechiae extravascular hemolysis (e.g. hyperbilirubinemia, hemoglobinuria, bilirubinuria)
Delayed non-immunologic	Infected donor	Disease transmission (e.g. FeLV, FIV)
Notes	• Fever is considered to be a > 1°C (2°F) increase over the pretransfusion temperature within 1–2 hours	

OXYGEN THERAPY

The objective of oxygen therapy is to provide adequate oxygen to the arterial blood and to remove carbon dioxide. Any acutely ill or injured patient has a higher demand for oxygen and should be provided supplemental oxygen until stabilized. Indications for its use are shock, wound repair, pulmonary edema, and lower cardiac output or hemoglobin concentration. Monitoring the patient who is receiving supplemental oxygen is crucial, as oxygen toxicity can occur along with hyperthermia, hypercapnia, and lower humidity.

Oxygen Administration

Oxygen administration requires the following equipment: an oxygen source, a humidifier, oxygen tubing, and Christmas tree adapters or syringe case.

Humidification

The normal function of the respiratory tract is to warm and humidify inspired gases. Providing humidified oxygen can reduce the risk of increased water loss and drying of the lower airway predisposing the patient to pneumonia. Humidification should be provided for all patients receiving long-term oxygen supplementation or when delivered directly into the nose, endotracheal tube, or trachea. The humidifier should be cleaned and dried after each patient.

Oxygen Flow Rates

Oxygen is toxic at high concentrations. One hundred percent oxygen should not be given for longer than 24 hours and 60% oxygen should not be given for more than 48 hours. After the patient is stabilized, the concentration should be reduced to the lowest level possible, with ideal concentrations less than 50%.

- Flow-by or oxygen mask: ≥ 5 l/minute, up to 100–150 ml/kg/minute, but many patients are intolerant of high flow rates.
- Oxygen hood: 200 ml/kg/minute.
- Nasal catheter: 50–150 ml/kg/minute.

Discontinuing Oxygen

Discontinuing oxygen can often begin once a patient is eupneic and has a pulse ox reading of over 90%. Weaning from the oxygen should be done slowly over 12–48 hours. Decrease the percentage of oxygen by small amounts every two to three hours and monitor the patient to ensure that oxygen therapy is no longer needed.

Immediate and Temporary Approaches to Respiratory Distress

The methods listed here are for immediate and temporary use. The patient tolerance is typically high.

Oxygen Flow-by

Connect the oxygen tube to the gas source and run at ≥ 5 l/minute. Place the open end of the tube about six inches from the patient's mouth/nose. Avoid directing the flowing into the nares as this can cause irritation.

Mask

Connect the oxygen tube to the gas source and run at ≥ 5 l/minute. Connect an anesthetic mask to the open end of the tube and place over the patient's mouth and nose. The mask can be kept in place with a muzzle. Be sure that the fit is loose enough to allow CO_2 to escape.

Oxygen Cage

Patients may be placed in an oxygen cage for both short- and long-term management, Commercial oxygen cages monitor the oxygen percentage and often have the capability to maintain temperature and humidity, as well as extracting carbon dioxide. Routine maintenance is imperative for these units to operate effectively.

Routes of Oxygen Administration

Skill Box 14.20 / Routes of oxygen administration: oxygen hood and nasal catheter.

	Oxygen hood	Nasal catheter
Indications	• Respiratory distress • Hypoxemia	• Respiratory distress • Hypoxemia
Contraindications	• Airway obstruction • Panting • Hyperthermia • ↑ Stress	• Airway obstruction, nasal or facial trauma • ↑ Stress • Epistaxis and coagulopathies • ↑ Intracranial pressure • Brachycephalic breeds
Setup	• Specialized oxygen hood E-collars (or E-collar and saran wrap) • Tape • Tie (e.g. gauze, collar) • Oxygen setup • Humidifier	• Red rubber catheter • Small patients: 3.5–5 Fr • Medium canines: 5–8 Fr • Large canines: 8–10 Fr • Topical anesthetic (e.g. proparacaine ophthalmic drops) • Permanent marker • Suture, non-absorbable • Needle holders • Oxygen setup • Humidifier • Lubricant • E-collar
Procedure	1. Tape Saran wrap to the outside of an E-collar to cover 50–80% of the opening. The opening at the top is for CO_2, heat, and condensation to escape 2. Place the E-collar over the patient's head and secure with gauze or using the patient's collar 3. Feed the oxygen tube in at the neck opening and secure near the front of the E-collar with tape	1. Place several drops of topical anesthetic in the nostril to be used and allow approximately 10 minutes to take full effect. Be sure to elevate the head to allow coating of the nasal passage. It may also be helpful to apply a drop to each eye 2. Measure the tube from the nostril to the medial canthus of the eye and mark 3. Place several more drops of anesthetic in the nostril 4. Place a simple interrupted suture at the lateral commissure of the nose and another somewhere between the eyes to on top of the head 5. Lubricate the tip of the tube with lidocaine gel 6. Using your thumb, push up on the nose into a pig position, then gently insert the tube ventrally and medially to the level of the mark on the tube 7. Use the sutures previously placed to connect with a Chinese finger-trap suture. Oxygen flow rate is 50–150 ml/kg/minute (see Skill Box 23.6, page 1073)
Complications	Hyperthermia, hypercapnia	Nasal passage irritation, sneezing; ↑ stress
Removal	Remove E-collar	Remove sutures and gently but swiftly remove the catheter
Tip	• Selecting a larger red rubber catheter for nasal catheters provides increased patient tolerance. The larger size fills the nasal cavity, eliminating movement and tickling and also eliminating the higher pressure hose effect when the O_2 is turned on	

Skill Box 14.21 / Routes of Oxygen Administration: Transtracheal Catheter and Tracheostomy

Method	Transtracheal catheter	Tracheostomy, emergency
Indications	• Upper airway obstruction • Head, facial, or nasal trauma • Epistaxis	• Airway obstruction • Laryngeal or pharyngeal collapse • Long-term PPV
Contraindications	• Tracheal trauma or injury • Airway obstruction distal to catheter placement	• Tracheal trauma or injury • Airway obstruction distal to tracheostomy site
Setup	• Surgical site preparation materials • Sedation or general anesthesia • Sterile surgical pack • Tracheal catheter or large bore over-the-needle catheter • Oxygen setup (not to exceed 0.5 l/minute) • Bandaging material	• Surgical site preparation materials • Sedation or general anesthesia • Tracheostomy tube (various sizes) • Sterile surgical pack • Suture material
Procedure	1. Place the patient is placed in dorsal recumbency and surgically prepare the neck from the ramus of the mandible to the thoracic inlet and dorsally to midline 2. Make an incision over the larynx and bluntly dissect down to the trachea 3. Insert the catheter along a groove director. Once in the trachea, remove the groove director and stylet and direct the catheter to the level of the carina. Secure the catheter to the skin with Chinese finger-trap sutures. Loosely bandage around the catheter. 4. If using an over-the-needle catheter, after aseptic preparation, insert the catheter percutaneously into the lumen of the catheter (between tracheal rings 4 and 5 or 5 and 6) 5. Once the stylet is in the trachea, advance the catheter and direct toward the carina 6. Oxygen can be administered via flow-by or a 3 mm endotracheal tube connector can be used to connect to an oxygen source. This method is difficult to secure and is typically more appropriate for short term intervention	1. Place the patient i in dorsal recumbency and surgically prepare the neck from the ramus of the mandible to the thoracic inlet and dorsally to midline 2. Make an incision over the larynx and bluntly dissect down to the trachea 3. Place two stay-sutures around the 4th and 5th tracheal rings and use to retract the opening 4. Make an incision between the rings while avoiding cutting > 35% of the circumference of the trachea 5. Retract the stay sutures and insert the tracheostomy tube 6. Secure the tube with tape.
Complications	• Tracheal trauma or injury • Tracheitis, SQ emphysema, catheter kink or obstruction, pneumomediastinum, and hematoma	• Tracheal trauma or injury
Maintenance	• All contact should be performed aseptically • Monitor respiratory rate, lung sounds, and all vital signs • Monitor site for infection, kinking, SQ emphysema, and dislodgement • Change bandages frequently	• All contact should be performed aseptically and the patient should be preoxygenated before any procedure • Monitor respiratory rate, lung sounds, and all vital signs • Suction 3–4 times every 30–60 minutes for 3–7 seconds; supplemental oxygen may be needed between suctioning • Clean the inner cannula every 2–4 hours • Instill sterile saline (1 ml/10 kg) every 3–4 hours • Nebulize and coupage 3–4 times a day • The tube should be changed daily
Removal	• Remove the tube and allow the wound to heal by second intention	• Remove the tube and stay sutures and allow the wound to heal by second intention

REFERENCES

1. Behrend, E., Holford, A., Lathan, P. *et al.* (2018). 2018 AAHA diabetes management guidelines for dogs and cats. *J Am Anim Hosp Assoc* 54: 1–21.
2. Wardrop, K.J., Birken heuer, M.C., Blais, M.B. et al. (2016). Update on canine and feline blood donor screening for blood-borne pathogens. *J Vet Intern Med* 30: 15–35.
3. Thrall, M.A. (2004). *Veterinary Hematology and Clinical Chemistry*. Baltimore, MD: Blackwell Publishing.

Chapter 15

Medical Calculations

Rebeccah Vaughan, CVT, VTS (Anesthesia/Analgesia), (Clinical Practice-C/F)

Veterinary Technician and Nurse's Daily Reference Guide: Canine and Feline, Fourth Edition. Edited by Mandy Fults and Kenichiro Yagi.

Companion website: www.wiley.com/go/fults/veterinary

Abbreviations

IV, intravenous
PCV, packed cell volume
RER, resting energy requirement

CALCULATING A DOSE BY PATIENT WEIGHT

The majority of our administered medications are dosed by weight, because our patients vary greatly in size. To calculate a dose by patient weight, we need to know two pieces of information: the recommended dose to be used, and the weight of the patient.

The recommended dose is usually given in a units/weight measurement. This is most commonly recorded in milligrams/kilograms (mg/kg), but can be demonstrated with other units such as grams (g), micrograms (μg), milliliters (ml) for fluid rates, or in pounds (lb) of body weight.

Example

Butorphanol 0.2mg/kg for "Duke" weighing 24kg

This states that for every kilogram of body weight, Duke should receive 0.2 mg of butorphanol, which can be arithmetically expressed as:

$$\frac{0.2\,\text{mg}}{1\,\text{kg}}$$

Since Duke weighs 24 kg, his weight can be expressed in the same manner:

$$\frac{24\,\text{kg}}{\text{Duke}}$$

Therefore, to calculate the dose for Duke, the 0.2 mg/kg is multiplied by the 24 kg of body weight. Using rules of unit conversion, kilogram units cancel out, leaving a milligram dose for the patient, Duke.

$$\frac{0.2\,\text{mg}}{1\,\cancel{\text{kg}}} \times \frac{24\,\cancel{\text{kg}}}{\text{Duke}} = \frac{4.8\,\text{mg}}{\text{Duke}}$$

CALCULATING A MEDICATION VOLUME BY PATIENT DOSE

Once a dose has been calculated for the patient, the volume of the drug must be determined. Most injectable drug concentrations are labeled as milligrams/milliliter, but can be displayed as many other units, including micrograms, grams, mg per vial, or percent solutions.

Example

Give 4.8 mg butorphanol to "Duke" intramuscularly. The butorphanol bottle states that the amount of drug in the vial is 10 mg/ml. This is the drug concentration.

Every 1.0 ml butorphanol in this vial contains 10 mg of drug. The calculated dose is divided by the concentration, after units are made equal. Since the dose and concentration are listed in the same units, the calculation can be expressed as:

$$\frac{4.8\,\cancel{\text{mg}}}{\text{Duke}} \times \frac{1.0\,\text{ml}}{10\,\cancel{\text{mg}}} = \frac{0.48\,\text{ml}}{\text{Duke}}$$

Tip: A mnemonic to remember which number to divide by the other is: "Divide what you want by what you have."

As the two previous equations are often performed in conjunction with one another to calculate administration volumes, they can be combined into a single equation which multiplies the dose by the patient weight, then divides the product by the concentration. Remember that this only works if all units have been converted to be equal:

$$\frac{\text{dose} \times \text{weight}}{\text{concentration}} = \text{drug volume or } \frac{0.2 \times 24}{10} = 0.48$$

CONVERTING PERCENT SOLUTIONS TO MILLIGRAMS/MILLILITERS

Percent solutions are equal to the number of grams per 100 ml of volume. Thus, the percent of the available solution can be converted by stating it as g/100 ml, then converting grams to milligrams and reducing the ratio from 100 ml to 1 ml.

Example

Lidocaine is available as a 2% solution. This means that this lidocaine contains 2 g/100 ml.

$$\frac{2\,\cancel{g}}{100\,ml} \times \frac{1000\,mg}{1g} = \frac{2000\,mg}{1g} \text{ reduced to } \frac{20\,mg}{1ml}$$

Thus, a 2% solution of lidocaine is equal to 20 mg/ml.

Tip: move the decimal point one place to the right, or multiply the percent by 10, to determine the mg/mL concentration.

CREATING PERCENT SOLUTIONS IN CRYSTALLOID FLUIDS TWO WAYS

Adding a medication to a volume of crystalloids to create a percent solution is sometimes ordered, particularly in the case of dextrose. A simple way to convert any volume of fluids into any percent solution is to create a set of comparative ratios, demonstrated as fractions, and cross multiplying to determine the amount of medication to add to the fluids.

Example:

Example: create a 5% dextrose solution for Scooter in his existing fluids. Scooter currently has a bag containing a remaining 600 ml Isolyte®. Dextrose is available as a 50% solution.

Calculation #1: Cross-Multiplication

We know that we currently have 600 ml fluids, and we want the final volume to contain 5% dextrose per milliliter of fluids. That 5% can be expressed as a fraction of 5 parts per 100 parts. But since we have 600 parts (ml) of fluids, we need to convert the fractions by making them equal to determine how much dextrose we need. This can be solving for our unknown variable (x) by cross-multiplying:

$$\frac{5}{100} = \frac{x}{600}$$

Cross-multiplying gives us the formula:

$$100x = 3000$$

Then, to solve for x, we divide both sides of the equation to allow x to "stand alone", giving us the result:

$$x = 30$$

This tells us that to make a 5% solution in 600 ml, we would need 30 units of dextrose. But since the solution is only 50% dextrose and not all drug, we need to double our volume of dextrose added to reach the proper concentration. This increases our 30 units to 60 units, which is expressed in milliliters. One would add 60 ml of 50% dextrose to 600 ml of Isolyte to reach a 5% dextrose concentration.

Calculation #2: Converting Units to Milligrams/Milliliters to Use Standard Calculations

Using the same example as above, we are being asked to make a percent solution. As we are also working with a drug available in a percent solution, one may find it easier to convert everything into a mg/ml form.

As percent solutions are stated as g/100 ml, we can deduce that to create a 5% solution, we want our final product to contain 50 mg/ml of dextrose. As dextrose is available as a 50% solution, we can convert that concentration to 500 mg/ml. In this case, our patient is not Scooter; rather, it is a bag of fluids containing 600 ml, in which we will use the milliliters of fluid rather than kg of body weight. So, for every ml, we want to add 50 mg. We can correlate this to our original formula of dose multiplied by the "weight" (in this case, 600 ml fluids) divided by concentration. This can be expressed as:

$$\frac{50\,\cancel{mg/ml} \times 600\,ml}{500\,\cancel{mg/ml}} = \frac{30000\,ml}{500} \text{ reduced to } 60\,ml$$

To create a 5% solution of 50% dextrose in 600 ml of Isolyte, one should add 60 ml to the bag.

Tip: Prior to adding the dextrose to fluids, always remove the same volume of crystalloid to create a more accurate dilution and not a ratio.

CONVERTING TEMPERATURE

To convert Celsius to Fahrenheit and back again, one must apply a ratio of 5 : 9 separate from the removal of the 32-unit difference. Compared with Celsius, Fahrenheit numbers have a 32-unit increase, so this must be subtracted prior to using the ratio, and it must be added afterward to a Celsius temperature. The 5: 9 ratio can be visualized as a fraction during calculation. This fraction will be relative to the direction of the conversion; from Fahrenheit to Celsius would multiply the number by 5/9, and from Celsius to Fahrenheit multiplies the value by 9/5. The formulas for conversion are:

$$\text{Celsius} = (F - 32) \times 5/9$$

$$\text{Fahrenheit} = C \times 9/5 + 32$$

DILUTION COMPARED WITH RATIO

Dilutions and ratios can be confusing, because they can both be expressed in writing using a colon to separate the numbers, but do not consist of the same volumes. A dilution expresses the number of parts to be added to a total volume, usually expressed in a solvent-in-solute form. A ratio expresses a comparison between two separate numbers. For example:

Create a 1:4 dilution of an IV antibiotic in sterile saline.

Reading this aloud, one would read "Create a one *in* four dilution . . .", which reminds you that the final product will have four total parts. In this case, one part of the solute (the antibiotic) would be added to sterile saline to create four total parts. This means that, for every one part antibiotic, three equal parts sterile saline are added.

The ratio of apples to oranges is 1:3

Reading this aloud, one would read "The ratio of apples to oranges is one *to* three". This states that for every one apple, three oranges are present. The components of the ratio are not dependent upon one another to create a total sum as in an expression of a dilution.

BLOOD VOLUME CALCULATIONS

Canine blood volume is usually 7–9% of total body weight. Dogs usually have 70–90 ml/kg of blood.[1]

Tip: Dogs have about 1 liter blood for every 12 kg/25lb body weight.

Feline blood volume is usually 6.5% of total body weight. Cats usually have 65 ml/kg blood.[1]

To calculate canine transfusion volume for specific packed cell volume (PCV) goals:[2]

$$VT(\text{ml}) = \text{kg BW} \times \text{blood volume}(90\,\text{ml}) \times \left[(\text{desired PCV} - \text{recipient PCV})/\text{Donor PCV}\right]$$

Resting energy requirement (RER) calculations for dogs and cats:[3]

- Most accurate: RER in kcal/day = 70 (ideal weight [kg])$^{0.75}$
- Quick calculation: RER in kcal/day = 30 (ideal weight [kg]) + 70

Varying metabolic energy requirements are shown in Table 15.1.

Table 15.1 / Metabolic energy requirements

Status	Canine	Feline
Neutered adult	1.6 × RER	1.2 × RER
Intact adult	1.8 × RER	1.4 × RER
Inactive/obese prone	1.2–1.4 × RER	1.0 × RER
Weight loss	1.0 × RER	0.8 × RER
Weight gain	1.2–1.4 × RER	1.2–1.4 × RER
Active/working	2.0–8.0 × RER	1.6 × RER

(*Continued*)

Table 15.1 / Metabolic energy requirements (Continued)

Status	Canine	Feline
Gestation (increase throughout pregnancy)	1.8–3.0 × RER	1.6–2.0 × RER
Lactation (varies based on number of puppies/kittens nursing)	3.0–8.0 × RER	2.0–6.0 × RER
Growth (weaning to 4 months)	3.0 × RER	2.5 × RER
Growth (4 months to adult)	2.0 × RER	2.5 × RER

COMMON FLUID RATES FOR DOGS AND CATS

- Resting energy requirement calculations for dogs and cats:[4]
  - Canine anesthetic maintenance: 5 ml/kg/hour
  - Feline anesthetic maintenance: 3 ml/kg/hour
- Correcting dehydration: kg × % dehydration = liters of replacement fluid required
- Correct continuing losses over 2–3 hours, but replace deficit volumes over 24 hours
- Canine crystalloid shock dose: 80–90 ml/kg, to be given in 25% increments over 15 minutes, then reassess after each quarter dose.
- Feline crystalloid shock dose: 50–55 ml/kg, to be given in 25% increments over 15 minutes, then reassess after each quarter dose.

Tip: A 25% shock dose in the canine can quickly be estimated by multiplying the patient's weight in pounds by 10. Example: 10 kg/22lb patient would receive 800–900 ml as a full shock dose, in 200–225 ml 25% increments. Weight (lb) 22 × 10 = 220 ml

KILOGRAMS TO BODY SURFACE AREA

Common equations used to calculate body surface area (m^2):[5]

- Canine: $\frac{10.1 \times (\text{weight in } g)2/3}{10000}$
- Feline: $\frac{10 \times (\text{weight in } g)2/3}{10000}$

Table 15.2 / Kilograms to body surface area (m^2): canine

kg	m^2
0.5	0.06
1	0.10
2	0.15
3	0.20
4	0.25
5	0.29
6	0.33
7	0.36
8	0.40
9	0.43
10	0.46
11	0.49
12	0.52
13	0.55

(Continued)

Table 15.2 / **Kilograms to body surface area (m^2): canine (Continued)**

kg	m^2
14	0.58
15	0.60
16	0.63
17	0.66
18	0.69
19	0.71
20	0.74
21	0.76
22	0.78
23	0.81
24	0.83
25	0.85
26	0.88
27	0.90
28	0.92
29	0.94
30	0.96
35	1.07
40	1.17

(Continued)

Table 15.2 / **Kilograms to body surface area (m^2): canine (Continued)**

kg	m^2
45	1.26
50	1.36
55	1.47
60	1.55
65	1.64
70	1.72
75	1.80
80	1.88
85	1.96

Table 15.3 / **Kilograms to body surface area (m^2): feline**

kg	m^2
0.5	0.063
1	0.1
1.5	0.131
2	0.159
2.5	0.184
3	0.208
3.5	0.231

(Continued)

Table 15.3 / **Kilograms to body surface area (m^2): feline (Continued)**

kg	m^2
4	0.252
4.5	0.273
5	0.292
5.5	0.311
6	0.330
6.5	0.348
7	0.366
7.5	0.383
8	0.400
8.5	0.416
9	0.432
9.5	0.449
10	0.464

CONVERSION CHARTS

Table 15.4 / **Metric units**

Prefix	Symbol	Power	Base 10
kilo	k	10^3	1000
hecto	h	10^2	100
deca	da	10^1	10
unity		1	1
deci	d	10^{-1}	0.1
centi	c	10^{-2}	0.01
milli	m	10^{-3}	0.001
micro	μ or r	10^{-6}	0.000001
nano	n	10^{-9}	0.000000001
pico	p	10^{-12}	0.000000000001

Table 15.5 / Weight conversions

Unit	Kilogram (kg)	Gram (g)	Milligram (mg)	Microgram (µg)	Pound (lb)	Ounce (oz)	Grain (gr)
Kilogram	1	1000	1 × 106	1 × 109	2.2	36	
Gram	0.001	1	1000	1 × 106	–	–	15
Milligram	1 × 10–6	0.001	1	1000	–	–	–
Microgram	1 × 10–9	1 × 10–6	0.001	1	–	–	–
Pound	0.454	454	–	–	1	16	–
Ounce	0.028	28.4	–	–	0.0625	1	–
Grain	–	0.065	65	–	–	–	1
Note	In cases in which the conversion is not useful, – has been included						

Table 15.6 / Liquid measure conversions

Unit	Liter (l)	Milliliter (ml)*	Gallon (gal)	Quart (qt)	Pint (pt)	Cup (c)	Tablespoon (Tbsp)	Teaspoon (tsp)	Ounce (oz)	Drop (gtt)	Dram
Liter	1	1000	¼	1	2	4	–	–	34	–	250
Milliliter	0.001	1	–	–	–	–	–	1/5	–	12	¼
Gallon	3.84	3840	1	4	8	16	–	–	128	–	–
Quart	0.960	960	¼	1	2	4	–	–	32	–	250
Pint	0.5	480	1/8	½	1	2	32	–	16	–	120
Cup	0.25	240	1/16	¼	½	1	16	48	8	–	60
Tablespoon	–	15	–	–	–	–	1	3	½	180	4
Teaspoon	–	5	–	–	–	–	1/3	1	1/6	60	1

(*Continued*)

Table 15.6 / **Liquid measure conversions (Continued)**

Unit	Liter (l)	Milliliter (ml)*	Gallon (gal)	Quart (qt)	Pint (pt)	Cup (c)	Tablespoon (Tbsp)	Teaspoon (tsp)	Ounce (oz)	Drop (gtt)	Dram
Ounce	–	30	–	–	–	–	2	6	1	360	8
Dram	–	4	–	–	–	–	1/3	1	1/8	60	1
Drop	–	–	–	–	–	–	–	–	–	1	–

Notes * Cubic centimeter (cc)
In cases in which the conversion is not useful, a "–" has been listed.

Table 15.7 / **Length**

Unit	Meter (m)	Centimeter (cm)	Millimeter (mm)	Yard (yd)	Feet (ft)	Inch (in)
Meter	1	100	1000	1.0936	3.2808	39.37
Centimeter	0.01	1	10	0.0109	0.03281	0.3937
Millimeter	0.001	0.1	1	0.0011	0.00328	0.03937
Yard	0.9144	91.44	914.40	1	3	36
Foot	0.3048	30.48	304.8	0.333	1	12
Inch	0.0254	2.54	25.4	0.0278	0.0833	1

REFERENCES

1. Cotter, S.M. (2019). Blod transfusions in animals. In: *Merck Veterinary Manual.* http://www.merckvetmanual.com/circulatory-system/blood-groups-and-blood-transfusions/blood-transfusions (accessed 26 July 2021).
2. Short, J.L., Diehl, S., Seshadri, R. *et al.* (2012). Accuracy of formulas used to predict post-transfusion packed cell volume rise in anemic dogs. *J Vet Emerg Crit Care (San Antonio)* 22: 428–434.
3. Gross, K.L., Jewell, D.E., Yamka, R.M. *et al.* (2010). Macronutrients. In: *Small Animal Clinical Nutrition*, 5e (ed. M.S. Hand, C.D. Thatcher, R.L. Remillard, *et al*), 49–105. https://s3.amazonaws.com/mmi_sacn5/2019/SACN5_5.pdf (accessed 26 July 2021).
4. Davis, H., Jensen, T., Johnson, A. *et al.* (2013). 2013 AAHA/AAFP Fluid Therapy Guidelines for Dogs and Cats. *J Am Anim Hosp Assoc* 49: 149–159.
5. Jack, C.M., Watson, P.M. and Heeren, V. Appendix: Metric units. *Veterinary Technician's Daily Reference Guide: Canine and Feline*, 3e. Ames, IA: Wiley Blackwell.

Chapter 16

Medical Procedures

Courtney Waxman, MS, CVT, RVT, VTS (ECC)

Veterinary Technician and Nurse's Daily Reference Guide: Canine and Feline, Fourth Edition. Edited by Mandy Fults and Kenichiro Yagi.

Companion website: www.wiley.com/go/fults/veterinary

Abbreviations

CNS, central nervous system
CPR, cardiopulmonary resuscitation
CRI, constant rate infusion
DABP, direct arterial blood pressure
ECG, electrocardiogram
EDTA, ethylenediaminetetraacetic acid
GDV, gastric dilation volvulus
IOP, intraocular pressure
IV, intravenous
LTT, lavender-top tube
RTT, red-top tube

ABDOMINAL PROCEDURES

Skill Box 16.1 / Abdominocentesis

Use	Supplies	Procedure	Comments
• To remove accumulation of fluid from the peritoneal cavity	• Clippers • Surgical preparation supplies (i.e. chlorhexidine scrub, sterile saline) • Sterile gloves • Analgesic/sedative drugs • Local anesthetic • Large-bore IV catheter (i.e. 14–16 gauge) or 22–20-gauge 1.5-inch needle • 5-, 10-, or 20-ml luer-lock syringe • 3-way stopcock • Fluid extension line • Collecting bucket/chamber/bowl • RTT • LTT	1. Administer analgesic/sedation drugs as needed. 2. Place the patient in lateral recumbency and shave a large area on the ventral aspect of the abdomen. 3. Administer a local anesthetic block as needed and surgically prepare the site. 4. Prepare the abdominocentesis set by attaching the luer-lock syringe to one end of the 3-way stopcock, and the fluid extension line to the other end, leaving an open end to the environment. 5. Turn the 3-way stopcock "OFF" lever toward the patient (i.e. toward the fluid extension line). 6. Insert the catheter/needle tip caudal to the umbilicus and lateral to the ventral midline. 7. Advance the catheter/needle into the peritoneal cavity slowly in 1-cm increments until fluid is seen in the catheter/needle hub. 8. Once the catheter/needle is in position, attach the fluid extension line (if using a catheter, the stylet must be removed first). 9. Aspirate the fluid by using a 3-way stopcock and syringe; open the 3-way stopcock to the environment to draw back fluid, then close it to the patient to push the fluid out to empty the syringe, repeating until the peritoneal cavity is adequately emptied. 10. Abdominocentesis may need to be repeated in all 4 quadrants.	• A sterile fluid sample should be saved in both RTT and LTT • Risks/complications include accidental laceration of internal organs

Note: Redirecting the catheter/needle dorsally or ventrally may be needed to help better direct fluid flow.

Skill Box 16.2 / Diagnostic Peritoneal Lavage

Use	Supplies	Procedure	Comments
To obtain abdominal fluid samples for evaluation	• Clippers • Surgical preparation supplies (i.e. chlorhexidine scrub, sterile saline) • Sterile gloves • Sterile fenestrated drape • Analgesic/sedative drugs • Local anesthetic • Surgical blade • Large-bore IV catheter (i.e. 14–16 gauge) • Warm sterile 0.9% NaCl 1-liter bag connected to an IV drip set • Sterile collection bowl • RTT • LTT	1. Administer analgesic/sedation drugs as needed. 2. Place the patient in lateral recumbency and shave a large area on the ventral aspect of the abdomen. 3. Administer a local anesthetic block as needed. 4. Surgically prepare the site and place the fenestrated drape so that it is centered at the umbilicus. 5. Using the surgical blade, cut fenestrations along the side of the large-bore IV catheter. 6. Insert the catheter caudal to the umbilicus on the lateral aspect of the ventral midline. 7. Gently twist the needle on insertion and advance the catheter into the peritoneal cavity slowly in 1-cm increments, gently twisting to move aside any hollow organs until fluid is seen in the catheter hub. 8. Once the catheter is in position, remove the stylet and attach the sterile saline fluid line to the catheter. 9. Using gravity, instill 10–20 ml/kg sterile saline over 3–5 minutes. 10. Gently agitate patient's abdomen to ensure movement of the sterile saline within the peritoneal cavity. 11. After several minutes, disconnect the fluid line and allow the fluid to drain via gravity into a sterile collection bowl. 12. Collect the sample fluid into RTT and LTT.	• Risks/complications include accidental laceration of internal organs

Note: Redirecting the catheter/needle dorsally or ventrally may be needed to help better direct fluid flow.

Skill Box 16.3 / Closed Suction (Jackson-Pratt™) Drain Management

Use	Supplies	Procedure	Comments
Drain care			
To allow for measurement of fluid production from the peritoneal cavity. These drains are typically placed following an abdominal surgical procedure (i.e. laparotomy)	• Exam gloves • Collection container153	1. Wear exam gloves when handling the drain bulb and tubing. 2. Examine the drain insertion site daily for signs of infection and/or inflammation (i.e. redness, swelling, bruising, bleeding, discharge). 3. To quantify drain fluid, open the bulb cap and pour the fluid into a collection container. 4. Squeeze the bulb then replace the cap to return negative pressure to the drain. 5. Record the volume of fluid in the medical record (i.e. treatment sheet). 6. Quantify the drain fluid every 4–6 hours.	• Drains are removed when fluid production has decreased to less than 2–5 ml/kg/day

(*Continued*)

Skill Box 16.3 / Closed Suction (Jackson-Pratt™) Drain Management (Continued)

Use	Supplies	Procedure	Comments
Fluid cytology collection			
To allow for cytological evaluation of peritoneal fluid	• Exam gloves • Collection container • Hemostats • Surgical preparation supplies (i.e. chlorhexidine scrub, sterile saline) • Surgical blade • Sterile 3-ml luer-lock syringe • RTT • LTT	1. While wearing gloves, empty the contents of the bulb into a collection container. 2. Clamp the drain tubing 2–3 inches away from the bulb with hemostats. 3. Surgically prepare the drain tubing in the area between the hemostat and bulb. 4. Using a sterile scalpel blade, slice the drain tubing over the surgically prepped area. 5. Attach a sterile 3-ml luer-lock syringe to the tubing line and unclamp the hemostat. 6. Draw back your fluid sample and put in LTT and RTT.	

Tip: Applying a stockinette to the patient or tying the drain tubing to the abdomen helps keep the drain secured.
Note: See Table 3.8: Fluid cytology, page 106.

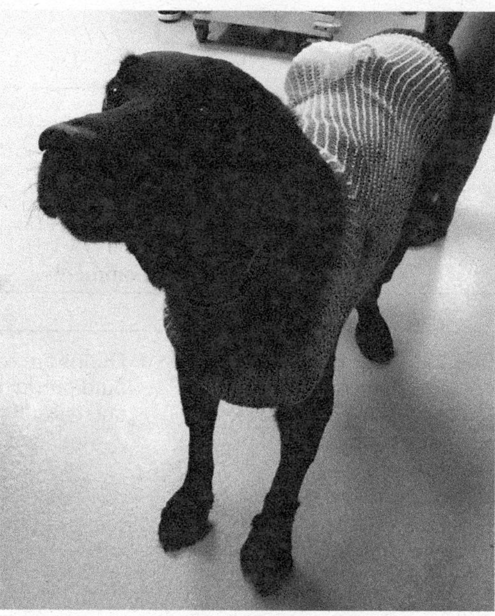

Figure 16.1 Patient with a Jackson–Pratt drain.

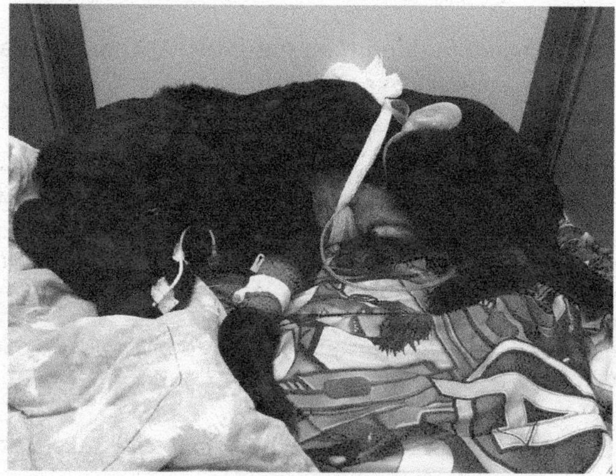

Figure 16.2 Patient with a Jackson–Pratt drain.

Skill Box 16.4 / Pericardiocentesis

Uses	Supplies	Procedure	Comments
• To remove accumulation of fluid from the pericardial sac • To stabilize a patient suffering from cardiac tamponade	• Clippers • Surgical preparation supplies (i.e. chlorhexidine scrub, sterile saline) • Sterile gloves • Analgesic/sedative drugs • Local anesthetic • Large bore IV catheter (i.e. 14–16 gauge) or 22–20-gauge 1.5″ needle • 5-, 10-, or 20-ml luer-lock syringe • 3-way stopcock • Fluid extension line • Collecting bucket/chamber/bowl • RTT • LTT • Flow-by oxygen therapy • ECG monitor	1. Administer analgesic/sedation drugs as needed. 2. Place the patient in sternal or lateral recumbency. Shave a large area on the lateral chest between the 7–9th intercostal space. 3. Administer a local anesthetic block as needed and surgically prepare the site. 4. Prepare the pericardiocentesis set by attaching the luer-lock syringe to one end of the 3-way stopcock, and the fluid extension line to the other end, leaving an open end to the environment. 5. Turn the 3-way stopcock "OFF" lever toward the patient (i.e. toward the fluid extension line). 6. Insert the catheter/needle tip between the 5th and 6th intercostal space, avoiding the intercostal arteries on the caudal aspect of each rib. 7. Advance the catheter/needle into the pericardial sac slowly in 1-cm increments until fluid is seen in the catheter/needle hub. 8. Once the catheter/needle is in position, attach the fluid extension line (if using a catheter, the stylet must be removed first). 9. Aspirate the fluid by using a 3-way stopcock and syringe; open the stopcock to the environment to draw back fluid, then close it to the patient to push the fluid out to empty the syringe, repeating until the pericardial sac is emptied.	• Flow-by oxygen should be provided to the patient during the procedure • An ECG should be used to monitor the patient during the procedure • The common ECG finding in a patient with pericardial effusion is electrical alternans, which shows different QRS complex amplitudes • A sterile fluid sample should be saved in both RTT and LTT • Risks/complications include accidental laceration of the heart wall

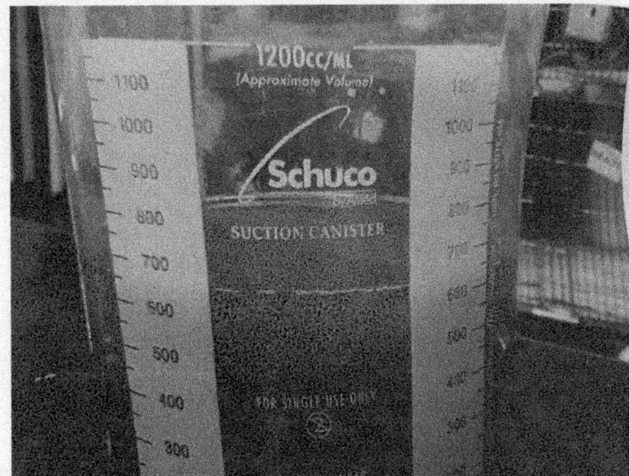

Figure 16.3 Pericardial fluid.

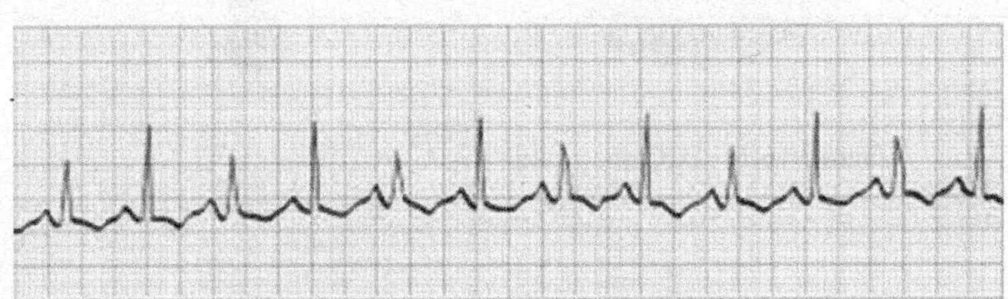

Figure 16.4 ECG showing electrical alternans.

Skill Box 16.5 / Telemetry

Uses	Supplies	Procedure	Comments
• Indicated in critically ill patients who require continuous ECG monitoring • Allows for constant assessment of a patient's heart rate and rhythm	• Clippers • ECG snap pads • ECG snap leads • Electrode gel • ECG monitor • 0.5–1″ nonporous tape • VetWrap®	1. Shave the fur on the caudodorsal aspect of the right forelimb, left forelimb, and left hindlimb just above the paw pads. 2. Apply a dime-sized amount of electrode gel to each snap lead, and stick to the dorsal aspect of the paw pad. 3. Secure each snap lead using either ½- or 1-inch nonporous tape. 4. Attached the snap ECG leads (black lead on left forelimb, white lead on right forelimb, red lead on left rear limb) to each snap pad. 5. Using VetWrap, lightly wrap each paw pad to ensure the snap lead stays attached to the snap pad.	Depending on the size of the patient, the snap pad may need to be cut along the edges to better fit on the paw pad

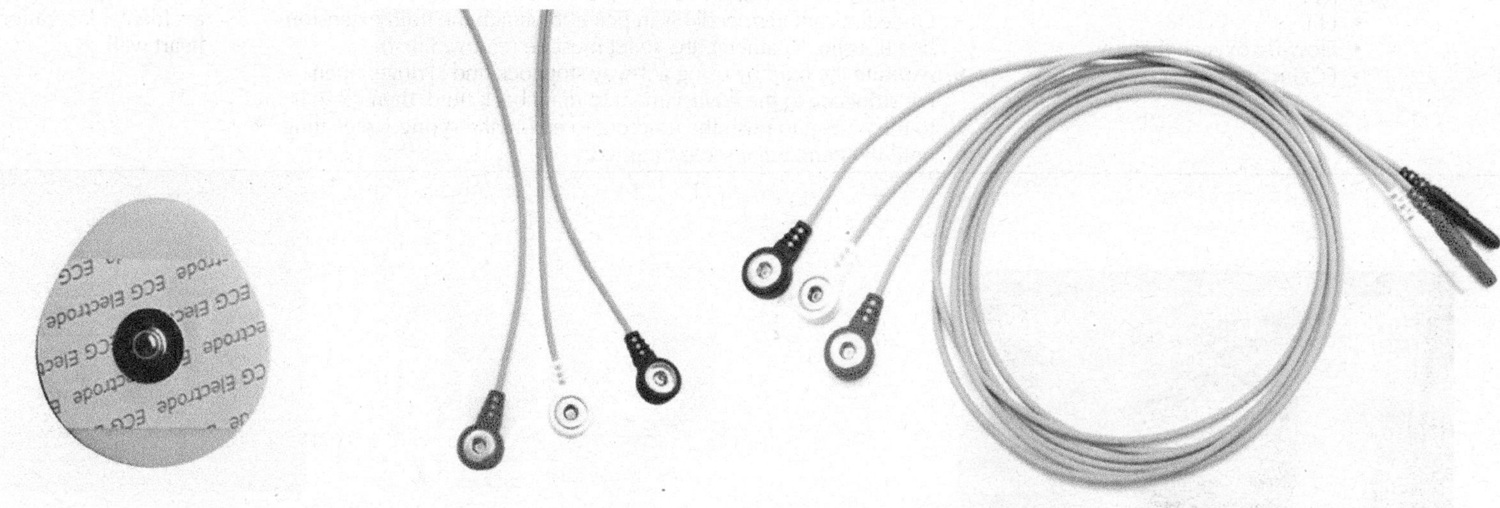

Figure 16.5 ECG snap pad.

Figure 16.6 ECG snap leads.

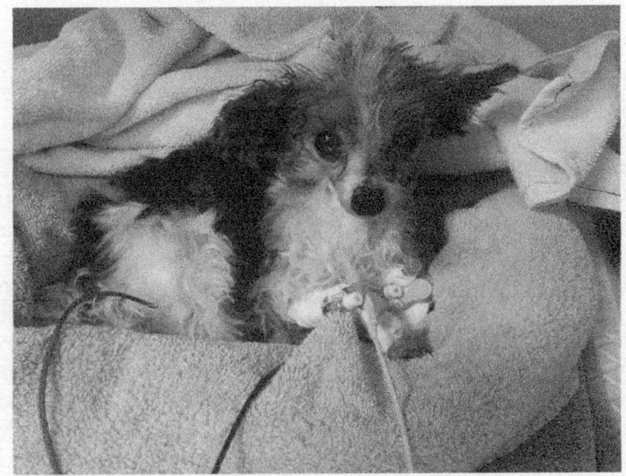

Figure 16.7 Telemetry setup.

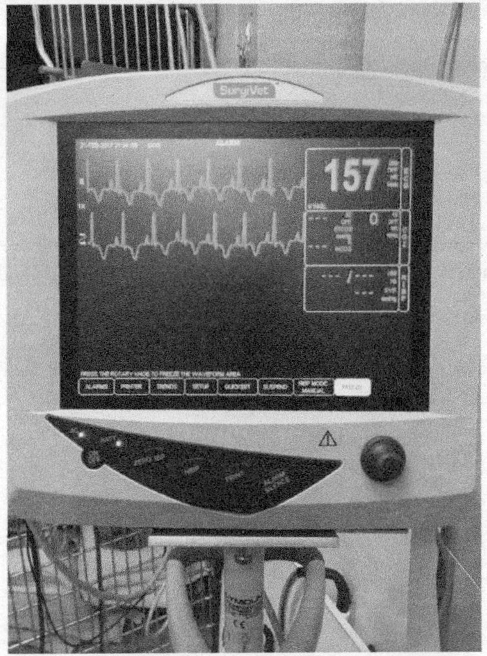

Figure 16.8 Telemetry ECG.

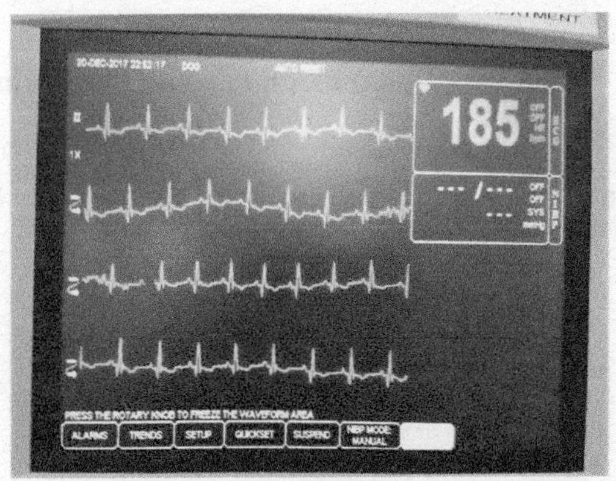

Figure 16.9 Telemetry ECG.

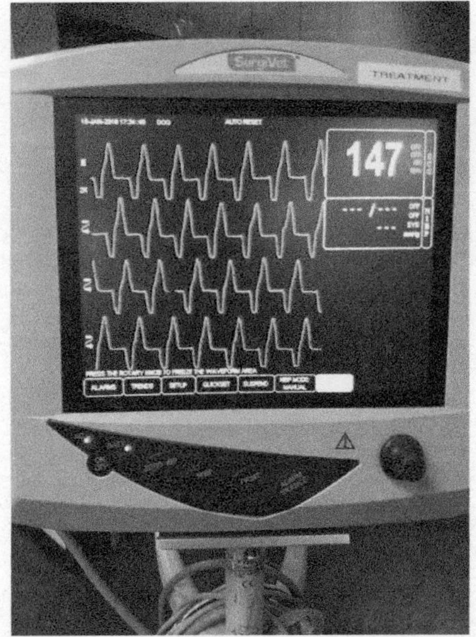

Figure 16.10 Telemetry ECG.

Skill Box 16.6 / Invasive (Direct) Blood Pressure Monitoring

Uses	Supplies	Procedure	Comments
• Indicated in critically ill patients who require continuous ECG monitoring • Provides second-by-second assessment of systolic, diastolic, mean arterial blood pressures • Gives direct insight to the cardiovascular status of the patient • Considered the "gold standard" for blood pressure monitoring	• Indwelling arterial catheter • Multiparameter monitor with DABP capability • Alcohol swab • Sterile gloves • 1 liter bag of 0.9% NaCl • 1000 U heparin • Pressure bag • Sterile pressure transducer integrated with fast flush device	1. Add heparin 1000 U to the 1-liter bag of 0.9% NaCl and appropriately label the bag. 2. Open the prepackaged pressure transducer set, turning the transducer stopcock "OFF" to the patient. 3. Insert the attached primary administration set with the roller clamp in the closed position into the fluid bag. 4. Insert the fluid bag into a pressure bag and inflate to a pressure of 300 mmHg. 5. Hang the pressurized bag in the area of the patient. 6. Once the fluid bag is connected to the pressure transducer setup and is pressurized, open the roller clamp to prime the line. It is imperative that all air is removed from the fluid line. 7. Using an alcohol swab, prepare the patient's arterial catheter port and flush the catheter to ensure patency. 8. Attach the pressure transducer/fluid bag line setup to the patient's catheter and turn on the multiparameter monitor; ensure all connections are tight. 9. Place the pressure transducer at the same level as the patient's level of the heart. 10. Turn the stopcock so that it is OFF to the patient, then press the "ZERO IBP" setting on the monitor. 11. Once the monitor reads a DABP of "0", open the stopcock so that it is OFF to the environment/air. 12. Observe the multiparameter monitor's blood pressure tracing.	• Standard dilution for the flush solution is 1 unit heparin per 1 ml saline – if otherwise directed, follow the veterinarian's orders • The pressure bag needs to be maintained at a constant pressure of 300 mmHg for the DABP reading to be accurate • The DABP setup may need to be calibrated based on patient movement and positioning. This is done by re-zeroing out the machine

Tip: Insert the pressure transducer into the tab of a food can (i.e. Hill's™ Prescription Diet™ a/d™) and secure with 1-inch non-porous tape. You can also use 1–3 cans of food (depending on the patient's size) to keep the pressure transducer at the level of the heart.

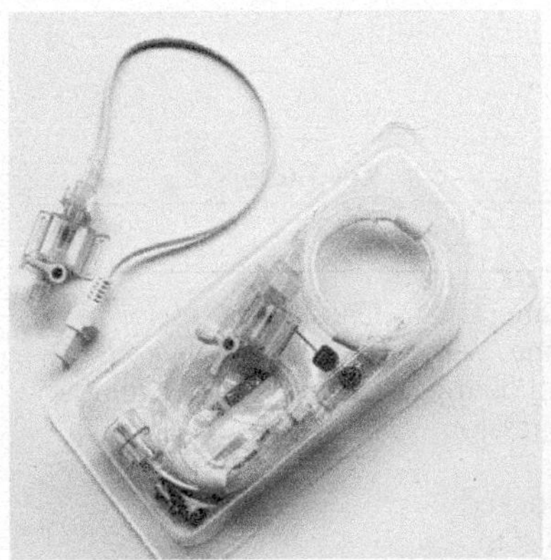

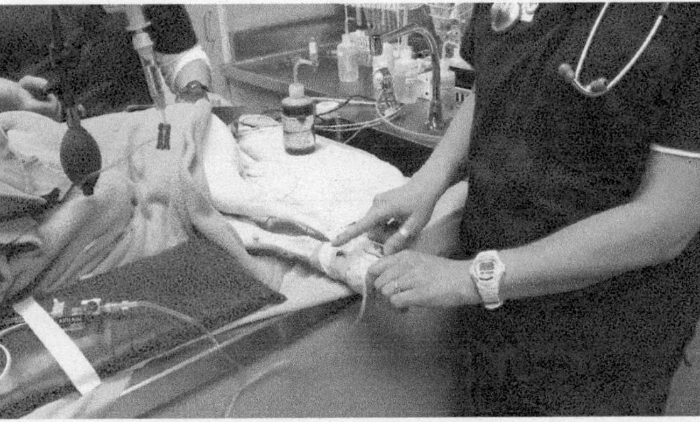

Figure 16.11 **Direct arterial blood pressure setup.**

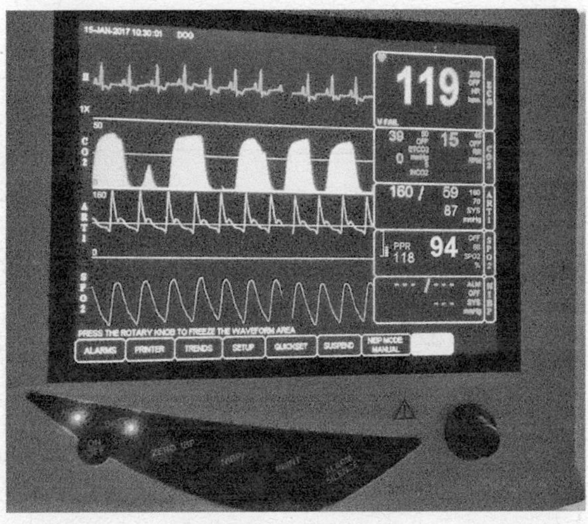

Figure 16.12 **Direct arterial blood pressure monitoring.**

Skill Box 16.7 / **Cardiopulmonary Resuscitation: Cardiac Compressions**

Uses	Indications	Technique	Posture	Key Factors
Cardiac pump theory				
To restore circulation in a patient in cardiopulmonary arrest	• Theory states that blood flow is generated from direct compression of the heart through the thoracic wall (simulates the systolic phase of a normal heartbeat) • Chest compression technique used in keel-chested dogs (i.e. Greyhound, Whippet), small dogs (weight < 7 kg), and cats	• Deliver chest compressions at a rate of 100–120 compressions/minute • Compression point is directly over the heart • Compress ½ to ⅓ the width of the chest, and allow for full chest-wall recoil	• Stand behind the patient • Place hand-over-hand, with your dominant hand on top, at the correct compression point • Keep your elbows locked and bend at the waist to drive the compression force from your core	Chest compressions should be delivered in uninterrupted 2-minute cycles

(Continued)

Skill Box 16.7 / Cardiopulmonary Resuscitation: Cardiac Compressions (Continued)

Uses	Indications	Technique	Posture	Key Factors
Thoracic pump theory				
To restore circulation in a patient that is in cardiopulmonary arrest	• Theory states that blood flow is generated from increased intrathoracic pressures during compressions (drives blood through the heart chambers) • Chest compression technique used in round-chested dogs (i.e. German Shepherd, Labrador Retriever, Golden Retriever, Rottweiler, Pit Bull) • Chest compression technique typically used in dogs weighing > 7 kg	• Deliver chest compressions at a rate of 100–120 compressions/minute • Compression point is over the highest (widest) part of the chest • Compress ½ to ⅓ the width of the chest, and allow for full chest-wall recoil	• Stand behind the patient • Place hand-over-hand, with your dominant hand on top, at the correct compression point • Keep your elbows locked and bend at the waist to drive the compression force from your core	Chest compressions should be delivered in uninterrupted 2-minute cycles

Tips:

- To perform chest compressions at a rate of 100–120 compressions/minute, sing a song such as "Stayin' Alive" by the BeeGees or "Another One Bites the Dust" by Queen in your head.
- Use a stool or stepladder if necessary to gain leverage to be above the patient.

Note: High-quality chest compressions still only produce 25–30% of normal cardiac output, so following correct compression technique, posture, and rate is essential.

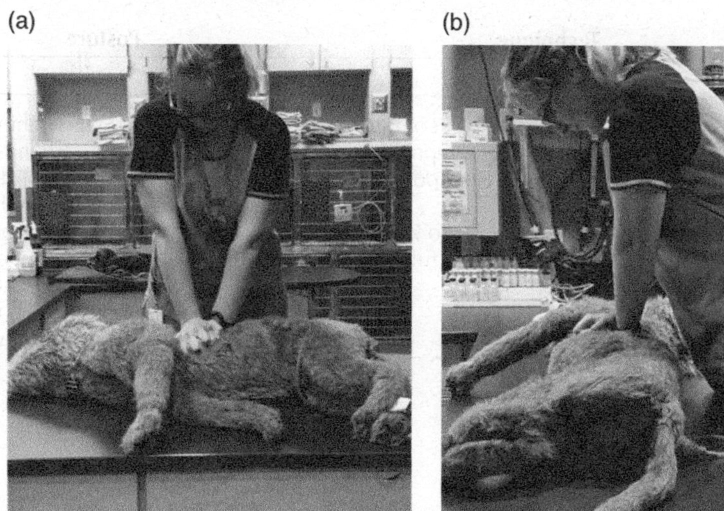

Figure 16.13 (a,b) Correct chest compression posture.

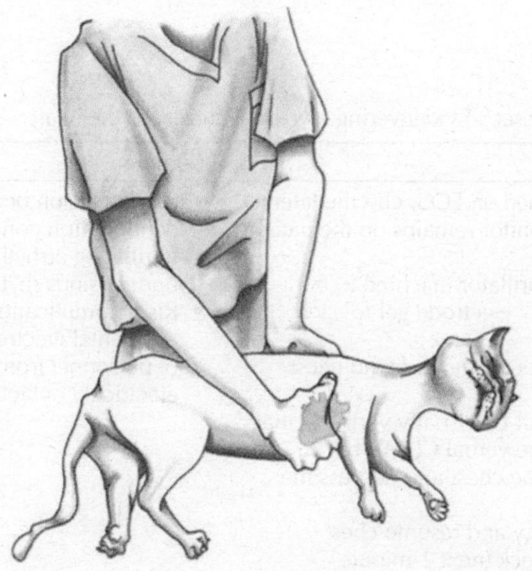

Figure 16.14 Cardiac theory compression point 1.

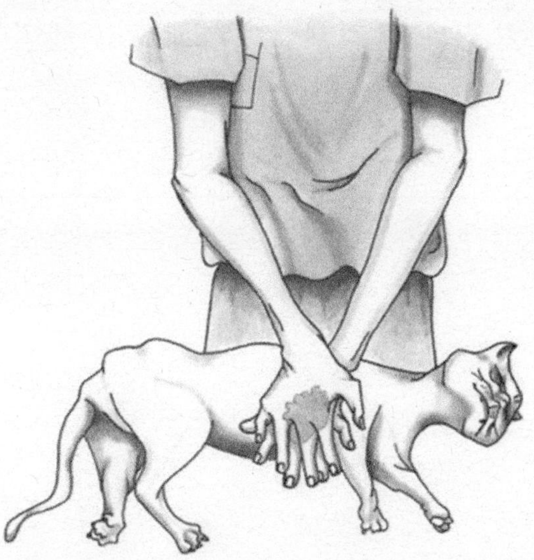

Figure 16.15 Cardiac theory compression point 2.

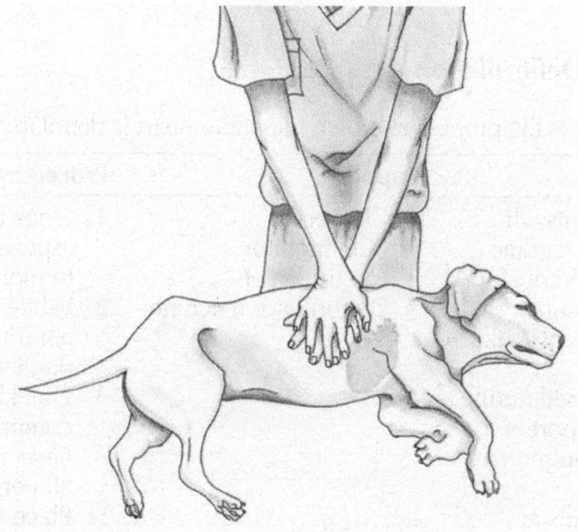

Figure 16.16 Thoracic pump theory compression point.

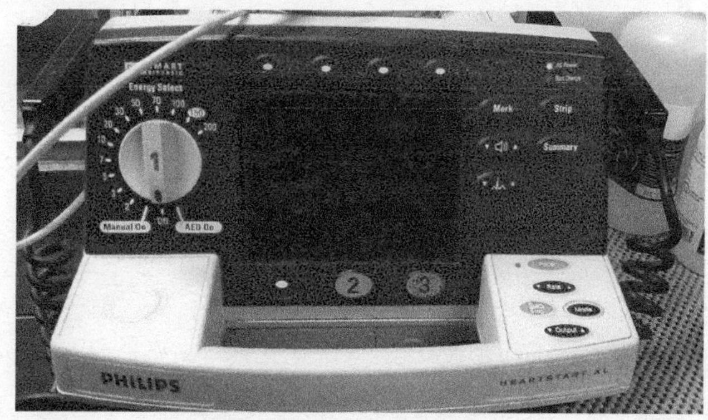

Figure 16.17 Defibrillator.

Skill Box 16.8 / Defibrillation

External defibrillation is the process in which the entire heart is depolarized simultaneously (i.e. the heart is "reset") by delivering electrical current to the heart.

Uses	Supplies	Procedure	Comments
• Indicated in patients who have a fibrillating cardiac arrhythmia (i.e. ventricular fibrillation, ventricular flutter, pulseless ventricular tachycardia) • Defibrillation is used during advanced life support of a patient in cardiopulmonary arrest • Dose typically starts at 2–5 J/kg, with the dose increasing by 50% for each defibrillation attempt	• Clippers • ECG monitor • Electrode gel • Defibrillator machine	1. Once a fibrillating rhythm has been confirmed on ECG, clip the lateral aspects of the chest. Ensure that an ECG monitor remains on the patient to monitor for cardioversion. 2. While holding the paddles, charge the defibrillator machine to the appropriate dose and have an assistant apply electrode gel to each paddle. 3. Quickly rotate the patient to dorsal recumbency and suspend chest compressions. 4. Give a verbal "CLEAR!" – confirm the CLEAR by visually verifying that all personnel are clear and have repeated the verbal CLEAR back. 5. Place the paddles on the lateral aspects of the chest and depress the buttons on the paddle. 6. Rotate the patient back to lateral recumbency and resume chest compressions until the next ECG rhythm check (next 2-minute CPR cycle).	• Cardioversion occurs when defibrillation converts the fibrillating arrhythmia back to normal sinus rhythm • Risks/complications include accidental electrocution of personnel from indirect electrical contact

Tip: Putting the patient in a trough helps to keep them in the dorsal recumbency position to perform the defibrillation procedure.
Note: Alcohol is considered flammable and should not be used as the conduction source for the defibrillator paddles.

Skill Box 16.9 / Gastrocentesis (Trocharization)

Uses	Supplies	Procedure	Comments
To remove the accumulation of air within the stomach from GDV	• Clippers • Surgical preparation supplies (i.e. chlorhexidine scrub, sterile saline) • Sterile gloves • Large-bore IV catheter (i.e. 14–16 gauge) or 22–20-gauge 1.5″ needle	1. Administer analgesic/sedation drugs as needed. 2. Place the patient in either semi-lateral recumbency, hips right side down. 3. Shave an area over the tympanic aspect of the left dorsolateral abdomen just caudal to the last rib. 4. Surgically prepare the site. 5. Don sterile gloves, and palpate for the most tympanic aspect. 6. Hold the large-bore IV catheter at a perpendicular angle to the abdominal wall and insert the catheter firmly and swiftly. 7. Remove the catheter stylet to allow the air (gas) to be expelled.	• Trocharization on the left side is preferred due to the location of the spleen • This procedure is often used as a stabilization method prior to surgical correction of GDV

Note: Once the stomach begins to decompress, you can gently push down around the catheter to help facilitate the release of gas from the stomach.

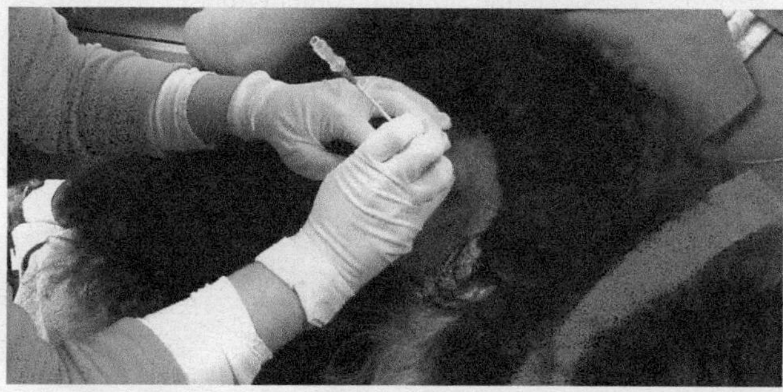

Figure 16.18 Gastrocentesis (trocarization).

Skill Box 16.10 / Orogastric Tube Passage and Gastric Lavage

Uses	Supplies	Procedure	Comments
Orogastric tube passage			
• Indicated to provide decompression of gastric dilation (i.e. GDV) • Decontamination from ingestion of toxins • Administration of medications (i.e. activated charcoal) • Perform gastric lavage	• Double lumen orogastric tube • Sterile lubricant • Roll of adhesive bandage material (i.e. VetWrap) • 1-inch non-porous tape • Collection bucket	1. Pre-measure the length of the tube from the nares to the last rib and mark the tube with 1-inch non-porous tape. 2. Place the roll of VetWrap into the patient's mouth so that the hole in the roll faces the pharynx. 3. Generously lubricate the end of the tube and, with the patient's mouth held closed, slowly advance the tube through the middle of the VetWrap roll. 4. Leave the other (distal) end of the tube at a level below the patient, terminating within a collection bucket.	• To remove the tube, you need to firmly kink the tubing and in the kinked position, slowly remove the tube – this is done to minimize potential fluid leakage into the airway
Gastric lavage			
• Decontamination from ingestion of toxins (i.e. large volume ingested, caustic toxin, when emesis is contraindicated) • Administration of medications (i.e. activated charcoal)	• Confirmed placement of orogastric tube • Collection bucket • Warm to room-temperature water • Sump pump	1. Fill the collection bucket with warm to room-temperature water. 2. Connect the second (ancillary) lumen of the orogastric tube to the sump pump. 3. Holding the sump pump in the water bucket, pump the lever up and down to instill 10–30 ml/kg of water into the stomach. 4. Let the stomach content fluid to passively drain. 5. Repeat the cycle of instilling water and allowing passive drainage as needed to completed lavage and empty the stomach contents.	• Following gastric lavage, medications such as activated charcoal can be administered via the orogastric tube • To remove the tube, you need to firmly kink the tubing and in the kinked position, slowly remove the tube – this is done to minimize potential fluid leakage into the airway

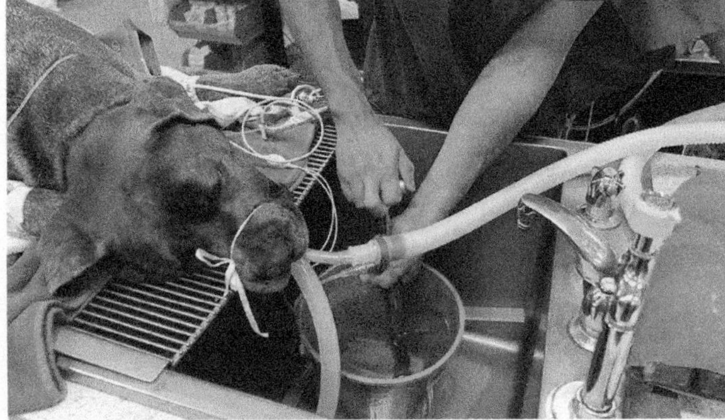

Figure 16.19 Gastric lavage.

Skill Box 16.11 / Nasoesophageal Tube Placement and Care

Uses	Supplies	Procedure	Comments
Tube placement			
• Minimally invasive means to provide enteral nutrition (bolus feeding or CRI) • Ideal for relatively short-term (3–14 days) feeding	• Topical anesthetic solution (i.e. proparacaine) • Feeding tube • Sterile lubricant • 1-inch non-porous tape • Marker pen • 2-0 or 3-0 non-absorbable suture • Needle holders	1. Instill 2–3 drops of a topical anesthetic into both nares, keeping the head elevated for a few minutes to allow for the local anesthetic to drain into the nasal passages. 2. Premeasure from the tip of the nose to the 7–8th rib (tube will terminate is the distal esophagus before reaching the cardiac sphincter) and mark the "exit" point with temporary piece of tape. 3. Gently hold the patient's muzzle with your non-dominant hand and press the nasal septum upward using your thumb (this diverts the nares dorsally to ease passing of the tube). 4. Lightly lubricate the tip and pass the tube, directing it ventromedially through the nasal cavity and advancing it to the premeasured piece of tape. 5. Remove the temporary piece of tape and mark the exit point with a marker pen. 6. Secure the tube using 2-0 or 3-0 non-absorbable suture in a finger-trap pattern.	• Typical nasoesophageal feeding tube sizes range from 5 to 12 Fr. • Some feeding tube brands are premarked with centimeter measurements • The patient should wear an Elizabethan collar while in hospital • Contraindications include patients who are actively vomiting, have no gag reflex, head trauma, nasal disease, or are comatose
Tube placement confirmation			
• Required prior to use of nasoesophageal tube	• 5- and 10-ml empty syringe • 5–10 ml sterile saline • Radiology	1. Aspirate the tube. If air is aspirated, the tube is in the trachea, if negative pressure is found, the tube is in the esophagus. 2. Instill 5–10 ml sterile saline into the tube. If the patient coughs, you are likely in the trachea. 3. Rapidly instill 5–10 ml air into the tube while auscultating where the tip of the tube should be. If you hear borborygmus, you are likely in the esophagus/gastrointestinal tract. 4. Obtain a right lateral radiograph to confirm placement; both cranial and caudal views should be taken to ensure that the tube enters the esophagus and has no dependent loops. 5. Tube placement should be confirmed by the attending veterinarian prior to use.	• Information regarding nasoesophageal tube placement is part of the medical record and must be appropriately documented
Tube care			
• Indicated for patients with indwelling nasoesophageal tubes	• Exam gloves • Room-temperature water	1. During each patient interaction, inspect the tube for kinks and ensure that the tube exit point mark is in place. 2. The tube should be flushed with room temperature water before and after administering medications and/or enteral nutrition to maintain patency. 3. If the tube becomes clogged, you can troubleshoot by either passing a stylet or instilling 3–5 ml of cola, or any type of soda (the acid in the soda unclogs the tube).	• If there is ever doubt about the placement of the tube (i.e. termination point), retake a lateral radiograph

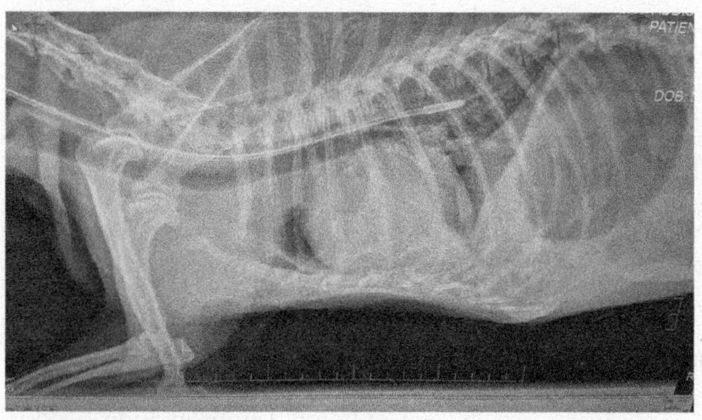

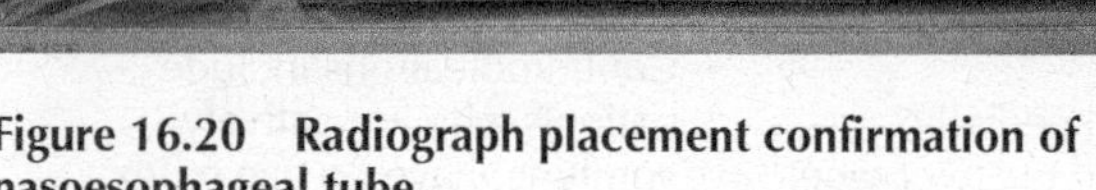

Figure 16.20 Radiograph placement confirmation of nasoesophageal tube.

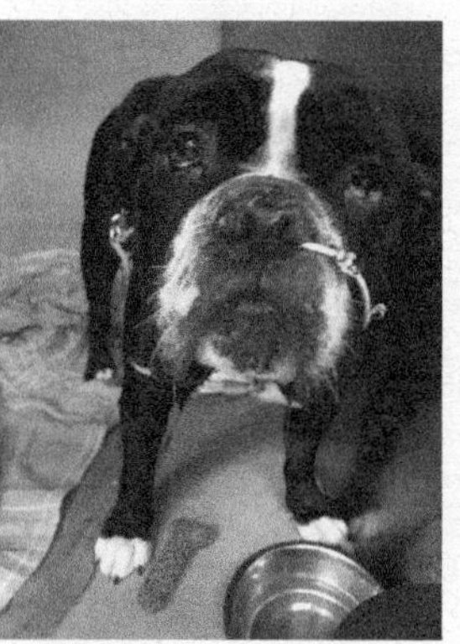

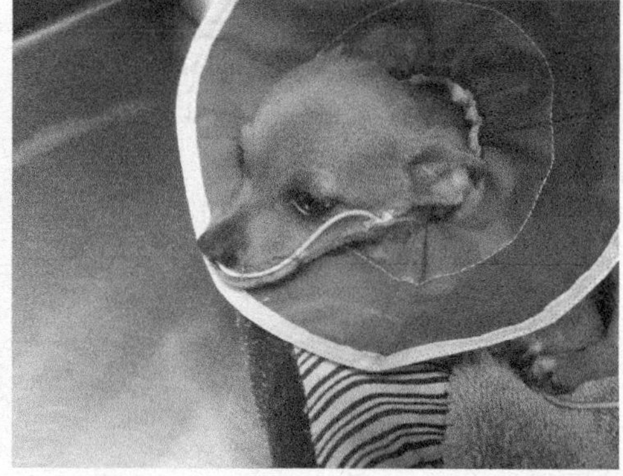

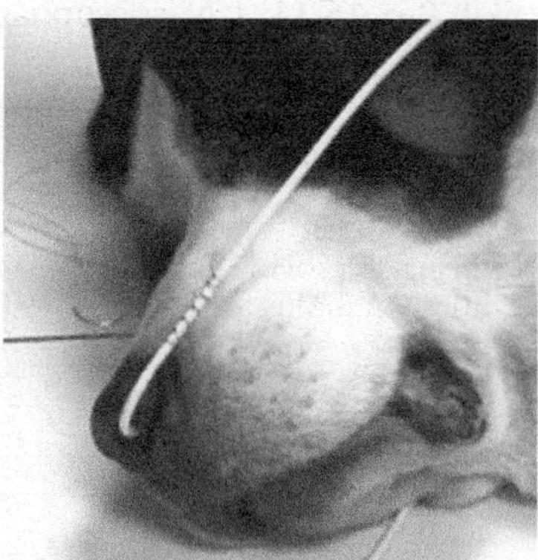

Figure 16.21 Patient with a nasoesophageal tube.

NASAL FEEDING TUBE PLACEMENT CHECKLIST			
Pre Placement (credentialed technician & assistant)	Placement (credentialed technician)	Post Placement (credentia led technician & DVM)	Documentation (credentialed technician)
Feeding tube guidelines have been reviewed? ❑ Yes Initials _____Initials _____	❑ Instill 2-3 drops of Proparacaine into each nostril, then gently tip the patient's nose upward Initials _____ Initials _____	❑ Aspirate the tube ❑ Instill sterile saline into the tube ❑ Rapidly instill air into the tube ❑ Obtain a right lateral radiograph ❑ Attending DVM interprets the radiograph to confirm placement ❑ Secure the tube using 2-0 to 3-0 suture in a finger-trap pattern	❑ Date & time ❑ Size & length of tube (i.e. 8Fr. x 42cm) ❑ Nostril it exits ❑ cm or Sharpie® mark where tube exits ❑ Type of suture used ❑ DVM who confirmed placement
Has the patient had a physical exam prior to tube placement? ❑ Yes Initials _____Initials _____	❑ Lubricate the tip of the tube with sterile lubricant Initials _____ Initials _____		
Sedation protocol (provided by DVM)? ❑ Yes Drug, dose (mg), route: _______________ (i.e. butorphanol 2mg IV) Level of consciousness: _______________ Gag reflex: _______________	Nasoesophageal: ❑ Measure from the tip of nose to 7-8th intercostal space ❑ Xyphoid process is another landmark ❑ Mark the tube with a temporary piece of tape		
Location for tube placement ❑ Radiology ❑ Treatment room Initials_____ Initials_____	Nasogastric: ❑ Measure from tip of nose to the last rib ❑ Mark the tube with a temporary piece of tape		
Supplies ready: ❑ Topical anesthetic (Proparacaine) ❑ Tube ❑ Sterile lubricant ❑ 1″ nonporous tape ❑ Sharpie® marker ❑ 2-0 or 3-0 non-absorbable suture ❑ Needle holders	Placement: ❑ Pass the tube while remaining ventral & medial ❑ Gently lift the nose up, similar to a pig nose, in order to promote tube passage ❑ Gently manipulate the head & neck, sometimes upward, to encourage passage into the esophagus ❑ Patient swallowing is a good sign ❑ Pass the tube to the pre-determined mark		

Figure 16.22 Nasal feeding tube checklist.

Skill Box 16.12 / Nasogastric Tube Placement and Care

Uses	Supplies	Procedure	Comments
Tube placement			
• Minimally invasive means to provide enteral nutrition (bolus feeding or CRI) • Ideal for relatively short-term (3–14 days) feeding	• Topical anesthetic solution (i.e. proparacaine) • Sterile lubricant • Feeding tube • 1-inch non-porous tape • Marker pen • 2-0 or 3-0 non-absorbable suture • Needle holders	1. Instill 2–3 drops of a topical anesthetic into both nares, keeping the head elevated for a few minutes to allow for the local anesthetic to drain into the nasal passages. 2. Premeasure from the tip of the nose to the 7–8th rib (tube will terminate in the stomach) and mark the "exit" point with temporary piece of tape. 3. Gently hold the patient's muzzle with your non-dominant hand and press the nasal septum upward using your thumb (this diverts the nares dorsally to ease passing of the tube). 4. Lightly lubricate the tip and pass the tube, directing it ventromedially through the nasal cavity and advancing it to the premeasured piece of tape. 5. Remove the temporary piece of tape and mark the exit point with a marker pen. 6. Secure the tube using 2-0 or 3-0 non-absorbable suture in a finger-trap pattern.	• Typical nasogastric feeding tube sizes range from 5 to 12 Fr. • Some feeding tube brands are premarked with centimeter measurements • The patient should wear an Elizabethan collar while in hospital • Contraindications include patients who are actively vomiting, have no gag reflex, head trauma, nasal disease, or are comatose
Tube placement confirmation			
• Required prior to use of nasogastric tube	• 5- and 10-ml empty syringe • 5–10 ml sterile saline • Radiology	1. Aspirate the tube. If air is aspirated, the tube is in the trachea, if negative pressure is found, the tube is in the esophagus. 2. Instill 5–10 ml sterile saline into the tube. If the patient coughs, you are likely in the trachea. 3. Rapidly instill 5–10 ml air into the tube while auscultating where the tip of the tube should be. If you hear borborygmus, you are likely in the stomach/gastrointestinal tract. 4. Obtain a right lateral radiograph to confirm placement; both cranial and caudal views should be taken to ensure that the tube enters the esophagus and has no dependent loops. 5. Tube placement should be confirmed by the attending veterinarian prior to use.	• Information regarding nasogastric tube placement is part of the medical record and must be appropriately documented
Tube care			
• Indicated for patients with indwelling nasogastric tubes	• Exam gloves • Room-temperature water	1. During each patient interaction, inspect the tube for kinks and ensure that the tube exit point mark is in place. 2. The tube should be flushed with room-temperature water before and after administering medications and/or enteral nutrition to maintain patency. 3. If the tube becomes clogged, you can troubleshoot by either passing a stylet or instilling 3–5 ml of cola.	• If there is ever doubt about the placement of the tube (i.e. termination point), retake a lateral radiograph

Note: nasogastric tubes are advantageous over nasoesophageal tubes in that they allow for aspiration of gastric residual volume, which is helpful in patients with gastrointestinal motility disorders.
See also Chinese finger trap – Skill Box 23.6: Suture patterns, page 1073.

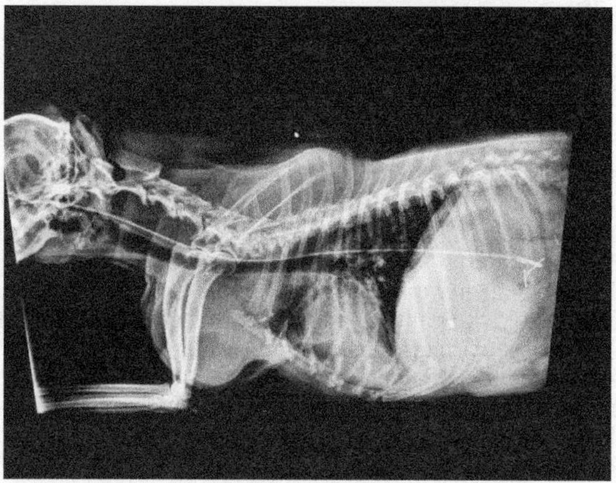

Figure 16.23 Radiograph placement confirmation of nasogastric tube.

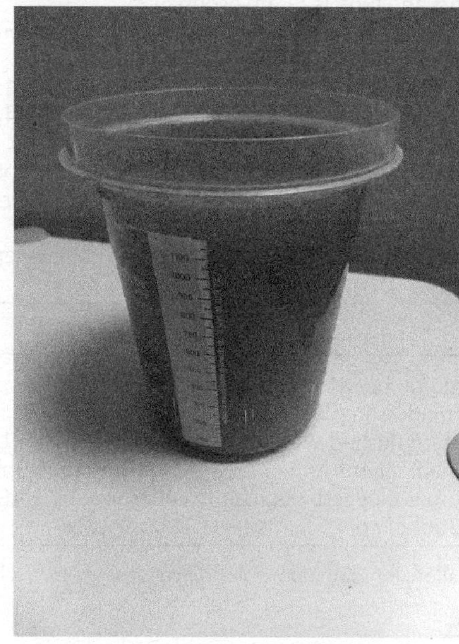

Figure 16.24 Gastric residual volume from a patient with a nasogastric tube.

Skill Box 16.13 / Esophagostomy Tube Placement and Care

Uses	Supplies	Procedure	Comments
Tube placement			
• Moderately invasive means to provide enteral nutrition (bolus feeding) • Ideal for relatively longer-term (weeks to months) feeding	• 8–20 Fr tube • Surgical preparation supplies (i.e. chlorhexidine scrub, sterile saline) • Surgical blade • Carmalt forceps • Marker pen • 0 to 2-0 non-absorbable suture • X-mas tree adapter • Injection cap • Bandage materials	1. Anesthetize and endotracheally intubate the patient. 2. Position the patient in right lateral recumbency. 3. Shave a moderate area around the left lateral neck, and surgically prepare the site. 4. Premeasure the E-tube from the neck to the 8–9th intercostal space and mark with a marker pen. 5. Insert the Carmalt forceps (locked closed) into the esophagus until the midpoint of the cervical neck, then push outwardly to "tent" the skin. 6. Using a surgical blade, make an incision through the skin/subcutaneous tissues at the tented point of the so that the Carmalt forceps tip can push through. 7. Open-hinge the Carmalt forceps and grasp the tip of the E-tube and pull through the skin, rostrally out through the mouth. 8. Release the Carmalt forceps and use them to redirect the E-tube caudally into the esophagus. 9. Once redirected, advance the E-tube down the esophagus to the point of the pen mark. 10. Take a right lateral radiograph to confirm placement of the E-tube (the tube should terminate in the distal esophagus). 11. Secure using 0 to 2-0 non-absorbable suture in a finger-trap pattern around the base of the E-tube entry site (stoma site). 12. Insert a X-mas tree adapter fitted with an injection cap into the open end of the E-tube.	• E-tubes allow for greater diet selection • E-tubes permit at-home feeding by pet owners
Tube care			
• Indicated for patients with indwelling nasoesophageal tubes	• Exam gloves • Dilute chlorhexidine • Bandage materials	1. During each patient interaction, inspect the tube insertion site for signs of mal-positioning and/or infection/inflammation. 2. The stoma site should be kept clean, dry, and covered with a non-absorbent pad (i.e. Telfa™). 3. The stoma site should be inspected daily for swelling, heat, or discharge. 4. The stoma site can be cleaned with dilute chlorhexidine solution and then thoroughly dried with gauze. 5. Place a non-absorbent pad wrapped in a light bandage (i.e. cast padding and VetWrap, Kitty Kollar®) to help better secure the tube.	

See also Chinese finger trap – Skill Box 23.6: Suture patterns, page 1073.

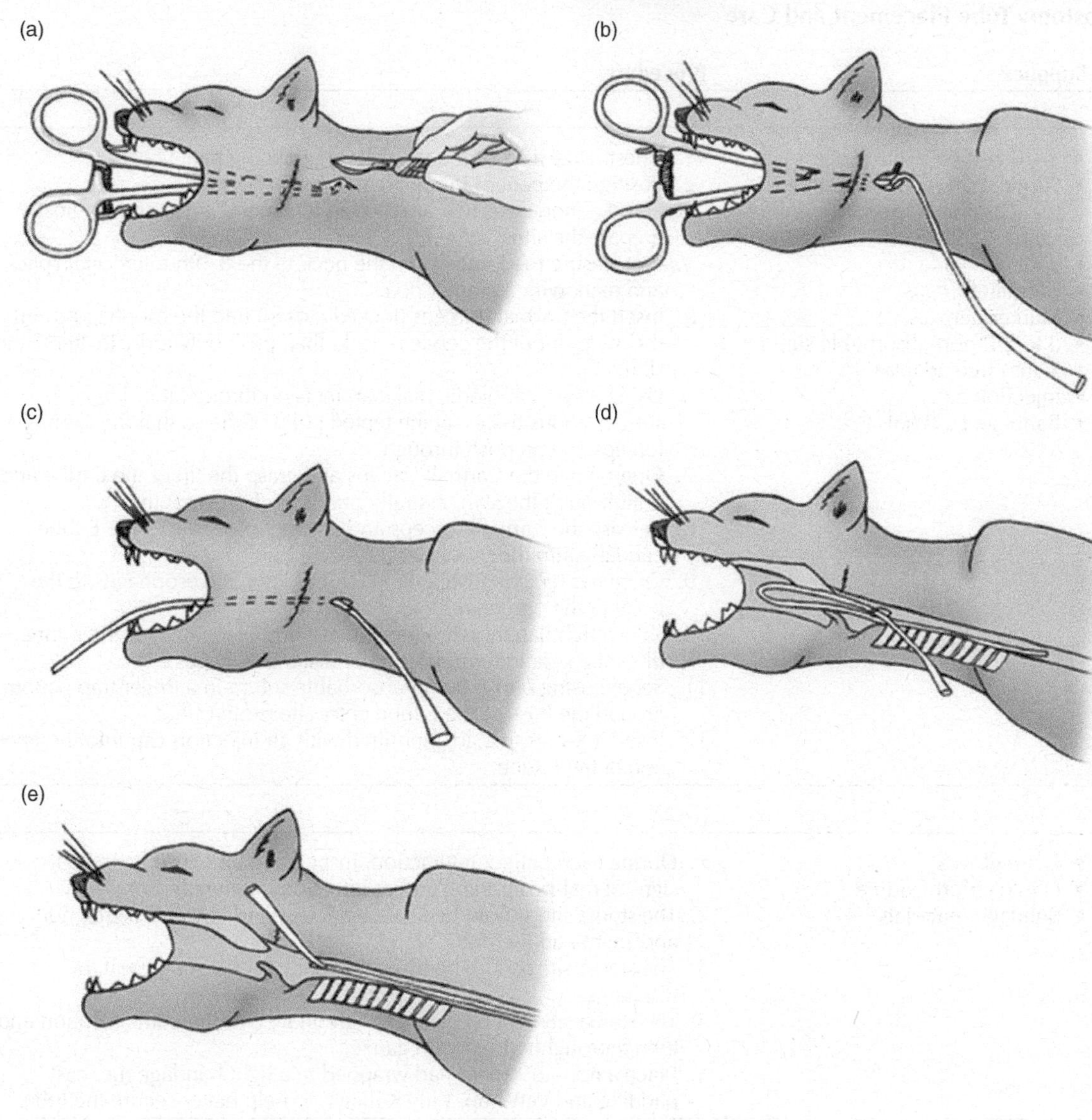

Figure 16.25 Esophagostomy tube placement.

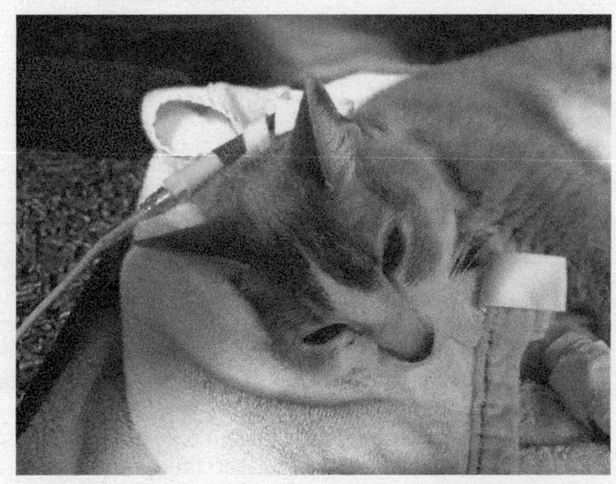

Figure 16.26 Esophagostomy tube feeding.

Skill Box 16.14 / Colonic Enema

Uses	Supplies	Procedure	Comments
• Indicated in constipated patients • Can be used as a decontamination technique to eliminate toxins from the lower gastrointestinal tract	• 12–14 Fr red rubber catheter • Sterile lubricant • Warm water • Dawn® dish soap and/or Pet-Ema™ • Bowl • Catheter tip syringe • Diaper pads	1. Place the animal in sternal or lateral recumbency. 2. Mix warm water and lubricant (± Dawn dish soap) in a bowl. 3. Draw up the dose of enema solution using a catheter tipped syringe and attach to the red rubber catheter (if using a luer-lock syringe, cut the end of the red rubber catheter until it will fit firmly on the luer-lock). 4. Lubricate the tip of the red rubber catheter and gently insert into the rectum to the level of the transcending colon (mid-abdomen). 5. Instill the enema solution at a moderate pace to irrigate the colon and expel colon remnants. 6. Once complete, kink the red rubber catheter and remove from the rectum.	• Colonic enemas are typically administered every 8–12 hours

NEUROLOGICAL PROCEDURES

Skill Box 16.15 / Cerebrospinal Fluid Collection

Uses	Supplies	Procedure	Comments
Cisternal collection			
• Part of the diagnostic evaluation of a patient with CNS disease	• General anesthesia • Surgical preparation supplies (i.e. chlorhexidine scrub, sterile saline) • Sterile surgical supplies (i.e. gloves, drapes) • 1.5–3 inch spinal needle • 3-ml luer-lock syringe • LTT (EDTA)	1. With the patient endotracheally intubated and under general anesthesia, position them in lateral recumbency (right lateral if veterinarian is right-handed, left lateral if left-handed). 2. Shave the area behind the neck between the ears and from about 2 cm rostral to the occipital protuberance to C2. 3. Arrange the patient's neck in a flexed position so that the median axis of the head is perpendicular to the spine. 4. The patient's nose should be slightly elevated so that the midline is parallel to the table surface. Surgically prepare the site. 5. The veterinarian will insert the spinal needle perpendicular to the spine.	• Once a CSF sample is collected, it should be placed in a LTT for analysis – the CSF fluid must be stored for a minimum of 1 hour prior to analysis
Lumbar collection			
• Part of the diagnostic evaluation of a patient with CNS disease	• General anesthesia • Surgical preparation supplies (i.e. chlorhexidine scrub, sterile saline) • Sterile surgical supplies (i.e. gloves, drapes) • Towel/foam cushions • 3.5-inch spinal needle • 3-ml luer-lock syringe • LTT (EDTA)	1. With the patient endotracheally intubated and under general anesthesia, position them in lateral recumbency with their trunk flexed. 2. Place towel/foam cushions between the limb and lumbar region so allow for a true lateral positioning. 3. Shave the area along the lumbar spine between L4–L7 intervertebral spaces. 4. Surgically prepare the site. The veterinarian will insert the spinal needle perpendicular to the spine.	• Once a CSF sample is collected, it should be placed in a LTT for analysis – the CSF fluid must be stored for a minimum of 1 hour prior to analysis

Notes:

- CSF collection is contraindicated in patients with risk of anesthesia, coagulopathy, or suspected increased intracranial pressure (i.e. head trauma, traumatic brain injury).

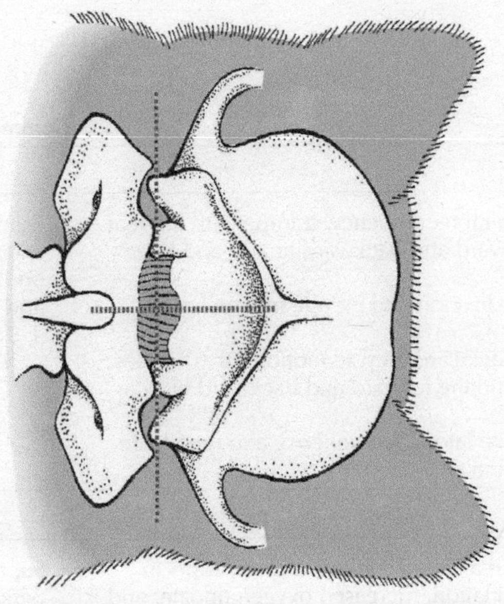

Figure 16.27 Cistern cerebrospinal fluid collection.

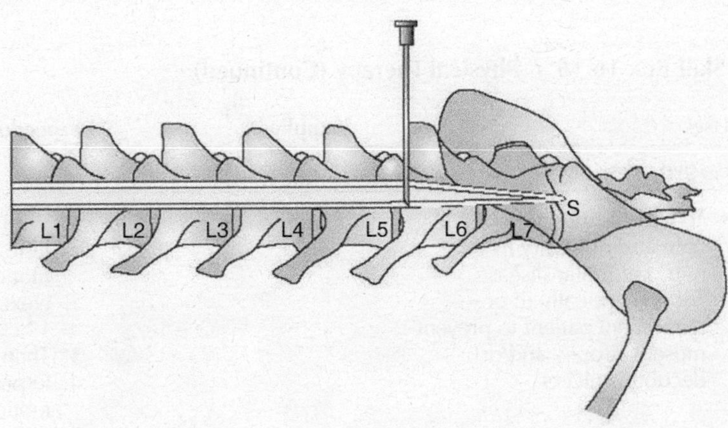

Figure 16.28 Lumbar cerebrospinal fluid collection.

Skill Box 16.16 / Physical Therapy

Uses	Supplies	Procedure	Comments
Soft-tissue mobilization			
• To address musculoskeletal pain and disability from neuromuscular disease • Manual manipulation of superficial and deep soft tissue layers with the goal of normalizing tissue function	None	1. Apply mild to moderate pressure in a massage-like motion along the major muscle groups of the rear limbs and fore limbs. 2. Perform limb massage on each affected limb for 5–10 minutes. 3. Following massage, gently flex and extend each limb at each joint point.	• Tissues addressed include muscle, tendon, ligament, and fascia. • Soft-tissue mobilization should be included on the patient's treatment sheet and should be performed every 4–8 hours

(Continued)

Skill Box 16.16 / Physical Therapy (Continued)

Uses	Supplies	Procedure	Comments
Passive range of motion			
• To address musculoskeletal pain and disability from neuromuscular disease • For any critically ill or recumbent patient to prevent muscle atrophy and/or decubitus ulcers	**None**	1. With the patient in left/right lateral recumbency, starting with the rear limb, gently move the limb forward and backward in a to-and-fro motion for 20 cycles. 2. Next, gently move the rear limb in a forward bicycle motion for 10 cycles. 3. Then move the rear limb in a backward bicycle motion for 10 cycles. 4. Repeat the to-and-fro motion and the forward and backward bicycle motion on the forelimb. 5. Rotate the patient to the opposite lateral recumbency and repeat the exercises on the rear and fore limbs.	• Passive range of motion exercises should be included on the patient's treatment sheet and should be performed every 4–8 hours.
Thermotherapy – heat			
• Application of heat for the purpose of changing soft tissue core temperature • Adjunctive treatment for musculoskeletal and soft tissue injuries in correlation with neuromuscular disease • Subacute and chronic traumatic and inflammatory conditions • Decreased range of motion • Pain relief	• Hot packs • Heat wraps • Whirlpools • Circulating warm water blankets	1. Increasing the temperature of an affected soft-tissue area results in increased blood via from vasodilation, increased oxygen update, and accelerated tissue healing. 2. Apply gentle pressure to the affected soft tissue area using your designated superficial heating device for a prescribed period of time (i.e. 10–15 minutes).	• Superficial heating agents penetrate up to approximately 2 cm of muscle/tissue depth
Thermotherapy – cold			
• Application of cold for the purpose of changing soft tissue core temperature • Adjunctive treatment for musculoskeletal and soft tissue injuries in correlation with neuromuscular disease • Minimize post-surgical swelling • Reduce pain and inflammation	• Cold packs • Ice massage • Cold water baths	1. Decreasing the temperature of an affected soft tissue area results in decreased blood flow via vasoconstriction, decreased tissue metabolism, decreased neuronal excitability, decreased tissue extensibility. 2. Apply gentle pressure to the affected soft tissue area using your designated superficial cooling device for a prescribed period of time (i.e. 10–15 minutes).	• Cold therapy mitigates the negative effects of inflammatory processes

Skill Box 16.17 / Laser therapy

Uses	Supplies	Procedure	Comments
• To address musculoskeletal pain and disability from neuromuscular disease • The application of light to modify a biologic process • To stimulate favorable tissue effects, such as enhanced wound healing and modulation of pain	• Laser therapy machine • Human safety goggles (laser specific) • Pet safety goggles (laser specific)	1. The laser probe should always be perpendicular to the target tissue area. 2. If using a low-level laser (laser that generates low heat), a point-to-point technique should be used: place the laser probe in direct contact with the patient's skin over the target tissue area and move in a point-to-point motion. 3. If using a high-level laser (laser that generates high heat), a scanning technique should be used: scan the laser over the target tissue area without being in direct contact with the patient's skin	• Laser therapy can affect all stages of wound healing (inflammation, proliferation, maturation). • Lasers have the ability to reflect if it comes into contact with metal, so the ideal location for laser therapy is on ground with the patient in a comfortable bed • Performing laser therapy is contraindicated for use over tumors (over areas with potential neoplastic cells), over the eye, over open growth plates, or over a pregnant uterus

Skill Box 16.18 / Bone marrow collection

Uses	Supplies	Procedure	Comments
Aspirate			
• Evaluates cell types and quantity • Estimates iron stores • Assess neoplastic conditions with bone marrow involvement • Identifies infectious agents	• Surgical preparation supplies (i.e. chlorhexidine scrub, sterile saline) • Sterile surgical supplies (i.e. gloves, drapes) • Analgesic/anesthetic drugs • Scalpel blade, no. 11 • Size 6-, 12-, or 20-ml syringe • Clean microscope slides • Hematocrit tubes • 10–20-ml syringe with 2–3% EDTA/isotonic fluid solution • Rosenthal or Illinois bone-marrow aspiration needle	1. Administer analgesic/sedation drugs as needed. 2. Place the patient in sternal or lateral recumbency. 3. Prepare the surgical site and block with a local anesthetic. 4. Make a stab incision with a no. 11 scalpel blade. 5. Position the needle on the periosteum and then gently, with a twisting motion, push into the marrow cavity. 6. Once the needle is positioned, remove the cap and stylet of the needle and attach a syringe with 0.5 ml of EDTA/isotonic solution. 7. Apply negative pressure. 8. Release pressure when bone marrow is visualized in the syringe. 9. Remove the syringe and make slides using smear techniques.	• Excessive negative pressure can contaminate the sample with peripheral blood • Monitor for hemorrhage or discomfort at the aspiration site.

(*Continued*)

ONCOLOGICAL PROCEDURES

Skill Box 16.18 Bone marrow collection (Continued)

Uses	Supplies	Procedure	Comments
Biopsy			
• Suspected bone marrow abnormalities (i.e. aplastic anemia, non-regenerative anemia, myelodysplasia, myelofibrosis)	• Surgical preparation supplies (i.e. chlorhexidine scrub, sterile saline) • Sterile surgical supplies (i.e. gloves, drapes) • Analgesic/anesthetic drugs • Scalpel blade, no. 11 • Size 6-, 12-, or 20-ml syringe • Jar containing 10% formalin • Jamshidi infant needle or pediatric bone-marrow biopsy needle	1. Administer analgesic/sedation drugs as needed. 2. Place the patient in sternal or lateral recumbency. 3. Administer a local anesthetic block as needed and surgically prepare the site. 4. Make a stab incision with a no. 11 scalpel blade. 5. Position the needle on the periosteum and then gently, with a twisting motion, push into the marrow cavity. 6. Once the needle is positioned, remove the stylet and advance the needle into the bone marrow to retrieve a core bone marrow sample. 7. Attach a syringe, apply negative pressure, and remove the instrument. 8. Remove the core sample and place in formalin jar.	• Monitor for hemorrhage or discomfort at the biopsy site

Tip: injecting 0.35 ml isotonic solution into a 7-ml EDTA blood collection tube produces a 0.42 ml of 2.5% EDTA/isotonic fluid solution.

Notes:

- The flat bones and extremities of long bones in adults and all long and flat bones of young animals have the greatest areas of hematopoiesis. Potential sites are the dorsal iliac crest, the femoral or humeral shaft, and the costochondral junction. Typically, a quality sample from any site will be representative to the overall bone marrow health.

OPHTHALMIC PROCEDURES

Skill Box 16.19 / Schirmer's Tear Test

Uses	Supplies	Procedure	Comments
Assessment of normal (> 15 mm) tear production	**Two Schirmer tear strips**	1. Place the notched end of the tear strip in the lower eyelid in the palpebral fissure (medial aspect of the eye). 2. Bend the tear strip so that the notched end remains within the eyelid. 3. Gently close the eyelids and hold them closed for 1 minute. 4. Remove the strip and record according to where the blue line is marked.	• When performing ophthalmic diagnostic tests (i.e. fluorescein stain, tonometry), the Schirmer tear test should be performed first, as instilling topical ophthalmic anesthetic solution (i.e. proparacaine), which is needed for the other tests, will skew the results • Results can be affected by discharge, inflammation, or corneal disease (i.e. ulceration)

Skill Box 16.20 / Fluorescein Stain

Uses	Supplies	Procedure	Comments
• Evaluation of the cornea for defects (i.e. abrasions, scratches, ulceration)	• Topical anesthetic solution (i.e. proparacaine) • Fluorescein stain strips • Empty 3-ml syringe with needle • Bag of sterile saline • Eyewash solution • 3 × 3 or 4 × 4 gauze squares • Ophthalmoscope with blue light attachment	1. Gently instill 2–3 drops of topical anesthetic solution into each eye. 2. Remove the plunger from the empty 3-ml syringe and carefully peel open the stain strip package into the syringe. 3. Replace the syringe plunger, then draw up 2–3 ml sterile saline. 4. Remove the needle from the syringe and gently instill 2–3 drops of the fluorescein stained saline into each eye. 5. Rinse each eye with sterile saline or eyewash solution. 6. Examine the eye with blue light ophthalmoscope observing for green stain, indicating a break in the corneal epithelium.	• It may be helpful to move the patient into a darkened room (i.e. radiology) to evaluate the eyes for fluorescein stain uptake

Skill Box 16.21 / Tonometry

Uses	Supplies	Procedure	Comments
• Assessment of IOP Normal IOP = 15–25 mmHg	• Topical anesthetic solution (i.e. Proparacaine) • Tonometer cover • Tonometer	1. Gently instill 2–3 drops of topical anesthetic solution into each eye. 2. Have the patient loosely restrained in a sitting position with the head in a normal position perpendicular to the floor/table. 3. Apply a sterile tonometer cover and calibrate the tonometer based on its user manual. 4. Hold the tonometer with your dominant hand, push the button, and gently tap the tip on the central cornea, keeping the tip perpendicular to the corneal surface. 5. The tonometer will "chirp" with each tap on the cornea until enough taps have occurred to have a reading displayed. Several readings (i.e. 2–5) should be taken to assure a consistent measurement.	• When restraining the patient, be careful not have excess pressure around the jugular veins or thoracic inlet, as this can falsely elevate IOP readings • When restraining the patient's head, be careful not to apply excessive pressure on the upper eyelid, as this can falsely elevate IOP readings

RENAL PROCEDURES

Skill Box 16.22 / Urine Collection: Voided, Manual Expression, Cystocentesis

Uses	Supplies	Procedure	Comments
Voided			
• To collect a urine sample for diagnostic testing	• Exam gloves • Collection container and/or litter box • Non-absorbable litter • 5–10-ml syringe • RTT	**Canine:** • Leash walk the patient to let them void naturally. • While wearing gloves, collect a urine sample midstream. • Draw up the urine from the collection container and inject into RTT. **Feline:** • Fill a litter box with non-absorbable litter and place the patient in a kennel to let them void naturally. • While wearing gloves, draw up the urine from the litter box and inject into a RTT.	
Manual expression			
• To collect a urine sample for diagnostic testing • To relieve bladder pressure in a patient with neurologic impairment	• Exam gloves • Collection container • 5–10-ml syringe	**Canine:** 1. With the patient standing, place one hand on either side of the caudal abdomen, palpate to isolate the bladder. 2. Apply steady, firm pressure on the bladder until a urine stream is produced. 3. With the patient in lateral recumbency, place your non-dominant hand along the patient's spine. 4. Using your dominant hand, palpate the caudal abdomen to isolate the bladder. 5. Apply a steady, firm pressure on the bladder, directing the pressure dorsally towards the spine, until a urine stream is produced. **Feline:** 1. With the patient in lateral recumbency, place your non-dominant hand along the patient's spine. 2. Using your dominant hand, palpate the caudal abdomen to isolate the bladder. 3. Apply a steady, firm pressure on the bladder, directing the pressure dorsally towards the spine, until a urine stream is produced.	

(*Continued*)

Skill Box 16.22 / Urine Collection: Voided, Manual Expression, Cystocentesis (Continued)

Uses	Supplies	Procedure	Comments
Cystocentesis			
• To collect a urine sample for diagnostic testing • To submit a urine sample for culture	• Exam gloves • Alcohol • 1–1.5-inch 22-gauge needle on a 5–10-ml luer-lock syringe • 22-gauge needle • Alcohol • Scanning ultrasound • RTT	1. Place the patient in lateral or dorsal recumbency; if in dorsal, a trough may be helpful to keep the patient in position. 2. Apply a generous amount of alcohol along the caudal abdomen. 3. Apply steady pressure of the ultrasound probe to the caudal abdomen until the bladder is visualized on the ultrasound screen. 4. Using a 1–1.5-inch 22-gauge needle (dependent on the patient's size) attached to a 5-10mL luer-lock needle, carefully insert the needle into the bladder, confirming its entry into the bladder on the screen. 5. Draw the urine sample into the syringe, then slowly remove the needle from the bladder. 6. Change the needle on the syringe to a new 22-gauge needle, then inject the urine sample into a red top tube. 7. If needing to submit a sample for culture, inject the urine in 2 × RTT.	• Risks: accidental puncture of internal organs, bladder hematoma, potential vagal response.

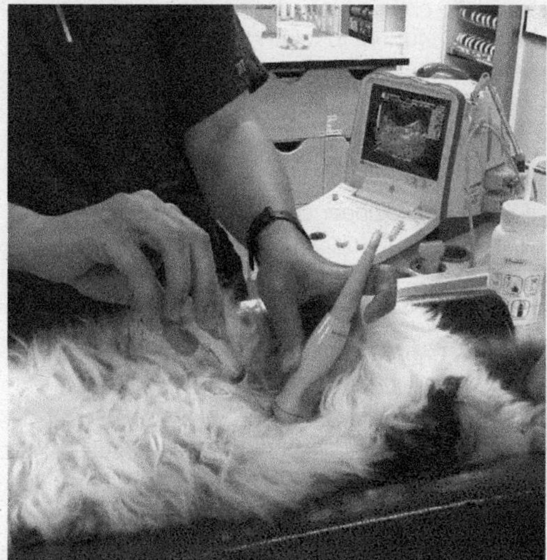

Figure 16.29 Cystocentesis.

Skill Box 16.23 / Canine Urinary Catheterization

Uses	Supplies	Procedure: Male	Procedure: Female
• To be able to more accurately quantify urine output • To relieve bladder pressure in a patient with neurologic impairment • To provide patency in an obstructed patient • As part of non-ambulatory and/or critical patient care	• Exam gloves • Clippers • Surgical preparation supplies (i.e. chlorhexidine scrub, sterile saline) • Red rubber or Foley catheter (± speculum for females) • Sterile gloves • Sterile lubricant • 5–10-ml sterile saline • X-mas tree adapter • 1-inch non-porous tape • 2-0 to 3-0 non-absorbable suture • Closed urinary collection system • Mal-adapter (for females)	1. Place the patient in lateral recumbency and clip the fur on around the tip of the prepuce. 2. Instill 5–10-ml dilute chlorhexidine into the prepuce to lavage. 3. Have an assistant extrude the prepuce, then surgically prepare the tip of the penis. 4. With the catheter still in the packaging, premeasure from the tip of the penis to the mid-bladder. 5. Don sterile gloves, keeping the sterile glove packaging accessible to use as your sterile field. 6. Have another assistant open the catheter and squeeze the sterile lubricant onto the sterile field. 7. If using a red rubber catheter, generously lubricate the end of the catheter; if using a Foley catheter, have an assistant instill sterile saline down the X-mas tree adapter port to lubricate the stylet, then generously lubricate the end of the catheter. 8. Insert the catheter into the urethral opening, being careful not to touch the penis. 9. Advance the catheter past the level of the os penis and the point where the urethral curves around the ischial arch. 10. Urine will begin to flow once the catheter has reached the bladder. 11. If using a red rubber catheter, cut the end until it will tightly fit into a urinary closed collection system. 12. Place two stay sutures on either side of the prepuce. 13. Apply a butterfly-winged piece of tape to the catheter about 1–2 cm from the prepuce opening. 14. Secure the catheter by suturing each wing of the tape to the stay suture. 15. If using a Foley catheter, fill the balloon with the correct amount of sterile saline, insert a X-mas tree adapter, and connect to a closed collection system.	1. Place the patient in sternal or lateral recumbency and clip the fur around the vulva. 2. Instill 5–10-ml dilute chlorhexidine into the vulva to lavage. 3. With the catheter still in the packaging, premeasure from the vulva to the mid-bladder. 4. Don sterile gloves, keeping the sterile glove packaging accessible to use as your sterile field. 5. Have another assistant open the catheter and squeeze the sterile lubricant onto the sterile field. 6. If using a red rubber catheter, generously lubricate the end of the catheter; if using a Foley catheter, have an assistant instill sterile saline down the X-mas tree adapter port to lubricate the stylet, then generously lubricate the end of the catheter. 7. Either place a speculum into the vagina to visualize the urethral opening, or insert your index finger of your dominant hand into the vagina to blindly palpate for the urethral opening. 8. The urethral orifice is 3–5 cm cranial to the vulva. 9. Insert the catheter into the vagina, following the speculum or your finger. If using your finger, point it downwards to direct the catheter into the urethral opening, then advance the catheter ventrally past the clitoral fossa. 10. 10.Urine will begin to flow once the catheter has reached the bladder. 11. If using a red rubber catheter, cut the end until it will tightly fit into a urinary closed collection system. 12. Place two stay sutures on either side of the vulva. 13. Apply a butterfly-winged piece of tape to the catheter about 1–2 cm from the vulva opening. 14. Secure the catheter by suturing each wing of the tape to the stay suture. 15. If using a Foley catheter, fill the balloon with the correct amount of sterile saline, insert a X-mas tree adapter, and connect to a closed collection system.

Note: see also Skill Box 16.25.

Skill Box 16.24 / Feline Urinary Catheterization

Uses	Supplies	Procedure	Comments
To provide urinary tract patency in an obstructed patient	• Exam gloves • Clippers • Sedation/analgesia • Surgical preparation supplies (i.e. chlorhexidine scrub, sterile saline) • Open/closed-end TomCat catheter (males) • Red rubber catheter • Sterile gloves • Sterile lubricant • 20–30-ml sterile saline • 1″ nonporous tape • 2-0 to 3-0 non-absorbable suture • Closed urinary collection system	*Male* 1. With the patient sedated or anesthetized, place them in dorsal or lateral recumbency. 2. Clip the fur on around the tip of the prepuce, then instill 3–5 ml dilute chlorhexidine into the prepuce to lavage. 3. Have an assistant extrude the prepuce, then surgically prepare the tip of the penis. 4. With the catheter still in the packaging, premeasure from the tip of the penis to the mid-bladder. 5. Don sterile gloves, keeping the sterile glove packaging accessible to use as your sterile field. 6. Have another assistant open the TomCat catheter, and red rubber catheter, and squeeze the sterile lubricant onto the sterile field. 7. First use the TomCat catheter to relieve the obstruction. This is done lubricating and advancing the TomCat in a rotary motion, then retropulsing sterile saline through the catheter into the urethra. 8. Once unobstructed, insert the red rubber catheter into the urethral opening, being careful not to touch the penis. 9. While advancing the catheter, gently hold and pull the penis and prepuce out to straighten the urethra. Urine will begin to flow once the catheter has reached the bladder. 10. Using a 12–20-ml syringe, empty the bladder by drawing out the urine. 11. Then instill 20–30 ml sterile saline into the bladder 2–3 times to lavage and empty the bladder again. 12. Cut the end of the catheter until it will tightly fit into a urinary closed collection system. 13. Place 2 stay sutures on either side of the prepuce. 14. Apply a butterfly-winged piece of tape to the catheter about 0.5 cm from the prepuce opening. 15. Secure the catheter by suturing each wing of the tape to the stay suture. 16. Use another piece of tape to secure the catheter to the tail while assuring enough space for normal movement.	• A local anesthetic block can be performed at the coccygeal region • If a urine sample is needed as part of the diagnostic work up, collect the sample in a RTT prior to lavaging the bladder with sterile saline

(*Continued*)

Skill Box 16.24 / Feline Urinary Catheterization (Continued)

Uses	Supplies	Procedure	Comments
		Female 1. With the patient sedated or anesthetized, place them in sternal or lateral recumbency. 2. Clip the fur around the vulva, then instill 3–5 ml dilute chlorhexidine into the vulva to lavage. 3. With the catheter still in the packaging, premeasure from the tip of the vulva to the mid-bladder. 4. Don sterile gloves, keeping the sterile glove packaging accessible to use as your sterile field. 5. Have another assistant open the catheter and squeeze the sterile lubricant onto the sterile field. 6. "Blindly" insert the red rubber catheter into the vulva, then advance the catheter through the urethral opening; the catheter should pass easily and directly. Urine will begin to flow once the catheter has reached the bladder. 7. Cut the end of the catheter until it will tightly fit into a urinary closed collection system. 8. Place 2 stay sutures on either side of the vulva. Apply a butterfly-winged piece of tape to the catheter about 0.5 cm from the vulva opening. 9. Secure the catheter by suturing each wing of the tape to the stay suture. 10. Use another piece of tape to secure the catheter to the tail while assuring enough space for normal movement.	• If a urine sample is needed as part of the diagnostic work up, collect the sample in a RTT prior to lavaging the bladder with sterile saline

Note: See also Skill Box 16.25.

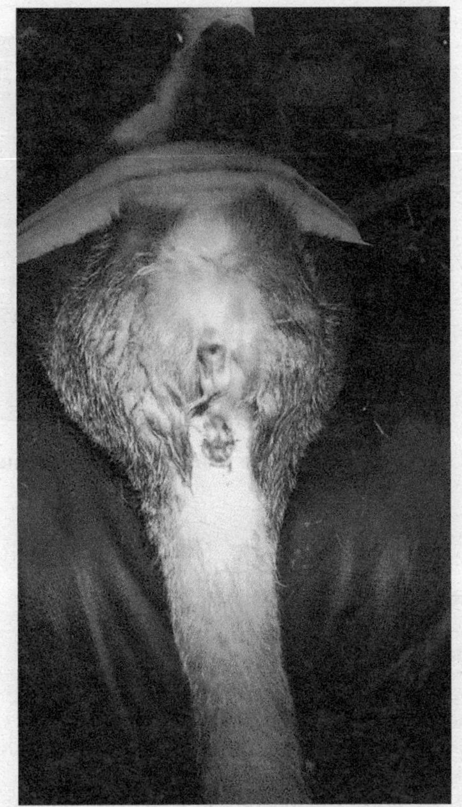

Figure 16.30 Male feline catheter placement 1.

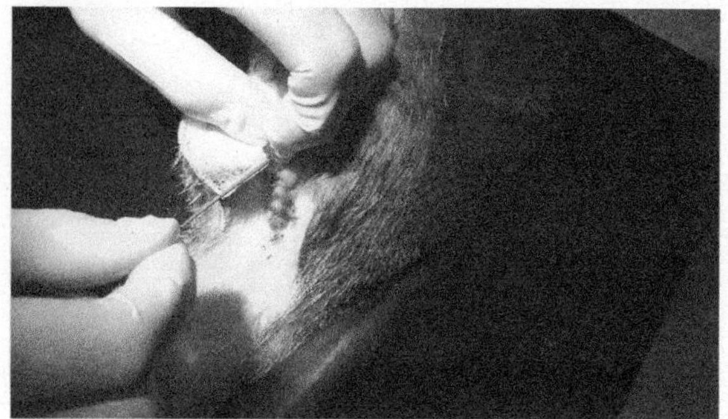

Figure 16.31 Male feline catheter placement 2.

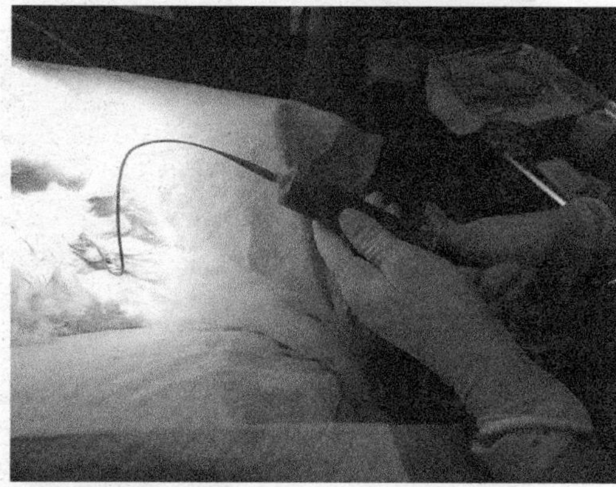

Figure 16.32 Male feline catheter placement 3.

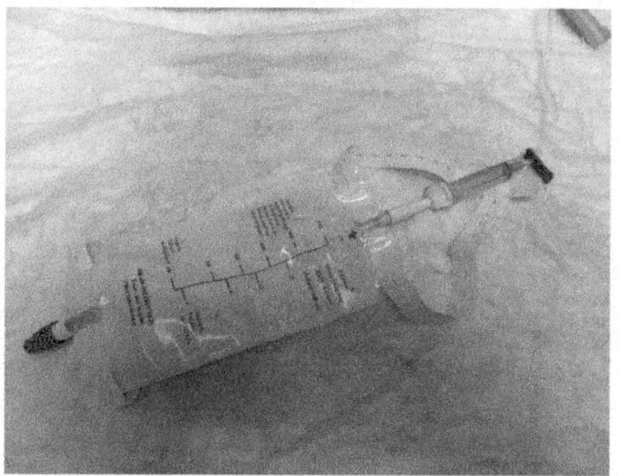

Figure 16.33 Urinary collection set 1.

Skill Box 16.25 / Urinary Catheter Care and Maintenance

Uses	Supplies	Procedure	Comments
Indicated for patients with indwelling urinary catheters	• Exam gloves • Diaper pad or cardboard tray • Alcohol preparation pad • 5–10-ml sterile saline • Curved-tip syringe filled with dilute chlorhexidine • Dry 4 × 4 gauze • Dilute chlorhexidine soaked gauze • Collection bowl/bucket • 20–60-ml syringe	1. Always wear exam gloves whenever handling the urinary catheter (u-cath), urinary collection set, or urine. 2. Place the urinary collection set at a level below the patient to prevent the backflow of urine to the patient. 3. Keep the urinary collection set on a clean surface (not directly in contact with the floor); use a diaper pad or cardboard litter tray to prevent bacterial contamination. **Patency:** 1. Evaluate u-cath patency every 4–8 hours. Observe the urinary collection set line for urine flow. 2. If patency is questionable, you will need to sterilely flush the line. 3. Using an alcohol preparation pad, wipe the urinary collection set line port. 4. Insert the syringe of sterile saline while occluding the line towards the patient, then flush 3–5 ml. 5. Occlude the line towards the collection bag and flush 3–5 ml.	• Urinary catheter care should be included on the patient's treatment sheet and should be performed every 8 hours • Normal urine output is 1–2 ml/kg/hour. Urine output should be quantified every 2–4 hours and recorded on the treatment sheet 3 ways: total ml, ml/hour, and ml/kg/hour

(*Continued*)

Skill Box 16.25 / **Urinary Catheter Care and Maintenance (Continued)**

Uses	Supplies	Procedure	Comments
		U-cath care: U-cath care consists of cleaning the vulva/prepuce, urinary catheter, and urinary catheter set connections. 1. Fill a curved tip syringe with dilute chlorhexidine. 2. While holding dry gauze under the prepuce/vulva, insert the curved tip into the prepuce/vulva and instill 10–12 ml dilute chlorhexidine. This flushes and cleans the prepuce/vulva. 3. Using dilute chlorhexidine soaked gauze, wipe the u-cath starting a few centimeters away from the prepuce/vulva and wiping away (down) the catheter towards the collection line/bag. 4. Ensure that each urinary collection set connection is tightly sealed. 5. Using chlorhexidine-soaked gauze, wipe each collection connection (i.e. u-cath to urinary collection line, urinary collection line ports, urinary collection line to urinary connection bag). **Urine output:** Urine output consists of quantifying and recording the urine in the collection bag. 1. While wearing gloves, carefully disconnect the collection bag from the collection line while maintaining sterility. 2. Pour the urine into a collection bowl, then resecure the collection bag to the collection line. 3. Measure the urine volume using a 10–60-ml syringe.	

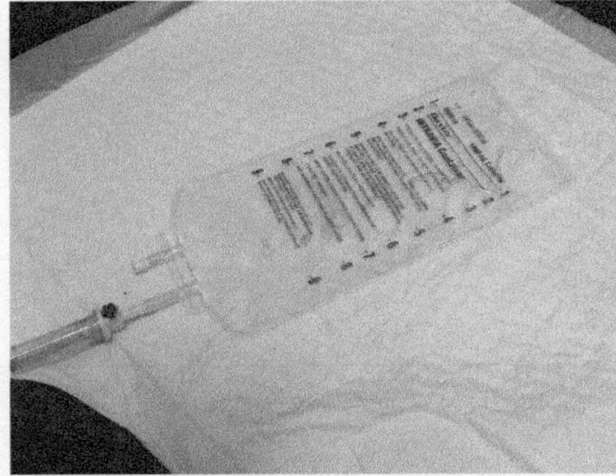

Figure 16.34 Urinary collection set 2.

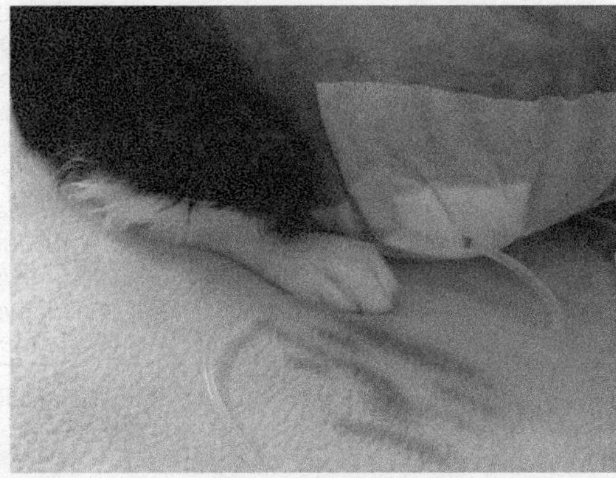

Figure 16.35 Peritoneal catheter insertion site.

Skill Box 16.26 / Peritoneal dialysis

Uses	Supplies	Procedure	Management & Care
Indicated for patients with acute kidney injury	• Peritoneal catheter placed • Urinary catheter placed and connected to a closed collection system • Sterile gauze • Bandage dressing (i.e. Hypafix®, Primapore®) • Sterile gloves • 3-way stopcock • Sterile closed collection set • Dialysate solution with primary IV line • 1-inch non-porous tape • Diaper pad or cardboard tray • Fluid infusion pump • Stopwatch/clock	1. Once the peritoneal catheter has been placed, don sterile gloves to cover the insertion site with sterile gauze, then apply bandage dressing over the sterile gauze. 2. While maintaining sterile technique, connect a 3-way stopcock between the peritoneal catheter and a sterile closed collection set. 3. Have an assistant connect the dialysate fluid line (roller clamp in the OFF position) to the third port on the 3-way stopcock and luer-lock the line into place. 4. Wrap sterile gauze over the 3-way stopcock setup, then secure with 1-inch non-porous tape. 5. Once all the lines have been connected following sterile technique, use 1-inch non-porous tape to label them as "inflow" and "outflow"; the inflow is the dialysate line, the outflow is the collection set line. Ensure that the inflow line is positioned at a level equal to the peritoneal insertion site and that it has no dependent loops. 6. Place the sterile closed collection set on a clean surface (not directly in contact with the floor); use a diaper pad or cardboard litter tray to prevent bacterial contamination. 7. Insert the dialysate solution line into a fluid infusion pump, then open the fluid line roller clamp. Input the prescribed volume (i.e. 100 ml) of dialysate to be infused over the prescribed time (i.e. 15–30 minutes) into the pump, then turn the 3-way stopcock so that the OFF position is toward the outflow line. 8. Once the dialysate infusion is complete, set a stopwatch/clock for the prescribed dwell time; the dwell period is how long the veterinarian wants the dialysate to dwell intra-abdominally. 9. At the end of the dwell time, turn the 3-way stopcock so that the OFF position is toward the inflow line, and allow the dialysate to drain via gravity into the collection set for a prescribed time (i.e. 15–30 minutes). 10. Repeat the infuse/dwell/drain process as directed by the DVM (typically every 1–4 hours). 11. For each cycle of peritoneal dialysis, record the following: 12. IV fluids in 13. Dialysate in 14. Dialysate out 15. Urine output.	• PD required a dedicated one-on-one credentialed technician. • PD should only be a service offered only in 24-hour hospitals • Dialysate is typically a hyperosmolar dextrose-containing solution. • Follow sterile technique (i.e. sterile gloves) whenever handling the patient or PD setup/lines. • Wipe down the PD catheter, inflow, and outflow lines every 4-8 hours with dilute chlorhexidine. • Following urinary catheter care guidelines for maintenance of the urinary catheter • Change the dialysate solution bag and inflow line every 24 hours; follow sterile technique. • Change the closed collection set (bag only) every 24 hours; follow sterile technique.

Tip: A recipe for a homemade dialysate solution is taking 1 liter lactated Ringer's solution and adding 30 ml 50% dextrose plus 1000 U/l heparin. Dextrose is used as the osmotic agent (yielding a 1.5% solution) and heparin is used to prevent clot occlusions of the peritoneal dialysis catheter.
Note: See also Skill Box 16.25.

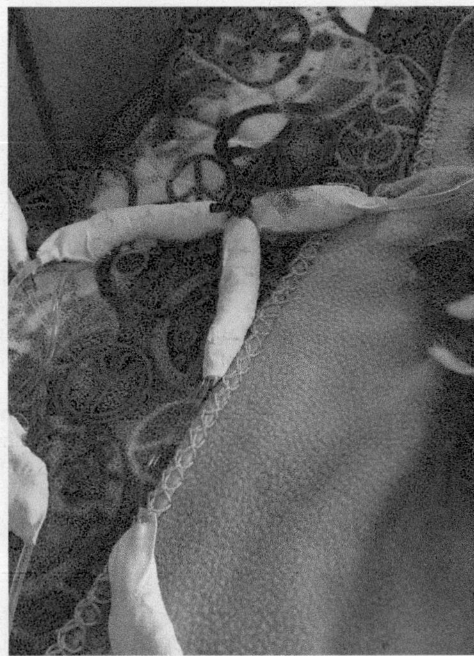

Figure 16.36 Peritoneal dialysis three-way stopcock.

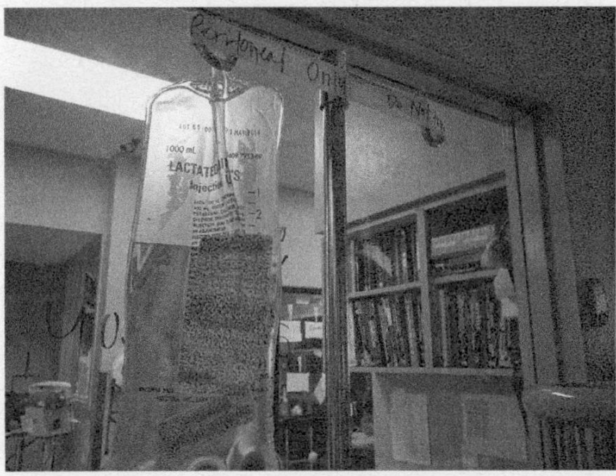

Figure 16.37 Peritoneal dialysate.

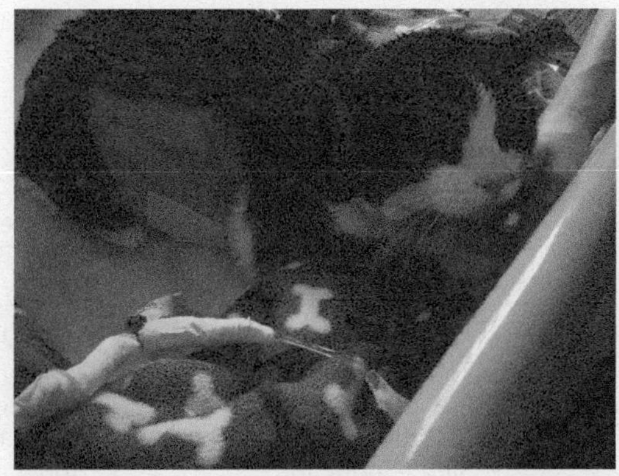

Figure 16.38 Patient receiving peritoneal dialysis.

RESPIRATORY PROCEDURES

Skill Box 16.27 / Nasal oxygen cannula placement

Uses	Supplies	Procedure	Comments
Nasal cannula placement			
To deliver supplemental oxygen therapy to patients in respiratory distress	• Exam gloves • Topical anesthetic solution (i.e. proparacaine) • Red rubber catheter • Sterile lubricant • Sharpie® marker • 2-0 or 3-0 non-absorbable suture • Needle holders	1. Instill 2–3 drops of topical anesthetic into each nares. 2. Measure the red rubber catheter from the tip of the nares to the medial canthus of the eye, then mark with a marker pen. 3. Apply a small amount of sterile lubricant to the tip of the catheter, then insert the catheter to the point of the medial canthus. 4. Secure using 2-0 or 3-0 non-absorbable suture in a finger-trap pattern. 5. Apply another single suture on the forehead area or on the side of the face for further securement.	• Instilling additional topical anesthetic into each eye will provide additional numbing via the nasolacrimal duct • Nasal oxygen cannulas can be placed unilaterally (one nares) or bilaterally (both nares) • Nasal oxygen should be delivered at a rate of 0.5–2 l/minute (unilateral) or 1–4 l/minute (bilateral) • Patients with nasal oxygen cannulas should wear an Elizabethan collar while in hospital to prevent them from accidental removal
Nasal prong placement			
To deliver supplemental oxygen therapy to patients in respiratory distress	• Exam gloves • Topical anesthetic solution (i.e. Proparacaine) • Scissors • Silicone nasal prongs • 1-inch non-porous tape	1. Instill 2–3 drops of topical anesthetic into each nares. 2. Based on the patient's size, cut each nasal prong to a length that will fit comfortably in the nares. 3. Insert the nasal prong and gently tighten behind the patient's ears. 4. Using 1-inch non-porous tape, make a "bridge" over the nose to better hold the nasal prongs in place.	• Instilling additional topical anesthetic into each eye will provide additional numbing via the nasolacrimal duct • Nasal oxygen should be delivered at a rate of 0.5–2 l/minute • Patients with nasal oxygen cannulas should wear an Elizabethan collar while in hospital to prevent them from accidental removal

Note: see also Chinese finger trap – Skill Box 23.6: Suture Patterns, page 1073.

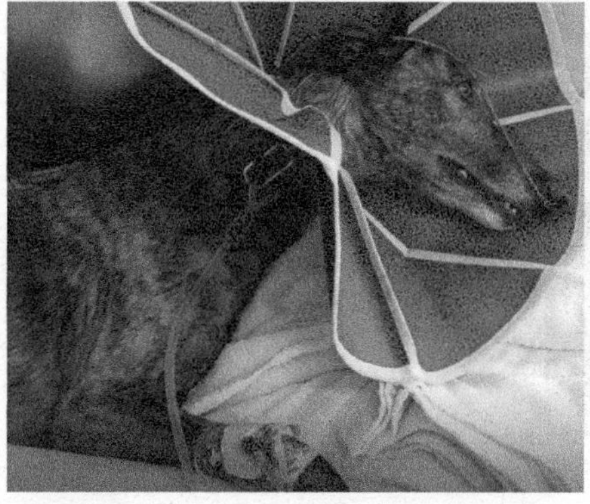

Figure 16.39 Nasal cannula placement.

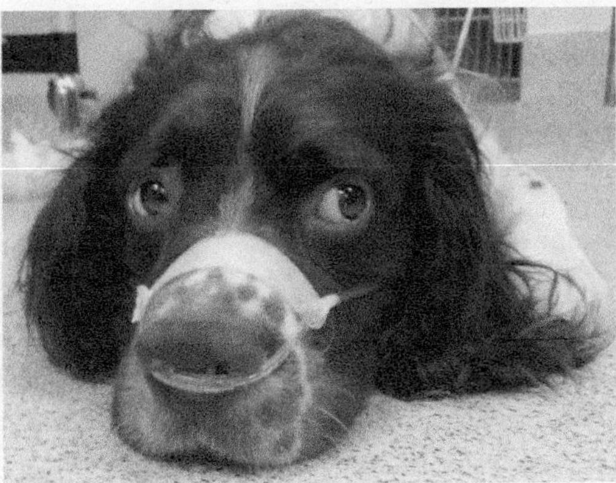

Figure 16.40 Nasal prong placement.

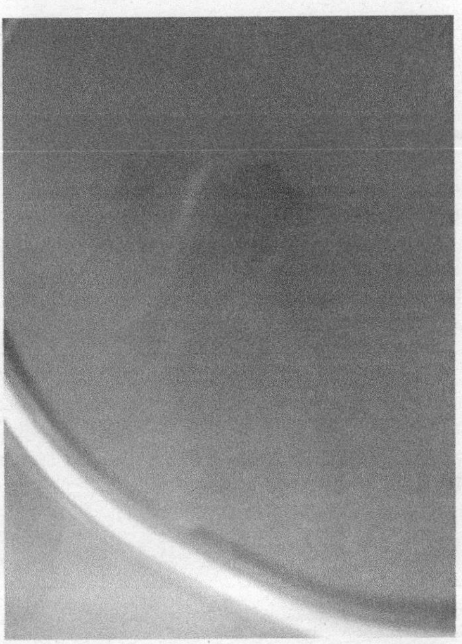

Figure 16.41 Patient being nebulized in an oxygen kennel.

Skill Box 16.28 / Nebulization, Coupage, and Inhalant Therapy

Method	Uses	Supplies	Procedure	Comments
Nebulization	• To deliver saline and/or medications (i.e. aminoglycosides) in a mist form that can be inhaled into the lungs • Commonly indicated for patients with upper airway disease (i.e. asthma, pneumonia, infectious causes) • Indicated in patients with tracheostomy tubes to keep airway moist	• Nebulizer machine • Nebulizer set • Sterile saline and/or medication • Oxygen source	1. Fill the nebulizer set with sterile saline and/or the prescribed medication. 2. For a patient in an oxygen kennel (Figure 16.42): 3. Insert the nebulizer set into the oxygen door system. 4. Turn on the nebulizer machine so the mist slowly fills the oxygen kennel. 5. Allow the animal to breathe normally; nebulizer treatments are typically 10–20 minutes. For a patient in a regular kennel: 1. Hold the nebulizer set i in front of the patient's mouth and nose, then turn on the nebulizer machine. 2. Allow the animal to breathe normally; nebulizer treatments are typically 10–20 minutes.	• Performing nebulization is contraindicated in patients that would sustain further injury/trauma from coughing • Each patient should have their own designated nebulizer set; sets should not be shared between patients

(Continued)

Skill Box 16.28 / Nebulization, Coupage, and Inhalant Therapy (Continued)

Method	Uses	Supplies	Procedure	Comments
Coupage	• Performed after nebulization • To break up intrapulmonary phlegm (i.e. secretions, infectious causes)	• None	1. Using a cupped hand on one or both sides of the chest, make repeated thumps against the chest wall, using firm and moderate force. 2. Work from back to front and lower to upper areas of the chest.	• Performing coupage is contraindicated in a patient with thoracic or chest-wall trauma • Performing coupage is contraindicated in patients that would sustain further injury/trauma from coughing
Inhalant therapy	• To administer inhalant medication in an aerosolized form that can be inhaled into the lungs	• Metered-dose inhaler • Inhaler spacer	1. Prime and shake the metered dose inhaler. Insert the inhaler into the inhaler spacer. 2. Place the inhaler spacer over the patient's face and press the metal canister down firmly and fully. 3. Hold the inhaler spacer in place for 5–10 seconds. 4. Repeat as needed according to the medication's dosing directions.	

Skill Box 16.29 / Thoracocentesis

Uses	Supplies	Procedure	Comments
• To remove accumulation of fluid from the pleural cavity (i.e. hemothorax, chylothorax, pyothorax) • To remove the accumulation of air from the pleural cavity (i.e. pneumothorax)	• Clippers • Surgical preparation supplies (i.e. chlorhexidine scrub, sterile saline) • Sterile gloves • Analgesic/sedative drugs • Local anesthetic • Large-bore IV catheter (i.e. 14–16 gauge) or 22–20-gauge 1.5-inch needle • 5-, 10-, or 20-ml luer-lock syringe • 3-way stopcock • Fluid extension line • Collecting bucket/chamber/bowl • RTT • LTT • Flow-by oxygen therapy	1. Administer analgesic/sedation drugs as needed. 2. Place the patient in sternal or lateral recumbency (whichever position is least stressful). 3. Shave a large area on the lateral chest between the 7–9th intercostal space. 4. Administer a local anesthetic block as needed and surgically prepare the site. 5. Prepare the thoracocentesis set by attaching the luer-lock syringe to one end of the 3-way stopcock, and the fluid extension line to the other end, leaving an open end to the environment. 6. Turn the 3-way stopcock "OFF" lever toward the patient (i.e. toward the fluid extension line). 7. Insert the catheter/needle tip between the 7–9th intercostal space, avoiding the intercostal arteries on the caudal aspect of each rib. 8. Advance the catheter/needle into the pleural space slowly in 1-cm increments while angling the catheter/needle flat against the chest wall with the bevel outward. 9. While moving the catheter/needle into the pleural space and along the chest wall, position the catheter/need dorsally to obtain air and ventrally to obtain fluid. 10. Once the catheter/needle is in position, attach the fluid extension line (if using a catheter, the stylet must be removed first). 11. Aspirate the fluid/air by using a 3-way stopcock and syringe; open the 3-way stopcock to the environment to draw back fluid/air, then close it to the patient to push the fluid/air out to empty the syringe, repeating until the pleural cavity is emptied. 12. Continue aspirating until the bevel of the catheter/needle can be felt "scraping" the lung.	• Flow-by oxygen should be provided to the patient during the procedure • If fluid is being removed from the pleural cavity, a sterile sample should be saved in both a RTT and LTT • Risks/complications include iatrogenic pneumothorax or intrathoracic hemorrhage from accidental laceration of the lung tissue

Skill Box 16.30 / Thoracostomy Tube Placement

Uses	Supplies	Procedure	Comments
• When multiple thoracocentesis procedures are required to achieve negative pressure • To better facilitate removal of the accumulation of fluid from the pleural cavity (i.e. hemothorax, chylothorax, pyothorax) • To better facilitate removal of the accumulation of air from the pleural cavity (i.e. pneumothorax)	• Clippers • Surgical preparation supplies (i.e. sterile gauze, chlorhexidine scrub, sterile saline) • Sterile surgical supplies (i.e. gloves, drapes) • General anesthesia or heavy analgesia/sedation • Local anesthetic • Surgical blade • Hemostats • Thoracostomy tube • Thoracostomy tube clamp • 0–2-0 non-absorbable suture • X-mas tree adapter • 3-way stopcock • Injection cap • Orthopedic wire and/or zip ties • Radiology • Bandage materials	1. With the patient either under general anesthesia or heavily sedation, place them in lateral or recumbency. 2. Shave the lateral thorax from the point of the shoulder to the last rib and from the dorsal spine to the ventral midline. 3. Make a small stab incision over the widest part of the thorax between the 9–10th intercostal space. 4. Have an assistant pull the skin cranially from the 9–10th intercostal space until it lies over the 7–8th intercostal space. 5. Administer a local anesthetic block. Using hemostats, bluntly dissect into the pleural space, then spread them wide enough to allow the tube to be passed. 6. Insert the thoracostomy tube, holding it parallel to the thoracic wall, and direct the tube cranioventrally into the thorax. 7. Have the assistant release the skin allowing a subcutaneous tunnel at the 7–8th intercostal space to be made. 8. Secure using 0–2-0 non-absorbable suture in a finger-trap pattern around the base of the thoracostomy tube entry site. 9. Slide a thoracostomy tube clamp of the end of the tube and clamp into place. 10. Insert a X-mas tree adapter fitted with a 3-way stopcock and an injection cap into the open end of the tube. 11. Secure the tube connections with orthopedic wire and/or zip ties.	• Take lateral and dorsoventral radiographs to confirm placement of the thoracostomy tube (the tube should terminate between the 7–9th intercostal space) • The tube insertion site should be covered with a sterile, non-absorbent dressing and a light bandage

Note: see also Chinese finger trap – Skill Box 23.6: Suture patterns, page 1073.

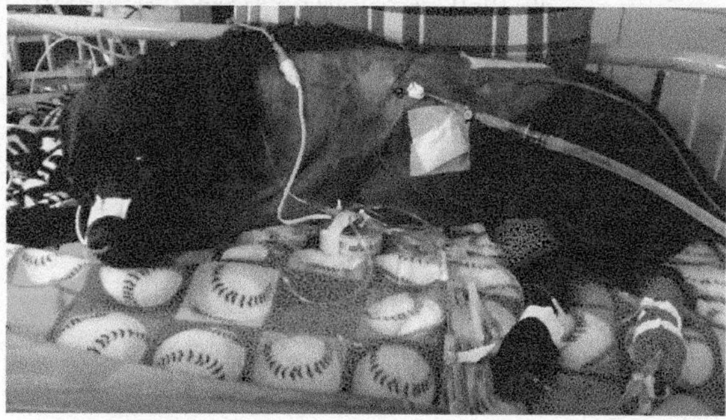

Figure 16.42 Patient with thoracostomy tube.

Skill Box 16.31 / Thoracostomy Tube Care

Uses	Supplies	Procedure	Comments
Indicated for patients with indwelling thoracostomy tube(s)	• Exam gloves • 5–20-ml luer-lock syringes • Collection bowl/ bucket	1. Keep tube connections as sterile as possible and inspect daily for appropriate securement/tightness. 2. Wear exam gloves when handling the tube. 3. Inspect the tube insertion site daily for redness, swelling, bruising, bleeding or discharge, as well as for any sign of tube migration. 4. Only use luer-lock syringes to aspirate the tube. During each manual tube aspiration, document the volume of air and/or fluid in the medical record. 5. Keep the 3-way stopcock in the "OFF" position whenever the tube is not in use. 6. Keep the thoracostomy tube clamped whenever the tube is not in use in the event that the 3-way stopcock becomes detached from the tube or is not kept in the OFF position.	• Management of thoracostomy tube requires 24-hour care and monitoring due to the risk of tube displacement and/or detachment • Appropriate analgesia must be provided, as thoracostomy tube(s) can be uncomfortable • Thoracostomy tube(s) should be manually aspirated every 2–6 hours until negative pressure is achieved • If negative pressure cannot be achieved, continuous pleural space drainage should be initiated

Skill Box 16.32 / Temporary tracheostomy tube placement

Uses	Supplies	Procedure	Comments
• To relieve life-threatening upper airway obstruction (i.e. foreign body, trauma, laryngeal paralysis, neoplasia) • When endotracheal intubation is not feasible (i.e. severe laryngeal edema, neoplasia) • For manual or mechanical intubation	• Clippers • Surgical preparation supplies (i.e. sterile gauze, chlorhexidine scrub, sterile saline) • Sterile surgical supplies (i.e. gloves, drapes) • General anesthesia • Surgical blade • Surgical instrument pack (towel clamps, scalpel handle, thumb forceps, Metzenbaum scissors, hemostats, needle holders, self-retaining retractor) • Sterile gauze • Tracheostomy tube • 0–2-0 non-absorbable suture • Umbilical tape	1. With the patient endotracheally intubated and under general anesthesia, position them in dorsal recumbency with a towel rolled under the neck. 2. Shave the ventral neck and surgically prepare the site. 3. Don sterile gloves and sterilely drape the patient. 4. Make a ventral midline cervical incision approximately 3–4 cm caudal to the larynx. 5. Apply a self-retaining retractor to hold open the skin edges. 6. Using Metzenbaum scissors, bluntly separate the muscles on the midline, then reposition the self-retaining retractor to hold open the musculature and skin. 7. Using a scalpel blade, incise between the second and third tracheal rings, using caution to not incise beyond 50% of the tracheal circumference. 8. Place stay sutures around the second and third tracheal rings, knotting them to create large loops, then hold them using hemostats. 9. Use the stay sutures to manipulate the intratracheal opening while the endotracheal tube is removed. 10. Quickly insert the tracheostomy tube (with or without an inner cannula). 11. Secure the tube by attaching umbilical tape to the flange eyelets and tying behind the neck.	• Most commercially available tubes are made of plastic or silicone – some contain a cuff, some contain an inner cannula • If/when a commercially available tube is not available, one can be fashioned from a standard. endotracheal tube • The tracheostomy tube should ideally be ½ to ⅓ of the tracheal diameter

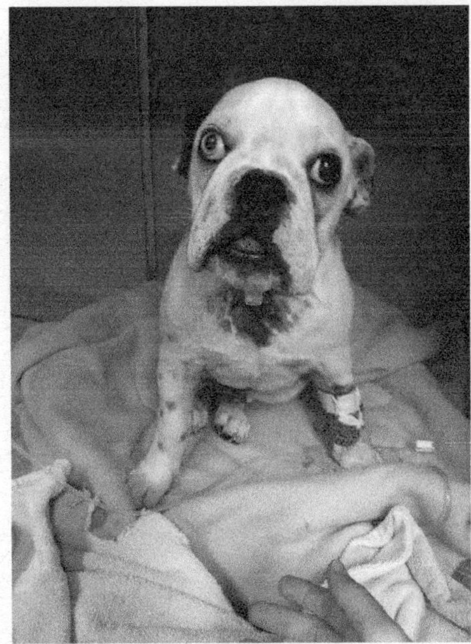

Figure 16.43 Canine patient with temporary tracheostomy tube.

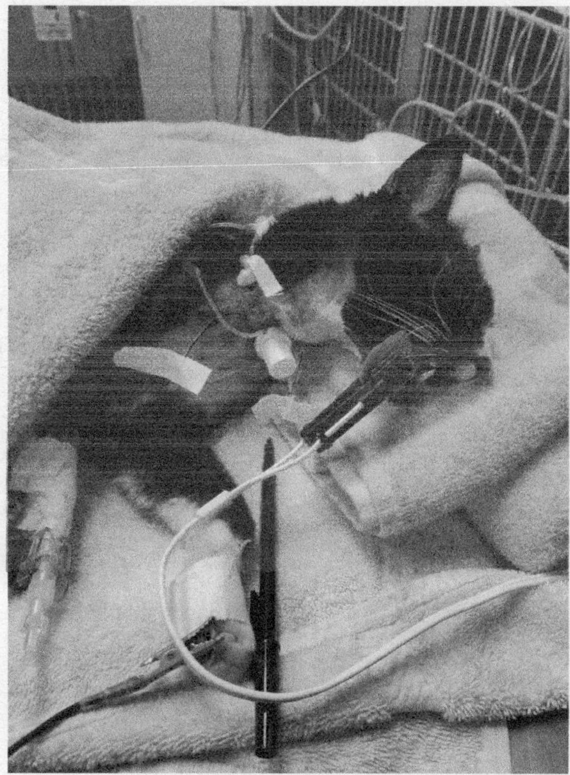

Figure 16.44 feline patient with temporary tracheostomy tube.

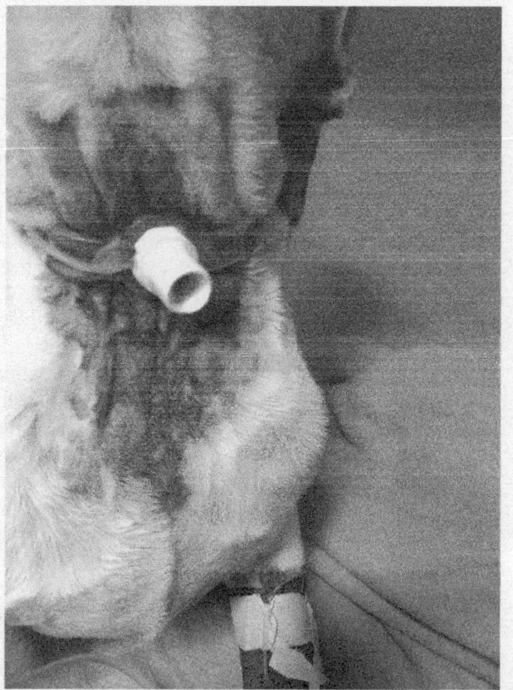

Figure 16.45 Tracheostomy tube in a canine patient.

Skill Box 16.33 / Temporary tracheostomy tube care

Uses	Supplies	Procedure	Comments
Indicated for patients with a temporary tracheostomy tube	• Exam gloves • Sterile gloves • Dilute chlorhexidine soaked gauze • 3–5-ml syringe • Humidified oxygen • 8–12 Fr sterile red rubber catheter • 1-l bottle 0.9% NaCl • Wall suction setup (wall unit, canister, tubing) • Sterile cotton-tipped applicators • Sterile bowl	1. Wear exam gloves when handling the outer aspects of the tracheostomy tube. 2. Wear sterile gloves when handling the inner aspects of the tracheostomy tube. 3. If the tube has a cuff, marginally inflate/deflate and reposition within the tracheal lumen every 6–8 hours to prevent pressure necrosis. 4. Inspect the tracheostomy tube insertion site for signs of redness, swelling, or bruising. 5. Gently cleanse the skin surrounding the incision with chlorhexidine-soaked gauze. 6. If the patient is receiving oxygen therapy (either flow-by or directly connected), humidify the oxygen to prevent drying out of airway secretions. 7. Suction the sterile tracheostomy tube every 1–4 hours, depending on the patient's secretions. 8. While wearing sterile gloves and following sterile technique, attach a red rubber catheter to suction tubing. 9. Have an assistant pour sterile saline into a sterile bowl. Have an assistant connect the suction tubing to wall suction, then turn on wall suction to "REGULAR". 10. Carefully insert the red rubber catheter into the tube lumen in a back-and-forth motion for about 5 seconds – the tip of the red rubber catheter should not surpass the tube by more than 3–5 inches. 11. Suctioning should be performed 2–3 times each treatment. 12. Between each suction, dip the red rubber catheter in the bowl of sterile saline. 13. If the tube has an inner lumen, it should be removed and cleaned following sterile technique, using saline in a sterile bowl and gauze/cotton-tipped applicator, every 4–6 hours.	• Management of tracheostomy tube requires 24-hour care and monitoring due to the risk of tube occlusion • Tracheostomy tube care should be performed at a minimum every 4–8 hours – additional care may be required based on the patient's respiratory status • In order to not rapidly deplete sterile supplies, rewrap/cover the red rubber catheter, bowl, and any remaining sterile gauze and cotton-tipped applicators for future use • Red rubber catheters should be changed every 8–12 hours; sterile bowls should be changed every 24 hours

Skill Box 16.34 / Cardiopulmonary Resuscitation: Airway and Ventilation

Uses	Supplies	Procedure	Comments
Airway			
To facilitate ventilation breaths	• Endotracheal tube • Laryngoscope • Endotracheal tube tie • 5–10-ml syringe	1. With the patient in lateral recumbency, place the laryngoscope blade into the oral cavity. 2. Depress the tongue with the laryngoscope blade and hold just rostral to the epiglottis. 3. Once the epiglottis is visualized, orient the endotracheal tube with the bevel to down. 4. Advance the tube over the epiglottis and through the arytenoids. 5. Secure the tube either around the muzzle (medium to large-sized dog) or behind the ears (small dog or cat). 6. Inflate the tube cuff using a 5–10-ml syringe.	• A laryngoscope should be used for direct visualization of the trachea • There should be minimal to no interruption of chest compressions • Intubating in lateral recumbency makes it so there is unnecessary manipulate of the spine, which would compromise cerebral perfusion
Ventilation			
To restore circulation in a patient in cardiopulmonary arrest	• Ambu bag • Anesthetic circuit	1. Deliver manual breaths at a rate of 10 breaths/minute. 2. If using an Ambu bag, squeeze firmly and quickly. 3. If using an anesthetic circuit (oxygen only) reservoir bag, close the pop-off valve, squeeze the bag up to 20 cm H_2O pressure, then re-open the pop-off valve	• Breaths should be delivered following the 1 : 2 inspiratory-to-expiratory ratio

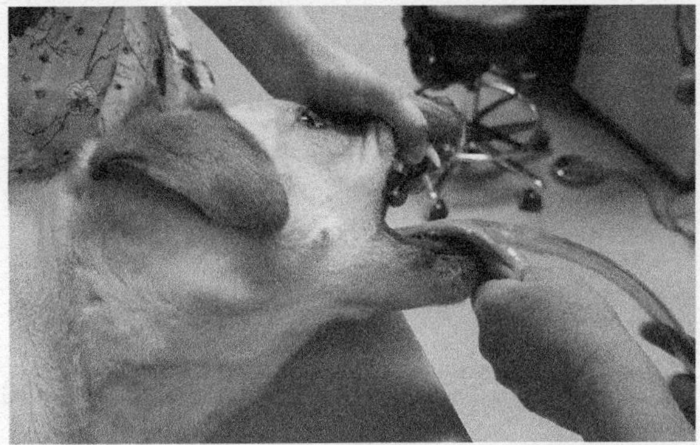

Figure 16.46 Lateral intubation technique.

REFERENCES

1. Jack, C.M. and Watson, P.M. (2014). *Veterinary Technicians Daily Reference Guide: Canine and Feline*, 3e. Ames, IA: Wiley Blackwell.
2. Creedon, J.M.B. and Davis, H. (2012). *Advanced Monitoring and Procedures for Small Animal Emergency and Critical Care*. Chichesterx: Wiley-Blackwell.
3. Norkus, C.L. (ed.) (2019). *Veterinary Technicians Manual for Small Animal Emergency and Critical Care*. Hoboken, NJ: Wiley.
4. Battaglia, A.M., Steele, A.M. and Battaglia, A.M. (2016). *Small Animal Emergency and Critical Care for Veterinary Technicians*. St. Louis, MO: Elsevier.
5. Silverstein, D.C. and Hopper, K. (eds.) (2015). *Small Animal Critical Care Medicine*, 2e. St. Louis, MO: Elsevier, Saunders.
6. Nelson, R.W. and Couto, C.G. (2014). *Small Animal Internal Medicine*, 6e. St. Louis, MO: Elsevier Mosby.
7. Goldberg, M.E. and Tomlinson, J. (2018). *Physical Rehabilitation for Veterinary Technicians and Nurses*. Hoboken, NJ: Wiley Blackwell.
8. Fletcher, D.J., Boller, M., Brainard, B.M. *et al.* (2012). RECOVER evidence and knowledge gap analysis on veterinary CPR. Part 7: clinical guidelines. *J Vet Emerg Crit Care* 22(Suppl 1): S102–S131.

Chapter 17

Nutrition

Ed Carlson, CVT, VTS (Nutrition)

Veterinary Technician and Nurse's Daily Reference Guide: Canine and Feline, Fourth Edition. Edited by Mandy Fults and Kenichiro Yagi.

Companion website: www.wiley.com/go/fults/veterinary

Abbreviations

AAFCO, Association of American Feed Control Officials
BCS, body condition score
CRI, constant rate infusion
CVM, Center for Veterinary Medicine
DER, daily energy requirement
IV, intravenous
kcal, kilocalories
ME, metabolizable energy
PEG, percutaneous endoscopic gastrostomy feeding
PER, partial energy requirement
RER, resting energy requirement
TPN, total parenteral nutrition
WSAVA, World Small Animal Veterinary Association

GENERAL NUTRITION

Proper nutrition is as important as physical examinations, vaccinations, and dental care in maintaining a healthy pet. It is now considered the fifth vital assessment after temperature, pulse, respiration, and pain. Unfortunately, not much time is usually given to the subject during client education. Obesity still remains the biggest nutritional challenge; it is estimated that over 50% of dogs and cats in the United States are overweight. The most important component to proper nutrition begins with a high-quality complete and balanced diet formulated to the appropriate life stage of the animal. Poor-quality, unbalanced, commercial diets, homemade diets which are not formulated by a veterinary nutritionist, indiscriminate mixtures of single food items, and variable supplements will lead to dietary imbalances. Together with proper nutrition, fresh, clean water must always be provided.

Owners often look to the veterinary healthcare team for a better understanding of the "right" diet to feed their pet. Many would like a concrete comparison between different foods, but unfortunately, this is virtually impossible to do. The information provided in the ingredient list and on the information panel appears at first glance to be consistent between products, but the variables that exist render comparison virtually impossible.

Some key points to look for when evaluating a pet food are:

- Read the Association of American Feed Control Officials (AAFCO) nutritional adequacy statement. Was the "complete and balanced" claim substantiated by preforming feeding trials or is the product formulated to meet the AFFCO standards? Feeding trials are designed to determine whether dogs or cats can metabolize the food and are the gold standard.[1]
- Is the food manufactured by the company? If the label reads "manufactured for" or "distributed by", the company does not actually make the food. Look for foods listing "manufactured by" on the label.
- Is the food for the life stage of the dog or cat you will be feeding? Especially for older dogs and cats, for example, diets formulated for all life stages are formulated for puppies, kittens, and pregnant/lactating animals; these diets are not appropriate for a senior pet or one that is overweight.
- Is the food 100% guaranteed? Is there a phone number to call for information? Is there a veterinary nutritionist, veterinarian, or credentialed veterinary technician on staff to answer your questions? Does the company have board-certified nutritionists on staff? Do they publish research?
- If the answer to any of these questions is no, consider continuing to search for a diet that meets these conditions.

For more information on selecting a pet food, visit the World Small Animal Veterinary Association (WSAVA) global nutrition toolkit "Recommendations on Selecting Pet Foods".[1]

PATIENT EVALUATION

To help the client choose the best diet, a nutritional assessment should be done, start with taking a full nutritional history, including any health issues and diagnostic testing if indicated. Perform a complete physical examination including determining the body condition and muscle condition scores of the patient. This baseline information will provide clues to the nutritional wellbeing of the dog or cat. A nutritional assessment and nutritional recommendation should be made on every pet, every time they visit the hospital.

Nutritional History

Obtaining a complete nutritional history is the foundation for assessing the nutritional needs of a pet. When taking a patient's nutritional history, ask the client the open-ended questions below about the pet's current diet. Open-ended questions are those that require more than a one-word or yes or no answer. They require more of an explanation or narrative to answer. For example, asking, "Does Lady like chicken-flavored canned food?" only requires a yes or no answer. Asking the open-ended question, "What flavor canned food does Lady like?" will provide you with more information on what Lady likes and possibly what she does not like.

Start by asking broad open-ended questions such as: "Tell me about Lady's typical day". "Tell me what Lady eats every day". After the client has answered these questions, ask additional questions to obtain more details as needed. For example:

- "When was the last time you changed Lady's diet?"
- "Why did you make the change?"
- "Tell me about any recent changes in Lady's appetite."
- "How many people, including children, reside in the household?"
- "Who is primarily responsible for feeding Lady?"
- "Who else feeds Lady?"
- "What treats does Lady enjoy?"
- "How many of these does she eat daily?"
- "What other pets live in the same house as Lady?"
- "What nutritional supplements do you give Lady?"
- "What medications does Lady get?"
- "How do you administer the medications?"

The goal of taking a nutritional history is to learn, in detail, what the patient is ingesting on a regular basis and what they eat occasionally.

Diet history forms are also a good tool for obtaining information for a complete nutritional history. They should not, however, be used to replace the client interview but rather to supplement it. An example of a diet history form is included as Figure 17.1. Other similar forms are available online on the WSAVA Global Nutrition Toolkit webpage.[2]

Diet History Form

Pet name: ____________ Owner's name: ____________

Breed: ____________ Age: ____________

Species: ❑ canine ❑ feline Gender: ❑ male ❑ female ❑ spayed/neutered

Current body weight: _____ lb _____ kg Ideal body weight: _____ lb _____ kg BCS: _______

Environment and Exercise

Environment: ❑ indoor ❑ outdoor ❑ both

If outdoor: ❑ fenced yard or kennel ❑ supervised ❑ free-roaming

Does your pet live with other animals? ❑ Yes (if yes, please specify animals and ages) ❑ No

____

Does your pet interact with other animals in your house? ❑ Yes ❑ No

Is your pet dominant? ❑ Yes ❑ No

Describe your pet's activity level: ❑ high ❑ medium ❑ low

Estimate the amount of exercise (explain duration and frequency):

❑ walks ____________ ❑ play time ____________

❑ swimming ____________ ❑ others ____________

Medical History

Have you observed changes in the following:

❑ appetite ❑ thirst ❑ chewing/swallowing ❑ salivation ❑ urination ❑ defecation ❑ activity level

If so, please explain: ____________

____

Have you noticed any of the following: ❑ weight loss ❑ weight gain ❑ vomiting ❑ dierrhea

If so, please explain amount, frequency, and duration: ____________

____

Does your pet have any allergies? ❑ Yes ❑ No

If so, please explain: ____________

Dietary History

Please list the brand or product name(s) of each item with an accurate amount or size and frequency it is given.

Current diet fed: ____________

Amount and frequency: ____________

Treats fed: ❑ biscuits ❑ rawhides ❑ dental chews ❑ ____________

Amount and frequency: ____________

Table scraps fed: ____________

Amount and frequency: ____________

Supplements given: ____________

Amount and frequency: ____________

Food to administer medication: ❑ cheese ❑ peanut butter ❑ others ____________

Amount and frequency: ____________

Feeding Practices

How often does your pet eat? ____________ Time of day: ____________

Who typically feeds the pet? ____________ What size cup? ________ What size bowl? ________

Is the food ❑ inhaled ❑ grazed ❑ others ________

Are other animals present during feeding? ❑ Yes ❑ No Are they fed the same diet? ❑ Yes ❑ No

____

Is there access to other food sources? ❑ neighbors ❑ hunting ❑ yard/trash ❑ others ________

Figure 17.1 Diet history form.

Body Condition Scoring

Part of evaluating the pet is to perform a complete physical exam and to assess the animal's body condition. The body condition score (BCS) system standardizes the interpretation of the overall physical appearance of the animal. It is an evaluation of body fat and should be a basic part of every examination and noted in the record for future comparison. This technique can be easily and quickly taught to clients as part of weight management at home. There are two scales that are most often used, a 1–5 scale and a 1–9 scale, with 1 being very thin or emaciated and 5 or 9 being extremely overweight. The 1–5 chart is shown in Figure 17.2. A BCS change by one value is an estimated 10% change in body weight. Other similar forms are available online on the WSAVA Global Nutrition Toolkit webpage.[3]

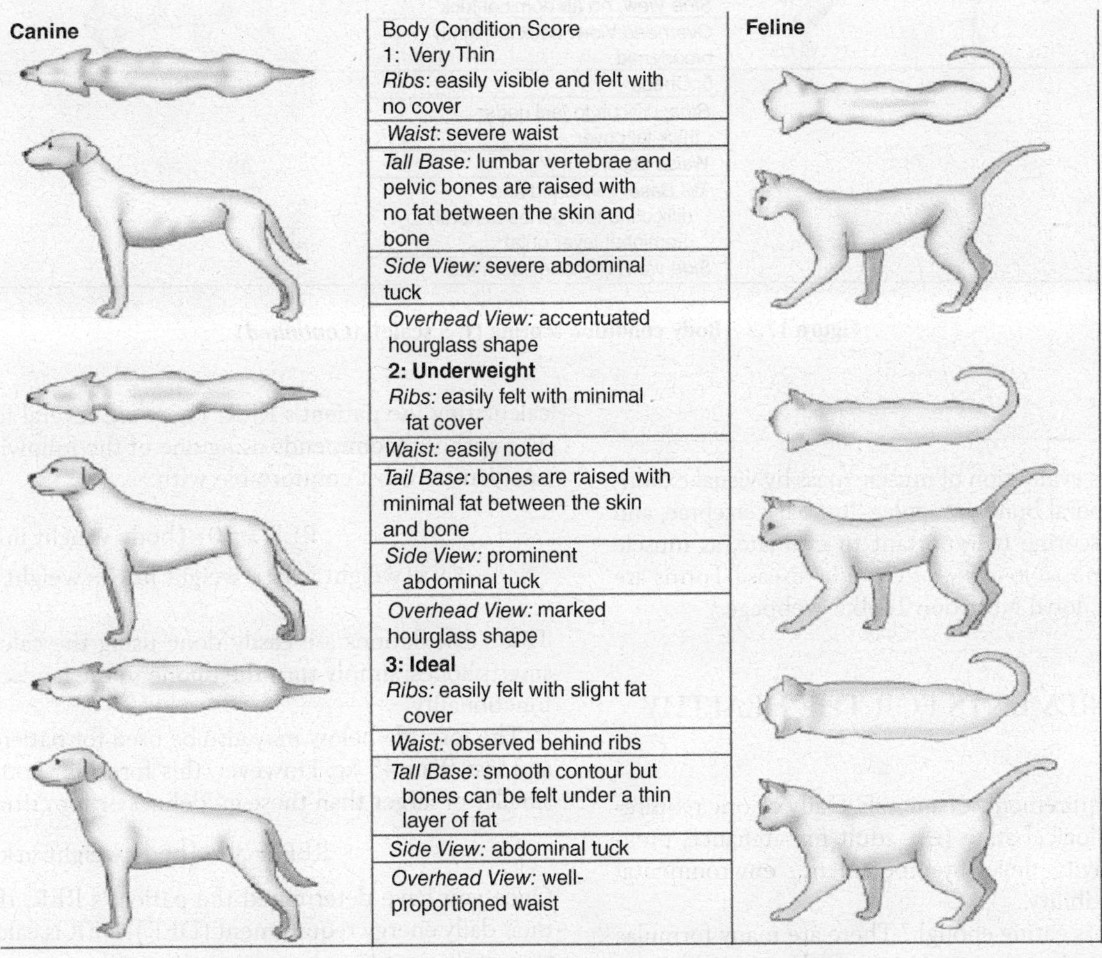

Figure 17.2 Body condition scoring (1–5 scale). (*Continued*)

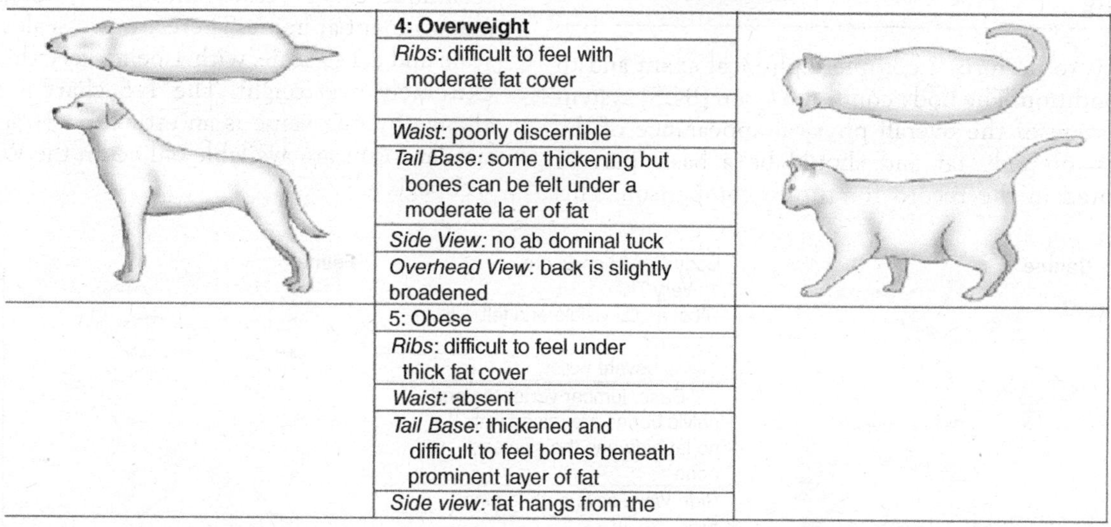

Figure 17.2 Body condition scoring (1–5 scale). *(Continued)*

Muscle Condition Scoring

Muscle condition scoring involves evaluation of muscle mass by visual examination and palpation of the temporal bones, scapulae, lumbar vertebrae, and pelvic bones. Muscle condition scoring is important to evaluate, as muscle loss can be an early indicator of possible acute or chronic disease. Forms are available online on the WSAVA Global Nutrition Toolkit webpage.[3]

DAILY CALORIC REQUIREMENTS FOR THE HEALTHY DOG AND CAT

Many factors affect the energy requirements of animals. Daily caloric requirements are altered by the physiological state (e.g. adult maintenance, pregnancy, lactation, growth), activity level, temperament, environmental temperature, and the diet's digestibility.

How do you know if a patient is eating enough? There are many formulas for calculating patient energy needs, for growth, weight loss, weight gain, extremely active individuals, and resting energy requirement (RER). Start by calculating the patient's RER. There are several formulas for calculating this. The author recommends using one of the following calculations, but use the one you are most comfortable with.

$$\text{RER} = 70 \times (\text{body weight in kg})^{0.75}$$

$$\sqrt{\sqrt{}}\,\text{x}(\text{weight in kg} \times \text{weight in kg} \times \text{weight in kg}) = \times 70 = \text{RER}$$

These calculations are easily done using the calculator application on most smartphones; simply turn the phone to the landscape view to access required functionality.

The formula below may also be used for patients weighting more the 2 kg and less than 45 kg. However, this formula should not be used for patients smaller or larger than these guidelines or for critical patients:

$$\text{RER} = 30 \times (\text{body weight in kg}) + 70$$

Once you have determined the patient's RER, the next step is to calculate their daily energy requirement (DER). DER is calculated by multiplying RER by a coefficient based on the patient's life stage and body condition. A list of coefficients for common life stages to determine DER is listed in Table 17.1.

Requirement	Canine	Feline
Growth	≤ Up to 4 months = 3 × RER	Growing kittens = 2.5 × RER
	> 4 months = 2 × RER	
Maintenance	Average neutered adult = 1.6 × RER	Normal neutered adult = 1.2 × RER
	Intact adult = 1.8 × RER	Intact adult = 1.4 × RER
	Obese prone = 1.4 × RER	Obese prone = 1.0 × RER
	Weight loss = 1.0 × RER	Weight loss = 0.8 × RER
Work	Light work = 2 × RER	
	Heavy work = 4 – 8 × RER	

Table 17.1 / Coefficients for common life stages to determine daily energy requirements[4]

It is important to remember that all caloric calculations are estimates of the average dog and cat's energy needs; actual caloric intake may vary from one individual to another. These calculations, however, are an excellent starting point for every nutritional recommendation.

Once the DER has been established, the amount of food required per day is calculated based on the specific diet to be fed. AAFCO guidelines require the calorie content to be listed on the packaging. The patient's daily calorie requirement is divided by number of calories in a can or cup of the selected to calculate the volume of food the dog or cat should be fed each day. This amount must be divided by the number of feeding the et will receive each day.

Note that the majority of pet owners treat their pets. Pet owners feel a connection through treating their pet and studies show owners believe treating is a way to connect with their pet and to demonstrate love for the pet. This strengthens the human–animal bond. Ask what treats are fed daily during the nutritional history to find out the type of treat, the amount of treat, and potential persons involved in treating. It is OK for owners to treat as long as the veterinary healthcare team realizes and calculates the treat calories into the DER. Treats should not constitute more than 10% of the daily caloric intake. Treat recommendations should come from the veterinary healthcare team.

Table 17.2 / Key nutritional requirements[4]

Condition	Energy Density (kcal ME/g)	Crude Fat and Essential Fatty acids (%)	Crude Fiber (%)	Crude protein (%)	Phosphorus (%)	Sodium (%)	Chloride (× Na)	Magnesium (%)	Antioxidants (Amount/kg food)		
									Vitamin E (iu)	Vitamin C (mg)	Selenium (mg)
Young adult dogs											
Normal body weight and condition	3.5–4.5	10–20	≤ 5	15–30	0.4–0.8	0.2–0.4	1.5	–	≥ 400	≥ 100	0.5–1.3
Inactive or obese prone	3.0–3.5	7–10	≥ 10	15–30	0.4–0.8	0.2–0.4	1.5	–	≥ 400	≥ 100	0.5–1.3
Mature dogs											
Normal body weight and condition	3.0–4.0	10–15	≥ 2	15–23	0.3–0.7	0.15–0.4	1.5	–	≥ 400	≥ 100	0.5–1.3
Inactive or obese prone	3.0–3.5	7–10	≥ 10	15–23	0.3–0.7	0.15–0.4	1.5	–	≥ 400	≥ 100	0.5–1.3

(*Continued*)

Table 17.2 / Key nutritional requirements (Continued)

Condition	Energy Density (kcal ME/g)	Crude Fat and Essential Fatty acids (%)	Crude Fiber (%)	Crude protein (%)	Phosphorus (%)	Sodium (%)	Chloride (× Na)	Magnesium (%)	Antioxidants (Amount/kg food)		
									Vitamin E (iu)	Vitamin C (mg)	Selenium (mg)
Young adult cats											
Normal body weight and condition	4.0–5.0	10–30	< 5	30–45	0.5–0.8	0.2–0.6	1.5	0.04–0.1	≥ 500	100–200	0.5–1.3
Inactive or obese prone	3.3–3.8	9–17	5–15	30–45	0.5–0.8	0.2–0.6	1.5	0.04–0.1	≥ 500	100–200	0.5–1.3
Mature cats											
Normal body weight and condition	4.0–5.0	18–25	< 5	30–45	0.5–0.7	0.2–0.4	–	0.05–0.1	≥ 500	100–200	0.5–1.3
Inactive or obese prone	3.5–4.0	10–18	5–15	30–45	0.5–0.7	0.2–0.4	–	0.05–0.1	≥ 500	100–200	0.5–1.3

All units are expressed as dry matter.

FEEDING METHODS

The method by which pets are fed should be evaluated as it can also affect their nutritional health. The chosen method will mostly affect the weight of the animal by the quantity of food that is eaten, leading to either obesity or anorexia.

Table 17.3 / Feeding methods.

Feeding method	Advantages	Disadvantages
Free choice	• Easy for owner • May be preferred by picky eaters • Those requiring multiple small meals a day • Ideal for animals during pregnancy and lactation	• 30–40% of animals become overweight on this method • Does not work with canned or semi-moist food due to spoiling • Medical problems or anorexia may be difficult to identify • May not be suited for multiple pet households
Time restricted	• Easy for owners • Allows owner to monitor eating and observe for medical conditions • Works with all food choices	• Encourages gluttony and aerophagia • Does not work well with cats or those not able to consume enough food in the given time
Meal feeding	• Allows owner to monitor eating and observe for medical conditions • Works with all food choices • Decreases likelihood of obesity	• Time commitment on the part of the owner

Feeding the Reluctant Eater

Caring for a pet that is reluctant to eat can be frustrating for owners, and owners often consider appetite an indication of quality of life in elderly and pets suffering from chronic disease. A complete physical examination including appropriate diagnostic testing and treatment initiated of any disease. Inappetence, including hyporexia (decreased eating), dysrexia (altered patterns of eating), and anorexia (complete lack of eating) may be indication of disease. Prolonged inappetence, if untreated, can be detrimental to the underlying condition. Once underlying heath issues have been ruled out, assessing feeding practices and recommending changes may improve food consumption in health pets.

Consider the following when trying to encourage pets to eat:

- Diet:
  - Preference for certain flavors, smells, and textures, which may change frequently.
  - Add top dressings such as baby food or canned food (intermittently, not intended for long term).
  - Separate foods with varying degrees of odors to determine preference (e.g. strong or mild odor).
  - Cold foods can decrease the odor.
  - Offer a variety of foods with differing flavors and textures, both canned and dry.
  - Preference for moist, warm, cold, or fresh food.
  - Warm the food; stir the food well before feeding to avoid hot spots.
  - Add water to either dry food (to moisten) or canned food (to make a slurry).
- Food container/bowl:
  - Determine the bowl shape based on head shape.
  - Flat plates may be required for brachycephalic breeds.
  - Use wide and shallow bowls for cats to avoid their whiskers touching the sides and causing irritation.
- Environment:
  - Place feeding dishes in easy-to-reach locations or on an elevated platform to avoid bending over (e.g. arthritic pet, deep-chested breeds).
  - Feed in a stress-free environment that is away from loud noises and other pets.
  - Avoid dominance/competition from other pets.
  - Spray the environment with feline facial pheromones (feline).
- Social:
  - Often animals, especially cats, are social eaters and prefer to have company and petting to stimulate eating.
- Medication:
  - Appetite stimulants may be indicated.

Feeding the Overexcited Eater

Dogs are sometimes overexcited eaters, inhaling their food without a second thought. Altering the feeding situation can either force them to eat more slowly or remove the urgency:

- Food container:
  - Place food in a food container/toy that slowly releases the food.
  - Feed in container designed for overexcited eaters with built-in obstacles to eat around.
  - Place a large rock or ball in the feeding bowl to provide an obstacle to eat around. *Important*, obstacles must be too large to fit in the dogs mouth so as not to be a choking hazard.
  - Portion out each meal into a muffin pan to increase difficulty and to reduce speed.
  - Offer small amounts multiple times over a period.
- Environment:
  - Feed in an area away from other pets to avoid dominance/competition.
  - Offer food only once the pet is calm.

PET FOOD EVALUATION

Pet Food Label Evaluation

Table 17.4 includes some of the guidelines that AAFCO has established. AAFCO establishes the nutritional standards for complete and balanced pet foods, but it is the pet food company's responsibility to formulate their products according to the appropriate AAFCO standard (AAFCO.org). Pet food regulations are enforced by the state feed control officials. For a complete description of the pet food labeling requirements, the AAFCO guidelines and state requirements should be reviewed.

Table 17.4 / Pet food label evaluation: association of american feed control officials guidelines

Product	Definition	Comments
Name		
Ingredient (usually meat, poultry, or fish)	• 95% of the ingredients listed in the product name must be of the product excluding water for processing	• Example: beef or chicken for cats • This does not include water added for processing • If two names are listed, they must total 95% when added together, but the first name must constitute a greater percentage than the second item listed • This rule only applies to products of animal origin
Dinner, platter, entrée	• Must be a minimum of 25% stated meat, excluding water for processing, and at least 10% of total weight	• Example: chicken dinner, chicken and liver entrée • This does not include water added for processing • With more than one product listed, they must total 25% when added together, but the first name must constitute a greater percentage than the second item listed • This rule applies to all ingredients listed in the product name, not just those of animal origin • Other words may be substituted for dinner such as "platter," "entrée," "nuggets," or "formula"
With	• The inclusion of the word "with" in the product names confirms there is 3% or more, excluding water, of the ingredient in the product	• Example: cat food with chicken
Flavor	• Must have stated ingredient in the ingredient list, generally less than 3%	• Example: salmon-flavored dog food
"in gravy" or "in sauce"	• May contain 78% or more moisture	• Canned foods may not be greater than 78% moisture • Foods with "in gravy" or "in sauce" in their name are allowed to have moisture of 78% or more
Claims		
Premium/super premium/ gourmet	• Marking term with no legal definition • Intended to imply a product of higher-quality ingredients but there is no guarantee of quality	• Does not currently have regulations to restrict its use

(Continued)

Table 17.4 / **Pet food label evaluation: association of american feed control officials guidelines (Continued)**

Product	Definition	Comments
Natural	• Consists of only natural ingredients without chemical alterations, except for added vitamins and minerals	• Is intended to imply a product without artificial flavors, colors, or preservatives • "Added vitamins and minerals" are not required to be natural
Organic	• Refers to the handling and processing of ingredients and products	• Pet food manufacturers are expected to comply with USDA National Organic Program to display USDA Organic Seal
Package information		
Ingredient list	• All products listed in order of descending weight before processing	• This includes their water content and can give a false perception when comparing two products of different water contents • Terminology used to describe ingredients are also regulated (e.g. meat, meat meal) • Name defines what can actually be included (e.g. meat meal: the rendered product from mammal tissues, exclusive of blood, hair, hoof, horn, hide trimmings, manure, stomach, and rumen contents except in such amounts as may occur unavoidably in good processing practices) • Refer to AAFCO guidelines for a complete list of ingredient list definitions
Guaranteed analysis	• Regulations require inclusion of the minimum percentages for crude protein and fat and the maximum percentages for crude fiber and moisture	• The term "crude" used in analysis refers to the method of testing, not the quality of the nutrient • Percentages between products are compared on a dry-matter basis, removing the moisture component • The dry matter of dry food is approximately 88–90% and 22–25% for canned food
Nutritional adequacy statement	• Products allowed to use the AAFCO nutritional adequacy statement must either meet the AAFCO nutritional nutrient profiles or have undergone the AAFCO feeding trial protocol (fed to the intended species with supporting data regarding the results on how the animal did while eating the specific food)	• The statement will also include the life stage the product is intended for: • *All life stages:* formulated to meet the needs of all animals, including those during growth and reproduction • *Maintenance:* will meet the needs of an adult, non-reproducing dog or cat of normal activity • *Puppy, kitten, or growth:* formulated to meet the needs of animals during growth • *Gestation and lactation:* formulated to meet the needs of reproducing females • Products labeled with the terms, "snack," "treat," or "supplement" must list "intended for intermediate or supplemental feeding only"

Comparing Nutrient Levels on a Dry-Matter Basis

When initially comparing the two diets, it appears as if the dry food diet has more protein than the canned diet. However, once the water content is removed and the diets are compared on a dry matter basis, it becomes apparent that the canned food has significantly more protein.

Table 17.5 / **Comparing nutrient levels on a dry-matter basis**

Estimating dry matter	Basis	Canned food	Dry food
Example		Guaranteed analysis: • crude protein (min.) 10.0% • crude fat (min.) 5.0% • crude fiber (max.) 1.0% • moisture (max.) 78.0% • ash (max.) 3.0% • taurine (min.) 0.05%	Guaranteed analysis: • crude protein (min.) 24.0% • crude fat (min.) 19.0% • crude fiber (max.) 3.0% • moisture (max.) 10.0% • ash (max.) 5.0% • taurine (min.) 0.08%
Step 1: determine the percentage of dry matter	Dry-matter: (100 – moisture content) ÷ 100	(100 – 78) ÷ 100 = 0.22 22% of diet is dry matter	(100 – 10) ÷ 100 = 0.90 90% of diet is dry matter
Step 2: determine nutrient levels on a dry-matter basis	(Nutrient % ÷ dry matter) × 100 = nutrient level on a dry-matter basis	Protein: (10% ÷ 22) × 100 = 45% Fat: (5% ÷ 22) × 100 = 23% Ash: (3% ÷ 22) × 100 = 14%	Protein: (24% ÷ 90) × 100 = 27% Fat: (19% ÷ 90) × 100 = 21% Ash: (5% ÷ 90) × 100 = 6%

Home-Prepared Diets

Home-prepared diets can be a valuable option to pet owners, for example, pets with adverse food reactions, those experiencing multiple medical conditions where a commercially prepared diet is not appropriate or when therapeutic diets are not accepted by the pet. The important factor to consider when feeding these diets is the nutritional adequacy. Diets must be those formulated by a board-certified veterinary nutritionist to guarantee that proper nutrients have been included and not altered. The most significant complication in home-prepared diets is the altering of ingredients and inadequacy of nutrients. Although these changes may seem insignificant to the owner, their health ramifications can be profound. Therefore, pets being fed a home-prepared diet should have a nutritional evaluation as recommended by a board-certified veterinary nutritionist to verify the health status of the pet and to verify the content of the specific diet being fed.

Dietary Supplements

In the early history of the commercially available dog and cat foods, dietary supplements were commonly used to supplement diets containing poor-quality ingredients and formulas that were not complete and balanced. Complete and balanced pet foods were introduced to the market during the 1960s, although some owners continued to use dietary supplements. A marked increase in types and quantity of dietary supplement sales has been reported over the past decade; these increases mirror similar trends in sales of human dietary supplements.

A large variety of products types are available for the pet owner; vitamins, minerals, herbal, botanicals, antioxidants, probiotics, and probiotics may be purchased in health food stores, pet supply stores, veterinary offices, and online. These products are often referred to as "nutraceuticals", a term with no formal definition.

A common misconception that there is no government regulation of dietary supplements is not accurate. However, it is likely that not all dietary supplement products are not completely in compliance with state and federal laws. Some commercial products may contain substances that are not listed on the product label, safety or dosing has not been established, and labels may contain unsubstantiated claims.

The Center for Veterinary Medicine (CVM) is responsible for the regulation of animal feed products including dietary supplements. "The Dietary Supplement and Health Education Act (DSHEA) of 1994, has affected the way FDA regulates" food for humans, "i.e. among other things, it restricts substances from being food additives or drugs if the product meets the definition of a dietary supplement. However, the agency's assessment of the law is that it was not intended and does not apply to animal feed, including pet food. This assessment was published in the Federal Register on April 22, 1996 (61 FR 17706). Thus, products marketed as dietary supplements or" feed supplements "for animals still fall under the FFDCA prior to DSHEA, i.e. they are considered" foods "or" new animal drugs "depending on the intended use (see below). The regulatory status of a product is determined by CVM on a case-by-case basis, using criteria provided in Guide 1240.3605 in Program Policy and Procedures Manual."[5] Malnutrition, with the exception of obesity, is infrequent in companion animals. Most receive ample nutrition to sustain a healthy life through their regular daily diet. Most dog and cat foods are rich in nutrients, either through the natural content of the ingredients or from manufacturer supplementation. Healthy animals on balanced rations do not require extra nutritional supplementation; in fact, excessive amounts of certain nutrients may cause health problems. The correct use of supplements is based on a diagnosis of a nutrient deficiency.[4]

Disease Nutritional Requirements

Nutritional management and support can have a positive effect on a great many diseases. Some would say nutritional support can have a positive impact on all diseases. The role nutrition plays on specific diseases varies. Sometimes it can reduce or eliminate clinical signs, extend life expectancy, improve quality of life, or even cause remission. Key points for nutritional support of a handful of diseases commonly seen in the veterinary hospital are provided below. It also bears mentioning that this is by no means intended to be an all-inclusive list of diseases that benefit from nutritional support; that would require writing a whole textbook.

Table 17.6 / Key nutritional factors in disease[4]

Key nutritional factors	Dogs	Cats
Chronic kidney disease		
Protein (%)	14–20	28–35
Phosphorous (%)	0.2–0.5	0.3–0.6

(Continued)

Table 17.6 / Key nutritional factors in disease (Continued)

Key nutritional factors	Dogs	Cats
Sodium (%)	≤ 0.3	≤ 0.4
Chloride	1.5 × sodium level	1.5 × sodium level
Potassium (%)*	0.4–0.8	0.7–1.2
Omega-3 fatty acids (%)	0.4–2.5	0.4–2.5
Omega-6 to omega-3 fatty acid ratio	1 : 1 – 7 : 1	1 : 1 – 7 : 1
Antioxidants		
Vitamin E (iu/kg)	≥ 400	≥ 500
Vitamin C (mg/kg)	≥ 100	100–200
Hepatic lipidosis or cholangitis		
Energy density (kcal/g)	≥ 4.0	≥ 4.2
Protein (%)	15–20	30–35
Protein (patients with hepatic encephalopathy) (%)	10–15	25–30
Arginine (%)		1.5–2.0
Taurine (%)	≥0.1	≥ 0.3
Sodium (%)	0.08–0.25	0.07–0.3
Copper (mg/kg)	≤ 5	
Zinc (mg/kg)	> 200	> 200
Iron (mg/kg)	80–140	80–140
Vitamin E (iu/kg)	≥ 400	≥ 500
Vitamin C (mg/kg)	≥ 100	100–200
Irritable bowel disease		
Highly digestible diets:		
Potassium (%)	0.8–1.1	0.8–1.1

(Continued)

Table 17.6 / **Key nutritional factors in disease (Continued)**

Key nutritional factors	Dogs	Cats
Energy density (kcal/g)	≥ 3.2	≥ 3.4
Fat (%)	8–12	9–18
Protein (%)	≥ 25	≥ 35
Protein (elimination diets) (%)	16–26	30–45
Crude fiber – increased fiber diets (insoluble preferred) (%)	7–15	7–15
Digestibility (increased fiber diets):		
Protein (%)	≥ 80	≥ 80
Fat (%)	≥ 90	≥ 90
Carbohydrate (%)	≥ 90	≥ 90
Chronic constipation or obstipation		
Water	> 75%	> 75%
Crude fiber (insoluble or mixed): chronic constipation and intermittent obstipation	≥ 7%	≥ 7%
Fiber: megacolon	≤ 5%	≤ 5%
Energy density (megacolon)		≥ 4%
Digestibility (megacolon):		
Fat		≥ 90%
Carbohydrate		≥ 90%
Protein		≥ 87%
Small bowel diarrhea		
Sodium (%)(%)	0.3–0.5	0.3–0.5
Chloride	0.5–1.3	0.5–1.3

(Continued)

Table 17.6 / **Key nutritional factors in disease (Continued)**

Key nutritional factors	Dogs	Cats
Potassium (%)	0.8–1.1	0.8–1.1
Fat (%)	8–12	9–18
Energy density (increased fiber diets)	≥ 3.2	≥ 3.4
Fiber (increased fiber diets, insoluble preferred)	7–15	7–15
Digestibility (increased fiber diets):		
Protein	≥ 80	≥ 80
Fat	≥ 90	≥ 90
Carbohydrate	≥ 90	≥ 90
Pancreatitis		
Fat (non-obese and non-hypertriglyceridemic) (%)	≤ 15	≤ 25
Fat (obese and/or hypertriglyceridemic) (%)	≤ 10	≤ 10
Protein (%)	15–30	30–40
Cardiovascular disease		
Sodium (%)	0.08–0.25	0.07–0.30
Chloride	1.5	1.5
Taurine (%)	≥ 0.1	≥ 0.3
L-carnitine (%)	≥ 0.2	
Phosphorus (%)	0.2–0.7	0.3–0.7
Potassium (%)	≥ 0.4	≥ 0.52
Magnesium (%)	≥ 0.06	≥ 0.04
Diabetes mellitus**		
Increased-fiber/high carbohydrate diet:		
Fiber (%)	7–18	7–18

(Continued)

Table 17.6 / **Key nutritional factors in disease (Continued)**

Key nutritional factors	Dogs	Cats
Fat (%)	< 25	< 25
Protein (%)	15–35	28–55
Low carbohydrate/high protein diet:		
Fat (%)	–	< 25
Protein (%)	–	28–55

* Lower in hyperkalemic patients.
** Avoid semi-moist foods.
All values listed are on a dry matter basis. Water should be available at all times.

OBESITY MANAGEMENT

The health risks associated with obesity are extensive including: diabetes mellitus, lower urinary tract disease, osteoarthritis, hypertension, hypothyroidism, hyperadrenocorticism, pregnancy complications, heart disease, skin disorders, hepatic lipidosis, higher anesthetic risk, some cancers, ruptured cruciate ligament, and pancreatitis (dogs) as well as many other conditions that have been associated with obesity.

Prevention Plan

Perhaps more important than weight loss for overweight and obese pets is working with clients to promote ideal weight for dogs and cats before they become too heavy. Here, communication is the key.

Begin at the first visit to the veterinary hospital educating clients how to score body and muscle condition. Handouts containing pictures of ideal and overweight dogs are useful tools for client education. Many people today are accustomed to seeing overweight dogs and often mistakenly confuse dogs in ideal weight as too thin. Having pictures of dogs in ideal weight and condition will help clients to better understand how to distinguish when their dog is beginning to become too heavy. Take photographs of each patient at its ideal body condition and use these images to illustrate the goal that the owner should try to achieve.

At each subsequent puppy or kitten and wellness visit, start with taking a nutritional history, documenting all changes including the patient's current weight. Ask the client to score the body and muscle condition of their own pet. If your assessment differs from the clients, explain how you arrived at your score. Remember to discuss the need to reduce the caloric intake of your patients at the time of neutering. Make a nutritional recommendation, based on the patient's BCS, MCS, and activity level. Discuss your recommendation at discharge from the surgical procedure, include your nutritional recommendation in your written discharge instructions, and in your follow-up call after discharge. Follow up with another call or email in a month after neutering. Communicate the importance of a healthy weight multiple ways and multiple times.

Consider starting a client education page on your hospital website and/or Facebook page. A new puppy/kitten group is also a great way to promote good feeding practices, as well as housebreaking and training education for clients. If your hospital offers puppy training or obedience classes, nutrition education can easily be added to the curriculum. Clients can be taught how to perform BCS and MCS on their own pets and can practice the techniques on each other's puppies and dogs.

Also consider starting a healthy weight educational campaign at your hospital. Invite new puppy and kitten owners to attend a "tips for keeping your puppy or kitten healthy" get-together. Explain the health benefits of keeping their pet at a healthy weight, risks of obesity, the importance of exercise, etc. Teach owners how to score their pet's body condition, have them practice scoring each other's pets. Discuss healthy treat options, types of human foods to avoid and the potential dangers of feeding food not made for dogs or cats. Provide handouts containing the information and links to your hospital website's "healthy weight" page.

Find local puppy training classes and ask to speak to the class, contact local shelters, rescue groups, humane societies, etc. Offer to hold healthy weight classes at their facility for the staff/volunteers and people adopting a dog or cat.

Weight Loss Plans

Support groups for clients with overweight pets, similar to groups people join when trying to lose weight, are also a good way to help facilitate weight loss for overweight pets. Clients can share tips and weight loss techniques that have worked for their pets with others that might not be having as much success. Each pet can be weighed at each group meeting, goals set and progress documented. Establish a nutritional history and make a nutritional recommendation focusing on weight loss before a new member joins the group. Provide clients with forms to document everything their pet eats, including the amount consumed, from one meeting to the next. Having clients record exactly what and how much their pet consumes each day gives a more accurate account of the number of calories consumed during the time period. A nutritional recommendation, revised if necessary, is given for each pet at each meeting. Incentivize participants to meet weight loss goals by offering such items as discounts on pet food or reduced calorie treats. Remember, however, that educating clients on the lifelong health benefits of pets in ideal body weight and condition is often the best motivation of all.

We must teach owners to perform BCS on their puppies and dogs. We must make a nutritional recommendation for every pet, at every visit, including the correct volume to feed and the total calories to feed per day. We all know that we all do that, but it is not working: we need other tools to help our clients succeed and make it easier for them to maintain their pets at a healthy weight.

Here are a few tips to try to set your clients up for success with their pets weight loss plan:

- Create a weight loss plan form and weight loss plan follow up form (Figure 17.3). List the food the pet is fed, calories per cup and/or can, the treats the client normally feeds, how many you recommend they feed, treats they sometimes feed, everything they feed, including the calorie content of everything. Use the form to document your nutritional recommendation.
- Give clients 8-oz measuring cups. Use a marker to indicate the amount their pet should be fed at each meal
- Use resealable plastic bags, branded with your hospital information, to send home individually portioned meals for the first few days or weeks. Use a permanent marker to indicate the correct amount to feed at each meal.
- Develop a weekly food log (Figure 17.1) and ask owners to record what they feed their pet every day. Owners will have a better understanding how "just feeding a little more" or giving "just a few more treats" can make a big difference in the number of calories their pet is consuming. Ask clients to share their feeding record with you weekly to start; the ones that do well and maintain their pet at a healthy weight for several months could perhaps share their success tips with others in the group at meetings. Emailing their feeding record to the clinic, sharing a Google document, or some other type of electronic document-sharing system are good, easy-to-manage options.
- Remember to discuss exercise. Encourage owners to walk their dogs more often, longer distances, and to use play in place of some treats. Food puzzles are a great option for both dogs and cats. Suggest that cat owners use the natural instinct to "hunt" their food by hiding small portions of their cat's meals around the house, placing some upstairs, downstairs, on a shelf or cat tree to encourage the cat climb.
- Warn cat owners about the dangers of hepatic lipidosis. If a cat is not eating, prolonged fasting due to refusal of a new diet is not recommended.

Educate your clients on the advantages of feeding a diet specifically designed for weight loss. These diets are formulated to avoid nutrient deficiencies and a reduced caloric density. Overly reducing the volume of a maintenance diet is not recommended and may lead to nutrient deficiencies. Canned cat food formulas are less calorically dense and have lower carbohydrate levels than dry formulations. Research has shown that a diet with low-energy density due to increased water content reduced weight gain and increased physical activity. Research has also shown L-carnitine to be beneficial in increasing lean muscle mass, fat utilization, and weight loss.[6]

Weight Loss Plan for ____________________

☐ **Examination**

☐ Physical exam ☐ Diagnostic testing

☐ **Complete Diet History Form**

☐ **Determine current caloric intake**

Determine the amount of calories the pet is currently consuming. If an accurate number is not possible, calculate the daily energy requirement for the pet with the process listed below.

Step 1: Calculate daily resting energy requirement (RER)

- The minimum calories that need to be consumed to maintain the weight and health of an animal at rest:

RER = 70 × (current body weight in kg)$^{0.75}$ = ______ kcal/day

or, for animals weighing between 2 and 30 kg:

RER = (30 × current body weight in kg) + 70 = ______ kcal/day

Tip: To calculate (BW kg)$^{0.75}$ without a scientific calculator, multiply the weight by itself three times, then take the square root twice.

Step 2: Calculate daily energy requirement (DER) by multiplying the RER by the activity factor.

- The minimum calories that need to be consumed to maintain weight and health considering their activity level.

DER = (RER × _____ activity factor) = _____ kcal/days

Adult activity factor	Canine	Feline
Inactive—neutered	1.6	1.2
Inactive	1.8	1.4
Active working	2.0–6.0	1.6

Adjust kcal based on visual and manual examination of animal.

☐ **Determine altered caloric intake**

DER X 60–80% = __________ total # of kcal/day to restrict to achieve a weight reduction of 1–2%/week

☐ **Determine diet and quantity**

- The kcal of the diet can be found on the bag, by contacting the manufacturer or following the equation below.

_____ kcal/day / _____ kcal/cup or can of food = _____ cup/can(s) of food/day

	Estimating Calorie Content	Example
	CP = crude protein, CF = crude fat, Fib = fiber, M = moisture, A = ash	Guaranteed analysis: crude protein (min) 10.0%, crude fat (min) 5.0%, crude fiber (max) 1.0%, moisture (max) 78.0%, ash (max) 3.0%, taurine (min) 0.05%. 1 can = 156 g
Step 1: Estimating carbohydrate content	100 –(CP% + CF% + Fib% + M% + A%)	100 – (10 + 5 + 1 + 78 + 3) = 3 3% of the diet is carbohydrates
Step 2: Estimating the calories from the macronutrients	Calories from protein = CP % × 3.5 kcal/g Calories from fat = CF % × 8.5 kcal/g Calories from carbohydrates = CHO % × 3.5 kcal/g	Protein: 10% × 3.5 = 0.35 kcal/g Fat: 5% × 8.5 = 0.425 kcal/g Carbohydrates: 3% × 3.5 = 0.105 kcal/g
Step 3: Estimating total calories	Total calories/100 g food = calories from protein + calories from fat + calories from carbohydrates	(0.35 + 0.425 + 0.105) = 0.88 calories/g food (35 + 42.5 + 10.5) = 88 cal/100 g food
	(Total calories/kg food = total calories/100 g food ×10)	0.88 cal/g × 156 g = 137.28 calories per can

☐ **Determine targeted program length**

- Each kg is equal to 7700 kcal.

(Amount to lose)kg × 7700 kcal/kg = ______ total # of kcal to restrict to reach targeted BW

(total # of kcal to restrict) / (# of kcal restricted per day) = _____ total # of days to reach targeted BW

☐ **Identify risk factors**

☐ Free feeding ☐ Lack of exercise ☐ Calorically dense diets ☐ Neutering

☐ Excessive treats ☐ Additional food sources

☐ **Protein**

- Verify the protein content of the food at the recommended calories is adequate for that particular pet (1 g protein/lb BW/day). Failure to verify protein content may lead to muscle loss along with fat loss.

☐ **Medication**

- The addition of microsomal triglyceride transfer protein inhibitors (e.g., Slentrol) may prove beneficial, as well as modifying feeding amounts and habits.

☐ **Follow up:**

- Weight check every 2–3 weeks to ensure a weight loss with a goal of 1–2% per week. (Weight loss >2% can be detrimental to the pet's health.) If this number is not obtained, verify all recommendations are being followed by the owner and then further restrict calories by 10%.

Figure 17.3 Example weight loss plan forms. (*Continued*)

Weight loss plan follow up

Pet name:____________ Owner's name: ____________

Current body weight:____ lb____ kg BSC:________

Program Goals

Target program weight:____ lb____ kg BSC:________

Daily calorie intake: ________ 10% adjusted: ________

Target program length: ________ week

Date	Week	Weight	BCS	Percent loss	Adjustment

Figure 17.3 Example weight loss plan forms. (*Continued*)

NUTRITIONAL SUPPORT

Many hospitalized patients are at risk of becoming severely malnourished because they lack the desire or ability to eat. In response to injury and illness, the body breaks down protein, depleting the body's protein stores. Providing protein, carbohydrate, fat, and other nutrients slows the breakdown of lean body mass and optimizes the patient's response to therapy. Injuries and illnesses can further increase a patient's caloric requirement, making nutritional support even more crucial. There are many ways to provide this support, both enterally and parenterally. The following sections give basic guidelines for choosing the correct method and administration protocols.

Enteral Nutrition

Enteral nutrition is the preferred way of providing nutrition. Providing nutrition to some portion of the gastrointestinal tract allows for the health and integrity of the tract to remain. Prolonged periods of non-use contribute to its mucosal barrier failure and systemic bacterial contamination. Patients that are unable or unwilling to eat at least 85% of their RER but are able to digest and absorb nutrients in the small intestines should be provided nutrition by this route. Depending on the patient's medical condition, there are many options for providing enteral nutrition.

Nasoesophageal and Nasogastric Feeding Tubes

Feeding tubes are generally tolerated well by most patients and most are relatively easy to place. Nasogastric tubes are inserted into the nostril, through the nasal cavity into the esophagus, terminating in the stomach and Nasoesophageal tubes are inserted into the nostril through the nasal cavity terminating in the distal esophagus, these tubes may be placed by technicians.

Nasogastric and nasoesophageal tubes are useful for patients who are unwilling to or are unable to eat but have normal gastrointestinal function. Placement does not require anesthesia and usually can be done without sedation, by using a topical anesthetic. They are used short term, usually for less than 14 days, and are sometimes used until the patient is stable enough to be anesthetized for a longer term feeding tube placement. Nasoesophageal/nasogastric tubes are contraindicated in patients that are actively vomiting, comatose, do not have a gag reflex, or have nasal tumor/nasal disease. Since these tubes are generally quite small (usually 8 French or smaller) patients may be fed only liquid food. Complications associated with the tubes include epistaxis caused by nasal mucosa irritation, aspiration pneumonia should the tube become dislodged due to vomiting or regurgitation, and esophageal stricture (although this is rare).

Nasogastric and Nasoesophageal Tube Placement

Materials needed for placement

- Tetracaine or proparacaine
- Sterile lubricant jelly
- Appropriately sized tube:

- 2.0 or 3-0 nylon suture material
- Scissors
- 22-gauge needle
- Permanent marker
- Empty 6-cc syringe
- 6-cc syringe of sterile water
- E-collar

Placement Procedure

- Elevate the patients muzzle and apply a few drops of a topical anesthetic, such as proparacaine hydrochloride ophthalmic solution 0.5% into the nostril you have selected for tube placement. Allow five minutes before attempting to insert tube.
- While you are waiting, place a stay suture as close to the nose as possible.
- An easy way to place a stay suture is quickly insert a 22-gauge needle through the skin at the point where the wing of the nostril meets the fur. With the needle in place insert a 2.0 or 3.0 nylon suture through the needle from the beveled tip and out the hub of the needle. While holding the suture remove the needle. Tie a square knot closely to the skin but loosely enough to allow passing another suture under it.
- Measure and mark tube
  - A nasoesophageal tube measures to the seventh or eighth intercostal space. The tip of the tube will fall in the distal esophagus, this will reduce likelihood of reflux esophagitis.
  - A nasogastric tube measures to the last rib. The tip of the tube will fall either slightly before or in the stomach.
- Apply a sterile lubricant to the tube.
- Holding the patients muzzle with your non-dominant hand, begin inserting the tube with your other hand. Press the patient's nose upward using the thumb of the hand that is holding the muzzle.
- Once you have inserted the tube about the length of the patient's muzzle, lower the patients head, pointing its nose downward slightly. These motions should help to guide the tube into the esophagus rather than the trachea.
- Continue to advance the tube until you have reached the mark you made when measuring the tube prior to placement. The patient may or may not swallow during placement. Gently stroking the throat may encourage swallowing which may assist the feeding tube to more easily pass down the esophagus.
- If the patient begins to cough at any time during placement, STOP, remove tube and try again. Lack of coughing *does not* ensure that the tube is not in the trachea.
- Attach a 6-ml syringe to the tube and check for negative pressure.
- If negative pressure exists, flush 5–6 ml sterile water into tube. If the patient coughs, the tube is in the trachea. If the patient does not cough, placement *may* be correct, confirmation with a radiograph is recommended.
- Cap the tube with an injection cap and temporally suture the tube to the stay suture, leaving long tails to secure tube in place once proper placement is confirmed.
- Confirm placement with a single left or right lateral post-procedural radiograph.
- Once proper placement is confirmed, secure the tube with a Chinese finger-trap suture.
  - The finger-trap suture is perfect for feeding tubes; it continues to tighten if the tube is tugged.
  - Pass a long piece of suture through the previously placed stay suture and secure with a square knot. Then begin the Chinese finger-trap pattern.
  - Wrap the suture around the tube, crisscrossed and tied into a square knot. Repeat a minimum of five crosses.
  - For red rubber tubes, each throw should be pulled tight enough to make a small indentation in the tube.
  - For silicone tubes, pull tightly; beware that indenting these tubes may cause them to become occluded.
- Secure the other end of the tube in a second location either on the cheek (the facial nerves run across this area of the cheek so the suture should go through the skin but be kept as superficial as possible) or on the top of the head. Tie a loose square knot near the skin then secure

the tube with a second square knot. This may also be done with the 22-gauge needle method described above. Smaller diameter tubes may also be attached in this second location with surgical staples.

- The patient may require an Elizabethan collar to prevent tube removal.

Esophageal Tubes

Esophageal tubes are surgically inserted in the neck and terminate in the distal esophagus. They are usually larger (often 14 Fr or larger), allowing for commercial complete and balanced diets blended with additional water. Esophageal tubes allow longer-term use and clients are able to use them to administer bolus feedings and medications at home. A minimum of 5–6 ml water should be flushed through the tube before use, to ensure that the tube has not become displaced, and after every feeding to prevent clogging. Surgical placement under brief general anesthesia is required.

Percutaneous Endoscopic Gastrostomy Feeding Tubes

Percutaneous endoscopic gastrostomy feeding (PEG) tubes are used for long-term cases and clients are able to administer bolus feedings and medications at home. General anesthesia is required and placement via an endoscope is recommended, although they may also be placed "blind". Feeding via the PEG tube can begin as early as 12 hours post-placement, although waiting 24 hours is usually recommended. Once a PEG tube is placed it should not be removed for 10–14 days, to prevent leakage of gastric contents into the abdominal cavity. This type of feeding tube can remain in place for months and maybe replaced with a low-profile tube for longer-term use. The incision site may require superficial cleaning for a few days post-insertion. A minimum of 10 ml water should be flushed through the PEG tube after every feeding to prevent clogging. After removal, the gastrocutaneous tract closes within 24 hours.

Other Less Common Feeding Tubes

Pharyngostomy requires anesthesia for placement. Care must be taken that the tube does not interfere with the laryngeal opening and epiglottis. Pharyngostomy tubes are not commonly used, as they are generally no large than nasoesophageal and nasogastric tubes (which do not require anesthesia to place) and thus only liquid diets may be used.

Jejunostomy tubes are normally 5–8 Fr and thus only liquid diets may be used. They are placed within the small intestine, surgically, or via laparotomy. Since the stomach is bypassed and the small intestine has limited storage space, constant rate infusion (CRI) feeding is ideal, although some patients tolerate frequent small bolus feedings quite well. Jejunostomy tubes are not often used unless the stomach must be bypassed. The cost is usually same or similar to gastrostomy tubes that can be used by owners at home and can be left in for much longer periods.

ENTERAL NUTRITION ADMINISTRATION

Nasogastric and Nasoesophageal Feeding

The general recommendation for feeding patients who have not been eating is to begin with one quarter of the patients total RER for the first 12 hours and, if well tolerated, to increase by one quarter of their total RER every 12 hours until full RER is reached. If at any time the patient vomits, discontinue feedings until vomiting has resolved, reduce the volume when feeding is resumed, and increase the volume more slowly.

Only liquid veterinary diets should be used for feeding through these tubes. The volume of water added can be varied dependent on the diameter of the feeding tube, but the caloric density is reduced as the volume of water is increased. Trickle feeding via CRI is most often used for hospitalized patients, although these tubes may also be used for bolus feedings and to administer oral liquid medications. Tablets should not be crushed and administered via these small tubes.

Liquid diets designed for people are also available. These diets are typically less expensive than veterinary liquid diets, but they are nutritionally inadequate, and some may contain ingredients that are inappropriate for dogs and cats. These human diets are especially inappropriate for cats as they are too low in protein, taurine, and arginine.

Esophageal Feeding

A calorically dense canned dog or cat food is blended with an appropriate amount of water to allow the mixture to be drawn into a feeding tip syringe and passed through a feeding tube of the same diameter as patients feeding tube. The volume of food to meet the patient's DER and the amount of water required to dilute to the required consistency for tube feeding should be recorded and used as a recipe for future use.

The mixture should be warmed to body temperature (100–102°F) before feeding by placing the can into a hot water bath for five minutes. Do not use a microwave, as the food may not heat evenly, leaving too cool and/or too hot areas. Water and liquid medications may also be administered through the tube. The patient's total daily caloric intake is normally split into three or four feedings per day. It is advisable to start by feeding small amounts for the first three or four days, gradually increasing to the desired daily total. Educate clients on feeding via tube and tube maintenance prior to discharge.

Feeding procedure

- Flush the tube with 5 ml water before and after food administration.
- Medications may be given with food. If administered separately without food, then flush 5–6 ml before and after administration of medication.
- Use a feeding tip syringe to pull up the food.
- Slowly feed over 15–20 minutes.
- If the patient starts to drool, lick their lips excessively or vomits then stop the feeding. Wait 5–10 minutes then try again more slowly.
- If this happens again, stop the feeding and wait at least one hour before resuming.
- If the tube becomes clogged:
  - Fill the tube with warm water, cap, and let set for 10–15 minutes. Try flushing the tube again.
  - If the clog has not been dislodged, flush the tube with cola (yes, that's right, cola, it works). Fill the feeding tube with cola (usually about 2–6 ml – the amount will vary depending on the tube size), leave it in for 20–30 minutes, and then try to flush with water again.

PEG Tube Feeding Procedure

- Before every feeding, aspirate the feeding tube by attaching a syringe to the end of the feeding tube and drawing back on the plunger. If a small amount of fluid is collected, then feeding can proceed. If an excessive amount is aspirated, do not feed; wait one hour and recheck. The quantity of fluid considered excessive is dependent on the size of the PEG tube.
- The prescribed amount of food should be feed over 20 minutes.
- Food should be warmed to body temperature (100–102°F) by placing the can into a hot water bath for five minutes. Do not microwave, as the food may not heat evenly leaving too cool or too hot areas. Mix the food with a spoon for three to five minutes until very soft and smooth. Water and liquid medications may also be administered through the tube. When warming always check the temperature to make sure it is not too hot.
- Start with feeding a small amount of food every six hours, then increase to one quarter of the patient's daily caloric requirement of food every six hours, if feedings are well tolerated, over the next one to two weeks.
- After the feeding, flush the feeding tube with 6 ml water and close the cap.
- If the patient is not drinking, water may be supplemented via the feeding tube every eight hours, not during feedings.

PARENTERAL NUTRITION

Parenteral nutrition supplies calories and nutrients to patients that cannot or should not have enteral nutrition. A balanced nutritional solution is compounded from components such as dextrose (carbohydrates), lipids (fats) and amino acids (proteins). While components can be used alone, it is usually not recommended because longer-term use can cause nutritional deficiencies.

Parenteral nutrition is administered through an aseptically placed intravenous catheter. Central and peripheral lines can both be used. A central line should be used for total parenteral nutrition because of its high osmolality. High osmolality solutions are irritating to the vein, and extravasation can lead to severe phlebitis. It is generally safe to administer solutions of less than 660 mOsm/kg osmolality through a peripheral vein. Unfortunately, this may limit the total calories and volume of the parenteral nutrition. Partial parenteral nutrition can be administered through a peripheral catheter only if the osmolarity is <660 mOsm/kg. It is typically calculated to provide 70% of the RER.

A dedicated catheter should be used for all parenteral nutrition solutions. To avoid contamination and precipitates, no other medications or fluids should be administered through the system. If a multilumen catheter is used, one lumen should be dedicated to parenteral nutrition, usually the proximal port. Once connected to the patient, the line should not be disconnected except in true emergency situations or to change out the administration/bag.

Parenteral nutrition and the IV administration system should be handled with clean exam gloves in an aseptic manner. Avoid contact with the open ends of IV lines and do not allow these lines to contact the floor or other contaminated surfaces. Daily examination of the IV catheter site and change of the IV catheter bandage are mandatory.

Parenteral nutrition should not be disconnected for walks or procedures except in a true emergency. If the line is disconnected from the patient intentionally or accidentally, it should be aseptically replaced above the disconnection point. Each bag of parenteral nutrition is formulated to last 24 hours and is usually calculated to be administered at a maintenance fluid rate.

Complications

Complications of parenteral nutrition can generally be grouped into three categories: metabolic, mechanical or infectious. Metabolic complications are most common, with hyperglycemia seen most frequently. The most important way to avoid mechanical or septic complications is proper prevention. Careful attention to asepsis at the time of IV catheter placement and continued daily catheter care are essential. An Elizabethan collar should be placed on animals receiving parenteral nutrition through peripheral catheters.

Parenteral nutrition is an excellent growth medium for bacteria. If sepsis/infection is suspected, the parenteral nutrition solution and tip of the IV catheter can be submitted for culture.

Skill Box 17.1 / Worksheet: Calculation of Total Parenteral Nutrition.

1. Resting energy requirement (RER)

$RER = 70 \times (\text{current body weight in kg})^{0.75}$

or, for animals weighing 2–30 kg:

$RER = (30 \times \text{current body weight in kg}) + 70 =$ ____ kcal/day.

2. Protein requirements

Requirement	Protein (g/100 kcal)	
	Canine	Feline
Standard	4	6
Decreased (hepatic/renal failure)	2	3
Increased (protein-losing conditions)	6	6

$(RER \div 100) \times$ ____ $\text{g/100kcal (protein req)} =$ ____ $\text{g protein required/day}$

3. Volume of nutrient solutions

a. *8.5% amino acid solution (0.085 g protein/ml)*

____ g protein required/day ÷ 0.085 g/ml

= ____ ml/day of amino acids

b. *Non-protein calories*

- The calories supplied by protein (4 kcal/g) are subtracted from the total calories needed to get the total non-protein calories needed:

  ____ g protein required/day × 4 kcal/g = ____ kcal from protein

  ____ total kcal required/day – kcal from protein

  = ____ total non-protein kcal needed/day.

(Continued)

Skill Box 17.1 / worksheet: calculation of total parenteral nutrition (continued)

c. *Non-protein calories are usually provided as a 50 : 50 mixture of lipid and dextrose.*

- This ratio may need to be adjusted if the animal is hyperglycemic or hypertriglyceridemic.

20% lipid solution (2 kcal/ml)
To supply 50% of non-protein calories ____ lipid kcal required ÷ 2 kcal/ml = ____ ml/day of lipid
50% dextrose solution (1.7 kcal/ml)
To supply 50% of non-protein calories ____ dextrose kcal required ÷ 1.7 kcal/ml = ____ ml/day of dextrose

4. Total daily requirements

____ ml 8.5% amino acid solution
____ ml 20% lipid solution
____ ml 50% dextrose solution (use half on first day)
____ ml total volume of TPN solution ÷ 24 hours = ____ ml/hours infusion rate

Be sure to adjust the animal's other intravenous fluids accordingly. TPN vitamins and trace metals can be added during formulation if indicated.

Skill Box 17.2 / Worksheet: Calculation of Peripheral or Partial Parenteral Nutrition.

1. Resting energy requirement (RER)

$RER = 70 \times (\text{current body weight in kg})^{0.75}$

or, for animals weighing between 2 and 30 kg:

$RER = (30 \times \text{current body weight in kg}) + 70 = RER =$ _____ kcal / day.

2. Partial energy requirement (PER)

To supply 70% of the patient's RER:

$PER = RER \times 0.70 = PER =$ _____ kcal / day.

3. Nutrient requirements

Patients 3–10 kg:

PER × 0.25 = ____ kcal/day from dextrose
PER × 0.25 = ____ kcal from amino acids
PER × 0.50 = ____ kcal/day from lipids

Patients 10–25 kg:

PER × 0.33 = ____ kcal/day from dextrose
PER × 0.33 = ____ kcal from amino acids
PER × 0.33 = ____ kcal/day from lipids

Patients >25 kg:

PER × 0.50 = ____ kcal/day from dextrose
PER × 0.25 = ____ kcal from amino acids
PER × 0.25 = ____ kcal/day from lipids

4. Volume of nutrient solutions 5% dextrose (0.17 kcal/ml)

____ kcal/day from dextrose ÷ 0.17 kcal/ml = ____ ml/day

5% amino acids (0.34 kcal/ml):

____ kcal/day from amino acids ÷ 0.34 kcal/ml = ____ ml/day

20% lipid (2 kcal/ml):

____ kcal/day from lipid ÷ 2 kcal/ml = ____ ml/day

5. Total daily requirements

_____ ml 5% dextrose
_____ ml 8.5% amino acids
_____ ml 20% lipid
_____ ml total volume of PPN solution ÷ 24 hours = _____ ml/hours infusion rate

This calculation should approximate a patient's maintenance fluid requirements. Be sure to adjust the animal's other intravenous fluids accordingly. The volume may be higher than maintenance fluid requirements for very small animals (< 3 kg) or in animals with cardiac disease. TPN vitamins and trace metals can be added during formulation if indicated.

REFERENCES

1. WSAVA Global Nutrition Committee. (2021). Guidelines on Selecting Pet Foods. Dundas, Ontario: World Small Animal Veterinary Association. https://www.wsava.org/WSAVA/media/Arpita-and-Emma-editorial/Selecting-the-Best-Food-for-your-Pet.pdf (accessed 28 July 2021).
2. WSAVA Global Nutrition Committee. (2021). Short Diet History Form. Dundas, Ontario: World Small Animal Veterinary Association. https://wsava.org/global-guidelines/global-nutrition-guidelines (accessed 28 July 2021).
3. WSAVA Global Nutrition Committee. (2021). Body condition score tools for dogs and cats. https://wsava.org/global-guidelines/global-nutrition-guidelines (accessed 28 July 2021).
4. Hand, M.S., Thatcher, C.D., Remillard, R.L. *et al.* (2010). *Small Animal Clinical Nutrition*, 5e. Topeka, KS: Mark Morris Institute. http://www.markmorrisinstitute.org/sacn5_download.html (accessed 28 July 2021).
5. US Food and Drug Administration. (2021). Product regulation. https://www.fda.gov/animal-veterinary/animal-food-feeds/product-regulation (accessed 29 July 2021).
6. Little, S. (2017). *Successful Weight Loss: Finding the inner cat.* Lakewood, CO: American Animal Hospital Association.

Chapter 18

Pain Management

Mary Ellen Goldberg, LVT, CVT, SRA, CCRVN, CVPP, VTS (Lab Animal), (Physical Rehabilitation), (Anesthesia and Analgesia-H)

Veterinary Technician and Nurse's Daily Reference Guide: Canine and Feline, Fourth Edition. Edited by Mandy Fults and Kenichiro Yagi.

Companion website: www.wiley.com/go/fults/veterinary

Abbreviations

CNS, central nervous system
CRI, constant rate infusion
DJD, degenerative joint disease
DMSO, dimethyl sulfoxide
FDA, US Federal Drugs Administration
IM, intramuscular
IV, intravenous
NK1, neurokinin-1
NMDA, N-methyl-D-aspartate
NSAIDs, non-steroidal anti-inflammatory drugs
OHE, ovariohysterectomy
PO, orally
SDS, simple descriptive scale
SQ, subcutaneously
SSNRI, selective serotonin-norepinephrine reuptake inhibitor
SSRI, selective serotonin reuptake inhibitor
UNESP, São Paulo State University

INTRODUCTION

What is pain and why do we care for our companion animal patients? This chapter attempts to answer this question to allow the veterinary technician to advocate for their patients that experience pain. We have definitive proof that untreated pain causes immediate changes in the neurohormonal axis, which in turn causes restlessness, agitation, increased heart and respiratory rates, fever, and blood pressure fluctuations, all of which are detrimental to the healing of the animal.

A catabolic state is created as a result of increased secretion of catabolic hormones and decreased secretion of anabolic hormones. The majority of neurohormonal changes produced is an increase in the secretion of catabolic hormones. Hyperglycemia is produced and may persist because of production of glucagon and relative lack of insulin. Lipolytic activity is stimulated by cortisol, catecholamines, and growth hormone. Cardiorespiratory effects of pain include increased cardiac output, vasoconstriction, hypoxemia, and hyperventilation. Protein catabolism is a common occurrence and major concern regarding healing.[1] Pain associated with inflammation causes increase in tissue and blood levels of prostaglandins and cytokines, both of which promote protein catabolism indirectly by increasing the energy expenditure of the body. In both human and veterinary medicine, pain is recognized as a disease. Pain encompasses the entire body and can often be the only thought that the patient can dwell upon.

Evidence indicates that multimodal analgesia may produce a modification of the responses to these physiologic changes. Variable reductions in plasma cortisol, growth hormone, antidiuretic hormone, beta-endorphin, aldosterone, epinephrine, norepinephrine, and renin are based on the analgesic technique and the drugs selected.[2] Prophylactic administration of analgesics blunts the response before it occurs. Analgesics administered following perception or pain are not as effective, and higher doses are generally necessary to achieve an equivalent level of analgesia. It is therefore prudent to use preoperative, intraoperative and postoperative analgesia. Multimodal pain management incorporates several classes of analgesics used at the same time with lower dosages. This makes it safer for the patient and allows the overall effect of pain to be less instead of using a high dose of just one class of medication.

PAIN DRUG CATEGORIES

Pain medications are drugs used to relieve discomfort associated with disease, injury, or surgery. Because the pain process is complex, there are many types of pain drugs that provide relief by acting through a variety of physiological mechanisms. Thus, effective medication for nerve pain will likely have a different mechanism of action than arthritis pain medication. The prescription arsenal against pain is extensive. It includes non-steroidal anti-inflammatory drugs (NSAIDs) and opioids. There are also some unconventional analgesics – drugs that were not originally developed as pain relievers but have been found to have pain-relieving properties in certain conditions, such as anticonvulsants, antidepressants like serotonin and norepinephrine reuptake inhibitors and N-methyl-D-aspartate (NMDA) receptor antagonists (Table 18.1).

Table 18.1 / Categories of pain medications

Class	Examples	Pain uses	Special considerations
Opioids:			
Short acting	Fentanyl, remifentanil	Anesthetic premedication, intra- and postoperative, trauma, medical treatment of acute pain	• Often via CRI rather than bolus
Longer acting	Morphine, hydromorphone, oxymorphone, methadone	Anesthetic premedication, intra- and postoperative, trauma, medical treatment of acute pain, chronic	• Adverse events include vomiting, respiratory depression, bradycardia; hydromorphone may cause hyperthermia (cats only)
Partial μ-opioid agonist, κ-opioid antagonist	Buprenorphine	Anesthetic premedication, intra- and postoperative, trauma, medical treatment of acute pain, chronic	• Less effective than full opioid agonists for analgesia
Partial κ-opioid agonist, mixed agonist/antagonist at μ-opioid receptor	Butorphanol	Anesthetic premedication, intra- and postoperative, trauma, medical treatment of acute pain, chronic	• Short acting; less effective than full opioid agonists for analgesia
Opioid and serotonin-affecting agent	Tramadol	intra- and postoperative, chronic, medical treatment of acute pain	• Oral formulation only; bitter taste
NSAIDs	Carprofen, meloxicam, deracoxib, Firocoxib, robenacoxib	intra- and postoperative, chronic, medical treatment of acute pain (cautious use), trauma	• Caution in animals with impaired renal, hepatic function; read data sheet carefully

(*Continued*)

Table 18.1 / **Categories of pain medications (Continued)**

Class	Examples	Pain uses	Special considerations
Local anesthetic agents	Lidocaine, bupivacaine	intra- and postoperative	• Useful for numerous local blocks and epidural; lidocaine may be administered via IV; must be careful with toxicity levels in cats
α2-adrenergic agonists	Medetomidine, dexmedetomidine, xylazine	Anesthetic premedication, intra- and postoperative	• Healthy patients only
NMDA antagonist	Ketamine	Anesthetic premedication, intra- and postoperative, trauma, medical treatment of acute pain (?)	• Dissociative anesthesia with analgesia; analgesic at subanesthetic doses
Anesthetic	Nitrous oxide	intraoperative	• Analgesic carrier gas used in combination with oxygen for inhalant anesthesia; do not exceed two-thirds N_2O by volume
Anticonvulsant	Gabapentin	Chronic	• Licensed for chronic pain management in humans
NMDA receptor antagonist	Amantadine	Chronic	• Amantadine is not expected to provide analgesic effects as a sole therapy, but may enhance the analgesic effects of NSAIDs, opioids, or gabapentin
Tricyclic anti-depressants	Amitriptyline	Chronic	• As a class, the most effective medications for neuropathic pain in humans
SS(N)RIs	Duloxetine, venlafaxine	Chronic	• has a chronic pain label in humans
Antiemetic	Maropitant®	Anesthetic premedication, chronic, medical treatment of acute pain, postoperative	• blockade of substance P to the NK1 receptor
Bisphosphonates	Pamidronate	Chronic	• exerts anti-osteoclast activity and can contribute to pain relief in dogs with bone cancer

(Continued)

Class	Examples	Pain uses	Special considerations
Corticosteroids	Glucocorticoid	Chronic, medical treatment of acute pain, trauma	• Glucocorticoids may have beneficial effects to reduce edema associated with CNS neoplasia
Glucosamine and chondroitin	Nutritional supplements	Chronic	• Current literature does not support the use of glucosamine and chondroitin supplements for the control of osteoarthritis pain in dogs
Polysulfated glycosaminoglycans	Adequan	Chronic	• the control of signs associated with noninfectious degenerative and/or traumatic arthritis of canine synovial joints
Anticonvulsant	Pregablin	Chronic	• an FDA-approved anticonvulsant and an analgesic for diabetic neuropathy, postherpetic, and fibromyalgia pain in humans

Table 18.1 / Categories of pain medications(Continued)

HISTORY OF THE SCIENCE OF PAIN

Rene Descartes, a French philosopher and scientist, can be credited with the first writings that attempted to describe the physiology of pain. Published in his *Treatise of Man* in 1664, Descartes depicted pain as the transmission of a stimulus (e.g. a burn from fire, from the skin through a single channel to the brain). In 1965, Melzack and Wall published a revolutionary theory about the physiology of pain, which proposed that pain sensations were "gated" within the spinal cord, where modulation could occur to either intensify or deintensify the painful stimulus as it was transmitted to the brain.[3] Thirty years later, Patrick Wall proposed that pain processing occurs as an integrated matrix, occurring at minimally three layers: peripheral, spinal, and supraspinal sites. Today, in the treatment of pain, strategies are employed that target these three sites in a multimodal approach to analgesia by using various classes of analgesics.

NOCICEPTION

Nociception (*nocer*, Latin, to injure or to hurt) or the pain "pathway" is the sensation of pain. Pain is "an unpleasant sensory and emotional experience associated with actual or potential tissue damage or described in terms of such damage".[4] Veterinary species may be unable to communicate that pain is being experienced, but this lack of evidence should never be interpreted that pain does not exist or does not warrant treatment.

Nociceptors are free (bare) nerve endings found in the skin, muscle, joints, bone and viscera. In the skin and deep tissues, there are additional nociceptors called "silent" or "sleep" nociceptors. These receptors are normally unresponsive to noxious mechanical stimulation but become "awakened" (responsive) to mechanical stimulation during inflammation and after tissue injury. One possible explanation of the "awakening" phenomenon is that continuous stimulation from the damaged tissue reduces the threshold of these nociceptors and causes them to begin to respond. This activation of silent nociceptors may contribute to the induction of hyperalgesia, central sensitization, and allodynia. Many visceral nociceptors are silent nociceptors.

Hyperalgesia is an increased painful sensation in response to additional noxious stimuli. One explanation for hyperalgesia is that the threshold for pain in the area surrounding an inflamed or injured site is lowered. An additional explanation is that the inflammation activates silent nociceptors and/or the damage elicits continuing nerve signals (prolong stimulation), which lead to long-term changes and sensitized nociceptors. These changes contribute to an amplification of pain or hyperalgesia, as well as an increased persistence of the pain. If one pricks normal skin with a sharp probe, it will elicit sharp pain followed by reddened skin. The reddened skin is an area of hyperalgesia.

Allodynia is pain resulting from a stimulus that does not normally produce pain. For example, a light touch to sunburned skin produces pain because nociceptors in the skin have been sensitized as a result of reducing the threshold of the silent nociceptors. Another explanation of allodynia is that when peripheral neurons are damaged, structural changes occur and the damaged neurons reroute and make connection also to sensory receptors (i.e. touch-sensitive fibers reroute and make synaptic connection into areas of the spinal cord that receive input from nociceptors).

Nociception refers to the processing of a noxious (harmful or damaging) stimulus resulting in the perception of pain by the brain. The components of nociception include transduction, transmission, modulation and perception (Figure 18.1).[5] Transduction is the conversion of a noxious stimulus (mechanical, chemical or thermal) into electrical energy by a peripheral

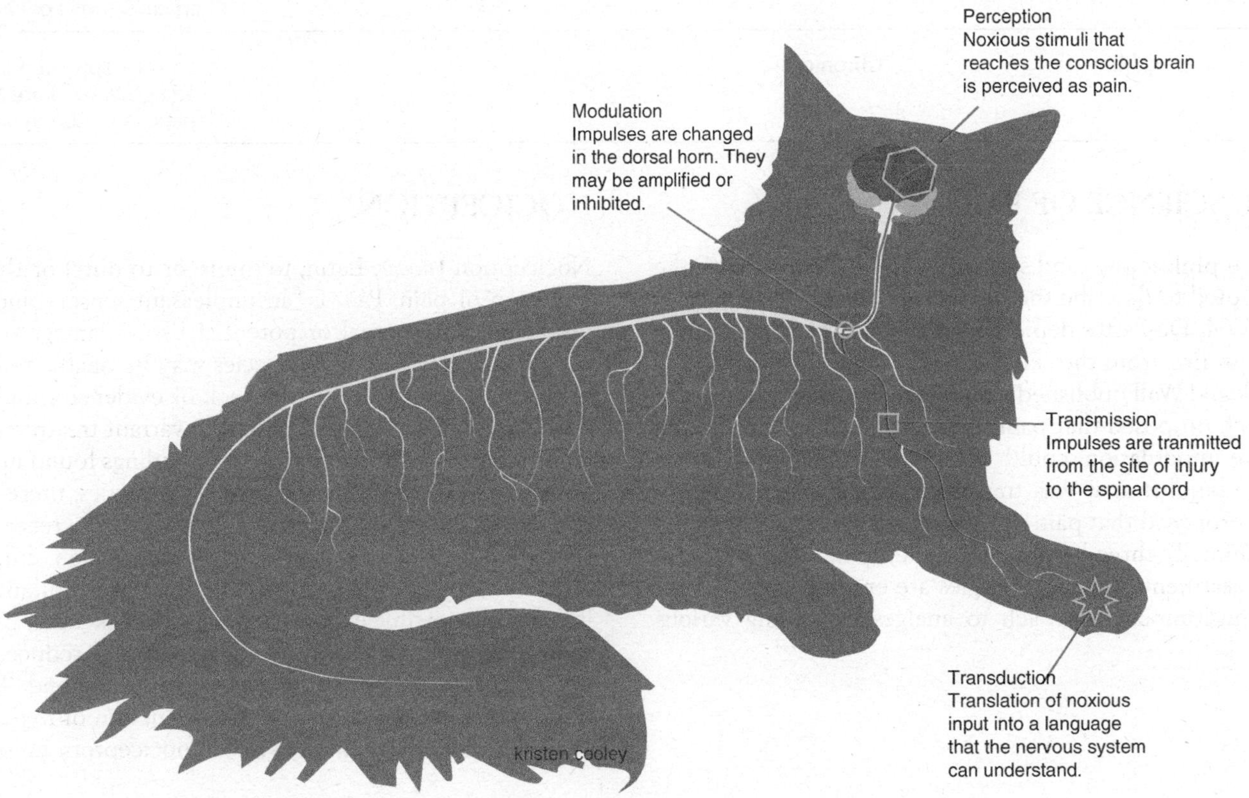

Figure 18.1 The nociceptive pathway. Source: courtesy of Kristen Cooley.

nociceptor (free afferent [conducting or conducted inward or toward] nerve ending). This is the first step in the pain process, and can be inhibited by NSAIDs, opioids and local anesthetics.

Transmission describes the movement through the peripheral nervous system via first-order neurons. Nerve fibers involved include A-delta (fast) fibers responsible for the initial sharp pain, C (slow) fibers that cause the secondary dull, throbbing pain, and A-beta (tactile) fibers, which have a lower threshold of stimulation. Transmission can be reduced by local anesthetics and alpha-2 agonists. Modulation occurs when first-order neurons synapse with second-order neurons in the dorsal horn cells of the spinal cord. Excitatory neuropeptides (including, but not limited to, glutamate, aspartate and substance P) can facilitate and amplify the pain signals in ascending projection neurons. At the same time, endogenous (opioid, serotonergic and noradrenergic) descending analgesic systems serve to dampen the nociceptive response. Modulation can be influenced by local anesthetics, alpha-2 agonists, opioids, NSAIDs, tricyclic antidepressants and NMDA receptor antagonists.

Perception is the cerebral cortical response to nociceptive signals that are projected by third-order neurons to the brain. It can be inhibited by general anesthetics, opioids and alpha-2 agonists.

Peripheral sensitization occurs when tissue inflammation leads to the release of a complex array of chemical mediators, resulting in reduced nociceptor thresholds. This causes an increased response to painful stimuli (primary hyperalgesia). Central sensitization refers to an increase in the excitability of spinal neurons, mediated in part by the activation of NMDA receptors in dorsal horn neurons (spinal cord). The net effect is expanded receptor fields (pain in neighboring areas not subjected to injury, or secondary hyperalgesia) and painful responses to normally innocuous stimuli (mediated by A-beta fibers and referred to as allodynia). The combination of peripheral and central sensitization results in an increase in the magnitude and duration of pain (Box 18.1).

Box 18.1 / What medications work where in the nociceptive pathway?

What drugs work in transduction?

- NSAIDS (e.g. carprofen, meloxicam, robenacoxib)
- Opioids (e.g. morphine, hydromorphone)
- Local anesthetics (lidocaine, bupivacaine)
- Corticosteroids (e.g. dexamethasone, methylprednisolone acetate, prednisone)

What drugs work on transmission?

- Local anesthetics (lidocaine, bupivacaine)
- Alpha-2-agonists (dexmedetomidine, xylazine)

What drugs work during modulation?

- Local anesthetics (lidocaine, bupivacaine)
- NSAIDS (e.g. carprofen, meloxicam, robenacoxib)
- Opioids (e.g. morphine, hydromorphone)
- Alpha-2-agonists dexmedetomidine, xylazine)
- NMDA antagonists (ketamine, amantadine)
- Tricyclic antidepressants (amitriptyline)
- Anticonvulsants (gabapentin)

What drugs work on perception?

- Opioids (e.g. morphine fentanyl)
- alpha-2-agonists (dexmedetomidine, xylazine)
- general anesthetics (isoflurane, sevoflurane)
- benzodiazepines (diazepam, midazolam)
- phenothiazines (acepromazine)

CLASSIFICATION OF PAIN

Pain has been classified into two major types (acute and chronic) with further subheading breakdowns.

Acute

Acute or pricking pain is pain caused by a needle, pin prick, skin cut, and so on. It elicits a sharp, pricking, stinging, pain sensation carried fast by the A delta fibers. The pain is precisely localized and of short duration. Pricking pain is also called fast pain, first pain, or sensory pain. Pricking pain is present in all individuals and is a useful and necessary component of our sensory repertoire. Without this type of protective pain sensation, everyday life would be difficult. Pricking pain arises mainly from the skin and carried mainly by A delta fibers which permits discrimination (i.e. permits the subject to localize the pain). Surgical pain is acute pain. Acute pain is often referred to as adaptive pain. This type of pain normally does not persist past three months. The term adaptive pain is defined as pain that triggers the initiation of responses and behaviors that contribute to animal survival and promote wound healing or prevent further injury.

Chronic

Chronic, burning pain, soreness pain, aching pain is pain caused by inflammation, burned skin, and so on. This pain is carried by the C fibers (slowly conducted pain nerve fibers). This type of pain is more diffuse, has slower onset, and is longer in duration. It is an annoying and often intolerable pain, which is not distinctly localized. Chronic, aching pain is a sore pain. This pain arises mainly from the viscera and somatic deep structures. Aching pain is carried by the C fibers from the deep structures to the spinal cord. Pain that persists longer than three months (chronic pain) is referred to as maladaptive pain. Maladaptive pain is defined as pain that is persistent or recurrent after healing and acts as a disease with abnormal sensory processing.

SUBCLASSIFICATIONS OF PAIN

Neuropathic

Neuropathic pain is a complex, chronic pain state that usually is accompanied by tissue injury or disease. With neuropathic pain, the nerve fibers themselves might be damaged, dysfunctional, or injured.[6] These damaged nerve fibers send incorrect signals to other pain centers. The impact of a nerve fiber injury includes a change in nerve function both at the site of injury and areas around the injury. Common qualities include burning or coldness, "pins and needles" sensations, numbness and itching.

Inflammatory pain results from tissue damage and trauma and can lead to inflammation or persistent inflammatory pain. The typical example is osteoarthritis. Acute inflammatory pain serves not so much as an alarm, but more as a reminder of recent injury, discouraging activities that risk reinjury so that recovery can proceed quickly. Unlike acute inflammation, chronic inflammation can have long-term and whole-body effects. Chronic inflammation is also called persistent, low-grade inflammation because it produces a steady, low-level of inflammation throughout the body, as judged by a small rise in immune system markers found in blood or tissue. This type of systemic inflammation can contribute to the development of disease.

Breakthrough pain can occur even with patients who appear to be well managed, they may still have episodes of breakthrough pain. Breakthrough pain is an acute pain episode that is not controlled by the current pain management plan and requires additional but typically short-term treatment. Clients should be educated about breakthrough pain and have a plan in place for treatment.

Wind-up pain can occur in patients who have been experiencing chronic pain, even low levels of chronic pain. Wind-up is an exaggerated response to pain resulting in hyperalgesia and allodynia. Wind-up can be prevented with the early identification and treatment of pain and with the use of constant rate infusions (CRI). The addition of microdose ketamine has shown to be very effective for the prevention and treatment of wind-up pain. Wind-up phenomenon not only increases pain intensity but also increases pain duration. This phenomenon is experienced through the NMDA receptors. The brain is even able to perceive pain in the absence of a painful stimuli.

In both humans and animals, neonates and pediatric patients do feel pain. Untreated pain in neonates can cause amplified pain sensation as the patient ages and may lead to chronic pain in adulthood.

PAIN MANAGEMENT MYTHS

1. *Analgesics Mask the Physiological Indicators of Patient Deterioration*

Evidence exists in both human and veterinary medicine showing that analgesics do not mask the physiological indicators of patient deterioration. In fact, if the patient were treated adequately for pain, any changes in physiological indicators would indeed be attributable to patient deterioration rather than a pain stress response.

2. *Potential for Toxicity or Adverse Reactions is Associated with Drug Administration*

With our current level of understanding, there is no longer an overpowering reason to avoid the use of analgesics. Many drug options exist for both canines and felines, with proven guidelines to allow safe administration.

3. *Pain is Hard to Recognize*

It is best to think of animal pain in terms similar to human pain. Treat for this level of pain, regardless of whether you think the animal is truly showing signs of pain. Assume that invasive procedures, trauma, and illness result in a need for analgesics. Merely being aware and observing for behavioral signs of pain will make recognition easier.

4. *Pain Keeps an Animal from Moving Around and Injuring Itself*

Research has shown that pain makes a patient more agitated and unable to relax and rest. Pacing, changing position, and chewing at the incision are behaviors that indicate pain rather than boredom or agitation. Continuous pain can also contribute to poor healing, decreased immune function, and increased inflammation. In cases of excessive activity, sedation and confinement can be used to control the activity level of the patient.

5. *The Breed is Just a Wimp*

Each animal and human experience and exhibit pain differently. Some breeds tend to show stronger reactions to pain, therefore having a lower threshold to pain. This additional knowledge can lead to better preemptive pain management in particular breeds.

CANCER PAIN

Pain in cancer is produced by pressure on, or chemical stimulation of, nociceptors (nociceptive pain), or it may be caused by damage or illness affecting the nerve fibers themselves (neuropathic pain). Between 40% and 80% of patients with cancer pain experience neuropathic pain.[7]

Tumors Associated with Pain

Tumors associated with pain include:[8,9]

1. Primary bone tumors such as osteosarcoma, fibrosarcoma, chondrosarcoma or hemangiosarcoma.
2. Tumors metastatic to bone, such as prostate carcinoma or mammary carcinoma.
3. Multiple myeloma.
4. Central nervous system tumors, particularly spinal tumors.
5. Inflammatory mammary carcinoma, although large mammary tumors may also be painful.
6. Lower urinary tract tumors and those involving the prostate may be painful.
7. Oral tumors, especially if invasive to bone.
8. Invasive cutaneous tumors.
9. Intrathoracic tumors, particularly if disseminated and involving the pleura.
10. Intra-abdominal tumors, particularly if placing traction on the root of the mesentery, causing complete or partial obstruction of the intestinal tract or resulting in distension of the capsule of solid organs.

THE ROLE OF THE VETERINARY TECHNICIAN IN PAIN MANAGEMENT

Veterinary technicians are in the unique position of being responsible for most of the quality of patient care.[10] They must advocate for patients that cannot speak for themselves.

Knowledge of the physiology of pain and pharmacology of analgesics is essential for good communication between veterinarians and veterinary technicians. The skilled technician is a source of vital information required to choose and administer appropriate analgesics. Familiarity with patient personalities and reactions to stimuli give additional insight into how particular patients may react when painful.

Advocating for the patient means looking for differences in expression between dogs and cats, and young and old, plus for variations among breeds. There are "grimace scales" showing facial expressions for mice,[11] rats,[12] rabbits,[13] ferrets,[14] cats,[15] horses,[16] cattle,[17] sheep,[18,19] goats,[20] and pigs.[21] These grimace scales rate pain in the animal facial expression.

Familiarity with the current principles of pain management, including preemptive and multimodal therapies and prevention of the "wind-up" phenomenon, are vital and must be put into practice.

The roles of the veterinary technician in pain management include:

1. Patient pain recognition and assessment.
2. Providing non-pharmacological comfort and care.
3. Differentiating pain from other stress.
4. Requesting appropriate analgesia and sedation.
5. Administering medications and performing analgesic techniques.
6. Monitoring and treating drug effects.
7. Assessing patients after surgery.
8. Communicating with clients about hospital and at-home care.
9. Logging controlled substances.

Communication among all members of the entire health care team, including veterinarians, veterinary technicians, assistants, and pet owners, is essential for consistent pain management. Veterinary technicians have the responsibility of continually monitoring their patients and often develop a sense of which analgesics seem to work best under various circumstances. Based on their interaction with patients, the technician may offer suggestions for adjustments in analgesic regimens, changes or additions to drug protocols, or the possible addition of sedatives, if needed. Technicians should provide as much feedback as possible as to which analgesic protocols are working well and which need to be improved to increase patient comfort (Box 18.2) Discussion about each case directly with the clinician should address concerns or expectations, potential for adjustments in analgesic regimens (as-needed injections to a constant rate infusion [CRI]), changes or additions to drug protocols (adding a NSAID or an adjunctive analgesic), or the possible addition of sedatives if needed. Pain management issues, such as the appearance and behavior of the patient that prompted the administration of analgesics; the type, dose, and timing of previous analgesic administration; and the response and any adverse reactions after administration, should be described to all those caring for the animal and recorded in the medical record.

Box 18.2 / "Do not quit until pain quits"

1. Pain medications prescribed by the patient's veterinarian need to be sent home with patients.
2. The owners must be educated to recognize signs of pain in their animal.
3. Owners must be educated in administering the medications.
4. Owners must be able to judge if the analgesic is effective and be encouraged to request additional analgesia if the pet's pain persists beyond the anticipated period.

PAIN ASSESSMENT AND RECOGNITION

The World Small Animal Veterinary Association (WSAVA) tenets of pain assessment and recognition are:[22]

- Pain is an illness, experienced by all mammals, and can be recognized and effectively managed in most cases.
- Pain assessment should accompany every patient assessment.
- Treat predictable pain – pain associated with surgery is 100% predictable (Table 18.2).
- Pain assessment is key to determining the degree and duration of pain treatment but should not replace the adage of treating predictable pain.
- Perioperative pain extends beyond 24 hours and should be managed accordingly.
- Practice preventive (preemptive) pain management – initiate appropriate treatment before a procedure to prevent the onset of pain, and continue this to prevent occurrence of pain for the duration of time commonly recommended for the problem or which the patient requires.
- Response to appropriate treatment is the gold standard to measure the presence and degree of pain.

Surgical procedures, illnesses, and injuries are known to cause pain in humans and the same pain is expected in animals. Table 18.2 can be used as a starting place to preemptively treat animals for an expected pain. Providing a pain management plan based solely on this information would be inaccurate as it would not account for the individual pain response of each patient. Understanding the expected pain level will also help to determine the correct drug or combination of drugs to administer, the route, and the duration.

Table 18.2 / Expected pain associated with illness, injury, and surgical and hospital procedures

	Mild to moderate	Moderate	Moderate to severe	Severe to excruciating
Illness	• Anal sac impaction • Chin acne, severe • Constipation/obstipation • Cystitis • Otitis • Urinary tract infections • Vaginitis	• Dental disease (tooth abscess, fractures or lesions, stomatitis, oral tumors or ulcers) • Diabetic neuropathy • Gastrointestinal obstruction • Pancreatitis (early or resolving) • Urethral obstruction	• Cancer • Corneal disease (glaucoma, uveitis) • Degenerative joint disease • Foreign body • Gastroenteritis, hemorrhagic • Osteoarthritis, acute polyarthritis • Peritonitis • Pleural effusion • Pruritis • Pulmonary edema • Renal failure, acute	• Meningitis • Bone cancer (especially after biopsy) • Inflammation, extensive (peritonitis, pleuritis, fasciitis, cellulitis) • Necrotizing cholecystitis • Necrotizing pancreatitis • Pathologic fractures • Thromboembolism

(*Continued*)

Table 18.2 / Expected pain associated with illness, injury, and surgical and hospital procedures (Continued)

	Mild to moderate	Moderate	Moderate to severe	Severe to excruciating
Injury	• Clipper burns • Laceration repair, minor • Muscle soreness • Removing cutaneous foreign bodies • Urine scalding	• Diaphragmatic hernia repair (acute, simple, with no organ injury) • Extracapsular cruciate repair • Fracture repair (radius, ulna, tibia, fibula) • Laceration repair (severe) • Soft-tissue injury (chronic wounds)	• Corneal abrasion or ulceration • Fracture repair (femur, humerus) • Frostbite • Mesenteric, gastric, testicular, or other torsions • Rewarming after accidental hypothermia • Trauma (orthopedic, extensive soft tissue injury, head injury) • Traumatic diaphragmatic hernia repair (organ and extensive tissue injury)	• Burns • Fracture repair (pelvis) • Multiple fracture repair with extensive soft tissue injury • Neuropathic pain (nerve entrapment, cervical intervertebral disk herniation, inflammation)
Surgical and hospital procedures	• Abscess lancing • Aural hematoma • Bandaging • Castration (young animals) • Chest drains • Dental cleaning • Ear examination and cleaning • Mass removal • OHE (young animals) • Restraint (exams, radiographs, sample collections) • Tracheotomy • Urinary/IV catheterization	• Anal sacculectomy • Castration (older or obese animals) • Cystotomy (inflamed) • Dental extractions • Enucleation • Fracture repair (radius, ulna, tibia, fibula) • Inguinal hernia repair • Laparotomy (short procedure with minimal manipulation and no inflammation) • Mass removal • OHE (older, obese, or pregnant animals)	• Disk surgery (thoracic, lumbar) • Exploratory laparotomy • Intra-articular surgical procedure (large canines or extensive manipulation) • Laminectomy • Mandibulectomy • Mastectomy • Onychectomy • Total ear ablation	• Disk surgery (cervical) • Ear resections • Limb amputation • Postsurgical pain (with extensive tissue injury or inflammation) • Thoracotomy

HOW CAN STRESS AFFECT PAIN?

The responses of humans to potential or actual tissue damage are parts of a complex experience that has sensory qualities and motivational and emotional consequences. The nervous system encodes the sensory features of tissue-damaging stimuli, such as their quality, intensity, location, and duration.

Pain and distress can be thought of in terms of a continuum of emotional and experiential states that may occur in an animal. On the left of Figure 18.2, "comfort" represents a state of wellbeing, where the animal is contented and comfortable. Stressors acting upon the animal in increasing severity cause the animal to progressively become uncomfortable (discomfort), then stressed (stress), and finally distressed (distress). Distress represents the extreme point in this continuum, on the far right. Stressors acting upon the animal may move the animal's experience along this continuum between the extremes of wellbeing and distress. Depending on the nature and severity of a stressor and on the animal's current state of being, the animal may adapt successfully to a stress (adaptive behaviors) or it may become distressed in a way that threatens its wellbeing or health (maladaptive behaviors). Maladaptive behaviors include abnormal feeding, absence or diminution of grooming, and changes in social interaction (aggression, withdrawal).

A departure from an animal's normal behavior can be an important indicator of pain and distress. It is therefore important to be aware of an animal's normal behavior, both as a species and individually. Responses to stress differ widely within and among species; often, signs of pain and distress are subtle and can be difficult to detect. Some of the more easily recognizable signs are listed below:

- Changes in temperament or attitude; a friendly, docile animal becomes aggressive or unresponsive.
- Restlessness; pacing, changing position frequently.
- Decreased activity; reluctance to move, does not respond normally when approached.
- Isolation; stays in the corner of the cage, does not interact with cage mates.
- Change in posture; hunching, huddling, crouching, stiff movement, head down.
- Protecting a part of the body; growls or attempts to bite when that body part is approached or touched.
- Abnormal vocalization, especially when a painful area is touched; whimpering, hissing, squealing, squeaking.
- Change in appetite and water consumption leading to weight loss and dehydration (in small rodents, dehydration causes rapid weight loss).
- Self-mutilation, excessive licking of the area, biting, scratching, rolling, kicking.
- Changes in hair coat appearance; decreased grooming leading to rough-looking coat, greasy appearance, piloerection (hair erect), loss of hair (baldness, hair shafts broken).
- Changes in facial expression; sleepy appearance, avoidance of light.
- Discharge from eyes (tears, pus, blood) or nose (runny).
- Changes in bowel movement or urination; diarrhea with soiling around the anus, or lack of bowel movements (constipation).
- Sores, reddened areas on the skin, open wounds.

Figure 18.2 Illustration of how pain can go from adaptive to maladaptive. Source: drawn by Mary Ellen Goldberg.

- Increased body temperature.
- Changes in respiration rate or character; rapid, shallow breathing.

SIGNS OF PAIN AND DISTRESS IN DOGS AND CATS

There are numerous stereotypical responses to stress or pain stimuli in animals, particularly in mammals. Nevertheless, species differences do exist. Recognition of changes in behavior and physical appearance in the species under study will allow early identification of an animal experiencing pain or distress.

Dogs

Dogs in pain generally appear quieter, less alert, and withdrawn, with stiff body movements and an unwillingness to move. In severe pain, the dog may lie still or adopt an abnormal posture to minimize its discomfort (Figure 18.3). In less severe states, it may appear restless; the immediate response to acute, but low intensity pain may be an increased alertness. There may be inappetence, shivering, and increased respirations with panting. Spontaneous barking is unlikely; the dog is more likely to whimper or howl, especially if unattended, and may growl without apparent provocation. A dog may lick or scratch at painful areas of its body. When handled, it may be abnormally apprehensive or aggressive. The animal exhibits anxious glances; it seeks cold surfaces. Its tail is often between its legs. Penile protrusion and frequent urination may also be noted. Key signs include inappetence, bites at pain regions, abnormally apprehensive.

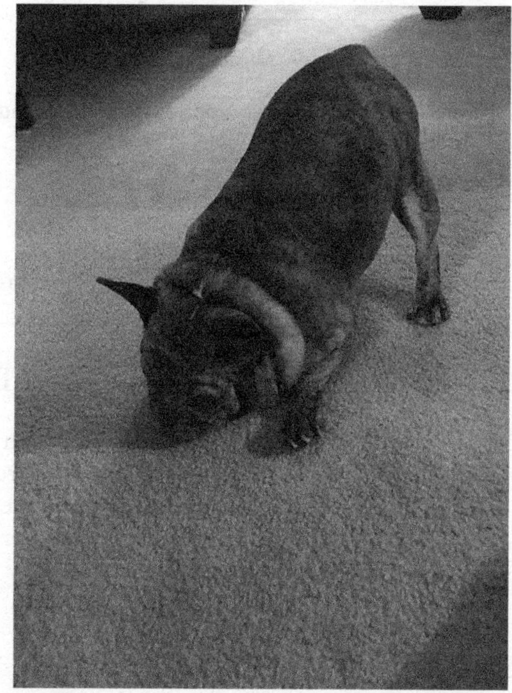

Figure 18.3 Acute abdominal pain – the prayer position. Source: courtesy of Mrs. Meredith White.

Cats

Cats in pain are generally quiet, with an apprehensive facial expression; the forehead may appear creased. There may be crying or yowling, and the cat may growl and hiss if approached or made to move. There is inappetence and a tendency to hide or to separate from other cats. The posture becomes stiff and abnormal, varying with the site of the pain. A cat with head pain may keep its head tilted. If the pain is generalized in the thorax and abdomen, the cat may be crouched or hunched. With thoracic pain alone, the head, neck, and body may be extended. In abdominal or back pain, the cat may lie in lateral recumbency with its back arched. If the animal is standing or walking, the back is arched, and the gait stilted. Incessant licking is sometimes also associated with localized pain. Pain in one limb usually results in limping or holding up of the affected limb.

A cat in severe pain may show demented behavior and make desperate attempts to escape. If a painful area is touched or palpated, there may be an instant and violent reaction. There may be panting, with an increased pulse rate and pupillary dilatation. A cat in chronic pain may have an ungroomed appearance and show a marked change from its normal behavior. The animal exhibits tucked in limbs, hunched head and neck, and utters a distinctive cry or hissing and spitting sound. Its ears are flattened. It shows fear of being handled and may cringe.

Key signs include stiff posture, demented behavior, lack of grooming, hunched head and neck, inappetence.

BEHAVIOR IS KEY

Animals are non-verbal, so they cannot self-report the presence of pain.[23] Pain assessment should be a routine component of every physical examination, and a pain score is considered the "fourth vital sign", after temperature, pulse, and respiration. When assessing an animal for pain, the following behavioral keys should be considered:

1. Maintenance of normal behaviors.
2. Loss of normal behaviors.
3. Development of new behaviors.

It is important to distinguish between pain and dysphoria in the postoperative period. Postoperatively signs in cats and dogs can be thrashing, restlessness, continuous activity, vocalization, self-mutilation, and tachypnea.[24,25] Knowing whether these behaviors are continuing pain/stress, or a reaction to opioids or general anesthesia is critical for the patient. Also described as emergence delirium, anesthesia-related behaviors should resolve within several minutes. Patients in pain can usually be soothed for a brief period when direct attention is paid to trying to calm them. The patient will usually make eye contact with the caregiver. Medium to large-sized dogs may need to relieve themselves and may feel claustrophobic after surgery. If the animal is in pain, palpating around the incisional area may elicit a painful response. Animals that are dysphoric or "delirious" because of opioid overdose rarely respond to soothing interaction or to light palpation of the painful area. These patients may benefit from sedation or partial opioid reversal using careful titration, which is usually reserved for patients who do not respond to distraction or sedation or have a physiologic condition that is of immediate medical concern.[24] Reversal of the opioid by 0.01 mg/kg naloxone or by 0.1 mg/kg butorphanol (both IV)[25] or small doses of either dexmedetomidine (0.5–2 μg/kg) or acepromazine (0.01–0.02 mg/kg) IV will generally improve the situation.[26]

Behavioral Considerations for Acute Pain in Cats

The type, anatomical location and duration of surgery, the environment, individual variation, age, and health status should be taken into consideration. The cat should be observed from a distance then, if possible, the caregiver should interact with the cat and palpate the painful area to fully assess the cat's pain. A good knowledge of the cat's normal behavior is very helpful as changes in behavior (absence of normal behaviors such as grooming and climbing into the litter box) and presence of new behaviors (a previously friendly cat becoming aggressive, hiding or trying to escape) may provide helpful clues. Some cats may not display clear overt behavior indicative of pain, especially in the presence of human beings, other animals or in stressful situations.

Behavioral changes associated with acute pain in cats include:[27]

- Reduced activity.
- Loss of appetite.
- Quietness.
- Hiding.
- Hissing and growling (vocalization).
- Excessive licking of a specific area of the body (usually involving surgical wounds).
- Guarding behavior.
- Cessation of grooming.
- Tail flicking.
- Aggression.

Cats in severe pain are usually depressed, immobile and silent. They will appear tense and distant from their environment.

Cats should not be awakened to check their pain status; rest and sleep are good signs of comfort, but one should ensure the cat is resting or sleeping in a normal posture (relaxed, curled up). In some cases, cats will remain very still because they are afraid, or it is too painful to move, and some cats feign sleep when stressed.[27]

Behavioral Considerations for Acute Pain in Dogs

Acute pain occurs commonly in dogs because of a trauma, surgery, medical problems, infections or inflammatory disease.[22] The severity of pain can range from very mild to very severe. The duration of pain can be expected to be from a few hours to several days (Table 18.3). Objective measures (such as heart rate, arterial blood pressure, plasma cortisol, and catecholamine levels) are unreliable because stress, fear and anesthetic drugs affect them. Therefore, evaluation of pain in dogs is primarily subjective and based on behavioral signs.

Table 18.3 / Behavioral signs of pain in dogs[28]

Category	Clinical signs
Attitude/ mentation	• Scared, submissive appearance • Unwilling to eat or interact with people • Inability to lay down
Body movement	• Constant trembling with/ without stimulation and/or handling • Flinching from fingertips lightly brushed over the body
Facial expression	• Tense facial muscles with furrowed brows • Lips drawn back • Grimace with unfocused or fearful look in eyes • Dilated pupils • Ears flattened against head
Guarding	• Guarding or biting at a painful area • Tensing abdomen when palpation is attempted • Growling when approached
Posture	• Back or abdominal pain: hunched up or tense appearance • severe abdominal pain: prayer position (standing on the hindlimbs, with sternum and forelimbs flat on the floor) • May move to back of cage or into corner
Respiratory pattern	• Short, shallow breathing pattern
Vocalization	• Crying, whining, whimpering

Behavioral Considerations for Chronic Pain in Cats

Since chronic pain is of long duration, the behavioral changes associated with chronic pain may develop gradually and may be subtle, making them most easily detected by someone very familiar with the animal (usually the owner; Figure 18.4).[28] Chronic pain in cats can be divided into degenerative joint disease (DJD)/osteoarthritis, Non-DJD, nonmalignant pain, and cancer pain.[29] This is a mixture of inflammatory, neuropathic and functional pain.[30] The most common cancers in cats are lymphoma (lymphosarcoma); alimentary (gastrointestinal); cranial mediastinal (chest); extranodal, which can occur at any site, including the nose, kidneys and central nervous system; squamous cell carcinoma, mouth, nose, ear, eyelid or other skin sites; soft-tissue sarcoma, injection sites, feline injection-site sarcoma.[29,31]

Behaviors that indicate chronic pain in cats include:[29]

- Decreased grooming.
- Reluctance to jump.
- Inability or reluctance to climb or descend stairs.
- Inability to jump as high as before.
- Urinating and soiling outside the litter tray.
- Increased or decreased sleep.
- Avoiding human interaction.
- Hiding.
- Dislike of being stroked or brushed.

Categories for Assessment of Chronic Pain in Cats

- General mobility (e.g. ease of movement, fluidity of movement).
- Performing activities (e.g. playing, hunting, jumping, using a litter tray).
- Eating, drinking.
- Grooming (e.g. scratching).
- Resting, observing, relaxing (how well these activities can be enjoyed by the cat).
- Social activities involving people and other pets.
- Temperament.

Feline Chronic or Neuropathic Pain Conditions

- Degenerative joint disease/osteoarthritis.
- Feline orofacial pain syndrome.[29,32]
- Post-amputation which includes onychectomy.[29,33]
- Diabetic neuropathy.[29,33]
- Feline hyperesthesia syndrome.[29,34]
- Feline interstitial cystitis.[29,33]
- Gingivostomatitis.[29,35]
- Inflammatory bowel disease.[33]
- Pancreatitis/pancreatic pain.[33]
- Spinal cord trauma/Intervertebral disc herniation.[33]
- Pelvic fractures.[33]
- Trauma: accidental or surgical.[33]

Feline cancer pain can be directly produced by the tumor, caused by the various treatment modalities, related to chronic debility, or due to unrelated, concurrent disease processes.[29,36]

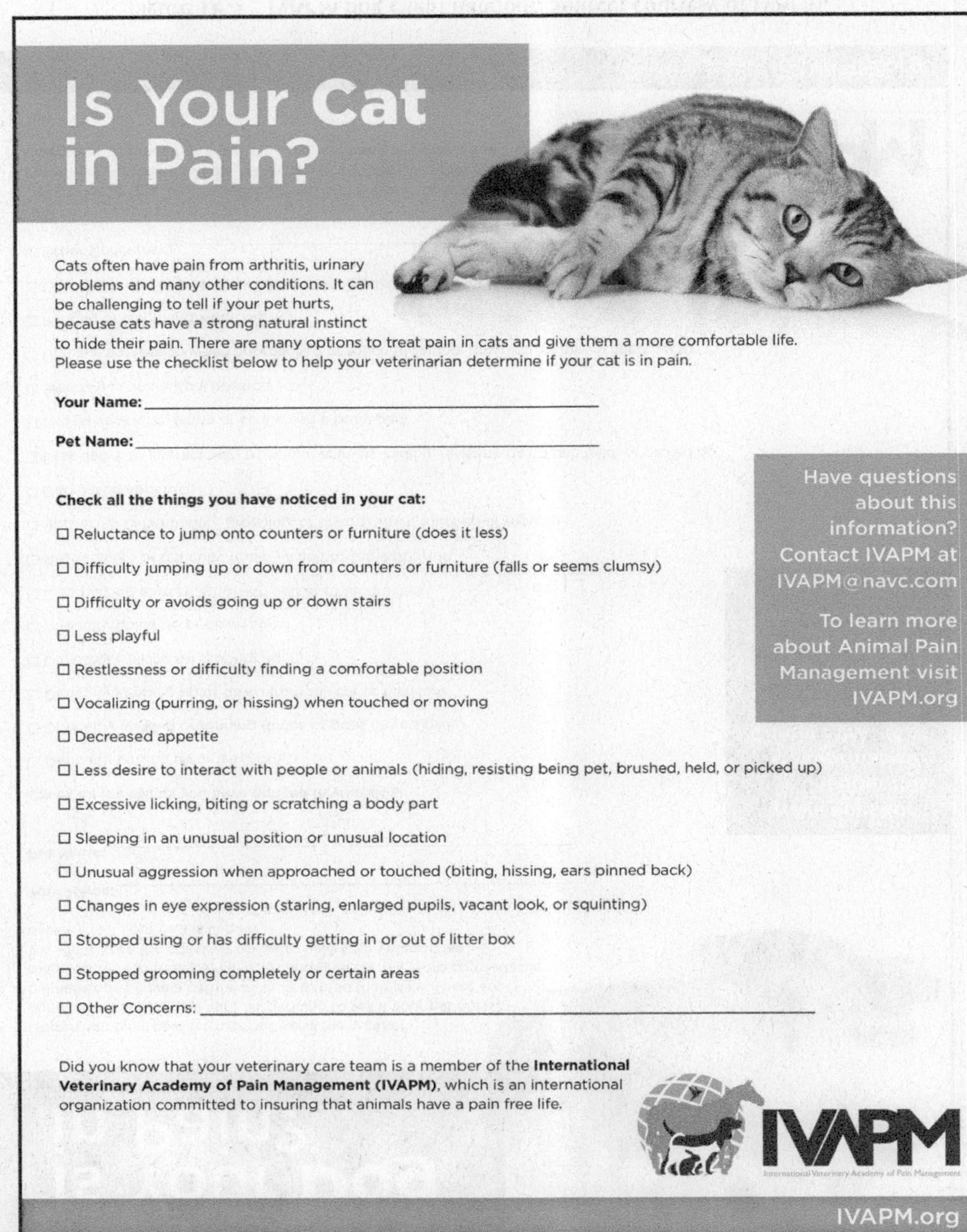

Is Your **Cat** in Pain?

Cats often have pain from arthritis, urinary problems and many other conditions. It can be challenging to tell if your pet hurts, because cats have a strong natural instinct to hide their pain. There are many options to treat pain in cats and give them a more comfortable life. Please use the checklist below to help your veterinarian determine if your cat is in pain.

Your Name: ______________________

Pet Name: ______________________

Have questions about this information? Contact IVAPM at IVAPM@navc.com

To learn more about Animal Pain Management visit IVAPM.org

Check all the things you have noticed in your cat:

- ☐ Reluctance to jump onto counters or furniture (does it less)
- ☐ Difficulty jumping up or down from counters or furniture (falls or seems clumsy)
- ☐ Difficulty or avoids going up or down stairs
- ☐ Less playful
- ☐ Restlessness or difficulty finding a comfortable position
- ☐ Vocalizing (purring, or hissing) when touched or moving
- ☐ Decreased appetite
- ☐ Less desire to interact with people or animals (hiding, resisting being pet, brushed, held, or picked up)
- ☐ Excessive licking, biting or scratching a body part
- ☐ Sleeping in an unusual position or unusual location
- ☐ Unusual aggression when approached or touched (biting, hissing, ears pinned back)
- ☐ Changes in eye expression (staring, enlarged pupils, vacant look, or squinting)
- ☐ Stopped using or has difficulty getting in or out of litter box
- ☐ Stopped grooming completely or certain areas
- ☐ Other Concerns: ______________________

Did you know that your veterinary care team is a member of the **International Veterinary Academy of Pain Management (IVAPM)**, which is an international organization committed to insuring that animals have a pain free life.

IVAPM
International Veterinary Academy of Pain Management

IVAPM.org

Figure 18.4 IVAPM Cat client pain handout. Source: courtesy of IVAPM.

Is Your Dog in Pain?

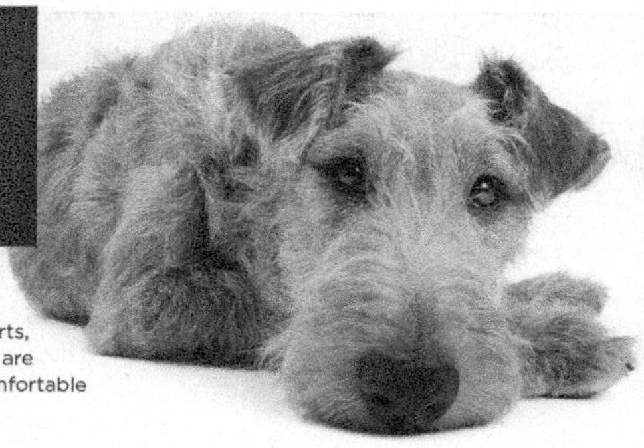

Dogs often have pain from arthritis and many other conditions but it can be very challenging to tell if your pet hurts, because dogs have a natural instinct to hide their pain. There are many options to treat pain in dogs and give them a more comfortable life. Please use the checklist below to help your veterinarian determine if your dog is in pain.

Your Name: ______________________

Pet Name: ______________________

Check all the things you have noticed in your dog:

- ☐ Difficulty getting up or lying down
- ☐ Difficultly walking or running (limps or goes more slowly)
- ☐ Difficulty jumping up or down from the car or furniture
- ☐ Difficulty walking on slippery floors
- ☐ Difficulty going up or down stairs
- ☐ Less playing or exercising with you or other animals
- ☐ Restlessness or difficulty finding a comfortable position
- ☐ Vocalizing (whimpering, groaning, or crying) when touched or moving
- ☐ Decreased appetite
- ☐ Less desire to interact with people or animals (hiding, resisting being pet, held, or picked up)
- ☐ Excessive licking, biting or scratching a body part
- ☐ Sleeping in an unusual position
- ☐ Unusual aggression when approached or touched (biting, growling, or ears pinned back)
- ☐ Panting or trembling when resting
- ☐ Changes in eye expression (staring, dilated pupils, vacant look, or squinting)
- ☐ Other Concerns: ______________________

Have questions about this information? Contact IVAPM at IVAPM@navc.com

To learn more about Animal Pain Management visit IVAPM.org

Did you know that your veterinary care team is a member of the **International Veterinary Academy of Pain Management (IVAPM)**, which is an international organization committed to insuring that animals have a pain free life.

IVAPM
International Veterinary Academy of Pain Management

IVAPM.org

Figure 18.5 IVAPM dog client handout. Source: courtesy of IVAPM.

Behavioral Considerations for Chronic Pain in Dogs

Chronic pain changes in dogs may develop gradually and may be subtle, so that they can only be detected by someone very familiar with the animal (usually the owner; Figure 18.5). The pet owner may see:

- Increasingly diminished function and mobility that indicate progressive disability.
- Diminished exercise tolerance and general activity.
- Difficulty standing, walking, taking stairs, jumping or getting up.
- Decreased grooming.
- Changes in urination or defecation habits.

Positive behaviors reduced in dogs with chronic pain include:[8]

- Decreased socialization/play with human family.
- Decreased socialization/play with other dogs.
- Decreased movement (quality and quantity).
- Decreased interest in hygiene/grooming.
- Decreased tail wagging.
- Hypo- or anorexic.
- Decreased curiosity.

Negative behaviors more frequent in dogs with chronic pain include:[8]

- Aggression toward humans and/or other dogs.
- More dependent on owner, jealous, "clingy".
- Sleeping more.
- Does not come up to greet owner.
- Fearful.
- Guarding behavior, guards body parts.
- Biting painful areas.
- Licking painful areas or dorsal aspects of front limbs.
- Sudden, excessive scratching.
- Sudden, excessive negative reaction (compulsive behavior).
- Under- or overactive.

Abnormal posture or movement seen in dogs with chronic pain include:[8]

- Reluctance to move (walk, trot, gallop, jump).
- Inability to turn in one or both directions.
- Hind legs tucked under abdomen.
- Tail between hind legs.
- Ears back.
- Restlessness, wandering, circling.
- Rigid posture and gait.
- Sitting or lying down in the middle of walks.
- Head hanging; will not lift or turn head (neck pain).
- Praying position (abdominal pain).
- Decreased weight bearing (limb pain).
- Sitting abnormally (e.g. knee out in stifle pain).
- Trembling or shaking.

Mental and physiological behavior seen in dogs with chronic pain includes:[8]

- Depressed, sad, and/or anxious demeanor.
- Visible white sclera around the iris (not always pain, some breeds show this all the time).
- Panting or tachypnea or tachycardia without exercise.

Canine Chronic of Neuropathic Pain Conditions

- Degenerative joint disease/osteoarthritis.[37]
- Intervertebral disc disease.[38]
- Post amputation.[33]
- Ocular conditions.[39]
- Otic conditions.[39]
- Trauma: accidental and surgical.[33]

PAIN SCALES

No single pain scoring system is right for all practices. In fact, it is not as important which system you choose as it is to simply choose one system to be used by the entire team. Once a pain scoring system is chosen, apply it! At every single outpatient visit, assess the animal for pain and record the finding in the medical record. Each individual pain assessment is important; for a patient with chronic pain, trends are even more important because they tell us whether the patient's pain is improving or worsening. Similarly, surgical patients with acute pain need to be assessed at regular intervals during hospitalization, with the results recorded in the medical record. Trends allow the practice team to understand the success of a perioperative pain management plan (Table 18.4).

The bottom line: pain hurts. Your clients know their pets feel pain. Make sure that your clients know you look for pain and that you treat it in their pets.

Table 18.4 / Various pain scales

Pain scale	Definition	Advantages	Disadvantages
Simple descriptive scale (SDS)	• Uses a numbering system based on the observation of the patient to indicate the level of pain: (0) indicating no pain and (4) indicating extreme pain	• Ease of use	• Observer bias • Failure to notice small changes
Preemptive scoring system	• Estimate of expected pain based on the procedure to be performed and amount of tissue trauma expected rated as none, mild, moderate, or severe	• Ease of use	• Individual patient extent of pain and response to therapy
Numerical rating scale	• A set of categories used to evaluate the patient on visual and physiological observations (e.g. vocalization, posture, movement, agitation)	• Ease of use • Encourages a thorough patient evaluation	• Similar to SDS • Limited validation
Visual analog scale	• A 100-mm straight line bracketed with *no pain* at one end and *worst pain possible* at other end • A vertical line is drawn across the line to indicate the patient's level of pain	• Ease of use • Visual indication that pain is improving or worsening.	• Subjective nature of where to stop the line • Uncertainty of what *worst pain possible* indicates, relating to all pain or pain for a specific procedure
Dynamic and interactive visual analog scale	• A 100-mm straight line bracketed with *no pain* at one end and *worst pain possible* at other end • A vertical line is drawn across the line to indicate the patient's level of pain • Assessments are taken at a distance, while handling the patient and encouraging movement, and palpation of the wound	• Ease of use • Visual indication if pain is improving or worsening • Includes additional assessments	

(*Continued*)

Table 18.4 / Various pain scales (Continued)			
Pain scale	Definition	Advantages	Disadvantages
Behavioral and physiological response scales			
Colorado State University Acute Pain Scale	• Evaluation of psychological and behavioral signs, responses to palpation, and body tension	• Limited observer bias • Observations clearly defined	• Limited validation
University of Melbourne Pain Scale	• Evaluation of psychological (e.g. heart rate, respiratory rate, pupil size, temperature) and behavioral signs (e.g. posture, activity, response to palpation, mental status, vocalization) each assigned to a value and then added for an overall pain score (0–27)	• Increased accuracy • Ability to weight the importance of different categories	• Limited validation
Glasgow composite pain tool	• Evaluation of six behavioral categories (e.g. vocalization, attention to painful area, mobility, response to touch, demeanor, posture/activity), each assigned a value and then added for an overall pain score (0–24) • Assessments are taken at a distance, while handling the patient and encouraging movement, and palpation of the wound	• Limited observer bias • Observations clearly defined • Avoids variable physiological responses	• Greater use for musculoskeletal

Acute Pain Scales for Dogs and Cats that Incorporate Behaviors

A behavior-based acute pain scoring system, the Glasgow Composite Measure Pain Scale (CMPS-Canine), was developed at the University of Glasgow.[28,40] The Glasgow Feline Composite Measure Pain Scale (CMPS-Feline) has been designed as a clinical decision-making tool for use in cats in acute pain.[41] The UNESP-Botucatu multidimensional composite pain scale for assessing post-operative pain in cats has also been validated.[42]

Multifactorial Clinical Measurement Instruments for Chronic Pain

Observation or reports, in a preexamination questionnaire, of behavioral changes or abnormalities are the first consideration in recognizing and assessing chronic pain. Such instruments are chronic pain indices that primarily use pet-owner observations and input. Ideally, patients with chronic pain should be evaluated with one of the multifactorial clinical measurement instruments.

Multifactorial clinical measurement instruments for chronic pain for dogs and cats that incorporate behaviors include:[23]

- Helsinki Chronic Pain Index[43]
- Canine Brief Pain Inventory[44]
- Cincinnati Orthopedic Disability Index[45]
- VetMetrica HRQL(health-related quality of life)[46]
- Liverpool Osteoarthritis in Dogs[47]
- Feline Musculoskeletal Pain Index.[48]

OWNER COMPLIANCE

When the veterinarian dispenses medication for in-home treatment of painful patients, owner compliance is a concern, owing to the unique challenges of administering medication.[23] Cats are usually more difficult to give medications than dogs. Palatability is also a huge factor, and most cats are finicky when it comes to food. Here are five ways to improve compliance:

1. Communication
2. Written information
3. Frequency of veterinary visits
4. Veterinarian continuity
5. Selection of medications.

Veterinarians or veterinary technician can demonstrate to owners how to administer a medication while still in the office. This helps avoid complications and promotes active discussion with the client. Written instructions should be provided. Follow-up calls from the veterinary clinic staff can help to increase owner compliance. This can facilitate identification of issues to be addressed with the clinical state of the patient and concerns with the treatment plan while offering an opportunity to set up a follow-up appointment if one is not already on the books. Prescribing medications that are easy and convenient to use can also improve owner compliance. If the patient is nauseated or vomiting, it is unlikely that medications will be easy to administer. Because of this, compounding of certain medications may be warranted. Clients should be encouraged to address their concerns about the pet's condition and treatment plan via email, phone or follow-up consultations.

Table 18.5 / **Pain management medication specifics**

Drug	Indications	Dose/route/duration	Comments
Opioids			
Buprenorphine HCl • Partial agonist at μ receptors	• Canine: mild to moderate pain • Feline: moderate to severe pain • Preoperative sedation, acute and perioperative pain	Dose (mg/kg): • Canine: 0.005–0.03 • Feline: 0.02–0.04 • Epidural: 0.03 • Sublingual: 0.01–0.02 Route: sublingual (felines only), SQ, IM, IV Duration (affected by dose): • Delayed onset of 45–60 minutes • 6–12 hours	• Very effective in felines, but ↓ appetite following several days of administration • Sublingual application is only acceptable for felines due to their unique oral pH • Will not usually achieve the same degree of analgesia as morphine, hydromorphone, or fentanyl • Virtually impossible to reverse due to its high affinity for the μ receptor
• Buprenorphine 1.8 mg/ml (Simbadol®)	• Control of postoperative pain in cats	• Feline only – SQ 0.12–0.24 mg/kg every 24 hours for up to 3 days	• Good analgesia especially when administered with local anesthesia and NSAIDs
Butorphanol tartrate • Pure antagonist at μ receptor and partial agonists at κ receptor	• Mild to moderate pain • Canine: visceral pain • Feline: skin pain	Dose (mg/kg): • Canine: 0.2–0.8 SQ IM; 0.1–0.4 IV • Feline: 0.1–0.4 SQ IM; 0.05–0.2 IV Route: SQ IM IV Duration: • Canine: 20 minutes SQ IM; 45 minutes IV • Feline: 4 hours SQ IM; 45–60 minutes IV	• Has an anesthetic ceiling effect in which an ↑ amount will not ↓ the pain further • Can be used to partially reverse pure agonist opioids at μ receptors • Will not usually achieve the same degree of analgesia as morphine, hydromorphone, or fentanyl • Can be given PO, but not highly effective for pain

(*Continued*)

Table 18.5 / **Pain management medication specifics (Continued)**

Drug	Indications	Dose/route/duration	Comments
Codeine/ acetaminophen	• Moderate to severe pain • Chronic pain	Dose (canine): 1–2 mg/kg codeine Route: PO Duration: 8–12 hours	• Do not use in felines • Available in 30 or 60 mg codeine and 300 mg acetaminophen (e.g. Tylenol No. 3®) • Chronic use: tolerance and constipation may occur

Fentanyl citrate
• Pure agonist at μ receptor
	• Moderate to severe pain	*Injection*
		Dose (μg/kg):
		• Canine: 10 SQ 2–5 IV
		• Feline: 1–2 IV
		Route: SQ (canine only), IV
		Duration:
		• Canine: 40–60 minutes (SQ)
		• Canine/feline 15–30 minutes (IV)
		Transdermal patch
		Dose (canine/feline): 3–5 μg/kg/hour
		• < 11 lb = 12.5 μg
		• 11–22 lb = 25 μg
		• > 22–44 lb = 50 μg
		• > 44–66 lb = 75 μg
		• > 66 lb = 100 μg
		Duration:
		• Delayed onset of 12–24 hours
		• Canine: minimum of 3 days
		• Feline: up to 4 days
			• Feline hyperthermia is often seen
			• May cause auditory sensitization, ↑ body temperature, bradycardia
			• Cotton in the ears and a quiet environment may alleviate sound sensitivity
			• Patch is inadequate when used alone with acute surgical pain or severe traumatic pain
			• Patch use with febrile patients or with a heating device can greatly ↑ rates of absorption and should be avoided
			• Mixed agonist/antagonist opioids will reverse the effects
			• Patch placement:
			  • Sites may be the neck, thorax, inguinal area, metatarsal/carpal areas, base of tail of canines and lateral thorax, inguinal area, metatarsal/carpal areas, base of tail of felines
			  • Clip hair over the desired area, clean with water, and allow to dry completely
			  • Apply the patch, hold in place with the palm of hand for several minutes to allow the patch to adhere, and cover with an adhesive bandage
			  • Label the bandage with the patch size, date, and time of placement

Hydromorphone • Pure agonist at μ receptor	• Moderate to severe pain	Dose (mg/kg): • Canine: 0.1–0.2 SQ IM; 0.03–0.1 IV • Feline: 0.05–0.1 SQ IM; 0.01–0.025 IV Route: SQ IM IV (slowly) Duration: • Delayed onset of 15–30 minutes • 3–4 hours SQ IM; 30–45 minutes IV	• Feline hyperthermia is often seen • Less likely to induce vomiting or hypotension than morphine • Constipation with long-term use

(Continued)

Table 18.5 / Pain management medication specifics (Continued)

Drug	Indications	Dose/route/duration	Comments
Methadone • Agonist at the μ receptor	• Mild to moderate pain	Dose (mg/kg): • Canine: 0.5–2.2 SQ IM; 0.1–0.5 IV • Feline: 0.1–0.5 mg/kg SQ IM 0.05–0.1 mg/kg IV • Transmucosal: 0.6 Route: transmucosal (felines) SQ IM IV Duration: • 4–6 hours SQ IM; 60 minutes IV	• May induce less vomiting and sedation than morphine • Less likelihood of developing tolerance
Morphine sulfate • Pure agonist at μ receptor	• Moderate to severe pain	Dose (mg/kg): • Canine: 0.5–4 PO; 0.5–2.2 SQ IM; 0.1–0.5 IV slowly • Feline: 0.25–1.0 PO; 0.1–0.5 SQ IM; 0.05–0.1 IV slowly • Epidural: 0.1 Route: PO SQ IM IV slowly Duration: • 3–4 hours PO • 3–6 hours SQ IM • 60 minutes IV	• Feline hyperthermia is often seen • High doses may cause excitement in felines; give lower doses combined with a tranquilizer • Avoid IV administration in canines that are not normovolemic and normotensive • Anorexia and constipation may occur with oral use
Oxycodone • Agonist at μ and κ receptors	• Moderate to severe pain	Dose: (canine) 0.3 mg/kg Route: PO Duration: 8–12 hours	• Often given in conjunction with an NSAID • Highly addictive with the potential for abuse, recommended for short-term use only
Oxymorphone HCl • Pure agonists at μ receptor	• Moderate to severe pain	Dose (mg/kg): • Canine: 0.05–0.2 • Feline: 0.02–0.1 Route: IM IV Duration • 2–6 hr	• Feline hyperthermia is often seen

(Continued)

Table 18.5 / Pain management medication specifics (Continued)

Drug	Indications	Dose/route/duration	Comments
α-2 agonists			
Dexmedetomidine	• Mild pain • Moderate to severe pain when combined with opioids	Dose • Canine: 375 μg/m² IV; 500 μg/m² IM • Feline: 40 μg/kg IM Route: IM Duration: 30–90 minutes	• 12-hour fast is recommended prior to administration • Used with opioids to enhance analgesic effects • Extremely excited and agitated dogs need 15–20 minutes of quiet rest time after the drug is given • Apply an eye lubricant to prevent corneal drying • Bottle labeled as μg/m² for dosing (see Appendix)
Medetomidine	• Mild pain • Moderate to severe pain when combined with opioids	Dose: (canine/feline) 5–10 μg/kg Route: IM IV Duration: 30–90 minutes	• Used with opioids to enhance analgesic effects • Extremely excited and agitated dogs need 15–20 minutes of quiet rest time after the drug is given • Use atropine or glycopyrrolate for bradycardia • Placement of cotton balls in the patient's ears and a quiet environment may alleviate sound sensitivity • Bottle labeled as μg/m² for dosing (see Appendix)
Xylazine	• Mild pain	Dose: (canine/feline) 0.05–0.1 mg/kg Route: IM IV Duration: 30–60 minute	• Sedation may outlast analgesia • Used with opioids to enhance analgesic effects • Use atropine or glycopyrrolate for bradycardia • Placement of cotton balls in the patient's ears and a quiet environment may alleviate sound sensitivity
Local			
Bupivacaine	• Eliminates all pain	Dose (mg/kg): • Canine/feline: 1–2 • Epidural: 0.1–0.75 Route: infiltration, epidural Duration: • Delayed onset of 15–20 minutes • 6–8 hours	• Avoid IV administration as cardiac arrest may result • Toxic dose is 4 mg/kg
Bupivacaine liposome injectable suspension (Nocita)®	• Dogs: for single-dose infiltration into the surgical site to provide local postoperative analgesia for cranial cruciate ligament surgery in dogs • Cats: for use as a peripheral nerve block to provide regional postoperative analgesia following onychectomy in cats	• Dogs: 5.3 mg/kg (0.4 ml/kg) administered by infiltration injection • Cats: administer 5.3 mg/kg per forelimb (0.4 ml/kg per forelimb, for a total dose of 10.6 mg/kg/cat) as a 4-point nerve block prior to onychectomy	• Dogs: single dose administered during surgical closure may provide up to 72 hr of pain control. • Cats: administration prior to surgery may provide up to 72 hours of pain control

(Continued)

Table 18.5 / **Pain management medication specifics (Continued)**

Drug	Indications	Dose/route/duration	Comments
Lidocaine	• Eliminate all pain	Dose: (canine/feline) 1–2 mg/kg Route: infiltration, epidural, IV Duration: • Onset of 3–10 minutes • 60 minutes	• Felines are very sensitive to the CNS effects—use with caution • Avoid IV administration in felines • Toxic dose is 10 mg/kg
Non-steroidal anti-inflammatory drugs			
Carprofen	• Mild to moderate (severe in some cases) • Treatment of inflammation	Dose (mg/kg): • Canine: 2.2 PO; 4.4 SQ IM IV • Feline: 1.2g SQ Route: PO SQ IM IV Duration: • Delayed onset of 60 minutes • 12 hours (PO, canine), 18–24 hours (SQ IM IV, canine), 48–72 hours (SQ, feline)	• Monitor blood values when using long term • NSAIDs are not recommended in hypovolemic or dehydrated patients or in patients with bleeding disorders, gastrointestinal, or renal disease • Discontinue if vomiting or diarrhea develops • Give with food
Deracoxib	• Mild to moderate (severe in some cases) • Post-op orthopedic pain • Treatment and pain associated with osteoarthritis	Dose (mg/kg): • Canine, postoperatively: 3–4 • Canine, osteoarthritis: 1–2 Route: PO Duration: 24 hours	• Monitor blood values when using long term • NSAIDs are not recommended in hypovolemic or dehydrated patients or in patients with bleeding disorders, gastrointestinal, or renal disease • Discontinue if vomiting or diarrhea develops • Give with food • Given for up to 7 days postoperatively
Etodolac	• Mild to moderate (severe in some cases) • Treatment of inflammation associated with osteoarthritis	Dose: (canine) 10–15 mg/kg Route: PO Duration: • Onset of 60 minutes • 24 hours	• Monitor blood values when using long term • NSAIDs are not recommended in hypovolemic or dehydrated patients or in patients with bleeding disorders, gastrointestinal or renal disease • Discontinue if vomiting or diarrhea develops • Very difficult to accurately dose canines < 5 kg
Firocoxib	• Mild to moderate (severe in some cases) • Treatment of inflammation associated with osteoarthritis	Dose: (canine) 5 mg/kg Route: PO Duration: 18–24 hours	• Monitor blood values when using long term • NSAIDs are not recommended in hypovolemic or dehydrated patients or in patients with bleeding disorders, gastrointestinal, or renal disease • Discontinue if vomiting or diarrhea develops

(*Continued*)

Table 18.5 / Pain management medication specifics (Continued)

Drug	Indications	Dose/route/duration	Comments
Ketoprofen	• Mild to moderate (severe in some cases) • Treatment of inflammation	Dose (mg/kg): • Canine/feline: 1 PO • Canine/feline 1–2 SQ Route: PO SQ Duration: 18–24 hours	• Monitor blood values when using long term • NSAIDs are not recommended in hypovolemic or dehydrated patients or in patients with bleeding disorders, gastrointestinal, or renal disease. • Discontinue if vomiting or diarrhea develops • May mask signs and symptoms of infection • Do not use preoperatively as it may cause intraoperative bleeding
Mavacoxib	• Mild to moderate pain • Treatment of degenerative joint disease	Dose: • Canine: 2 mg/kg PO initially, repeated in 14 days and then every 30 days thereafter Route: PO Duration: 30 days	• Not yet approved in the United States • Give right before or with a large meal • Monitor blood values when using long term • NSAIDs are not recommended in hypovolemic or dehydrated patients or in patients with bleeding disorders, gastrointestinal, or renal disease • Discontinue if vomiting or diarrhea develops
Meloxicam	• Mild to moderate (severe in some cases) • Treatment of chronic inflammatory disease of the musculoskeletal system, hip dysplasia, and chronic osteoarthritis (canine)	Dose (mg/kg): • Canine: 0.2 PO on first day of treatment; then 0.1 every 24 hours • Feline: 0.2 PO on first day of treatment; then 0.1 every 24 hours for 2–4 days Route: PO Duration: 18–24 hours	• Monitor blood values when using long term • NSAIDs are not recommended in hypovolemic or dehydrated patients or in patients with bleeding disorders, gastrointestinal, or renal disease • Discontinue if vomiting or diarrhea develops • Small canines and felines: place drops into the animal's food, not directly into the mouth
Robenacoxib	• Mild to moderate pain • Feline: musculoskeletal disorders	Dose (mg/kg): • Canine: 1–2 PO for up to 10 days • Feline: 1–2 PO for up to 6 days; 2 SQ once Route: PO SQ Duration: 18–24 hours	• Given on an empty stomach or with small amounts of food • Monitor blood values when using long term • NSAIDs are not recommended in hypovolemic or dehydrated patients or in patients with bleeding disorders, gastrointestinal, cardiac, hepatic, or renal disease • Tablets should not be broken or crushed
Adjuvants			
Amantadine • Antiviral • NMDA antagonist	• Mild to moderate chronic pain	Dose • Canine/feline: 3–5 mg/kg Route • PO Duration • 24 hr	• Used in conjunction with an opioid or NSAID to prevent or treat wind-up • Effects may not be seen for up to 1 week • Treatment is often only 21 days • Should not be used with tricyclic antidepressants

(*Continued*)

Table 18.5 / Pain management medication specifics (Continued)

Drug	Indications	Dose/route/duration	Comments
Gabapentin Anticonvulsant	Mild to moderate neuropathic pain • Prevents allodynia and hyperalgesia	Dose • Canine/feline: 5–10 mg/kg • PO • 8–12 hr	• Evaluate patients frequently for response and adjust as needed • Sedation may be seen • Taper dose at withdrawal
Tramadol • Synthetic μ receptor opiate agonist	• Moderate to severe chronic pain	Dose • Canine: 5–10 mg/kg • Feline: 2–5 mg/kg Route • PO Duration • 6–12 hr	• Most effective when used in conjunction with an NSAID • Do not use along with tricyclic antidepressants. • Taper dose at withdrawal.
Cannabis[49]	• Moderate to severe chronic pain	Dose • Canine: 2 mg/kg • Feline: 1–2 mg/kg Route • PO Duration • 8–12 hr	• 2 mg/kg has better ½ life
Misc. Analgesic			
Acetaminophen	• Breakthrough pain	Dose: (canine) 10–15 mg/kg Route: PO Duration: 12 hours	• Do not use in felines • Can be used for short periods of time in canines; treatment up to 5 days • Alternative option when other NSAIDs are contraindicated

LOCAL ANESTHETICS

Local anesthetic techniques are the only analgesic techniques that produce a complete blockade of the peripheral nociceptive input. They are, therefore, the most effective way to prevent sensitization of the central nervous system and development of pathological pain.[49] We use local blockade because it permits a reduction of general anesthetic requirements, which is safer for patients. The requirements for postoperative pain medications are also lowered.[50] Patients can awaken comfortably from anesthesia.

There are fewer unwanted effects from systemic opioids that could cause sedation or respiratory depression.[51] Local anesthesia can have anti-inflammatory effects (reduced production of eicosanoids, thromboxane, leukotriene, histamine, and inflammatory cytokines;[52] and scavenging of oxygen free radicals) and antibacterial, antifungal, and antiviral effects.[53] Patients return to activity faster and there is a decreased chance of chronic pain establishment. See Chapter 20: Anesthesia for information regarding local and regional anesthetics.

CONSTANT RATE INFUSIONS

CRIs were developed to maintain constant plasma concentration of drugs such as analgesics and general anesthetics. The technique allows a steady state of drug to be maintained, without the over- and under-dosing associated with the administration of boluses (T. Grubb, personal communication). CRIs can only be provided using a syringe driver or an infusion pump; using a free-flow drop technique (in which the rate of infusion is determined by the number of drops per minute) can lead to under- or over-dosage and may be dangerous for the patient. Initially, a loading dose is given to rapidly achieve therapeutic levels, then a maintenance dose is started to maintain those established therapeutic levels. Avoiding the loading dose will greatly delay the amount of time for pain control to be achieved. As with any analgesic plan, pain assessments and monitoring must continue during the CRI and the plan or rate adjusted as needed to control pain. See Table 18.6 to review problems that can occur with CRIs and Tables 18.7 and 18.8 for dosages of CRI pain medications.

You can expand your flexibility by running two separate fluid lines through two different IV fluid pumps. In the two-pump model, the CRI drugs would be delivered at a very low rate (for example, 1 ml/kg/hour) while the patient's additional fluid needs are separately managed through the second line (Table 18.9). This allows for total flexibility of drug and fluid delivery but requires two pumps and double IV access.

CRIs can be used to:

- Provide analgesia and anesthesia.
- Smoothen recovery from anesthesia.
- Decrease the requirements of inhalant anesthetic agents.
- Provide sedation in recovery.
- Indirectly improve hemodynamics.

Skill Box 18.1 / Constant Rate Infusion Tips

1. To allow easy adjustment of the fluid rate without the risk of overhydration or dehydration, piggyback the CRI drugs into the main fluid line via another fluid bag or a syringe pump.
2. CRIs containing an opioid or lidocaine can be protected from light by being wrapped with a dark towel or bandaging material.

Conversions:

To convert micrograms (μg) to milligrams (mg), divide the μg by 1000.
To convert milligrams (mg) to micrograms (μg), multiply the mg by 1000.
To convert μg/kg/hour to μg/kg/minute, divide by 60. For example, 10-kg patient 5 μg/kg/hour = (5 μg)(10 kg) = 50 μg/h ÷ 60 minutes = 0.83 μg/minute.
To convert μg/kg/minute to μg/kg/hour, multiply by 60. For example, 20-kg patient 2 μg/kg/minute = (2 μg)(20 kg) = 40 μg/minute × 60 = 2400 μg/hour.
To convert μg/kg/minute to mg/kg/hour, multiply by 16.67 (1000 ÷ 60).

Skill Box 18.2 / Calculations of Constant Rate Infusion Dosages

Generally, dosing tables or individualized spreadsheets should be used for constant rate infusions. These sheets greatly improve the speed at which CRIs can be initiated and greatly decrease the chance of mathematical errors (see Table 18.9 for calculations in dogs). However, CRI dosages can also be easily calculated using the formula:

$$A = \text{desired dose in microg / kg / minute}$$

$$B = \text{body weight in kg}$$

$$C = \text{Diluent volume in ml}$$

$$D = \text{Desired fluid rate in ml / hour}$$

$$E = \text{Drug concentration in mg / ml}$$

$$A \times B \times C \times 60 / D \times E \times 1000 = \text{ml of drug to add to diluent}$$

Online Calculators

- The calculator available from the International Veterinary Academy of Pain Management (https://ivapm.wildapricot.org/CRI-Calculator) is accessible to members only. If you do calculations regularly, it is well worth becoming a member of IVAPM to have access to this calculator.
- The Veterinary Anesthesia and Analgesia Support Group (www.vasg.org) has a free veterinary calculator.
- The Veterinary Support Personnel Network has a calculator for members (https://www.vin.com/vspn).

Table 18.6 / Potential problems related to the use of constant rate infusions, and measures to prevent or treat them[54]

Problem	Actions to prevent problem
Catheter disconnection/kinking	• Ensure connection of the catheter and patency of the catheter at each check of the patient
Extravasation	• Assess the catheter at least once a day and each time the infusion pump or syringe driver alarm sounds for high pressure • In the event of extravasation of drugs that cause pain on extravasation, saline flush or lidocaine can be administered
Power failure	• Most syringe drivers and infusion pumps have a battery that can sustain delivery of the drugs for several hours; ensure that batteries are fully charged
Air embolism	• Accurately flush the delivery set initially, and assess for disconnection periodically
Rate of infusion of concomitant drugs	• Do not administer boluses through the same intravenous fluid line as the CRI, especially if the 3-way tap or injection port is distant from the patient's intravenous cannula
Cumulative effects of drugs	• Reassess patient's clinical parameters periodically and titrate the infusions accordingly
Synergic adverse effects of drugs	• Titrate the dose to the clinical effects on the patients and try to reduce the dose of each individual drug whenever possible
Inadequate labelling of syringes/bags of fluids containing drugs for CRI (a bolus can prove fatal in some circumstances)	• Make sure each syringe or bag with added drug for CRI is adequately labeled and visible • The CRI infusion rate should be added on the patient's chart • Ensure that there are clear instructions on dilution and dose rates

Table 18.7 / Dosages for constant rate infusions used in cats[50]

Drug	Loading Dose	CRI dose	Quick calculation	Comments
Morphine*	0.5 mg/kg IM (or 0.25 mg/kg slowly IV)	0.12–0.3 mg/kg/hour (2.0–5.0 μg/kg/minute)	Add 60 mg to 500 ml fluid and run at 1 ml/kg/hour for 0.12 mg/kg/hour	• May cause sedation; can be combined with ketamine and/or lidocaine
Hydromorphone	0.05–0.1 mg/kg IV	0.01–0.05 mg/kg/hour	Add 5–24 mg to 500 ml fluid and run at 1 ml/kg/hour	• May cause sedation; can be combined with ketamine and /or lidocaine

(Continued)

Table 18.7 / Dosages for constant rate infusions used in cats (Continued)

Drug	Loading Dose	CRI dose	Quick calculation	Comments
Fentanyl	0.001–0.003 mg/kg IM or IV (1–5 μg/kg IV)	Postoperative: 0.002–0.010 mg/kg/hour (0.03–0.2 μg/kg/minute) Intraoperative: 0.003–0.04 mg/kg/hour (0.05–0.7 μg/kg/minute	For 5 μg/kg/hour, add 2.5 mg to 500 ml fluid and run at 1 ml/kg/hour	• 2.5 mg = 50 ml fentanyl, remove 50 ml lactated Ringer's solution before adding fentanyl • Can be combined with ketamine and /or lidocaine • Intraoperative dose can be up to 20–40 μg/kg/hour
Methadone	0.1–0.2 mg/kg IV	0.12 mg/kg/hour	Add 60 mg to 500 ml fluid and run at 1 ml/kg/hour	• May cause sedation • Can be combined with ketamine and /or lidocaine
Butorphanol	0.1 mg/kg IV	0.1–0.2 mg/kg/hour	Add 50 mg to 500 ml fluid and run at 1 ml/kg/hour for 0.1 mg/kg/hour	• Only moderately potent and has ceiling effect • Use as part of multimodal protocol
Ketamine*	0.25–0.5 mg/kg IV	0.12–0.6 mg/kg/hour (2–10 μg/kg/minute)	Add 60 mg to 500 ml fluid and run at 1 ml/kg/hour for 0.12 mg/kg/hour	• Generally combined with opioids; may cause dysphoria • Postoperative dose may be higher
Lidocaine	0.5–1.0 mg/kg IV	1.5–3.0 mg/kg/hour (25–50 μg/kg/minute)	Add 750 mg to 500 ml fluid and run at 1 ml/kg/hour for 25 μg/kg/μg	• 750 mg = 37.5 ml, remove 37.5 ml lactated Ringer's solution before adding lidocaine • Can be combined with opioid and/or ketamine
Medetomidine or dexmedetomidine	1–5 μg /kg medetomidine; 1–2 μg/kg dexmedetomidine; can be IV or IM; may not be necessary	0.001–0.004 mg/kg/hour medetomidine (1–4 μg/kg/hr) 0.0005–0.002 mg/kg/hour dexmedetomidine	Add 500 μg medetomidine or 250 μg dexmedetomidine (0.5 ml of either) to 500 ml fluid and run 1–4 ml/kg/hour	• Provides analgesia and light sedation • Excellent addition to opioid CRI or can be administered as solo drug CRI
Morphine*/ ketamine*	Morphine: 0.5 mg/kg IM; ketamine: 0.25–0.5 mg/kg IV	0.12 mg/kg/hour morphine and 0.12 mg/kg/hour ketamine	Add 60 mg morphine and 60 mg ketamine to 500 ml fluid and run at 1 ml/kg/hour	• Can be administered up to 3 ml/kg/hr but sedation or dysphoria may occur • Can substitute hydromorphone, fentanyl or methadone for morphine
Morphine/ ketamine/ lidocaine	Morphine 0.5 mg/kg IM; ketamine 0.25–0.5 mg/kg IV; lidocaine 0.5 mg/kg IV	0.12 mg/kg/hour morphine, 0.12 mg/kg/hour ketamine; 1.5 mg/kg/hour lidocaine	Add 60 mg of morphine, 60 mg ketamine and 750 mg lidocaine to 500 ml fluid and run at 1 ml/kg/hour	• Can substitute hydromorphone, F or methadone for morphine • Dr. Muir's dose is 3.3 μg/kg/μg morphine, 50 μg/kg/minute lidocaine; 10 μg/kg/min ketamine

* Any of the drug amounts in the bag of fluids can be decreased and the fluids administered at a higher rate if necessary. For example, for morphine, ketamine and morphine/ketamine infusions, 7.5 mg morphine and 30 mg ketamine can be used and the CRI administered at 2 ml/kg/hour if more fluids are needed.

Table 18.8 / **Dosages for constant rate infusions used in dogs**[50]

Drug	Loading Dose	CRI dose	Quick calculation	Comments
Morphine*	0.5 mg/kg IM (or 0.25 mg/kg slowly IV)	0.12–0.3 mg/kg/hour (2.0–5.0 μg/kg/minute	Add 60 mg to 500 ml fluid and run at 1 ml/kg/hour for 0.12 mg/kg/hour	• May cause sedation • Can be combined with ketamine and/or lidocaine
Hydromorphone	0.05–0.1 mg/kg IV	0.01–0.05 mg/kg/hour	Add 5–24 mg to 500 ml fluid and run at 1 ml/kg/hour	• May cause sedation • Can be combined with ketamine and/or lidocaine
Fentanyl	0.001–0.003 mg/kg IM or IV (1–5 μg/kg IV)	Postoperative: 0.002–0.010 mg/kg/hour (0.03–0.2 μg/kg/m) Intraoperative: 0.003–0.04 mg/kg/hour (0.05–0.7 μg/kg/minute	For 5 mic/kg/hr, add 2.5 mg to 500 ml fluid and run at 1 ml/kg/hour	• 2.5 mg = 50 ml fentanyl, remove 50 ml lactated Ringer's solution before adding fentanyl • Can be combined with ketaimne and/or lidocaine • Intraoperative dose can be up to 20–40 μg/kg/hour
Methadone	0.1–0.2 mg/kg IV	0.12 mg/kg/hour	Add 60 mg to 500 ml fluid and run at 1 ml/kg/hr	• May cause sedation • Can be combined with ketamine and/or lidocaine
Butorphanol	0.1 mg/kg IV	0.1–0.2 mg/kg/hour	Add 50 mg to 500 ml fluid and run at 1 ml/kg/hour for 0.1 mg/kg/hour	• Only moderately potent and has ceiling effect • Use as part of multimodal protocol
Ketamine*	0.25–0.5 mg/kg IV	0.12–0.6 mg/kg/hour (2–10 μg/kg/minute)	Add 60 mg to 500 ml fluid and run at 1 ml/kg/hr for 0.12 mg/kg/hr	• Generally combined with opioids • May cause dysphoria • Postoperative dose may be higher
Lidocaine	0.5–1.0 mg/kg IV	1.5–3.0 mg/kg/hour (25–50 μg/kg/minute)	Add 750 mg to 500 ml fluid and run at 1 ml/kg/hour for 25 μg/kg/minute	• 750 mg = 37.5 ml • Remove 37.5 ml lactated Ringer's solution before adding lidocaine • Can be combined with opioid and/or ketamine
Medetomidine or dexmedetomidine	1–5 μg/kg medetomidine; 1–2 μg/kg dexmedetomidine; can be IV or IM; may not be necessary	Medetomidine 0.001–0.004 mg/kg/hour (1–4 μg/kg/hour) Dexmedetomidine 0.0005–0.002 mg/kg/hour	Add 500 μg medetomidine or 250 μg dexmedetomidine (0.5 ml of either) to 500 ml fluid and run 1–4 ml/kg/hour	• Provides analgesia and light sedation • Excellent addition to opioid CRI, or can be administered as solo drug CRI

(*Continued*)

Table 18.8 / Dosages for constant rate infusions used in dogs (Continued)

Drug	Loading Dose	CRI dose	Quick calculation	Comments
Morphine*/ ketamine*	Morphine 0.5 mg/kg IM Ketamine 0.25–0.5 mg/kg IV	0.12 mg/kg/hour morphine and 0.12 mg/kg/hour ketamine	Add 60 mg morphine and 60 mg ketamine to 500 ml fluid and run at 1 ml/kg/hour	• Can be administered up to 3 ml/kg/hour but sedation or dysphoria may occur • Can substitute H, F or methadone for M
Morphine/ ketamine/ kidocaine	M: 0.5 mg/kg IM K: 0.25–0.5 mg/kg IV L: 0.5 mg/kg IV	0.12 mg/kg/hour morphine; 0.12 mg/kg/hour ketamine; 1.5 mg/kg/hour lidocaine	Add 60 mg morphine, 60 mg ketamine and 750 mg lidocaine to 500 ml fluid and run at 1 ml/kg/hour	• Can substitute hydromorphone, fentanyl or methadone for morphine • Dr. Muir's dose is 3.3 μg/kg/minute morphine, 50 μg /kg/minites lidocaine; 10 μg/kg/minute ketamine

* Any of the drug amounts in the bag of fluids can be decreased and the fluids administered at a higher rate if necessary. For example, for morphine, ketamine and morphine/ketamine infusions, 30 mg morphine and 30 mg ketamine can be used and the CRI administered at 2 ml/kg/hour if more fluids are needed.

Table 18.9 / SAMPLE chart for adding analgesic drugs to intravenous fluids for dogs[50]

Fluid rate*	Maintenance (50 ml/kg/24 hours)*	½ Maintenance	2 × Maintenance	Surgical (5–10 ml/kg/hour)
Lidocaine dose:	Amount of lidocaine (20 mg/ml) to add to a 1-liter fluid bag (ml):			
25 μg/kg/minute	36	72	18	15 (5 ml/kg/hour) 7.5 (10 ml/kg/hour)
50 μg/kg/minute	72	144	36	30 (5 ml/kg/hour) 15 (10 ml/kg/hour)
75 μg/kg/minute	108	216	54	45 (5 ml/kg/hour) 22.5 (10 ml/kg/hour)
Before adding the lidocaine, remove the same volume of lactated Ringer's solution as you will be adding of lidocaine. Lower dosages (25–50 μg/kg/minute) are used for analgesia while all 3 dosages are used for antiarrhythmic therapy.				
Quick calculation: You can split the difference on the two analgesic dosages and administer 36 μg/kg/minute: add 50 ml 2% lidocaine to 1 liter lactated Ringer's solution and run at 1 ml/lb/hour (0.5 ml/kg/hour).[50]				
Morphine dose:	Amount of morphine (15 mg/ml) to add to a 1-liter fluid bag (ml):			
0.5 μg/kg/minute (cat dose)	0.96	1.92	0.48	0.40 ml (5 ml/kg/hour) 0.20 ml (10 ml/kg/hour)

(Continued)

Table 18.9 / SAMPLE chart for adding analgesic drugs to intravenous fluids for dogs[50] (Continued)

Fluid rate*	Maintenance (50 ml/kg/24 hours)*	½ Maintenance	2 × Maintenance	Surgical (5–10 ml/kg/hour)
1 μg kg/minute	1.92	3.83	0.96	0.80 ml (5 ml/kg/hour) 0.40 ml (10 ml/kg/hour)
2 μg/kg/minute	3.84	7.68	1.92	1.60 ml (5 ml/kg/hour) 0.80 ml (10 ml/kg/hour
Quick calculation: ketamine CRI, add 60 mg (0.6 ml of 100 mg/ml) ketamine to a 1-liter bag and run at 2 ml/kg/hour to provide 2 μg/kg/minute or at surgical fluid rate (10 ml/kg/hour) to provide 10 μg/kg/minute (intraoperative dose).				
Quick calculation: morphine/lidocaine/ketamine:				
To a 500 ml bag of lactated Ringer's solution add:			Administer at 10 ml/kg/hour to provide:	
10 mg morphine (0.66 cc)			morphine 0.2 mg/kg/hour	
120 mg lidocaine (6 cc 2%)			lidocaine 2.5 mg/kg/hour	
100 mg ketamine (1 cc)			ketamine 2 mg/kg/hour	

* Most veterinarians consider maintenance to be 40–60 ml/kg/24 hr, with the lower end of that rate used in cats. If the infusion rate is halved, the amount of lidocaine in the bag should be doubled to keep the dose constant.Source: Appropriate if you do not need to change the IV fluid rate – if the patient might need a fluid bolus it is better to have the CRI in a separate fluid bag or syringe.

NON-PHARMACEUTICAL APPROACHES TO PAIN MANAGEMENT

A multimodal approach to pain management includes not only using different classes of drugs but also incorporating non-drug forms of treatment. Although many of these treatment options can at times stand on their own, using a combination of drug and non-drug options provides the most thorough control of pain (Figure 18.6; Table 18.10).

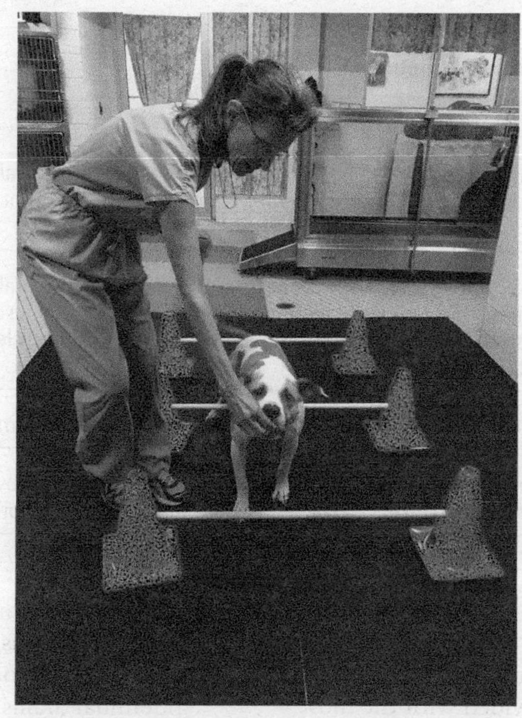

Figure 18.6 Author performing proprioceptive therapeutic exercise over cavaletti rails.

Table 18.10 / Non-pharmaceutical approach to pain management

Modality	Definition	Additional benefits
Acupuncture	• Dry needles, electroacupuncture, aqua-acupuncture, moxibustion, and low-intensity laser therapy	• Postoperative nausea and vomiting and adverse effects of chemotherapy
Chondroprotectants	• Polysulfated glycosaminoglycan, pentosan polysulfate, and sodium hyaluronate	• ↑ Joint health
Environmental enrichment	• Exercise and movement (e.g. cat towers, toys, hiding food) • Grooming	• Provides a possible distraction to pain • Assists with weight management and overall general wellbeing

(Continued)

Table 18.10 / **Non-pharmaceutical approach to pain management (Continued)**

Modality	Definition	Additional benefits
Nutraceuticals	• Glucosamine, chondroitin, manganese ascorbate, superoxide dismutase, DMSO, bioflavonoids, methyl-sulfonyl-methane, omega-3 fatty acids	• Overall ↑ of general wellbeing • ↑ Joint health
Physical rehabilitation	• Therapeutic exercise, passive and active range of motion exercises, electrotherapy, manual therapeutic techniques • Therapeutic laser therapy, shock wave therapy, therapeutic ultrasound, heat and cold therapy	• Overall ↑ of general wellbeing • ↑ Muscle strength and joint range of motion and ↓ edema and muscle spasms
Radiation	• Local or whole-body radiation to decrease tumor size	• Treatment can be curative for some tumors
Weight management	• Maintaining an optimum body conditioning score • Reducing obesity with diet and exercise	• Improves mobility and ↓ continuing damage to ligaments and tendons

PATIENT CARE TO DECREASE PAIN AND ANXIETY

Veterinary technicians/nurses can institute numerous non-pharmacological methods available to ensure that a painful patient is provided with the most comfort possible, in addition to judicious use of analgesics.[55] The technician/nurse needs to assess the patient's pain level and implement plans to help achieve maximum comfort for the patient. Nursing interventions for patient comfort can include:

- House cats away from barking dogs. Consider strategies such as boxes in the cage for the cat to hide within, with an opening large enough for observation.
- Keep barking to a minimum by asking the veterinarian to provide an "as needed" basis.
- Providing bedding, toys, food dishes, or owners' clothing from home can be soothing for the pet that is having trouble adjusting to the hospital environment.
- Tender loving care and extra attention for the patient that is anxious or stressed will be comforting.
- Ensure that adequate sleep is occurring for the patient to aid in healing and reduce stress/pain.
- Certain monitoring devices are invasive. These can contribute to stress/pain. Intravenous, arterial, nasal and urinary catheters, as well as other tubes such as esophagostomy/gastrostomy tubes, thoracic drains and abdominal drains all need to be recognized as causing stress and pain. Therefore, care in checking these devices needs to be taken to keep the patient comfortable. Consideration of additional pain medications during checking these devices or removal of them should be thought of before it is needed.
- Positional comfort needs to be examined for postoperative recovery, and especially for geriatric patients, where extra padding and cushioning may be needed. Patients that have paralysis or shock need to be adjusted and turned so they do not develop decubital ulcers from being in one position too long. Changing the position of these patients, even from lateral to sternal, will often allow the patient to relax without increasing anesthetic/analgesic doses.
- Be aware of urinating and defecating needs. Placing a temporary or indwelling urinary catheter may be beneficial to relieve the anxiety of needing to urinate, and to prevent urine scalding. The patient that is eating and has normal stool should produce a bowel movement daily. Occasionally, the act of taking a temperature will stimulate a bowel movement, so having a diaper pad handy is advisable. Using assist

devices such as slings or harnesses may allow the patient to assume an elimination posture more easily without risk of a fall.

- Temperature and humidity need to be evaluated. Is the patient panting and does it have a heavy coat? If so, maybe a fan or cooling gel pads may be beneficial. Is the patient shivering and struggling to control hypothermia? If so, warm blankets and padding or warming devices may be what is needed.
- Be ready to address patient thirst and hunger by providing water in a syringe or moving their water bowl within reach if they are unable to reach it by themselves. A nutritional plan needs to be assessed prior to hospitalization. To begin eating, some patients may need coaxing with extra fragrant "sauces" added to their meals, such as chicken or beef baby food, juice from a can of tuna or sardines, gravy or other flavor enhancers.
- Visits from owners or nursing care go a long way in improving the health and relieving stress/pain for the hospitalized patient.

CONCLUSION

The veterinary technician is the primary advocate for their patients in pain because they are unable to "speak". Advanced knowledge about the pain process, pain behaviors, stress, pain medications, non-pharmacologic pain relief and patient comfort are often required. It is the duty of every technician to be the "voice" for their patients so that premium care is provided for all painful patients.

REFERENCES

1. Middleton, C. (2003). Understanding the physiological effects of unrelieved pain. *Nurs Times* 99: 28–31.
2. Muir, W.W. and Woolf, C.J. (2001). Mechanisms of pain and their therapeutic implications. *J Am Ved Med Assoc* 219: 1346–1356.
3. Melzack, R. and Wall, P. (1965). Pain mechanisms: a new theory. *Science* 150: 971–979.
4. Merskey, H., Bogduk, N. (1994). *Classification of Chronic Pain*. Seattle, WA: International Association for the Study of Pain Press.
5. Thompson, D. (2004). The pain process. Veterinary Anesthesia and Analgesia Support Group. http://www.vasg.org/the_pain_process.htm (accessed 30 July 2021).
6. Bouhassira, D., Lantéri-Minet, M., Attal, N. *et al.* (2008). Prevalence of chronic pain with neuropathic characteristics in the general population. *Pain* 136: 380–387.
7. Kurita, G.P., Ulrich, A., Jensen, T.S. *et al.* (2012). How is neuropathic cancer pain assessed in randomised controlled trials? *Pain* 153: 13–17.
8. Goldberg, M.E. (2017). A look at chronic pain in dogs, *Vet Nurs J* 32: 37–44.
9. Lucroy, M.D. (2013). Cancer pain management. In *A Color Handbook of Small Animal Anesthesia and Pain Management* (ed. J. Ko), 305–310. Boca Raton, FL: CRC Press.
10. Goldberg, M.E. (2020). Pain management. In: *Mosby's Comprehensive Review for Veterinary Technicians*, 5e (ed. M.M. Tighe and M. Brown), 495–526. St. Louis, MO: Elsevier.
11. Langford, D.J., Bailey, A.L., Chanda, M.L. *et al.* (2010). Coding of facial expressions of pain in the laboratory mouse. *Nat Methods* 7: 447–449.
12. Sotocinal, S.G., Sorge, R.E., Zaloum, A. *et al.* (2011). The rat grimace scale: a partially automated method for quantifying pain in the laboratory rat via facial expressions. *Mol Pain* 7: 55
13. Keating, S.C.J., Thomas, A.A., Flecknell, P.A. *et al.* (2012). Evaluation of EMLA cream for preventing pain during tattooing of rabbits: changes in physiological, behavioural and facial expression responses. *PLoS One* 7: e44437.
14. Reijgwart, M.L., Schoemaker, N.J., Pascuzzo, R. *et al.* (2017). The composition and initial evaluation of a grimace scale in ferrets after surgical implantation of a telemetry probe. *PLoS One* 12: e0187986.
15. Holden, E., Calvo, G., Collins, M. *et al.* (2014). Evaluation of facial expression in acute pain in cats. *J Small Anim Pract* 55: 615–621.
16. Dalla Costa, E., Minero, M., Lebelt, D. *et al.* (2014). Development of the horse grimace scale (HGS) as a pain assessment tool in horses undergoing routine castration. *PLoS One* 9: e92281.
17. Gleerup, K.B., Andersen, P.H., Munksgaard, L. *et al.* (2015). Pain evaluation in dairy cattle. *Appl Anim Behav Sci* 171: 25–32.
18. Abu-Serriah, M., Nolan, A.M., Dolan, S. (2007). Pain assessment following experimental maxillofacial surgical procedure in sheep. *Lab Anim* 41: 345–352.
19. McLennan, K.M., Rebelo, C.J.B., Corke, M.J. *et al.* (2016). Development of a facial expression scale using footrot and mastitis as models of pain in sheep. *Appl Anim Behav Sci* 176: 19–26.
20. Muri, K. and Valle, P.S. (2012). Human–animal relationships in the Norwegian dairy goat industry: assessment of pain and provision of veterinary treatment (part II). *Anim Welfare* 21: 547–558.
21. Di Giminiani, P., Brierley, V.L.M.H., Scollo, A *et al.* (2016). The assessment of facial expressions in piglets undergoing tail docking and castration: toward the development of the piglet grimace scale. *Front Vet Sci*, 3: 100.

22. Mathews, K.A., Kronen, P.W., Lascelles, D. *et al.* (2014). WSAVA guidelines for recognition, assessment and treatment of pain, *J Small Anim Pract* 55: E10–E68.
23. Epstein, M.E., Rodan, I., Griffenhagen, G. *et al.* (2015). AAHA/AAFP pain management guidelines for dogs and cats, *J Feline Med Surg* 17: 251–272.
24. Shaffran, N. (2008). Pain management: the veterinary technician's perspective, *Vet Clin Small Anim* 38: 1415–1428.
25. Karas, A. (2011). Pain, anxiety, or dysphoria – how to tell? A video assessment lab. *Proc Am Coll Vet Surg* 2011: 509–512.
26. Maher, J. (2016). Wakin' up is hard to do [blog post]. *VetBloom* 6 September. http://blog.vetbloom.com/anesthesia-analgesia/wakin-up-is-hard-to-do ().
27. Taylor, P.M. and Robertson, S.A. (2004). Pain management in cats: past, present and future. Part 1. The cat is unique. *J Feline Med Surg* 6: 313–320.
28. Balakrishnan, A. and Benasutti, E. (2012). Pain assessment in dogs and cats. *Today's Vet Pract* 2(3): 68–74.
29. Goldberg, M.E. (2017). A look at chronic pain in cats. *Vet Nurs J* 32: 67–77.
30. Monteiro, B. and Lascelles, D. (2018). Assessment and recognition of chronic (maladaptive) pain. In: *Feline Anesthesia and Pain Management* (ed. P. Steagall, S. Robertson and P. Taylor), 241–256. Ames, IA: Wiley.
31. Adams, V. (2016). Approach to the companion animal cancer patient part 1: an overview. *Vet Nurse* 7: 318–325.
32. Heath, S., Rusbridge, C., Johnson, N. *et al.* (2010). Feline orofacial pain syndrome. In: Proceedings of the Australian Veterinary Association (AVA) Annual Conferences. Proceedings of the 3rd AVA/NZVA Pan Pacific Veterinary Conference, Dental Stream, Brisbane, Queensland, Australia, June 2010.
33. Mathews, K. (2008). Neuropathic pain in dogs and cats: if only they could tell us if they hurt. *Vet Clin N Am Small Anim Pract* 38: 1365–1414.
34. Ciribassi J. (2009). Understanding behavior: feline hyperesthesia syndrome. *Compend Contin Educ Vet* 31: E10.
35. Cannon, M. (2015). Feline chronic gingivostomatitis. *Comp Anim* 20: 616–623.
36. Fox, S.M. (2014). Cancer pain. In: *Pain Management in Small Animal Medicine*, 267–284. Boca Raton, FL: CRC Press.
37. Hielm-Björkman, A.K., Rita, H., and Tulamo, R.M. (2009). Psychometric testing of the Helsinki chronic pain index by completion of a questionnaire in Finnish by owners of dogs with chronic signs of pain caused by osteoarthritis. *Am J Vet Res* 70: 727–734.
38. Fingeroth, J.M. and Thomas, W.B. (eds.) (2015). *Advances in Intervertebral Disc Disease in Dogs and Cats*. Ames, IA: Wiley/Blackwell.
39. Fox, S.M. Chronic pain in selected physiological systems: ophthalmic, aural, and dental. In: *Chronic Pain in Small Animal Medicine*, 202–208. Boca Raton, FL: CRC Press.
40. Reid, J., Nolan, A.M., Hughes, J.M.L. *et al.* (2007). Development of the short-form Glasgow composite measure pain scale (CMPS-SF) and derivation of an analgesic intervention score. *Anim Welfare* 16: 97–104.
41. Reid, J., Scott, E.M., Calvo, G. *et al.* (2017). Definitive Glasgow acute pain scale for cats: validation and intervention level. *Vet Rec* 180: 449.
42. Brondani, J.T., Mama, K.R., Luna, S.P. *et al.* (2013). Validation of the English version of the UNESP-Botucatu multidimensional composite pain scale for assessing postoperative pain in cats. *BMC Vet Res* 9: 143.
43. Hielm-Björkman, A.K., Rita, H. and Tulamo, R.M. (2009). Psychometric testing of the Helsinki chronic pain index by completion of a questionnaire in Finnish by owners of dogs with chronic signs of pain caused by osteoarthritis. *Am J Vet Res* 70: 727–734.
44. Brown, D.C. (2017). The Canine Brief Pain Inventory. https://www.vet.upenn.edu/research/clinical-trials-vcic/our-services/pennchart/cbpi-tool (accessed 29 July 2021).
45. Gingerich, D.A. and Strobel, J.D. (2003). *Vet Ther* 4: 56–65. http://www.thek9rehabcenter.com/wp-content/uploads/2015/09/CODI.pdf (accessed 29 July 2021).
46. University of Glasgow. (2018). VetMetrica HRQL. https://www.newmetrica.com/vetmetrica-hrql (accessed 29 July 2021).
47. University of Liverpool. (2014). Liverpool Osteoarthritis in Dogs (LOAD) owner questionnaire for dogs with mobility problems. https://dspace.uevora.pt/rdpc/bitstream/10174/19611/2/liverpool%20OA%20in%20dogs%20-%20load.pdf (accessed 29 July 2021).
48. Comparative Pain Research Laboratory. (2015). Feline Musculoskeletal Pain Index. North Carolina State Univeristy. https://painfreecats.org/the-fmpi (accesssed 29 July 2021).
49. Barker, M. (2013). Local anaesthesia; part 1 regional anaesthesia of the head. *Vet Nurs J* 28: 396–399.
50. MacDougall, L.M., Hethey, J.A., Livingston A. *et al.* (2009). Antinociceptive, cardiopulmonary, and sedative effects of five intravenous infusion rates of lidocaine in conscious dogs. *Vet Anaesth Analg* 36: 512–522.
51. McCarthy, G.C., Megalla S.A. and Habib, A.S. (2010). Impact of intravenous lidocaine infusion on postoperative analgesia and recovery from surgery: a systematic review of randomized controlled trials. *Drugs* 70: 1149–1163.
52. Cassuto, J., Sinclair, R., and Bonderovic, M. (2006). Antiinflammatory properties of local anesthetics and their present and potential clinical implications. *Acta Anaesthesiol Scand* 50: 265–282.
53. Goldberg, M.E. (2017). Be the pain-attacking offensive midfielder – local anaesthetic blocks every practice can utilize. *Vet Nurs J* 32: 329–338.
54. Zoff, A. and Bradbrook, C. (2016). Constant rate infusions in small animal practice. *Comp Anim* 21: 516–522.
55. Steele, A. (2018). Optimal Nursing Care for the Management of Pain. In: *Analgesia and Anesthesia for the Ill or Injured Dog and Cat* (ed. K.A. Mathews, M. Sinclair, A.M. Steele et al.), 219–229. Hoboken, NJ: Wiley.

Chapter **19**

Wound Care and Bandaging

Danielle Browning, LVMT, VTS (Surgery)

Veterinary Technician and Nurse's Daily Reference Guide: Canine and Feline, Fourth Edition. Edited by Mandy Fults and Kenichiro Yagi.

Companion website: www.wiley.com/go/fults/veterinary

Abbreviations

EDTA, ethylenediaminetetraacetic acid
NaCl, sodium chloride
psi, pounds per square inch
SSD, silver sulfadiazin

Inevitably, pets end up with wounds, either self-inflicted or caused by another source. These wounds may be intentional, such as a surgical incision, or an accident. A technician plays a valuable role in the setup, preparation, cleaning, and the actual bandaging of these wounds. An understanding of the wound healing process, objective descriptions of the wound, supplies to use, and the expected final outcome is necessary for proper treatment and care. These items are included in this chapter to facilitate excellent nursing care by the technician.

STAGES OF WOUND HEALING

Wound healing is a continuous process, where several phases occur simultaneously with subtle transitions. The rate and quality of the healing is dependent on many factors, such as nutritional status, current medications (e.g. steroids, cytotoxic drugs), infection, and additional treatments (e.g. radiation).

Table 19.1 / Stages of wound healing

Inflammatory phase (3–5 days)	Proliferative (repair) phase (4–20 days)	Maturation (remodeling) phase (weeks to 2 years)
1. Hemorrhage cleans the wound and platelets aid in the formation of a fibrin clot which serves as a scaffold for cells. 2. Vasoconstriction occurs initially to stop bleeding, followed by vasodilation. 3. Vasodilation causes an increase in blood flow and permits the leakage of plasma and proteins necessary to establish an immune barrier. 4. Neutrophils leak out (around 6 hours after initial trauma) to engulf and remove bacteria and necrotic tissue. 5. Monocytes fill the wound (around 12 hours after initial trauma) and participate in tissue formation remodeling. 6. Monocytes become macrophages (around 24–48 hours after initial trauma) and continue to phagocytize bacteria, foreign material, and necrotic tissue. 7. "Lag phase" refers to the lack of wound strength during this phase of healing. 8. Classic signs of inflammation; heat, redness, pain and swelling may be noted.	9. The proliferative phase is characterized by angiogenesis, fibroplasia, contraction and epithelialization 10. Fibroblasts and new capillaries make up granulation tissue, which protects the wound from infection and provides a surface for the migration of epithelial cells. 11. New epithelial cells reproduce at the wound edge, and migrate across the wound covering the granulation bed. Epithelialization will occur one to two days after injury, but is often not visible seen in open wounds until day 4–5. Epithelialization can take place under a scab. 12. Fibroblasts transform into myofibroblasts to pull together the wound edge. Contraction has been reported to occur at a rate around 0.6–0.8 mm/day (beginning around 6 days after initial trauma and continue the following 2 weeks). 13. Collagen plays a key role in proliferation and remodeling and is a major component of the wounds extracellular matrix.	14. Remodeling of collagen, type I replaces type III collagen and wounded tissue strengthens (begins around 4 weeks after initial trauma). 15. The wounded tissue may continue to gain strength over years but will remain 15–20% weaker than surrounding normal skin.

CLASSIFICATION OF WOUNDS

Table 19.2 / Classification of wounds

Classification	Characteristics
Tissue integrity	
Open	• Lacerations or skin loss
Closed	• Crushing injuries and contusions
Etiologic force	
Abrasion	• Loss of epidermis and portions of dermis; usually attributable to shearing between two compressive surfaces or friction from blunt trauma
Avulsion/degloving	• Tearing of tissue from its attachment and the creation of skin flaps • Avulsions with extensive skin loss on extremities are degloving injuries • Forces similar to those causing abrasion but of greater magnitude
Thermal burn	• A partial or full thickness skin injury caused by extreme heat • Extent of tissue damage is difficult to predict and needs to declare over days
Laceration/incision	• Created by a sharp object • Wound edges are smooth and minimal tissue trauma is present in surrounding tissue • An irregular wound caused by tearing of tissue with variable damage to superficial and underlying tissue
Puncture	• Skin penetration by a missile or sharp object (e.g. bite wound) • Superficial damage may be minimal, but damage to deeper structures may be considerable • Contamination by hair and bacteria with subsequent infection is common
Decubital ulcer	• Result of skin compression over a bony prominence or hard surface. • Common locations affected are: greater trochanter, elbow, and hock • Thin, recumbent animals are at high risk
Degree of contamination	
Clean	• Surgically created under aseptic conditions; no invasion of respiratory, alimentary, or genitourinary tracts or of the oropharyngeal cavities
Clean contaminated	• Minimal contamination where the contamination can be effectively removed; includes operative wounds involving the respiratory, wound alimentary, and genitourinary tracts
Contaminated wound	• Open traumatic wound with heavy contamination and possibly foreign debris; includes operative wounds with major breaks in aseptic technique, and incisions in areas of acute non-purulent inflammation adjacent to inflamed or contaminated skin
Dirty/infected wound	• Older, traumatic wounds with clinical infection or perforated viscera

WOUND CHARACTERISTICS

When evaluating a wound, it is important to record pertinent information in the patient's medical record. When detailed descriptions of wound parameters are provided, they can help guide a veterinarian to choosing their next course of action. Creating a wound evaluation sheet can help the team record valuable information in a well-organized and consistent manner.

Parameters that should be included on a wound evaluation sheet are the amount of wound fluid, fluid color, nature of fluid, wound odor, peri-wound status, wound character, granulation tissue, and epithelialization. Identify the type, location, and size of the wound. Measure the length, width, and depth of the wound, indicating if it is an actual or estimated value and the units of measurements used (i.e. centimeters or inches).

Additional information that should be recorded on a wound evaluation sheet include discomfort on dressing removal, sedation required, and the appearance of the bandage prior to the dressing change.

Table 19.3 / Descriptions of wound characteristics

Wound characteristic	Description
Wound fluid[1]	• None/absent • Minimal (+) – wet wound tissue or 5 cc of exudate in 24 hours • Moderate (++) – saturated wound tissue or 5–10 cc of exudate in 24 hours • Excessive/high (+++) – wound tissue bathed in wound fluid or > 10 cc every 24 hours
Fluid color	• Clear, pink/red, brown, yellow, green
Nature of fluid	• Serous/gel: clear, amber, thin and watery • Serosanguineous: clear, pink, thin and watery • Sanguineous: reddish, thin and watery • Fibrinous: cloudy and thin, which strands of fibrin • Purulent: opaque, milky; sometimes green • Hemorrhagic: presence of blood, red, thick
Wound odor	• yes or no (may also indicate amount of odor present and pungency)
Peri-wound status (indicate all that apply)	• Normal tissue • Maceration: to become soft from excessive moisture • Irritation: redness, sore, abraded skin • Inflammation: heat, redness, swelling and pain • Desiccation: to dry out
Wound character (indicate all that apply)	• No apparent healing • Desiccated • Necrosis • Partially granulated • Fully granulated

(Continued)

Table 19.3 / Descriptions of wound characteristics (Continued)

Wound characteristic	Description
Granulation tissue	• None • Healthy red and granular • Dark red and granular • Purple and friable • Pale and fibrous • Exuberant (when the above adjacent skin surface)
Epithelialization	• None • < 25%, the wound edges • 25% to < 50% • 50% to < 75% • 75% to < 100% • 100% wound coverage (surface intact)
• Additional information that should be recorded on a wound evaluation sheet, include discomfort upon dressing removal, sedation required and the appearance of the bandage prior to the dressing change. • Appearance of the bandage: dry and clean, dry and stained, moist, wet, strike-through	
Discomfort upon dressing removal	• None • Mild irritation (twitches upon removal, turns head) • Moderately painful (yelps, flinches at each touch) • Marked pain (screams, tries to bite and/or flee)
Sedation administration	• Indicate the medication(s), dosage and route given
• **When possible take a photo with a measurement ruler of the wound**	

FACTORS AFFECTING THE HEALING PROCESS

Table 19.4 / Factors affecting the healing process

Factor	Effect on healing
Age of patient	• An older patient may require more nursing care and good nutrition for healing to occur • These patients are often arthritic and muscle wasted, requiring therapeutic bedding to provide additional padding • Wound closure is generally preferred over open wound management in geriatric patients
Wound perfusion	• Blood supply is responsible for the delivery of oxygen and metabolic substrates that promote wound healing • Dehydration, trauma to the area, tight bandages, or location of the wound may have an effect on this factor • Avoid drugs that cause peripheral vasoconstriction • Avoid perioperative hypothermia
Dead space	• Separation of tissue can result in fluid accumulation (e.g. seromas), producing a hypoxic state impairing cell migration • Fluid accumulation mechanically inhibits adhesion (e.g. flaps and grafts) to the granulation bed • Sutures, drains and bandages are used to reduce the dead space
Diseased or debilitated patients	• Diseased, debilitated, or stressed organs hinder the healing process • Delayed wound healing with diabetes, hepatic disease, hyperadrenocorticism, neoplasia, and uremia • Geriatrics often heal slower, potentially due to concurrent disease or debilitation • Uremia/azotemia: increases the time formation of granulation tissue occurs
Foreign material	• Foreign material (e.g. foreign debris or suture material) results in prolonged inflammatory phase of healing and ↑ risk of infection
Hemostasis	• If bleeding is not stabilized effectively, a seroma or hematoma may form • Extra fluid in a wound slows down the healing process as the body must reabsorb and break down old blood and fluid during the inflammatory phase • Can predispose to sepsis of wound
Incision	• A surgical incision is a wound created in a controlled environment • Skin sutures may need to remain in place longer (14–21 days until removal) in locations of known neoplasia (e.g. mast cell tumor)
Infection	• Overgrowth of bacteria prolongs the inflammatory phase and may lead to a systemic infection (sepsis)
Mechanical	• High tension, motion, and pressure will prolong the wound healing process • A tension-relieving suture can be used to pull skin edges closer and stretch intact skin • Bandages and splints can minimize motion • Donut bandages are used to eliminate pressure over bony prominences
Medications	• Medications may inhibit connective tissue building and epithelial cell turnover rate • Corticosteroids delay the entire wound healing process and ↑ the risk of infection • Aspirin may affect blood clotting during the early phase of wound healing • Anti-inflammatory drugs affect inflammation • Chemotherapeutic drugs and radiation can drastically inhibit wound healing (e.g. postoperative interval 10–14 days desirable between surgery and adjunct antineoplastic treatment)

(*Continued*)

Table 19.4 / **Factors affecting the healing process (Continued)**

Factor	Effect on healing
Moisture	• A moist environment allows for optimal healing • Allows for cell migration and subsequent healing, ↑ rate of epithelialization, and limits infection and penetration of topical medications • Bandaging helps to keep a wound warm and moist • Excessive moisture can be detrimental to the wound and macerate the surrounding skin • Use absorptive dressings to manage moderate to heavy exudative wounds • Skin barrier film (Cavilon®, 3M)
Necrotic Tissue	• Non-viable tissue prolongs the inflammatory phase and predisposes the animal to infection. • An eschar is a hard, black piece of dead tissue that occurs in burn wounds, covering the wound surface. This dead tissue will trap in exudate that is detrimental to healing
Nutrition	• Malnutrition and serum albumin < 1.5–2.0 g/dl delay wound healing and diminish wound strength • Vitamin supplementation (e.g. vitamins A and E) and aloe vera can ↑ wound healing

WOUND CARE

Care for an open or superficial wound should begin immediately after trauma. The wound should be covered with a clean, dry cloth or bandage to prevent further hemorrhage or contamination. Ideally, wounds should be treated within the first six hours before bacteria has multiplied and the risk of infection increases. Infected wounds, rather than contaminated wounds, are often characterized by a thick, purulent (viscous) exudate and visually appear unhealthy, as seen with abscesses. However, not all infected wounds will have purulent exudate.

Before any procedure involving wound care, clean exam gloves should be worn by those in contact with the wound to avoid environmental bacteria translocated to the wounds. Gloves should be changes after bandage removal, and prior to the application of a new bandage.

Skill Box 19.1 / **Wound care**

Setup

- Antiseptic or antimicrobial solution (2% chlorhexidine: diluted 1: 40 with water or saline)
- Wound irrigation fluids or sink tap
- 4 × 4 gauze
- Suture material (size and type depends on need)
- Surgical instruments needed to debride, explore and suture the wound
- Electric clippers and #40 clipper blade, clipper cleaner with a brush
- Non-sterile and sterile gloves (multiple pairs)
- Multiple absorbent potty pads or towels to keep workspace clean and dry
- Trash bin
- Vacuum
- Wet-sink table (optional)
- Sterile water-soluble lubricant
- Dressing and bandaging material
- Surgical drain (optional)

Step I: wound preparation

1. Clean out any large, obvious debris.
2. Protect the wound from further contamination with sterile water-soluble lubricant, (e.g. K-Y Jelly™) saline-soaked gauze, or temporarily close with sutures, towel clamps, or staples.
3. Clip a wide margin of the hair from around the wound with electric clippers.

(Continued)

Skill Box 19.1 / Wound care (Continued)

4. When shaving patients with multiple bite wounds, it is important to account for all the puncture sites that may have occurred from both the top and bottom jaw of the attacker.
5. Prepare the clipped skin as a surgical preparation; avoid using alcohol directly on the wound bed.
6. Remove any wound protectant (e.g. water-soluble lubricant, saline-soaked gauze, or temporarily close with sutures, clamps, or staples).

Step II: wound cleaning

- For acute traumatic or highly contaminated wounds, copious lavage is important.
- Lavage the wound to reduce the bacterial count and remove additional contaminants and necrotic debris.
- For heavily contaminated or infected wounds, antimicrobial scrub soaps can be used directly on the wound. *Important:* all the soap must be thoroughly lavaged out of the wound bed.
- Scrub soaps are cytotoxic to wound cells and generally should be avoided.
- It is recommended to only use diluted antimicrobial solutions after the inflammatory phase.

Lavage solutions

- Warm, balanced electrolyte solutions (e.g. lactated Ringer's solution)
- Sterile saline
- 0.05% chlorhexidine solution(add 25 ml 2% chlorohexidine solution to 1 liter water or saline)
- 1% diluted povidone-iodine solution (color of weak tea)
- Tap water (ideal for large heavily contaminated wounds)
- Hydrochlorous acid (e.g. Vetericyn®) wound and skin care solution

Lavage method

- Ideal fluid pressure is 7–9 psi
- Best method to provide 7–9 psi: fluid administration set with a 16–22-gauge needle, attached to a 1-liter fluid bag that is placed inside a pressure bag and filled to 300 mmHg 16–22-gauge needle. This moderate pressure is used to thoroughly clean the wound; all debris should be removed.
- An alternative method is to use an 18-gauge needle to puncture the cap of a 1-liter saline bottle; this method is low pressure (< 7 psi), but can be effective in high volume.
- Using the hose on the wet sink(pressure can vary).
- Bowl and bulb syringe (low pressure).

Step III: wound debridement

Debridement is the removal of necrotic tissue and debris that has adhered to the wound surface impeding wound healing.

Debridement method

- Autolytic: maintaining a moist wound environment with hydrophilic, occlusive, or semiocclusive bandaging, to allow the body's enzymes to debride away necrotic tissue (e.g. honey).
- Larval therapy: medicinal maggot therapy to remove necrotic tissue, and to promote granulation. Ideal for chronic wounds infected with a multidrug resistant organism. Use care to protect the intact epithelium.
- Enzymatic: agents (e.g. trypsin, chymotrypsin) used to break down necrotic tissue.
- Excisional (surgical): sharp removal of devitalized tissue (e.g. skin, muscle, contaminated fat) and bone sequestra. This can be performed en bloc (complete excision) or layered (sequential removal repeated as necessary).
- Mechanical: wet-to-dry and dry-to-dry dressings adhere to the wound surface and are removed when dry. These dressings are unfavorable because of their non-selective nature and pain associated with removal. Recommended to use only during the early stage of healing.

Step IV: wound closure

The type of closure is dependent on time lapse, degree of contamination, tissue damage, thoroughness of debridement, blood supply (viability), animal's health, available tissue, closure without skin tension or dead space, and location of wound (function).

Primary wound closure

- First-intention wound healing; wound is sutured closed.
- Used when wounds are six to eight hours old, with minimal tissue damage and minimal contamination or cleaned wounds.
- Contaminated wound can be flushed and primarily closed over a drain.
- Following en bloc debridement

(*Continued*)

Skill Box 19.1 / Wound care (Continued)

Contraction and epithelialization (second-intention wound healing)

- Wound is left to heal open, with epithelialization and skin defect contraction over time (days to weeks).
- Used when wounds are ≥ 5 days old, have significant tissue damage and loss, or are excessively contaminated.
- The new skin may not contain hair follicles and result in a scar.

Delayed primary closure

- Closure before the formation of granulation tissue, usually within three to five days after wounding.
- Used when wounds are greater than six hours old, were mildly contaminated, infected or needed a few days to declare (e.g. burns).
- Allows controlled debridement and optimal drainage.

Secondary wound closure (third-intention wound healing)

- The wound is sutured closed after the granulation tissue has formed and a thin layer of epithelium has appeared along the wound edges, typically three to five days after wounding.
- Used for severely contaminated, infected or traumatized wounds.

Drain placement

- Used to eliminate dead space and to provide drainage of potentially harmful body fluids (e.g. blood, pus, serum).
- Passive drains (e.g. Penrose drains) allow drainage by gravity and are most commonly used for subcutaneous spaces. When shaving the patient, these drains will always exit ventral to the wound. Wounds can be partially closed.
- Active drains (e.g. Jackson-Pratt) allow drainage with an intermittent or continuous negative pressure that remains closed to the environment and are most commonly used for deep pocketing wounds. Active drains allow for a more precise measurement of the volume and characteristics of the drainage. Wounds must be completely sutured closed to hold negative pressure.
- Ascending infection is an associated complication of drains (especially Penrose drains) and should therefore be covered with a sterile dressing; change as needed.

Step V: drain care and assessment

Monitoring

- Visual inspection for fluid accumulation, tension, infection, dehiscence, and necrosis.
- Ultrasound evaluation for fluid accumulation, scar formation, granulation tissue, blood clots, edematous regions, and epidermis can be performed.
- Record the volume of drainage collected each day.
- Protect the intact skin from maceration by applying a barrier film to protect the skin from fluid maceration.

Drain care

- Monitor for drainage as tissue fragments, viscous exudates, or fibrin may occlude the tube.
- Apply warm compresses to the drainage area two to three times daily to improve drainage and to keep passive drainage sites open.
- Drain removal is dependent on the fluid quantity and quality; typically, a drain remains in place for three to five days, but may be needed longer.

Suture care

- Keep clean and dry. Avoid patient molestation.
- Suture removal is 7–14 days; with longer use, suture material may become a foreign material.
- Prevent patient molestation of the incision by using head and neck-collars, t-shirts or bandages.

Client Education: Drain Care

Surgical drains (e.g. Penrose drains) are often placed in wounds to eliminate dead space and to allow drainage of the contaminated fluid. The latex tubing is a passive drain that allows gravity or a capillary action to draw fluid out of the wound around the outside of the tube. Fluid will not be seen flowing through the center as the tube is used to only maintain a drainage path. As easily as the contaminated fluid drains from the wound, potentially pathogenic bacteria can enter the wound, which is the most common complication of passive drains. Keeping the area clean and dry will decrease this likelihood.

Drain care is often required two to three times per day and includes bandage changes and hot compressing.

Skill Box 19.2 / Client education: drain care

Surgical drains (e.g. Penrose drains) are often placed in wounds to eliminate dead space and to allow drainage of the contaminated fluid. The latex tubing is a passive drain that allows gravity or a capillary action to draw fluid out of the wound around the outside of the tube. Fluid will not be seen flowing through the center as the tube is used to only maintain a drainage path. As easily as the contaminated fluid drains from the wound, potentially pathogenic bacteria can enter the wound, which is the most common complication of passive drains. Keeping the area clean and dry will decrease this likelihood.

Drain care is often required two to three times per day and includes bandage changes and hot compressing.

Supplies

- Gloves
- Warm water
- Clean towels
- Petroleum jelly or skin barrier film

Warm compress procedure

1. Wearing gloves, wet a clean towel with very warm water (not too hot, ensure that you can tolerate it on your own skin), and place it directly over the wound and drain exit holes.
2. Place gentle pressure over the towel for 5–10 minutes, rewarming the towel as needed.
3. Remove the towel and clean away any exudate at the drain exit holes and on the skin or fur.
4. Gently tug back and forth on the tube to verify the tract is clear and not adhering to the tube to allow continued drainage.
5. Use a clean towel to dry off the drain area and reapply the bandage if necessary.

Tip: Apply ointment or skin barrier film (Cavilon®, 3M) at the exit holes to prevent skin irritation.

Notes

- Patients with incisions and drains placed should be kept indoors and the use of an Elizabethan collar is recommended.
- All towels should be laundered after each use to avoid contamination of the environment.
- After the drain has been removed, the exit holes can continue to be warm compressed. The exit holes are not sutured closed and should heal by second intention.

Table 19.5 / Wound cleaning solutions

Solution	Indications	Comments
0.9% NaCl	Grossly contaminated, burns, lacerations, dermal ulcers, abrasions	• Isotonic solution • No antimicrobial activity
Balanced Electrolyte Solution (lactated Ringer's solution, Normosol®)	Grossly contaminated, burns, lacerations, dermal ulcers, abrasions	• Ideal isotonic solution that is the least cytotoxic • No antimicrobial activity
Tap water	Grossly, contaminated wounds, lacerations, acute traumatic wounds	• Hypotonic • Has been reported to cause cell swelling, leading to destruction and delayed wound healing • No antimicrobial activity • No difference of wound infection rates when compared to sterile saline

(*Continued*)

Table 19.5 / Wound cleaning solutions (Continued)

Solution	Indications	Comments
Chlorhexidine (Nolvasan®)	Grossly contaminated or infected wounds, burns, lacerations, dermal ulcers, abrasions, bite wounds	• Wide spectrum of antimicrobial activity and residual activity for up to two days • A 0.05% solution (25 ml 2% chlorhexidine + 1 l saline or tap water) is recommended as higher concentrations are cytotoxic • Precipitates that form in lactated Ringer's solution and NaCl do not affect the antimicrobial efficacy • Complications: resistance in some bacteria, corneal drying, toxic to meninges and not recommended for arthritic joints
Chloroxylenol (Technicare®)	All wound care	• Effective against all Gram-negative and -positive organisms within 30 seconds, antiviral, antifungal • Apply to the wound and gently scrub with a gauze sponge for 2 minutes to cleanse and stimulate antimicrobial action and rinse • Safe and effective for mucous membranes and around ears and eyes • Do not leave in the wound bed
Povidone-iodine (iodopovidone; Betadine®)	Grossly contaminated	• Wide spectrum of antimicrobial activity and residual activity for 4–8 hours • A 0.1% solution (1 ml povidone-iodine +99 ml lactated Ringer's solution) is recommended • Scrubbing of wounds can damage tissues and ↑ infections • Complications: intensifies metabolic acidosis, excessive systemic iodine, inactivated by organic debris, and contact hypersensitivities
Diluted sodium hypochlorite solution 0.5% (Dakin's solution)	Wounds infected with bacteria or fungi; promotes granulation tissue	• 0.5% solution can be applied over the wound for > 7 days • Modified solution of 0.25% can be used as a fluid dressing • High germicidal activity
Tris-EDTA	Otitis externa, abscess, rhinitis, cystitis	• Keeps solution slightly basic and allows entry of antibiotics through the cell wall of Gram-negative bacteria, leaving them more susceptible to destruction • Increases effectiveness of antiseptics and antibiotics
Hypochlorous acid (Vetericyn®)	All wound care	• Safe to treat any wounded area • Broad antimicrobial spectrum • No known microbial resistance

TOPICAL WOUND MEDICATIONS

The use of topical medications allows direct contact of the medication with the wound bed. While each topical medication has its benefits, they can cause deleterious effects (e.g. cytotoxicity, delaying epithelialization), and care should be taken when choosing the medication. Topical medications used on wounds heavily contaminated will not be able to penetrate the deeper tissues; therefore, the wound should be debrided and cleaned prior to the use of the medication.

Table 19.6 / **Topical wound medications**

Medication/therapy	Stage of healing	Anti-bacterial	Hydro-philic*	Promotes Granulation	Promotes Epithelialization	Comments/Indications
Acemannan (Carravet® gel)	• Inflammatory • Repair		X	X	X	• Derived from the aloe vera plant • Acts as a growth factor and reduces edema • Best used for partial and full-thickness burns, lacerations, dermal ulcers, abrasions, slow healing wounds • Applied under a non-adherent bandage
Alginate	• Inflammatory • Repair	X	X	X	X	• Made from kelp (seaweed) • Promotes a moist wound environment, autolytic debridement, and wound healing • Alginates are best used in the early stages of healing heavy to moderate exudative wounds • They are secured under a moisture-retentive dressing and can be left in place for up to 7 days • Alginates will wick exudate vertically into the absorbent layer, protecting the peri-wound skin • The bandage is changed when strikethrough has occurred. Wounds covered in alginate may have a foul odor or appearance similar to that of infection; however, this "exudate" is easily rinsed from the site • They are not recommended for use on wounds with > 25% necrotic tissue
Antimicrobial impregnated gauze	• Inflammatory • Secondary bandage layer	X				• When the gauze is saturated, an antimicrobial, seeps from the gauze creating an antimicrobial environment • Can be applied as the primary (contact) or secondary bandage layer • If used as a primary layer can either be used as a dry layer if the wound is effusive or with honey for infected or heavily contaminated wounds
Cefazolin	• Infected	X				• Provides high levels of antibiotics in the wound fluid • Local administration directly on wound
Gentamicin sulfate 0.1% ointment	• Repair • Maturation	X		X		• Effective against Gram-negative bacteria found in wounds • Apply a thin layer on wound bed under a low adherent pad • Apply to the wound bed 24 hours prior to grafting • ideally for Gram-negative and *Staphylococcus* organisms and can promote wound contraction but may inhibit epithelialization

(*Continued*)

Table 19.6 / **Topical wound medications (Continued)**

Medication/therapy	Stage of healing	Anti-bacterial	Hydro-philic*	Promotes		Comments/Indications
				Granulation	Epithelialization	
Honey, (raw and unpasteurized), sugar, maltodextrin (D-glucose polysaccharide)	• Inflammatory • Repair	X**		X	X	• Enhances debridement, granulation bed formation, epithelialization, improves wound nutrition, reduces edema and inflammation and is antibacterial-like • Increasing the level of growth factors, reducing odor, and provide a local energy source to the wound • Excellent for necrotic wounds and can be applied until healed • Commonly used in the inflammatory phase to the presence of granulation tissue, although some of these products can be used until the wound is healed • Absorption factor of the bandage is important • Daily bandage changes are often required, owing to the amount of fluid production • With newer advanced absorbent dressings you can keep these types of bandage on longer • Monitor electrolyte levels when used in large wounds • When using granulated sugar it needs to have a 1-cm deep layer over the wound bed • Medical-grade honey is unpasteurized honey and has been sterilized with gamma radiation
Hydrogels (80–90% water or glycerin base sheets)	• Inflammatory • Repair	X			X	• Promote a moist wound environment and autolytic debridement • Best used in dry to low exudative wounds, in the late stages of healing, or when the wound has a healthy granulation bed and evidence of epithelialization • Can potentially macerate the skin around the wound, so the sheet should have minimal to no contact on surrounding healthy skin. It is secured under a bandage and can be left in place for up to five days. They are available in a felt-like sheet that may be cut to size and turns to gel after contact with an open wound
Hydrocolloids	• Repair	X		X	X	• Stimulate angiogenesis, collagen synthesis, enhance epithelialization • Form a gel over the wound and have an impermeable backing • Used for wounds with low to moderate effusion • Can use on top of another dressing to create an occlusive bandage • Warm sheet in hands *before* opening to make it pliable

(Continued)

Table 19.6 / Topical wound medications (Continued)

Medication/therapy	Stage of healing	Anti-bacterial	Hydro-philic*	Promotes		Comments/Indications
				Granulation	Epithelialization	
Medicinal maggots	• Inflammatory • Debridement • Early repair	x		X	X	• Use disinfected fly larvae (*Lucilia sericata*, green bottle fly) • Care must be taken to secure the edges of the wound with adhesive drapes or pads to provide an area of containment for the maggots • A mesh or porous bandage is placed over the maggots followed by a few layers of gauze always maintaining air flow • The absorbent layer is changed every 12 hours and the wound is flushed at 36–48 hours; the maggots are disposed of in a biohazard container
Nitrofurazone	• Inflammatory	X	X			• Effective against Gram-positive organisms • Promotes a moist environment but may inhibit wound epithelialization • Not effective against *Pseudomonas*
Silver (1% sulfadiazine cream)	• Infected (any stage) • Inflammatory • Early repair	X			x	• Effective against most Gram-positive and -negative bacteria and fungi • Can have a negative effect on fibroblasts and slow wound contraction • Ability to penetrate eschar and necrotic tissue • Apply a thin layer SSD on wounded area and cover with a low adherent bandage • Slow-release nano particles, ionic silver dressings, and silver impregnated dressings have been shown to provide a more consistent antimicrobial activity compared traditional SSD cream
Triple antibiotic ointment	• Inflammatory	X	X			• Bacitracin, neomycin, polymyxin • Reduces surface microbial burden • Anaphylactic reactions (feline, rare) • Poor activity against *Pseudomonas* • Not very effective on infected wounds • Poor absorption by the tissues • used over dry wounds to help promote a moist environment

(*Continued*)

Table 19.6 / **Topical wound medications (Continued)**						
Medication/therapy	**Stage of healing**	**Anti-bacterial**	**Hydro-philic***	**Promotes**		**Comments/Indications**
				Granulation	**Epithelialization**	
Tripeptide-copper complex (lamin®)	• Repair • Maturation	X	X	X		• A hydrogel that enhances growth factors • It will speed epithelialization and contraction, making it ideal for partial and full-thickness wounds • Non-adherent dressings (such as a Telfa pad) are used to cover the wound after a thin layer of this dressing is applied to the wound bed
Liquid skin barrier film	• Peri-wound skin • Minor abrasions					• Waterproof, vapor-permeable liquid acrylate • Protects surrounding skin from maceration and adhesive stripping during bandage removal • Helps prepare the skin surface so adhesives and tape may adhere better

* Moisture retentive dressing.
** The osmotic effects help decrease wound edema and create a bactericidal and bacteriostatic environment.
Epithel., epithelialization; Granul., granulation.

WOUND THERAPY

Table 19.7 / **Wound therapy**

Medication/therapy	Definition	Indications	Comments
Extracorporeal shock wave therapy	Shock waves in the form of sound energy are released causing ↑ superficial blood perfusion and tissue regeneration	Musculoskeletal conditions (e.g. chronic tendinopathies, osteoarthritis pain)	• Increases bone, tendon, and ligament healing • May cause mild bruising of the treated area and may result in transiently increasing pain and lameness following treatment • Contraindicated on neoplasias, open physis, or used over the chest and abdomen
Hyperbaric oxygen therapy	Inhalation of 100% oxygen at ↑ atmospheric pressure resulting in up to 17 times the oxygen concentration to injured tissues	Wounds with delayed healing, anaerobic infections, radiation burns, edema, tissue ischemia, envenomations, severe soft tissue inflammation	• Avoid use in patients with fevers, pacemakers, untreated pneumothorax, and those receiving doxorubicin or cisplatin • ↑ perfusion so medication dosages should be adjusted • Hyperbaric chambers can be highly combustible and extreme care should be taken with their use • Remove all collars and leashes, cover staples and vet wrap, and avoid use of lubricants and topical ointments • Static electricity should be controlled with the use of 100% cotton towels and dampening of the pet's hair

(Continued)

Table 19.7 / **Wound therapy (Continued)**

Medication/therapy	Definition	Indications	Comments
Negative pressure wound therapy vacuum-assisted closure	Application of sub-atmospheric pressure (vacuum) at the wound site	Traumatic wounds after surgical debridement (e.g. degloving injuries, burns, dehiscence, cytotoxic sloughs)	• Contributes to granulation tissue formation, ↑ local circulation and perfusion, ↓ edema, exudate and infectious material; contraindicated in wounds that may contain neoplastic cells or necrotic tissue • Change the bandage every 38–72 hours (may need to be changed every 24 hours for traumatic or highly contaminated wounds)
Therapeutic lasers, cold laser therapy (low-level laser therapy)	Application of low light lasers to affect cellular function through photostimulation	Cutaneous wounds and tissue	• Benefits are control of inflammation and pain relief, improved tissue healing and regeneration, ↑ strength of the repaired tissue, and improvement of immune function • Contraindicated in wounds that may contain neoplastic cells, over a pregnant uterus or over growth plates • Not recommended for use around the eyes

WOUND BANDAGING

Wound healing is a process involving many different stages, each requiring a specific environment for optimal results. Bandaging most often can provide the changing environment needed for each stage. Bandaging provides cleanliness, immobility, control of wound environment, elimination of dead space, hemostasis, decreased edema and pain, moisture, and warmth. Bandaging can also increase the acidity of the wound environment, resulting in an increase in oxygen dissociation from hemoglobin, thereby increasing oxygen to the wound, which promotes healing.

The patient should be more comfortable after bandage placement. A patient that is very upset with a bandage should be evaluated for incorrect bandage placement, skin irritation, or worsening of the wound. Some keys to successful bandaging are the following:

- Pressure should be applied over and distal to the wound as proximal pressure will impede blood and lymphatic return with subsequent swelling and edema.
- Avoid wrinkles in the bandaging material as these may become areas of discomfort.
- Ensure the areas to be bandaged (e.g. surrounding skin, hair, between toes) are dry as these areas may develop moist dermatitis.
- Almost all bandages and splints should be applied with the limb at a normal functional angle, seen when the animal is at rest in lateral recumbency. Wounds over joints may need to be bandaged in extension to avoid contracture deformity and subsequent limited joint use.

Record the type and size of contact (primary) layer used as well as the secondary and tertiary layers applied. It will be important that all pieces of the bandage material are accounted for at the next bandage change. Provide a list of all the current medications that are being administered by the owner at home, medications may need to be refilled or discontinued. Finally, indicate when the next bandage change is due in the patient record, so a recheck appointment may be scheduled. Many veterinary practices employ multiple veterinarians and having a routine way of evaluating each wound can allow for consistent and effective medical treatments.

Table 19.8 / **Wound bandaging**

Bandage layer	Purpose	Material type	Comments
Primary (contact layer)	• Protects the wound and in some cases for debridement	See below	• Should remain in contact even during movement
Adherent: promotes debridement in the inflammatory stage			
Dry/dry • Dry gauze is placed over the wound and bandaged	• Absorbs exudate, necrotic tissue, and foreign material • Debris adheres to the material and is removed with bandage change	Gauze pads, cling gauze	• Not highly recommended due to unselective debridement and damage during the proliferative stage of wound healing • Painful to remove, rewetting the gauze with warm saline may facilitate removal • Change daily
Wet/dry • Dry gauze is soaked in saline or Diluted chlorhexidine and placed over the wound, then bandaged	• Loosens dried exudate, necrotic tissue, and foreign material by rehydration of wound • Absorbed by the secondary layer	Gauze pads or cling gauze, saline or 0.05% chlorhexidine	• Not highly recommended due to unselective debridement and damage during the proliferative stage of wound healing • Painful to remove; rewetting the gauze with warm saline may facilitate removal • Disadvantage: bacterial proliferation and strike through • Change daily
Film	• Provides a barrier to the wound surface from bacteria, water, environmental contaminants (e.g. urine, feces) • Mimics normal skin • Waterproof and vapor permeable	Polyurethane film sheet	• May be used alone or over other dressings • Change every 3–4 days
Low adherent (nonadherent) • Used over dry wounds and incisions • Promotes moisture retention and epithelialization with minimal disruption of granulation bed • Switched from adherent dressing when the granulation bed is forming and drainage is serosanguineous			
Occlusive	• Used when no exudate is present, in the repair stage	Hydrocolloid dressing, hydrogel, hydrophilic beads, polyurethane films	• Impermeable to air, which can lead to trapping excessive moisture and subsequent skin damage • Change every 2–7 days, depending on product
Semi-occlusive	• Prevents tissue dehydration but allows fluid absorption	Telfa pads, gauze-coated with petrolatum, polyethylene glycol, petrolatum-based antibiotic ointment, calcium alginate	• Used once epithelialization begins • Change every 1–3 days, dependent on product

(*Continued*)

Table 19.8 / **Wound bandaging (Continued)**

Bandage layer	Purpose	Material type	Comments
Foam	• To protect the wound from further impacts and trauma • Promotes moist wound environment and autolytic debridement • absorptive	Polyurethane foam, hydrophilic foam Impregnated with silver, dextrans and alginates (Algidex Ag® DeRoyal)	• Non-adherent to wound surface but adhesive to surrounding skin • Can be used dry or moistened with saline or medications • Used for all types of wounds, cut to fit • Change every 1–7 days depending on the product

Secondary layer (intermediate layer)

- To protect the wound from further impacts and trauma and to draw away and store heavy secretions and exudates
- Heavy padding: rolled cotton
- Moderate padding: cast padding
- Light padding: stretch bandage
- Super-absorbent dressings
- Xtrasorb® (DermaSciences)
- Enough pressure needs to be applied to avoid spaces between the wound, primary layer and secondary layer
- Excessive pressure impairs blood supply and impairs wound healing (e.g. contraction)
- Thickness is determined on the expected amount of drainage needing to be absorbed

Tertiary layer (outer layer)

- To provide consolidation of the secondary layer
- Stretch gauze
- Enough pressure needs to be applied to avoid spaces between the wound, primary layer, secondary layer, and tertiary layer
- Excessive pressure impairs blood supply and impairs wound healing (e.g. contraction)
- Splints and supports are incorporated into the tertiary layer
- Protective layer
- To protect the bandaging from outside contamination
- Apply pressure, conform, and immobilize the bandage.
- Elastic wrap (Coban™, VetWrap™)
- Adhesive tape
- Can create an occlusive bandage leading to trapped excessive moisture and subsequent skin damage

Notes

- Record the type and size of contact (primary) layer used as well as the secondary and tertiary layers applied. It will be important that all pieces of the bandage material are accounted for at the next bandage change.
- Provide a list of all the current medications that are being administered by the owner at home, medications may need to be refilled or discontinued.
- Finally, indicate when the next bandage change is due in the patient record, so a recheck appointment may be scheduled.
- Many veterinary practices employ multiple veterinarians and having a routine way of evaluating each wound can allow for consistent and effective medical treatments.

Skill Box 19.3 / General bandaging tips

Prepare all needed supplies prior to beginning in a quiet part of the hospital:

- Gloves, clippers, rolled cotton, cotton balls, nail trimmers, bandage scissors, tape, marker pen
- Select bandaging materials that are appropriately sized for your patient (generally, cats and small dogs = 2 or 3-in. materials; medium dogs = 3–4 in. materials; and large dogs = 4-in. materials).
- Select appropriate wound cleaning solutions, medications, and dressings.

Use proper technique:

- Knowing the absorptive properties of a dressing is essential in preventing "strike-through" before the next bandage change. The two most common dressings, in the author's opinion, used in most veterinary practices are Telfa™ pads (Medtronic Minneapolis, MN) and a wide mesh gauze square or roll. The Telfa pad is most ideal for dry or low exudative wounds, such as a healthy granulation bed or closed incision. Wide mesh gauze is most useful to aid in debridement of wound beds, due to its adherence to wounds.
- The secondary layer provides absorption, compression and stabilization. Cast padding, followed by two to three layers of rolled gauze comprises this layer. This layer should be thick enough that strikethrough (wound drainage penetrating the tertiary layer) does not occur prior to the next scheduled bandage change.
- Some key points to remember when placing the secondary layer of a soft padded limb bandage include:
  - Always begin at the toes, leaving the toenails of digit three and four exposed.
  - Choose a wider size material (4 inches instead of 2 inches) when applicable to avoid the tourniquet effect.
  - Apply layers in a spiral fashion, beginning at the most distal area working proximal.
  - 50% overlap of the previous layer.
  - Avoid excessive wrinkles in the bandage.
  - Cotton cast padding material will often tear before it is too tight.
  - Always use even tension (not too tight) when applying the rolled gauze layer over the cotton cast padding.
- A wide-mesh rolled gauze may be used over the cast padding to add compression and hold a splint in place. When using a splint, be sure to have proper placement and adequate layers of padding to avoid pressure sores associated with poor placement. Sponges, foams and cast padding can be used to make a "donut" to protect bony prominences.
- Cotton can be placed between toes and to fill in depressions (see Skill Box 19.7).

Monitor tension throughout the process:

- Bandage material is to be unrolled from the bottom to eliminate excessive tension.
- The tertiary layer can be unrolled and then rerolled to eliminate excessive pressure prior to use.

General tips:

- Proper skin preparation is key to ensure good adherence of the tape or transparent film. Keeping the peri-wound intact skin healthy will keep the patient more comfortable and reduce the risk of infection. Using a silicone medical adhesive remover to remove tape and adhesive from the skin.
- Place a hand over adhesive tape once applied to fur. This warmth of the palm and the patient's body will result in better adherence, especially to hair.
- Using pretorn strips of the tertiary layer (e.g. adhesive tape) can eliminate excessive tension (e.g. respiratory restriction).
- Windows can be marked and cut into bandages to allow access to the wound without having to remove the entire bandage.

Skill Box 19.4 / Client education: bandage care

Pets with bandages must be frequently monitored while they are healing. Bandages are meant as a temporary coverage to a wound or injury.

Bandage care

- Bandages should be checked twice daily for wetness, dirt or contamination, odor, destruction, slippage, or change in bandage tension (e.g. too loose or too tight).
- Bandages that become wet or soiled must be changed immediately as these conditions may compromise and possibly worsen the healing process.
- Chewing the bandage should be controlled to avoid causing further damage.
- Mechanical deterrents: collars (e.g. Elizabethan collar, BiteNot® collars, inflatable collars, towel collars), muzzles, side braces, clothing, commercial boots (e.g. Medipaw®).
- Chemical or electrical deterrents (e.g. foul-tasting sprays or tapes, electronic patches, pepper-impregnated tape).
- Adhesive bandage removal.
- Commercial silicone adhesive removers are ideal in preventing skin irritation and pain associated with bandage removal.

Patient care:

- The area above and below the bandage should be checked twice daily for swelling, redness, discharge, odor, or change in temperature.
- Restrict activity: all outside activity should be on leash and cats should remain indoors.
- A plastic bag should be secured over a bandage when outside but should be removed within a 30-minute period to reduce a buildup of moisture.
- Follow instructions of the veterinarian for bandage changes and removal.
- Instruct owners to check the patient toenails for separation, which would indicate swelling

Tip: If your pet becomes agitated with the bandage where previously was not affected by it, it may be a sign of discomfort or a developing problem. Schedule a recheck appointment with your veterinarian.

Skill Box 19.5 / Head or ear bandage

Use

Bandaging following auricular hematomas, total ear ablation, traumatic wounds, and tumor removals

Procedure

For bandaging the ear on top of the head:

- Place two adhesive tape strips on ear edges and another two on the underside of the pinna that line up with the previous two strips and extends 3 inches past the pinna (to prevent bandage slippage).
- Place the padding on top of the head to provide a level surface to lay the pinna.
- Lay the pinna on top of the head with the strips of tape laid on either side of the opposite ear.
- Flex the patient head (avoid flexion in atlantoaxial luxation). Wrap secondary layer around the head alternating in the front and back of the opposite ear. A mark is placed on each layer to identify the ear canal.
- Wrap the tertiary in the same way as the secondary layer. Be very careful to avoid excessive tension or restriction of the neck area.

Tips

- A small hole can be cut into the bandage over the ear canal if medications need to be applied. As the bandage is being placed, an identifying mark to the location of the ear canal can be made on each layer to assist with hole placement.
- Drawing the outline of the ear on the outside of the bandage will assist with removal and inadvertent laceration of the pinna.

Skill Box 19.6 / Chest/abdominal bandage

Use

To control abdominal bleeding (effective for one to two hours and should be removed before four hours) and to cover and protect wounds, surgical incisions, or drains

Procedure

1. Apply a primary bandage layer over the wound if necessary.

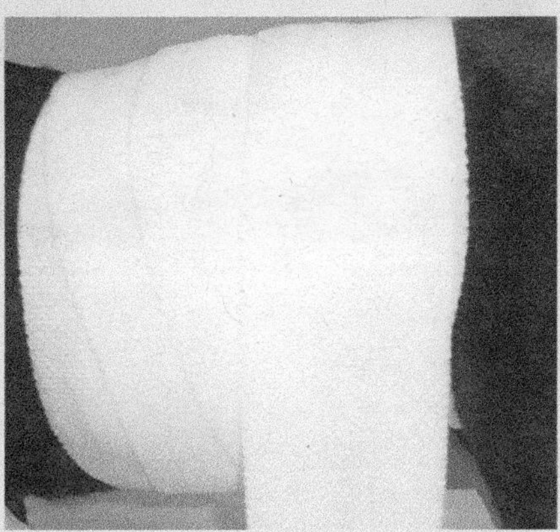

2. Apply a secondary bandage layer, starting mid-thorax, such that the layers overlap one another by 50% and are taut but not constricting. The bandage should extend to the pelvis. On male dogs, be sure to leave the animal's prepuce exposed. Care must be taken to ensure that the bandages are not too tight to restrict thoracic movement. The amount of secondary layer is determined by the expected amount of drainage.

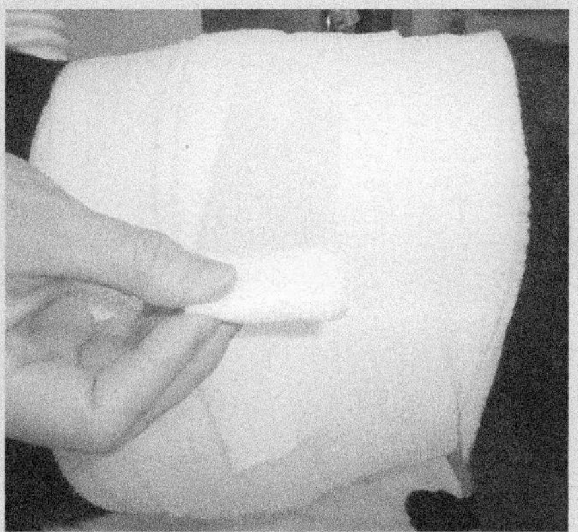

(*Continued*)

Skill Box 19.6 / Chest/abdominal bandage (Continued)

3. Apply a tertiary layer around the torso, then through the legs and over the shoulders in a crisscross fashion (or figure eight) to prevent slippage.
4. Place a protective layer of elastic wrap.
5. Place adhesive tape around the cranial aspect of the bandage, partially adhering to fur.

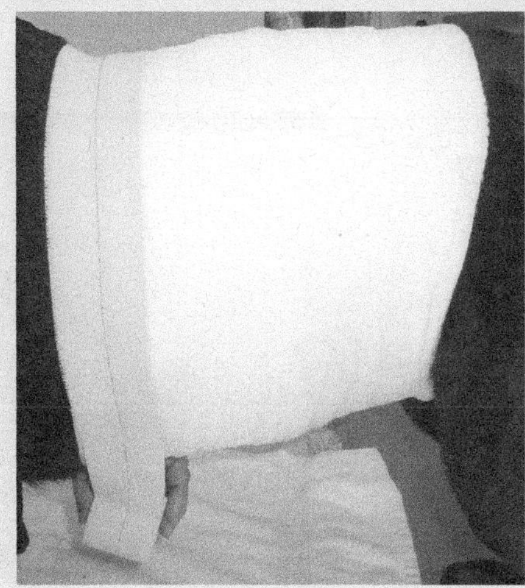

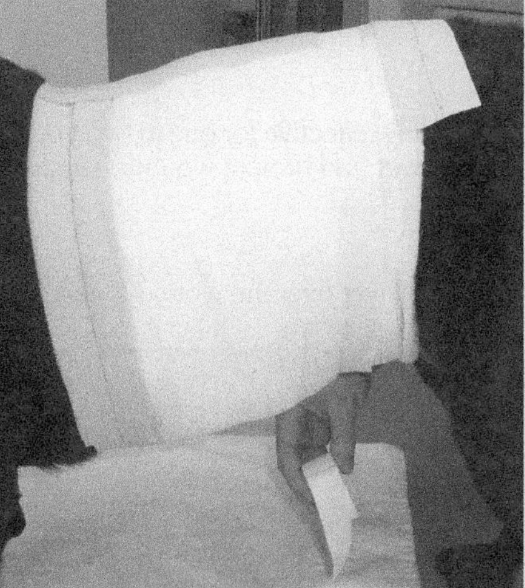

Skill Box 19.7 / Extremity bandage

Use

Bandaging of basic wounds and incisions

Procedure

1. Pad prominences as needed to provide a uniform surface.

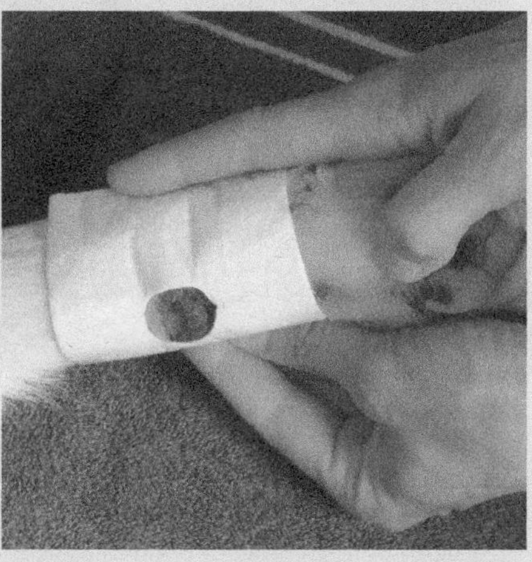

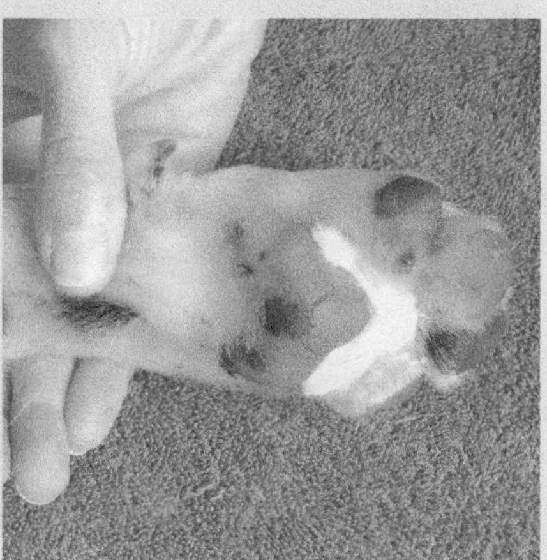

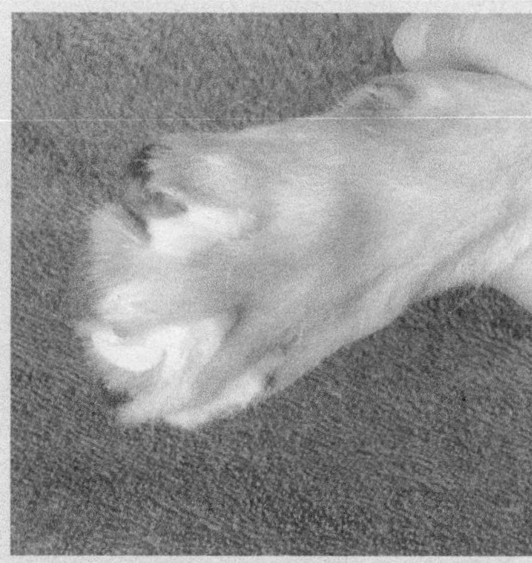

2. Place two adhesive tape strips on either side of the wound along the limb extending 6 inches past the paw (helps to prevent bandage slippage).
3. Stirrup tape strips are used to hold the bandage in place, and are first applied directly to the skin, then folded over attaching to the last layer gauze layer. Stirrup tape strips should never be placed directly on the wound, graft, and incision or over the accessory carpal pad since excessive traction may result in tissue necrosis

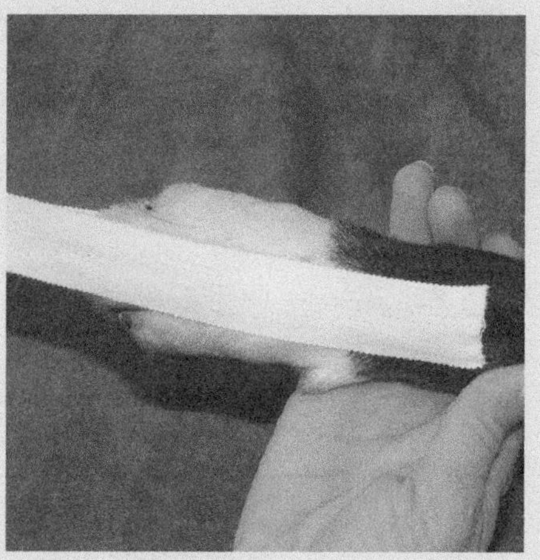

(*Continued*)

Skill Box 19.7 / Extremity bandage (Continued)

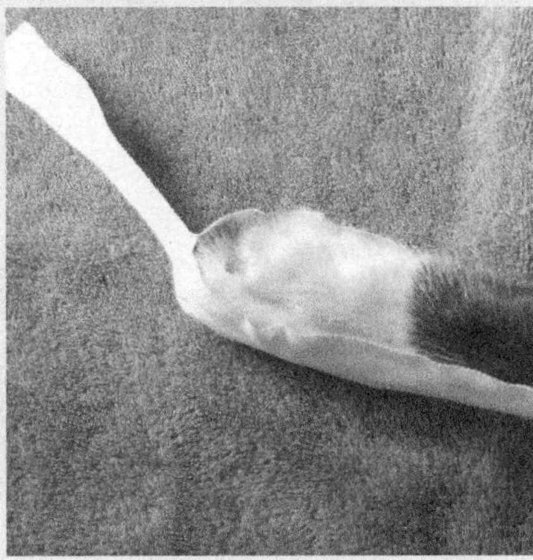

Tips

- A tongue depressor may be placed at the distal end to temporarily adhere the tape ends and to avoid tape entanglement.
- Apply tape laterally when the wound is at the distal end of the extremity (e.g. onychectomy, toe amputation).
- Small pieces of cotton or gauze can be placed in depressions (e.g. between toes, metatarsal–metacarpal pad) to smooth out bandaging area.

4. Apply primary bandage layer over the wound.

5. Apply secondary bandage layer starting at the distal end and working up the limb such that the layers overlap one another by 50% and are taut but not constricting. Place extra padding over the depression areas and be careful not to permit wrinkles.

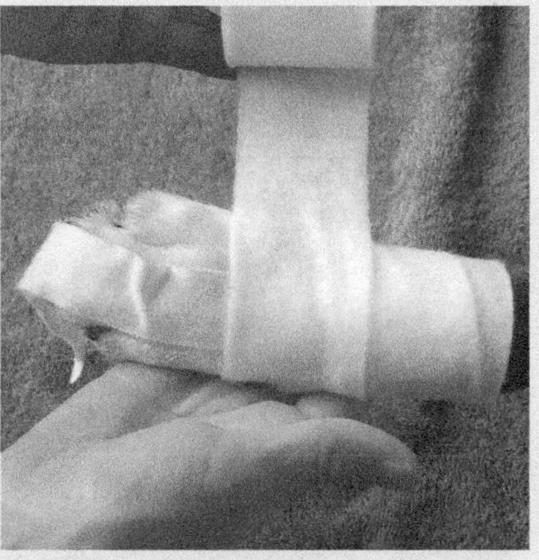

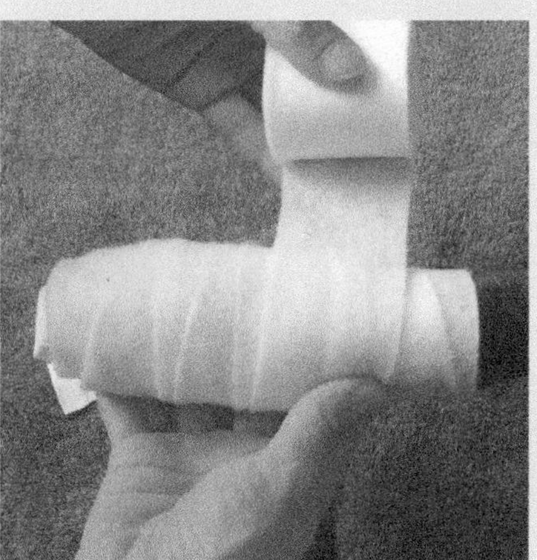

(*Continued*)

Skill Box 19.7 / Extremity bandage (Continued)

Toes can be covered to inhibit edema (the secondary layer is brought over the toes dorsal to ventral and then reflected back, ventral to dorsal) or can be left exposed to check on the temperature of the limb, permit drainage of fluids, and permit assessment of the healing environment (wrap the secondary layer obliquely at the distal end to keep the third and fourth digits exposed).

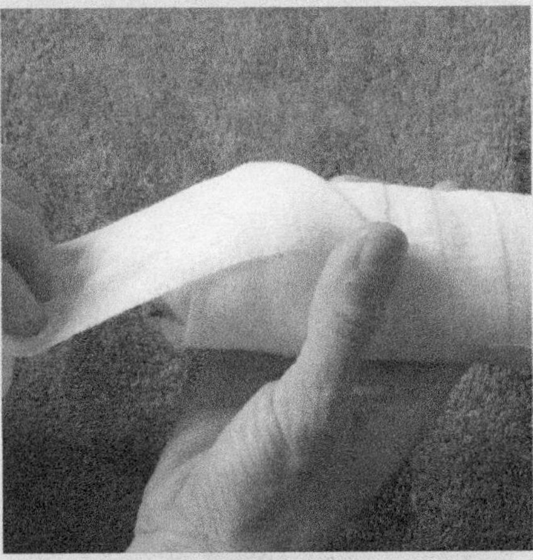

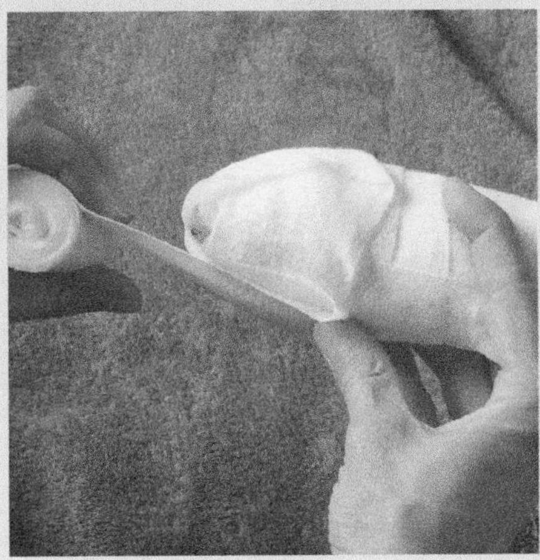

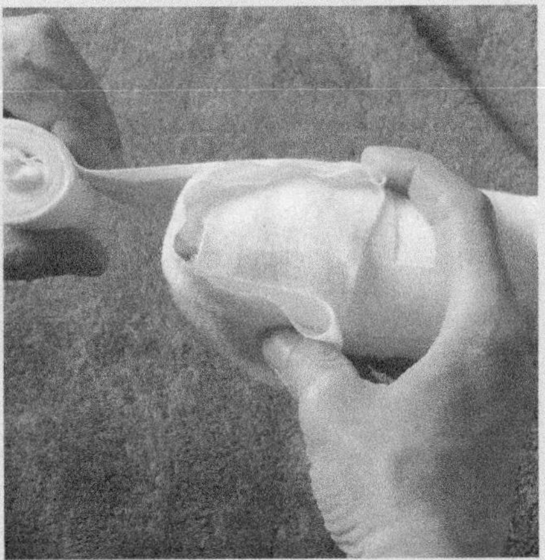

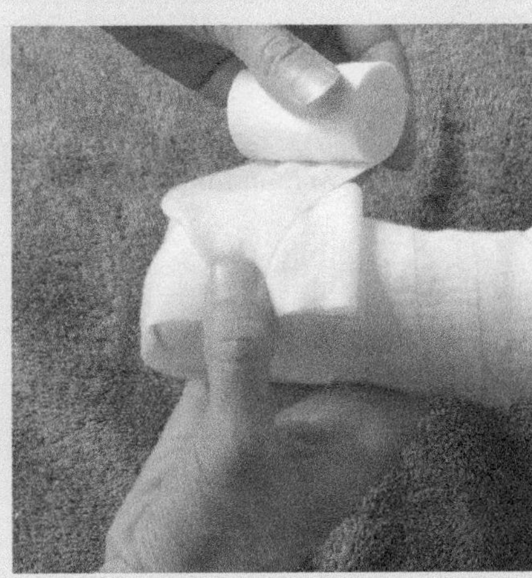

(*Continued*)

Skill Box 19.7 / Extremity bandage (Continued)

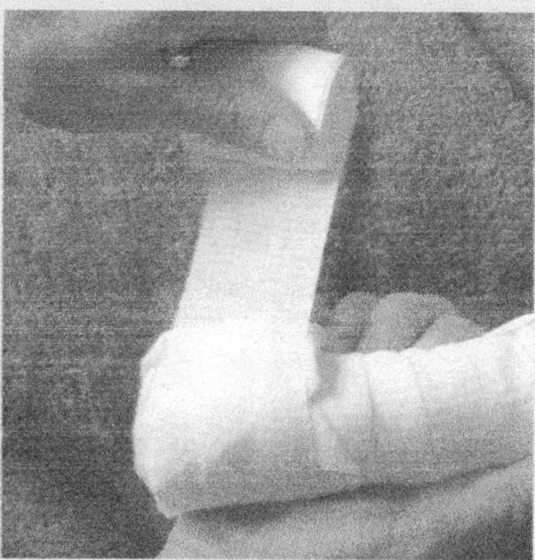

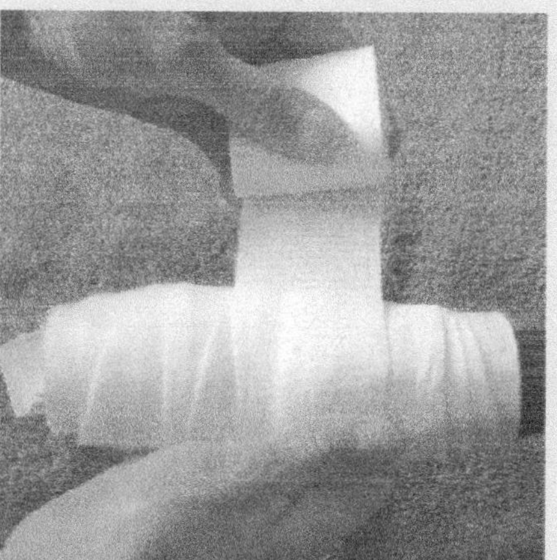

Tip: Always end the bandage at the bottom of the area to alleviate pressure.

6. Place one layer of tertiary bandage layer (as described in step 3), twist and reflect adhesive strips back over this layer, and finish with the final layer of tertiary bandage.

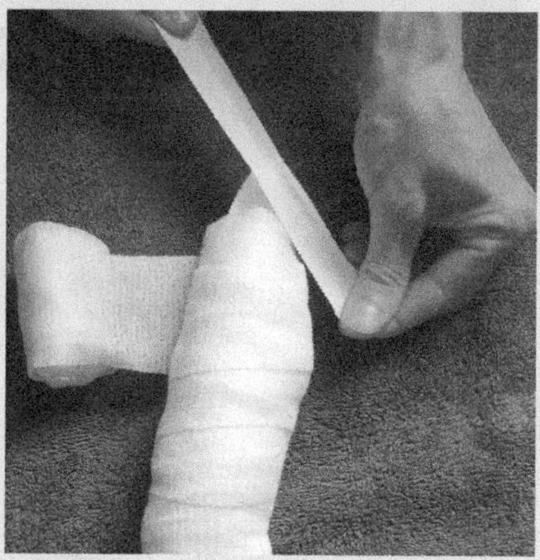

(*Continued*)

Skill Box 19.7 / **Extremity bandage (Continued)**

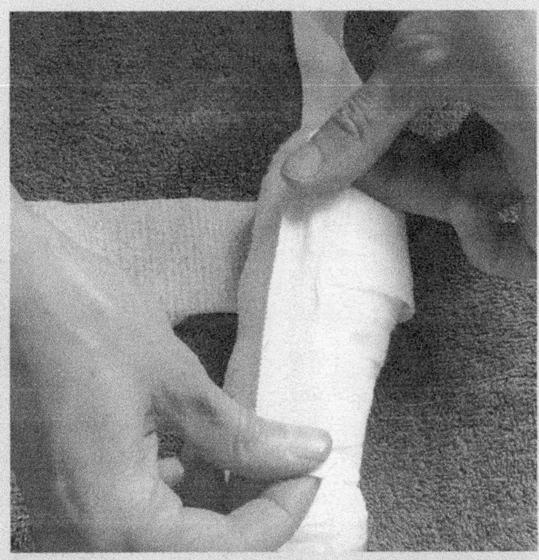

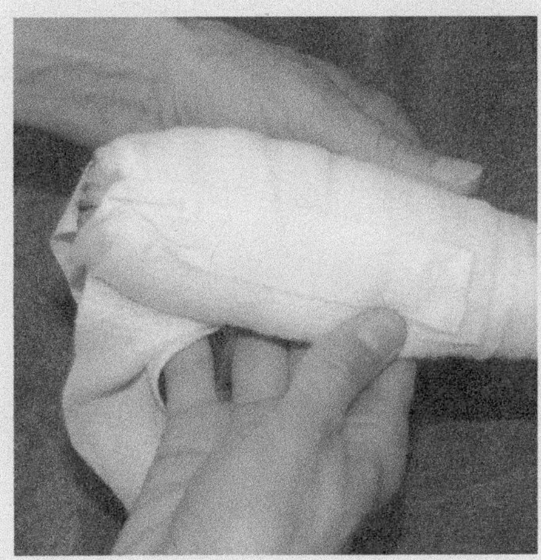

7. Place a protective layer of elastic wrap (as described in step 3).

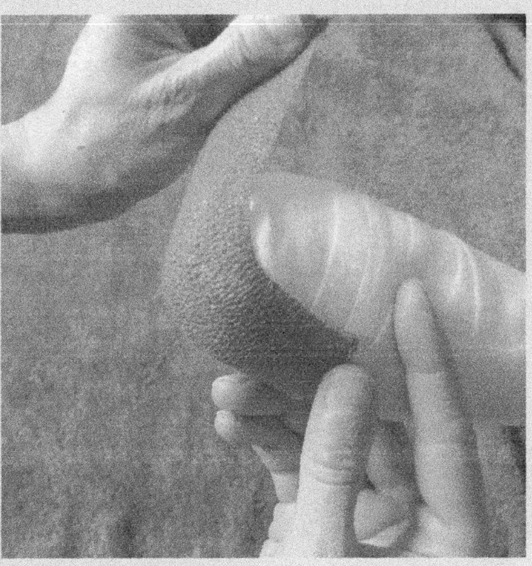

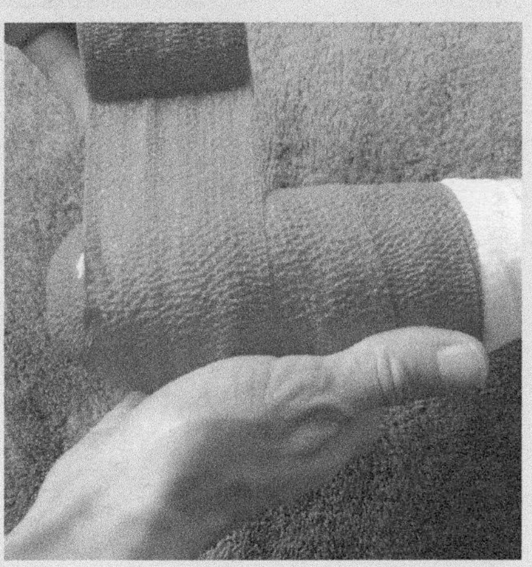

(Continued)

Skill Box 19.7 / Extremity bandage (Continued)

8. Place adhesive tape around the top of the bandage, partially adhering to fur and covering the bottom of the bandage for reinforcement of the toe area.

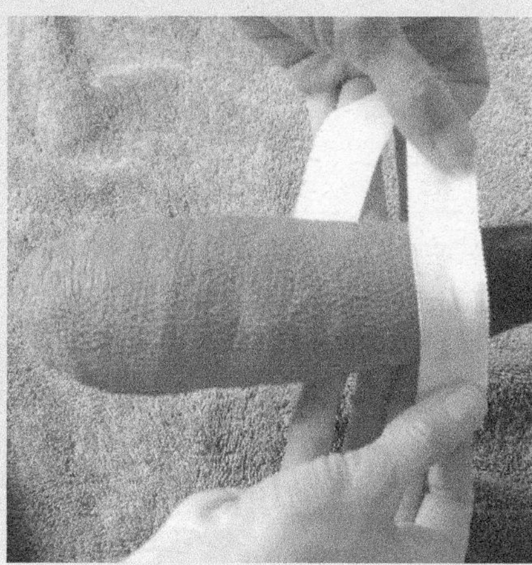

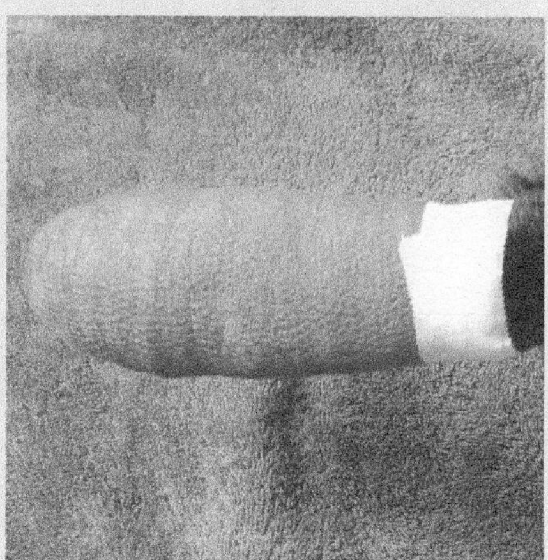

Skill Box 19.8 / Robert Jones bandage

Use

- Temporary immobilization of fractures below the stifle or elbow joint before or after surgery by providing rigid stabilization
- Remove after one day

Procedure

1. Place two adhesive tape strips on either side of the wound, if present, from where you expect the bandage to extend to the distal portion of the limb.
2. There is no primary layer unless sutures or wounds are present. If so, then a non-adherent dressing can be placed over that area.
3. While maintaining normal flexion of the limb, wrap a thick roll of cotton (4–6 inches thick) around the limb from the mid-femur/mid-humerus to toes to constitute the secondary layer. Additional cast padding can be placed to smooth out depressions.

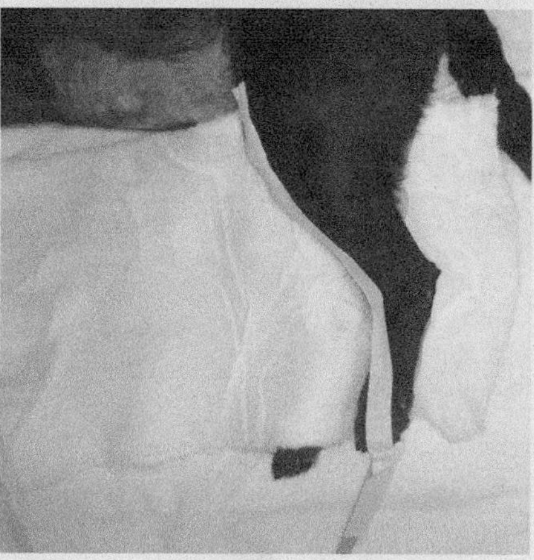

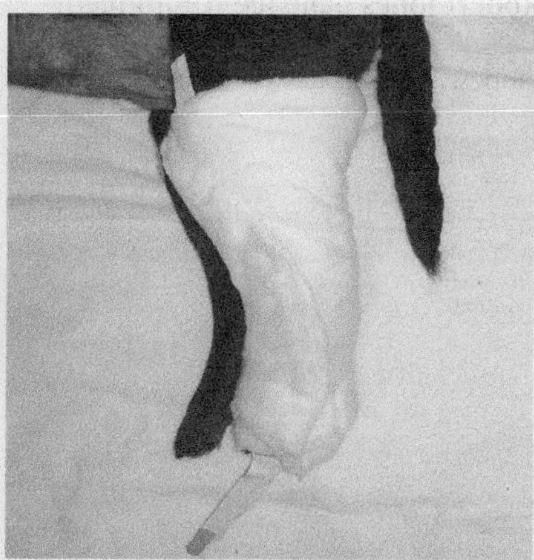

4. Compress with at least two to three layers of a conforming gauze (3–4 inch width) secondary layer. Apply sufficient compression on the conforming gauze throughout application to achieve a smooth, even tension.

(Continued)

Skill Box 19.8 / Robert Jones bandage (Continued)

5. Twist and reflect adhesive strips back over the secondary layer.

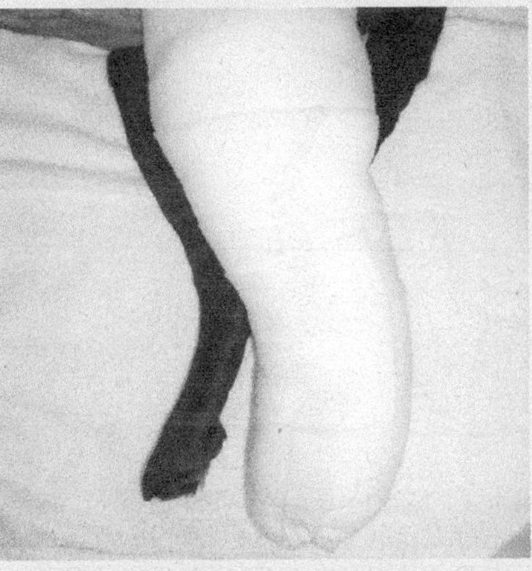

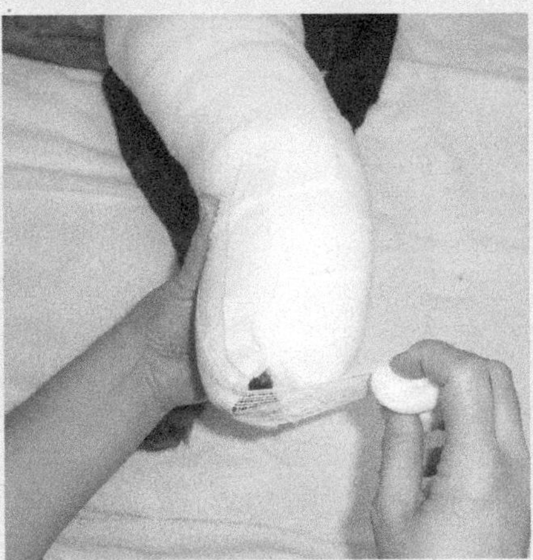

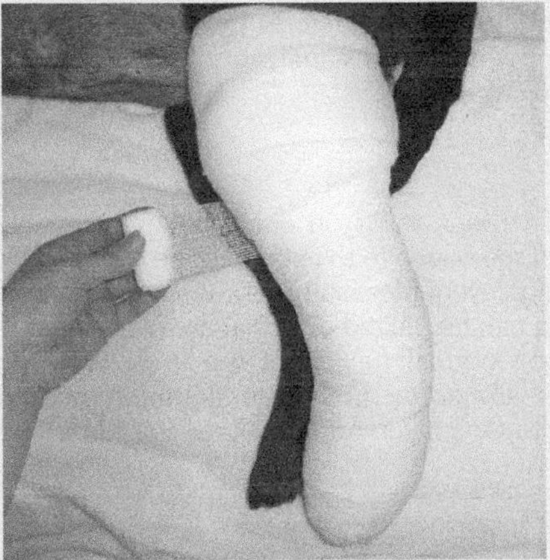

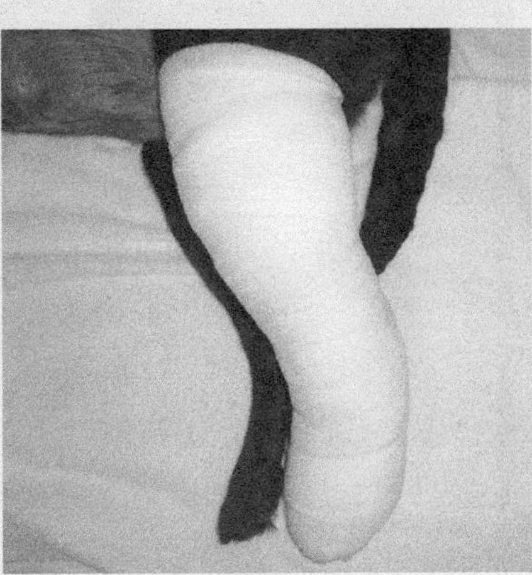

(Continued)

Skill Box 19.8 / Robert Jones bandage (Continued)

6. Place protective layer of elastic wrap as the tertiary layer.
7. Place adhesive tape around the top of the bandage, partially adhering to fur and around the bottom of the bandage for reinforcement.

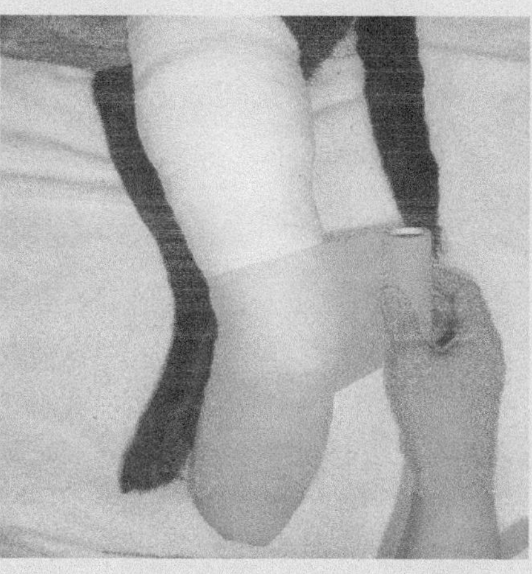

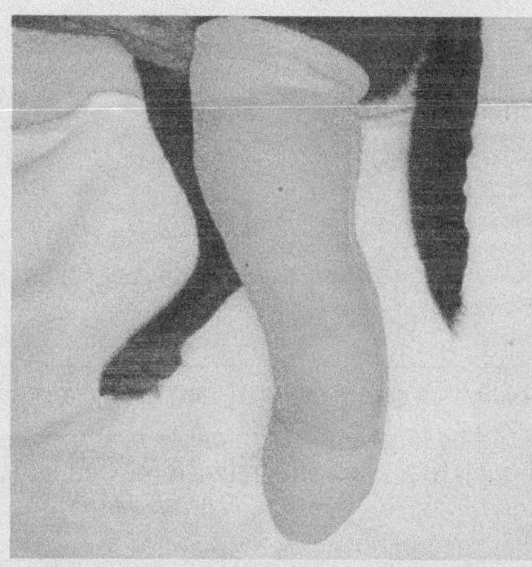

Tip: A well-applied Robert Jones bandage should make a dull thudding sound when tapped.

Alternative: A modified Robert Jones bandage is placed following the instructions above while using less than half of the cotton padding to place a less bulky bandage. Their use is to reduce postoperative swelling of a limb.

Skill Box 19.9 / Tail bandage

Use

Protection of tail injuries

Procedure

- Apply a primary bandage layer of the wound and secure with tape around the circumference of the tail.
- Place two adhesive tape strips on either side of the tail being sure to extend into the hair and past the tip of the tail for further anchoring.
- Apply a light secondary bandage layer around the tape and reflect back the tape strips and then around the circumference of the tail at the top.
- Apply an additional adhesive tape layer to cover the entire bandage. Long hair from the tail can be incorporated into the taping by laying it on top of an already placed tape and then taping over the top to provide additional security.

Tip:Bandage should be applied with minimal padding and lightweight. A syringe case or other similar item can be placed over the tip for added protection.

Skill Box 19.10 / Tie-over bandage

Use

Covering of open wounds over a large surface area or wounds in difficult to bandage areas

Procedure

1. Place multiple, loose, simple interrupted sutures (≥ 5) in the healthy skin, 3–4 mm from the wound edges.

Tip: Use a large monofilament suture material with strong knot security (e.g. 0 or 2–0).

Tip: Suture loops should be large enough to easily pass the umbilical tape (¼ inch) through but small enough to allow enough tension when tying.

2. Apply the primary dressing (e.g. adherent or nonadherent) to fill the open wound followed by a protective outer layer (e.g. laparotomy pad).
3. Secure the outer bandage layer by lacing umbilical tape through the preplaced suture loops and tying it to itself.
4. Adhesive tape or other tertiary bandage material may be placed over the top for additional stability.
5. Subsequent bandage changes only require the removal of the umbilical tape and placement of new wound dressing and secondary layer.

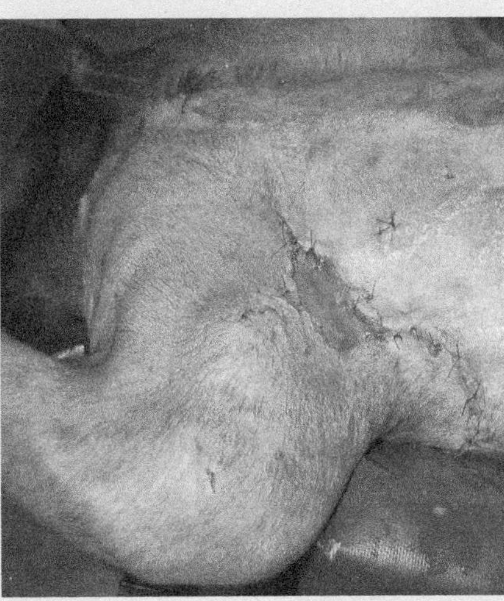

Tip: Initial placement of sutures and bandage may need to be under sedation or with a local anesthetic; however, subsequent bandage changes are often well tolerated.

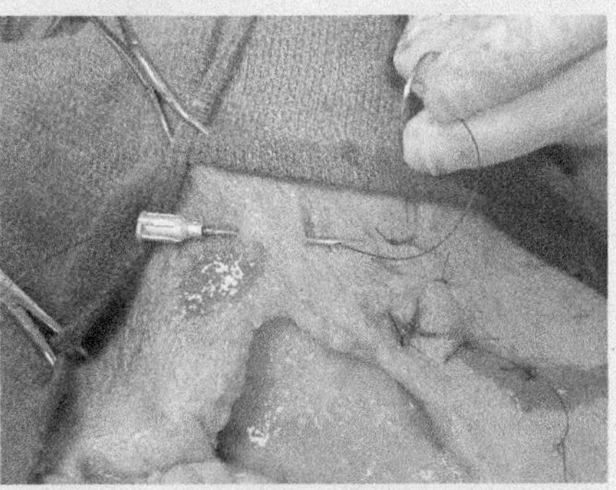

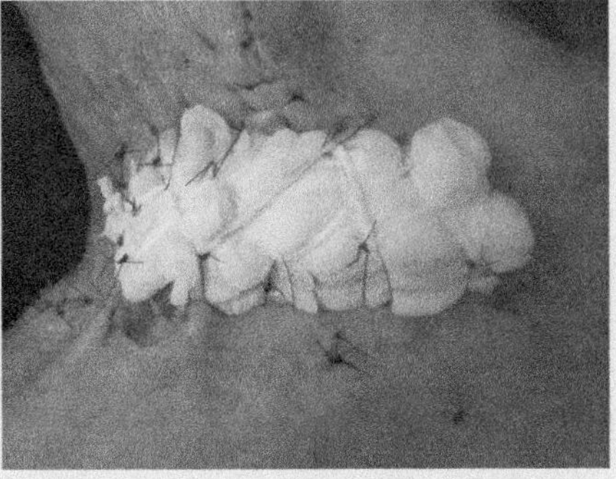

Skill Box 19.11 / Distal limb splint

Use

Temporary immobilization or definitive stabilization for distal extremity fractures or luxations

Procedure

1. Place two adhesive tape strips on either side of the wound, if present, from where you expect the bandage to extend proximally to the distal portion of the limb.
2. Apply primary bandage layer over the wound or suture line if necessary.
3. While maintaining normal flexion of the limb, firmly wrap a secondary bandage layer (e.g. cast padding) around the limb to 1 in. above the proximal end of the splint. Apply enough material to cover bony prominences to ensure comfort from pressure sores and abrasions while limiting material bulk.
4. Apply a conforming gauze tertiary bandage layer compressing the secondary bandage layer. Place the appropriate sized splint on the caudal aspect of the limb, ensuring there are no gaps between the tertiary layer and splint. Twist and reflect adhesive strips onto the splint. Continue with a final layer of the tertiary layer.

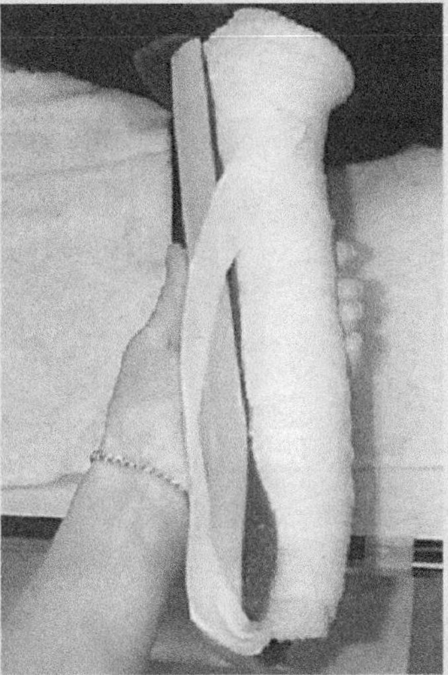

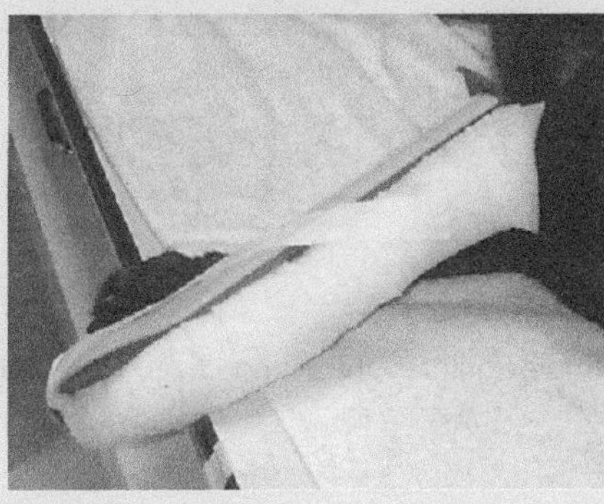

(Continued)

Skill Box 19.11 / Distal limb splint (Continued)

5. Place a protective layer of elastic wrap.
6. Place adhesive tape around top of bandage, partially adhering to fur and covering the bottom of bandage for toe reinforcement.

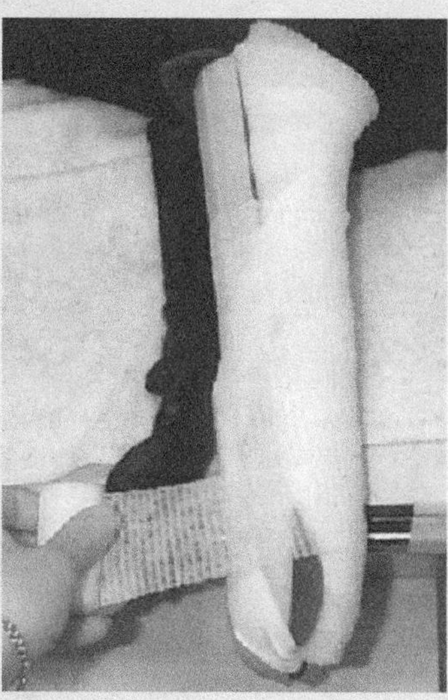

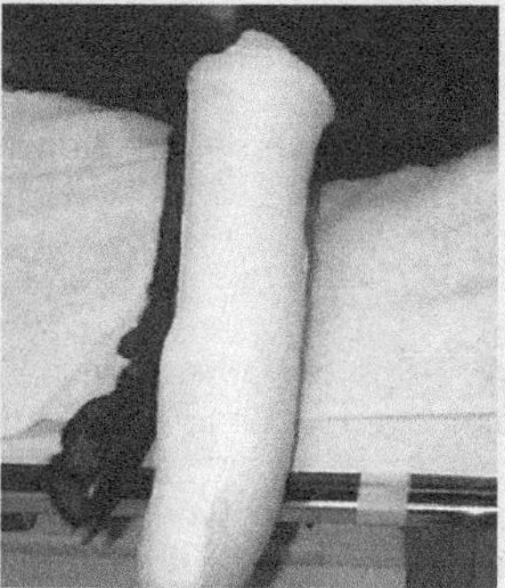

Skill Box 19.12 / Casts

Use

For stabilization of simple fractures and immobilization of limbs (typically for four to five weeks)

Procedure

1. Have a bowl of hot water ready for the cast material and examination gloves ready for the application process.
2. Place two adhesive tape strips on either side of the wound or incision line from where you expect the bandage to start to the distal portion of the limb.
3. Apply a stockinette as a primary layer (smooth with wrinkles).
4. Apply a secondary bandage layer, starting two-thirds up from the expected bottom of the bandage such that the layers overlap one another by 50% and are taut but not constricting. Pad the prominences on the leg, not the depressions. Toes can be covered to inhibit edema or they can be left exposed to check on the temperature of the limb, permit drainage of fluids, and permit assessment of the healing environment.
5. The cast material is used as the tertiary layer. Cast materials vary, and the manufacturer's guidelines should be followed.
6. Twist and reflect adhesive strips and stockinette edges back over the top layer of the cast material.
7. Protective tape is applied over the ends of the cast.

Skill Box 19.13 / Ehmer sling

Use

Immobilization of the hind limb after reduction of a craniodorsal coxofemoral luxation and prevention of weight bearing after pelvis surgery (change every five to seven days)

Procedure

1. Place minimal padding on the metatarsal area using a secondary layer material.
2. Using 2-inch adhesive tape, wrap the tape around the medial aspect of the metatarsal and attach the tape end to the tape roll. Continue medially around the flank and back around the metatarsus. Keep the limb with stifle and hock in maximum flexion for one to two passes.
3. On next pass, go around the flank and twist behind the hock.

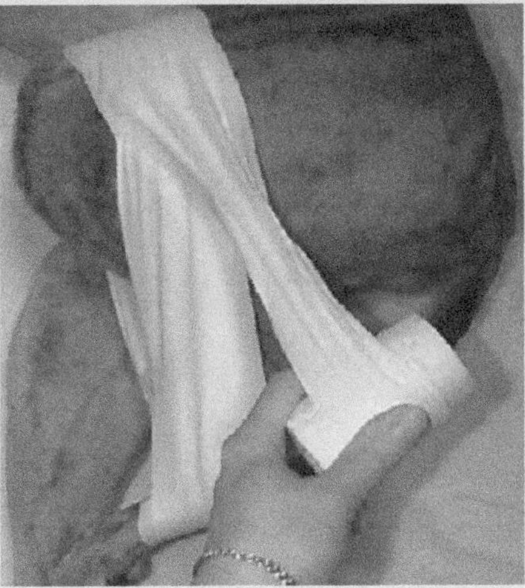

4. Pass over the front of the metatarsal area.
5. Repeat steps 3 and 4 for three to four passes.

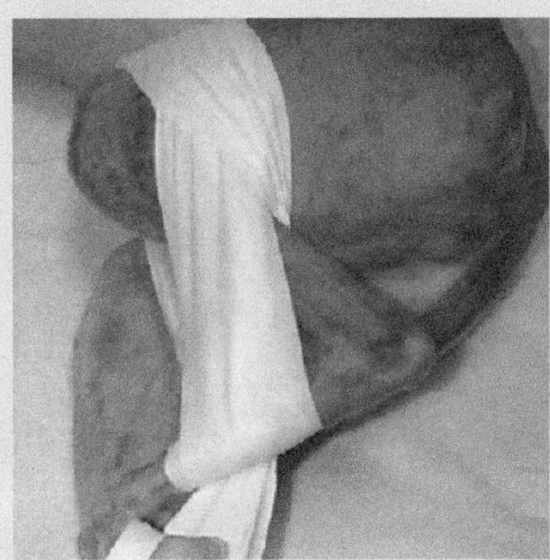

(*Continued*)

Skill Box 19.13 / Ehmer sling (Continued)

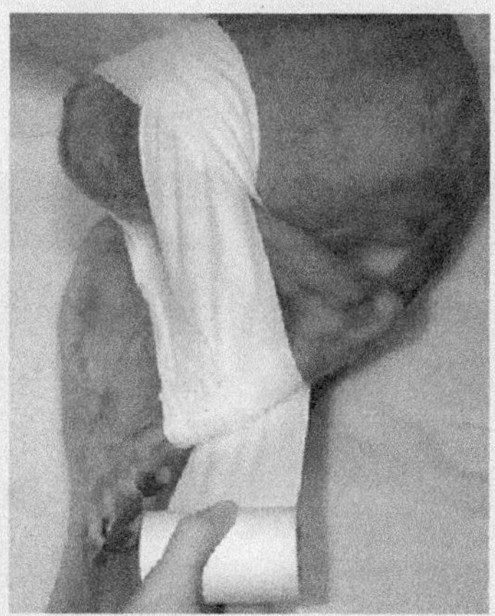

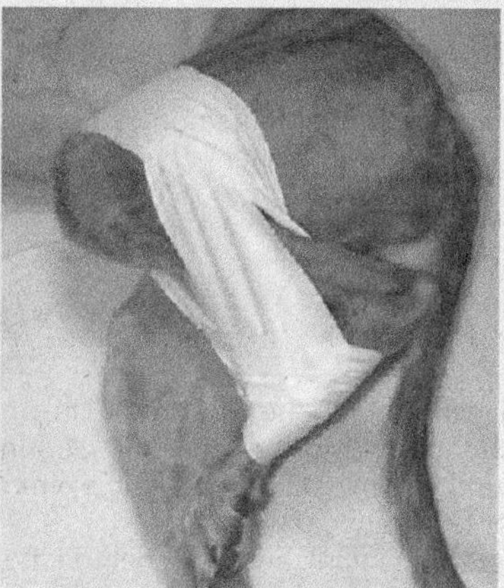

Note

- Correct application results in the internal rotation and adduction of the coxofemoral joint.
- Alternative: use gauze in place of adhesive tape followed by a final layer of elastic adhesive.

Skill Box 19.14 / 90–90 flexion

Use

After distal femoral fracture surgery in young patients and for prevention of weight bearing after hind limb surgeries

Procedure

1. Stifle and hock are in a 90-degree flexion. No attempt to adduct or internally rotate the coxofemoral joint is made.
2. Place minimal padding on the metatarsal area.
3. Same as Ehmer sling, step 2.
4. The tape is passed horizontally around the tibia to hold the layers in place.

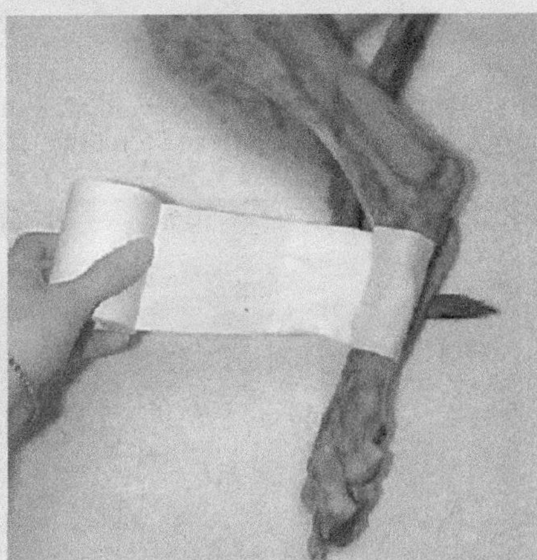

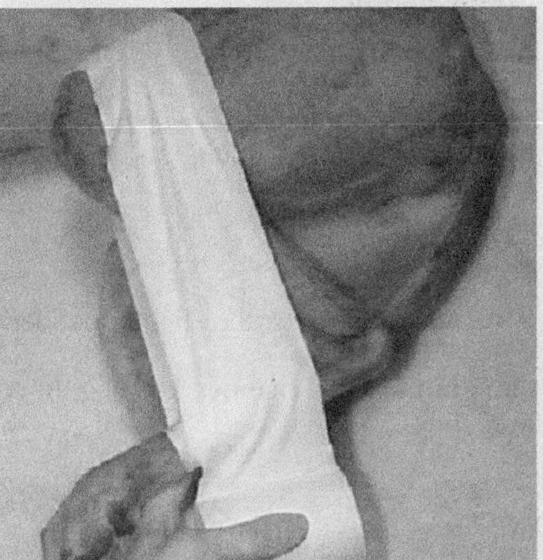

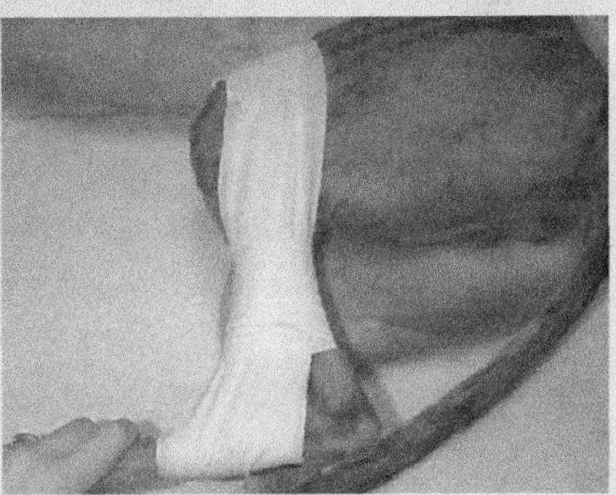

Skill Box 19.15 / Velpeau Sling

Use

Holds flexed forelimb against the chest; non-weight-bearing sling for the forelimb, reduction of scapulohumeral joint luxation, and immobilization of a scapular fracture

Procedure

1. Cover the chest wall and shoulder with a lightly padded secondary layer and gauze tertiary layer.
2. Bandage the forelimb in the same manner, keeping the foot exposed, and pad the depressions of the limb.

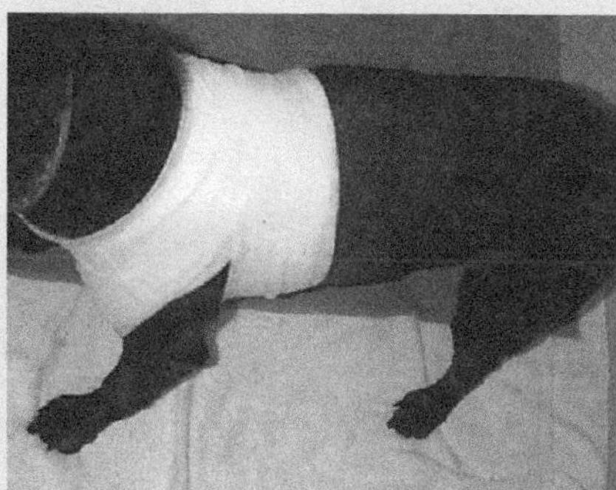

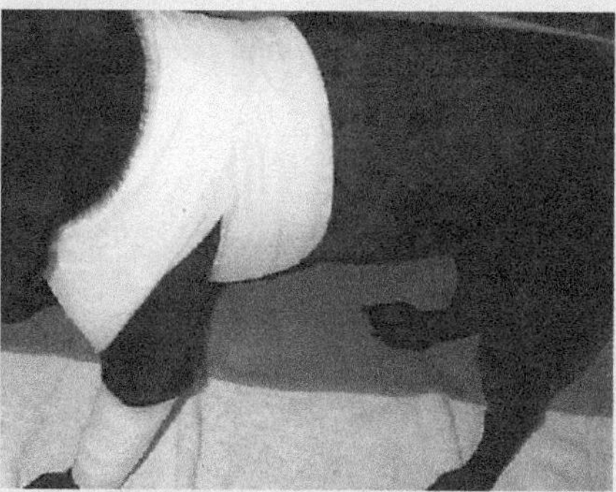

3. Gently flex the forelimb against the chest wall and attach adhesive tape (2–4 inches wide) around the chest and flexed forelimb, creating a sling.

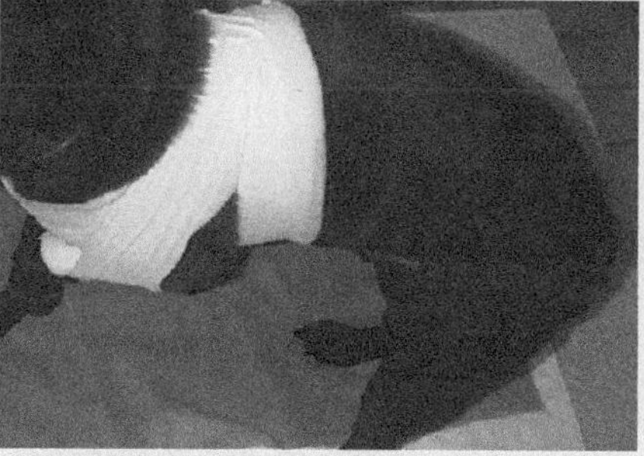

Skill Box 19.16 / Hobbles

Use

To prevent excessive abduction of the hind limbs; specifically indicated after reduction of ventral coxofemoral luxation, to relieve excessive tension in the inguinal region, to prevent excessive activity after pelvic fracture repair, or nonsurgical, conservative management of pelvic fractures

Procedure

1. Stand the animal with the hind limbs equally distant to the width of the pelvis.
2. Pass the adhesive tape (which needs to be wide enough to cover half of the metatarsal area) around the two limbs. Press the tape together in the area between the two limbs.

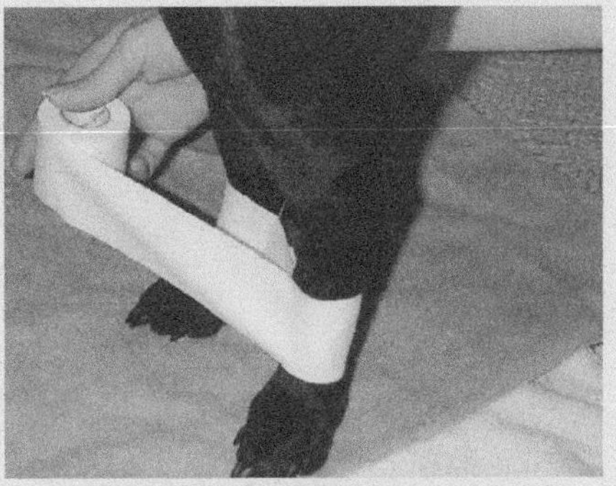

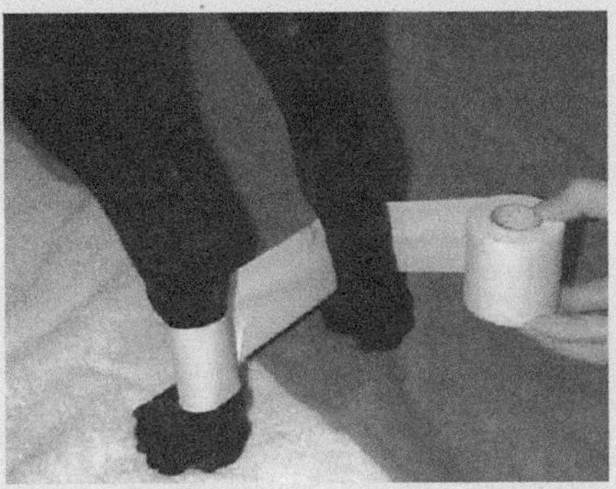

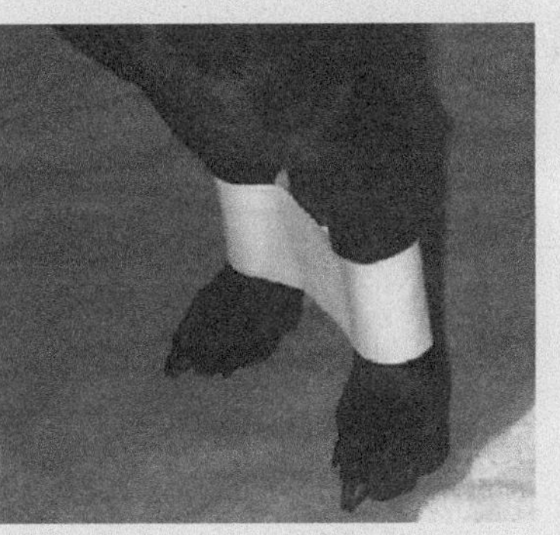

REFERENCE

1. Ratcliff, C.R. (2008). Wound exudate: an influential factor in healing. *Adv Nurse Pract* 16:32–36.

RECOMMENDED READING

Johnston, S.A. and Tobias, K.M. (2018). *Veterinary Surgery: Small Animal*, 2e. St Louis, MO: Elsevier Saunders.

Pavletic, M. (2018). *Atlas of Small Animal Wound Management and Reconstructive Surgery*, 4e. Hoboken, NJ: Wiley Blackwell.

Swaim, S., Renberg, W.C. and Shike, K.M. (2011). *Small Animal Bandaging, Casting, and Splinting Techniques*. Ames, IO: Wiley Blackwell.

Welch, J.A., Gillette, R.L. and Swaim, S.F. (2015). *Management of Small Animal Distal Limb Injuries*. Jackson, WY: Teton NewMedia.

Section Six

Anesthesia and Anesthetic Procedures

Chapter 20

Anesthesia and Anesthetic Procedures

Heather A. Sidari, RVT, VTS (Anesthesia & Analgesia)

Veterinary Technician and Nurse's Daily Reference Guide: Canine and Feline, Fourth Edition. Edited by Mandy Fults and Kenichiro Yagi.

Companion website: www.wiley.com/go/fults/veterinary

Abbreviations

ABG, arterial blood gases
ALP, alkaline phosphatase
ALT, alanine aminotransferase
aPTT, activated partial thromboplastin time
ASA, American Association of Anesthesiologists
AV, atrioventricular
BUN, blood urea nitrogen
CNS, central nervous system
CRI, constant rate infusion
CRT, capillary refill time
CSF, cerebrospinal fluid
CT, computed tomography
CVP, central venous pressure
DJD, degenerative joint disease
ECG, electrocardiogram
ETCO2, end tidal CO2
GABA, γ-aminobutyric acid
GDV, gastric dilation volvulus
IPPV, intermittent positive pressure ventilation
IBP, intra-arterial blood pressure
IV, intravenous
IM, intramuscular
MAP, mean arterial pressure
MDR1, multidrug resistance mutation 1
NaCl, sodium chloride
NMDA, N-methyl-D-aspartate
NSAIDs, non-steroidal anti-inflammatory drugs
PCV, packed cell volume
PEEP, positive end expiratory pressure
RBC, red blood cells
SpO2, peripheral capillary oxygen saturation
SQ, subcutaneously
T4, tetraiodothyronine
TPP, total plasma protein

GUIDELINES FOR SAFE ANESTHESIA

Anesthesia is a controlled loss of sensation and/or consciousness To provide this loss safely and effectively, many factors must be known and understood by the anesthetist. The anesthetist must consider multiple factors including the signalment of the patient, their history, the evaluation of the current condition, comorbidities, together with knowledge of the anesthetic equipment, anesthetic drugs, monitoring techniques, recovery, and emergency protocols. It is only through this knowledge that the inherent risks of anesthesia can be lessened and anticipated.

The anesthetist should follow a methodical and stepwise approach with each patient to ensure that all precautions and evaluations have been reviewed to obtain the most desirable outcome.

Potential Problems Associated with All Anesthetic Procedures

- Hypothermia
- Hypotension
- Hypoventilation
- Hypoxemia
- Discomfort or pain

Patient Admissions

- Review of medical record.
- Review the following with the owner:
  - 6–10-hour fast (patients < 4 months of age, 4-hour fast)[1]
  - Medication history
  - Anesthetic history
  - New health concerns
  - Vaccination history
  - Reviewed and signed surgical release form and estimate
  - Client contact information
  - Resuscitation code

Patient Evaluation

- Signalment (species, breed, sex and reproductive status, age)
- History
- Weight
- Temperament[2]
- Diet
- Vital signs (temperature, pulse, respiratory rate/mucous membranes/ capillary refill time)
- Physical examination
- Laboratory workup
- Diagnostic tests
- ASA physical status
- Preoperative pain score
- Anticipated postoperative pain score

Patient Preparation

- Premedication
- Venous access
- Providing a calm, relaxed, and pain-free state
- Intravenous fluid choice and rate

Machine Preparation

- Check/fill vaporizer
- Check oxygen supply
- Choose breathing circuit and reservoir bag
- Leak test

Drug Protocol

- Calculate all emergency drugs or prepare an emergency drug reference sheet.
- Create an anesthetic and analgesic plan based on the ASA status, the procedure being performed, and the preanesthetic evaluation.

Induction preparation

- Endotracheal tube selection (typically three sizes)
- Endotracheal tube tie
- Eye lube
- Laryngoscope

- Sterile lube for endotracheal tube cuff
- Emergency drugs/crash cart
- Suction unit for esophageal/tracheal suction with supplies[2]

Induction

- Provide pre-oxygenation if indicated for a minimum of three to five minutes and as long as it does not create undue stress for the patient.
- Provide a rapid loss of consciousness to obtain quick control of the airway.

Perioperative

- Monitor the patient for physiologic support and pain management as needed.
- Maintain an appropriate surgical plane of anesthesia.

Recovery

- Allow a smooth recovery without excitation, distress, or struggling.
- Maintain normal vital signs.

PREANESTHESIA

A complete review of the list in Table 20.1 should be conducted on each patient prior to the administration of any drugs. These initial assessments will prove valuable in choosing the correct drug protocol and in monitoring the patient during and following the anesthetic procedure. Potential complications and plans to correct them are projected during this step. Patients with known health concerns or those revealing abnormalities with the tests that follow should have a specific anesthesia plan put in place. Guidelines for specific health conditions can be found in Table 20.15.

Table 20.1 / Preanesthetic evaluation

Category	Parameters to evaluate
Signalment	• Species, breed, age, sex, reproductive status, and temperament of the patient can have direct implications on the type of drugs used during the anesthetic procedure, together with the type of monitoring used
History	• Both recent and past history of anesthetic episodes, medications, meals, and continuing diseases will affect the anesthetic protocol
Weight	• A current weight in both kilograms and pounds
Vital signs (see Table 2.1: Initial examination, page 30)	• Temperature • Pulse • Heart rate • Respiration • Capillary refill time • Mucous membrane color
Physical examination (see Table 2.2: Physical examination, page 33)	• A complete physical exam including the patients emotional wellbeing must be performed to help acquire a baseline for the patient • This initial exam must be performed prior to the administration of any drugs for accurate results • Any variations from normal should be followed up with additional diagnostics and then evaluated in regard to drug choice and monitoring

(Continued)

Table 20.1 / Preanesthetic evaluation (Continued)	
Category	**Parameters to evaluate**
Laboratory workup (see Chapter 3: Clinical Pathology; Chapter 14: Patient Care Skills in Clinical Practice)	• A wide range of protocols exist for preanesthetic laboratory workup. However, all patients should have a minimum of a PCV, total protein, BUN, creatinine, ALT, ALP, and blood glucose prior to any anesthetic procedure. Additional tests would be warranted based on the above-mentioned results, with obvious signs of disease or with increased age • PCV/total protein • Serum chemistry panel • Complete blood count • Electrolytes • Urinalysis • Coagulation profile • Buccal mucosal bleeding time • Activated clotting time • prothrombin time/aPTT assays • Platelet count • Venous or arterial blood gases
Additional diagnostic testing	• Radiography is used to detect and evaluate congenital or acquired cardiopulmonary disease or conditions associated with traumatic injuries; for example, pulmonary contusions, diaphragmatic hernia, or pneumothorax. Abdominal radiographs can detect and evaluate congenital or acquired organ disease, for example, hepatic, urinary, or gastrointestinal diseases • Electrocardiography should be performed in patients with suspected or known heart disease, those with recent trauma, possible myocarditis, and patients with electrolyte abnormalities • Ultrasound/echocardiography can be an additional tool used to evaluate the degree of many diseases or traumatic states
ASA physical status[3]	• The ASA classification system adapts to small animal medicine with ease. It allows a system to evaluate the patient based on the presence and severity of systemic disease present • Excellent anesthetic risk; patients with no underlying disease, undergoing elective surgeries • Good anesthetic risk, mild disease changes • Fair anesthetic risk, severe disease changes • Poor anesthetic risk, severe disease changes that are a constant threat to life • Critical anesthetic risk; moribund, not expected to survive without surgery • E Denotes an emergency surgery

Preanesthetic Drugs

The preanesthetic drug is the first part of a complete anesthetic drug protocol. The desirable effects of premedication include decreasing stress and anxiety on the patient, preemptive analgesia, decreasing the doses of induction and maintenance anesthetic agents, aid in a smoother maintenance and recovery phases of anesthesia, and aid in preventing nauseousness.

Premedicating a patient for an anesthetic event can start at home the night before and the morning of the procedure. This is especially needed for fearful, stressed, or anxious animals. Oral sedatives such as gabapentin, trazodone, alpha-2 agonists, acepromazine, or benzodiazepines will aid in reduction of the sympathetic responses seen in these patients. Challenging anesthesia can occur when the wind up of the "flight or fight" response has not been addressed.[4]

Further preanesthetics are needed once the patient has been evaluated on the day of the anesthetic event. They typically consist of a combination of drugs that will provide additional sedative and tranquilizing effects (alpha-2 agonists, phenothiazines, or benzodiazepines) and analgesics for any procedure where a mild to moderate level of pain is expected (opioids, alpha-2 agonists, NMDA antagonists). A combination of a sedative/tranquilizer and an opioid is termed a neuroleptanalgesic. These combinations have a synergistic effect that provides better sedation while using less of each drug and subsequently producing fewer adverse effects.

Anticholinergics are a class of drugs with a history of being added to the premedication, but their routine use has now proven unnecessary for most procedures. These drugs cause an increase in heart rate and cardiac output, decreased oral, pharyngeal, and respiratory tract sections, and gastrointestinal tract motility, pupil and bronchial dilation, and block vagal nerve stimulation. They may be added to the preanesthetic for brachycephalic patients, those less than four months of age, bronchoscopies, or any other procedures with an expected vagal response.

Before the administration of any medication, all laboratory work should be completed as drugs can alter certain values (e.g. packed cell volume can be lowered by 30% by the preadministration of acepromazine: splenic sequestration). An emergency drug reference sheet should be prepared specifically for each patient, with all drugs available and ready. All syringes must be clearly labeled with the patient's name, drug name, and amount. Subcutaneous preanesthetics are typically given 30–45 minutes before the procedure, whereas intramuscular preanesthetics are only given 15–20 minutes before the procedure. You can also give intravenous premedications, which produce a more rapid onset, allowing for decreased time between premedication and catheter placement.

Table 20.2 / Steps to choosing a preanesthetic combination

Steps	Level of coverage	Drug choice
1: What level of sedation is required? (Dose is important when deciding level of sedation)	None	Opioid alone (buprenorphine)
	Mild	Gabapentin, trazodone, butorphanol, ± buprenorphine or methadone
	Moderate	Acepromazine dexmedetomidine with opioid
	Profound	Medetomidine, dexmedetomidine with opioid
2: What level of analgesic is required?	Mild	Butorphanol
	Mild to moderate	Buprenorphine
	Significant	Hydromorphone, oxymorphone, morphine, fentanyl, methadone
3: Is an anticholinergic required?	Moderate/ significant	Atropine, glycopyrrolate

Anesthetic Equipment and Setup

Table 20.3 / **The anesthetic machine**

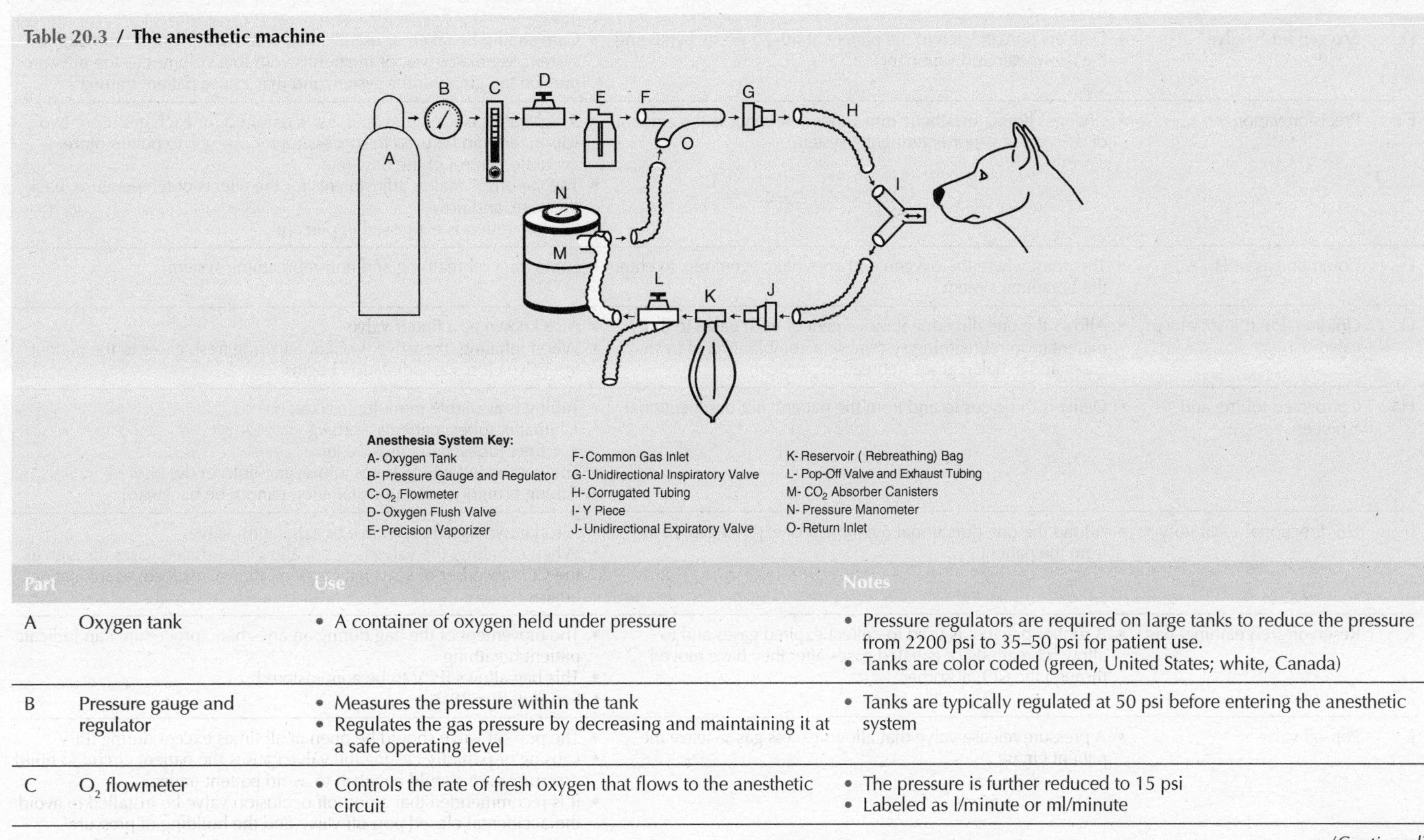

Part		Use	Notes
A	Oxygen tank	• A container of oxygen held under pressure	• Pressure regulators are required on large tanks to reduce the pressure from 2200 psi to 35–50 psi for patient use. • Tanks are color coded (green, United States; white, Canada)
B	Pressure gauge and regulator	• Measures the pressure within the tank • Regulates the gas pressure by decreasing and maintaining it at a safe operating level	• Tanks are typically regulated at 50 psi before entering the anesthetic system
C	O_2 flowmeter	• Controls the rate of fresh oxygen that flows to the anesthetic circuit	• The pressure is further reduced to 15 psi • Labeled as l/minute or ml/minute

(*Continued*)

Table 20.3 / **The anesthetic machine (Continued)**

Part		Use	Notes
D	Oxygen flush valve	• Delivers pure oxygen to the patient at 40–70 psi by bypassing the flowmeter and vaporizer	• Care should be taken or use avoided when using a non-rebreathing system, ventilator use, or in circuits with low volumes as the pressure may be too great for the system and may cause patient trauma
E	Precision vaporizer	• Changes liquid anesthetic into vapor and controls the amount of delivery of vapor entering the system	• A separate gas-specific vaporizer is required for each gas used; two vaporizers can be used in succession for one gas to obtain more accurate control of the flow rate • The vaporizer makes adjustments for the effects of temperature, back pressure, and flow • Concentration is expressed in percent
F	Common gas inlet	• The point where the oxygen and anesthetic agent mix to enter the breathing system	• Same for a rebreathing and non-rebreathing system
G	Unidirectional inspiratory valve	• Allows the one directional movement of fresh gases to the patient (non-rebreathing system) or a combination of fresh gases and exhaled gases (rebreathing system)	• Also known as a flutter valve • When inhaling, the valve is open, allowing fresh gases to the patient; the valve closes as exhalation begins

H/I	Corrugated tubing and Y-piece	• Delivers the gases to and from the patient; not unidirectional	• Tubing is available in multiple sizes:
			  • Smaller tubes: patients 7–20 kg
			  • Larger tubes: patients > 20 kg
			• The corrugated tubing helps to prevent kinks in the line
			• Tubing is unidirectional; installation cannot be backward

J	Unidirectional expiratory valve	• Allows the one directional movement of expired gases away from the patient	• Also known as a flutter valve or exhalation valve • When exhaling, the valve is open, allowing exhaled gases through to the CO_2 absorber or scavenger system; the valve closes as inhalation begins
K	Reservoir (rebreathing) bag	• A rubber bag that is used to collect expired gases and to allow rebreathing of exhaled gases after they have moved through the CO_2 absorber	• The movement of the bag during an anesthetic procedure can indicate patient breathing • This bag allows IPPV to be administered • See Skill Box 20.2
L	Pop-off valve	• A pressure release valve that allows excess gas to leave the patient circuit	• The pop-off valve should be open at all times except during IPPV • Closing or partially closing the valve causes the patient circuit to build pressure; care should be taken to avoid patient trauma • It is recommended that a pop-off occlusion valve be installed to avoid the accidental closed pop-off valve and the building of pressure

(*Continued*)

Table 20.3 / **The anesthetic machine (Continued)**

	Part	Use	Notes
M	CO_2 absorber	• Absorbs the CO_2 in the expired gases from the patient	• Determining exhausted granules and the need to change • A visible color change is seen to light purple; this color change can disappear after isoflurane use is discontinued • Fresh crystals easily crumble and exhausted crystals are hard and brittle • ½ inch should be left at the top of the canister for proper air movement • Follow the manufacturer's directions on which absorber to use with certain inhalant anesthetics
N	Pressure manometer	• Measures the pressure within the system • Aids anesthetist when administering IPPV	• Pressure not to exceed 20 cm H_2O when connected to a patient • A reading of 0 cm H_2O is expected when the pop-off valve is open
O	Return inlet	• The point where the used anesthetic gases are returning to the system	• Part of a rebreathing system • CO_2 has been removed in the CO_2 absorber canisters

Anesthetic Machine Setup

Before the administration of every general anesthetic, the equipment must be checked over to assure it is in proper working condition. Many anesthetic complications can be avoided by taking this important step.

Verify the following:

- Adequate amount of inhalant in the vaporizer; the cap is tightly closed.
- Adequate oxygen supply.
- Fresh CO_2 absorber (expired absorber will not absorb CO_2, leading to hypercarbia and rebreathing of CO_2 by the patient)
- Equipment is connected correctly:
  - Oxygen supply tube is connected.
  - Machine is set up for the correct breathing system (Skill Box 20.2).
  - Correct sized reservoir bag is attached.
  - Pop-off occlusion valve is installed or the pop-off valve is open.
  - Scavenger tube is connected and the evacuation fan is activated or connected to an activated charcoal container.
- Adequate pressure test (entire system):
  - Once the machine is properly connected, close the pop-off valve, occlude the patient end of tubing, fill the system with oxygen from the O_2 flush, and monitor the pressure gauge.
  - No leaks will maintain a constant pressure.
  - Leaks in the system will show a dropping pressure.
  - Test for leak detection by spraying with diluted soapy water at the system junctions and observing for bubble formation.
  - Common leak areas are any machine joint, connection of rebreathing bag, seal of absorber canister, valve caps, and tubing or hoses.
  - Open pop-off valve before releasing pressure. This ensures that the pop-off is open and slowly decreases pressure in the system. Fast release of pressure can cause soda-sorb from the cannister to enter breathing circuits.
- Inhalation valves:
  - Once the machine is properly connected; close the pop-off valve, occlude the patient end of the tubing, fill the system with oxygen

from the O_2 flush, release patient tubing, squeeze reservoir bag and observe for movement of inhalation valves.

- Exhalation valves:
  - Once the machine is properly connected and while wearing a surgical mask, exhale into the patient tubing to observe for movement of exhalation valves.
- Test the inner tubing on a non-rebreathing or f-circuit systems (Pethick test).
- Once the machine is properly connected; occlude the patient end of the tubing with the O_2 flowing at 1–2 liters/minute. The float in the flowmeter should fall if no leaks are present.

Dead Space

Dead space is an important part of consideration for all patients undergoing an anesthetic procedure. It refers to areas within the patient or the anesthetic machine that are not participating in gas exchange. Increased dead space decreases the patient's ability to receive fresh gases and the subsequent retention of carbon dioxide. Physiologic dead space is always present and makes up 35% of an awake animal's tidal volume. This increases to 50% in a healthy anesthetized animal and refers to the nasal passages, nasopharynx, larynx, trachea, and alveoli that are not perfused by the pulmonary circulation. Mechanical dead space refers to areas within the anesthetic machine and equipment and includes any space where gas is being held such as the endotracheal tube from the patient's mouth to the tubing connector, the "Y" piece at the terminal end of the anesthetic tubing, anesthetic masks, any attached adaptors (monitoring devices, humidification management exchangers, and positioning adaptors), exhausted CO_2 absorbers, malfunctioning one-way valves, defects in tubing, and low flow rates on non-rebreathing systems.

Skill Box 20.1 / Dead space

The consideration of dead space is important in all patients, but is especially of concern in those weighing less than 6 kg. The addition of just two adaptors can add enough dead space to reduce spontaneous alveolar ventilation up to 95%.

Steps to take to reduce mechanical dead space

- Properly sized endotracheal tubes; not to extend no more than 1 inch past the patient's incisors.
- Properly functioning anesthetic equipment: one-way valves, fresh carbon dioxide absorbers, no defects in tubing.
- Use of minimal positional adaptors, especially in smaller patients.
- Use of properly selected anesthetic set-up; pediatric equipment.

Skill Box 20.2 / Anesthetic breathing systems

Rebreathing–circle system

- Patient rebreathes its own exhaled gases after the CO_2 has been filtered out by the CO_2 absorber and fresh O_2 and anesthetic gases have been added.

Types	Indications for use	Oxygen flow rates	Comments
• Total rebreathing/closed • Pop-off valve is completely closed	• Patients > 15 lb (standard circuit) • Patients < 15 lb (pediatric circuit) • Patients must have lungs strong enough to push gases through the machine	• 4–6 ml/kg/minute • O_2 flow equals the patient's metabolic O_2 consumption	• Do not use with nitrous oxide • The relative low gas rates used result in slow changes in anesthetic depth • Ventilation is readily observed and controlled by the rebreathing bag • Minimal heat loss and airway drying as recycled gas is warmer and more humidified • ↑ Resistance to ventilation • Flow rates must be closely monitored to avoid barotraumas
• Partial rebreathing/semi-closed • Pop-off valve is partially or fully open	• Patients > 15 lb (standard circuit) • Patients < 15 lb (pediatric circuit)	• 20–40 ml/kg/minute	• Much higher gas rates need to be used • Ventilation can be observed by the rebreathing bag

Non-rebreathing system

- Patient receives fresh O_2 and anesthetic gases with each breath.
- CO_2 is removed by the high gas flow rates that push all exhaled gases into the scavenger system.

Types	Indications for use	Oxygen flow rates	Comments
• Open • Pop-off valve is completely open	• Any size patients, typically those < 8 kg • Minimal resistance to breathing	• 200–400 ml/kg/minute[2]	• Much higher gas rates needed to eliminate exhaled gases • Minimal or no rebreathing of expired gases by the patient, which can lead to hypothermia and drying of respiratory tract • Minimal resistance to gas flow and breathing • Allows rapid alterations in anesthetic concentrations • Risk of barotrauma with use of oxygen flush valve

(Continued)

Skill Box 20.2 / Anesthetic breathing systems (Continued)

Rebreathing bag size

Types	Calculations	Comments
< 15 lb = 1-liter bag > 15 and < 40 lb = 2-liter bag > 40 and < 120 lb = 3-liter bag > 120 and < 300 lb = 5-liter bag	• Patient tidal volume is calculated at 10–15 ml/kg (5–7 ml/lb) and then multiplied by 6 • 60 ml/kg • (Weight in kg × V_T 15) 5 = ml ÷ 1000 = liter of bag needed	• Bags size is always chosen by rounding up • If bag too small, cannot take an adequate breath • If bag too big, ↑ in dead space, slow changes in anesthetic depth, inability to monitor respiration by observing bag movement

Compressed gas cylinders

- Green tank = oxygen
- Blue tank = nitrous oxide

VENTILATION

One of the key elements to successful anesthesia is monitoring and providing adequate ventilation. Even though respirations can be seen by the rising and falling of the chest and observing movement of the reservoir bag, this does not always ensure adequate ventilation is taking place. Manual or mechanical intermittent positive pressure ventilation (IPPV) can ensure that the patient is receiving proper delivery of oxygen and gas inhalant. This approach is essential for certain surgical procedures when spontaneous ventilation is compromised. Prior to setting patients up to a ventilator, the anesthetist must be comfortable with the equipment and has performed an equipment and pressure check. Patients should also have arterial blood gas analysis or capnograph monitoring to adequately monitor the levels of CO_2. Hypocapnia (hyperventilating) can lead to respiratory alkalosis and hypercapnia (hypoventilating) to respiratory acidosis.

Uses of ventilation include:

- Animals with compromised respiration (e.g. obese or debilitated animals).
- Thoracic surgery (e.g. diaphragmatic hernia, pericardiectomy, lung lobectomy)
- Head, chest, or nerve trauma.
- Procedures needing neuromuscular blocking agents.
- Inadequate gas exchange leading to improper plane of anesthesia.
- Hypoventilation.
- Drug overdose.

Table 20.4 / Ventilation	
	Description
Normal values	
Tidal volume	The amount of gas exchanged in one respiratory cycle
	10–20 ml/kg
Airway pressure	15–20 cm H_2O in awake animals and when ventilator is in use
	20–30 cm H_2O when ventilator is in use during thoracic surgery
Inspiratory time	1 second in awake animals
	< 1.5 seconds when ventilator is in use
Ventilatory rate	Canine: 8–14 breaths/minute
	Feline: 10–14 breaths/minute
Minute ventilation	200 ml/kg/minute[5]
Controls	
Volume preset	Delivers a preset constant volume of gas despite changes in the lungs during anesthesia
	Volume is variable and depends on the following: lung compliance, airway resistance, pressure within the thorax, and the number of functioning alveoli
	Allows for development of high airway pressures and for small leaks that cannot be compensated for, compromising the patient's tidal volume
Pressure preset	Delivers a gas at a preset volume during the inspiratory phase
	Does not allow a buildup of high pressure and compensates for leaks in the system
	Pressure may need to be increased to compensate for volume variability.
Time cycled	Delivers gas at a preset frequency or respiratory rate, inspiratory: expiratory ratio (I : E), or inspiratory flow rate
Associated risks	Thoracic blood flow impairment, leading to ↓ blood pressure, stroke volume, and cardiac output
	Hyperventilation, leading to respiratory alkalosis and ↓ cerebral blood flow
	Barotrauma, leading to pneumothorax, pneumomediastinum, pulmonary hemorrhage, and air embolism
	Improper setup of ventilator or ventilator malfunction
	In-circle vaporizers can cause ↑ amounts of vaporized anesthetics; leading to deepened anesthetic states
	Ventilator equipment can be a source of microbial contamination for the patient

Ventilator Machine Setup

Before the administration of each procedure requiring a ventilator, the equipment must be checked over to ensure that it is in proper working condition. Many complications can be avoided by taking this important step. Verify the following:

- The power to the unit.
- Equipment is connected correctly.
  - Connections on both ventilator and anesthetic machine; oxygen supply, exhaust, driving gas and supply gas.
  - Select the correct size of bellow, and ensure that it is in good working condition (e.g. tears, dirt), and install.
  - Pop-off valve is open or closed depending on the unit.
- Adequate pressure test.
- Entire system:
  - Once the machine is properly connected, connect a reservoir bag to the patient end of the tubing, close the pop-off valve, fill the system with oxygen until the bellow is inflated, turn on the volume to minimum setting, set the rate and turn on; adjust the volume until the peak pressure is at 30 cm H_2O, and depress the inspiratory hold button to check that no leaks are present (no drop is pressure is seen).
  - Leaks in the system will cause a drop in pressure and deflating bellows.

Ventilation Administration

There are numerous types of ventilators used in veterinary medicine, each with varying complexity of controls. The manufacturer's guidelines for instructions should be referred to for proper use. Prior to each use, the ventilator function should be verified with a leak check and a general function test.

When a patient is trying to breath against the ventilator, it is termed "bucking" the ventilator. This is a normal process when initially switching the patient to the ventilator or when weaning at the end of the procedure. Bucking during the procedure warrants investigation as to plane of anesthesia, health of the patient, and equipment failure.

Skill Box 20.3 / Ventilation administration

Type	Definition	Uses	Initiating method	Ending method
Manual				
Assist	• Patient's breathing is assisted by manual compressions of the reservoir bag • Often referred to as giving a "sigh" or as manual IPPV (Skill Box 20.4)	Any healthy, anesthetized animal	• The pop-off valve is closed and pressure is applied to the reservoir bag to a manometer reading of 10–15 (feline and canine < 22 lb) and 15–20 (canine) cm H_2O to inflate the lungs (holding for no more than one s) and then slowly released for exhalation	• Normal procedure of discontinuing inhalant anesthetics
Controlled	• Patient's breathing is controlled by manual compressions of the reservoir bag	Animals with compromised respiration (e.g. obese or debilitated animals)	• Reduce vaporizer setting initially and begin bagging (as described earlier) at a rate of 12–16 breaths/minute • If the chest cavity is open, the manometer reading should be ↑ to 20–30 cm H_2O. • Spontaneous breathing should cease after 3–5 minutes; if it does not, a neuromuscular agent may need to be used • Once control of respiration has been established, a rate of 8–12 breaths/minute should be maintained • Inspiratory time should be 1–1.5 seconds with an expiratory time twice as long • The pop-off valve should be closed during compressions but should be opened every 2–3 breaths to allow escape of back pressure	• Discontinue the use of the inhalant anesthetic and nitrous oxide while continuing to ventilate with O_2 • Administer the reversal if a neuromuscular agent and an opioid were used • The rate of respiration should be gradually ↓ to 5 breaths/minute while the animal is observed for spontaneous breathing • Spontaneous breathing may take several minutes to resume, especially in older or debilitated animals or in those undergoing a long anesthetic procedure • Once spontaneous respiration is seen, the anesthetist should switch to manual-controlled ventilation • The rate can continue to ↓ to 1–4 breaths/minutes • Bagging can be stopped altogether when the rate and tidal volume are back to normal

(*Continued*)

Skill Box 20.3 / Ventilation administration (Continued)

Type	Definition	Uses	Initiating method	Ending method
Mechanical				
Assist	• Patient-initiated ventilation • The initiation of a breath from the patient triggers a preselected tidal volume from the ventilator • The patient determines frequency of ventilation and minute volume	Animals with compromised respiration (e.g. obese or debilitated animals), animals with prolonged anesthetic procedures	• Refer to the ventilator's manual for complete instructions • Connect the ventilator to the patient's breathing system • Adjust the controls • Turn the ventilator on • Make minor adjustments to the controls based on the patient's monitored values	• See Manual controlled: ending method above
Assisted-Controlled	• The initiation of a breath from the patient triggers a preselected tidal volume from the ventilator • The anesthetist sets a minimal respiratory rate, which the animal may override by initiating spontaneous respiratory efforts at a faster rate	See above	• See Mechanical assist: initiating method above	• See Manual controlled: ending method above
Controlled	• The anesthetist sets the ventilator to control the rate and volume of the animal's respiratory cycle	See above; thoracic surgery (e.g. diaphragmatic hernia or pneumothorax), head trauma	• See Mechanical assist: initiating method above	• See Manual controlled: ending method above

Intermittent Positive Pressure Ventilation

IPPV is the manual compression of the reservoir bag to provide adequate ventilation to the lungs.

Skill Box 20.4 / Intermittent positive pressure ventilation

- Perform every 5 minutes on an anesthetized patient with no complications.
- Perform frequently (every 6 seconds to deliver 10 breaths/minute) in place of a mechanical ventilator.
- Certain medical conditions may require increased pressure to adequately ventilate the patient (e.g. diaphragmatic hernias, thorax or abdominal tumors, or fluid in the thorax and abdomen).
- IPPV may cause ↓ blood pressure because of the pressure placed on the venous return to the heart; the amount of pressure may need to be ↓ if this poses an additional risk to the patient:
  - Smaller (15 cm H_2O), more frequent shallow breaths may need to be performed to avoid this complication.
- Technique:
  - Assess depth of anesthesia:
    - If the animal is adequately anesthetized, turn down the vaporizer before giving IPPV.
    - If the animal is too lightly anesthetized, leave the vaporizer at current setting, thereby increasing inhalant agent in alveoli.
  - Close pop-off valve and gently and consistently squeeze the reservoir bag for ≤ 1 second to a pressure reading of 15 cm H_2O while monitoring the rising chest of the patient; if the chest is not rising sufficiently, increase to no more than 20 cm H_2O.
  - Release the bag and open the pop-off valve.

Note: because of the risk of barotrauma and possibly death from failure to open the pop-off valve and release pressure in the system, it is recommended that all anesthetic machines have a pop-off occlusion valve in place. These valves allow closing of the pop-off valve with the use of a button that, once released, immediately releases pressure and eliminates the risk of patient injury.

ANESTHETIC ADMINISTRATION

The administration of anesthesia allows necessary veterinary procedures to commence without difficulty by immobilizing the patient and eliminating pain. The proper administration of anesthesia ensures the comfort of the patient during administration, the procedure, and following the procedure. Prior to the induction of any anesthetic, an intravenous catheter should be placed. This allows for titration of the induction agent, emergency intravenous access, intravenous fluid administration, and to avoid the risk of a perivascular injection.

Table 20.5 / General anesthesia induction

Method of induction	Common drugs used	Procedure	Uses	Associated risks	Patient contraindications
Oral	• Ketamine	• Draw up a single dose of the drug into a syringe and squirt into the patient's mouth	• Uncooperative animals • Animals where injections are difficult	• Aspiration • Poor administration	• Animals with gastrointestinal disease or injury
Intramuscular	• Ketamine • Ketamine and midazolam • Tiletamine and zolazepam	• Draw up a single dose of the drug into a syringe and administer by an IM injection	• Uncooperative animals • Animals where IV injections are difficult (e.g., puppies, kittens)	• Delayed recovery • Overdose	• Old and debilitated animals that would benefit from induction to effect (e.g. lower dosing) • Brachycephalics, as no rapid control of airway
Intravenous	• Opioid and diazepam/midazolam (canine) • Etomidate • Ketamine and diazepam/midazolam • Propofol • Alfaxalone • Thiopental • Tiletamine and zolazepam	• Place an IV catheter and administer the drug by one of the following methods: • Bolus ¼ dose; wait 30–45 seconds, then repeat • Bolus over 10–15 seconds • Slow injection over 1–2 minutes • IV fluid drip	• Minor anesthetic procedures • Induction to general anesthesia with inhalant anesthetics • Animals where rapid control of the airway is needed (e.g., laryngeal collapse, and brachycephalic)	• Perivascular injection • Accumulation of drug with repeated dosing (e.g. delayed recovery)	• Obese animals where locating a vein may not be possible • Fractious animals
Face mask*	• Isoflurane • Sevoflurane	• With adequate restraint, place an anesthetic mask over the mouth and nose tightly to minimize waste gas and dead space • Run 100% oxygen at 3 l/minute for5 minutes to allow adjustment to mask then begin anesthetic flow slowly over a few minutes to a level of 3–4%	• Induction to general anesthesia with inhalant anesthetics • Premedicated animals, moribund animals, or tractable dogs	• Inability to adequately monitor • No airway control • Requires an ↑ concentration of inhalant anesthetic leading to hypotension and hypoventilation • Not a balanced anesthetic plan; no sedative or analgesic effects • Environmental anesthetic pollution • waste anesthetic gas exposure to staff • Extremely stressful for the patient • Stress-induced cardiac arrhythmias increasing morbidity and mortality[6]	• Brachycephalic dogs or nasal or pharyngeal tumor present • Animals with respiratory or cardiovascular disease • Excited animals, ventricular arrhythmias or any cardiovascular disease • Animals that have not been fasted
Chamber*	• Isoflurane • Sevoflurane • Desflurane	• Place the animal in a chamber large enough to allow lying down and extension of the neck. • Run oxygen at 3–5 l/minute and the anesthetic flow at 4–5% • Once the animal has lost its righting reflex, remove them from the chamber and place an endotracheal tube	• Induction to general anesthesia with inhalant anesthetics • Intractable, fractious cats		

* Mask or chamber inductions should be strictly avoided and only used as a last resort.

Skill Box 20.5 / Endotracheal intubation

Setup

Size

1. Palpate the neck of the awake patient and view thoracic radiographs if available.
2. Select the estimated size based on the chart below and then one size larger and smaller (two sizes smaller with brachycephalic breeds). Endotracheal tubes are based on lean body weight, as trachea size is independent of body weight.
3. Use the largest tube that will fit into the trachea without strain.

Weight		Tube size, internal diameter (mm)	
(kg)	(lb)	Canine	Feline
1	2.2	4.0–4.5	3
2	4–5	4–5.0	3.5
3	6–7	4.5–5.0	4.0
4	8–9	5.5	4.5
6	13–14	6.5	
8	17–18	7	
10	22–23	7.5	
12	26–27	8	
14	31–32	8.5	
16	35–36	9	
18	39–40	9.5	
20	44–45	10	
25	55–56	11	
30	66–67	12	
40–60	88–132	14–16	

Length

- The length of the tube should extend from the thoracic inlet to no more than 1 inch past the incisors.
- Tubes must be cut if they do not fall within these guidelines to avoid dead space and endobronchial intubation.

Function

1. Fill the cuff with air to observe for any leaks. Suggest letting sit inflated for 10 minutes as there can be a slow leak.
2. Acquire supplies for intubation:
   a. Laryngoscope
   b. Endotracheal tubes
   c. Gauze squares (for assistant to hold tongue)
   d. Endotracheal tube tie (rolled gauze, IV tubing)
   e. Packet of sterile lube
   f. Stylet
   g. Syringe for inflation of tube cuff

Technique

1. Roll inflated cuff in sterile lubricant. Then deflate cuff for intubation. This improves the seal to reduces risk of aspiration.[2,7]
2. Place patients in sternal recumbency; patients can be placed in lateral recumbency for intubation with the right training and practice.
3. Have the assistant open the patient's mouth while simultaneously gently grasping the tongue with a 3 × 3 gauze pad (to prevent slipping).
4. Have the assistant extend the tongue for a clear view of the larynx.
5. Place laryngoscope so the tip of the blade depresses the base of the tongue, which aids in pulling down the epiglottis. Take care to not use the blade to pull down the epiglottis.[6]
6. Insert the tube over the epiglottis between the arytenoid cartilages into the larynx, rotating from 0 to 90 degrees to facilitate passage.
7. Confirm placement immediately with capnograph by attaching and administering manual breaths.
8. Confirm depth of tube by either palpating at thoracic inlet and feeling for end of tube or by measuring against another tube (line up cm marks)
9. Tie the tube in place with gauze or tubing to prevent slippage.
10. Perform leak check to ensure proper seal of endotracheal tube:
    a. Attach a clean syringe full of air to the tubing of the cuff. Depress the occlusion valve or close the pop-off valve and place the ear next to the mouth of the patient to listen for escaping air while gently squeezing the

(Continued)

Skill Box 20.5 / Endotracheal intubation (Continued)

reservoir bag (the pressure manometer should read less than 20 cm H_2O). Depress the plunger of the syringe and fill the cuff with air just until no air can be heard escaping around the tube. Remove the syringe and open the pop-off valve. Record the volume of air used to inflate the cuff.

b. Another way to ensure seal is by closing the pop-off valve, squeeze the reservoir bag and watch the manometer. If there is a leak, the needle will drop, and the reservoir bag will deflate in your hand. Administer a small amount of air into the cuff and repeat until manometer needle holds steady at 15–20 cm H_2O and the reservoir bag does not deflate.

11. Turn on the vaporizer.

Note: wait to turn on vaporizer until leak check is performed to decrease exposure of waste anesthetic gases to yourself and others around.

To ensure proper use

1. Verify placement
2. Capnography
   a. Immediately after intubation, attach capnograph and breathing circuit. Give manual IPPV (at least 2–3 breaths) and conform placement by visualizing capnogram.
   b. If no waveform or number present, esophageal placement.
   c. Palpate the throat region.
   d. One hard structure assures tracheal placement.
   e. Two hard structures indicate esophageal placement.
3. Thoracic auscultation:
   a. Auscultate the lungs bilaterally during a breath and listen for lung sounds:
      – Unilateral lung sounds indicate endobronchial intubation.
      – No lung sounds indicates esophageal intubation.
   b. Absence of vocalization.
   c. Condensation of respiratory gases on the inside of the tube during exhalation.
   d. Movement of reservoir bag with each breath.
4. Verify seal:
   a. Check for leaking air
   b. See inflating cuff mentioned earlier.

Tips:

- A stylet can be used for small floppy tubes. Polypropylene urinary catheter (5 Fr) can be used as a "guidewire" to lead the tube between the arytenoid cartilages. This technique can facilitate rapid intubation or aid in difficult cases such as in patients with pharyngeal tumors.
- Laryngospasm (felines):
  - Provide a level of anesthesia deep enough to allow intubation.
  - Apply lidocaine (0.1 ml) to the glottis.
  - Wait for the glottis to relax and open and then insert the tube; attempting when closed may increase spasms or cause severe trauma to the trachea.
  - Consider a supraglottic airway device for felines (Figure 20.2).

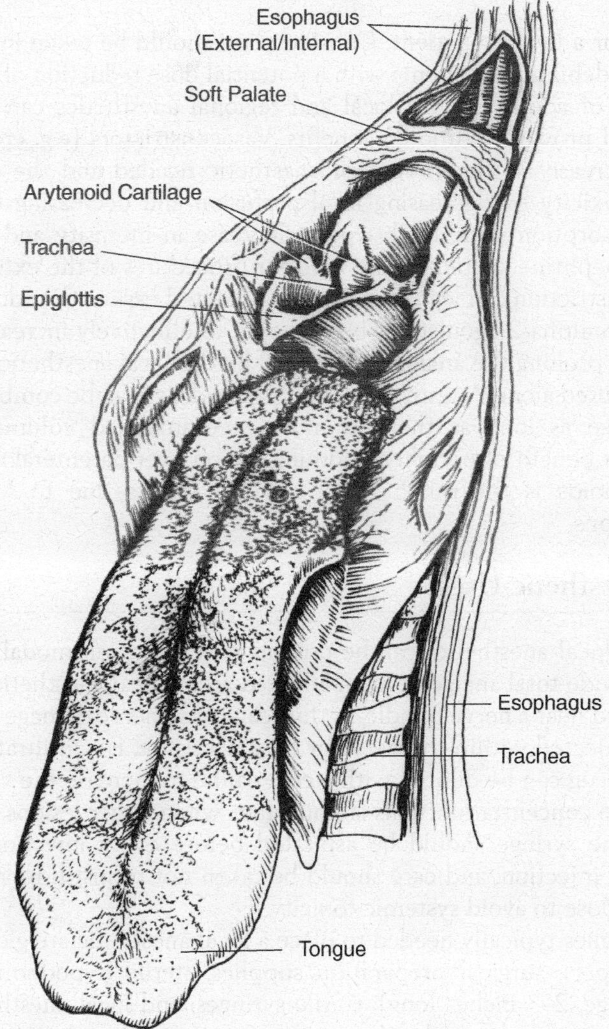

Figure 20.1 Endotracheal intubation.

Induction complications

A common complication of anesthetic administration is the inability of the patient to reach a surgical plane of anesthesia.

Difficulty with induction can be related to the patient's excitement prior to the procedure. Administer a balanced preanesthetic drug combination and avoid excessive handling to reduce patient's excitement.

Table 20.6 / Anesthetic induction complications

Clinical sign	Treatment
Patient will not stay anesthetized	• Check patient respiration; breath holding or rapid, shallow breaths inhibit gases from getting into the lungs • Verify proper placement of the endotracheal tube and the properly inflated cuff (Skill Box 20.5) • Verify that vaporizer and oxygen flow rates are correct • Verify the anesthetic level in vaporizer • Verify the anesthetic machine setup; follow the system from the machine to the patient checking each connection • Verify that one-way valves are not warped and there are no leaks along the machine setup, allowing the rebreathing of expired gases and ↓ anesthetic concentration
Light plane of anesthesia	• Verify proper placement of the endotracheal tube and the properly inflated cuff • Verify that vaporizer and oxygen flow rates are correct • Administer additional induction drugs
Patient is able to vocalize	• Verify proper placement of the endotracheal tube
Exaggerated breathing motions	• Verify proper placement of the endotracheal tube, possible endobronchial intubation

LOCAL AND REGIONAL ANESTHESIA

The use of local anesthetics should be considered as part of the patient's anesthetic/analgesic plan whenever possible. The potential for their use is extensive and they can be applied to numerous surgical and nonsurgical procedures. Besides the analgesic effects, additional benefits are seen, such as decreased requirements of anesthetics, smoother anesthetic recovery,[8] decreased "wind-up," quicker return to normal activity, and decreased chance of establishing chronic pain.

Local anesthetic drugs can vary in many ways including on onset of action, duration of action, concentration, dosages, and safety. That is why choosing a local anesthetic drug for your clinic or practice should be geared for the type of locoregional anesthesia you will be performing. Although mixing a combination of local anesthetics, such as lidocaine and bupivacaine, had been previously thought to help with increasing the onset of action and prolonging the duration of action, it has been shown that results are variable and may actually decrease the efficacy and duration of both drugs. What has been shown to increase efficacy and duration of action is to add other analgesic drugs, such as opioids or alpha-2 agonists. Table 20.7 shows differences among drugs and dosages that are commonly used for local anesthetic administration. Specific factors should be taken into consideration for each patient and procedure being performed. The facts listed as follows are generally accepted protocols for a healthy patient. Consideration should be taken into account for aged or debilitated patients with a potential dose reduction of 30–40%.

Table 20.7 / **Commonly used local anesthetics**

Drug	Dose (mg/kg)	Rate of onset (minutes)	Duration (hours)	Uses
Bupivacaine[6]	Canine: 1–2 Feline: 1 Toxic dose: 4	10–20	4–6	Splash, infiltration, nerve blocks, and epidurals
Lidocaine[6]	Canine: 1–2 Feline: 1 Toxic dose: Canine: > 8 Feline: > 2	2–5	1–2	Splash infiltration, nerve blocks, intra-articular, and epidural
Mepivacaine[6]	Canine: 1–5 Feline: 1–2.5 Toxic dose: 20	5–10	2–3	Infiltration, nerve blocks, intra-articular, and epidural
Ropivacaine[6]	Canine:1–2 Feline: 1 Toxic dose: 5	10–20	3–5	Infiltration, nerve blocks, and epidural
Liposome-encapsulated bupivacaine	5.3	30	72	Infiltrative (canine), nerve blocks (feline); off label both blocks used in canines and felines

The use of additives with local and regional anesthetics can alter their efficacy and provide additional benefits. Vasoconstrictors (e.g. epinephrine) allow a decrease in the amount of anesthetic needed and the chance for potential toxicity by decreasing local perfusion and decreasing the rate of vascular absorption with a subsequent increase in intensity and anesthetic depth. Epinephrine should not be used for procedures of the extremities, as the vasoconstriction can lead to ischemia. As stated earlier, the addition of an opioid or an alpha-2 agonist has been shown to effectively increase the efficacy and to prolong the analgesia provided by the local anesthetic compared with when used alone. Anesthetic and analgesic drugs can be combined in the same syringe as long as the maximum recommended volumes are not exceeded. A benefit of peripheral administration over parenteral administration of opioids is the much lower adverse effects due to low plasma concentrations.

Local Anesthetic Uses

In general, local anesthetics can be used as part of a multimodal anesthetic plan to provide total analgesia to an affected area. Local anesthetics are typically injected near a nerve bundle, as they can cause nerve damage and can be painful if injected within the nerve or nervous tissue. For infiltration procedures, the drug can be diluted with sterile saline to increase the volume and decrease the concentration. This is important when larger lesions need to be blocked. The syringe should be aspirated before every injection to avoid intravenous injection, and care should be taken not to instill more than the maximum dose to avoid systemic toxicity.

The supplies typically needed to place a local anesthetic are gloves, sterile gloves, clippers, surgical preparation supplies, sterile hypodermic needles (20–25 gauge, 2–3 inches long), sterile syringes, and local anesthetic drugs. Placement of a local anesthetic requires strict aseptic technique. The area should be clipped and surgically prepared, which can often take place during prep for surgery. Many of the techniques listed further require minimal skill, while others can be mastered with proper instruction.

Table 20.8 provides a brief description of local anesthetic techniques. Please review a text dedicated to this subject for more complete technique descriptions.

Table 20.8 / **Local anesthetic uses**

Area and nerves blocked	Uses	Drug and dose	Equipment and method	Notes
Brachial plexus block				
• Block distal to and including the elbow • Radial, ulnar, median, musculocutaneous and axillary nerves	Surgery below the elbow	Drug: • Lidocaine 2% • Bupivacaine 0.5% Dose (mg/kg): • Lidocaine 2–5 • Bupivacaine 1–2	• Equipment: 22-gauge, 2- to 3-inch spinal needle, sterile syringe • Method: instill the drug into the axillary space at the level of the shoulder joint, parallel to the vertebral column, the distal end of the needle should lie caudal to the distal end of the spine of the scapula[6]	• Avoid insertion into a blood vessel or thoracic cavity • Complication is failure to obtain complete anesthesia with unreliable results (e.g. overweight dogs) • A nerve locator is recommended for accuracy and safety
Brachial plexus block, paravertebral				
• Blocks entire forelimb • Spinal nerves C6–C8 and thoracic nerve T1	Surgery of the forelimb	Drug: • Bupivacaine 0.25–0.5% • Ropivacaine 0.2–0.5% Dose: 1–2 mg/kg	Equipment: 22-gauge, 2–3-inch spinal needle, sterile syringe Method: • Animal is placed in lateral recumbency and the scapula moved caudally to expose C6 and first rib • The nerves are blocked at a close proximity to the intervertebral foramina as possible	• Avoid insertion into a blood vessel or thoracic cavity • Complication is failure to obtain complete anesthesia with unreliable results (e.g., overweight dogs) • A nerve locator is recommended for accuracy and safety

(Continued)

Table 20.8 / Local anesthetic uses (Continued)

Area and nerves blocked	Uses	Drug and dose	Equipment and method	Notes
Radial/ulnar median/musculocutaneous (RUMM) block				
Blocks distal to the elbow	Surgery below the elbow	Bupivacaine 0.25–0.5%	Equipment: 22-gauge spinal needle, sterile syringe Method: • Clip lateral and medial area around humerus • Radial nerve: patient placed in lateral recumbency with affected limb up • Pull brachialis muscle cranial and rest thumb on humerus. Insert 22 g needle caudally midway to one third distally on humerus until it makes contact with the bone. Withdraw slightly of the bone and inject. Always aspirate prior to injecting • Ulnar/musculocutaneous/median nerves • Patient placed in lateral recumbency with affected limb down. The nerves are located medially • Position with elbow in flexion at a 90-degree angle • Palpate mid-humerus and insert 22-gauge needle at a 45-degree angle caudally, running perpendicular to length on humerus • After making contact with bone, back out slightly, aspirate and inject half the volume • Start pulling back to inject the rest of the volume as the needle is withdrawing • Aspirate occasionally as the needle is being pulled out	• Avoid insertion into a blood vessel • Complication is failure to obtain complete anesthesia with unreliable results

(*Continued*)

Table 20.8 / **Local anesthetic uses (Continued)**

Area and nerves blocked	Uses	Drug and dose	Equipment and method	Notes
*Epidural anesthesia**				
• Blocks caudal to the umbilicus • Central neuraxial block • Depending on dose, block up to T5	• Animals that are severely depressed, in shock, or need of immediate hindquarter surgery • Aged animals, those at high risk, or those where anesthetics agents are contraindicated • To provide analgesia after abdominal surgery or hindquarter surgery • Rear limb lacerations or fractures, abdominal surgery, perianal surgery, cesarean sections, surgical procedures of the tail, perineum, vulva, vagina, rectum, and bladder, urethrostomies, obstetrical manipulations	Drug: • Lidocaine 2% • Bupivacaine 0.5% • Mepivacaine 3% Dose (mg/kg): • Lidocaine 3–5 • Bupivacaine 1–2.5 • Mepivacaine 3–4.5 Opioid: • Morphine preservative free (onset of action epidurally is 1–2 hours) 0.1 mg/kg	Equipment: 2–4 inch, 20–22-gauge short bevel with stylet spinal needle; 1, 3, 5, and/or 10 ml syringe (weight dependent); sterile gloves Method: • In the "hanging drop" technique the patient is placed in sternal recumbency with the hind legs pulled cranially. This technique will not work in lateral recumbency • In lateral recumbency, use "loss of resistance" technique with hind legs pulled cranially. • Deposit a small amount of SQ 2% lidocaine and then apply a surgical prep to the site • Palpate midline depression caudally to L7, cranially to S1 • Insert spinal needle just into the skin/subcutaneous space • Remove stylet • Administer sterile saline into the hub of the spinal needle until a meniscus is formed • Insert the spinal needle between L7 and S1. Push the needle in a slight cranial or caudal angle as needed until a distinct "pop" is felt or resistance is met • Remove the stylet and observe for blood or CSF and inject 1–2 ml air to assure correct placement. If SQ crepitus is felt, the needle is incorrectly placed; no resistance should be felt • Inject the drug over 60 seconds to achieve the correct level of anesthesia. • Elevate the head for 5 minutes after administration to ↓ cranial movement	• Duration is prolonged 1–1.5 hours with the addition of epinephrine • Do not use in patients with skin infections, septicemia, coagulation defects, pelvic fractures, and spinal inflammation • Respiratory depression and paralysis with drug overdose or improper placement; drug needs to migrate to C5 or C7 for this effect • Felines and young or small dog's dural sac terminates further caudally increasing risk of spinal or intrathecal epidural. Cut dose by ⅓ or ½ • Abort epidural if blood is present in hub of spinal catheter. Can attempt again • Anesthetic placement in vertebral sinuses: vomiting, tremors, hypotension, convulsions, and paralysis • IV injection may result in systemic toxicity (e.g., convulsions, cardiovascular, and respiratory depression) • Monitor for hypothermia and malignant hyperthermia for susceptible animals • Opioids may cause urine retention; express bladder and monitor urine production

(Continued)

Table 20.8 / **Local anesthetic uses (Continued)**

Area and nerves blocked	Uses	Drug and dose	Equipment and method	Notes
*Epidural analgesia**				
• Same as epidural anesthesia • Relieves somatic and visceral pain	• Intraoperative and postoperative pain • Critical care patients	Drug (preservative free): • Morphine (M) • Oxymorphone (O) • Hydromorphone (H) • Buprenorphine (B) Dose (mg/kg): • M = 0.5–1.5 • O = 0.025–0.15 • H = 0.1 • B = 0.005–0.015 Duration (hours): • M = 10–24 • O = 7–10 • H = 10–24 • B = 16–24	• Same as epidural anesthesia • Can be administered as a continuous rate infusion if epidural catheter is placed	• Toxicity (e.g., respiratory depression, urine retention, delayed gastrointestinal motility, vomiting, and pruritus) • Do not use drugs containing preservatives
Intercostal and interpleural block				

• Block cranial and caudal to incision or injury site
• Intercostal nerves
	Thoracotomy, chest tube placement, rib fractures, and pleural drainage	Drug:
		• Bupivacaine 0.25%/0.5%
		Dose (mg/kg):
		• Intercostal:
		  • Canine: 1–4
		  • Feline: 1–2
		• Interpleural
		  • Canine: 1.5
		  • Feline: 0.5
			Equipment: 22–25-gauge needle; sterile syringe
			Method (intercostal):
			• Block the two nerves cranial and two nerves caudal to the incision site
			• Instill the drug at the caudal border of the rib near the level of the intervertebral foramen
			Method (interpleural):
			• Instill the drug into the thoracic cavity during a thoracotomy, chest tube, or catheter placement.
			• Instill 2–5 ml sterile saline to flush the drug into the interpleural space
				• Complication of inadvertent pneumothorax, potentially several hours post-injection
				• Contraindicated with an open pericardium, pulmonary disease (canine), and not effective in pyothorax
				• Bupivacaine may sting when administered through the chest tube
				• When using a chest tube, allow the patient to lay with that side down for 15 minutes
				• Greater risk of toxicity due to high blood concentrations

(*Continued*)

Table 20.8 / Local anesthetic uses (Continued)

Area and nerves blocked	Uses	Drug and dose	Equipment and method	Notes
Intra-articular block				

• Variable, dependent on joint
• Block tissues surrounding the joint capsule
	• Arthroscopy
	• Joint surgery; stifle, elbow, shoulder
		Drug:
		• Lidocaine 2%
		• Bupivacaine 0.5%
		Dose (mg/kg):
		• Lidocaine:
		  • Canine: 5
		  • Feline: 2.5
		• Bupivacaine:
		  • Canine: 1.0–2.0
		  • Feline: 1.0
			Equipment: 22–25-gauge needle; sterile syringe
			Method:
			• With the patient in lateral recumbency and the affected stifle up, flex the stifle and apply digital pressure to the medial side of the straight patellar ligament
			• Insert the needle on the opposite side of the straight patellar ligament midway between the patella and the tibial tuberosity and direct it obliquely and distally toward the intercondylar space of the tibia
				• Morphine may also be used in inflamed joints at 0.1–0.3 mg/kg

Intratesticular block				
• Areas surrounding the spermatic cord	Neuter	Drug: • Lidocaine 2% • Bupivacaine 0.5% Dose (mg/kg): • Lidocaine 1.0 • Bupivacaine 1.0	Equipment: 22–25-gauge needle; sterile syringe Method: • Isolate one testicle and insert the needle from the caudal aspect directing the needle proximal toward the spermatic cord • Aspirate with negative pressure for several seconds due to the dense tissue of the testicle, then slowly inject ⅓ dose while withdrawing the needle • Repeat with the other testicle	• Testicle will feel firm with the addition of the local
Intravenous regional block, "Bier block"				

• Extremity distal to tourniquet
• Nerve endings in peripheral tissues
	• Biopsies
	• Foreign bodies from the paw or other minor surgical procedures of an extremity
		Drug:
		• Lidocaine 1%
		• Mepivacaine 1%
		Dose (mg/kg):
		• Lidocaine:
		  • Canine: 2.5–5
		  • Feline: 2–3
		• Mepivacaine:
		  • Canine: 1–2
		  • Feline: 1
			Equipment: 22-gauge needle, 1½ inch
			Method:
			• Place an IV catheter in a vein distal to the tourniquet
			• Apply a pressure bandage to exsanguinate the limb prior to placing the tourniquet. Remove bandage once the tourniquet is placed
			• Inject lidocaine intravenously. Full effects are seen in 5–10 minutes
			• Following the procedure, the tourniquet should be removed (ideally after 30 minutes) slowly over a five-min period to prevent overdose of local anesthetic agents (especially in felines)
				• Do not use bupivacaine
				• Do not use epinephrine as the vasoconstriction as it can lead to ischemia
				• Diluted lidocaine (0.25–0.5%) can be used
				• Tourniquet left on over 90 minutes can lead to tourniquet-induced ischemia; 4 hours can lead to reversible shock and over eight hours can lead to sepsis, endotoxemia, and death
				• Malignant hyperthermia in susceptible animals
				• Injection should begin as distal as possible as the anesthesia progresses proximally

(Continued)

Table 20.8 / Local anesthetic uses (Continued)

Area and nerves blocked	Uses	Drug and dose	Equipment and method	Notes
Line block				

• Tissues immediately proximal to target area
• Placed between the target area and the spinal cord
	• Surgery on an area of tissue served by many nerves
	• Analgesia involving superficial tissues
	• Skin biopsies and small skin tumors
	• Repair of minor lacerations
		Drug:
		• Lidocaine 2%
		• Bupivacaine 0.5%
		Dose (mg/kg):
		• Canine: 5
		  • Feline: 2.5
		• Bupivacaine:
		  • Canine: 1.0–2.0
		  • Feline: 1.0
		• Volume of total dose can be diluted with sterile saline up to 50% for greater coverage
			Equipment: 23- or 25-gauge needle; sterile syringe
			Method:
			• Apply a surgical prep to surgery site
			• Visualize a line of infiltration that is proximal to the surgery site
			• Insert the needle along the proposed line of infiltration and aspirate to verify placement is not in a blood vessel
			• Inject small amounts of drugs as the needle is gradually withdrawn. The drug will then diffuse through the tissues to reach the target tissues
				• Avoid injecting directly into a nerve as temporary or permanent nerve loss can occur.
				• Avoid IV injection as CNS or cardiovascular effect may occur
				• Do not inject into inflamed areas
				• Cats are more sensitive to systemic effects of lidocaine; avoid using > 1 ml/10 lb

Nerve block				
Any nerve with direct visualization	Amputations	Drug: • Lidocaine 2% • Bupivacaine 0.5% Dose (mg/kg): • Lidocaine: Canine: 5 Feline: 2.5 Bupivacaine: Canine: 1.0–2.0 Feline: 1.0	Equipment: 23- or 25-gauge needle; sterile syringe Method: visualize and directly infiltrate the nerve to be severed (e.g. amputation)	• Do not attempt to inject the nerve; rather, bathe the nerve by applying the drug to the immediate area

(*Continued*)

Table 20.8 / Local anesthetic uses (Continued)

Area and nerves blocked	Uses	Drug and dose	Equipment and method	Notes
Ring block				

• Block of the distal radial, median, dorsal, and palmar branches of the ulnar nerve	• Onychectomy, digit or tail amputation, laceration of lower extremity	Drug:
		• Lidocaine 2%
		• Bupivacaine 0.5%
		Dose (mg/kg):
		• Lidocaine:
		  • Canine: 5
		  • Feline: 2.5
		• Bupivacaine:
		  • Canine: 1.0–2.0
		  • Feline: 1.0
			Equipment: 20- or 22-gauge needle; sterile syringe
			Method:
			• Insert the needle subcutaneously along the lateral aspect of the paw proximal to the carpus
			• Slowly withdraw the needle while instilling the local anesthetic
			• Repeat on the medial side
				• Do not attempt to inject the nerve; rather, bathe the nerve by applying the drug to the immediate area
				• Doses do not exceed 2 mg/kg
				• Do not perform in the presence of an infection

Splash block				

• Tissues in contact with the drug	• Open surgical incision line
	• Ear ablation
		Drug:
		• Lidocaine 2%
		• Bupivacaine 0.5%
		Dose (mg/kg):
		• Lidocaine:
		  • Canine: 5
		  • Feline: 2.5
		• Bupivacaine 2
			Equipment: 20- or 22-gauge needle; sterile syringe
			Method: spray/drip a surgical area with the drug and allow it to remain in contact for 15–20 minutes
				• Fluids (e.g., blood) will negate the effect of this block
				• Not as effective as blocking prior to incision
				• Do not flush area after administration

* Preservative-free fentanyl, buprenorphine, and morphine are required for epidurals (see Skill Box 21.3: Local Dental Nerve Blocks, page 977).

PERIOPERATIVE

Anesthetic Monitoring

Anesthesia monitoring requires the frequent and vigilant observation of the anesthesia patient. Monitoring should include recording monitored parameters at least every five minutes for uncomplicated cases and as frequent as continuous monitoring for more complicated cases. Recording provides a legal record of the anesthetic event and also allows trends or unusual values to be recognized and addressed. Monitoring consists of visual and hands-on monitoring by the anesthetist, together with the use of monitoring equipment. There is a variety of sophisticated and complex monitoring devices available for monitoring. The monitor must be used in conjunction with a skilled anesthetist to make the best decisions for the patient.

Together with knowledge of the individual patient and the drugs being used, awareness of the connection between the patient and the equipment used is important to avoid complications.

Table 20.9 / **Patient care**

Procedure		Complication	Treatment
Patient			
Induction	Inducing anesthesia	• Bodily injury when losing consciousness • Stress-induced catecholamine release with subsequent potential for harmful cardiac arrhythmias • Hypoxia due to dose dependent respiratory depression of certain induction drugs	• Support all body parts when inducing • Try to avoid stage II anesthesia level; rapidly induce to stage III • Reduce stress by premedication • Induction environment should be quiet, and technique chosen according to patient sensitivity to stress • Pre-oxygenate 3–5 minutes with 100% oxygen when indicated (e.g. brachycephalic, felines) • Rapid security of airway with endotracheal tube
Body positioning	Positioning	• Overextension or hyperflexion of the neck and limbs, causing permanent neurological injury. • Neuropathies from Trendelenburg positioning • Hyperflexion of the neck may occlude the endotracheal tube • Geriatric patients becoming sore or stiff postoperatively due to musculoskeletal pain. Also consider DJD or osteoarthritis patients	• Assure the patient maintains as normal of a position as possible • Provide significant padding under hips and upper thighs • Be aware of any restrictions due to orthopedic or neurological conditions • Provide support to shoulders, hips, and knees when possible
Hydration	Fluid administration: • Feline: 3 ml/kg/hour • Canine: 5 ml/kg/hour (decrease if patient has cardiac concerns)	• Overhydration • Hemodilution • ↑ Lung sounds and respiratory rate • Dyspnea • Chemosis • Ocular and nasal discharge	• ↓ Fluid rate • Oxygen administration • Drug administration (e.g. diuretics)
		• Dehydration • Hypovolemia • Hypotension • Tacky or dry mucous membranes • Oliguria or anuria	• Bolus fluids • ↑ Fluid rate (and colloid or blood administration)
Thermoregulation	Heat administration	• Hypothermia • Thermal injury	• Do not use excessive alcohol or saturate the patient's fur during surgical preparation • Preinduction warming significantly reduces the heat loss during the first hour of surgery; use of a heated air blanket prior to induction • Do not place the patient on a cold metal surface; insulate with a circulating warm water blanket (avoid the use of heating pads). • Avoid warming bags of fluids in the microwave as it can create pockets of intense heat and cause thermal injury. Use a regulated heating source such as a fluid warmer • See Table 13.5: Temperature therapy, page 627

(Continued)

Table 20.9 / **Patient care (Continued)**

Procedure		Complication	Treatment
Ocular	Eye lubricant	• Corneal drying	• Instill an eye lubricant every 90 minutes and at recovery
Equipment			
Endotracheal tube	Intubation	• Incorrect placement (e.g. esophageal or endobronchial placement) • Incorrect size • Malfunctioning tube • Traumatic placement into the glottis (laryngitis)	• See Skill Box 20.5
	Rolling or turning the patient	• Kinked endotracheal tube resulting in airway obstruction • Tracheal trauma or tear • Removal of the endotracheal tube	• Disconnect tube from circuit before moving. • Armored tubes (spiral wire embedded in tube wall) to prevent kinking
Anesthetic hoses	Placement of anesthetic hoses	• Tracheal trauma • Removal of the endotracheal tube • Kinked endotracheal tube	• Correct support of anesthetic hoses to prevent weight placed on the endotracheal tube. • Correct position of anesthetic hoses to prevent a kink or bend in the tube
Instruments	Placement of instruments	• Compression of chest cavity of small patients	• Avoid placing heavy instruments directly on the chest of small patients
Table	Tilted table, restraining devices, positioning	• Abdominal organs compressing the diaphragm and compromising heart and lung function • ↓ Peripheral blood circulation • Neuropathies	• Do not tilt more than 15 degrees • IPPV • Avoid tight limb restraints or avoid using ties if not needed • Provide padding under shoulders in dorsal recumbency. Pad between limbs in lateral recumbency

Stages of Anesthesia

Anesthesia is divided into four stages depending on the physical response of the patient. Understanding these different levels and when patients should be entering or leaving each one is an important aspect of induction and recovery. Stage I is characterized by excitement and struggling accompanied by epinephrine release with associated increased heart and respiratory rate. Stage II is the beginning of unconsciousness and involuntary movement. Vomiting may happen in this stage, along with breath holding and self-injury. Stage III consists of four different planes of anesthesia with plane 1 as light anesthesia to plane 4 as deep anesthesia (early overdose). Stage IV is irreversible anesthesia often leading to death within one to five minutes.

Table 20.10 / Stages of anesthesia

System affected	Characteristic observed	Stage I	Stage II	Stage III				Stage IV
				Plane				
				1	2	3	4	
				Light	Medium		Deep	
Cardiovascular	Heart rate	Normal	Increased	90–120 beats/ minute	Dog: 80–120 beats/minute Cat: 120–160 beats/minute	Decrease	Decrease	Cardiac arrest
		Tachycardia		Progressive bradycardia				Weak or imperceptible
	Pulse	Normal	Normal	Regular and strong	Relatively strong	Weakened	Weakened	
	Blood pressure	Hypertension		Normal	Increasing hypotension			Shock level
	Capillary refill time	1 s or	less		Progressive delay			3 s or more
	Dysrhythmias probability	+ + +	+ + +	+ +	+		+ +	+ + + +
Respiratory	Respiratory rate	Irregular or increased		Progressive decrease			Slow irregular	Ceased, may gasp terminally
	Respiratory depth	Irregular or increased		Progressive decrease			Slow irregular	Ceased
				12–20 breaths/ minute	Dog: 12–16 breaths/minute Cat: 20–40 breaths/minute			
	Mucous membrane, skin color	Normal					Cyanosis	Pale to white
	Respiratory action	May be breath holding		Regular and smooth rhythm	Irregular rate and pattern thoracoabdominal, abdominal		Variable pattern diaphragmatic	Ceased
	Cough reflex	+ + + +	+ + +	+	Lost			
	Laryngeal reflex	+ + + + May vocalize		Lost				
	Intubation possible	No		Yes				

(*Continued*)

Table 20.10 / Stages of anesthesia (Continued)

System affected	Characteristic observed	Stage I	Stage II	Stage III				Stage IV
				Plane				
				1	2	3	4	
				Light	Medium		Deep	
Gastrointestinal	Salivation	+ + + +	+ + +	+	Diminished, absent			Absent
	Oropharyngeal reflex	+ + + +	+ + +	+	Lost			
	Vomiting probability	+ + +		+	Very slight			
	Reflux potential	None		Increases with relaxation				+ + + +
Ocular	Pupils	Constricted	Dilated	Constricted	Progressive dilation			Fully dilated
					Moderately dilated		Widely dilated	
	Corneal reflex	Normal	+ + +	Diminishes, lost				Absent
	Lacrimation	Normal	+ + +	+	Diminished, absent			Absent
	Photomotor reflex	Normal		Responsive	Sluggish response	Minimal or absent response	Unresponsive	Absent
	Palpebral reflex	Normal	+ + +	+	Diminished, absent			Absent
	Eyeball position	Variable	Central	Third eyelid prolapsed		Centrally fixed		
				Rotated medially	Slight medial, rotation			
	Nystagmus	Normal	Possible nystagmus	Possible slight nystagmus or absent		Absent		
Musculoskeletal	Jaw tone	+ + + +		Decreased, minimal				Lost
	Limb muscle tone	+ + + +		Decreased, minimal				Lost
	Abdominal muscle tone	+ + + +		+ +	Decreased, minimal			Lost
	Sphincters (anus, bladder)	May void		Progressive relaxation				Control lost

(*Continued*)

Table 20.10 / **Stages of anesthesia (Continued)**

System affected	Characteristic observed	Stage I	Stage II	Stage III				Stage IV
				Plane				
				1	2	3	4	
				Light	Medium		Deep	
Nervous	Pedal reflex	+ + + +		Decreased	Absent			
	Reaction to surgical stimulus	Increased respiratory rate and heart rate				No response		Absent
		Limb movement			Traction reflexes			

Anesthesia Monitoring

There are many parameters to monitor with the anesthetized patient. They are broken up into four categories, with cardiovascular and respiratory providing the most information about how the patient is handling the anesthetic procedure. Reflexes are an excellent determinate for anesthetic depth and thermoregulation plays an overall role in the patient's ability to metabolize drugs, recovery, and heal appropriately .

Table 20.11 / **Anesthesia monitoring**

System	Significance	Values	Equipment and technique	Complication and treatment
Cardiovascular				
Heart rate	• Cardiac function • ↓ Rate is often seen in an anesthetized animal • Acute intraoperative blood loss can trigger compensatory tachycardia	Normal: • Canine: 70–180 bpm • Feline: 110–220 bpm Abnormal: • Canine: < 70 and > 160 bpm • Feline: < 100 and > 200 bpm	• Direct palpation of chest wall or pulse • Auscultation of chest with a stethoscope • See Skill Box 2.1: Cardiac examination, page 43 • Esophageal stethoscope • Monitors heart rate, rhythm, and pulse deficits • A thin tube attached to a stethoscope is placed in the esophagus of the patient until an audible heartbeat is heard • Allows auscultation even when the patient's chest is covered during surgery • ECG • See also Skill Box 14.5: Electrocardiogram procedure, page 649 • Doppler pulse monitor • See also Skill Box 14.1: Blood pressure procedure, page 642 • Used to monitor heart rate indirectly	*Bradycardia* Cause: • ↑ Anesthetic depth • ↑ Vagal tone • Opioid induced • Reflex bradycardia caused by alpha-2 agonist administration Treatment: • Drug administration of anticholinergics if patient is also hypotensive • Reverse alpha-2 agonist if patient is bradycardic with hypotension. If longer than 2 hours from time of administration of alpha-2 agonist, administer glycopyrrolate *Tachycardia* Cause: • Pain • ↓ Anesthetic depth • Preexisting disease • Hypoxemia, hypercapnia, hypovolemia, or hyperthermia • Anesthetic drug adverse effects • Sympathetic response Treatment: • Evaluate anesthetic depth and/or treat pain • Assess oxygenation • Provide IPPV to decrease CO_2 • Administer fluid bolus (5–10 ml/kg) if indicated

(*Continued*)

Table 20.11 / **Anesthesia monitoring (Continued)**

System	Significance	Values	Equipment and technique	Complication and treatment
Blood pressure*	• Blood pressure is the product of cardiac output and systemic vascular resistance • Cardiac output is the result of heart rate and stroke volume • Stroke volume is dependent on preload, contractility, and afterload • Blood pressure reflects perfusion throughout the body	*Normal (mmHg)* Canine: • Systolic: 110–160 • Diastolic: 60–100 • Mean: 80–120 Feline: • Systolic: 120–170 • Diastolic: 70–120 • Mean: 80–120 *Abnormal (mmHg)* Canine: • Systolic: < 80 and > 160 • Mean: < 60 and > 120 • Systolic: < 80 and > 160 • Mean: < 60 and > 120	• Strength of peripheral pulse (note: palpation of metatarsal pulse does not always indicate adequate blood pressure)[9] • Direct palpation of femoral, lingual, carotid, or dorsal pedal arteries • Indirect monitoring (non-invasive) • Doppler: a cuff with a crystal sensor to measure the systolic blood pressures is placed on the limb of the patient • Stethoscope: same steps are taken as for Doppler use except a stethoscope is used to listen for the returning pulsating artery • Oscillometric: a cuff with an incorporated device to measure and calculate the systolic, diastolic, and mean blood pressures is placed on the limb of the patient • IBP monitoring: arterial catheter placed in an artery (e.g. pedal artery) and connected to a pressure transducer to determine the diastolic, systolic, and MAP at the catheter tip • See Skill Box 14.1: Blood pressure procedure, page 642	*Hypotension* Cause: • Hypovolemia • ↓ Cardiac output (e.g., bradycardia, tachycardia, arrhythmia, or valvular disease) • Peripheral vasodilation (e.g., sepsis, drugs, hypoxemia, hypercapnia, or hyperthermia) • Anesthetic drug side effects • ↓ Venous return to the heart (e.g., hypovolemia, ↑ intra-abdominal pressure, controlled ventilation, or change in posture) • Bradycardia Treatment: • ↓ Anesthetic depth if appropriate • Rapid fluid administration (e.g., bolus or ↑ rate) • Colloids and RBC administration • Drug administration of sympathomimetics (e.g., dopamine, dobutamine, or ephedrine) • Anticholinergic: atropine or glycopyrrolate *Hypertension* Cause: • Anesthetic drug adverse effect (alpha-2 agonist) • Pain • Light plane of anesthesia • Hypercarbia or malignant hyperthermia syndrome Treatment: • Evaluate anesthetic depth • Evaluate ventilation • IPPV • Discontinue drugs causing adverse effects • Drug administration (e.g., dobutamine, dopamine, or sodium bicarbonate) • IV fluid administration adjustment

(Continued)

Table 20.11 / Anesthesia monitoring (Continued)

System	Significance	Values	Equipment and technique	Complication and treatment
Capillary refill time (CRT)	Reflects the perfusion of tissues with blood	Normal: 1–2 seconds Abnormal: > 2 seconds	• Direct palpation • Direct digital pressure is applied to the mucous membranes until blanched and then time for blood (pink color) to return	↑ *CRT/hypoperfusion* Cause: • Hypovolemia, hypothermia, and pain • ↑ Anesthetic depth • Drug adverse effects (e.g., alpha-2 agonists) Treatment: • Evaluate anesthetic depth • Correct underlying condition • See Hypotension ↓ *CRT/hypoperfusion* • Distributive shock Treatment: • Correct underlying shock
CVP	Allows assessment of blood return to the heart and how well the heart can receive and pump blood	Normal: • < 8 cm H_2O Abnormal • > 12–15 cm H_2O • Monitor trends over time, not a single reading	• Central venous catheter • A long catheter is inserted percutaneously or by cutdown into the anterior vena cava • The catheter is inserted close to the right atrium of the heart • The catheter is then connected to a water manometer to obtain a measurement • The manometer should be positioned at the approximate level of the heart • See Skill Box 14.2: Central venous pressure, page 644	↑ *CVP* • Hypervolemia, venoconstriction or ↓ cardiac output Treatment: • ↓ or stop IV fluid administration • Drug therapy (e.g., dobutamine or furosemide) ↓ *CVP* • Hypovolemia, ↑ cardiac output or vasodilation Treatment: • ↑ IV fluid administration (and/or colloid or blood administration)

(*Continued*)

Table 20.11 / **Anesthesia monitoring (Continued)**

System	Significance	Values	Equipment and technique	Complication and treatment
ECG	• To assess the rate and rhythm of myocardial contractions • Abnormal size, duration, shape, and regularity of ECG tracing offer information on electrical impulse conduction and myocardial function • Identification of arrhythmias	Normal: See Table 14.10 Electrocardiogram interpretation, page 651 Abnormal: See Table 14.11: Common heart rhythm abnormalities, page 654	• See Skill Box 14.5: Electrocardiogram procedure, page 649	*Ventricular premature contractions* Causes: • Preexisting heart disease • Catecholamine release (e.g., ↓ anesthetic depth, hypoxemia, hypercapnia, or hypotension) • Anesthetic drug adverse effects • Electrolyte abnormalities • See Table 14.11: Common heart rhythm abnormalities, page 654 Treatment: • Evaluate potential anesthetic administration problems. • IPPV • Rapid fluid administration • Correct electrolyte abnormalities • Administration of an antiarrhythmic (e.g. lidocaine, procainamide or propranolol) if indicated by frequency, or if causing decrease in cardiac output)
Blood Loss	• Circulation • Blood pressure • Cardiac output • Peripheral perfusion	Normal: < 15% loss Abnormal: > 15% loss PCV < 20–25% Tip: To calculate normal blood volume: • Canine: 88 ml/kg • Feline: 56 ml/kg	• Visual observation • Free blood in surgical site, suction bottle, soaked gauze, and drapes • Tachycardia, hypotension, white mucous membranes, and labored breathing	*Hypovolemia* • Hemorrhage • Rapid IV crystalloid administration • IV hetastarch administration • IV fluid colloid administration • Blood transfusion

(*Continued*)

Table 20.11 / **Anesthesia monitoring (Continued)**

System	Significance	Values	Equipment and technique	Complication and treatment
Respiratory				
Respiratory rate	Ability to take in oxygen and eliminate carbon dioxide from the blood	Normal: • Canine: 10–30 breaths/minute • Feline: 25–40 breaths/minute	• Movement of the reservoir bag or thorax • Direct visualization of the bag or thorax • Auscultation of the thoracic cavity • A normal chest cavity has almost inaudible sounds • Harsh noises, whistles, squeaks, crackles, or wheezes may indicate narrow or obstructed airways in the presence of fluid or secretions. • See Skill Box 2.2: Pulmonary examination, page 45 Capnography: • Measures the CO_2 at the end of an exhalation and respiratory rate • The capnograph, capnogram, or capnometer is placed between the endotracheal tube and breathing circuit	*Bradypnea* Cause: • ↑ Anesthetic depth • Hypercapnia • Patient position Treatment: • Manual or mechanical IPPV • Correct patient positioning to assist ventilation *Tachypnea* Cause: • Pain • ↑ or ↓ Anesthetic depth • Hypercapnia, hypoxemia, hypotension, hyperthermia, airway obstruction, pleural or pulmonary disease Treatment: • Administer analgesic drugs and/or gas inhalant • IPPV (with anesthetic gas flowing) to correct level of anesthesia • Evaluate anesthetic depth and/or pain *Hypercapnia* Cause: • ↑ Anesthetic depth • Obesity • Patient positioning • Upper airway obstruction Treatment: • Evaluate anesthetic depth. • Manual or mechanical IPPV to increase RR or tidal volume • Correct patient positioning to assist ventilation *Hypocapnia* Cause: • ↓ anesthetic depth • Pain • Overzealous IPPV • Decreased body temperature or cardiac output

(*Continued*)

Table 20.11 / Anesthesia monitoring (Continued)

System	Significance	Values	Equipment and technique	Complication and treatment
Respiratory action	Reflects anesthetic depth	Normal: regular and smooth rhythm Abnormal: rocking motion of the abdomen and chest; thoracoabdominal or abdominal breathing	• Movement of the reservoir bag or thorax • Direct visualization of the thorax	*Irregular respiratory rate and pattern* Cause: • ↑ or ↓ anesthetic depth Treatment: • IPPV (with anesthetic gas flowing) to correct level of anesthesia • Evaluate anesthetic depth
$ETCO_2$	• A measure of carbon dioxide at the end of exhalation using capnography, capnogram, or a capnometer • Measures adequacy of ventilation, and indirectly measures cardiac output, pulmonary perfusion, and systemic metabolism	Normal: 35–45 mmHg (otherwise healthy patients can be permissively hypercapnic to c. 60 mmHg under general anesthesia)	Capnograph: • Monitors ventilation by measuring exhaled CO_2 • A sensor is placed between the breathing circuit and the ET tube. • See also Table 20.12	*Hypocapnia* Cause: • Hyperventilation form overzealous IPPV • Endobronchial intubation • Decreased cardiac output • Hypothermia • Cardiovascular collapse Treatment: • Decrease IPPV • Evaluate tube placement • Assess blood pressure • Warm patient *Hypercapnia* Cause: • ↑ Anesthetic depth • Obesity • Patient positioning • Upper airway obstruction Treatment: • Evaluate anesthetic depth. • Manual or mechanical IPPV to increase respiratory rate or tidal volume • Correct patient positioning to assist ventilation

(*Continued*)

Table 20.11 / **Anesthesia monitoring (Continued)**

System	Significance	Values	Equipment and technique	Complication and treatment
Blood gases	• Alterations in acid–base status and respiratory function and oxygenation • Venous blood determines metabolic acidosis and alkalosis • Arterial blood determines metabolic and respiratory acidosis and alkalosis	*Normal* • pH: 7.35–7.45 • $paCO_2$: 35–42 mmHg • paO_2: 85–105 mmHg • Base excess: −4 to +4 Venous: • pH: 7.35–7.45 • paCO2: 40–50 mmHg • paO2: 30–42 mmHg • Base excess: −4 to +4 *Abnormal* Single or multiple alterations from above	• Blood gas analysis equipment • Arterial blood draw • See Skill Box 14.3: Blood gas analysis, page 645 • Follow the manufacturer's directions	See Table 14.8: Acid–base disturbances, page 648 *Alkalosis* Cause: • Drugs effects • Brain damage, thoracic disease or trauma, pulmonary disease, excessive emesis, gastrointestinal obstruction, or obesity Treatment: • Evaluate IV fluid administration. • Drug administration (e.g., potassium chloride) *Acidosis* Cause: • Anxiety, fear, endotoxemia, or pneumonia • Hypoxemia or heart failure Treatment: • Drug administration (e.g., sodium bicarbonate) • IV fluid administration
Mucous membranes	Blood loss, anemia, and poor perfusion	*Normal* Pink *Abnormal* • Pale: blood loss, anemia, hypoxia, pain, or poor perfusion • Dark pink: vasodilation, sludging of capillaries, or ↑ CO_2, shock • Cyanotic: severe hypoxia	• Visual observation • Observed at the gingival, tongue, buccal mucous membranes, conjunctiva of the lower eyelid, mucous membrane lining the prepuce or vulva	*Cyanosis* Cause: • Shock or cardiac arrest • Methemoglobinemia • Hypotension • Apnea • Improper endotracheal tube placement or obstruction Treatment: • Oxygen administration and IPPV • Discontinue further anesthetics. • Evaluate endotracheal tube position

(*Continued*)

Table 20.11 / **Anesthesia monitoring (Continued)**

System	Significance	Values	Equipment and technique	Complication and treatment
Reflexes	Assessment of anesthetic depth	Normal See Skill Box 2.6: Neurological examination, page 49	Corneal: • Touch the cornea with a sterile cotton swab, sterile drop of water, or ophthalmic ointment and observe for blinking and withdrawal of the eye into the orbital fossa Ear flick: • Gently touch the hairs on the inside of the pinna and observe for movement Eye position: • Visual observation Muscle tone: • Open the jaw to observe for jaw tone • Flex and extend the foreleg and observe for resistance • Observe the size of the anal orifice for anal tone Palpebral: • Tap the lateral or medial canthus of the eye to observe for blinking Pedal: • Pinch or squeeze a digit or pad and observe for resistance • Visual observation Pupillary light reflex: • Shine a penlight to observe constriction of the pupil Salivary/lacrimal secretions: • Visual observation • Tactile estimate Surgical stimuli: • Visual observation of body movement, lacrimation, salivation, and sweating on foot pads Swallowing: • Observe neck/throat for typical movements	• Alter the level of anesthesia

(*Continued*)

Table 20.11 / Anesthesia monitoring (Continued)				
System	**Significance**	**Values**	**Equipment and technique**	**Complication and treatment**
Thermoregulation	• Circulation • Hypothermia causes delayed recovery from anesthesia due to slow rate of anesthetic drug metabolism by the liver • Hypothermia can produce arrhythmias and coagulation problem • Malignant hyperthermia can be a fatal condition and should be tended to immediately	Normal: 100.5–102.5°F Abnormal: < 101°F and > 103°F	• Direct palpation of paws and ears • Rectal thermometer • Temperature probe (e.g. rectal or esophageal) • Temperature should be monitored at a minimum of every 30 minutes	*Hypothermia* Cause: • Anesthetic drug adverse effects • Exposure to cold solutions, cold table surfaces, or open body cavities Treatment: • Warmed IV fluids, hot water circulating heating pads, warm air blanket, insulated hot water bottles, bubble packing, foil wraps, thermal blankets and regular blankets • See Skill Box 13.5: Temperature therapy, page 627 *Hyperthermia* Cause: • ↑ Metabolic rate due to ↑ muscle activity, ↓ depth of anesthesia, bacteremia, or endotoxemia • Insulation due to drapes and obesity • Malignant hyperthermia syndrome • Anesthetic drug adverse effect Treatment: • Rapid fluid administration • Drug administration (e.g., corticosteroids and sodium bicarbonate) • Alcohol or cold-water baths/compresses • Ice-water enemas or gastric lavage • Administration of antipyretics (e.g. aminopyrine, dipyrone or phenylbutazone) • See Skill Box 13.5: Temperature therapy, page 627

* To calculate MAP: MAP = diastolic + ⅓ (systolic–diastolic).
Note: Warm air blankets placed over the head of patients can lead to corneal drying and ulceration.
Note: Afterdrop – the core temperature will continue to drop after cooling techniques have been stopped. Aggressive techniques should be stopped when the core temperature reaches 104°F.

Table 20.12 / Capnograph waveforms

Waveform	Cause	Definition	Graph
Normal	• Described as one elephant following another	• A–B: baseline • B–C: expiratory upstroke • C–D: expiratory plateau • D: end-tidal concentration • D–E: inspiration	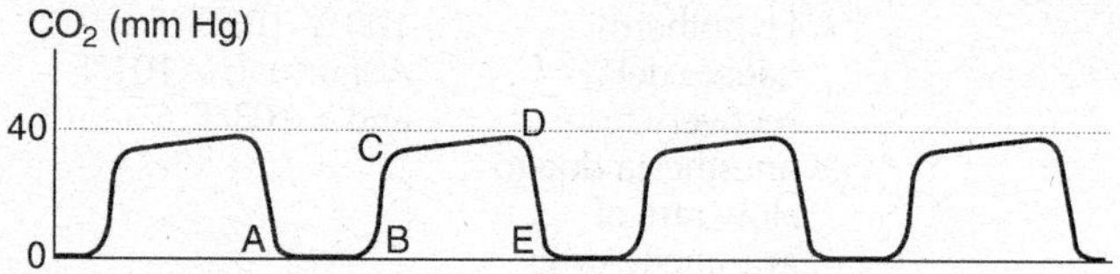
Esophageal intubation		• No detection or very minimal detection of CO_2 and lose of waveform right after intubation	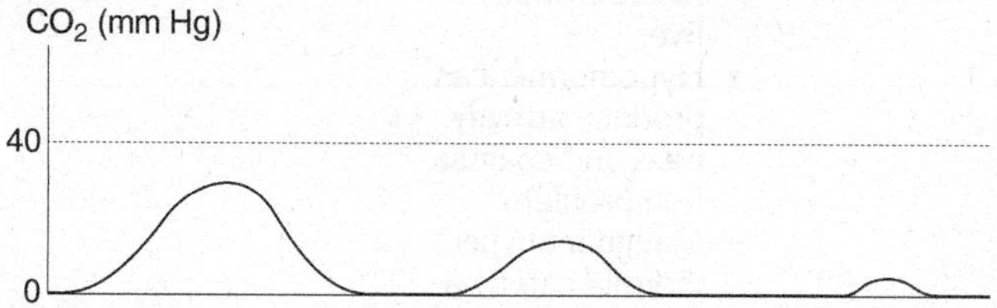
Rebreathing of exhaled gases	• Inadequate inspiratory flow • Faulty expiratory valve • Partial rebreathing circuits • Insufficient expiratory time • Exhausted CO_2 absorbent • Significant mechanical dead space	• Increase of baseline above zero	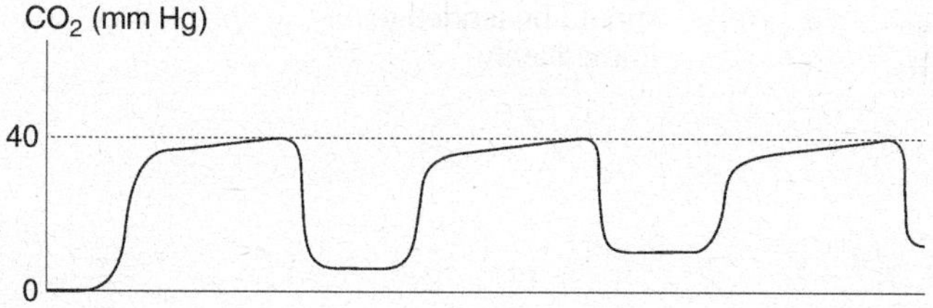
Hyperventilation (↑ in rate or tidal volume)	• Hypothermia • Vasoncontriction • Overzealous "bagging" or breathing for patient	• Gradual decrease	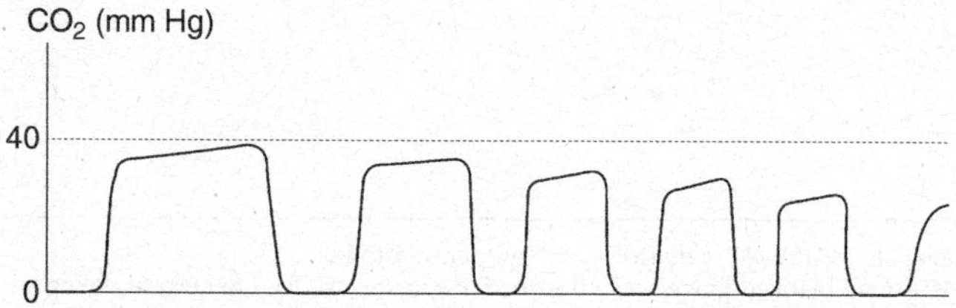
Hypoventilation (↓ in rate or tidal volume)	• Anesthetic/analgesic drugs decreasing ventilatory drive • Obesity or patient positioning decreasing patient's ability to ventilate • Exhausted soda lime	• Increase of waveform and/or number above 45 mmHg	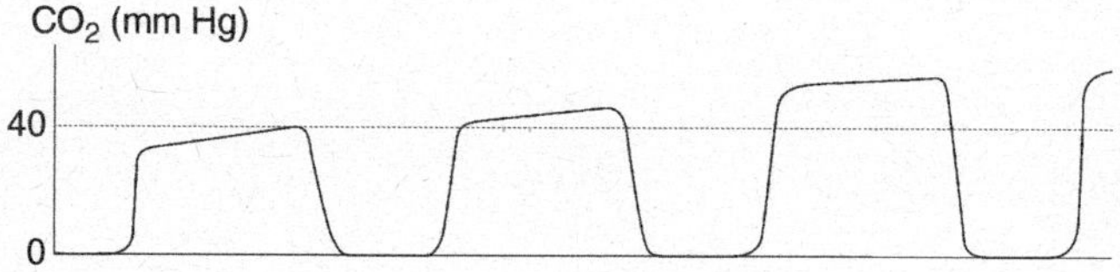

(Continued)

Table 20.12 / Capnograph waveforms (Continued)

Waveform	Cause	Definition	Graph
Partial or complete obstruction	• Asthmatic patient	• Gradual rise without a plateau • Often called a "shark fin" waveform	
Airway or breathing circuit obstruction	• Large leak in breathing circuit • Disconnection • Bronchospasm • Extubation • Cardiac or respiratory arrest	• Sudden drop and eventual no detection of CO_2 and lose of waveform	
Cardiogenic oscillations	• Caused by the pulsation of the heartbeat transmitting to the lung parenchyma	• "Stair step" appearance on inspiratory downstroke. Aligns with heartbeat	
Endotracheal tube leak		• Abnormal plateau, "hill-like" slope on inspiratory downstroke	

POSTANESTHETIC

Recovery

The postanesthetic period begins when the procedure(s) end and the anesthetic inhalant has been discontinued. Monitoring should be continuous until the patient is extubated and sternal. Temperature, pulse, and respirations should be closely monitored for the first three hours post-extubation as this is the most critical time in which morbidity occurs. Pain and anxiety assessment should also be continued through the recovery period and through patient discharge.

The patient should remain connected to the anesthetic machine with oxygen flowing and for 5–10 minutes following the procedure. This will help to provide oxygen to a depressed respiratory system and will allow the exhaled gases to be scavenged and avoid environmental contamination. All oral monitoring devices should be removed (e.g., temperature probe, esophageal stethoscope) in case of rapid return to consciousness.

Owing to decreased ventilatory drive, performing 21% room air trials is recommended after each anesthetic event. After 5–10 minutes of post-procedure oxygen supplementation, remove the breathing circuit that is administering 100% oxygen and monitor oxygenation via pulse oximetry. If a patient is unable to compensate on their own, a drop in their SPO_2 will occur. The patient should then be hooked back up to 100% oxygen until they are able to compensate on their own.

If the patient is able, the urinary bladder should be emptied at the end of surgery and the amount of urine noted. The patient should be monitored for normal urine production postoperatively.

A rectal temperature should be taken immediately to set a baseline for postoperative heat support. Temperatures should be taken every 15–30 minutes and maintained between 99 and 102.5 degrees F. Patients need to be closely monitored for hypothermia and hyperthermia. Post-heat removal temperature should continue to be checked as it can start decreasing again.

Intravenous fluids should be continued postoperatively, depending on the veterinarian's requests. The intravenous catheter should be flushed with saline if fluids are disconnected and should remain in place for a minimum of one hour postoperatively.

Once patients have adequately recovered from anesthesia, they are moved to a dedicated recovery area in view of numerous nursing staff for close observation. This location should be warm, quiet, and comfortably padded. The patient should be positioned in such a way to protect surgical incisions and airways.

Pediatric patients should be offered food as soon as they are able to eat to reduce hypoglycemia.

Each patient will differ on their recovery, so use best judgment on when they eat.

Extubation

It is best to get into the practice of visualizing the back of the oral cavity for incidences of regurgitation prior to extubation. The endotracheal tube should remain in place until the swallowing reflex has returned. That will vary patient to patient. The rule of thumb is to extubate after three swallows, but the anesthetist should be able to evaluate and make that judgment based on each patient. For example, a patient can swallow three times and still be too sedated for extubation. On the other hand, a patient can swallow once and then chew on their tube the next second. It is vital that the patient has control over their swallowing reflex so that their airway can be protected in cases in which regurgitation or vomiting occur.

Particular breeds and certain disease processes require the endotracheal tube be maintained as long as possible. Commonly, brachycephalic breeds have soft palate tissue that overlaps the epiglottis. They benefit from prolonged endotracheal tube retention postoperatively to hold their airway open. Keeping the patient in a subdued, quiet area without physical stimulation will help facilitate tube retention. In most patients, when the patient is removed from the anesthetic machine, the cuff should be completely deflated, and the tie used to secure the tube should be untied. The tie should also be arranged out the front of the mouth to assure it will not get tangled upon extubation. In some cases, the cuff should only be slightly deflated if there is fear that fluids may be resting on the top of the tube. Slow removal of the tube with a partial deflated cuff will remove the fluids.

Stimulating the patient to wake up or swallow should be avoided. By over-stimulating the patient, they can experience a rapid recovery in which extubation occurs relatively fast. Rapid extubation from stimulation gives a false sense of security that the patient was ready to be extubated. The patient could fall back asleep and respiratory depression or airway obstruction can occur. Use best judgment during extubation.

When extubated, inspect the end of the tube for material (e.g. blood, stomach content). If found, the patient's head should be hung down over the end of the table to allow the contents to drip out. The patient should be evaluated to determine if action is required to clear or rinse the throat of the material and reintubate. The coughing reflex may return well in advance of the swallowing reflex. Complete protection against aspiration may not be assured until several hours after the patient has regained consciousness.

The period following extubation presents a good point for assessing pain management and the need for additional postoperative analgesics as the patient regains sensation and control of its body.

Stages of Anesthesia Recovery

Similar to the four stages of anesthesia, there are four stages that patients move through as they recover from anesthesia. For the most part, it is the reverse of the anesthetic stages, but often they move through them slower and experience each one more fully.

Table 20.13 / **Stages of anesthesia recovery**

Stage	Definition	Monitoring	Considerations
4	• Patient in lateral recumbency and is unconscious to semiconscious • Patient is likely still intubated	• The patient is continuously monitored; recorded every 5 minutes • All areas are monitored (Table 20.10): cardiovascular, respiratory, ocular, musculoskeletal, nervous, urogenital, thermoregulatory	• Follow instructions for recovery and extubation
3	• Patient is beginning to regain the ability to right itself and is conscious • Patient is likely extubated or soon will be • All reflexes are present	• The patient is continuously monitored; recorded every 10–15 minutes • Administration of additional analgesics if necessary	• Transition from stages 4 to 3 can be rapid and unexpected. Patients should be closely monitored at all times • Aggressive or fractious animals may begin to be difficult to handle • Patients may become excited or may vocalize; a quiet recovery area or sedatives may be necessary
2	• Patient is able to walk or move around but may be unsteady	• Hydration, thermoregulation, pain levels, and surgical sites are closely monitored	• Patients under 4 months of age should be offered canned food
1	• All patient functions are normal	• Pain levels are monitored • Food and water may be offered	• Catheter may be removed • The patient is discharged if all parameters are within normal limits including eating, drinking, pain levels

Prolonged Recovery

If a patient experiences slow recovery, it should be investigated and treated. Hypothermia can prolong recovery so heat support should continue if other options are not the reason for prolongation. If prolongation is due to anesthetic or analgesic drugs, consider reversing those drugs. Titrating butorphanol can reverse pure mu opioids without taking away all of the analgesia. Reversing benzodiazepines with flumazenil or reversing alpha-2 agonists with atipamezole can also facilitate recovery. Hypoglycemia in pediatric patients should be evaluated as this can play a role in prolonged recoveries.

Emergence Delirium, Pain, and/or Dysphoric Recoveries

Part of patient recovery is being able to be ready for "rough" recoveries. Rough recoveries can occur due to pain, dysphoria or emergence delirium.

Emergence delirium is an unconscious dissociated state. The patient does not know what is occurring around them. This can be displayed as vocalization, thrashing, paddling, or agitated. Emergence delirium can happen with any patient, but it is prevalent in anxious or cognitively impaired patients. It can also occur if a patient is awoken too fast from stimulation.

Patients experiencing emergence delirium should be treated with a sedative such as acepromazine or dexmedetomidine if they do not calm down right away. The choice depends on the health and comorbidities of the patient and should be determined prior to the anesthetic event in preparation for such an incidence.

Patients in pain will often be vocal, agitated, or sometimes aggressive. Assess heart rate and evaluate the last time an analgesic was given. Patient's that are in pain usually will be cognitive enough to understand their name or being talked to. This can help differentiate between emergence delirium and pain. Sometimes talking to patients will calm them down but they can still be in pain. Never withhold pain medications. If differentiation is hard to determine, a gentle palpation of the surgical site can be performed. If the patient is reactive to the palpation, they are typically painful. If pain is found to be part of the patients recovery, an appropriate analgesic should be administered or an analgesic constant rate infusion should be set up and started (see Chapter 18: Pain Management).

A patient can be anxious or stressed from its experience, including the unfamiliarity of its surroundings or the use of cage confinement. If the patient cannot be soothed and quieted (e.g. being held, resting in a controlled environment outside of the cage), an anxiolytic or sedative should be administered (e.g. trazodone, dexmedetomidine).

Note: empty the bladder following surgery as the need to urinate may cause additional stress or anxiety.

Dysphoria can be caused by the over administration of opioids. Patients will tend to have a glassy-eyed look and be unaffected by palpation of the surgical site or injured part of the body. They can be vocalizing, paddling, or agitated. Reversal of the opioids by incremental administration of naloxone or an opioid μ-antagonist such as butorphanol can alleviate this dysphoria. Complete reversal of the opioid will take away all analgesic effects of the drug as well as the dysphoria. Sedatives or tranquilizers can also be used.

Postanesthetic Monitoring

Monitoring an animal recovering from anesthesia continues through stage 1, until monitoring parameters return to normal for that particular patient (see Table 20.11).

Table 20.14 / Postanesthetic monitoring

System affected	Vital signs monitored	Complication and potential cause	Clinical signs	Treatment

Cardiovascular	• Heart rate
	• Capillary refill time
	• Electrocardiograph
	• Pulse
		• Dysrhythmias
		  • Drug adverse effect
		  • Pain
		  • Disease condition (e.g. GDV)
			• Irregular ECG tracing
			• Tachycardia
			• Pulse deficits
				• Continuous or intermittent ECG tracing
				• Drug administration (e.g. antiarrhythmics)
				• Manage pain

		• Pain
		  • surgical procedure
		  • (see Chapter 18: Pain Management)
			• Tachycardia
			• Tachypnea or hypoxemia
			• Hypertension
			• Vomiting, regurgitation, or ileus
			• Prolonged recumbency
			• Behavioral changes
				• Evaluate analgesic plan and adjust as needed using pain score/index
				• Provide heat support
				• Provide a clean, dry cage in a peaceful and quiet environment
				• Provide reassuring contact
				• Provide acupuncture, acupressure, massage as indicated

		• Circulatory shock
		  • Anaphylactic shock
		  • Drug administration or vaccines
		  • Cardiogenic shock
		  • Heart disease, pulmonary embolus, dysrhythmias, hypoxia, and hypercarbia
		  • Hypovolemic shock
		  • Hemorrhage, excessive vasodilation, inadequate fluid administration
		  • Septic shock
		  • Portocaval shunt, intestinal spillage or gastric volvulus
		  • See Table 10.5: Types of shock, page 547
			• Tachycardia or bradycardia
			• Weak or irregular pulses and hypotension
			• ↑ Capillary refill time
			• Pale mucous membranes
			• Cold extremities
			• Oliguria/anuria
				• Check the airway and supply oxygen.
				• ↑ IV fluid administration
				• Blood transfusion
				• Drug administration (e.g., corticosteroids, anesthetic antagonist, dopamine, atropine, sodium bicarbonate)
				• Monitor urine output

(Continued)

Table 20.14 / **Postanesthetic monitoring (Continued)**

System affected	Vital signs monitored	Complication and potential cause	Clinical signs	Treatment
Respiratory	• Respiratory rate • Mucous membranes • Oropharyngeal reflex • Pulmonary auscultation	• Airway obstruction • Upper airway swelling due to prolonged head down position, allergic reaction, or pharyngeal surgery • Tongue swelling • Soft palate entrapment • Trauma from intubation • Breed predisposition (e.g. brachycephalics) • Foreign body • Laryngeal paralysis • Collapsing trachea	• Cyanotic • Bradypnea or apnea • Excessive chest wall or abdominal movement • Anxious behavior • Noise during inspiration (e.g. stridor)	• Oxygen therapy • Position the head to extend the neck and tongue. • Recover in a dark, quiet room. • Drug administration (e.g., dexamethasone sodium phosphate) • Reinduce/reintubate • Tracheotomy/tracheostomy
		• Pulmonary edema • ↑ Pulmonary capillary pressure • Acute respiratory failure • Hypoproteinemia • Rapid expansion of collapsed lung • Seizures	• Anxiety, restlessness • Dyspnea, coughing • Cyanosis • Pulmonary rales • Froth in endotracheal tube or at the nostrils	• Oxygen therapy • Sedation and controlled ventilation • Drug administration (e.g. furosemide, aminophylline)
Ocular	• Pupils • Palpebral reflex • Eyeball position	• Blindness • Cerebral hypoxia	• Mouth gag use in feline patients • Blindness	• Supportive therapy to return the vital signs to normal as quick as possible • Drug administration (e.g. corticosteroids)

Musculoskeletal	• Jaw tone
	• Limb muscle tone
	• Sphincters (anus and bladder)
		• Rigidity
		  • Drug adverse effect
		  • ↓ Anesthetic depth
			• Extended and stiff extremities	• Supportive care

		• Flaccid • ↑ Anesthetic depth	• Lack of any muscle tone	• Supportive care

(*Continued*)

Table 20.14 / Postanesthetic monitoring (Continued)

System affected	Vital signs monitored	Complication and potential cause	Clinical signs	Treatment

Nervous	• Pedal reflex
	• Reaction to stimulus
	• Behavior
	• Comfort
		• Seizures
		  • Epilepsy
		  • Hypoglycemia, hypoxemia, or thromboembolism
		  • ↑ Intracranial pressure
		  • Drug adverse effect (e.g., ketamine)
		  • Radiographic contrast media parenteral or intrathecal
		  • Secondary hyperthermia
			• Seizure activity
			• Hyperthermia
				• Maintain adequate oxygen levels
				• Monitor hypoglycemia
				• Maintain or administer IV fluids
				• Administer seizure medications (e.g. diazepam or phenobarbital)
				• Drug administration (e.g. methylprednisolone and mannitol)

		• Behavior change
		  • Drug administration (e.g. oxymorphone-acepromazine, fentanyl, droperidol, ketamine)
		  • Hypoglycemia
			• Emergence delirium
			• Excitement
			• Hyperreflexia
			• Disoriented
			• Depression
			• Restlessness
			• Aggression
			• Listlessness and lethargy
				• Manage pain
				• Provide postoperative sedation
				• Holding the patient when safe
				• Provide a dark, quiet place for recovery

		• Pain • See Chapter 18: Pain Management	• See above	• See above

Urogenital	• Urine output	• Oliguria or anuria
		  • Hypoperfusion
		  • Renal dysfunction
		  • Nephrotoxicity
		  • Hypovolemia
			Urine output (ml/kg/hour):
			• < 0.5 in recovery
			• 1–2 normally
				• Verify patent urethra and check bladder size.
				• Placement of a urinary catheter
				• Drug administration (e.g. furosemide, dopamine, mannitol)

(Continued)

Table 20.14 / **Postanesthetic monitoring (Continued)**

System affected	Vital signs monitored	Complication and potential cause	Clinical signs	Treatment
Thermoregulatory	• Temperature	• Hypothermia • Drug adverse effect • Inadequate heat support • Pediatric or geriatric	• Rectal temperature < 101°F • Shivering • Curled-up resting position or hiding	• Warmed IV fluids from fluid warmer, not microwave, hot water circulating heating pads, warm air blanket, insulated hot water bottles form fluid warmer, bubble packing, foil wraps, and blankets • See Skill Box 13.5: Temperature therapy, page 627
		• Hyperthermia • Excessive heat application • ↑ Metabolic rate • Drug adverse effect • Malignant hyperthermia syndrome	• Rectal temperature > 103°F • Panting • Patient hot to the touch • Injected mucous membranes or flushed skin	• Rapid IV fluid administration if clinically indicated • Wet towels over patient • Ice-water enemas or gastric lavage • Administration of antipyretics (e.g. aspirin, aminopyrine, dipyrone, phenylbutazone) • See Skill Box 13.5: Temperature therapy, page 627

Discharge Instruction

The effects of anesthesia can often be seen for 24 hours following the event. Patients should be kept quiet during this time and should be observed closely. Patients are often unstable and slightly disoriented and normal activities should be delayed until the patient is back to themselves.

Patients should be offered small amounts of water and food as soon as they are clinically able to take them. If they are up and moving around postoperatively and are able to eat or drink, it should be slowly offered to them. It has been shown that the sooner the patient eats and drinks the faster the gastrointestinal tract heals and returns to normal function.[10]. If the patient tolerates small amounts, they may return to a normal feeding schedule.

Clients should leave feeling comfortable about the home care they will be providing and the medical follow-up care. These include suture removal, drain care, analgesic plan, activity plan, Elizabethan collar use, medications, and recheck appointments (see Skill Box 23.7: Standard postoperative care instructions, page 1074).

CASE-BASED ANESTHESIA

Together with the basic preanesthetic evaluation, patients presenting with an existing health concern should be further evaluated and should have a specific anesthetic plan designed for them.

Table 20.15 / **Case-based anesthesia**

Preoperative exam and diagnostic tests	Potential complications	Recommended anesthetic protocols	Anesthetic alterations	Special surgical care and recovery
Brachycephalic (English Bulldog, French Bulldog, Pug, Boston Terrier, Boxer, Shar-Pei, Pekingese)				
• Evaluate the degree of respiratory compromise. • Baseline oxygen saturation (SpO_2) reading on room air • Thoracic radiographs	• ↑ Vagal tone • Airway obstruction • Bradycardia • Cyanosis • Difficulty or failure to intubate (e.g. laryngeal collapse, small tracheal lumen size, difficult visualization) • Dyspnea and apnea	*Preanesthetic* • Prokinetic (metoclopramide or cisapride). Oral/injectable prior to premedication. Best starting night prior to surgery • Maropitant • Butorphanol • Methadone *Induction* • Ketamine and diazepam or midazolam • Propofol • Propofol and ketamine • Propofol 1 mg/kg wait 30 seconds, then midazolam 0.3 mg/kg, wait 30 seconds. If unable to intubate after this, administer additional propofol as needed • Alfaxalone • Alfaxalone 1 mg/kg, wait 30 seconds, then midazolam 0.3 mg/kg, wait 30 seconds. If unable to intubate after this, administer additional alfaxalone as needed	• Avoid deep sedation. • Preoxygenate for 3–5 minutes • Rapid IV induction with subsequent intubation • Prepare for a tube 1–2 sizes smaller than anticipated • Prepare for possible tracheostomy tube placement if presenting for respiratory distress	• Maintain the endotracheal tube as long as possible in recovery • Possibly sedate to reduce stress during recovery and allow the tube to remain in longer • Possibly continue oxygen administration after extubation via flow-by • Closely monitor respiration for at least 3 hours following recovery • Recover in sternal recumbency with head elevated or propped up on towel
Congenital heart disease				
• Echocardiogram • ECG • Obtain the resting heart rate and respiratory rate (this should be standard for every case) • Thoracic radiographs	• Bradycardia • Cardiac arrhythmias • Pulmonary edema	• Special considerations depend on cardiac disease	• Preoxygenate • Avoid anticholinergics, barbiturates, alpha-2 agonists, halothane • Fluid rate 2.5 ml/kg/hour	• Observe for overhydration (fluid overload)

(*Continued*)

Table 20.15 / **Case-based anesthesia (Continued)**

Preoperative exam and diagnostic tests	Potential complications	Recommended anesthetic protocols	Anesthetic alterations	Special surgical care and recovery
Impaired cardiac function				
• Echocardiogram • Blood pressure • ECG • Chemistry panel/PCV/ total protein • Electrolytes • Thoracic radiographs • Urinalysis	• Arrhythmias • Bradycardia • Hypovolemia • Pulmonary edema • Tachycardia	Preanesthetic: • Opioid • ± acepromazine, low dose if sedation is needed Induction: • Etomidate with benzodiazepine • Propofol 1 mg/kg wait 30 seconds, then midazolam 0.3 mg/kg, wait 30 seconds. If unable to intubate after this, administer additional propofol as needed • Alfaxalone 1 mg/kg, wait 30 seconds, then midazolam 0.3 mg/kg, wait 30 seconds. If unable to intubate after this, administer additional alfaxalone as needed • Ketamine and diazepam; avoid with hypertrophic cardiomyopathy	• Preoxygenate 3–5 minutes • Avoid induction by inhalation gases • Avoid drugs producing tachycardia (anticholinergics and cycloheximides), except with congestive cardiomyopathy where ↑ heart rate may be beneficial • Avoid alpha-2 agonists, and halothane • Fluid rate 2.5 ml/kg/hour	• Monitor body temperature • Observe for overhydration • Continuous ECG, blood pressure, heart rate, rhythm monitoring
Anemia/hypoproteinemia				
• Complete blood evaluation • Urinalysis	• Anesthetic drug overdose • Delayed recovery • Fluid overload • Hypoxemia • Pulmonary edema	• No special considerations	• Avoid general anesthesia with a PCV < 25% if acute and < 20% if chronic if possible • Preoxygenate • Highly protein-bound drugs will give an ↑ effect but proper pain management should be standard. Use reversible drugs to do this • Avoid alpha-2 agonists and halothane	• Anesthesia causes a 3–5% ↓ in PCV • Blood transfusion pre- and intraoperatively if PCV is < 20% • Intermittent monitoring of PCV and total protein should be done intra- and postoperatively • Conservative fluid therapy to avoid pulmonary edema due to reduced vascular oncotic pressure (especially crystalloids) • Supplemental oxygen postoperatively

(Continued)

Table 20.15 / **Case-based anesthesia (Continued)**

Preoperative exam and diagnostic tests	Potential complications	Recommended anesthetic protocols	Anesthetic alterations	Special surgical care and recovery
Heartworm disease				
• Complete blood evaluation • Thoracic radiographs	• ↓ Cardiac output • Cardiac dysrhythmias • Pulmonary dysfunction	• No special considerations	• No special considerations	• No special considerations
Cesarean, emergency				
• PCV and total protein • Serum calcium • Thorough history	• ↑ Cardiac output • Dyspnea • Hypertension • Hypotension • Neonatal depression from anesthetic agents • Tachycardia • Uterine hemorrhage • Vomiting	Preanesthetic: • Buprenorphine, although best to give after pups/kittens have been delivered Induction: • Propofol At closure: • Incision block with bupivacaine or a liposomal bupivacaine	• Preoxygenate • Consider drugs that can be antagonized or are rapidly metabolized • Avoid pentobarbital because of its close to 100% mortality in neonates • Avoid phenothiazines, benzodiazepines, cycloheximides, alpha-2 agonists • Regional anesthetics as the sole anesthetic or in conjunction with inhalants • IPPV to compensate for the distended abdomen	• Surgical preparation should be done in an awake animal in left lateral recumbency to remove pressure from the vena cava • Drug selection must consider transfer into the milk; careful use of opioids and NSAIDs for pain control is recommended • See Chapter 23, Neonatal Resuscitation Post-cesarean, page 1063

(*Continued*)

Table 20.15 / **Case-based anesthesia (Continued)**

Preoperative exam and diagnostic tests	Potential complications	Recommended anesthetic protocols	Anesthetic alterations	Special surgical care and recovery
Endocrine				
Diabetes mellitus				
• Blood glucose • Urinalysis	• Delayed recovery • Hyperglycemia • Hypoglycemia • Higher infection risk	• No special considerations	• Consider drugs that can be antagonized or are rapidly metabolized. • Caution with alpha-2 agonist can inhibit secretion of insulin, but is reversible and can be closely monitored with glucometer • Caution with ketamine	• Do not withhold water[6] • Patient should be stabilized and regulated if possible • Delay procedure if blood glucose is > 300 mg/dl if possible • Should be first anesthetic patient of the day. • Possibly ↓ insulin dose by 50% on day of surgery due to fasting • Intermittent blood glucose monitoring every 30–60 minutes • IV fluid administration of 5% dextrose if needed • Maintain IV fluids to counteract diuresis caused by hyperglycemia
Hyperadrenocorticism (Cushing's disease)				
• Blood pressure • Thoracic radiographs • CT • Abdominal ultrasound • Electrolytes	• Hypertension • Hypoventilation, hypercapnia • Pulmonary thrombosis • Hypoxemia[6]	• No special considerations	• Gentle handling as prone to bruising and delayed healing[6] • Ventilatory support[6] • IBP and keeping MAP at 70–90 mmHg for patients with previous hypertension[6]	• Monitor ventilation (e.g. $ETCO_2$, pulse oximetry, arterial blood gases) due to pendulous abdomen • Predisposed to poor wound healing and infection • Heparin therapy 72 hours post-adrenalectomy surgery[6] • Avoid NSAIDs[6] • Adequate analgesia with frequent walks for blood flow and ventilation.[6]

(Continued)

Table 20.15 / **Case-based anesthesia (Continued)**

Preoperative exam and diagnostic tests	Potential complications	Recommended anesthetic protocols	Anesthetic alterations	Special surgical care and recovery
Hyperthyroidism				
• Cardiac ultrasound • Complete blood evaluation • ECG • T4 level • Thoracic radiographs • Blood pressure	• Airway obstruction • Bradycardia • Hypoglycemia • Hyper- or hypotension • Hypoxemia • "Thyroid storm" (tachycardia, atrial fibrillation, ventricular tachycardia, congestive heart failure, pleural effusion, pulmonary edema, hypertension, hyperthermia, shock or sudden death)[6]	Opioid: • ± acepromazine, low dose • ± benzodiazepine • ± alfaxalone *Induction* Propofol: • If unable to intubate after this, administer additional propofol as needed Alfaxalone: • Alfaxalone 1 mg/kg, wait 30 seconds, then midazolam 0.3 mg/kg, wait 30 seconds • If unable to intubate after this, administer additional alfaxalone as needed Etomidate and diazepam/midazolam: • If significant cardiac dysfunction is present	• Fluids may need glucose supplementation • Avoid alpha-2 agonists, anticholinergics, cycloheximides, and halothane • Avoid phenothiazines and barbiturates with complicated disease • ↑ Oxygen consumption • Due to the thyroid tumor, intubation may be more difficult, leading to airway obstruction (canines)	• Continue to decrease stress and anxiety • Patient should be stabilized and regulated before an anesthetic procedure • Beta-blockers for severe tachycardia may be necessary • Continuous ECG, $ETCO_2$, SPO_2 and blood pressure monitoring • Intermittent blood glucose monitoring • Calcium and potassium concentration checks • ± O_2 supplementation • Tracheomalacia or trachea collapse can occur after tumor removal • Be prepared for reintubation or tracheostomy
Hypoadrenocorticism				
• Electrolytes • Dehydration correction	• Arrhythmias • Hypocortisolemia • Hypotension • Shock	• No special considerations	• Avoid phenothiazines and etomidate	• Patient should be stabilized and regulated before an anesthetic procedure • IV fluid and glucocorticoids administration pre-, intra-, and postoperatively to avoid an Addisonian crisis • Fluid of choice is 0.9% NaCl but use caution to not rapidly correct hyponatremia[6]

(*Continued*)

Table 20.15 / Case-based anesthesia (Continued)

Preoperative exam and diagnostic tests	Potential complications	Recommended anesthetic protocols	Anesthetic alterations	Special surgical care and recovery
Hypothyroidism				
• PCV and total protein • Electrolytes • Glucose	• Bradycardia • Delayed recovery • Hypotension • Hypothermia • Respiratory difficulty • Hypoventilation/ hypercapnia • Hypoxemia • Hyponatremia	• *Preanesthetic* • Opioids • ± alpha-2 agonist • *Induction* • Propofol • Propofol and ketamine • Alfaxalone	• Pre-oxygenation 3–5 minutes • Consider drugs that can be antagonized or are rapidly metabolized • Avoid phenobarbital, benzodiazepines, NSAIDs	• Patient should be stabilized before an anesthetic procedure if possible • Heat support • Redosing schedules of opioids may be prolonged as well as recovery • Monitor ventilation during surgery (capnography, ABG) • Be prepared to provide ventilatory support (manual or mechanical IPPV) • Continuous ECG monitoring • Glucose monitoring • Monitor oxygenation and respiratory system post-anesthesia
Gastrointestinal				
Gastric dilatation volvulus				
• Arterial gases • Complete blood evaluation • Coagulation profile • Lactate • ECG • Hypovolemic status	• Cardiac arrhythmias • Septic shock • Metabolic acidosis • Hypokalemia • Peritonitis	*Preanesthetic* • Maropitant SQ/IV • Pure mu opioid • ± benzodiazepine *Induction* Propofol: • Propofol, lidocaine, fentanyl • Propofol, lidocaine, midazolam • Propofol, lidocaine, ketamine • Fentanyl, benzodiazepine • Pure mu, benzodiazepine, lidocaine • Propofol 1 mg/kg wait 30 seconds, then midazolam 0.3 mg/kg, wait 30 seconds • If unable to intubate after this, administer additional propofol as needed Alfaxalone: • Alfaxalone 1 mg/kg, wait 30 sec, then midazolam 0.3 mg/kg, wait 30 s. If unable to intubate after this, administer additional alfaxalone as needed.	• Stabilize shock before anesthesia. • Preoxygenate 3–5 minutes • 2 peripheral IV catheters • Avoid the use of emetics (e.g., morphine, acepromazine, and xylazine) • Avoid nitrous oxide • ± manual or mechanical IPPV throughout surgery • Continuous CRI lidocaine	• IBP monitoring and ABG sampling • PCV and TPP monitoring • Continuous ECG and blood pressure monitoring intra- and postoperatively • Heart rate, SpO_2, and body temperature monitoring • IV antibiotics • Avoid the use of morphine due to its tendency to cause vomiting • Serial lactate

(*Continued*)

Table 20.15 / **Case-based anesthesia (Continued)**

Preoperative exam and diagnostic tests	Potential complications	Recommended anesthetic protocols	Anesthetic alterations	Special surgical care and recovery
Pancreatitis				
• Complete blood evaluation • Blood pressure	• Hypotension • Hypokalemia • Hypocalcemia • Acid/base disturbances • Fluid imbalances	• No special considerations	• Very painful, recommend multi-modal analgesic plan • Avoid the use of alpha-2 agonists and halothane	• Monitor and care for the underlying condition • Pain control (e.g. epidural or interpleural local anesthetics)
Obesity				
• Complete blood evaluation • Estimate lean body weight • SPO_2 • Blood pressure	• Airway obstruction • Delayed recovery • Drug overdose • Hyperthermia • Hypoventilation • Hypoxemia • Respiratory difficulty	• No special considerations	• Preoxygenate 3–5 minutes due to potential Pickwickian syndrome • Dose IV drugs on lean weight to prevent overdosing • Preoxygenate • Prepare to administer manual or mechanical IPPV throughout surgery • Drugs that distribute to the body fat will have longer recovery times (halothane)	• Avoid dorsal recumbency with head positioned down if possible • Monitor ventilation via capnography or ABG • Maintain endotracheal tube as long as possible • Continue to monitor SPO_2 oxygenation post-anesthesia

(*Continued*)

Table 20.15 / Case-based anesthesia (Continued)

Preoperative exam and diagnostic tests	Potential complications	Recommended anesthetic protocols	Anesthetic alterations	Special surgical care and recovery
Geriatric (a patient who has reached 75% of its expected life span)				
• Complete blood evaluation • ECG • Thoracic radiographs • Thorough history and medications • Thyroid hormone levels • Urinalysis • Assessment of exercise intolerance	• ↓ Organ function • Hypotension • Hypothermia • Hypoventilation	Preanesthetic: • Opioids • Neuroleptanalgesics Induction: • No special considerations	• Pre-oxygenation 3–5 minutes • Avoid phenothiazines and alpha-2 agonists • Allow longer time for response to drugs	• Heat support • Monitor fluid rate to ensure adequate hydration and urine production (e.g. enlarging bladder, skin tenting, mucous membranes) • Local and regional anesthetics for pain control • Provide cushioning between limbs when laterally recumbent, provide padding/cushion under shoulders in dorsal recumbency, provide hip support when in sternal recumbency • Fasting no longer than 6 hours[6] • Post-anesthesia oxygenation monitoring via SPO_2
Hepatic disease: portal-caval shunt				
• Coagulation profile • Complete blood evaluation	• Delayed recovery • Further hepatic disease • Hypoglycemia • Hypokalemia • Hypotension • Hypothermia • Pulmonary edema • Seizures • Hypoalbuminemia	Preanesthetic: • Opioid and diazepam or midazolam • Remifentanil IV Induction: • Propofol • Propofol, remifentanil • Alfaxalone • Alfaxalone, remifentanil	• Avoid phenothiazines, and halothane • Consider local anesthetics to ↓ systemic drugs • Sevoflurane and desflurane have the least effect on hepatic blood flow • Avoid seizurogenic drugs • Preoxygenate 3–5 minutes • Can use alpha-2 agonists and benzodiazepines but will likely need reversal. Monitor blood glucose if using alpha-2 agonist	• Heat support • Intermittent PCV, TPP, blood glucose intraoperative monitoring • Blood pressure and CVP monitoring • Arterial blood gases in portacaval shunts monitoring • Caution with dosing intra-op analgesics due to ↓ liver metabolism • Liver function tests post-operatively • Avoid large boluses with crystalloids • May need blood transfusion if hemorrhage occurs during surgery • Monitor for portal hypertension for 48 hours post-surgery

(*Continued*)

Table 20.15 / Case-based anesthesia (Continued)

Preoperative exam and diagnostic tests	Potential complications	Recommended anesthetic protocols	Anesthetic alterations	Special surgical care and recovery
Neonatal (patient under three months of age)				
• PCV and TPP • BUN and creatinine • Glucose • Temperature	• Bradycardia • Hypoglycemia • Hypothermia • Hypotension • Hypovolemia • Hypoxemia • Inadequate organ function • Pulmonary edema	Preanesthetic: • Opioid, diazepam and atropine or glycopyrrolate • Neuroleptanalgesics Induction: • Ketamine and benzodiazepine • Propofol • Alfaxalone • Opioid, benzodiazepine	• ↓ drug dose by 30–50% • Allow longer time for response to drugs • Neonates have a higher oxygen consumption, yet anesthetic concentrations are the same as for adults • ↑ Sensitivity to protein-bound anesthetics • Due to immature organ systems, drugs may have a prolonged effect • Nonrebreathing systems and properly sized endotracheal tubes should be used	• Heat support • Blood transfusion should be considered after 10% blood loss. • Preoperative fasting of no more than 2–4 hours for those on a diet of solids and no withholding of water • Traditional monitoring parameters are unreliable (e.g. eye position). • Monitor blood glucose perioperatively • Local and regional anesthetics for pain control • Monitor fluid rate to ensure adequate hydration and urine production (e.g. enlarging bladder, skin tenting, mucous membranes)

(*Continued*)

Table 20.15 / Case-based anesthesia (Continued)

Preoperative exam and diagnostic tests	Potential complications	Recommended anesthetic protocols	Anesthetic alterations	Special surgical care and recovery
Renal disease				
• Blood pressure • Complete blood evaluation • ECG • Urinalysis	• Dehydration • Delayed recovery • Further renal disease • Hyperkalemia • Hypotension • Renal hypoperfusion	*Preanesthetic* • Opioid • Opioid and alfaxalone (small dogs or felines) IM • Opioid, benzodiazepine/alfaxalone (small dogs or felines) IM *Induction* Propofol: • Propofol 1 mg/kg wait 30 seconds, then midazolam 0.3 mg/kg, wait 30 seconds • If unable to intubate after this, administer additional propofol as needed Alfaxalone: • Alfaxalone 1 mg/kg, wait 30 seconds, then midazolam 0.3 mg/kg, wait 30 seconds • If unable to intubate after this, administer additional alfaxalone as needed Benzodiazepine and opioid Ketamine and benzodiazepine	• Azotemic animals have ↑ CNS drug sensitivity. • Acidotic animals have ↑ sensitivity to protein-bound anesthetics	• Avoid preoperative fasting • RBC transfusion if PCV is < 18% in felines and < 20% in canines • 12–24 hours IV diuresis prior to anesthetic event • Proper positioning and padding is needed to avoid pressure necrosis. • Blood pressure, arterial gases, CVP, and $ETCO_2$ monitoring • Continuous ECG monitoring if any risk of hyperkalemia (e.g. acute renal failure) • Continue IV fluids postoperatively and monitor fluid rate to ensure adequate hydration and urine production (e.g. enlarging bladder, skin tenting, mucous membranes) • Pain is managed with opioids

(Continued)

Table 20.15 / **Case-based anesthesia (Continued)**

Preoperative exam and diagnostic tests	Potential complications	Recommended anesthetic protocols	Anesthetic alterations	Special surgical care and recovery
Respiratory disease (pleural effusion, diaphragmatic hernia, pneumothorax, pulmonary contusions, pneumonia, tracheal collapse, and pulmonary edema)				
• Arterial blood gases • Complete blood evaluation • Complete respiratory exam • ECG • Thoracic radiographs	• Hypoventilation • Hypoxemia • Tachypnea, dyspnea, and apnea • Worsening pneumothorax	*Preanesthetic* Opioid: • Opioid and alfaxalone in felines • Opioid and benzodiazepine in appropriate patients *Induction* • Ketamine and diazepam • Propofol 1 mg/kg wait 30 econds, then midazolam 0.3 mg/kg, wait 30 seconds • If unable to intubate after this, administer additional propofol as needed Alfaxalone: • Alfaxalone 1 mg/kg, wait 30 seconds, then midazolam 0.3 mg/kg, wait 30 seconds • If unable to intubate after this, administer additional alfaxalone as needed	• Postpone any anesthesia for a few days if possible • Avoid nitrous oxide • Preoxygenate • Mild preanesthetic may be needed to reduce stress • Rapid induction with injectable anesthetic agents to obtain control of airway • Avoid deep planes of anesthetic and their respiratory depressant effects. • IPPV ↓ pressure to reduce the chance of a tension pneumothorax • PEEP valve in circuit to maintain slight positive pressure	• Prepare for thoracocentesis and chest tube placement • Monitor breathing during surgery for worsening pneumothorax (e.g. respirometry, capnography or pulse oximetry) • Supplemental oxygen pre- and postoperatively • Maintain endotracheal tube as long as possible. • Place nasal catheter postoperatively to continue oxygen administration • Provide adequate analgesia to assist with ease of breathing
Sighthounds (Greyhound, Saluki, Afghan Hound, Whippet, Russian Wolfhound)				
• No special considerations	• Death	Preanesthetic • Opioid and diazepam or midazolam • ± acepromazine or (dex)medetomidine Induction • Propofol • Alfaxalone	• Do not use barbiturates (except methohexital)	• Monitor body temperature. • Proper positioning and padding are needed to avoid pressure necrosis • Recover in a quiet area to ↓ excitement

(Continued)

Table 20.15 / **Case-based anesthesia (Continued)**

Preoperative exam and diagnostic tests	Potential complications	Recommended anesthetic protocols	Anesthetic alterations	Special surgical care and recovery
Trauma (hit by car, head trauma, thoracic and abdominal trauma, thermal/burn trauma)				
• Arterial gases • Complete blood evaluation • ECG • Lactate • Thoracic radiographs • Urine output and concentrating ability	• Cardiac dysrhythmias • Dyspnea or tachypnea • Internal injuries • Pneumothorax • Seizures (e.g. head trauma) • Shock • Tachycardia	Preanesthetic: • Opioid and diazepam or midazolam Induction: • Ketamine and diazepam • Propofol and diazepam • Etomidate and diazepam • Alfaxalone and diazepam • Opioid and diazepam, alternating IV injections Maintenance: • ↓ Inhalant with supplemental narcotic	• Postpone any anesthesia for a few days if possible. • ↓ drug doses • Avoid phenothiazines, barbiturates, alpha-2 agonists, and N_2O • Preoxygenate • IPPV ↓ pressure to reduce the chance of a tension pneumothorax	• Monitor body temperature • Intensive patient monitoring; blood pressure, $ETCO_2$, CVP, heart rate and rhythm • Continuous ECG monitoring • Intermittent PCV and TPP monitoring • Local and regional anesthetics for pain control • Contraindicated in patients that are septic or with coagulopathy
Urinary obstruction				
• Complete blood evaluation • ECG • Evaluate hydration, heart rate and rhythm, CNS depression	• Bradycardia • Cardiac dysrhythmias • Cardiac failure • Hyperkalemia	Preanesthetic: • Opioid and midazolam • Alfaxalone with benzodiazepine and/or opioid Induction: • Ketamine and diazepam • Propofol • Alfaxalone	• Avoid alpha-2 agonists if renal values elevated	• Do not administer fluids until after the obstruction has been relieved (unless patient is in shock) • Cystocentesis may be required preoperatively to relieve bladder tension • Careful positioning is needed in animals with urethral obstruction to avoid rupture • Continuous ECG monitoring if any risk of hyperkalemia ($K^+ > 7.0$)

ANESTHETIC DRUGS

Preanesthetic Drugs

Table 20.16 / Anticholinergics, general information

Drug class	Anticholinergics
Drug (proprietary name)	• Atropine sulfate • Glycopyrrolate (Robinul-V)
Mode of action	• Works on muscarinic receptors of the parasympathetic nervous system by blocking the action of the neurotransmitter, acetylcholine • Antagonizes the effects of the parasympathetic nervous system
Physical effects	• ↑ Heart rate and cardiac output • ↓ Oral, pharyngeal, and respiratory tract secretions and gastrointestinal tract motility • Pupil and bronchial dilation • Blocks vagal nerve stimulation
Uses	• Preanesthetic • Treatment of sinus bradycardia, sinoatrial arrest, incomplete atrioventricular block, and bronchoconstrictive disease • Antidote of organophosphate poisoning
Monitoring	• Heart rate and rhythm • Mouth/secretions and dryness • Thirst/appetite, urination/defecation compatibility
Notes	• Counters bradycardia that develops from laryngeal or ocular stimulation and other vasovagal stimulation • Glycopyrrolate has a ↓ chance of tachycardia over atropine as well as a ↓ chance of cardiac dysrhythmias, and it suppresses salivation more thoroughly • Glycopyrrolate does not cross the blood–brain or placental barriers

Table 20.17 / Anticholinergic drugs

Drug	Administration	Anesthetic precautions	Toxicity
Atropine	Dose: 0.02–0.04 mg/kg Route: SQ, IM, IV Duration: 60–90 minutes	• ↑ Risk of cardiac dysrhythmias and sinus tachycardia in dogs • ↓ Serous portion of salivary secretions, leaving the thicker, ropey mucoid portion (especially in felines) • ↓ Tear production (eyes should be protected with an ophthalmic ointment to prevent corneal drying especially if using ketamine) • Bronchodilation (↑ dead space) • Do not mix with diazepam. • Mydriasis (especially in felines, can cause retinal damage if exposed to bright light for an extended period of time due to reduced pupillary light reflex) • Urine retention	• Canines are more susceptible to toxicity than felines • Drowsiness, dry mucous membranes, thirst, excitability, dilated pupils, tachycardia, vomiting, seizures, and depression
Glycopyrrolate	Dose: 0.005–0.01 mg/kg Route: SQ, IM, IV Duration: 2–3 hours for major effects; 7 hours for salivation		

Table 20.18 / Phenothiazines, general information

Drug class	Phenothiazines
Drug (proprietary name)	• Acepromazine maleate (Promace®), acetylpromazine, promazine (Sparine®) and chlorpromazine (Thorazine®)
Mode of action	• Depresses the reticular activating center of the brain • Inhibits action of dopamine as a neurotransmitter in CNS
Physical effects	• Calming effect • Muscle relaxant • ↓ Motor activity • ↑ Threshold for responding to external stimuli and analgesic effects of other drugs, even though they are not personally noted for producing any analgesic qualities • Antiemetic effect is very obvious at low doses during the anesthetic period, gastrointestinal tract upset, or motion sickness • Depress respiratory system (dose dependent and an additive effect with hypnotics or narcotics) • Vasodilator (may exacerbate anesthetic-induced hypotension) • Protects against catecholamine induced arrhythmias
Uses	• Preanesthetic agent • Tranquilizer • Antiemetic • Antispasmodic • Antidysrhythmic effects
Monitoring	• Blood pressure • Body temperature • Cardiac rate and rhythm • Degree of tranquilization
Notes	• Protect from light • Minimal effects on the cardiac system • ↓ Seizure potential in myelogram cases • More effective when used in combination with an opioid agent

Table 20.19 / Phenothiazine drugs

Drug	Administration	Anesthetic precautions	Toxicity
Acepromazine	*Preanesthetic* Dose: • Canines: 0.03–0.05 mg/kg (max dose of 3 mg) • Felines: 0.02–0.1 mg/kg Route: PO, SQ, IM, IV (cautiously) Duration: 4–8 hours *Sedative* Dose (mg/kg): • Canines: 0.025–0.2 IV (max dose 3 mg) • 0.1–0.25 IM • Felines: 0.05–0.1 IV (max dose 1 mg) Route: SQ, IM, IV (cautiously) Duration: 4–6 hours	• Excitement rather than sedation (paradoxical aggression from CNS stimulation) • Peripheral vasodilation (possibly leading to hypothermia or hypotension) • Prolonged recovery in aged animals, portocaval shunts, or ↓ hepatic function	• Seizures, hypotension, hypothermia, and hypoventilation

Table 20.20 / Benzodiazepines: general information

Drug class	Benzodiazepines
Drug (proprietary name)	• Diazepam (Valium®, Vazepam®) • Midazolam HCl (Versed®)
Mode of action	• Releases an inhibitory neurotransmitter in the brain, GABA
Physical effects	• Antianxiety and calming effect • Skeletal muscle relaxation • Anticonvulsant activity
Uses	• Preanesthetic • Sedative • Anticonvulsant, those undergoing procedures that commonly show seizures postoperatively (cerebrospinal fluid taps or myelograms), or with drugs that lower the seizure threshold (ketamine, opioids, and local anesthetics) • Oral diazepam may be used to curb inappropriate urination in cats • IV diazepam may be used as an appetite stimulant (feline); however, it is transient and dose dependent
Monitoring	• Level of sedation • Respiratory and cardiac signs
Notes	• Class IV controlled substance • Protect from light • Diazepam should not be stored in plastic syringes, bags, or tubing; it is readily absorbed into the plastic • Diazepam may increase the effects of digoxin • Minimal adverse effects on the cardiovascular and respiratory systems • Oral diazepam is a controlled drug that is not licensed for use in animals in the United States • Benzodiazepines should be given IV slowly to prevent hypotension associated with the propylene glycol carrier (diazepam) and to ↓ the apnea response

Table 20.21 / **Benzodiazepines**

Drug	Administration	Anesthetic precautions	Toxicity	Notes
Diazepam	Dose (mg/kg): • 0.1–0.5 • Status epilepticus 0.5–1 IV, IN, or rectally • CRI for status epilepticus 0.1–2 mg/kg/hour Route: • PO, IV (slowly) Duration: • Canines: 3–5 hours • Felines: 5 hours Reversal: • Flumazenil • 0.01 mg/kg IV (shorter duration than diazepam, may need to redose every 1 hour as required)	• Rapid IV administration may cause bradycardia, short-term arrhythmias, hypotension, and apnea • Do not administer IM • Best not used as a sole anesthetic agent because it does not produce sedation; combine with opiates or ketamine • Avoid in patients with liver dysfunction	• Ataxia • Central nervous system depressant • Confusion, coma, and decreased reflexes • Hypotension • Oral use in cats linked to liver failure	• Avoid in nursing mothers (readily crosses into milk) • Do not draw up until ready to use (absorbs into plastic) • If administering CRI only draw up 4 hours' worth at a time due to plastic absorption • Use dedicated line if administering as CRI (incompatible with most fluids and medications) • Do not dilute • Protect from light
Midazolam	• 0.1–0.3 mg/kg • IM, SQ, IV (slowly) • Can go up to 0.5 mg/kg for seizures • CRI 0.05–0.5 mg/kg/hour Duration: 1–2 hours Reversal: • Flumazenil • 0.01 mg/kg IV every 1 hour as required (may need to redose due to shorter duration of action than midazolam)	• Crosses the placenta • Protect from light • Rapid IV administration may cause bradycardia and respiratory depression • Best not used as a sole anesthetic agent because it does not produce sedation; combine with opiates or ketamine • May cause either sedation or excitement • May cause behavior modification in cats; irritability, dysphoria, agitation, depression, and difficult restraint	• Ataxia • Central nervous system depressant • Confusion, coma, and ↓ reflexes • Respiratory depression	• Cannot give rectally

Table 20.22 / **Alpha-2 agonists: general information**

Drug class	Alpha-2 agonists
Drug (proprietary name)	• Dexmedetomidine (Dexdomitor®) • Xylazine (Rompun®, AnaSed®)
Mode of action	• Stimulates alpha-2 receptors, causing a decrease in the level of the neurotransmitter norepinephrine released in the brain
Physical effects	• Calming and sedation • Muscle relaxation • Suppresses salivation, gastric secretions, and gastrointestinal motility; can trigger emesis
Uses	• Preanesthetics • Sedation • Short anesthetic procedures • Chemical restraint • Short periods of analgesia • Induce vomiting in cats after ingestion of toxins • Stimulate appetite in low doses
Monitoring	• Body temperature • Cardiovascular function including oxygenation and blood pressure • Level anesthesia and analgesia • Respiratory function-ventilation
Notes	• Xylazine has the highest rate of anesthetic complications and death. • Medetomidine is more potent than xylazine with fewer adverse effects. • Dexmedetomidine is twice as potent as medetomidine. • Do not administer anticholinergic to counter bradycardia. If necessary, reverse with atipamezole. • Affects glucose values after drug administration; suppresses insulin release causing ↑ plasma glucose concentration and glucosuria; use with caution in non-insulin-dependent diabetics – transient and often not clinical. • Decreases cardiac output: monitor blood pressure. • Vasoconstriction will cause pale/gray mucous membranes. • Great benefit when added to local anesthetics.

Table 20.23 / **Alpha-2 agonist drugs**

Drug	Administration	Anesthetic precautions	Toxicity	Notes
Dexmedetomidine	Dose: • Doses greatly depend on route of administration and can be reduced and work synergistically with other drugs • 1–10 μg/kg IV or IM) • CRI 0.5–3 μg/kg/hour • Loading dose for CRI 1–3 μg/kg IV Route: • SQ, IM, IV Duration: • 1–2 hour Reversal: • Atipamezole (Antisedan®) • For each 1 μg/kg used, use 10 μg/kg atimpamizole IM • IV use only during CPR	• Vasoconstriction causing a reflex bradycardia; normal physiologic effect • Do not administer anticholinergic unless severely hypotensive • Contraindicated in patients with cardiovascular disease, shock, severe debilitation and/or renal disease • Use caution in patients with liver disease • Patients can override the sedation if stimulated • Best reserved for patients that are healthy and having procedures in which reversing is appropriate	• Cardiac arrhythmias • Respiratory depression	• Best used in conjunction with an opioid such as butorphanol or hydromorphone • Atipamezole: Give an equal volume (milliliter per milliliter) as dexmedetomidine IM • Patients should be allowed to sit in a quiet location for 10–15 minutes with full affect seen at 30 minutes if given IM • Apply an eye lubricant • Occasional AV block • Hypothermia • Vomiting (extralabel emetic in felines) • Mucous membranes cannot be used as a vital sign for oxygen saturation; they may appear blanched or cyanotic • Transient hyperglycemia • During sedation procedures monitor SPO_2, ECG and provide oxygen supplementation
Xylazine	Dose (mg/lb): • 0.2–0.5 IV • 0.05–1 SQ, IM Route: • SQ, IM, IV, epidurally and subarachnoidally Duration: • 20–40 minutes Reversal (mg/lb): • Yohimbine: 0.05 IV slowly • Tolazoline: 1–2 IV slowly	• Vomiting (50% of canines and 90% of felines) usually seen within 3–5 minutes; do not induce further anesthesia until after this time period to prevent aspiration • Severe respiratory depression • Hypotension (initial ↑ and then subsequent ↓) • Bradyarrhythmias • Cardiac output possible ↓ of 30–50% • Depresses thermoregulatory mechanism	• Cardiac arrhythmias • Hypotension • Profound CNS depression • Respiratory depression • Seizures	• Can be absorbed through skin abrasions and mucous membranes (handle carefully)

Table 20.24 / **Opioids: general information**

Drug class	Opioids
Drug (proprietary name)	• Butorphanol (Torbutrol®, Torbugesic®) • Buprenorphine (Buprenex®) • Fentanyl (Sublimaze®) • Hydromorphone • Morphine sulfate • Remifentanil • Oxymorphone (Numorphan®) • Methadone
Mode of action	• Acts on one or more of three different receptors (μ, κ, and σ) found within the brain
Physical effects	• CNS depression or excitement • Respiratory depression • Gastrointestinal function; nausea, vomiting, hypermotility, and defecation • Bradycardia • Hypotension • Cough suppression, except oxymorphone • Miosis in dogs and mydriasis (feline) • ↑ Response to noise • Excessive salivation • Histamine release (morphine)
Uses	• Preanesthetics • Induction agents • Analgesia • Epidurals
Monitoring	• Respiratory and cardiovascular function • Ventilation (ETCO$_2$, PaCO$_2$) • Provide anti-emesis and anti-nausea medications
Notes	• Reverse pure μ opioids with naloxone: canine: 0.04 mg/kg SQ, IM, IV, and feline: 0.05–0.1 mg/kg SQ, IM, IV. Butorphanol can partially reverse pure μ opioids without taking away all analgesic effects and endogenous endorphins. Start with 0.05–0.1 mg/kg (can dilute and give to effect) IV • Naloxone can partially reverse butorphanol • Rapid IV administration in canines can cause excitement and histamine release (morphine) • Meperidine usually does not cause vomiting and defecation and fentanyl usually does not cause vomiting • Opioids can be combined with local anesthetics to provide spinal analgesia for several hours or in CRI solutions • Store away from light

Table 20.25 / Opioid drugs

Drug	Administration	Anesthetic precautions	Toxicity

Butorphanol	Dose: 0.2–0.4 mg/kg
	Route: SQ, IM, IV (use lower dose if IV)
	Duration:
	• Canines: 30–60 minutes
	• Felines: 1–3 hours
		• Apnea
		• Poor analgesia, mild pain only
		• MDR1 mutation: decrease dose in heterozygous dogs by 25% and decrease dose in homozygous dogs by 30–50%
		• Ataxia and incoordination
		• Excitement, dysphoria
		• Mild bradycardia
		• Mild hypotension
		• Rarely causes anorexia and diarrhea
		• SQ injection absorption can be unpredictable
		• Note:
		  • Antitussive
		  • Partial reversal for pure μ opioids
		  • Naloxone will partially reverse
			• CNS effects
			• Cardiovascular changes
			• Profound respiratory depression
			• Seizures
			• Diuretic response

Buprenorphine	Dose (mg/kg): • Canines: 0.01–0.03 • Felines: 0.01–0.03 • Epidural: 0.03 Route: • Sublingual, SQ, IM, IV, epidural Duration (affected by dose): • 3–12 hours • Delayed onset of 30–60 minutes	• Mild to moderate analgesia • Bradycardia, rare • Respiratory depression, rare • Behavior changes in felines • Hyperthermia in felines • SQ injection absorption can be unpredictable • Cannot be reversed. Consider before administration	• Cardiovascular changes • Profound respiratory depression • ↑ bile duct pressure (caution in cholestasis)
Fentanyl	Dose (μg/kg): • Felines: 1–3 IV • CRI surgical doses 2–6 μg/kg/hour • Postoperative maintenance analgesia 1–5 μg/kg/hour Route: • IM, IV (bolus or CRI) Duration: • < 30 minutes (bolus) Reversal: • Naloxone 0.04 mg/kg SQ, IM, IV • Butorphanol 0.05–0.2 mg/kg IV diluted with saline and given to effect for partial reversal to treat dysphoria or prolonged recovery	• Ataxia • Bradycardia • Exaggerated response to loud noises • Panting • Respiratory depression, may persist for several hours • Urine retention and constipation • Contraindicated in myasthenia gravis patients • Hypothermia • Dysphoria	• Bradycardia • Cardiac arrhythmias • Cardiovascular collapse • Profound respiratory and CNS depression • Tremors, neck rigidity, and seizures

(Continued)

Table 20.25 / Opioid drugs (Continued)

Drug	Administration	Anesthetic precautions	Toxicity
Hydromorphone	Dose: 0.05–0.2 mg/kg Route: SQ, IM, IV (slowly) • Duration: 2–4 hours • Delayed onset of 15–30 minutes Reversal: • Naloxone 0.04 mg/kg SQ, IM, IV • May have to redose as duration of action is shorter than hydromorphone • Butorphanol 0.05–0.2 mg/kg diluted with saline and given to effect for partial reversal to treat dysphoria or prolonged recovery	• ↓ Gastrointestinal tract motility with resultant constipation • Nausea • Bradycardia • Panting • Respiratory and CNS depression • Vomiting and defecation • Dysphoria • Hyperthermia in felines	• Cardiovascular collapse • Hypothermia • Muscle hypotonia • Profound respiratory and CNS depression
Morphine	Dose (mg/kg): • Canines: 0.5–1.0 SQ, IM; 0.2 IV • Felines: 0.25–0.5 SQ, IM Route: • SQ, IM, IV (slowly) Duration: • 4–6 hours Reversal – naloxone (mg/kg): • Canines: 0.04 SQ, IM, IV • Felines: 0.05–0.1 SQ, IM, IV	• ↓ Cough reflex and tidal volume and drying of respiratory secretions • ↓ Gastrointestinal motility/constipation • Bradycardia • Histamine release with IV administration • May cause bladder hypertonia • May cause CNS depression, hypothermia, panting and miosis in dogs • May cause stimulatory effects and hyperthermia in cats • Respiratory depression • Vomiting and defecation after administration	• Cardiovascular collapse • Hypothermia • Muscle hypotonia • Profound respiratory and CNS depression • CNS excitability and seizures in felines
Methadone	Dose (mg/kg): • Canines: 0.5–1 SQ, IM, IV • Felines: 0.25–0.5 SQ, IM, IV Route: • SQ, IM, IV (slowly) Duration: • 4–6 hours • Reversal – naloxone: • Canines/felines: 0.04 mg/kg SQ, IM, IV • Short acting (as short as 45 minutes), may need to redose	• Respiratory depression • ↓ Gastrointestinal motility/constipation • Bradycardia • Less histamine release than morphine • Less sedating than morphine • Least likely opioid to cause vomiting/nausea, but still can • Panting • Whining • Mild sedation with heavy doses • Hyperthermia in feline patients • NMDA antagonist, μ, κ agonists, and some δ agonist effects	• Cardiovascular collapse • Hypothermia • Profound respiratory and CNS depression • CNS excitability, head trauma, and seizures • *Do not* use in patients stung by scorpions, may potentiate the venom

(*Continued*)

Table 20.25 / Opioid drugs (Continued)

Drug	Administration	Anesthetic precautions	Toxicity
Oxymorphone	Dose: • Canines 0.05–0.4 mg/kg IM, IV • Felines 0.2–0.5 mg/kg IV, IM • Epidural Route: • SQ, IM, IV Duration: • 2–4 hours IV • Epidural 8 hours • Reversal – naloxone: • Canines: 0.04 mg/kg SQ, IM, IV • Felines: 0.05–0.1 mg/kg SQ, IM, IV	• Rapid IV administration in cats may cause excitement in felines • Bradycardia • Crosses placenta • Hyperthermia in felines • Panting after initial administration in dogs • Respiratory depression • Contraindicated in which emesis is not a desired effect	• Cardiovascular collapse • Hypothermia • Muscle hypotonia • Profound respiratory depression • Effects may last longer than the initial dose of naloxone
Remifentanil	Dose: • 3–5 μg/kg IV; followed by CRI of 0.2–0.6 μg/kg/minute Route: • IV Duration: • 5–10 minutes • Reversal: naloxone	• Half as potent as fentanyl • Ultra-short acting even after sustained CRIs • Apnea • Bradycardia/bradyarrhythmias • Hypotension • Hyperthermia (feline) • Respiratory depression • Elimination by non-specific protein esterases in blood and tissues	• Apnea • Cardiovascular collapse • Hypothermia • Profound respiratory and CNS depression

Injectable Induction Anesthetics

Table 20.26 / Cyclohexamines: general information

Drug class	Cyclohexamines
Drug (proprietary name)	• Ketamine (Ketaset®, Ketalean®, Vetalar®)
Mode of action	• Acts by disruption of the nervous system pathways within the cerebrum and a stimulation of the reticular activating center of the brain • Induce a state of anesthesia and amnesia by overstimulating the CNS or inducing a cataleptic state
Physical effects	• ↓ Corneal reflex • ↑ Heart rate and blood pressure • ↑ Sensitivity to sound, light, and other stimuli, especially with large doses • Confusion, agitation and fear • Excessive salivation • Hallucinations • Normal to ↑ muscle tone and rigidity • Respiratory depression at high doses
Uses	• Restraint • Unconsciousness • Analgesia, somatic pain • Inhibits NMDA receptors in CNS (↓ "wind-up" effect) • Induction agent
Monitoring	• Body temperature • Cardiovascular function • Level of anesthesia and analgesia • Monitor eyes to prevent drying or injury (lubrication recommended) • Respiratory function
Notes	• This agent is a dissociative anesthetic that produces catalepsy • Ocular, oral, and swallowing reflexes are only weakened • The use of a premedication like a tranquilizer, barbiturate, opioid, or benzodiazepine is recommended to relieve ↑ muscle tone, ↓ salivation and lacrimation, and to produce visceral analgesia • Its use as an induction agent is enhanced when mixed with a benzodiazepine and given IV

Table 20.27 / Cyclohexamine drugs

Drug	Administration	Anesthetic precautions	Toxicity
Ketamine	Dose: • 1–5 mg/kg depending on route of administration and if mixing with other anesthetics/analgesics Route: • Canines: IV, IM • Felines: PO, SQ, IM, IV (onset 50–60 seconds) Duration: • 10–30 minutes	• Eyes remain open, central, and dilated during anesthesia; use an ophthalmic ointment to prevent corneal drying • Pinnal, palpebral, pedal, laryngeal, and pharyngeal reflexes remain when used alone • Emesis • Produces apneustic breathing, can induce significant respiratory depression at high doses or if given too rapidly IV • Recovery is hyperresponsive with ataxia. • Repeated doses can accumulate in the tissues prolonging recovery and ↑ the chance of convulsions during the recovery period • Respiratory depression • Spastic jerking movements, seizures, muscular tremors, and hypertonicity • Tachycardia, hypertension, hypersalivation, hyperthermia, and nystagmus • Tissue irritation and pain on IM injection • Cautioned use in: hypertension, heart failure, hypertrophic cardiomyopathy, hyperthyroidism, hepatic dysfunction, seizure disorders, shock, congestive heart failure, pheochromocytoma	• Profound respiratory depression/apnea • Cardiac arrest

Table 20.28 / Propofol: general information

Drug class	Propofol, propofol 28
Drug (proprietary name)	• Propofol (Diprivan®, Rapinovet®, PropoFlo®, Propoflo® 28)
Mode of action	• Induces depression by enhancing the effects of the inhibitory neurotransmitter GABA and ↓ the brain's metabolic activity • It is a short-acting hypnotic agent
Physical effects	• ↓ Intraocular pressure • Antiemetic properties • Bradycardia (especially with opiate preanesthetics) • Hyperkinesis during induction (e.g. paddling, myoclonic twitching) • Hypotension • Respiratory depression and apnea
Uses	• Sedation/short anesthesia (up to 20 minutes) • Induction agent • Total/partial intravenous anesthesia

(*Continued*)

Table 20.28 / **Propofol: general information (Continued)**

Drug class	Propofol, propofol 28
Monitoring	• Level of anesthesia • CNS effects • Respiratory depression • Cardiovascular status
Notes	• Propoflo 28 formulation has a 28-day shelf life after opening • Propoflo 28 contains benzyl alcohol which can be toxic to cats in high doses, but formulation has been used anecdotally in healthy cats with no indications of toxicity • No analgesic properties • Short duration due to rapid redistribution from CNS to peripheral tissue • Preoxygenate

Table 20.29 / **Propofol**

Drug	Administration	Anesthetic precautions	Toxicity
Propofol/propofol 28	Dose: • Induction: 2–8 mg/kg IV • CRI 0.1–0.6 mg/kg/min IV Route: • IV slowly; onset of 20 seconds Duration: • 2–5 minutes for each single bolus (titrate)	• Direct myocardial depression and arterial hypotension • Bradycardia • Crosses placenta • Epilepsy • Heinz body production in felines with multiple day usage • Hypotension • Respiratory depression and dose dependent apnea • Hypothermia	• Respiratory depression • Cardiovascular depression

Table 20.30 / Alfaxalone: general information

Drug class	Alfaxalone
Drug (proprietary name)	• Alfaxalone (Alfaxan®)
Mode of action	• Modulation of neuronal cell membrane chloride ion transport, induced by binding to GABA receptors • Short and rapid durations of action with minimal adverse effects
Physical effects	• Hypotension • ↑ Heart rate • Mild tachycardia • Respiratory depression, minimal
Uses	• Sedation/short anesthesia (up to 20 minutes) • Induction agent • Constant rate infusions
Monitoring	• Respiratory parameters
Notes	• Protect from light, refrigerate, shake well, and use within seven days to prevent iatrogenic sepsis • Little to no analgesic properties • Can be safely given with preanesthetics, opioids, and NSAIDs, but do not combine in the same syringe • Little to no effect on neonates for cesarean section • Can be used for sight hounds and high-risk patients • Patients should be not handled or disturbed during recovery to avoid stimulation and violent movements • Premedication is advised to facilitate a smooth recovery • IV injections are given slowly to reduce the period of apnea, although less commonly seen than with propofol

Table 20.31 / Alfaxalone

Drug	Administration	Anesthetic precautions	Toxicity
Alfaxalone	Dose: • Induction: 1–3 mg/kg (canines) and 2–5 mg/kg (felines) depending on sedation • Maintenance: 4–7 mg/kg/h (canines) and 5–8 mg/kg/hour (felines) Route: • IM, IV slowly; give in a slow continuous injection over 60 seconds Duration: • 10 minutes for each single bolus	• Respiratory depression and initial apnea • Provide oxygen supplementation during induction and maintenance • Decrease dose and dosing interval by 20% with patients showing hepatic insufficiencies • Psychomotor excitement may be seen during recovery, especially without appropriate preanesthetics	↓ Cardiac output

Table 20.32 / **Etomidate: general information**

Drug class	Etomidate
Drug (proprietary name)	• Etomidate (Hypnomidate®, Radenarcon®, Sibul®)
Mode of action	• Not well understood • Causes minimal hemodynamic changes along with minimal effects on the cardiovascular and respiratory systems • ↓ Cerebral blood flow and oxygen consumption, intraocular pressure, and intracranial pressure
Physical effects	• Excitement or myoclonus during induction or recovery • Eye movements • Postoperative retching/vomiting • Suppresses adrenocortical function for 3 hours after administration • Hemolysis due to propylene glycol
Uses	• Cardiac dysfunction (e.g. dilated cardiomyopathy) • Critically ill patients
Monitoring	• Level of consciousness • Respiration rate and rhythm • Cardiovascular function
Notes	• Protect from light • Adequate premedication is highly recommended due to excitatory effects • Give injection in the fluid line to ↓ injection site pain • Little to no analgesic properties

Table 20.33 / **Etomidate**

Drug	Administration	Anesthetic precautions
Etomidate	Dose (mg/kg): • Canines: 0.5–2 rapidly IV or 1 and diazepam 0.5 IV • Felines: 0.5–2 Route: • IV; administer 50% of calculated dose over 15 seconds and then to effect Duration: • 3–5 minutes	• ↓ Cerebral blood flow and oxygen consumption • ↓ Intraocular and intracranial pressure • Excitement or myoclonus during induction or recovery • Eye movements • Hypoproteinemia • Postoperative retching/vomiting • Suppresses adrenocortical function for three h after administration • When using the propylene glycol preparation, give slowly IV or give with IV fluids to minimize pain on injection and to minimize hemolysis due to the propylene glycol

Inhalant Anesthetics

Table 20.34 / Inhalant anesthetics: general information

Drug class	Inhalants
Drug (proprietary name)	• Nitrous oxide • Isoflurane (AErrane®, Isoflo®, Florane®) • Sevoflurane (Sevoflo®, Ultane®) • Desflurane (Suprane®)
Mode of action	• True mode of action is unknown; the following are two possibilities: • Inhibits the breakdown of GABA, an inhibitory neurotransmitter • Causes the membrane to lose its ability to conduct nerve impulses by dissolving in the nerve cell membrane
Physical effects	• Muscle relaxation
Uses	• General anesthesia
Monitoring	• Level of anesthesia • Respiratory and ventilatory status • Cardiac rate and rhythm • Blood pressure; all inhalants are potent vasodilators and overdose will lead to blood pressure decrease
Notes	• Store isoflurane in a tight, light resistant container

Table 20.35 / **Inhalant anesthetic agents: isoflurane and sevoflurane**

Drug class	Inhalants	
Drug (proprietaryname)	• Isoflurane (AErrane®, IsoFlo®, Florane®)	• Sevoflurane (Sevoflo, Ultane)
Attributes	• Extremely rapid induction and recovery • Mask and chamber induction • Used for animals with cardiac disease, liver and kidney disease, and neonatal and geriatric animals • Excellent muscle relaxation	• Extremely rapid induction and recovery • Mask and chamber induction • Produces muscle relaxation and analgesia • Non-pungent odor
Dose	• Induction: 5%	• Induction: 5–7%
	• Maintenance: 0.5–2.5%	• Maintenance: 2–4%
Metabolism	• 99% eliminated unchanged by the alveoli • 0.17% metabolized by the liver	• Rapid elimination through the lungs • 3% metabolized by the liver
Precautions	• ↑ Cerebral blood flow • ↓ Smooth muscle tone and motility • Arrhythmias (ventricular premature contractions) • Crosses placenta • Gastrointestinal effects (e.g. nausea, vomiting, and ileus) • Hypothermia • Progressive vasodilation and hypotension occurs with deeper levels of anesthesia. • Rapid recovery and no analgesia postoperatively can lead to pain and excitement (e.g., emergence delirium). • Respiratory and CNS depression • Slight ↓ in cardiac output	• ↑ Cerebral blood flow • ↑ Concentration may cause rapid hemodynamic changes (e.g. hypotension) • Bradycardia • Crosses placenta • Gastrointestinal effects (e.g. nausea, vomiting, and ileus) • Hypotension, bradycardia, shivering, and nausea • Hypothermia • Myocardial depression • Not stable in moist soda lime and may release carbon monoxide • Respiratory and CNS depression • The safety of this agent has not been evaluated in geriatric, debilitated, breeding, or neonate animals • Vasodilation
Contraindications	• History of malignant hyperthermia • Use with caution in animals with ↑ CSF, head injury, or myasthenia gravis • Concurrent use with angiotensin-converting enzyme (**ACE**) inhibitors can cause ↓ blood pressure	• History of malignant hyperthermia • ↑ CSF and head injury • Renal compromise/insufficiency

REFERENCES

1. Griffin, B., Bushby, P.A., McCobb, E., et al. (2016). The Association of Shelter Veterinarians' 2016 veterinary medical care guidelines for spay-neuter programs. *J Am Vet Med Assoc* 249(2): 165–181.
2. Bednarski, R., Grimm, K., Harvey, R., et al. (2011). AAHA Anesthesia Guidelines for Dogs and Cats. *J Am Anim Hosp Assoc* 47(6): 377–385.
3. American Society of Anesthesiologists. (2020). *ASA Physical Status Classification System*. Schaumburg, IL: ASA. https://www.asahq.org/standards-and-guidelines/asa-physical-status-classification-system (accessed 31 July 2021).

4. Ko, J., Krimins, R. (2012). Anesthetic monitoring: your questions answered. *Today's Vet Pract* January/February: 23–29.
5. Congdon, J. (2012). At-home medications to smooth the "in-hospital" experience. In: Proceedings of the NAVC Conference, January 14–18, 2012, Orlando, Florida. Book 1: Small Animal and Exotics: Disciplines A-R. Gainesville, FL: North American Veterinary Conference.
6. Duke-Novakovski, T., Seymour, C. (eds.). (2016). *BSAVA Manual of Canine and Feline Anesthesia and Analgesia*, 3e. Gloucester: British Small Animal Veterinary Association.
7. Blunt, M.C., Young, P.J., Patil, A., Haddock, A. (2001). Gel lubrication of the tracheal tube cuff reduces pulmonary aspiration. *Anesthesiology* 95(2): 377–381.
8. Schroeder, C. (2020). Regional anesthesia and pain management in veterinary medicine. American Society of Regional Anesthesia and Pain Medicine. https://www.asra.com/guidelines-articles/original-articles/article-item/asra-news/2020/04/30/regional-anesthesia-and-pain-management-in-veterinary-medicine (accessed 25 September 2021).
9. Ateca, L.B., Reineke, E.L., Drobatz, K.J. (2018). Evaluation of the relationship between peripheral pulse palpation and Doppler systolic blood pressure in dogs presenting to an emergency service. *J Vet Emerg Crit Care* 28(3): 226–231.
10. Corbee, R.J., Van Kerkhoven, W.J.S. (2014). Nutritional support of dogs and cats after surgery or illness. *Open J Vet Med* 4: 44–57.

Chapter 21

Dentistry

Tammi Smith, MEd, CVT, VTS (Dentistry)

Veterinary Technician and Nurse's Daily Reference Guide: Canine and Feline, Fourth Edition. Edited by Mandy Fults and Kenichiro Yagi.

Companion website: www.wiley.com/go/fults/veterinary

Abbreviations

A complete list of American Veterinary Dental College approved abbreviations and nomenclature is available on the AVDCwebsite.[1]

ALARA, as low as reasonably achievable
AVDC, American Veterinary Dental College
AT, attrition
AB, abrasion
AVDC, American Veterinary Dental College
B/E, excisional biopsy
B/I, incisional biopsy
CA, caries
CCF, complicated crown fracture
CCRF, complicated crown root fracture
CI, calculus index
DR, digital radiograph
DTC, dentigerous cyst
E/H, enamel hypoplasia
E/HM, hypomineralization
F, furcation exposure
FS, fibrosarcoma
GH, gingival hyperplasia
GI, gingivitis index
GR, gingival recession
M, tooth mobility
MAL 1, Class 1 malocclusion
MAL 2, Class 2 malocclusion
MAL 3, Class 3 malocclusion
MM, malignant melanoma
NV, non-vital
OM, oral mass
ONF, oronasal fistula
P, pocket
PD, periodontal disease
RD, retained deciduous tooth
RPC, root plane closed
RPO, root plane open
RTR, retained root
SCC, squamous cell carcinoma
SN, supernumerary
ST, stomatitis
T/I, impacted tooth
T/NV, non-vital tooth
TR, tooth resorption
UCF, uncomplicated crown fracture
UCRF, uncomplicated crown root fracture
X, simple extraction (one root)
XS, sectioned extraction (2–3 roots)
XSS, surgical extraction (gingival retraction)

The basic definition of periodontal disease is infection of the hard and soft support systems of the tooth. These tissues include the gingiva, periodontal ligament, and alveolar bone. The impact of periodontal disease reaches far beyond the immediate area surrounding a particular tooth. The vehicle of the infection is plaque and the ultimate control of the disease is anchored in control of plaque. Plaque contains oral bacteria, saliva, and food products. These bacteria form a biofilm that is resistant to antibiotics and antiseptics. As these bacteria cause inflammation, the body will mount an immune response. It is the combination of the bacterial toxins and the immune response that causes the destruction that ultimately leads to tooth loss. There are local and systemic complications associated with this process. Local manifestations include oronasal fistulas, pathologic fractures, endodontic disease, and ocular complications.[2] Renal, hepatic, pulmonary, and cardiac systems are also affected. The inflammation caused by periodontal disease can make it difficult to regulate diabetes.[3]

The earliest detectable sign of periodontal disease is bleeding on probing. Unfortunately, this cannot be accomplished on conscious patients. The first visible sign for conscious patients is gingivitis. Both veterinary staff and owners tend to focus on calculus as the sign that intervention is necessary. Calculus may not be present in the early stages of periodontal disease. Since the only stage of disease that can be cured is gingivitis, treatment will be most effective early in the disease process.

Periodontal disease is the most common condition encountered in small animal patients. Studies have shown that, by two to three years of age, 80–85% of both cats and dogs are affected.[4] Unfortunately, most patients will never exhibit clear signs of the pain they may be experiencing, and some signs may be attributed to old age or other disease processes. Possible signs of pain include drooling, changes in food preference, swallowing food without chewing, chewing only on one side of the mouth, jaw chattering, lip smacking, tooth grinding, blood in bowls or on toys, rubbing face, dropping food, facial hair loss, and various behavior changes.[5]

Education of veterinary staff and pet owners is the key to gaining acceptance to veterinary dentistry. Veterinary staff need to recommend dental care early in the disease process. Following a dental procedure, home care is essential. Plaque begins building up within 24 hours of the procedure and without continuing home care the patient can return to preprocedure levels of disease relatively quickly. The combination of preventative and therapeutic dental care will positively impact the quantity and quality of life of our veterinary patients.

ANATOMY

Figures 21.1–21.5 illustrate the anatomy of the canine and feline mouth.

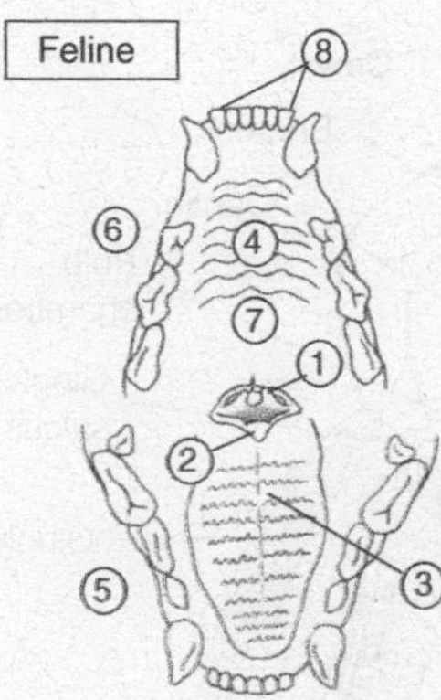

Anatomy of the mouth

1 – Arytenoid cartilage
2 – Epiglottis
3 – Frenulum (under tongue)
4 – Hard palate
5 – Mandible
6 – Maxilla
7 – Soft palate
8 – Incisors

Deciduous teeth = 26
Dental formula
2 × i 3/3 : c 1/1 : p 3/2
Permanent teeth = 30
Dental formula
2 × I 3/3 : C 1/1 : P 3/2 M : 1/1

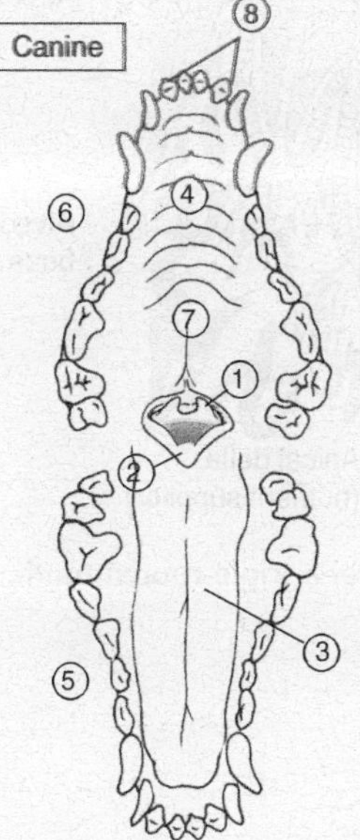

Deciduous teeth = 28
Dental formula
2 × i 3/3 : c 1/1 : p 3/3
Permanent teeth = 30
Dental formula
2 × I 3/3 : C 1/1 : P 4/4 M : 2/3

Figure 21.1 Dentition: canine and feline.

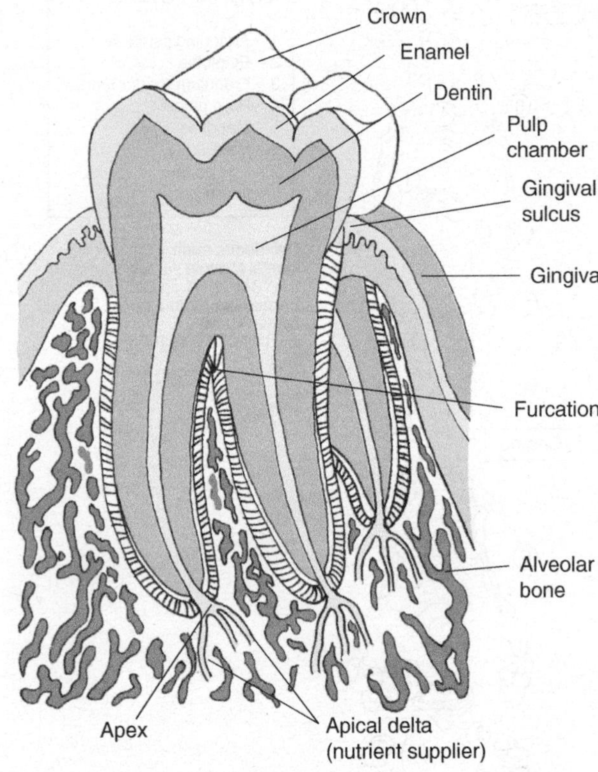

Figure 21.2 Cross-section of a triple-rooted tooth.

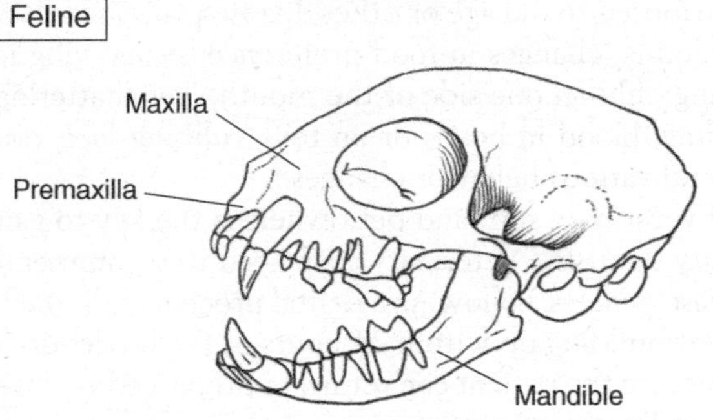

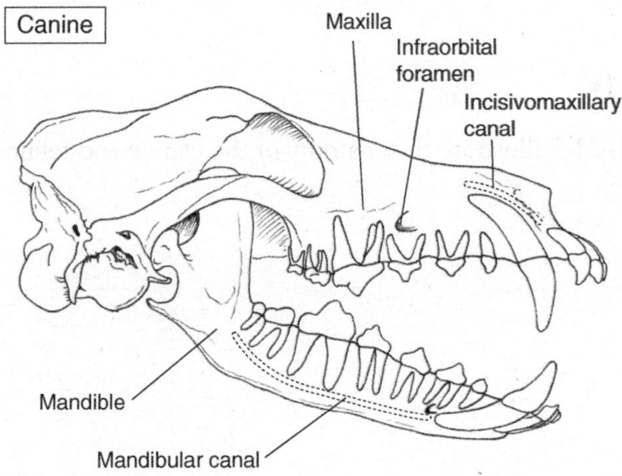

Figure 21.3 Skeletal structure: canine and feline.

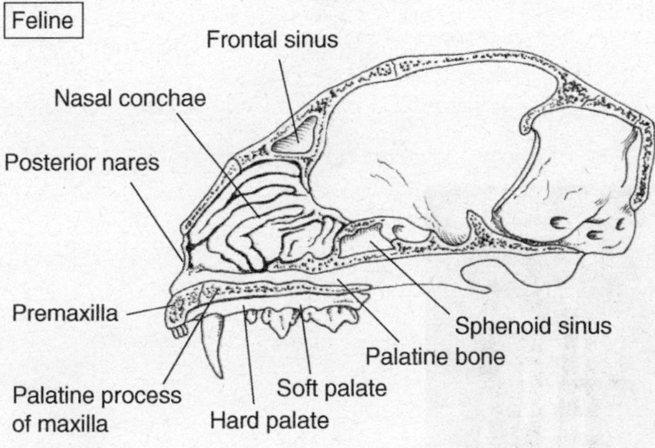

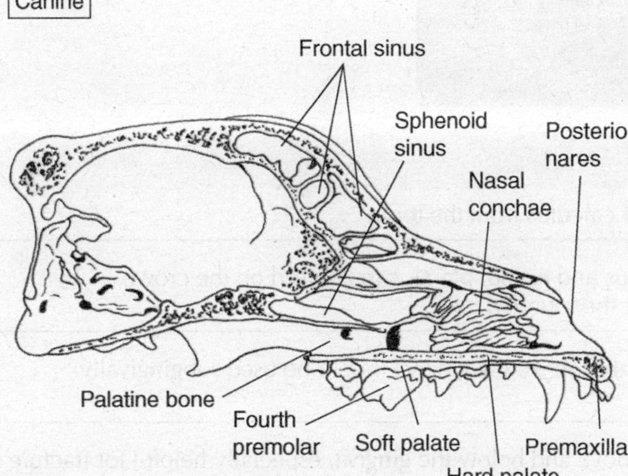

Figure 21.4 Cross-section of facial structures: canine and feline.

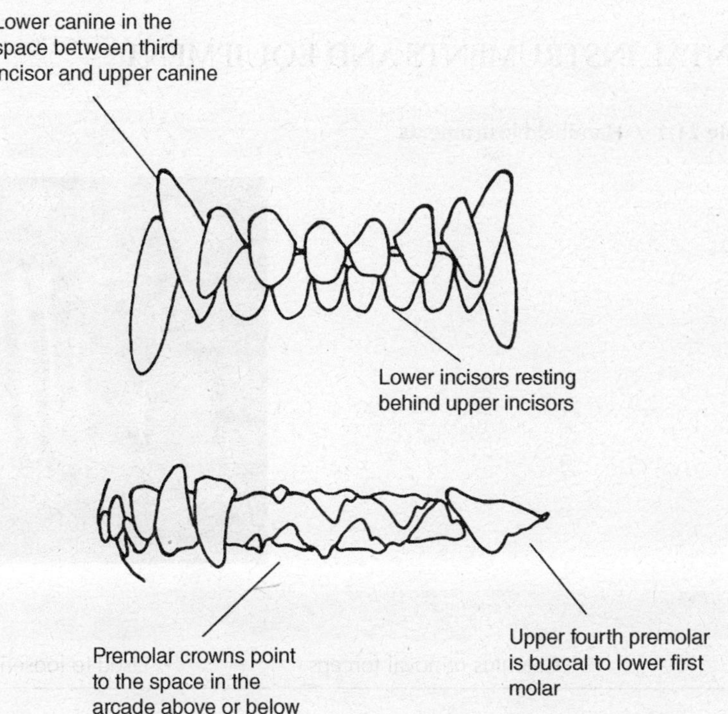

Figure 21.5 Normal occlusion of the canine; feline occlusion is very similar. Artist: Mark Smith.

DENTAL INSTRUMENTS AND EQUIPMENT

Table 21.1 / Handheld instruments

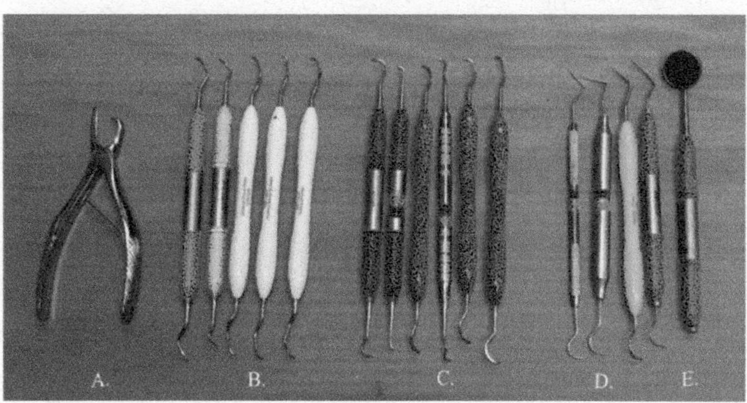

	Instrument	Usage
A	Calculus removal forceps	• Used to loosen and remove large chunks of calculus from the tooth
B	Curette (subgingival)	• Used beneath the gingiva to remove calculus and to root plane, can be used on the crown • Has a rounded toe, cutting surface is inside the rounded toe
C	Hand scaler	• Used on the exposed tooth to remove calculus above the gingiva (not to be used subgingivally) • Has a triangular face and 2 sharp edges
D (lower end)	Explorer	• Used to examine the tooth's surface both above and below the gingiva, especially helpful for fracture sites, tooth resorption, attrition, abrasion and caries • Normal tooth structure should feel glass-like, any roughness is a sign of pathology
D (upper end)	Periodontal probe	• Used to measure the depth of the gingival sulcus, furcation exposure, gingival recession and gingival hyperplasia in millimeters • Probe a minimum of 4–6 locations around each tooth
E	Dental mirror	• Used to view parts of the teeth not easily visible
	Spring-loaded mouth gags (not in picture)	• Not recommended for use on any patient • Use pieces of syringes, endotracheal tubes, wedges, etc.

Table 21.2 / **Extraction instruments**

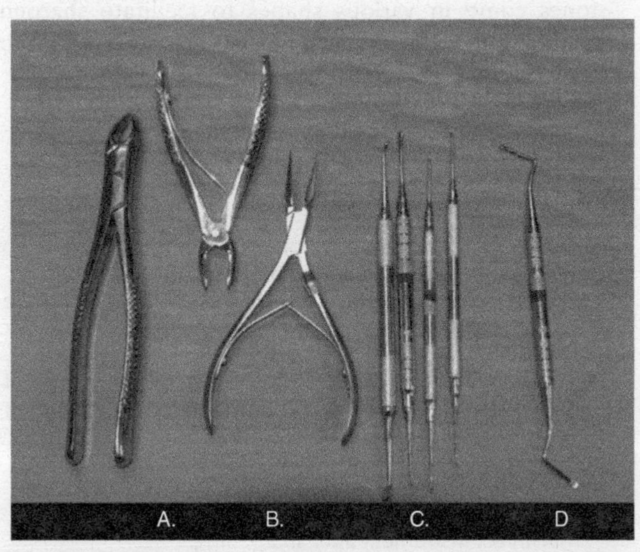

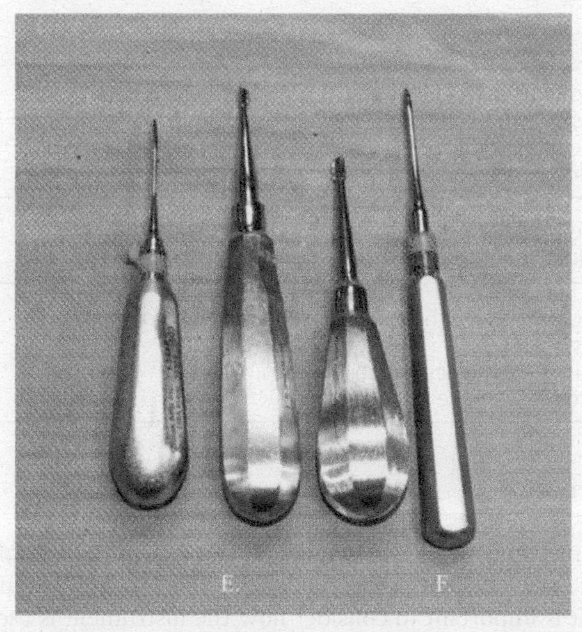

	Instrument	Usage
A	Dental extraction forceps	• Used to remove tooth from its socket • Long-handled and small breed varieties are shown • Small-breed forceps are preferred
B	Fragment forceps	• Used similar to extraction forceps but narrow grasp allows access to smaller areas
C	Periosteal elevators	• Used to reflect mucoperiosteum to expose bone over tooth root • Various sizes available for smaller and larger patients
D	Miller bone curette	• Used to clean alveolus after tooth has been removed
E	Dental elevators and luxators	• Used to cut the periodontal ligament and displace the tooth from the socket • Various sizes are available • Short handles are preferred
F	Root tip pick	• Used to delicately tease fractured root tips from the alveolus

Table 21.3 / Bur types

Type	Use
Round	• Used to remove alveolar bone • Various sizes available, the larger the number the larger the round cutting surface • Cuts along the entire round surface of the bur
Crosscut	• Used to section teeth • Cuts along the side of the bur
Diamond	• Used for smoothing the alveolus after extraction to remove rough surfaces • Come in many shapes and roughness • Most common shape is football

Instrument Maintenance

Sharpening is important to keep the instruments in top performing condition. This will allow for more efficient dental procedures, less operator fatigue, and better sensitivity. It is important to consider how the instrument is used and not change how the instrument functions by sharpening improperly. Improper sharpening may also shorten the life of the instrument. If instruments are sharpened on a routine basis, the process will not take very long and the instrument will be maintained for optimum functionality.

Table 21.4 / Instrument maintenance

Sharpening stones	Type/lubricant required	Use
India	Fine/medium/ coarse—oil lubricant	To sharpen extremely dull instruments or reshape damaged instruments
Arkansas	Fine—oil lubricant	Routine sharpening or to finish sharpening after a medium coarse stone was used
Ceramic	Fine/medium—water lubricant or dry	Same as the other two, but uses water as its lubricant

Sharpening Technique

Handheld instruments need to be sharpened on a regular basis. Sharpening stones come in various shapes to facilitate sharpening. Common shapes include round, flat, conical, wedge, and various combinations (Figure 21.6).

Skill Box 21.1 / Sharpening technique

Flat Stone: Hand Instruments

1. Place small amount of oil onto the stone and wipe to cover the stone face.
2. Place the stone on a flat surface parallel to the floor.
3. Place the instrument to be sharpened on the oiled stone with the tip facing the operator and the face of the instrument on the surface of the stone.
4. Care should be taken so as not to damage the surface of the instrument.
5. Move the instrument up and down on the stone, ending with a down stroke.
6. Check for sharpness by visual inspection or by using an acrylic stick:
    a. Dull edges look rounded and reflect light
    b. Sharp edges give off no light reflection
7. Disinfect instrument after sharpening.

Conical Stone: Hand Instruments

1. Place the instrument in hand with tip pointing outward, wrapped around the oiled conical stone.
2. As you rotate the stone, slide the stone toward the tip of the instrument.
3. This technique may cause more wear to the instrument and shorten its effective life.

Note: In either technique, safety glasses are recommended.

Elevators

1. Using a flat stone, place the instrument in your dominant hand with your index finger at the tip.
2. Place the instrument on the stone at a 45-degree angle. Starting at one side of the rounded sharp edge move the instrument in a smile shaped motion.
3. Use a conical stone or rounded edge on the center of the blade to remove any burrs that may have occurred during the sharpening process.

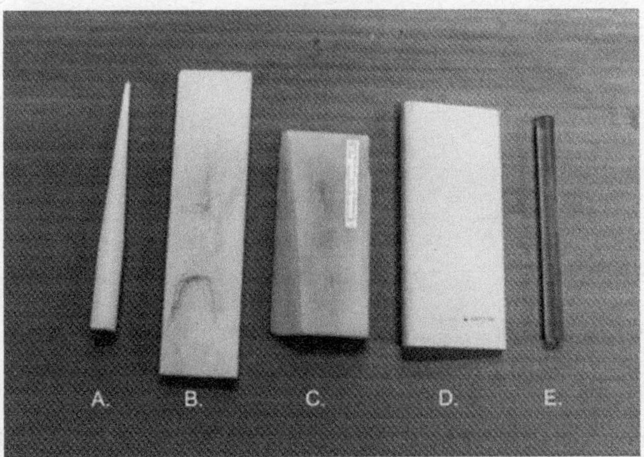

Figure 21.6 Sharpening stones: A) conical; B) flat; C) flat with angled edge; D) angled with rounded edge; E) acrylic stick for testing sharpness.

Mechanical Instruments

Purchasing of dental equipment should be a clinic-directed process, including reviewing the current types of equipment available, an assessment of who will be using it, and what procedures will be performed. Manufacturer's care and maintenance should be followed for all instruments. All power scaler tips should be checked periodically to ensure that they remain in working condition. Some manufacturers recommend replacing the tips every six months while others provide a chart that can be used to measure the length of the tips. The power scaler will not work correctly if the tips are worn or damaged. This will result in a longer procedure.

Table 21.5 / Mechanical instruments (power scalers)

Equipment	Description
Ultrasonic	• Converts energy to sound waves, which results in a mechanical vibration of the handpiece • When water passes over the tip, a scouring property known as cavitation is produced • Follow manufacturer's maintenance guidelines
Magnetostrictive	• Tip vibrates in an elliptical motion; has a working tip on all sides; uses metal stacks
Piezoelectric	• Tip vibrates in a linear motion; only one side of the tip is used against the tooth • Uses crystals in handpieces
Polishers/drilling units	• Two types are available, electric or air driven • Various heads are available • Follow manufacturer's maintenance guidelines
High- and low- speed handpieces	• Ensure that maintenance is performed for proper operation, all handpieces require either oil or conditioning as per manufacturer's instructions

ORAL EXAMINATION, SCALING AND POLISHING

Skill Box 21.2 / Oral examination, scaling and polishing procedure

Step	Method	Comments

1. Setup
• Technician:
  • Face shield or glasses, gloves, surgical mask, optional smock for dental use only, surgical cap
  • Dental equipment and supplies
  • Adjustable stool
• Patient:
  • Appropriate measures to maintain patient's temperature and towels to cushion patient
  • Appropriate monitoring equipment
  • IV catheter/fluids if necessary
  • Pain management protocol
  • Anesthesia protocol
  • Gauze sponges in back of throat to absorb excess water and debris
  • Head positioned downward to permit proper drainage
	See:
	• Heat (thermotherapy) (see Skill Box 13.5: Temperature therapy, page 627)
	• IV catheter placement (see Skill Box 14.9, Intravenous catheter placement: peripheral and jugular, page 663)
	• Fluid therapy (Chapter 14)
	• Pain management (Chapter 18)
	• Anesthetic administration (see Table 20.5: General anesthesia induction, page 872)
	• Anesthesia monitoring (see Table 20.11: Anesthesia monitoring, page 889)
		• Proper setup reduces risk of cumulative trauma disorders (include carpal tunnel syndrome and any trauma caused by repetitive motions) to technicians
		• It is important to perform dentistry procedures from a seated position at the proper height
		• Heating pad with proper cover to ↓ chance of burning, warmed towels, warmed fluid bags, or Baer hugger blanket
		• Doppler or other blood pressure device, pulse oximetry, ECG, and/or apnea monitor

2. Oral examination • Perform a thorough examination of the patient's mouth, charting all abnormal conditions. The veterinarian should be consulted on any abnormality noted	• External examination: check for symmetry of the animal's head and face, halitosis, nasal or ocular discharge or swelling, problems with occlusion, anomalies of lips, mouth or tongue • To evaluate occlusion, note six relationships: incisor, canine, premolar, maxillary fourth premolar/mandibular first molar, head symmetry, and each individual tooth location, this is difficult to do after intubation (see Figure 21.5 for normal occlusion) • Internal examination: inspect the oropharynx during intubation, chart the entire oral cavity including the degree of gingivitis/calculus, missing teeth and any abnormalities that can be visualized at this time; check lips, oral tissues, and tongue for any abnormalities (see Chapter 20: Anesthesia; Table 20.6: Anesthesia induction complications, page 875; Table 20.10: Stages of anesthesia, page 886; Table 20.4: Ventilation, page 867) • Make sure to visualize under the tongue, inside the cheeks, and the palate • Document mouth condition and, if available, take a "pre" and "post" digital photograph (Tables 21.7 and 21.8) • If periodontal disease is identified, administer appropriate nerve blocks (Skill Box 21.3)	• Be gentle with any manipulation of the tongue • Follow a systematic approach to ensure that all teeth are checked, cleaned, and charted

(*Continued*)

Skill Box 21.2 / **Oral examination, scaling and polishing procedure (Continued)**

Step	Method	Comments
3. Full-mouth radiographs	• Radiograph all dentition (Tables 21.11 and 21.12) • Taking radiographs at this point allows the veterinarian to begin designing a treatment plan while the cleaning portion of the procedure is taking place. They can also be taken later in the process	
4. Brushing of teeth	• Brush with chlorhexidine toothpaste and/or irrigate with 0.1–0.2% chlorhexidine solution	• Decreases bacterial load before cleaning. This will reduce the amount of bacteria that is available to enter the patient's bloodstream and aerosolized into the treatment area
5. Removal of gross calculus	• Use a heavy calculus tip for your power scaler to remove heavy calculus. Alternatively, calculus removal forceps may be employed with caution for this task; extraction forceps should not be used for this task • Do not grasp the entire tooth and squeeze but use the forceps along the face of the crown • The blade of the heavy scaler tip can be applied toward the tooth, unlike other scaler tips that should not be placed with the point into the enamel • A hand scaler can be employed using a modified pen grasp, place the scaler at a 45–90-degree angle on the tooth, such that the tip conforms to the curve of the tooth and the cutting edge of the scaler is beneath the calculus. Use a pull stroke away from the gumline • This stroke should use the shoulder muscles and not the wrist • The hand scaler is only used supragingivally	• Power scalers can be used to complete the removal of any remaining calculus • Cautious power scaling is preferred to reduce the possibility of carpal tunnel from hand scaling
6. Power scaling	• Using the same grasp as on a scaler, use light brush stroke touches on the tooth. Keep the tip moving to prevent overheating of the tooth and remain no longer than 10 seconds on any tooth at any one time. If additional calculus remains, allow the tooth to cool before returning • Never apply the point of the scaler tip to the tooth. This will damage the enamel very quickly • Scaler tips are not to be used below the gingiva unless they are specifically designed for that purpose. The design of a standard tip will not allow water to be delivered if the tip is inserted below the gingiva • Scaler tips designed for subgingival use are available and will greatly reduce the amount of time required for the procedure. Ensure that they are used as per the manufacturer's recommendation (i.e. do not insert a tip that is designed for up to a 3-mm pocket in a 5-mm pocket)	

(*Continued*)

Skill Box 21.2 / Oral examination, scaling and polishing procedure (Continued)

Step	Method	Comments

7. Subgingival cleaning and root planing	• Preliminary removal of subgingival calculus can be achieved with specially designed perio tips. They are designed for insertion below the gingiva. Use hand curettes at a 45–90-degree angle with a sharp, firm, pulling stroke in areas beyond the reach of the power scaler tip. Check removal effectiveness with an explorer
	• Root plane, using a curette, on teeth with pocketing of 3–5 mm. Use 10–20 short overlapping strokes (horizontal, vertical, and oblique) to achieve a glassy smooth surface. This can be accomplished without surgery in some cases (pocketing of 4–5 mm) and is noted as RPC; in other cases (pocketing of 5–6 mm), the root will need to be exposed by cutting a flap in the gingiva, which is considered surgery, and charted as RPO
		• Used when pocket depths are:
		  • Canine: 3–5 mm
		  • Feline: 2–4 mm
		• Care must be taken so as not to be too aggressive in these techniques
		• Removing cementum will damage the tooth

8. Air drying of the teeth or using a plaque disclosing solution	• Direct a stream of compressed air to each tooth to inspect for remaining calculus. When dried it will have a chalky appearance • The air will also reflect the unattached gingiva allowing visualization of the gingival sulcus	• Plaque disclosing products are available and can be used but may stain the coat of lighter-colored dogs
9. Polishing the teeth	• Using plenty of fine paste with a light touch (enough to make the cup flare) and a setting according to the manufacturer's guidelines, place the prophylaxis cup on the tooth at the gumline and move smoothly downward. Ensure that every surface of the tooth is polished • Coarse paste does not give a smooth enough surface	• A smooth surface deters plaque accumulation • Make sure an adequate amount of prophy paste is used
10. Irrigation	• Use the air/water syringe to flush prophy paste and debris from the oral cavity	
11. Oral cavity and tooth evaluation	• Measure and chart the gingival sulcus for each tooth, tooth mobility, and general gingival health (Table 21.6) • Probe around the circumference of each tooth in 4–6 locations and note any pocket depths or gingival recession • Make sure all findings are recorded	
12. Adjust patient to the other side and repeat steps 3–10 if cleaning laterally	• Disconnect the endotracheal tube • Rotate the patient to the other side and reconnect the endotracheal tube and start the dental routine	• If the patient is positioned dorsally, the entire mouth can be cleaned without turning the patient

(Continued)

Skill Box 21.2 / Oral examination, scaling and polishing procedure (Continued)

Step	Method	Comments
13. Oral surgery and extractions	• While state laws may vary,[12] the AVDC has recommendations on oral surgery and who should perform it[6] • The AVDC considers operative dentistry to be any dental procedure which invades the hard or soft oral tissue including, but not limited to, a procedure that alters the structure of one or more teeth or repairs damaged and diseased teeth. A veterinarian should perform operative dentistry and oral surgery • The AVDC considers the extraction of teeth to be included in the practice of veterinary dentistry. Decision making is the responsibility of the veterinarian, with the consent of the pet owner, when electing to extract teeth. Only veterinarians shall determine which teeth are to be extracted and perform extraction procedures • See Table 21.15 for order of instrumentation	
14. Optional barrier sealant application	• Apply a barrier sealant to each tooth following the manufacturer's guidelines	• Plaque can reattach to the tooth as soon as 24 hours after cleaning, barrier sealants can slow this process • Apply a barrier sealant to each tooth following the manufacturer's guidelines • There are 2 commercially available products
15. Clean up animal and continue with anesthesia recovery	• Inspect the animal's mouth for blood and debris or gauze and remove if found • Dry off the animal's head with a towel or hair dryer	• Each clinic should set up and follow a cleaning routine for the dental area and equipment
16. Home care instructions	• Home care is critical for all patients, since plaque can reattach to the tooth as soon as 24 hours following a cleaning • There are multiple products available either active or passive • Active homecare is more effective to the mesial teeth • Passive home care is more effective for the distal teeth • Tooth brushing is considered the gold standard, but some studies show that passive homecare may be more effective since owners will do it more consistently • The best care for the patient may ultimately be a combination of active and passive home care • Depending on what oral surgery was performed, the owner should be advised of the next recheck and food recommendations (see Skill Box 2.9: Grooming, page 60)	• Active homecare would involves brushing or applying oral rinses • Passive homecare would involve giving treats or food

DENTAL CHARTING

Table 21.6 shows some generally used charting abbreviations. Your clinic may have adapted their own abbreviations.

The triadan numbering system is the most commonly used system to indicate teeth (Figure 21.7). It works well with digital systems, translates well across languages and adapts to all species. The first number indicates the quadrant. The following two numbers indicate the tooth position in the arcade starting with the central incisor. Canines are always tooth 04 and first molars are always tooth 09.

Full page dental charts are recommended to ensure that there is adequate space for all diagnoses and treatments. Figures 21.8 and 21.9 show dental assessment charts for dogs and cats, respectively.

Table 21.6 / **Dental charting**

Area of concern	Method	Charting symbol	Description
Abrasion	Visual examination, radiograph	AB	• Wear indicated by brown staining in the center with no access to the pulp cavity by an explorer • All teeth with wear require a radiograph to evaluate for infection and pain • Abrasion is wear on a tooth or teeth from anything other than another tooth • Attrition is wear on a tooth or teeth from another tooth, make sure to evaluate the occlusion
Attrition		AT	
Calculus index	Determined visually	CI1	• Calculus covers ½ of the crown
		CI2	• Calculus covers ¾ of the crown
		CI3	• Calculus covers all the crown and is found subgingivally
Enamel hypoplasia	Visual examination	E/H	• Enamel is thin, missing or flaking off
Hypomineralization	Radiograph	E/HM	
Extractions	Radiograph	X	• Simple extraction (1 root)
		XS	• Sectioned extraction (2–3 roots)
		XSS	• Surgical extraction (requires gingival flap)
Furcation exposure	Visual examination	F1	• Periodontal probe can be inserted into the furcation but less than half way under the tooth
	Periodontal probe	F2	• Probe extends more than half way but not through the tooth
	Radiograph	F3	• Probe passes through the furcation

(Continued)

Table 21.6 / **Dental charting (Continued)**

Area of concern	Method	Charting symbol	Description
Gingivitis index	Visual examination and periodontal probe	GI0	• Normal: gum tissue is shrimp color; sharp gingival margins
		GI1	• Marginal gingivitis: mild inflammation, slight color change
		GI2	• Moderate gingivitis, gingiva bleeds upon probing
		GI3	• Severe gingivitis, gingiva bleeds with mild contact
Gingival hyperplasia	Periodontal probe, radiograph	GH + the mm of tissue above the normal gingival margin (e.g. GH2)	• Indicates the presence of a pseudopocket; this will cause periodontal disease: veterinarian should be consulted • Should be confirmed with biopsy
Gingival recession	Periodontal probe used to measure the distance between the enamel or normal gingival margin and the cementum, radiograph	GR + mm of recession (e.g. GR5)	• Indicates periodontal disease and attachment loss; veterinarian should be consulted
Missing teeth	Visual examination, radiograph	Circled on chart	• Radiograph to see whether tooth is impacted or root is retained
Non-vital tooth	Visual examination, radiograph	T/NV	• Most discolored teeth are NV • May have a larger pulp chamber than the contralateral tooth
Oronasal fistula	Visual examination, periodontal probe, radiograph	ONF	• There may be a visible hole if the tooth has exfoliated • There may be nothing visible on radiograph, probing the palatal side if the tooth will detect inapparent ONF
Periodontal disease Index	Periodontal probe, radiograph	PD0	• Normal
		PD1	• Gingivitis only
		PD2	• Up to 25% attachment loss, early periodontitis
		PD3	• 25–50% attachment loss, moderate periodontitis
		PD4	• Over 50% attachment loss, severe periodontitis

(Continued)

Table 21.6 / **Dental charting (Continued)**

Area of concern	Method	Charting symbol	Description
Pocketing	Periodontal probe placed in gingival sulcus and walked around the tooth, radiograph	P + the mm depth (e.g. P5)	• Normal: 1–3 mm (canine) and 0.5–1 mm (feline) • ↑ Pocketing depths indicate periodontal disease and attachment loss; the veterinarian should be consulted
Retained root	Visual examination, periodontal probe, radiograph	RTR	• Tooth crown is missing, but roots are still present • Use the probe to determine if there is a draining tract from the root into the oral cavity
Root planing		RPC	• Closed root planing
		RPO	• Open root planing
Supernumerary	Radiograph	SN and draw tooth and/or root	• Mark on chart where the extra tooth or root is located
Tooth fractures	Visual examination, explorer, radiograph		• Use the explorer to feel the fracture site for an opening into the pulp • *Every* tooth fracture requires a radiograph; the dentin is porous and even uncomplicated fractures can result in infection and pain
Complicated crown fracture		CCF	• Fracture extends through the enamel and the dentin into the pulp
Uncomplicated crown fracture		UCF	• Fracture extends through the enamel into the dentin but not into the pulp
Complicated crown root fracture		CCRF	• Fracture extends through the enamel and dentin into the pulp chamber but also involves the root surface
Uncomplicated crown root fracture		UCRF	• Fracture is through the enamel and dentin but not into the pulp, also involves the root surface

(*Continued*)

Table 21.6 / **Dental charting (Continued)**

Area of concern	Method	Charting symbol	Description
Tooth mobility	Periodontal probe, radiograph	M0	• Normal physiologic movement up to 0.2 mm
		M1	• Slight mobility: 0.2 mm → 0.5 mm movement
		M2	• Moderate mobility: 0.5 → 1.0 mm movement
		M3	• Marked mobility: > 1.0 mm of movement, any axial movement[7]
Tooth resorption	Visual examination, explorer, radiograph	TR1	• Enamel, cementum or both are the only structure(s) affected
		TR2	• Dentin affected; lesion does not enter pulp
		TR3	• Pulp penetration
		TR4	• Significant structure has been lost, pulp penetration
		TR5	• Crown is gone, gingiva covers lesion[8]

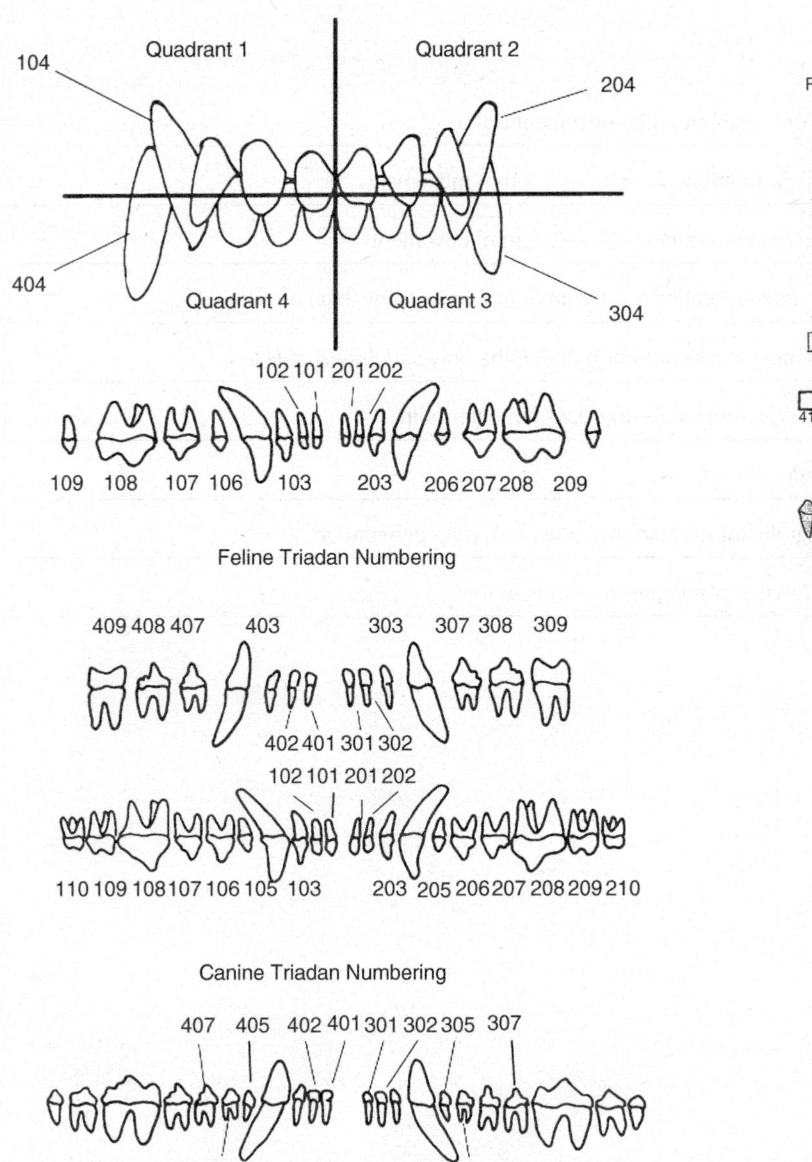

Figure 21.7 Triadan numbering system.

Canine Dental Chart

Patient Name______________________ Date________

110 109 108 107 106 105 104 103 102 101 201 202 203 204 205 206 207 208 209 210

411 410 409 408 407 406 405 404 403 402 401 301 302 303 304 305 306 307 308 309 310 311

Right Occlusal Left

Intraoral Regional Nerve Blocks ______________________

Middle Mental	R	L	_____ml
Inferior Alveolar	R	L	_____ml
Infraorbital	R	L	_____ml
Maxillary	R	L	_____ml

ABBREVIATIONS
AB abrasion (1-3)
AT attrition (1-3)
BG bone graft
B/I biopsy incisional
B/E biopsy excisional
CA caries
CI calculus index (1-3)
CRA crown amputation
CRR crown reduction
CWD crowding
ED enamel defect
EH enamel hypo plasia/calcif
F furcation exposure (1-3)
GH gingival hyperplasia
GI gingivitis index
GR gingival recession
GV gingivectomy
M mobility (1-3)
MN/FX mandibular fracture
MX/FX maxillary fracture

O missing tooth
OM oral mass
ONF oronasal fistula
P (#) periodontal pocket (#=mm)
PCT perioceutic
PDI periodontal disease index
PH pulp hemorrhage
RC root canal therapy
R/C restoration composite
RD retained deciduous
ROT rotated
RPC root planing closed
RPO root planing open
RR internal root resorption
RRT retained root tip
RTR retained tooth root
SC subgingival curettage
SN supernumerary
SYMP symphysis

T/FX tooth fracture
EI enamel infraction
EF enamel fracture
UCF uncomplicated crown fx
CCF complicated crown fx
UCRF uncomplicated crown root fx
CCRF complicated crown root fx
TR –Tooth resorption
1-enamel only
2-enamel and dentin
3-into pulp
4–extensive damage
4a crown & root equally affected
4b crown more affected than root
4c root more affected than crown
5 crown missing
VP vital pulp therapy
X simple closed extraction
XS extraction with tooth sectioning
XSS surgical extraction

GI _____
CI _____
PDI _____

MIDMARK

Figure 21.8 Canine dental assessment chart. Source: courtesy of Midmark Corporation (www.midmark.com).

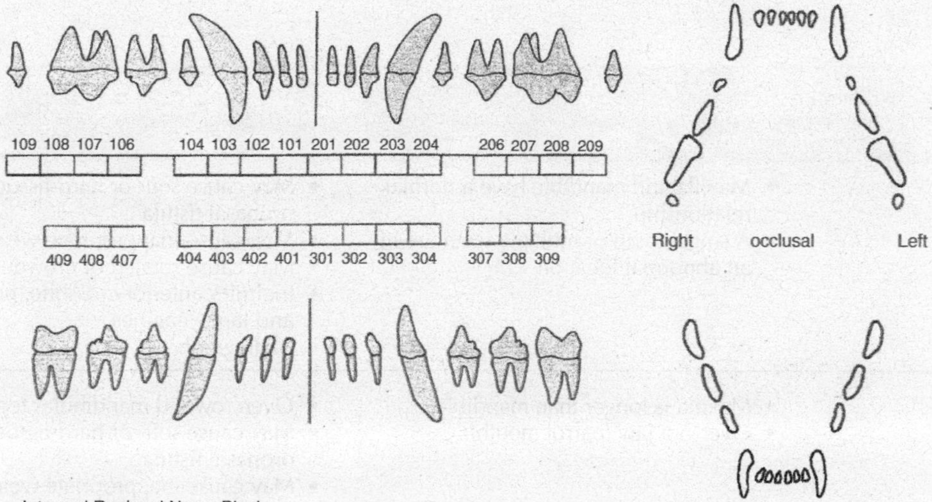

Feline Dental Chart

Patient Name ________________ Date _______

109 108 107 106 104 103 102 101 201 202 203 204 206 207 208 209

409 408 407 404 403 402 401 301 302 303 304 307 308 309

Right occlusal Left

Intraoral Regional Nerve Blocks

Inferior Alveolar RL ______ ml

Infraorbital RL ______ ml

Maxillary RL ______ ml

ABBREVIATIONS

AB abrasion (1-3)
AT attrition (1-3)
BG bone graft
B/1 biopsy incisional
B/E biopsy excisional
CA caries
CI calculus index (1-3)
CRA crown amputation
CRR crown reduction
CWD crowding
ED enamel defect
EH enamel hypo plasia/calcif
F furcation exposure (1-3)
GH gingival hyperplasia
GI gingivitis index
GR gingival recession
GV gingivectomy
M mobility (1 -3)
MN/FX mandibular fracture
MN/FX maxillary fracture

O missing
OM oral mass
ONF oronasal fistula
P (#) periodontal pocket (#=mm)
PCT perioceutic
PDI periodontal disease index
PH pulp hemorrhage
RC root canal
R/C restoration composite
RD retained deciduous .
ROT rotated therapy
RPC root planing closed
RPO root planing open
RR internal root resorption
RRT retained root tip
RTR retained tooth root
SC subgingival curettage
SN supernumerary
SYMP symphysis

TIFX tooth fracture
EI enamel infraction
EF enamel fracture
UCF uncomplicated crown fx
CCF complicated crown fx
UCRF uncomplicated crown root fx
CCRF complicated crown root fx
TR – Tooth resorption
1- enamel only
2- enamel and dentin
3- into pulp
4 –extensive damage
4a crown & root equally affected
4b crown more affected than root
4c root more affected than crown
5 crown missing
VP vital pulp therapy
X simple closed extraction
XS extraction with tooth sectioning
XSS surgical extraction

GI ______

CI ______

PDI ______

MIDMARK

Figure 21.9 Feline dental assessment chart. Source: courtesy of Midmark Corporation (www.midmark.com).

COMMON DENTAL DISORDERS

While it is the veterinarian's responsibility to diagnose the following problems, the technician can assist the veterinarian by being aware of the following conditions and their presentation.

Table 21.7 / Anatomical disorders

Disorders	Charting symbol	Description	Comments
Class 1 malocclusion, neutroclusion	MAL1	• Maxilla and mandible have a normal relationship • A single tooth or multiple teeth are in an abnormal location	• May cause soft- or hard-tissue damage and possible formation of oronasal fistula • May cause inappropriate wear on teeth due to contact • May cause rotated or crowded teeth • Includes anterior crossbite, posterior crossbite, base narrow canines and lance canines • Radiograph
Class 2 malocclusion, mandibular distoclusion	MAL2	• Maxilla is longer than mandible • Overshot jaw (parrot mouth)	• Overcrowded mandibular teeth; ↑ chance of periodontal disease • May cause soft- or hard-tissue damage and possible formation of oronasal fistula • May cause inappropriate wear on teeth due to contact • May cause rotated or crowded teeth • Radiograph
Class 3 malocclusion, mandibular mesioclusion	MAL3	• Maxilla is shorter than mandible • Upper incisors are distal to the lower incisors	• May cause inappropriate wear on teeth due to contact • May cause soft- or hard-tissue damage • May cause rotated or crowded teeth • Radiograph
Class 4 malocclusion, maxillomandibular asymmetry	MAL4	• One quadrant develops unevenly from other quadrants	• May cause inappropriate wear on teeth due to contact • May cause soft- or hard-tissue damage • May cause rotated or crowded teeth • Radiograph
Dental interlock	–	• Caused when mandibular canines are distal to maxillary canines	• Prevents forward growth of the mandible • May cause soft- or hard-tissue damage • May cause inappropriate wear on teeth due to contact • Requires early intervention (removing deciduous teeth) for best result • Radiograph

(*Continued*)

Table 21.7 / **Anatomical disorders (Continued)**

Disorders	Charting symbol	Description	Comments
Impacted tooth	T/I	• Teeth did not erupt correctly • May cause formation of a dentigerous cyst	• Any tooth that appears to be missing requires a radiograph to determine if it is impacted • Radiograph
Missing tooth	–	• Should be circled on the dental chart	• Radiograph to ensure the tooth is not impacted
Oligodontia	–	• Fewer teeth than considered normal	• Typically, incisors or premolars but can be any tooth
persistent deciduous	RD	• Permanent teeth erupt, and deciduous teeth fail to exfoliate	• Can cause malocclusion • Can cause periodontal disease • Deciduous teeth should be removed as soon as adult teeth are visible
Polydontia (supernumerary)	SN	• More teeth than considered normal	• ↑ Chance of PD

Table 21.8 / **Pathological disorders**

Disorders	Charting symbol	Description	Comments
Caries	CA	• Occur on molars	• Always use explorer to examine dark staining on molars, normal tooth structure will feel glass-like, a cary will feel "sticky" • Radiograph
Enamel hypoplasia	E/H	• Sections of enamel are reduced or missing	• Radiograph
Gingival hyperplasia	GH	• Overgrowth of gingival tissue	• Can be drug-induced (e.g. cyclosporine) • Breed predilection – Boxers • Radiograph as pseudopockets can cause periodontal disease
Oral mass	OM	• Numerous types and can involve any tissue • Can be malignant or benign • Numerous abbreviations for the different types once a biopsy is completed	• B/E or B/I • Radiograph

(*Continued*)

Table 21.8 / **Pathological disorders (Continued)**

Disorders	Charting symbol	Description	Comments
Oronasal fistula	ONF	• Abnormal opening between the oral and nasal cavities; can be visible or inapparent • Possible clinical signs: inappetence, halitosis, nasal discharge and/or sneezing but can be present with no apparent symptoms • A periodontal probe will extend from the palatal aspect of the maxillary canine to the nasal cavity	• Typically caused by periodontal disease or trauma • Always probe the palatal aspect of the maxillary canines to detect inapparent ONF • Radiograph
Periodontal disease	PD	• Infection of hard and soft support systems of the tooth	• Can result in the loss of teeth and changes in the pet's overall systemic health • Radiograph to identify disease not apparent in the oral cavity
Stomatitis	ST	• An inflammation of the soft tissue of the oral cavity	• Causes severe pain
Tooth fractures		• Can occur with any tooth	• Can be infected and painful • Can cause swelling or draining tracts • Radiograph
Tooth resorption	TR	• Breakdown of the structure of the tooth, can be enamel, dentin, cementum or all • Previously known as osteoclastic resorptive lesions, external odontoclastic resorption, cervical line lesions, cervical neck lesions, feline odontoclastic resorption lesions	• Painful to animal • Radiographs should be taken prior to extraction
Tumors, malignant[9]		• Benign and malignant masses can appear very similar	• Radiograph
Malignant melanoma	OM/MM	• Canine: orally a very aggressive tumor • Can be pigmented or unpigmented	• Metastases common • Most common malignant tumor in canines (rare in felines) • New cancer treatment is available (e.g. melanoma vaccine)
Squamous cell carcinoma	OM/SCC	• Canine: Locally invasive; metastases is rare. • Feline: Locally invasive, rapid growing cancer; metastases is rare	• Second most common malignant tumor in canines and most common in felines
Fibrosarcoma	OM/FS	• Locally invasive • High recurrence rate	• Metastases uncommon • Third most common malignant tumor in canines.

(Continued)

Table 21.8 / Pathological disorders (Continued)			
Disorders	**Charting symbol**	**Description**	**Comments**
Benign oral masses:			
Oral cysts		• Various types including dentigerous cysts, which form around unerupted teeth	• Radiograph all "missing" teeth
Eosinophilic granuloma complex		• Cause unknown • Various manifestations including what is commonly called a rodent ulcer • Treatment varies	

RADIOLOGY

The importance of radiography in dentistry cannot be underestimated. It provides information that cannot be obtained by any other method. Studies have shown that 27.8% of lesions in dogs and 41.7% of lesions in cats will not be identified without dental radiographs.[10] Full-mouth dental radiography is rapidly becoming standard of care since many conditions cannot be diagnosed properly without radiography. Radiographs assist in the determination of complete root remnant removal after a tooth extraction, identifying unerupted and/or impacted teeth, the status of periodontal disease, the presence of endodontic disease and/or the progress of a therapeutic program. Radiographs also assist in the diagnosis of fistulas, cysts, tumors, and neoplasms. Radiographs are critical in evaluation and treatment of feline tooth resorption and treatment of these patients should not be attempted without radiography.[11] See Chapter 4: Diagnostic Imaging for an in-depth discussion of radiology.

Radiographic Anatomy

Technicians need a basic understanding of radiographic anatomy to ensure that they acquire all of the information that the veterinarian will need to make a diagnosis. At a minimum, the image should include everything not visible in the oral cavity. The image of the root must extend 3 mm past the apex. With a size-2 sensor obtaining all of the crown and all of the root may require multiple images.

It is important to orient dental radiographs correctly when viewing. The standard is viewing as if the viewer were looking at the face of the dog. Therefore, the right of the patient is to the viewers left and the crowns of the maxillary teeth point downward (Figures 21.10–21.12).

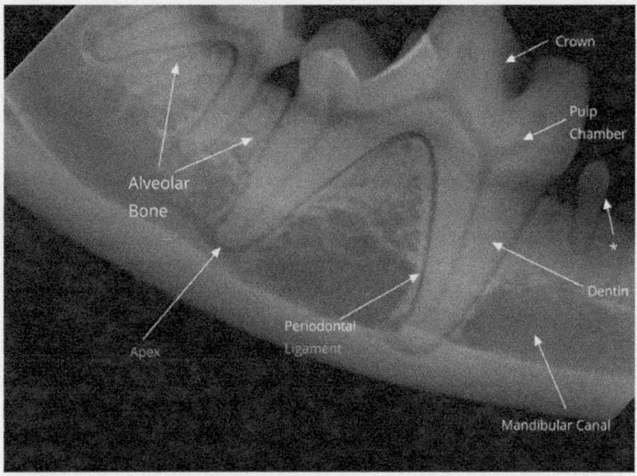

Figure 21.10 Canine mandible *This patient has microdontia. Tooth 408 is very small and does not have the normal number of roots.

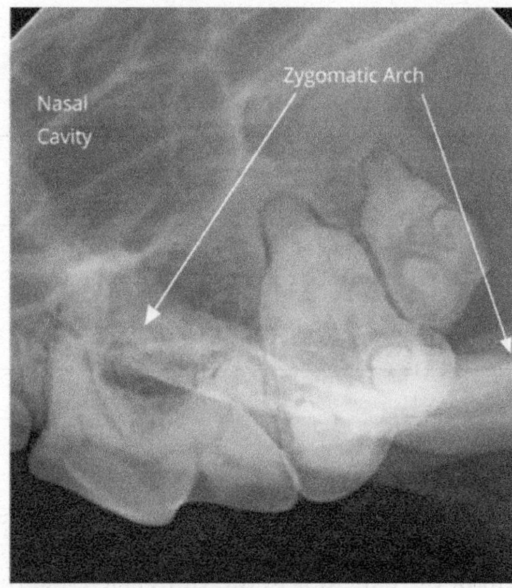

Figure 21.11 Canine maxilla.

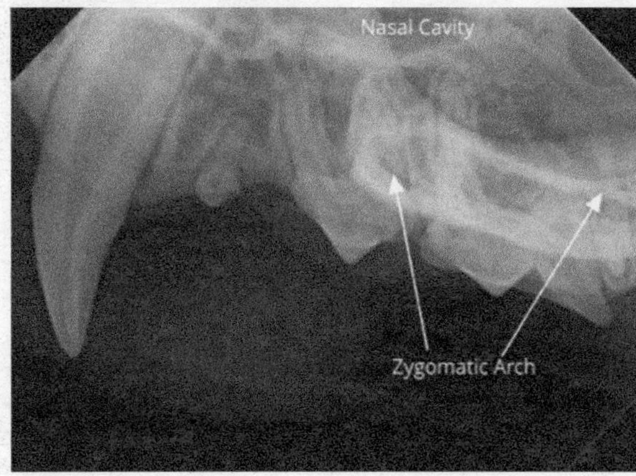

Figure 21.12 Feline maxilla. Various methods can be used to decrease the appearance of the zygomatic arch in feline patients. An extraoral image can be taken or the angle between the tube head and the sensor can be decreased.

Radiographic Equipment

There are a variety of suppliers and configurations of dental x-ray equipment. The preferred configuration is to have a wall-mounted unit but that is not ideal for every situation. Other options include mobile and hand held units. Using the clinic's whole-body x-ray in an attempt to produce dental radiographs is time consuming and does not generate the same quality radiograph. Various positioning aids can be employed to generate the radiographs. The operator should remain a minimum of six feet from the generator and/or wear safety apparel. Dosimetry badges must be worn while obtaining dental radiographs.

Table 21.9 / Radiographic equipment

Type of equipment	Advantages	Disadvantages
Wall mounted	• Preferred • Does not require floor space	• Reinforced wall space must be available • Can only be used in one location
Mobile	• Can be used in multiple locations	• Requires floor space in a usually crowded area
Handheld	• Requires no floor or wall space • Can be used in multiple locations	• Heavy • Can be damaged if dropped • Does not allow the operator to maintain the minimum distance

Table 21.10 / Radiographic media

Type of media	Advantages	Disadvantages
Film • Handling: side with the raised dot always faces the x-ray beam. Raised dot should always be placed in the mouth in the same orientation	• Minimal initial expense • Various sizes available	• Toxic chemicals must be used and disposed of and staff is exposed • Films must be stored and can degrade over time • Difficult to send for consultation • Becoming obsolete
Sensor-based (DR)	• Image is rapidly available • Sensor can be left in place and adjustments made if the image is unacceptable • Images store in original quality with no degrading over time • No toxic chemicals required • Easy to send for consultation • Require less exposure, better compliance with ALARA • Faster learning curve for positioning	• Sensor is very expensive, and care must be taken to ensure that the patient does not "bite" the sensor • Initial investment is high • Requires back up system
Phosphor plate (computed radiography)	• Various size plates available • Cost of plates is less than DR sensors • Images store in original quality with no degrading over time • No toxic chemicals required • Easy to send for consultation • Require less exposure, better compliance with ALARA	• Plates can be scratched or damaged • Initial investment is high • Requires a backup system

Radiographic Techniques

Table 21.11 / Radiographic techniques

Technique	Description	Usage
Parallel	• Place patient in dorsal, sternal, or lateral recumbency • Position media parallel to the long axis of the tooth, but as close to the tooth as possible • X-ray beam is positioned perpendicular (90-degree angle) to the film and the axis of the tooth	• Evaluating distal mandibular premolars, molars, or nasal cavity • Positions where the media may be positioned next to the structure to be imaged
Bisecting angle	• Place patient in dorsal, sternal, or lateral recumbency • Film is placed intraorally • The beam is placed over the root of the tooth of interest and perpendicular to an imaginary bisecting line located between the plane of the tooth axis and the plane of the film • Tip: a tongue depressor can be used to help visualize the bisecting angle	• Evaluating maxillary premolars and molars, and both maxillary/mandibular canines, mesial premolars and incisors • The goal is accurate angles that minimize distortion of the teeth

(*Continued*)

Table 21.11 / Radiographic techniques (Continued)

Technique	Description	Usage
Simple method	• Various simple methods are available. Bisecting angle can be difficult to visualize and time consuming to calculate • Simple methods involve placing the patient in the same orientation every time and will provide set angles for each type of tooth • This allows the operator to become fast at obtaining the radiographs since they are taking the same views over and over	• The goal is accurate angles that minimize distortion of the teeth • In this type of system parallel technique is also used in the distal mandible

Radiographic Positioning

Table 21.12 / Radiographic positioning

View		Positioning	Visualization diagram for bisecting angle	Radiograph
Incisor teeth	Rostral maxillary view	• Patient: sternal or lateral recumbency • Media: placed against the canine and premolar tips • Beam: centered over the midline of the nose and perpendicular to the bisecting line. On small canines and felines, the beam will need to be centered more over the nose • Simplified: media placement would be the same, but patient would be positioned with palate parallel to the tabletop if sternal or perpendicular to the table top if lateral, tube head should be angled 60–70 degrees from the media if sternal or 29–30 degrees if lateral • Beam: centered over the midline of the nose and perpendicular to the bisecting line. On small canines and felines, the beam will need to be centered more over the nose	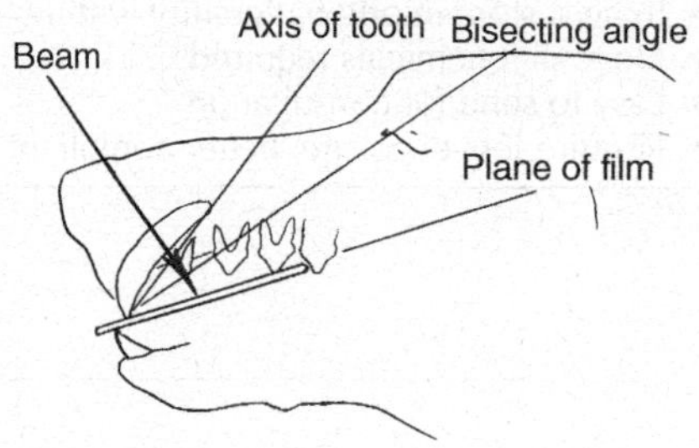	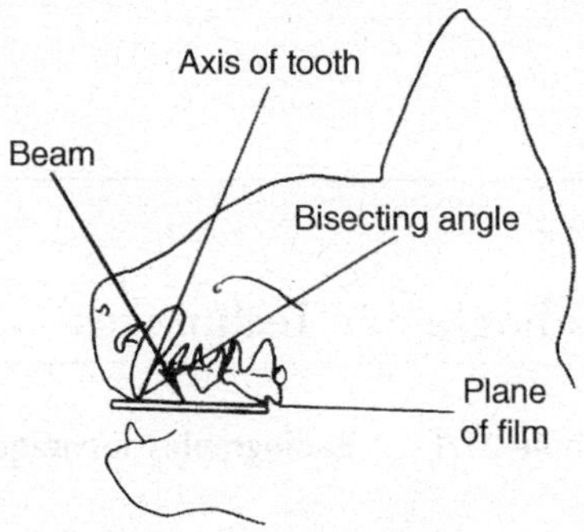

(Continued)

Table 21.12 / **Radiographic positioning (Continued)**

	View	Positioning	Visualization diagram for bisecting angle	Radiograph
Canine teeth	Rostral maxillary view	• Patient: sternal or lateral recumbency • Media: placed against the canine and premolar tips • Beam: centered over the canine tooth and perpendicular to the bisecting line. The beam will be more lateral than for the incisor view • Simplified: media placement would be the same, but patient would be positioned with palate parallel to the tabletop if sternal or perpendicular to the table top if lateral, tube head should be angled 60–70 degrees from the media if sternal or 20–30 degrees if lateral • The view taken straight from the front of the patient is not considered diagnostic for the canine due to superimposition of the premolars on the canine root	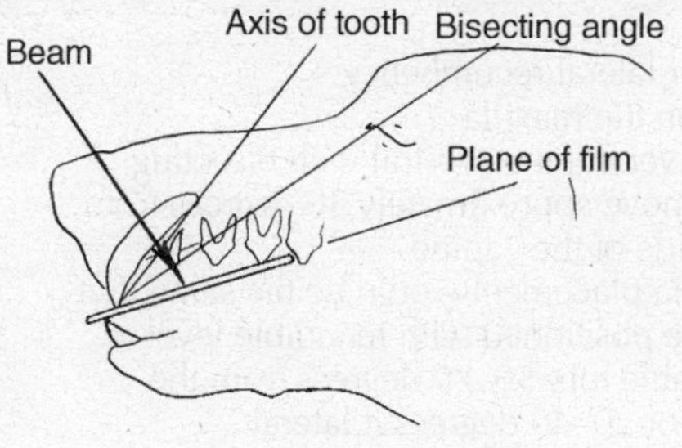	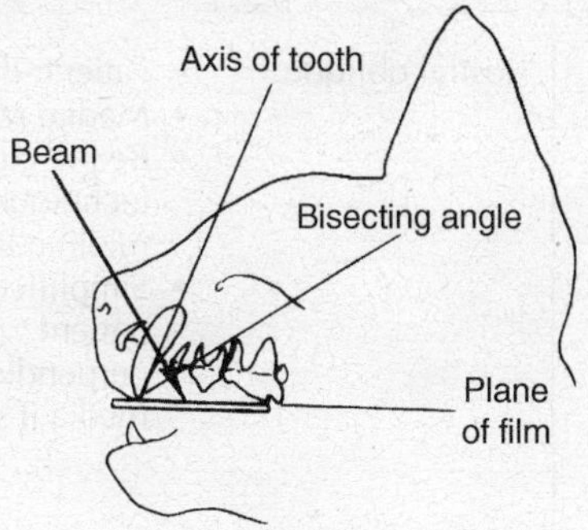
	Rostral mandibular view	• Patient: dorsal or lateral recumbency • Media: placed against the canine and premolar tips of the maxilla • Beam: directed rostrocaudally, centered over the chin perpendicular to the bisecting line • Simplified: media placement would be the same, but patient would be positioned with mandible parallel to the tabletop if sternal or perpendicular to the table top with nose raised if lateral, tube head should be angled 45–70° from the media if sternal or 20–45° if lateral	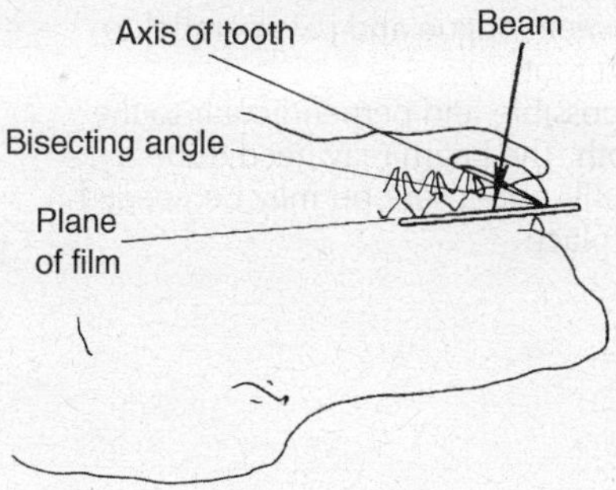	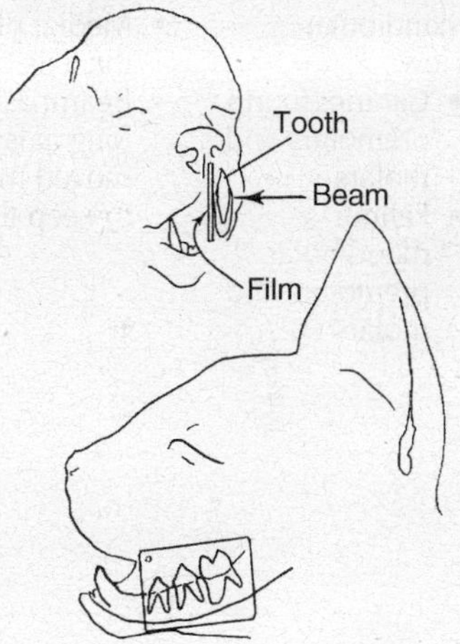

(Continued)

Table 21.12 / Radiographic positioning (Continued)

	View	Positioning	Visualization diagram for bisecting angle	Radiograph
	Rostral oblique	• Patient: dorsal or lateral recumbency • Media: resting on the maxilla • Beam: closer to ventral than rostral with bisecting technique, but move approximately 30 degrees from midline to the side of the canine • Simplified: media placement would be the same, but patient would be positioned with mandible level or perpendicular table top, 50–70 degrees from the media if sternal or 20–40 degrees if lateral		
Premolar and molar teeth	Caudal mandibular view: • Canine: fourth premolars and molars • Feline: mandibular premolars and molars	• Patient: any • Media: placed between tongue and jaw; parallel to the axis of the tooth roots • Beam: as close as possible and perpendicular to the long axis of the tooth. The beam may need to be moved more ventrally, and a support may be needed to keep the film in place		

(*Continued*)

Table 21.12 / **Radiographic positioning (Continued)**

View	Positioning	Visualization diagram for bisecting angle	Radiograph
Rostral mandibular view: • Canine: premolars	• Patient: dorsal or lateral recumbency • Media: vertical to table in mouth, placed at the crown of near lower canine and base of opposite lower canine • Beam: centered over premolars and bisecting lower canine • Simplified: media placement on the maxilla, positioned with mandible parallel to the tabletop if sternal or perpendicular to the table top if lateral, tube head should be angled 50–70 degrees from the media if sternal or 20–40 degrees if lateral	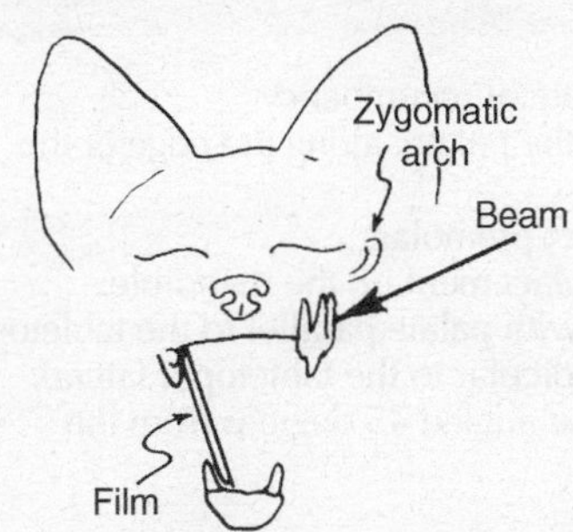 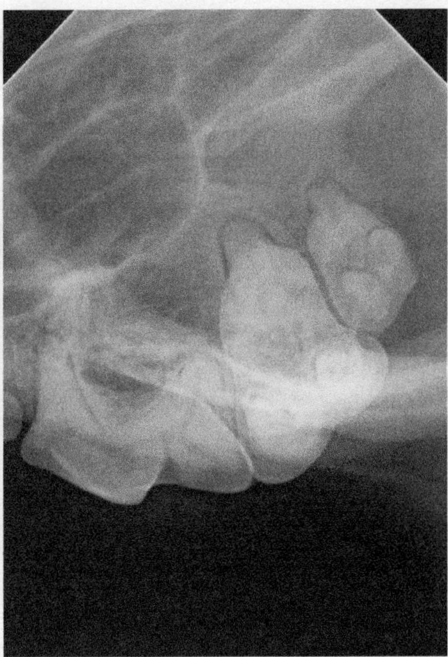	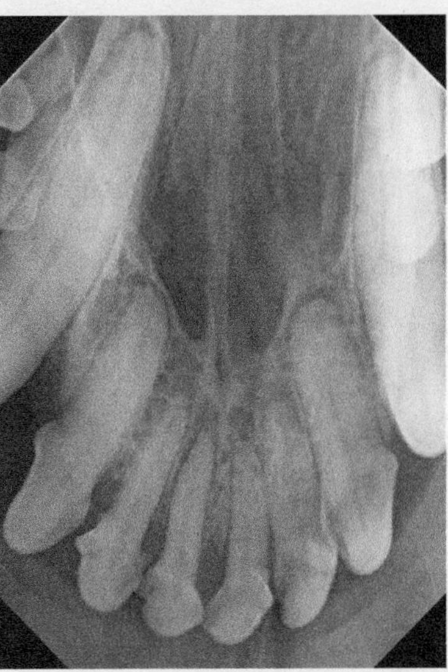

(*Continued*)

Table 21.12 / **Radiographic positioning (Continued)**

View	Positioning	Visualization diagram for bisecting angle	Radiograph
Rostral maxillary view: • Canine: canines and premolars	• Patient: sternal or lateral recumbency • Media: laid across the palate, along the edge of the crowns • Beam: centered over premolars • Simplified: media placement on the mandible, patient positioned with palate parallel to the tabletop if sternal or perpendicular to the tabletop if lateral, tube head should be angled 45 degrees from the media	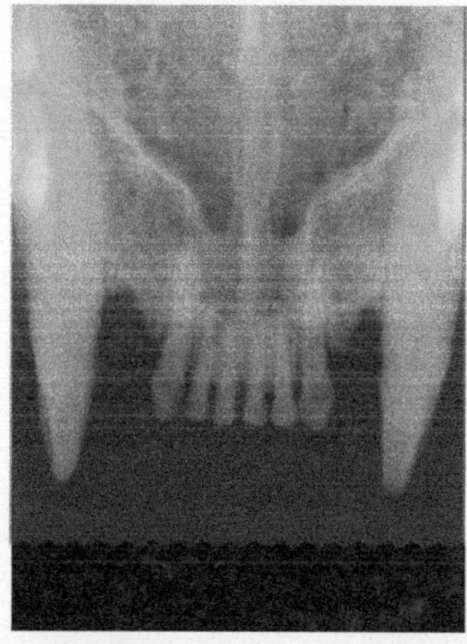 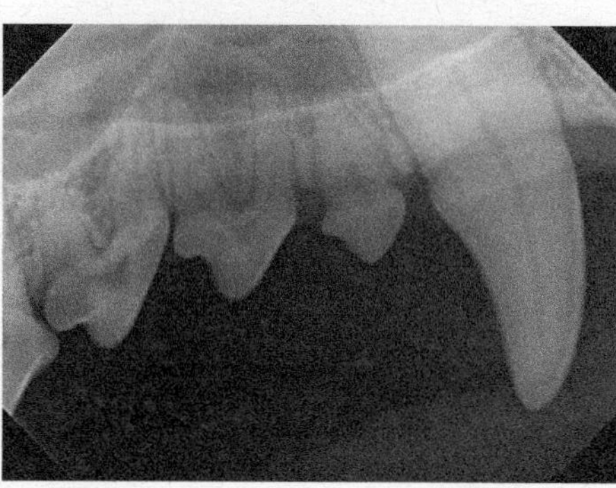	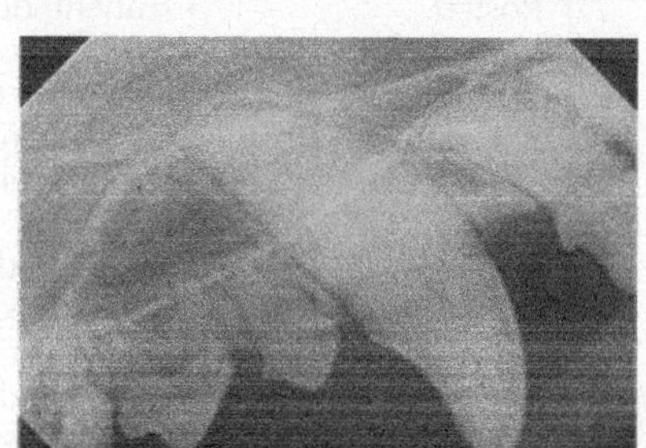

(*Continued*)

Table 21.12 / **Radiographic positioning (Continued)**

View	Positioning	Visualization diagram for bisecting angle	Radiograph
Caudal maxillary view: • Canine: fourth premolar and molars	• Patient: sternal or lateral recumbency • Media: laid across the palate • Beam: directed at the middle of the fourth premolar • Simplified: media placement would be the same, but patient would be positioned with palate parallel to the tabletop if sternal or perpendicular to the tabletop if lateral, tube head should be angled 60 degrees from the media if sternal or 30 degrees if lateral	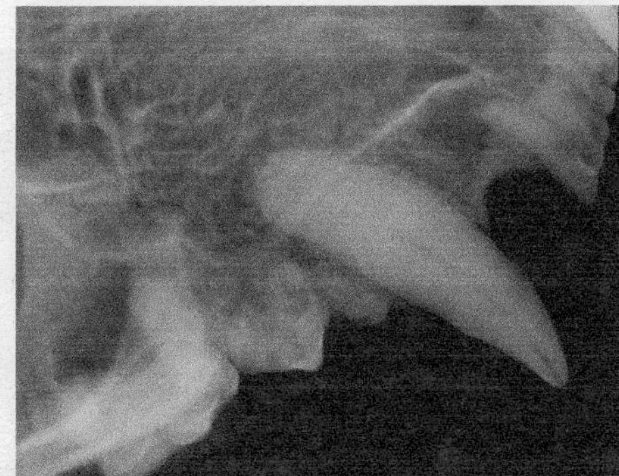 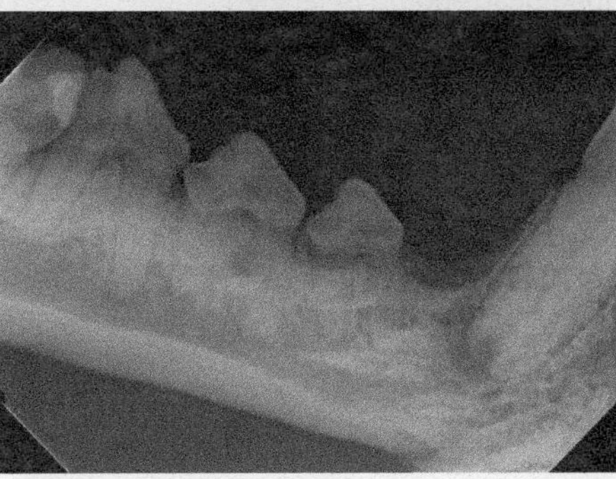	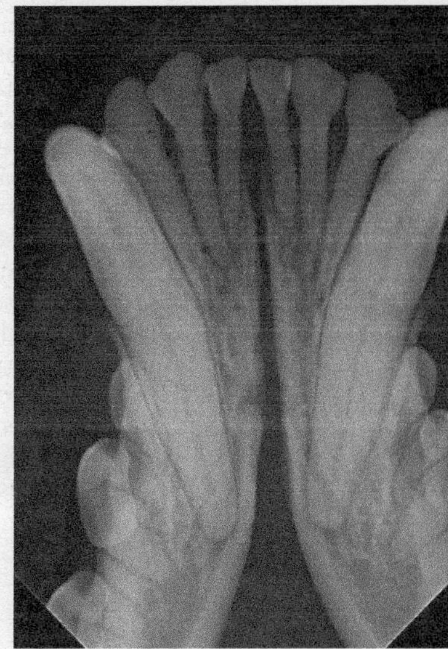

(*Continued*)

Table 21.12 / Radiographic positioning (Continued)

View	Positioning	Visualization diagram for bisecting angle 	Radiograph
Maxillary view: • Feline: premolars and molars • Alternate	• Patient: lateral or sternal recumbency with the mouth propped open • Media: vertically in the mouth, resting on the far side lingual teeth; parallel to tooth roots • Beam: modified parallel technique, directed at the base of the root in question • Patient: lateral or sternal recumbency • Media: on the mandible along the arcade • Beam: bisecting angle technique • Simplified: Simplified: media placement on the mandible, patient positioned with palate parallel to the tabletop if sternal or perpendicular to the table top if lateral, tube head should be angled 30–45 degrees from the media if sternal or 45–60 degrees if lateral	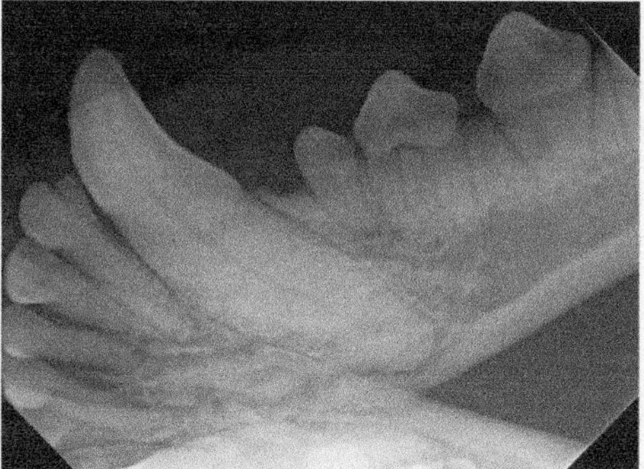	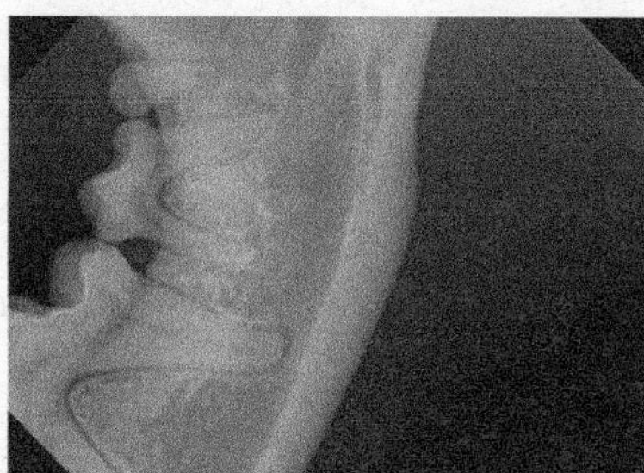 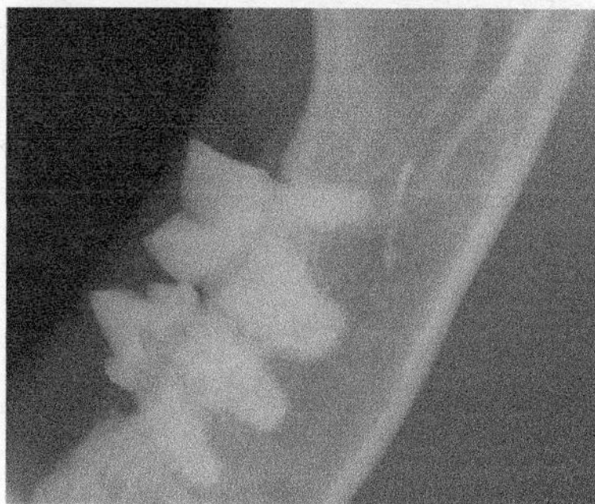

Positioning Errors and Corrections

Table 21.13 / Positioning errors and corrections

Error	Cause and correction	Image
Cone cutting	• Tube head is not centered over the media leaving a white area on the media • Adjust the tube head to expose the entire plate/film/sensor (For size 4 media this may require pulling the tube head further from the patient to allow the beam to spread out.)	 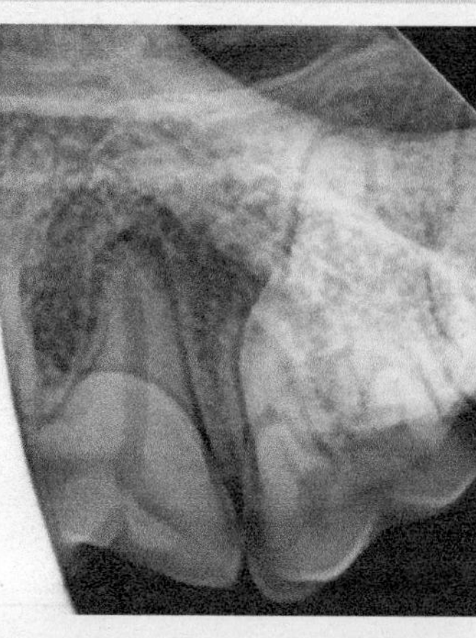
Elongation	• Tube head is too shallowly angled to the media and the image is lengthened • Adjust the tube head to a more perpendicular position or increase the angle	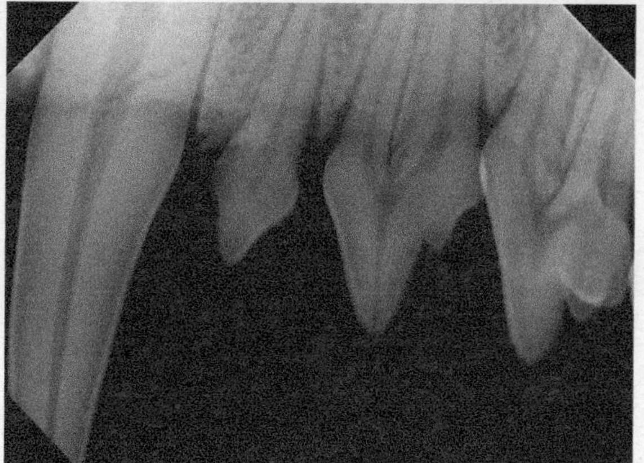

(*Continued*)

Table 21.13 / **Positioning errors and corrections (Continued)**

Error	Cause and correction	Image
Foreshortening	• Tube head is too steeply angled to the media and the image is shortened • Adjust the tube head to a more lateral position or decrease the angle	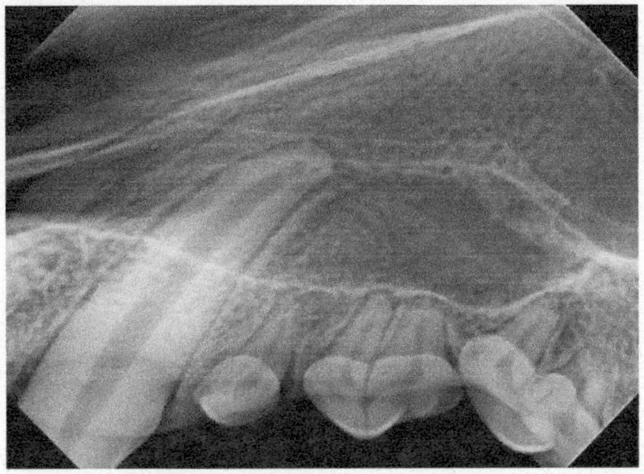
Distortion	• Tube head is angled causing the image to be distorted • Straighten the tube head	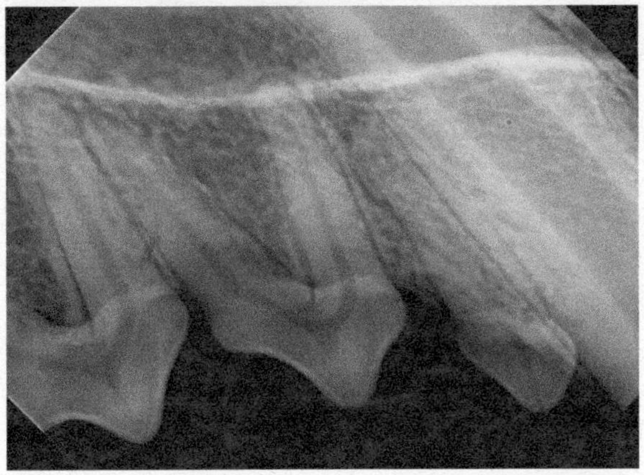

(*Continued*)

Table 21.13 / **Positioning errors and corrections (Continued)**

Error	Cause and correction	Image
Overexposure	• Exposure time is too long causing the image to be dark • Decrease the time	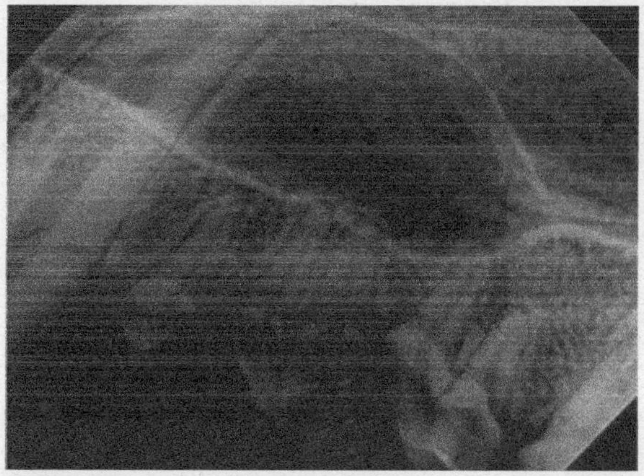
Underexposure	• Exposure time is too short causing the image to be light • Increase the time	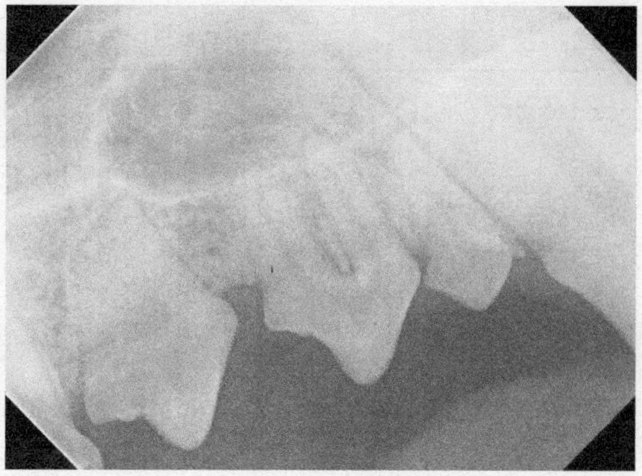

Basic Radiologic Pathology

Table 21.14 / Basic radiographic pathology

Pathology	Charting symbol	Causes	Image
Horizontal bone loss		• Periodontal disease • The level of the bone is dropped across these teeth	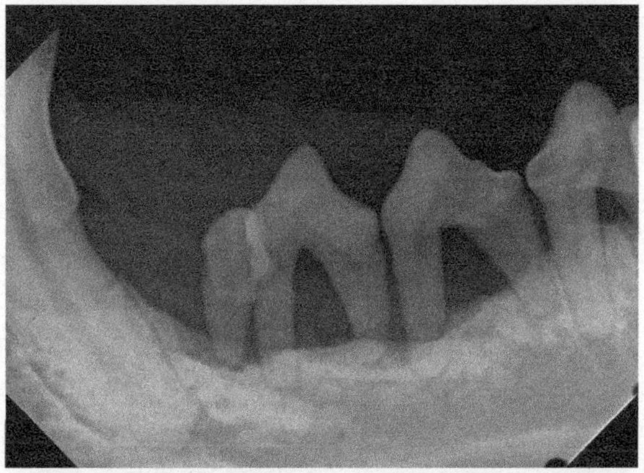
Impacted tooth	T/I	• Tooth did not erupt correctly • Impacted teeth can result in the formation of a DTC • All apparently missing teeth should be radiographed	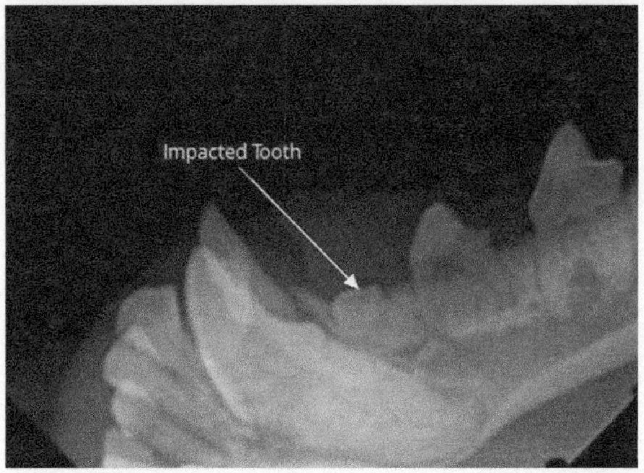

(*Continued*)

Table 21.14 / Basic radiographic pathology (Continued)

Pathology	Charting symbol	Causes	Image
Nonvital tooth	T/NV	• Teeth continue to lay down dentin as the pet ages causing pulp chambers to get smaller • In this radiograph the tooth with the larger pulp chamber is no longer vital • The best comparison is to the contralateral tooth	

(Continued)

Table 21.14 / Basic radiographic pathology (Continued)

Pathology	Charting symbol	Causes	Image
Periapical lucency	T/NV	• A sign of infection inside the tooth (endodontic disease) • Can occur in teeth with complicated and uncomplicated crown fractures • Can occur in teeth with no fracture • Illustrates why it is important to radiograph 3 mm past the apex of the tooth	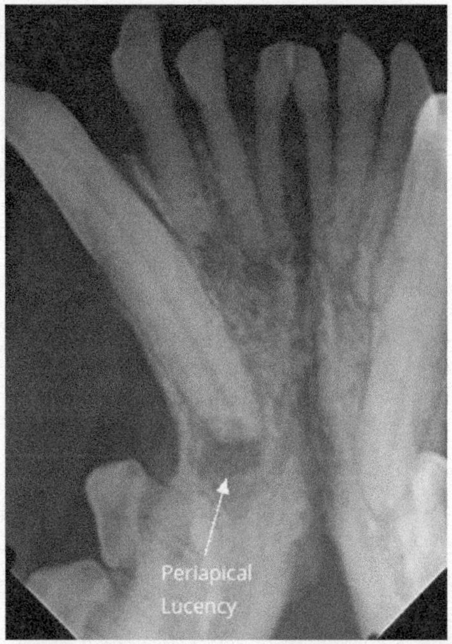
Tooth resorption	TR	• Tooth is being broken down • Root may be present or may be remodeled into alveolar bone • Radiographs are the only way to determine the condition of the root • Occurs in cats and dogs	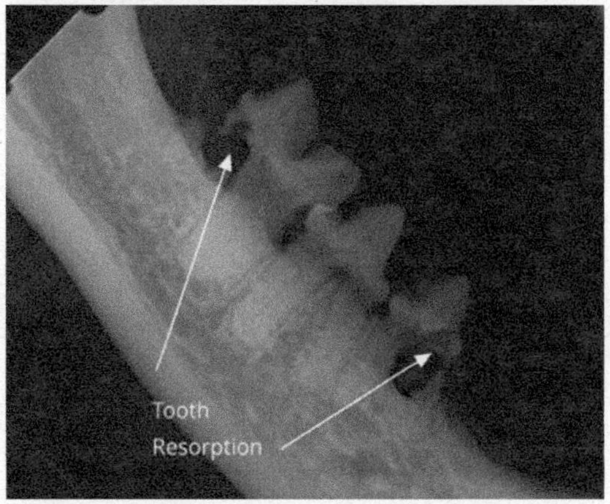

EXTRACTIONS

Depending upon the laws governing technicians in your state, extractions may only be performed by a veterinarian.[12] Table 13.11 indicates the instruments typically used and the general procedure so that the technician will be better able to assist the veterinarian.

The American Veterinary Dental College (AVDC) considers operative dentistry to be any dental procedure which invades the hard or soft oral tissue including, but not limited to, a procedure that alters the structure of one or more teeth or repairs damaged and diseased teeth. A veterinarian should perform operative dentistry and oral surgery. The AVDC considers the extraction of teeth to be included in the practice of veterinary dentistry. Decision making is the responsibility of the veterinarian, with the consent of the pet owner, when electing to extract teeth. Only veterinarians shall determine which teeth are to be extracted and perform extraction procedures. General extraction complications include fractured socket or jaw, fractured or broken root tips that could enter the mandibular canal or nasal cavity, hemorrhage, endocarditis, secondary infection, oronasal fistula, soft tissue trauma, ocular trauma, osteomyelitis, alveolitis, and gingival laceration.[5]

Tip: Post-extraction care:

- Medication: pain management with or without antibiotic therapy.
- Feed soft food.
- Schedule a surgical recheck in two weeks.

Table 21.15 / Extraction procedures

Extraction	Instruments	Order of instrumentation	Cautions
Simple: (X) • Involves elevation of the tooth	• Dental elevators and/or luxators • Extraction forceps • Miller bone curette • Gauze sponges • Dental radiography equipment • Scissors: periodontal and suture • Needle holder • Thumb forceps • Absorbable suture (4–0 or 5–0)	1. Pre-extraction dental radiograph 2. Appropriately sized dental elevator or luxators 3. Extraction forceps 4. Miller bone curette (some will use a periosteal elevator) 5. High-speed handpiece if needed 6. Post extraction radiograph 7. Suture, needle holders, forceps and suture scissors if site is to be sutured	• Elevation may cause gingival and bone damage • Root breakage caused by improper use or force • Suturing of small extraction sites may cause additional trauma; second intention wound healing may be the best approach
Sectioned: (XS) • Target tooth is sectioned at the furcation to produce single root pieces	• Simple extraction instruments	1. Pre-extraction dental radiograph 2. High-speed handpiece with crosscut bur 3. Follow above order from simple extraction starting at 2	• Fracture of adjacent teeth if they are used for leverage • Avoid getting air from drill or air water syringe into the bone as it can cause an air embolus in the patient's system
Surgical: (XSS) • Alveolar bone is exposed and then removed to expose the tooth root prior to extraction	• Simple extraction instruments • Surgical blade (#15 or #15C) on scalpel handle • Periosteal elevator	1. Pre-extraction dental radiograph 2. Scalpel handle with attached blade 3. Periosteal elevator 4. High-speed handpiece with round bur 5. High-speed handpiece with crosscut bur 6. Follow above order from simple extraction starting at 2	• Technique used when there is no access to the root, danger to the adjacent structures, tooth root fragility, or ankylosis of the bone to the root is present • Must always be sutured

(Continued)

Table 21.15 / **Extraction procedures (Continued)**

Extraction	Instruments	Order of instrumentation	Cautions
Crown amputation: (XSS)	• Dental radiography equipment • Periosteal elevator • High speed handpiece with small round or diamond bur • Surgical blade (#15 or #15C) on scalpel handle • Periosteal elevator • Scissors: periodontal and suture • Needle holder • Thumb forceps • Absorbable suture (5–0)	1. Pre-extraction dental radiograph 2. Periosteal elevator 3. High-speed handpiece with round or diamond bur 4. Post-crown amputation radiograph 5. Suture, needle holder, thumb forceps, scissors	• Technique used when there is no evidence of root structure • Must always be sutured • Must never be performed without dental radiographs [10]
Complications	• Root tip picks • Fragment forceps	• Used as needed for fractured root tip removal	

Local Dental Nerve Blocks

Local dental nerve blocks prior to extractions have been found to decrease the amount and depth of general anesthetic used during the procedure, to create a smoother recovery, and to decrease the need for immediate postoperative narcotics for pain management. Training on proper placement of these blocks is essential.

It is critical to aspirate prior to injection of the anesthesia to avoid improper injection into the bloodstream. Intravenous injection of the local anesthetic may cause cardiac and/or nervous system toxicosis (total dose should not exceed 2 mg/kg). Make sure to calculate the total dose for the patient weight and do not exceed that amount. Ensure that you include any lidocaine that is used at intubation in the calculations. Local complications can occur including hematoma and ocular trauma. Always aspirate before injecting and do not inject if resistance is encountered. Do not use in areas of infection, irritation or neoplasia.

Epinephrine may be added for its vasoconstrictive effects. Local anesthetics cause a vasodilation effect, which removes the drug from the intended area quicker. With the addition of epinephrine and its vasoconstrictive effects, the duration of the local anesthetic effect is extended. Its use is contraindicated in patients with cardiac arrhythmias, uncontrolled hyperthyroidism, or asthma.

Opoids such as buprenorphine (0.003–0.005 mg/kg) may also be added. This may decrease the amount of inhalant required over bupivacaine alone.[13]

Note: see also Table 4.8: Directional terms, page 222, and Chapter 4: Anatomy.

Skill Box 21.3 / Local Dental Nerve Blocks

Types	Area and Nerves Blocked	Drug and Dose*	Injection Site and Method†	Associated Risks
Infraorbital	• Infraorbital nerve and rostral maxillary alveolar nerve • Maxillary incisors, canines, premolars one through three, adjacent bone and soft tissue	Drug: • Lidocaine 2% • Bupivacaine 0.5% Dose: • Lidocaine 1.0 mg/kg • Bupivacaine 0.2–0.5 mg/kg Volume per block: • Canine: 0.2–0.4 ml • Feline: 0.1–0.2 ml	• Injection site • Infraorbital foramen • Canine: palpated at the distal root of the maxillary third premolar • Feline: typically, not palpated; located dorsal to the furcation of the maxillary third premolar • Method • Insert needle into the foramen approximately 1 mm, aspirate, then inject slowly, placing digital pressure over the injection entrance and maintaining pressure 30–60 seconds after injecting.	**Feline: needle advancement into the foramen is not recommended due to possible orbital trauma**
Caudal maxillary	• Maxillary nerve (middle and caudal superior alveolar nerve) • All maxillary teeth, bone, and soft tissues on the blocked side of the head	Drug: • Lidocaine 2% • Bupivacaine 0.5% Dose: • Lidocaine 1.0 mg/kg • Bupivacaine 0.2–0.5 mg/kg Volume per block: • Canine: 0.2–0.4 ml • Feline: 0.1–0.15 ml	• Injection Site • Infraorbital foramen • Canine: directly behind the second molar • Method • Canine: insert the needle perpendicular to the hard palate. Advance the needle up to 3 mm in small patients, up to 5 mm in large patients • Feline: This nerve block is not recommended due to proximity of the eye.	**Use caution in brachycephalic patients due to the position of the eye**
Middle mental	• Rostral alveolar nerve • Mandibular incisors, canines, and soft tissues	Drug: • Lidocaine 2% • Bupivacaine 0.5% Dose: • Lidocaine 1.0 mg/kg • Bupivacaine 0.2–0.5 mg/kg Volume per block: 0.1–0.3 ml	• Injection site • Middle mental foramen • Canine: caudal to mandibular labial frenulum palpated at the mesial root of the mandibular second premolar • Feline: not easily palpated; at or just caudal to the apex of the mandibular canine tooth • Method • Canine: insert needle into just rostral to the frenulum, advance needle into the foramen, aspirate, apply digital pressure at needle insertion site and inject slowly as the needle is gradually withdrawn. • Feline: insert needle at the rostral border of the mandibular labial frenulum at or just caudal to the apex of the mandibular canine tooth, aspirate, apply digital pressure at insertion site and inject slowly	**Rarely performed**

(*Continued*)

Skill Box 21.3 / Local Dental Nerve Blocks (Continued)

Types	Area and Nerves Blocked	Drug and Dose*	Injection Site and Method†	Associated Risks
Caudal mandibular	• Inferior alveolar nerve • All mandibular teeth and associated soft tissue of the ipsilateral hemimandible	Drug: • Lidocaine 2% • Bupivacaine 0.5% Dose: • Lidocaine 1.0 mg/kg • Bupivacaine 0.2–0.5 mg/kg Volume per block: 0.25–0.5 ml if nerve is well palpated from the intraoral approach; more volume is needed when extraoral approach is used	• Injection site • Mandibular foramen • Lingual aspect of mandible above mandibular notch; palpated caudal to the last molar • Method • Extraoral: insert needle perpendicular to mandible through skin and walk it off ventral mandible; then advance dorsally to the mandibular foramen, aspirate, inject. • Intraoral: draw a mental line between the last molar and the angular process of the mandible; insert needle just rostral to the midpoint of this line, aspirate, inject [11]	

*In mm/km as a total dosage, all blocks cumulative: bupivacaine 0.5%, lidocaine 2%.
†Use tuberculin syringe with 25–27 gauge, ¾ to 1-inch needle, or via Teflon IV catheter (over the needle type).

Advanced Procedures

Table 21.16 / Advanced procedures: typically referral cases

Procedure	Indications	Definition	Comments
Root canal (RCT)	• Fractured tooth with pulp exposure • Non-vital tooth • Endodontically compromised tooth • Contraindicated in the presence of periodontal disease	• Removes infected or dead pulp tissue, shapes the canal then seals and fills the tooth	• Less painful than extraction • Allows the patient to retain the functionality of the tooth • Commonly performed in working dogs • Follow-up radiograph needed in 1 year
Vital pulpotomy (VPT)	• Fractured tooth with pulp exposure within a short period of time (not often performed) • To shorten a tooth that is causing soft tissue trauma	• Allows the tooth to remain alive and retain functionality • Keeps the majority of the pulp alive, a treatment is placed to stimulate the formation of tertiary dentin	• Most commonly done to treat MAL2 with palatal trauma

REFERENCES

1. American Veterinary Dental College. (2019). AVDC abbreviations for use in case logs: equine and small animal. https://avdc.org/technician-services (accessed 3 August 2021).
2. Niemiec, B. (2013). Local and regional consequences of periodontal disease. In: *Veterinary Periodontology* (ed. B. Niemiec), 69–80. Ames, IO: Wiley Blackwell.
3. Niemiec, B. (2013). Systemic manifestations of periodontal disease. In: *Veterinary Periodontology* (ed. B. Niemiec), 81–90. Ames, IO: Wiley Blackwell.
4. Stepaniuk, K. (2018). Periodontology. In: *Wiggs's Veterinary Dentistry: Principles and Practice*, 2e (ed. H. Lobprise and J. Dodd), 81–108. Hoboken, NJ: Wiley Blackwell.
5. Niemiec, B., Gawor, J., Nemiec, A. *et al.* (2020). World Small Animal Veterinary Association Global Dental Guidelines. *J Small Anim Pract* 16: E36–E161.
6. American Veterinary Dental College. About AVDC. https://avdc.org/about (accessed 18 August 2021).
7. Lobprise, H. *and* Dodd, J. *(*2018*). Wiggs's Veterinary Dentistry: Principles and Practice*, 2e. Hoboken, NJ: Wiley Blackwell.
8. Bellows, J. (2011). *Feline Dentistry*. New York, NY: Wiley.
9. Niemiec. (2011). Part C: Periodontal radiography. In: *Small Animal Dental, Oral and Maxillofacial Disease: A color handbook*. Boca Raton, FL: CRC Press.
10. Gawor, J. (2018). *Practical Veterinary Dental Radiography* (ed. B. Niemiec, J. Gawor and V. Jekl), 128–142. Boca Raton, FL: CRC Press.
11. Niemiec, B. (2018). The importance of and indications for dental radiography. In: *Practical Veterinary Dental Radiography* (ed. B. Niemiec, J. Gawor and V. Jekl), 5–30. Boca Raton, FL: CRC Press.
12. American Veterinary Medical Association. (2021). Authority of veterinary technicians and other non-veterinarians to perform dental procedures. https://www.avma.org/Advocacy/StateAndLocal/Pages/sr-dental-procedures.aspx (accessed 3 August 2021).
13. Beckman, B. (2016). Dental nerve blocks in dogs and cats enhance anesthesia safety. International Veterinary Dentistry Institute. https://veterinarydentistry.net/dental-nerve-blocks-dogs-cats (accessed 3 August 2021).

Chapter 22

Disinfection and Sterilization in Veterinary Healthcare Facilities

Heidi Reuss-Lamky, LVT, VTS, (Anesthesia/Analgesia), (Surgery), CFVP

Veterinary Technician and Nurse's Daily Reference Guide: Canine and Feline, Fourth Edition. Edited by Mandy Fults and Kenichiro Yagi.

Companion website: www.wiley.com/go/fults/veterinary

Abbreviations

AAMI, Association for the Advancement of Medical Instrumentation
ANSI, American National Standards Institute
ECG, electrocardiogram
FDA, Food and Drug Administration
HLD, high-level disinfectant
LCS, liquid chemical sterilant
OPA, orthophthaldehyde
OSHA, Occupational Safety and Health Administration
PPE, personal protection equipment
SV, stated value

TRANSMISSION OF INFECTIONS

Hospital-acquired infections require the presence of infectious organisms, a viable route of transmission, and a population of susceptible individuals. Understanding how infections occur will enable the healthcare team to develop and implement policies and procedures to help mitigate this risk.

A hospital-acquired infection, also known as a nosocomial infection, is an infection acquired in a hospital or other healthcare facility. This type if infection may not only involve patients, but also others present in the hospital, including the healthcare team.

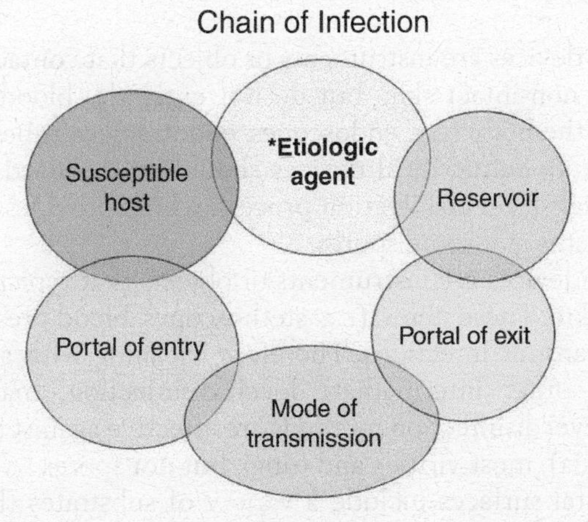

Figure 22.1 Components of the infectious disease process. Source: In: Fiutem, C. Risk Factors Facilitating Transmission of Infectious Agents. In Boston K.M., et al, eds. APIC Text Online. Published October 3, 2014. Available at https://text.apic.org/toc/microbiology-and-risk-factors-for-transmission/risk-factors-facilitating-transmission-of-infectious-agents. Accessed [Month Day, Year]. Used with permission of the Association for Professionals in Infection Control and Epidemiology.

There are six elements in the chain of infection: the etiologic agent, a reservoir, the portal of exit, the mode of transmission, the portal of entry, and a susceptible host (Figure 22.1). Each factor must be present for an infection to occur.[1]

Chain of Infection

Etiologic Agent

The etiologic agent itself is considered to be the first link in the chain of infection. These agents may be bacterium, virus, fungus, or other microorganism. Prions are considered the smallest infectious particle, and do not contain genetic material. Prions are responsible for degenerative diseases involving the brain, such as Creutzfeldt-Jakob disease, variant Creutzfeldt-Jakob disease (also bovine spongiform encephalopathy or "mad cow" disease), and fatal familial insomnia, among others. A microorganism must be able to invade the tissues of the body. Organisms capable of penetrating the body's intact barrier are generally more concerning than those lacking this ability. However, not all microorganisms need to directly attack intact body tissues to cause disease. Additionally, enough microorganisms must be present to constitute an "infectious dose". The infectious dose can vary, not only from organism to organism, but also from host to host.[1]

Reservoir

The second factor in the chain of infection is a reservoir, or source(s) that facilitate the etiologic agent's survival and/or replication. There are a multitude of reservoirs in a typical hospital environment, and may include supplies and equipment used during patient care, food and drink, linens, or other inanimate objects. Nevertheless, these items play a comparatively small role when measured against one of the biggest reservoirs of all; man himself. The human body harbors well over a trillion microorganisms, and it is a well-documented fact that most hospital-acquired infections are caused by the patient's own microbial flora.[1]

Portal of Exit

The third factor in the chain of infection requires a source from which the etiologic agent can appear. Portals of exit may include the skin, respiratory or vascular systems, mucous membranes, gastrointestinal or genitourinary tracts. Moreover, diseases can further spread once a contaminated patient contacts supplies and equipment used again on an uninfected patient.[1]

Mode of Transmission

Although other modes of transmission exist for etiologic agents, main transfer methods involve either indirect or direct contact with a patient, or through contact with conjunctival, oral or nasal mucous membranes, or respiratory secretions. Indirect-contact transmissions may occur when a contaminated object (e.g. catheter, surgical instrument) comes into contact with an uninfected hospitalized patient. An example of direct-contact transmission may occur when the unwashed hands of a healthcare worker come into contact with an uninfected hospitalized patient. Droplet spread may also occur, primarily during coughing, sneezing, or talking. Other forms of disease transmission include airborne, vehicular (e.g. contaminated medications – eye drops, multidose vials, food, or water), and vector (e.g. insect or rodent) transmission.[1,2]

Portal of Entry

The fifth factor in the chain of infection involves a suitable portal of entry. The routes for gaining entry into the body are identical to the portals of exit. Most infectious diseases require very specific portals of entry and exit. For example, Hepatitis B is transmitted via the hematogenous route, while influenza is transmitted only via the respiratory tract.

Susceptible Host

The last link in the chain of infection is a susceptible host, lacking the ability to resist any given etiologic agent. Predisposing host factors may include breaches in the integrity of the skin, gastrointestinal tract, or upper respiratory tract, the inability to mount a local inflammatory response, or immunocompromised individuals.[1]

A thorough understanding of the chain of infection also validates the importance of hand hygiene. Although hand washing alone will not eliminate all microorganisms present on the skin, it can decrease their numbers enough to prevent the transfer of most diseases.[1]

SPAULDING CATEGORIES

In 1972, Earle H. Spaulding created a system that divided medical instruments and equipment into three categories, based on the risk of infection from contact with a contaminated item. The Centers for Disease Control and Prevention recognizes the three Spaulding categories, and a fourth category that encompasses environment surfaces:[1,3]

- Critical devices
- Semicritical devices
- Non-critical devices
- Environmental surfaces.

Critical devices are instruments or objects that are introduced either into or in contact with the bloodstream, or other normally sterile areas of the body (e.g. surgical instruments, needles, catheters, implants). Critical devices present a high degree of risk of the potential to spread infection if contaminated and must be sterilized before use.

Semicritical devices are instruments or objects that contact intact mucous membranes or non-intact skin, but do not enter the bloodstream or other sterile areas of the body (e.g. endoscopes, endotracheal tubes, laryngoscopes, urinary catheters). Semicritical devices should be sterilized (if possible), or exposed to a high-level disinfection process, which provides lethality against all microorganisms and some spores.

Non-critical devices are instruments or objects that typically contact only intact patient skin. These items, (e.g. stethoscopes, blood pressure cuffs, ECG leads) rarely transmit infections. Therefore, cleaning with a mild detergent and water, or other intermediate level disinfection, may be adequate. Intermediate level disinfection methods are effective against bacteria (including mycobacteria), most viruses and fungi, but not spores.

Environmental surfaces include a variety of substrates that normally do not come into direct contact with patients or contact intact skin. These surfaces carry minimal risk of infection, but may contribute to secondary contamination via direct contact with the hands of healthcare providers or other surfaces that subsequently come into contact with patients. Low-level disinfection, which involves inactivation of bacteria and some viruses, but not mycobacteria or spores, is indicated for environmental surfaces. These surfaces are further divided into two subcategories:

- Medical equipment surfaces (e.g. adjustment knobs on monitoring devices, instrument cart handles, and dental machines).
- Housekeeping surfaces (e.g. floors, walls, tables, and window sills).

Depending on the surface and the degree of contamination, medical equipment surfaces may require cleaning with mild soap and water, cleaning with a chemical disinfectant agent, or cleaning with mild soap and water followed by application of a chemical disinfectant. Housekeeping surfaces have the least potential for causing infections, and should be kept visibly clean by using water and detergent or a hospital-grade disinfectant designed for this purpose. Blood and other potentially infectious fluid spills should be cleaned with an intermediate-level chemical disinfectant.[1]

Other areas of the veterinary hospital that can pose unique disinfection challenges include rehabilitation equipment (e.g. underwater treadmills, mats, or balls), surgical or dentistry procedural areas, resuscitation, obstetrics, and burn treatment areas, or areas housing patients that are immunocompromised, have multidrug-resistant organisms or are fed a raw meat diet (Box 22.1).[2]

Box 22.1 / Pathogens of greatest infection control concern for a small animal hospital[2]

- *Adenovirus* (canine)
- *Bordetella bronchiseptica*
- *Calicivirus* (feline)
- *Chlamydophila* (feline)
- Distemper virus (canine)
- *Herpesvirus* (feline)
- Influenza viruses (canine, novel)
- *Leptospira interrogans*
- *Microsporum canis*
- Parainfluenza virus (canine)
- Parvoviruses (canine, feline)
- Respiratory coronavirus (canine)
- *Salmonella* spp.
- Multidrug-resistant organisms:
  - *Acinetobacter* spp.
  - *Escherichia* coli
  - *Enterococcus* spp.
  - *Staphylococcus* spp.
  - *Pseudomonas* spp.

A four-tiered hierarchy should be implemented to perform effective infection control, prevention and biosecurity, including:

- Eliminating sources of pathogen exposure by preventing or removing pathogens.
- Engineering controls are structural designs and/or equipment that help remove hazardous sources or improve infection control compliance.
- Administrative controls that compel compliance for new practices, procedures, or policies, by providing the staff with information, training, and supervision surrounding infectious agents moving throughout the hospital.
- The availability and proper use of personal protection equipment (PPE); checklists, or a list of key tasks surrounding cleaning and disinfection, have been shown to improve compliance and reduce the incidence of hospital-acquired infections.[2]

PERSONNEL CONSIDERATIONS

The Association for the Advancement of Medical Instrumentation (AAMI) sets forth extensive guidelines and rationalizes recommended practices for disinfection and sterilization in human healthcare facilities. Relevant content from this preeminent resource has been included in this chapter. It is important that only qualified personnel are engaged in sterile processing duties and understand how to minimize bioburden and environmental contamination. Written policies should be developed and communicated to all personnel involved, as part of the hospital's standard operating procedures.

Personnel should have a thorough understanding of all phases of instrument and equipment preparation and sterilization, including decontamination, inspection, packaging, sterilization principles and sterilizing systems, storage and distribution, and handling biohazardous materials (OSHA standard 29 CFR 1910.1200).[4] Infectious waste should be discarded as per OSHA regulations (29 CFR 1910.1030)[5] and other applicable federal, state, and local regulations.

- Training should be given on all new instrumentation, devices and equipment.
- Access should be provided to information on protective work practices, the use of PPE and emergency procedures. Never reuse PPE.[2]
- Hand hygiene techniques, as related to washing after visible soil or as part of decontamination using alcohol-based, waterless hand sanitizers containing emollients should be followed. Fingernails must be kept short. Jewelry on the hands or wrists, nail polish, and artificial nails are prohibited (Table 22.1).[2]
- Wear clean clothes, sturdy shoes (no open toes); all head and facial hair should be covered (except eyebrows and eyelashes).
- Minimize injuries and use caution when handling sharp objects; wear appropriate PPE.
- Do not eat, drink, smoke, apply cosmetics, lip balm or handle contact lenses in areas where occupational exposure to chemical or biological materials is possible.
- Supervisors should be experienced and should stay current in pertinent education and training, including local and federal regulations, and infection prevention and control.

- More information is available from the Certification Board for Sterile Processing and Distribution (www.sterileprocessing.org), and the International Association of Healthcare Central Service Materiel Management (www.iahcsmm.org).[1]

Table 22.1 / **Protocol for hand hygiene**[2]

Hand wash (soap and water)	Hand rub (alcohol-based hand sanitizer)
Turn on water	–
1. Wet hands	–
2. Dispense appropriate amount of product directly onto hands (e.g. 1–2 pumps from dispenser)	1. Dispense appropriate amount of product directly onto hands (e.g. 1–2 pumps from dispenser)
3. Apply product to all surfaces of hands; minimum 15 seconds' contact time: • Palms • Back of hands • Between fingers • Finger tips • Thumb and thumb web • ± wrists	2. Apply product to all surfaces of hands; minimum 15 seconds' contact time • Palms • Back of hands • Between fingers • Finger tips • Thumb and thumb web • ± wrists
4. Rinse all surfaces with water	–
5. Dry hands thoroughly with single-use towel	4. Rub hands until dry
6. Turn water off, using drying towel to avoid direct contact with faucet handles (unless automatic faucet present)	–
7. Discard towel	–
Total time around 30–60 seconds	Total time around 20–30 seconds

LIQUID CHEMICALS FOR DISINFECTION AND STERILIZATION

In the United States, the US Environmental Protection Agency and US Food and Drug Administration (FDA) regulate liquid chemical germicides (also known as disinfectants, such as alcohols, phenolic compounds, and quaternary ammonium compounds, QUATs) used on environmental surfaces in healthcare settings. The FDA also regulates the labeling of liquid chemical sterilants (LCS)/high-level disinfectants (HLD) (e.g. glutaraldehyde, hydrogen peroxide, and peracetic acid) used as part of a final processing step for reusable critical and semicritical medical devices (Tables 22.2 and 22.3).[6] Understanding the Spaulding categories and a base knowledge of antimicrobial activity for various types of products will guide appropriate product selection.

Liquid chemical sterilization methods should be selected based on:

- Manufacturer's written instructions for use.
- How the equipment or device will be used in the next patient.
- Physical configuration (cleanability) of the equipment or device.
- Type and degree of contamination after the equipment or device is used.
- Physical and chemical stability of the equipment or device.
- Ease or difficulty in removing the LCS after the necessary exposure time.
- Ability to completely submerge the item for the necessary time and temperature.

Liquid chemicals are classified as high, intermediate, or low level disinfectants, based on their ability to destroy various microorganisms. Published descriptions of the efficacy of various LCS products (active ingredients) can be confusing, since the ability of a specific LCS to kill or inactivate microorganisms may be impacted by factors such as the concentration of the product, contact time, and temperature during exposure.[1] The label conditions required for HLD to occur is the time and temperature needed to achieve a six-log reduction of an appropriate *Mycobacterium* species, when used as per the manufacturer's instructions.[2,7]

Liquid chemicals used for LCS or HLD must not be used at concentrations below the minimum recommended concentration or minimum effective concentration. Remove excess moisture from items after the cleaning process to prevent accidental dilution of the disinfectant. Agent-specific test strips should be used regularly to monitor the concentration of the active ingredient(s) and ensure continued efficacy during product use or reuse (Figure 22.2).

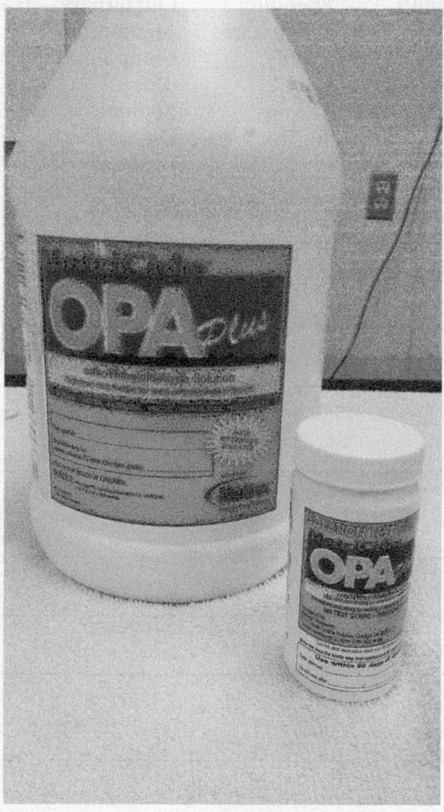

Figure 22.2 Agent-specific test strips are used to determine whether a solution has maintained effective concentration levels after prior use or storage. Do not use solutions that appear discolored or turbid. Source: photograph courtesy the author.

Actual reuse life may be shorter than label claims because of the presence of organic material contamination (e.g. serum, pus, blood, feces), residual detergents, or interference from cotton, wool, cellulose sponges or minerals found in hard water.[1] Some products do require heated solutions for maximal efficacy. Use a thermometer to monitor the temperature of these solutions throughout the required exposure time period.

Table 22.2 / **Chemical germicide classes and activity levels**

The Antimicrobial Spectrum of Disinfectants Chemical Disinfectants

Note: Removal of organic material must always precede the use of any disinfectant

	Acids hydrochloric acid, acetic acid, citric acid	**Alcohols** ethyl alcohol, isopropyl alcohol	**Aldehydes** formaldehyde, paraformaldehyde, gluteraldehyde	**Alkalis** sodium hydroxide, ammonium-hydroxide, sodium-carbonate	**Biguanides** chlorhexidine, Nolvasan®, ChlorHex®, Virosan	**Oxidizing Agents** Peroxygens accelerated hydrogen peroxide (Rescue®), potassium peroxymonosulfate (Virkon-S®), peroxyacetic acid, (Oxy-Sept® 333)	**Phenolic Compounds** (Lysol®, Osyl®, Amphyl®, TekTrol®, Pheno-Tek II®)	**Quaternary Ammonium Compounds** (Roccal®, Zepharin®, DiQuat®, Parvosol®, D-256®)	**Halogens** hypochlorite	Iodine
Most Susceptible										
mycoplasmas	+	++	++	+	++	++	++	++	++	+
gram-positive bacteria	+	++	++	+	++	+	+	+	++	++
gram-negative bacteria	+	++	++	+	++	+	+	+	++	+
pseudomonads	+	++	++	+	+/-	+	+	+	++	×
rickettsiae	+/-	+	+	+	+/-	+	+	+	+	+/-
enveloped viruses	+	+	++	+	+/-	+	+	+	+/-a	+/-
chlamydise	+/-	+/-	+	+	+/-	+	+	+	+-	×
non-enveloped viruses	×	×	+	+/-	×	+	+/-	+/-	×	×
fungal spores	+/-	+/-	+	+	+/-	+	+	+/-	+	+-

(*Continued*)

Table 22.2 / Chemical germicide classes and activity levels (Continued)

The Antimicrobial Spectrum of Disinfectants Chemical Disinfectants										
Note: Removal of organic material must always precede the use of any disinfectant										
	Acids hydrochloric acid, acetic acid, citric acid	**Alcohols** ethyl alcohol, isopropyl alcohol	**Aldehydes** formaldehyde, paraformaldehyde, gluteraldehyde	**Alkalis** sodium hydroxide, ammonium-hydroxide, sodium-carbonate	**Biguanides** chlorhexidine, Nolvasan®, ChlorHex®, Virosan	**Oxidizing Agents** Peroxygens accelerated hydrogen peroxide (Rescue®), potassium peroxymonosulfate (Virkon-S®), peroxyacetic acid, (Oxy-Sept® 333)	**Phenolic Compounds** (Lysol®, Osyl®, Amphyl®, TekTrol®, Pheno-Tek II®	**Quaternary Ammonium Compounds** (Roccal®, Zepharin®, DiQuat®, Parvosol®, D-256®)	**Halogens** hypochlorite Iodine	
picornaviruses (i.e. FMD)	+	N	+	+	N	N		+	N	N
parvoviruses	N	N	+	N	N	+	N	+/-	N	×
acid-fast bacertia	×	+	+	+	×	+	+	+/-	+/-	×
bacterial spores	+/-	×	+	+/-	×	+	+	+b	×	×
coccidia	×	×	×	+c	×	×	×	×	+d	×
prions	×	×	×	×	×	×	×	×	×	×
Most Resistant										

++ Highly Effective	× No Activity
+ Effective	N Information Unavailable
+- Limited Activity	

a–varies with compositon
b–peracetic acid is sporicidal
c–ammonium hydroxide
This table provides general information for selected disinfectant chemical classes. Antimicrobial activity may vary with formulation and concentration. The use of trade names does not in any way signify endorsement of a particular product. They are provided as examples.

LIQUID CHEMICAL GERMICIDES FOR ENVIRONMENTAL SURFACES

Alcohols

Ethanol (ethyl alcohol, C_2H_5OH) and 2-propanol (isopropyl alcohol, $(CH_3)_2CHOH$) share similar disinfectant properties. Aqueous alcohol solutions do not leave a residue on treated items. Alcohols have demonstrated efficacy against vegetative bacteria, fungi, and lipid-containing viruses, but are not effective against spores. Alcohols have variable efficacy against non-lipid viruses. A 70% concentration has shown the highest effectiveness; higher or lower concentrations may not perform as well as a germicide. Alcohol is often mixed with other agents to increase the spectrum of activity (e.g. 70% alcohol and100 g/l formaldehyde). A 70% aqueous ethanol solution may be used on skin, work surfaces, or to soak small instruments. Alcohol-based hand rubs are advised for decontaminating mildly soiled hands where performing a proper hand wash was inconvenient or impossible. Ethanol alcohol can dry skin and is often mixed with emollients. Alcohols are volatile, flammable, and can evaporate if not stored in the appropriate containers, but can also harden rubber and dissolve some types of glue (see the Centers for Disease Control and Prevention guideline for more information and recommended contact times).[8]

Biguanides

Chlorhexidine solution is popular in veterinary medicine, through versatility that ranges from veterinary oral hygiene applications to disinfecting equipment. It is important to note that using chlorhexidine at higher than clinically recommended concentrations (e.g. > 0.5% vs. 0.15%) has been associated with oral ulcers, pharyngitis, and tracheitis from endotracheal tubes that were not thoroughly rinsed after chlorhexidine disinfection. Furthermore, biguanides are easily inactivated by organic matter, so items must be meticulously clean prior to use.[3]

Sodium Hypochlorite Solutions

Chlorine and chlorine-releasing agents such as household bleach have a long history of use for antisepsis of the skin, hands, and wounds, as well as for disinfection of hospitals, water and sewage, and textile bleaching. Sodium hypochlorite (NaOCl) is the most commonly used chlorine-releasing agent in healthcare facilities as a hard surface and environmental disinfectant. Sodium hypochlorite and related solutions rapidly lose effectiveness in the presence of organic matter (e.g. blood, feces, tissue), or light exposure. Household bleach solutions contain 50 g/l available chlorine, and therefore must be diluted. Chlorine concentrations of 1 g/l (1 : 50 dilution) to 5 g/l (1 : 10 dilution) are advised for general purpose disinfectant use, with stronger concentrations recommended for handling biohazardous spills with large amounts of organic matter involved. Diluted bleach loses potency quickly and should be made fresh and used within the same day prepared. Bleach should be diluted with cold water to prevent breakdown of the disinfectant.

Although chlorine compounds are biocidal to a broad spectrum of microorganisms, most chlorine-releasing preparations are not intended for HLD or sterilization of medical devices because of their highly corrosive effects on metals. Mixing chlorine-releasing agents with acids can cause the release of toxic chlorine gas. The byproducts of chlorine-releasing agents can be harmful to humans and the environment, so indiscriminate use of these products should be avoided. Chlorine-releasing agent should be stored and used only in well-ventilated areas.[9,10]

Iodine and Iodophors

The action of iodine and iodophors is similar to chlorine, albeit slightly less impacted by the presence of organic matter. Iodine can stain fabrics and environmental surfaces, making it unsuitable for disinfection. Conversely, iodophors (0.1–0.2%) and iodine tinctures are good antiseptics, with a low to intermediate activity level. Povidone-iodine is often used as a safe and reliable surgical scrub or preoperative skin antiseptic. Iodine can be toxic and should not be used on aluminum or copper.[9]

Hydrogen Peroxide and Peracids

Hydrogen peroxide (H_2O_2) and peracids are strong oxidants with potent broad-spectrum germicidal effects. Hydrogen peroxide is available as a ready-to-use 3% solution or 30% aqueous solution that is diluted 5–10 times in volume with sterilized water. However, 3–6% hydrogen peroxide solutions offer limited value as a germicide due to prolonged exposure times. Newer accelerated hydrogen peroxide products (e.g. 4.25% Rescue™ Concentrate, Virox Animal Health) offer greater stability and are associated with less corrosion and more rapid germicidal activity (e.g. 5 minutes at 1 : 16 dilution – bactericidal and fungicidal; 5 minutes at 1 : 16–1 : 64 –virucidal; 3 minutes at 1 : 128 dilution –broad-spectrum non-food contact surface sanitizer)).

Stronger hydrogen peroxide solutions are suitable for disinfecting heat-sensitive medical and dental devices, but can be corrosive to metals (e.g. aluminum, copper, brass, and zinc), and decolorize fabrics, hair, skin and mucous membranes. Always rinse articles treated with hydrogen peroxide-based agents thoroughly before contact with mucous membranes or ocular tissue.[9]

Phenolic Compounds

Phenolic compounds were among the earliest germicides and encompass a broad group of agents. They are active against vegetative bacteria and lipid-containing viruses, with some activity against mycobacteria, but demonstrate variable efficacy against non-lipid viruses and are not effective against spores. Phenolic products are used for decontaminating environmental surfaces, or may be commonly used as antiseptics (e.g. triclosan and chloroxylene). Triclosan is active against vegetative bacteria and may be safely used on skin and mucous membranes. Some phenolic compounds may be inactivated by water hardness, requiring dilution with distilled or deionized water. Phenolics are not advised for use on food contact surfaces and may be absorbed by rubber. Phenolics are also known to penetrate skin, and require following national chemical safety regulations.[9]

Quaternary Ammonium Compounds

QUATs are often used as mixtures or in combination with other germicides such as alcohols. They are effective against some vegetative bacteria and lipid-containing viruses. Some QUAT types are used as an antiseptic (e.g. benzalkonium chloride). The germicidal activity of certain QUATs is reduced considerably in the presence of organic matter, hard water, or anionic detergents, so careful selection of a precleaning agents is important. QUATs have also been demonstrated to grow potentially harmful bacteria, and may accumulate in the environment due to their low biodegradability properties.[9]

Table 22.3 / **Characteristics of selected disinfectants**

Characteristics of Selected Disinfectants	This table provides general information for each disinfectant chemical classes. Antimicrobial activity may vary with formulation and concentration. Always read and follow the product label for proper preparation and application directions.							
Disinfectant Category	Alcohols	Alkalis	Aldehydes	Oxidizing Agents			Phenols	Quaternary Ammonium Compounds
				Halogens: Chlorine	Halogens: Iodine	Peroxygen Compounds		
Common Active Ingredients	• ethanol • isopropanol	• calcium hydroxide • sodium carbonate • calcium oxide	• formaldehyde • glutaraldehyde • ortho-phthalaldehyde	• sodium hypochlorite (bleach) • calcium hypochlorite • chlorine dioxide	• providone-iodine	• hydrogen peroxide/accelerated HP • peracetic acid • potassium peroxymonosulfate	• ortho-phenyl/phenol • orthobenzyl/para-chlorophenol	• benzallonium chloride • alkyldimethyl ammonium chloride
Sample Trade Names*			*Synergize®*	*Clorox®, Wysiwash®*		*Rescue®, Oxy-Sept 333®, Virkon-S®*	*One-Stroke Environ®, Pheno-Tek II®, Tek-Trol, Lysol®*	*Roccal-D®, DiQuat®, D-256®*
Mechanism of Action	Precipitates proteins; denatures lipids	Alters pH through hydroxyl ions; fat saponification	Denatures proteins; alkylates nucleic acids	Denatures proteins	Denatures proteins	Denature proteins and lipids	Denatures proteins; disrupts cell wall	Denatures proteins; binds phospholipids of cell membrane
Characteristics	• Fast acting • Rapid evaporation • Leaves no residue • Can swell or harden rubber and plastics	• Slow acting • Affected by pH • Best at high temps • Corrosive to metals • Severe skin burns; mucous membrane imitation • Environmental hazard	• Slow acting • Affected by pH and temperature • Irritation of skin/mucous membrane • Only use in well ventilated areas • Pungent odor • Noncorrosive	• Fast acting • Affected by pH • Frequent application • Inactivated by UV radiation • Corrodes metals, rubber, fabrics, • Mucous membrane Irritation	• Stable in storage • Affected by pH • Requires frequent application • Corrosive • Stains clothes and treated surfaces	• Fast acting • May damage some metals (e.g., lead, copper, brass, zinc) • Powdered form may cause mucous membrane irritation • Low toxicity at lower concentrations • Environmentally friendly	• Can leave residual film on surfaces • Can damage rubber, plastic; non-corrosive • Stable in storage • Irritation to skin and eyes	• Stable in storage • Best at neutral or alkaline pH • Effective at high temps • High concentrations corrosive to metals • Irritation to skin, eyes, and respiratory tract

(*Continued*)

Table 22.3 / Characteristics of selected disinfectants (Continued)

Characteristics of Selected Disinfectants				This table provides general information for each disinfectant chemical classes. Antimicrobial activity may vary with formulation and concentration. Always read and follow the product label for proper preparation and application directions.				
Disinfectant Category	**Alcohols**	**Alkalis**	**Aldehydes**	**Oxidizing Agents**			**Phenols**	**Quaternary Ammonium Compounds**
				Halogens: Chlorine	**Halogens: Iodine**	**Peroxygen Compounds**		
Precautions	Flammable	Very caustic	Carcinogenic	Toxic gas released if mixed with strong acids or ammonia			May be toxic to animals, especially cats and pigs	
Bactericidal	+	+	+	+	+	+	+	+
Virucidal	±[a]	+	±	+	+	+	+	+ Enveloped
Fungicidal	+	+	+	+	+	±	+	±
Tuberculocidal	+	±	+	+	+	±	+	—
Sporticidal	—	+	+	+	±	+	—	+
Factors Affecting Effectiveness	Inactivated by organic matter	Variable	Inactivated by organic matter, hard water, soaps and detergents	Rapidly inactivated by organic matter	Rapidly inactivated by organic matter	Effective in presence of organic matter, hard water, soaps, and detergents	Effective in presence of organic matter, hard water, soaps, and detergents	Inactivated by organic matter, hard water soaps and anionic detergents

+ = effective; ± = variable or limited activity; — = not effective   a - slow acting against nonenveloped viruses (e.g., norovirus)

*DISCLAIMER: **The use of trade names serves only as examples and does not in any way signify endorsement of a particular product.***

REFERENCES: Fraise AP, Lambert PA et al. (eds). *Russell, Hugo & Ayliffe's Principles and Practice of Disinfection, Preservation and Sterilization*, 5th ed. 2013. Ames, IA: Wiley-Blackwell; McDonnell GE. *Antisepsis, Disinfection, and Sterilization: Types, Action, and Resistance*. 2007. ASM Press, Washington DC. Rutala WA, Weber DJ, Healthcare Infection Control Practices Advisory Committee (HICPAC). 2008. Guideline for disinfection and sterilization in healthcare facilities. Available at: *http://www.cdc.gov/hicpac/Disinfection_Sterilization/toc.html*; Quinn PJ, Markey FC et al. (eds). *Veterinary Microbiology and Microbial Disease*. 2nd ed. 2011. West Sussex, UK: Wiley-Blackwell, pp 851-889.

LIQUID CHEMICALS FOR HIGH LEVEL DISINFECTION AND STERILIZATION

In general, cold sterilization is not recommended for disinfecting high-quality surgical instruments.[7] In fact, prolonged immersion of surgical instruments in any solution can be damaging. Furthermore, immersing surgical instruments containing tungsten carbide inserts (e.g. gold-handled instruments) in solutions containing benzyl ammonium chloride can cause loosening of the tungsten carbide.[7]

Glutaraldehyde Solutions

Glutaraldehyde ($OHC(CH_2)_3CHO$) is a major component of LCS/HLD products. Two-percent glutaraldehyde in alkaline aqueous solution was discovered in the 1960s. Alkaline glutaraldehyde products are usually supplied in two parts and require mixing to become activated, while acid glutaraldehyde usually does not. Activated glutaraldehyde solutions may be reused for one to four weeks, based on formulation and use frequency. Discard solutions if they become turbid. Depending on the glutaraldehyde formulation and concentration, conditions for HLD generally range from 5 to 90 minutes, at temperatures ranging from 20°C to 35°C (68–95°F). The contact time for sterilization is 10 hours, at temperatures of 20–25°C (68–77°F), or 7 hours and 40 minutes at 35°C (95°F). Glutaraldehyde is effective against vegetative bacteria, spores, fungi, and both lipid- and non-lipid-containing viruses. However, evidence suggests that some types of microorganisms demonstrate resistance to the antimicrobial effects of glutaraldehyde. Glutaraldehyde is toxic and irritating to skin and mucous membranes, and must be used in well-ventilated areas. Always follow national chemical safety regulations when using glutaraldehyde.[9,10]

Hydrogen Peroxide Solutions

Ready-to-use hydrogen peroxide HLD solutions are used primarily for heat-sensitive and submersible medical devices (e.g. flexible or rigid endoscopes.) A 2% hydrogen peroxide has contact conditions of 8 minutes at 20°C (68°F), has a reuse life of 21 days at or above 1.5% concentration; 7.5% hydrogen peroxide is labeled for an HLD contact time of 30 minutes at 20°C (68°F), and a sterilization contact time of 6 hours at 20°C (68°F), with a similar 21-day reuse life if the solution concentration remains above 6%.

Orthophthaldehyde Solutions

Orthophthaldehyde (OPA) is FDA cleared for use as an HLD for reprocessing heat sensitive medical devices. It is especially active against particular strains of *Mycobacteria*, but some strains have shown high level resistance to it, as have some cyst and vegetative forms of protozoa. Products containing 0.55–0.6% OPA have been cleared for use as an HLD during manual reprocessing at 12 minutes and 20°C (68°F), and has a reuse life of 14 days. OPA should not be used to process urological instrumentation for humans with a history of bladder cancer, as it has been associated with anaphylaxis-like reactions in these patients.

Peracetic Acid Hydrogen Peroxide Solutions

Peracetic acid solutions have strong microbial effects and a broad spectrum of activity, and can be used for HLD and sterilant applications. Peracetic acid solutions can vary significantly, ranging from 35% peracetic acid and 6% hydrogen peroxide to 5% peracetic acid and 26% hydrogen peroxide. Based on composition, typical HLD contact times range from 5 to 30 minutes, with sterilant contact times of 6 minutes to 8 hours at 20°C (68°F). Ready-to-use formulations can be reused for up to 14 days.

Vaporized hydrogen peroxide or peracetic acid (CH_3COOOH) requires the use of specialized equipment.

Additional resources are available from the FDA.[11]

SAFE HANDLING OF LIQUID CHEMICAL STERILANT PRODUCTS

It is important to fully understand the product label, and to always read the product insert and follow the manufacturer's instructions for use. Product labels contain information surrounding the safe and effective use of the product including active ingredients, concentrations, or any dilution or activation requirements, expiration dates, required exposure time and temperature.[2,12]

The OSHA has established occupational exposure limits for LCS, and employers are required by law to comply with safe work practices, generate monitoring and surveillance programs, and implement adequate engineering controls. Always consult the Material Safety Data Sheets supplied by the disinfectant manufacturer for a complete list of potential precautions and hazards. General safety precautions are:

- Ensure adequate engineering controls are in place, including adequate ventilation and/or a vented hood to evacuate chemical vapors.
- Use covered containers to store previously prepared or diluted solutions, as appropriate.
- Use PPE, such as gloves, eye protection, face masks or liquid-resistant gowns, and shoe covers, as appropriate (OSHA requirement 29 CFR 1910.1030).[5]
- Ensure adequate rinsing of items after disinfection using sterile distilled water.
- An LCS/HLD spill containment "response team" should be established to ensure accidental spills can be safely resolved.

Occupational exposure limits for chemical agents are commonly categorized as maximum amounts over specified time periods. For example, the OSHA mandates permissible exposure limits in both "short-term exposure limits", defined as a 15-minute exposure period, and an 8-hour time-weighted average. More information regarding OSHA limits for airborne contaminants, LCS and other gas sterilant chemicals can be found in OSHA air contaminants standard (29 CFR 1910.1000).[13]

THERMAL DISINFECTION

Thermal disinfection processes use hot water at 60–95°C, (140–203°F) to decontaminate or disinfect reusable medical devices. Thermal disinfection selectively kills some microorganisms, depending on the exposure time and temperature. Vegetative bacteria are the easiest to destroy using this method, while bacterial spores and certain fungi and viruses are considered resistant. Use temperature-sensitive indicators to assure appropriate internal temperatures were achieved.

SURGICAL INSTRUMENT DECONTAMINATION AND CLEANING

Adequate sterile processing depends on the performance of people, processes, and equipment to achieve the highest level of sterility assurance all the time. Observance of the principles of infection prevention and control will help stop the spread of potentially infectious microorganisms and ensure that all items are safe for handling during all phases of the sterilization process, as part of an essential element in achieving sterilization. The goals for individuals participating in a sterile processing program include:

- Ensuring that every item in each load is sterile.
- Minimizing the risk of hospital acquired infections.
- Meeting regulatory requirements using best industry practices.
- Assuring quality outcomes.

All reusable medical devices should be meticulously washed by hand or mechanically immediately after use. Thorough cleaning and rinsing is the first and most important step in reprocessing surgical equipment and instrumentation (medical devices). Cleaning removes organic and inorganic matter as well as microorganisms. It is important to note that cleaning does not kill microorganisms (decontamination). The level of decontamination required may be dictated by the circumstances surrounding the device's use, the type of patient contact, and the threat of the biological hazard exposure to personnel.[1]

During decontamination, a microbicidal process is meant to render a device safe for handling and subsequent processing, but this step alone is not considered sufficient processing for reuse (such as the case with surgical instruments requiring sterilization). Subsequent disinfection or a sterilization process may be necessary to render the item completely safe for reuse (see Thermal Disinfection section).[1]

If medical devices cannot be cleaned immediately, they should be presoaked or kept moist until such time, preferably using products approved for this purpose (such as Spectra-Moist®, Integrated Medical Systems International). Presoaking products are intended to augment cleaning regimens by serving to moisten and loosen soil.

Medical devices placed in presoaking solutions should be thoroughly rinsed to remove blood, residues, and potentially infectious materials. Always follow the manufacturer's instructions for the recommended dilution, temperature, and contact time. Presoaking should not be performed if it is contraindicated in the instrument manufacturer's written instructions for use. Saline or other solutions may cause corrosion, and alcohol or other disinfectants may cause biofilms to affix to surfaces, thereby making cleaning more difficult.[1]

Items should be pretreated with an initial cold water rinse with running tap water or an initial cold water soak to remove the majority of blood contamination, prior to hand or mechanical washing.[1]

Only designated pH balanced detergents and enzymatic cleaners approved for surgical devices are used for washing, following the manufacturer's instructions.

- Laundry soap, Lysol®, chlorhexidine, dish soap, hand scrubs, bleach, or any other unapproved chemicals are not recommended for cleaning surgical instruments.
- Most surgical instruments can be cleaned with a detergent specifically designed for this purpose. Enzymatic cleaners differ from detergents as they contain biological catalysts that help remove proteins or biofilms from instruments such as an endoscope. There are also dual role enzymatic detergents available (e.g. Cetyl-Zyme ProAm®).

Use dedicated surgical instrument cleaning brushes to access small nooks and crannies such as box locks, channels, or any other area considered difficult to clean. Stainless steel bristle brushes designed for cleaning surgical instruments do not harm the instruments they are cleaning, but should not be used on insulated or coated instruments. Store brushes while clean and dry when not in use (Figure 22.3).[10,14]

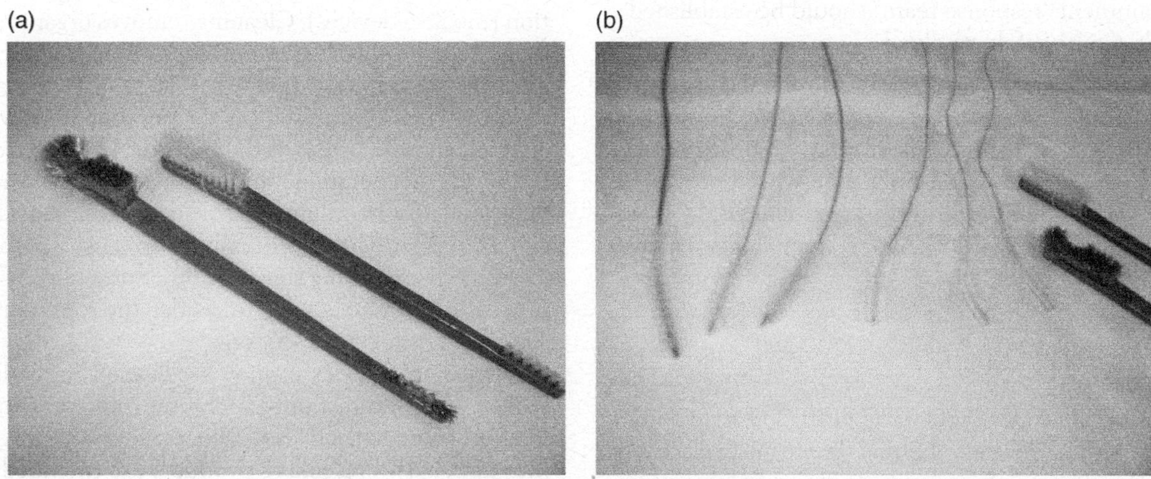

Figure 22.3 (a) Cleaning brushes for surgical instruments. Brushes should be checked for visible soil and damage after each use, and replaced as needed. (b) Left to right: cut-to-length Flexistem brushes and Flexistem (007A Healthmark) wavy brushes contain embedded nylon bristles which aid in the cleaning of small bore lumens and channels. Single-use features limit cross-contamination between instruments. Commercially available cleaning brushes can be labeled for a sole purpose (e.g. endotracheal tubes vs. bloody suction tip cleaning) and reused many times. This type of brush requires periodic cleaning and disinfection. Source: photographs courtesy of the author.

All cannulated items (e.g. Frazier or Poole suction tips, endoscopic or arthroscopic equipment) should be cleaned using a three-step process:

1. Flush (using copious amounts of water).
2. Brush (with an appropriate diameter brush).
3. Rinse.

Use the correct brush size for the lumen to create effective cleaning friction against the lumen walls, and ensure that the brush exits the distal tip of the instrument being cleaned (Figure 22.4).[1,14]

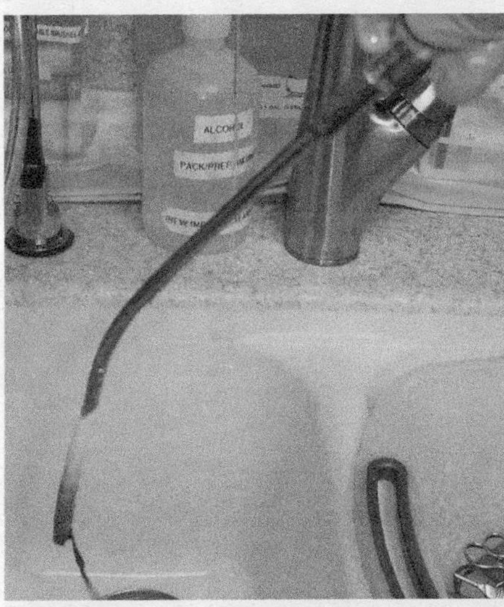

Figure 22.4 Use a three-step cleaning process for cannulated items; flush, brush, and rinse. Ensure that the cleaning brush is long enough to exit the distal tip of the instrument. Source: photograph courtesy of the author.

Ultrasonic Cleaners

Ultrasonic cleaners are growing in popularity, predominantly due to their ease of use, efficiency and effectiveness. Ultrasonic cleaning units are a vital processing tool, capable of cleaning 99.9% of residual blood contamination after three minutes.[15] Ultrasonic cleaning is created by high frequency sound waves produced by a generator located within the unit. A unique vibration pattern occurs as the result of alternating high and low pressures during the cleaning cycle as the sound waves are carried throughout the liquid in the tank. Millions of tiny bubbles form cavities during the low-pressure stage, resulting in a process called cavitation. These bubbles collapse or implode during the high-pressure stage and release enormous amounts of energy. The bubbles invade all surfaces, nooks, and crannies in every direction, thereby removing debris from the objects being cleaned.

Generally speaking, heated ultrasonic cleaning solutions have not demonstrated measurable improvement in cleaning or timing, so a heated tank feature is not imperative when choosing an ultrasonic cleaner.[16] Assess proper cavitation energy in ultrasonic cleaners using SonoCheck™ test ampoules or perform the aluminum foil test.

A test object surgical instrument can be used to verify the cleaning efficacy of mechanical cleaning equipment such as ultrasonic cleaners or automated instrument washers and protolytic detergents in a water bath. The test object surgical instrument consists of "soil" on a scratched stainless steel substrate covered with a clear plastic holder to mimic a contaminated box lock. The soil is composed of blood proteins in proportions similar to human blood (95% water soluble hemoglobin/albumin and 5% insoluble fibrin; Figure 22.5).

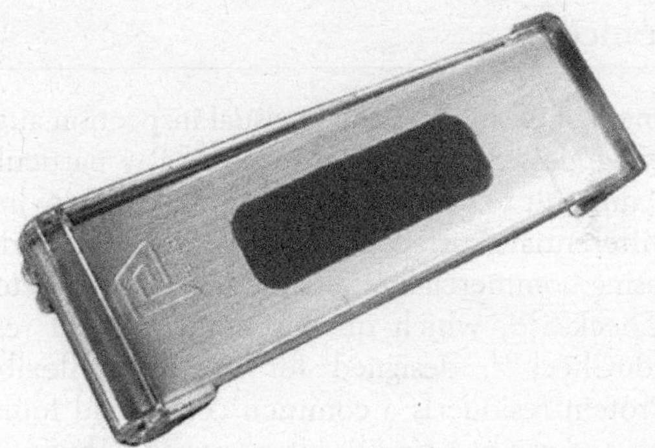

Figure 22.5 A test object surgical instrument mimics a blood-contaminated box lock, and is used to verify the cleaning efficiency of ultrasonic cleaners and/or automated instrument washers. Source: photograph courtesy of Healthmark.

- Use only solutions specifically designed for use in ultrasonic cleaners.
- Degas stagnated or freshly made ultrasonic cleaning solutions by running the tank empty for a specified time, as per the manufacturer's

instructions. Degassing helps to eliminate gas bubbles that could impede the cavitation process.

- After manual cleaning, place items into the ultrasonic cleaning basket with box locks in the open position. Try to avoid mixing instruments of varying metal content in the same ultrasonic cleaning cycle to prevent cross-plating, which results in stubborn bluish-black surface stains. See Table 22.4 for other causes of staining on surgical instruments. Fill the ultrasonic cleaning basket two thirds to three quarters full. Do not overfill the tank.
- Run the ultrasonic cleaning cycle for 10–20 minutes, following the manufacturer's instructions. Ultrasonic cleaning solutions should be changed daily, or sooner if the solution appears cloudy or dirty.
- Instruments should be thoroughly rinsed once removed from the ultrasonic cleaner. A distilled water rinse may be preferred since tap water can contain high concentrations of minerals that contribute to staining.
- Never allow water to dry onto surgical instruments, as residual water spots can result in stains.[14]

Quality Assurance

Assess thoroughness of cleaning via keen visual inspection augmented by the use of a magnifying glass and good light source. Pay particular attention to areas considered difficult to clean, such as box locks, screw heads and hinges (Figure 22.6). Differentiate surface stains from residual blood contamination on surfaces by using commercially available peroxidases detection products such as HemoCheck-S™, which quickly detects blood residue down to 0.1 μg, or EndoCheck™, designed for use with flexible endoscopes (Figure 22.7). Protein residue is a common compound found on contaminated instruments and can be a significant source of bioburden. ProChek-II™ detects residual amounts of protein (sensitive to 1 μg) using clinical chemistry techniques that evolved from the pyrogallol-red method. Repeat the cleaning process for any instruments found still dirty at this juncture.

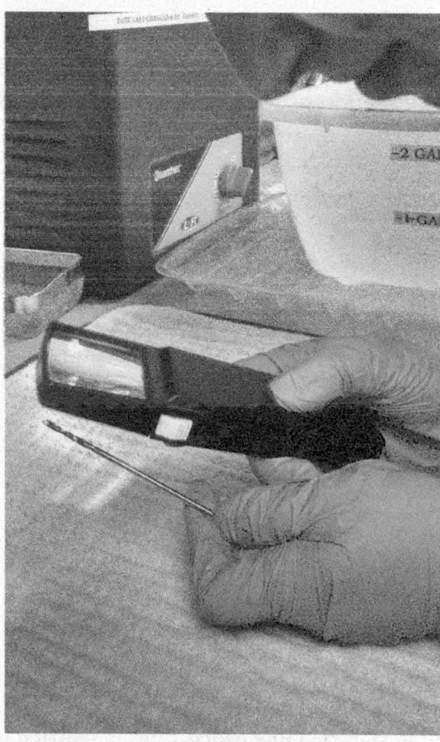

Figure 22.6 Use a magnifying glass with a good light source to identify residual debris or damage on clean surgical instruments. Source: photograph courtesy of the author.

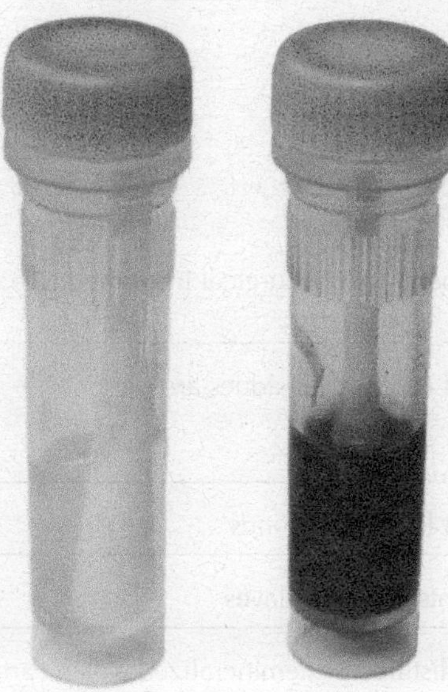

Figure 22.7 A HemoCheck-S detection kit quickly detects residual blood contamination on surgical instrumentation. A positive result (pictured right) is evident by a strong bluish color change. A negative test result is pictured left. Source: photograph courtesy of Healthmark.

Once the surgical instruments are scrupulously clean, they should be carefully inspected for stains, wear or damage, and repaired or replaced, as indicated (Table 22.4). Scissors, osteotomes, and rongeurs should be assessed for sharpness, bending, cracks, or damage. Ratchet testing should be performed on hemostats and needle holders. Box locks should be examined for cracks, instrument jaws inspected for excessive wear and proper alignment; verify that self-retaining mechanisms are functional.[14]

Table 22.4 / **Common surgical instrument stains: potential causes and resolutions**

Instrument Stain Identification Chart		
Stain Color	Reason	Action
Orange-Brown to Reddish stain (looks like rust)	Do eraser test, if stain rubs off and no pitting exists, problem is most likely from:	• Change to Neutral pH detergent. Recommend Miltex Surgical Instrument Cleaner.
	• Detergent residue on towels or High Alkaline >8 pH detergent is being used leaving a phosphate surface deposit	• Check pH of towels with litmus to verify if detergent residues are present.
	• Dried blood	• Rinse the instruments in warm water for at least 30 seconds
	• Iodine or Betadine residue	• Use a stain remover on both the instruments and autoclaves
		• If problem persists, consider changing to distilled or demineralized water. Particularly if local water supply is high in Iron or other minerals.
Black, Brown & Pitting	Subjected to an Acidic Low <6 pH substance such as:	• Change to Neutral pH detergent. Recommend Miltex Surgical Instrument Cleaner.
	• Low pH detergent residues on instrument surface or from towels	• Check pH of towels with litmus to verify if detergent residues are present.
	• Exposed to other chemical compounds from “cold soaking”	• Eliminate exposure to chemicals or bleach
	• Exposure to Bleach	• Rinse thoroughly and consider using distilled or demineralized water. Particularly if local water supply is high in Iron or other minerals.
		• Use stain remover on both the instruments and autoclaves • Eliminate any use of bleach.
		• If pitting remains, send instrument back to manufacturer for evaluation.
Rainbow or Multi-Color	• Heat compromised, tensile strength is compromised	• Check the autoclave for proper temperature
Bluish-Green Bluish-Black	• Cross contamination between dissimilar metals	• Separate instruments by type before cleaning or autoclaving

(*Continued*)

Table 22.4 / Common surgical instrument stains: potential causes and resolutions (Continued)

Instrument Stain Identification Chart		
Stain Color	**Reason**	**Action**
Bluish-Gray (w/ possible pitting)	• Improper preparation of cold sterilization solutions	• Follow solution manufacturer's directions closely, particularly temp. & soak times.
		• Use distilled or demineralized water
		• Change solution per mfg's instructions
Rust	• Sterilizing instruments of dissimilar metals in the same cycle.	• Separate instruments by metal types prior to sterilization. • Use neutral pH detergents and change to distilled or demineralized water. Particularly if local water supply is known to contain Iron or other minerals.
	• Chemicals in detergents or excess amounts of Iron or other minerals from local water supply.	• Wipe off as much residue leaving shiny metal underneath. Use a stain remover on both the instruments and autoclaves.
	• New Instruments may be slightly magnetized during the manufacturing process.	• After several autoclaving sequences, the instruments lose their magnetic property
Spotting Light or Dark colored	• Slow evaporation of water drops with mineral content	• Eliminate water droplets and moisture by adhering to autoclave manufacturer's operating instructions.
	• Instrument wraps & towels may contain detergent residue	• Use Miltex Stain Remover on both the instruments and autoclaves
		• Change to distilled or demineralized water. Particularly if local water supply is known to contain Iron or other minerals.
		• Thoroughly wash & rinse wraps & towels with a neutral pH detergent.
Chart recreated: https://www.integralife.com/file/general/stains.pdf		

Source: courtesy of Miltex.

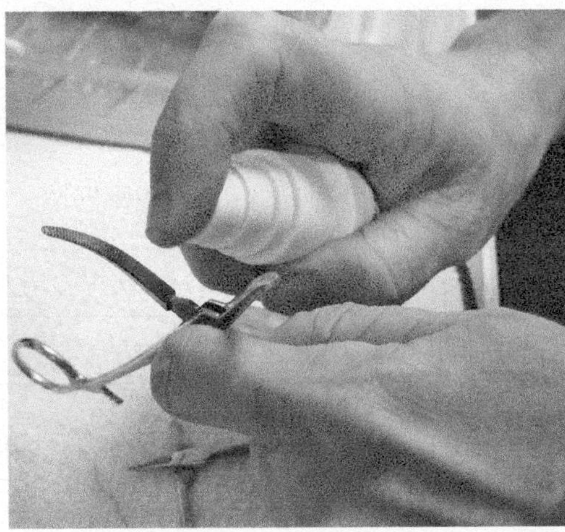

Figure 22.8 Surgical instruments containing moving parts, such as joints, box locks, ratchet and screws should be lubricated. Source: photograph courtesy of the author.

Lubrication

Lubrication should be done after surgical instruments have been thoroughly cleaned and dried.[17] Proper lubrication of surgical instruments prevents rubbing and scraping and helps ensure that dulling and staining are minimized. The use of lubricant sprays may be preferred over lubricant baths due to the presence of bacteria from previously dipped instruments lingering in bathing solutions. Additionally, lubricant sprays are associated with decreased costs and spray bottles use less counter space than most lubricant bath containers.[7,18]

Instrument lubricants should be specifically formulated for the intended use and must be compatible with the processing and sterilization methods used. Lubricant manufacturers can provide documentation to support compatibility and biocompatibility (e.g. lack of tissue toxicity) with devices requiring lubrication. Always use lubricants used according to the manufacturer's instructions.[1]

PACK ASSEMBLY

Ensure that all instruments are in working order (e.g. clean and rust free, moveable hinges, proper alignment). Surgical instrument packs should be assembled following specific steps to assure a uniform approach every time. Instrument checklists can be customized for each pack, and should contain the type and number of instruments unique to that pack, as well as specific gauze counts and chemical indicators. Instrument stringers should be used to safeguard instrument handling, help audit and organize pack contents, ensure all ratchets stay open during sterilization, and expedite set up of the sterile field (Figure 22.9).[14] Instruments from various pack types can be easily identified using colored instrument marking tape.

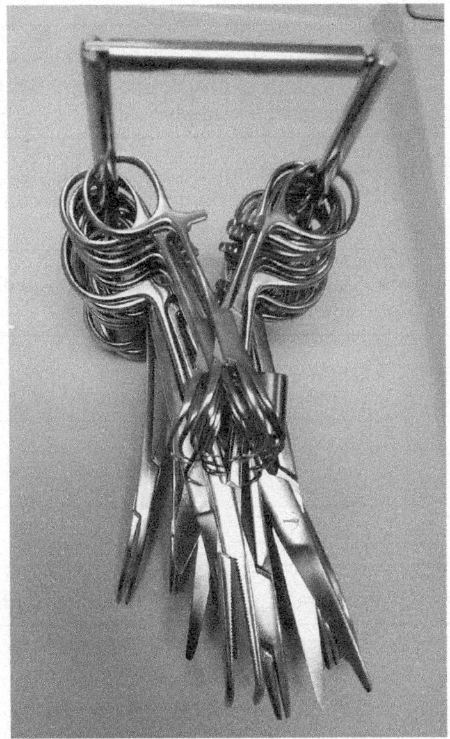

Figure 22.9 Surgical instrument stringer. Instruments are often organized from largest to smallest, and curved to straight (e.g. large curved hemostat, large straight hemostat, small curved hemostat, etc.). Source: photograph courtesy of the author.

Instrument marking tape should be applied as follows:

1. Clean your fingers with alcohol to remove grease, oils and dirt.
2. Wipe the tape application site with an alcohol swab to remove residual lubricant.
3. Using firm pressure, place the instrument tape 1–1.5 times around the shank of the surgical instrument. This amount of tape should not interfere with closing the tips of most scissors.
4. Avoid placing the tape around the rings of the instrument.
5. Autoclave the instrument after the tape is applied to help bond the tape in place.

Be sure to label the indicator tape on the outside of each pack with the contents (e.g. general surgical pack, thoracic pack), date, and initials of the person assembling the pack.

Instruments that are used only on occasion should be set aside in separate packages. Instruments can weaken with constant scrubbing and autoclaving, and therefore, should not be subjected to unnecessary and repeated sterilization.

Packaging Surgical Instruments

It is imperative to ensure that all items to be wrapped for sterilization are dry and inspected for cleanliness and damage prior to packaging. Surgical instruments with multiple parts should be disassembled prior to sterilization. Ensure that instruments are completely dry prior to packaging, as water droplets can interfere with steam sterilization or cause dilution of liquid chemical sterilants. The drying phase can be accelerated using towel drying or canned air. Hot air drying is contraindicated, especially prior to ethylene oxide sterilization.

All packaging materials should be equilibrated for at least two hours at room temperature 20–23 degrees C (68–73.4°F) and at a relative humidity of 30–60% prior to use.[10]

Peel Pouches

Peel-pouch wraps should allow adequate penetration and removal of both the sterilants and air, should resist tearing and prevent contamination of the contents. They should also be easy to seal, simple to open beyond the chevron seal without tearing, and able to withstand the conditions of the sterilization process. When labeling peel pouches, use an indelible (permanent) marker, and write only on the film (transparent) part of the pouch or on the designated area beneath the adhesive strip. Never write on the paper or breathable side of the pouch. Sterilization processes such as hydrogen peroxide gas plasma are not compatible with cellulose (paper based) pouch materials. Always follow the manufacturer's instructions.[16]

- Ensure that the item is inserted into the pouch so that only the handle or "grasping end" will be accessible when the item is issued to the surgeon.
- Remove as much air as possible to ensure proper sealing conditions are met (e.g. prevent wrinkles and air bubbles.)
- When heat sealing tubing, always leave about 1.5–2 inches beyond the seal to assure the item can be easily opened after the sterilization process. Use cut-to-size sterilization tubing for pouching long items.
  - To prevent "blow out" or a ruptured pouch due to items being packaged too tightly, allow at least 1 inch of space between the item being sterilized and the pouch/chevron seals on all four sides. Items that can rupture the pouch due to size, weight, or shape should be packaged using another method, such as wrapping in drape material.
  - Items packaged in excessively large pouches may allow shifting during processing or require additional space for sterilization and storage.
- Sharp tips and delicate instruments (e.g. ophthalmic instruments, pointed scissors, skin hooks, cutting edges of osteotomes) should have protector tips applied to prevent damage and provide cushioning during the sterilization process. Protector tips may be either vented (fenestrated) or non-vented.
  - Protector tips used to cushion or secure instruments in peel pouch wraps should be loosely applied so the sterilant can easily penetrate the surface area underneath it.
  - Do not use rubber bands and/or latex tubing to secure items together.
- Double pouching may be considered when multiple small items must be sterilized or to facilitate aseptic presentation to the sterile field (Figure 22.10). Never fold a pouch before or after sterilization, as folding can interfere with the sterilization process or compromise the material.
- Peel pouches should never be used inside of another wrapped sterile instrument set or pack.[10]

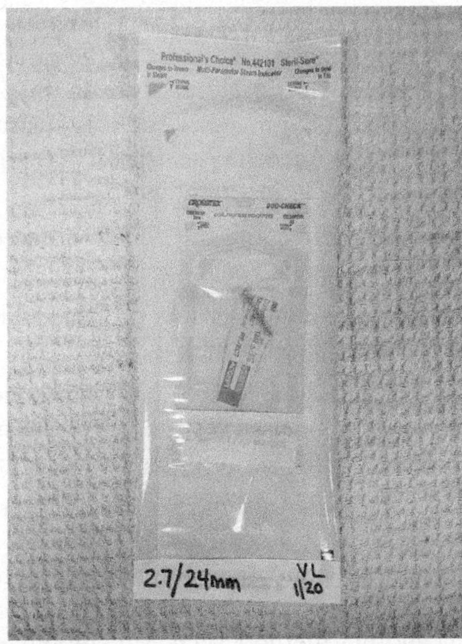

Figure 22.10 To ensure adequate sterilant penetration, double-pouched items should be wrapped so that the paper side of the inner pouch faces the same side as the paper side of the outer pouch. The chemical indicator should be placed inside of the innermost pouch. Source: photograph courtesy of the author.

Central Sterilization Drapes

Packaging materials used for sterilization should be engineered to allow sterilants to pass through readily while blocking bacteria. Although no stringent FDA standard exists for class II sterilization drapes, manufacturers have agreed that each type of packaging material developed must demonstrate appropriate scientific evidence that:

1. Material is specifically designed and suitable for the recommended sterilization methods and cycles.
2. Material provides an effective barrier to contamination when used according to the manufacturer's written instructions.
3. Manufacturer should provide adequate in-service education and instructions for use/reuse.[16]

Two different methods determine how central sterilization drapes filter bacteria. Linen and paper drapes function as sieve-type filters. The sieve filter concept illustrates that excessively washed or old linen wraps lose effectiveness as threads wear away, and the space between the threads("sieve" holes) become so large that bacteria pass through freely. Sterilization drapes made of SMS polypropylene (i.e. Kimberly-Clark wraps) act as a probability-type filter, and consist of dense microfibers that create a tortuous path. This type of filter provides a more reliable barrier against dust particles and microorganisms (Figure 22.11).

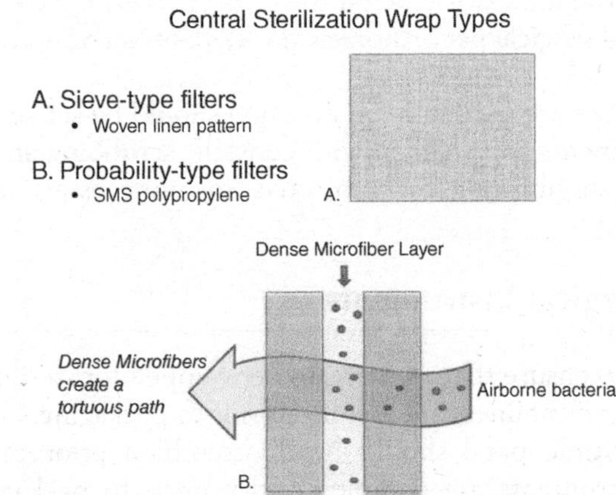

Figure 22.11 Wrap types. Source: courtesy of 3M and the author.

- Always follow the manufacturer's instructions regarding paper drape materials.
- Paper drape materials should never be reused.
- Cloth drapes should be washed and carefully inspected for wear, holes, or residual soil. Do not use cloth drapes beyond the manufacturer's instructions.(see Surgical Huck Towel, Gown and Cloth Drape Care section).

Steps to folding surgical huck towels or drapes for sterilization include (Figure 22.12a):

1. Place a clean, lint free surgical huck towel (or drape) on a clean table.
2. Fold the huck towel in half lengthwise and reflect the top layer back and forth (e.g. accordion style) to a width that is less than that of the final pack (Figure 22.12b).
3. Continue the accordion fold for the bottom half of the huck towel (Figure 22.12c).
4. Fold the accordioned huck towel in half and reflect back the top half once (Figure 22.12d).
5. Flip the huck towel over and repeat step 4 for the bottom half (Figure 22.12e).

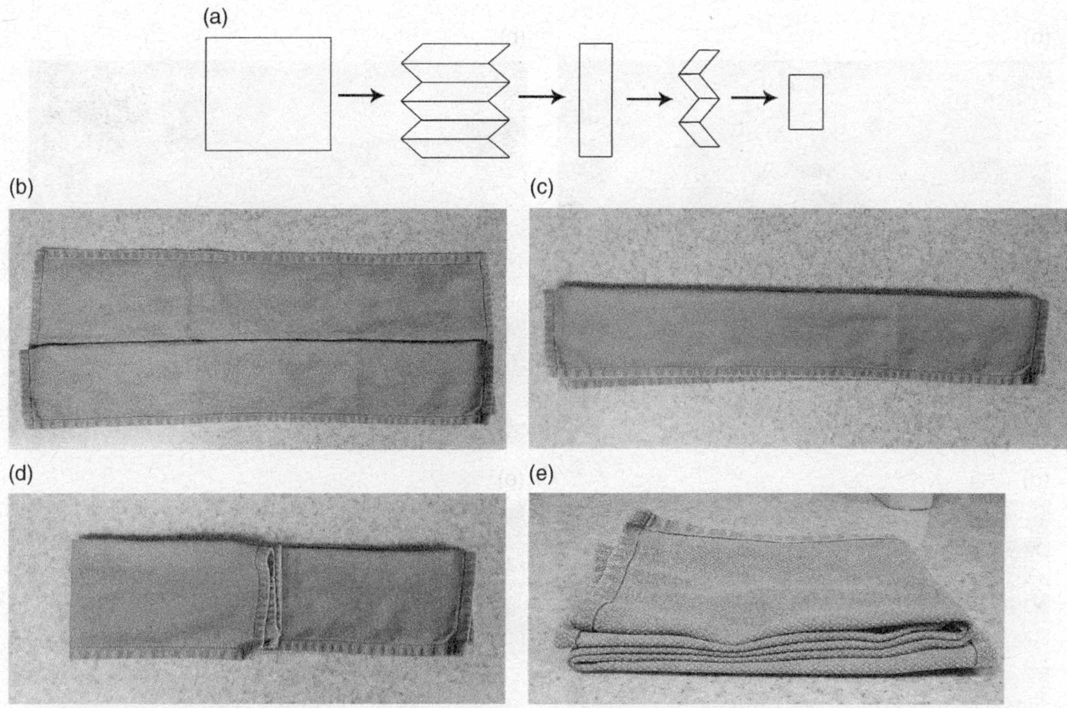

Figure 22.12 **(a) Steps to folding surgical huck towels or drapes for sterilization. (b) Place two drapes (one on top of the other) on the table, with the bottom corner facing the technician. Then center the pack perpendicularly on the drape with a chemical indicator strip. (c) Fold the bottom corner of the top drape over the pack and then fold the corner back down toward the technician to create tabs that will make the pack easier to open. (d, e) Repeat the step above for the corners to the left and right. Before folding the corner over, tuck the drape material down along the sides of the pack to eliminate air pockets and excess wrinkles. The envelope fold. Steps to double wrapping packs for sterilization.**

Wrapping Packs for Sterilization

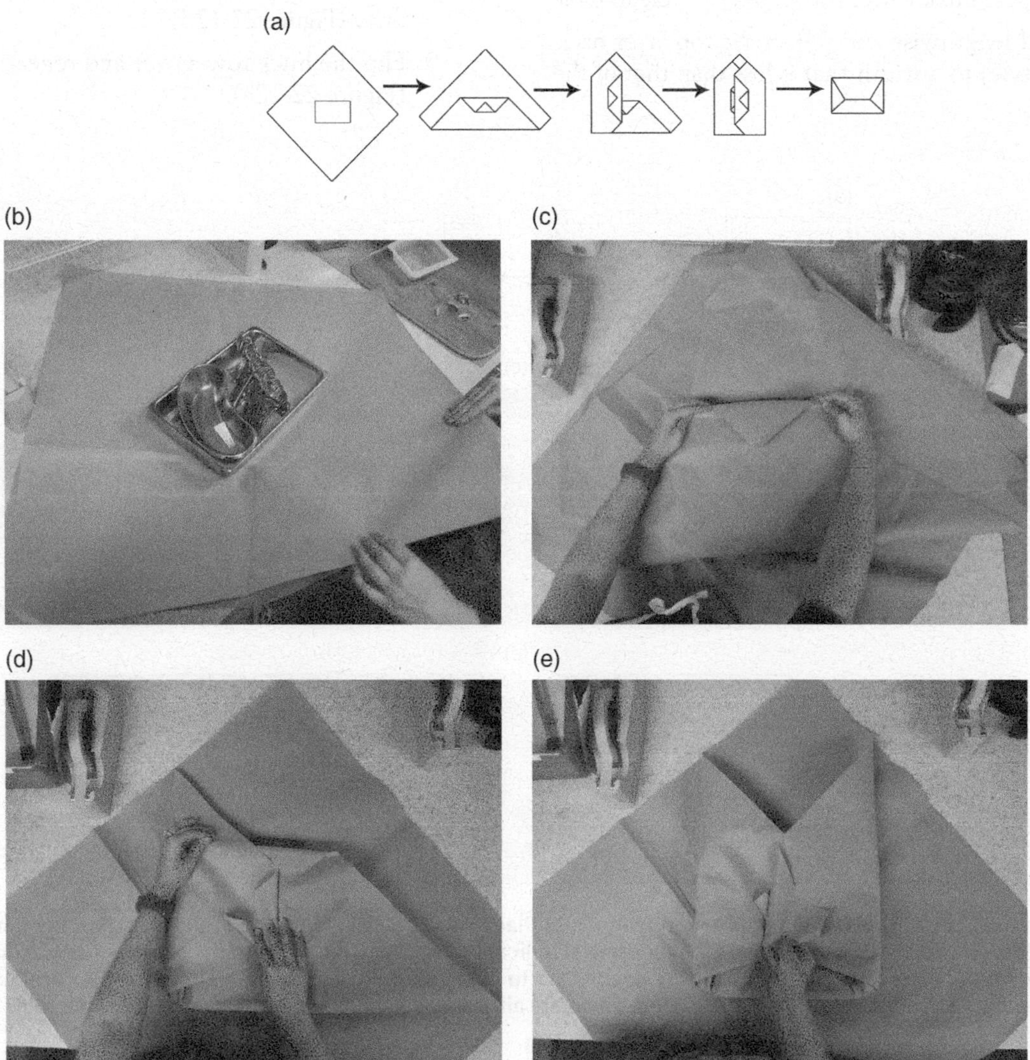

Figure 22.13 (a) The envelope fold. Steps to double wrapping packs for sterilization. (b) Place two drapes (one on top of the other) on the table, with the bottom corner facing the technician. Then center the pack perpendicularly on the drape with a chemical indicator strip. (c) Fold the bottom corner of the top drape over the pack and then fold the corner back down toward the technician to create tabs that will make the pack easier to open. (d, e) Repeat the step above for the corners to the left and right. Before folding the corner over, tuck the drape material down along the sides of the pack to eliminate air pockets and excess wrinkles.

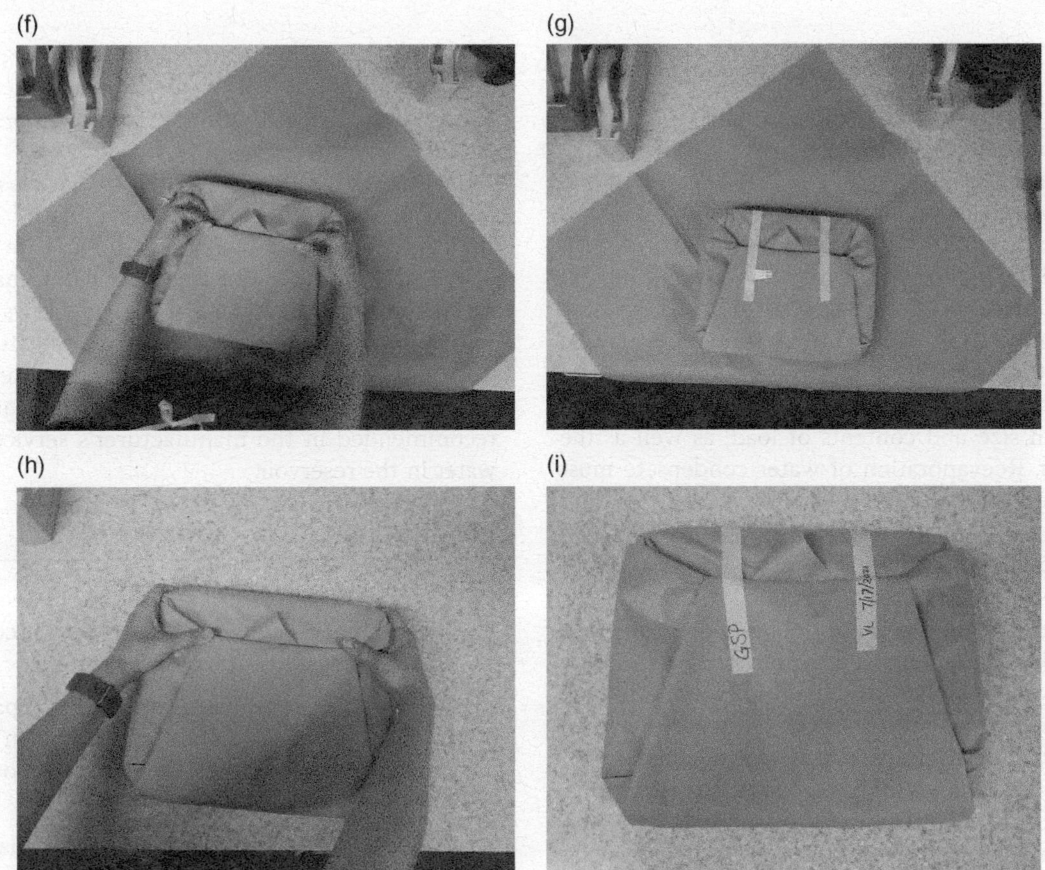

Figure 22.13 **(Continued) (f) Fold the top (last) corner over the pack and tuck into the side flaps, leaving an access tab for opening. (g) Secure the inside drape using steam sterilization indicator tape, with or without a second chemical indicator strip. (h) Repeat the folding process above with the second drape to complete a double wrapped pack. (i) Steam sterilization indicator tape is used to secure the pack prior to autoclaving. The tape should be labeled with the technician's identification, pack type, and date.**

STEAM AUTOCLAVES

Direct saturated steam contact (moisture), heat, time, and pressure are the basis of the steam sterilization process. Death by moist heat (steam) occurs via the denaturation and coagulation of protein or the enzyme-protein system within the cells. After pressurized steam enters the sterilizer chamber, it condenses upon contact with cold items. This condensation liberates heat, simultaneously heating and wetting all items in the load. No living thing can survive direct exposure to saturated steam at 250 degrees F (120°C) for more than 15 minutes. As the temperature is increased, exposure time may be decreased. A minimum temperature–time relationship must be maintained throughout the entire cycle to achieve effective sterilization. The actual exposure time may depend upon size and contents of load, as well as the temperature within the sterilizer. Reevaporation of water condensate must effectively dry the contents of the load to maintain sterility at the conclusion of the cycle.

There are several types of steam autoclaves. The gravity displacement autoclave is commonplace in most veterinary facilities, owing to its small size and economy. Once this sterilizer is loaded and the door is closed, steam is pumped into the chamber containing ambient air. Steam has a lower density than air and rises to the top of the chamber, eventually displacing the air. Once the air is removed, the steam can directly contact the surface of all items in the load and the sterilization cycle begins. A typical standard for steam sterilization is achieved at 121 degrees C (250°F) after 20–30 minutes at 15 psi. It is important to refer to the manufacturer's instructions for operation, since exposure times can vary according to the design of the particular sterilizer or items being sterilized.

The prevacuum steam sterilizer was designed to minimize trapped air in the chamber. The speed and efficiency of the steam sterilizer is augmented by removing air from the chamber with a pump, thereby creating an efficient vacuum prior to steam being introduced into the chamber. Full heating of the loads is faster in the prevacuum sterilizer than in the gravity displacement sterilizer. For example, wrapped instruments can be sterilized at 131 degrees C (270°F) after four minutes exposure in a prevacuum steam sterilizer.

Another design in steam sterilization is a steam flush, pressure pulse process, which removes air rapidly by repeatedly alternating a steam flush and a pressure pulse above atmospheric pressure. Air is rapidly removed from the load as with the prevacuum sterilizer, but air leaks do not affect this process because the steam in the sterilizing chamber is always greater than atmospheric pressure. Typical sterilization temperatures are 132–135 degrees C (269.6–275°F) with three to four minutes exposure time for porous loads and instruments.

"Flash" sterilization is also referred to as an emergency sterilization cycle. Single, unwrapped instruments are placed on a perforated metal tray and sterilized as per the instructions for use for a flash cycle, then immediately delivered to the operating room using detachable tray handles. Do not sterilize metal implants such as bone plates and screws using a flash sterilization cycle.[1,19]

It is imperative to follow the manufacturer's instructions regarding the care and maintenance of steam autoclaves. Steam autoclaves should be cleaned regularly, and worn door gaskets and filters should be changed as recommended in the manufacturer's service manual. Always used distilled water in the reservoir.

Loading the Steam Autoclave

- Every item to be sterilized should be loosely packed in the autoclave. Ensure that all contained items do not come into contact with either the inside walls or top of the chamber.
- Peel pouches should be loosely placed paper-to-plastic (resulting in all pouches facing the same direction or "in line"), so that the sterilant can easily reach all surfaces. Do not stack pouches on top of one another during sterilization (Figure 22.14).[16]
- Surgical packs wrapped in drape materials should be placed in the autoclave so that steam can freely circulate around all items in the sterilizer. Pans or trays used for sterilizing surgical packs should ideally be fenestrated to enable better steam sterilization and more effective drying.
- For most efficient sterilizing, place heavier instruments on the bottom shelving and lighter, more delicate instruments on upper shelving.
- The sterilization cycle for each medical device is dictated by the manufacturer's instructions. General use surgical instruments may require a different sterilization cycle parameters than other types of medical devices, such as nitrogen powered orthopedic equipment (Table 22.5).

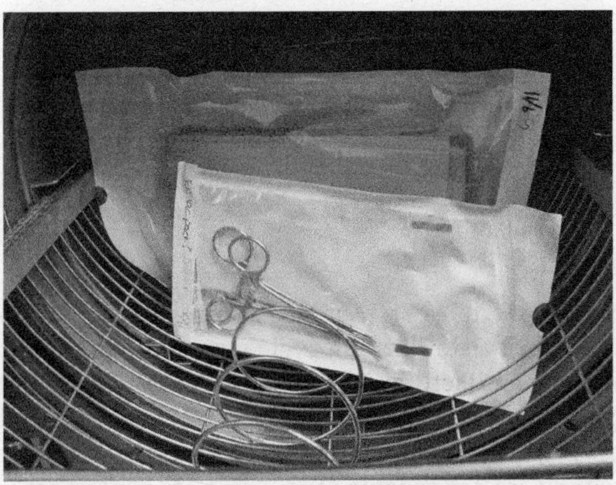

Figure 22.14 Using a spiral metal "letter holder" standing aid facilitates proper steam flow for peel pouches loaded in an autoclave chamber. Source: photograph courtesy of the author.

Table 22.5 / Minimum sterilization cycle times for gravity displacement autoclaves

Item	Exposure time (minutes)			Drying time (minutes)
	At 250°F (121°C)	At 270°F (132°C)	At 275°F (135°C)	
Wrapped instruments	30	15		15–30*
			10	30
Textile packs	30	25		15
			10	30
Wrapped utensils	30	15		15–30
			10	30
Unwrapped non-porous items (e.g. instruments)		3	3	0–1
Mixed load*		10	10	0–1

* Unwrapped non-porous and porous items.
Note: this table represents the variation in sterilizer manufacturers' recommendations for exposure at different temperatures. For a specific sterilizer, consult only that manufacturer's instructions.

How to Operate a Gravity Displacement Steam Autoclave

1. Open the door and load the autoclave as indicated above.
2. Fill the reservoir with distilled water. Once the reservoir is full, set the sterilizer knob to STERILIZE.
3. Set the desired cycle TEMPERATURE.
4. Set the desired cycle TIME.
5. Lock the autoclave door.
6. Once the designated time elapsed, open the door immediately to VENT the autoclave.
7. Unlock the door and leave it only slightly ajar. Residual heat from the autoclave chamber will facilitate the drying process.
8. Remove contents once they are completely dry. Sterile goods removed from the autoclave at this time may feel damp, but there should never be water droplets or wet areas present on the sterile packages.

It is important to allow items to cool at the end of the sterilization cycle and prior to handling to avoid compromising the barrier properties of the packaging materials and contaminating the contents. Furthermore, avoid placing warm or hot processed items on cool or cold surfaces since the formation of condensation may cause breaches in the packaging materials.[16]

Sterilization Process Monitoring

Variations that occur in the sterilization cycle may be due to independent factors such as the condition of the sterilizer equipment, the frequency (or infrequency) of equipment use, the expertise of the sterilizer operator or other factors such as steam quality or purity. As such, proof that adequate sterilization has been achieved is not easy to verify with the naked eye. The rationale behind utilizing monitoring devices to assure adequate sterilization is as follows:

- Ensure the probability of the absence of all living organisms on medical devices being processed.
- Detect failures as soon as possible.
- Verify failures as soon as possible.
- Remove medical devices involved in failures before used in the patient.
- Improve patient outcomes and safety.
- Control costs.

Physical Monitors

Physical monitors (previously referred to as mechanical monitors) can verify that the parameters of a sterilization cycle were met to within the guidelines established by the manufacturer.[20] These physical monitors may include unit-specific devices such as recording charts, printouts, gauges, or digital displays. However most physical monitors only record the conditions of one location in the sterilizer and are not capable of assessing other physical conditions that may impact the sterility of the load, such as whether or not proper packaging and loading protocols were achieved.[16]

Chemical Indicators

Chemical indicators are used to monitor the presence or attainment of one or more parameters required for a successful sterilization process, or used during specific tests of steam sterilization equipment. Chemical indicators may be used either externally or internally. Class 1 external indicators are predominantly used to differentiate between processed and unprocessed units. Internal indicators should be placed inside the pack in an area considered most difficult for the sterilant to penetrate. While internal indicators do not guarantee sterility, they do represent an indication of whether or not sterilization conditions were met within a package.[16]

There are six classes of chemical indicators that are used to assess parameters identified as being essential or "critical" to the steam sterilization process (Table 22.6). For example, the variables considered critical for effective steam sterilization may include parameters such as time, temperature and water (as delivered by saturated steam), but those considered critical for effective ethylene oxide sterilization may consist of time, temperature, relative humidity and ethylene oxide concentration. It is imperative to use only chemical indicators intended for each particular sterilization method. For example, a class 1 steam indicator tape will not change color after exposure to ethylene oxide and vice versa.[6]

Table 22.6 / Classes of chemical indicators

Class	Indicator	Description
1	Process	• Used externally as an exposure control (e.g. indicator tapes) and are used with individual units to distinguish between processed and unprocessed items • Relatively simplistic and designed to react to one or more of the critical process variables
2	Test sterilizer performance during a specific test procedure, such as a Bowie–Dick test	• Bowie–Dick testing can detect anomalies such as air leaks, inadequate air removal, inadequate steam penetration or the presence of non-condensable gases (air or gases from boiler additives) in vacuum-assisted sterilizers
3	Single variable	• Designed to react to one of the critical variables and indicate exposure to a sterilization process at an SV of the chosen variable • For example, the SV of 121°C (250°F) must be > 16.5 minutes
4	Multivariable indicators, usually paper strips	• Designed to react to two or more of the critical variables • This type of chemical indicator indicates exposure to a sterilization cycle at a SV of the chosen variables
5	Integrating	• Designed to react to all critical variables • SV for class 5 indicators are equivalent to the performance requirements for biologic indicators (ISO 11138 series: 2006) • Their response must correlate to a biologic indicator at 3 × temperature relationships • For example, 121°C (250°F), 135°C (275°F), and at one or more temperatures in between, such as 128°C (263°F). Stated values must be listed on the product or provided on the label/instructions for use (Figure 22.16)
6	Emulating	• Emulating indicators are cycle verification indicators that shall be designed to react to all critical variables for specified sterilization cycles • SV are generated from the critical variables of the specified sterilization process • Cycle specific: must pass an appropriate dry heat test, and the response does not correlate to a biologic indicator

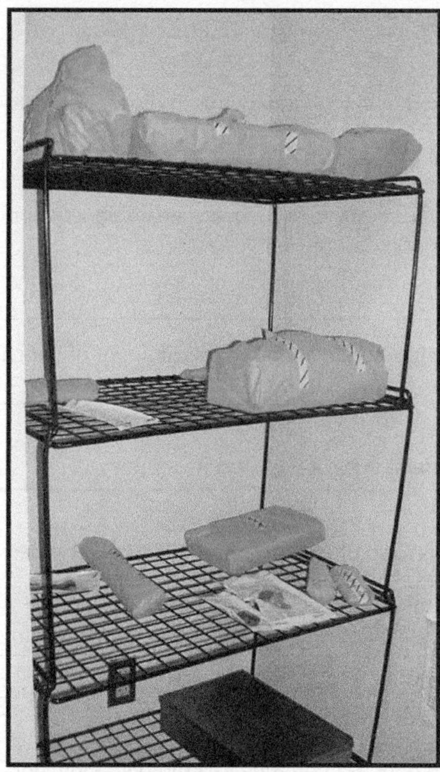

Figure 22.15 Allow items removed from the autoclave to completely cool prior to storing. Source: photograph courtesy of the author.

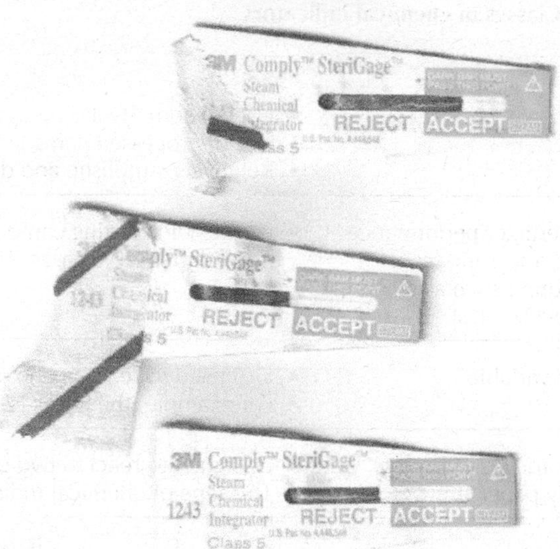

Figure 22.16 This class 5 (integrating) indicator is designed to correlate with the performance of a biologic indicator at three time/temperature relationships. Ink migration allows for easy-to-read "accept" or "reject" results. Even though the black ink line does not extend all the way to the end, the indicator on top is acceptable, while the two indicators pictured beneath it are from a failed cycle and should be rejected. Source: photograph courtesy of the author.

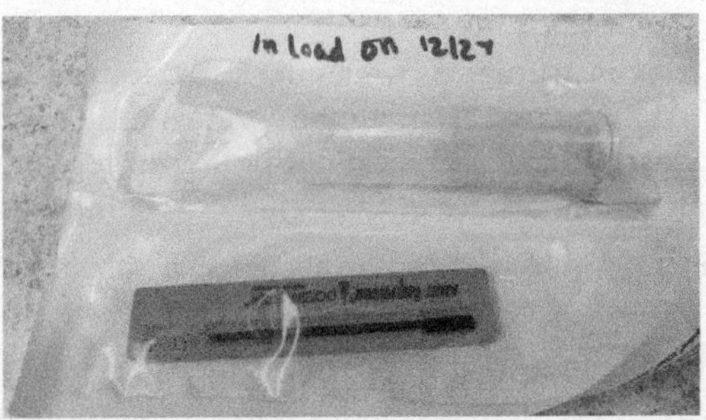

Figure 22.17 The Steritest combines a dosimeter and a bacterial spore preparation (*Bacillus atrophaeus*). The yellow material in the dosimeter column will turn blue in proportion to the dose of sterilizing gas detected. The blue column must pass the triangular pointer on the dosimeter to indicate an appropriate gas dose was present during the sterilization cycle. Source: photograph courtesy of the author (Andersen Products).

Some chemical indicators function by using reactive ink technology that produces a chemical reaction driven by exposure to process variables and results in a color change. The moving front style of chemical indicators possess tablets that melt in response to steam and temperature and wick down a paper path.

Biologic Indicators

Biologic indicators contain more than 100 000 viable spores of a highly resistant organism (e.g. *Geobacillus stearothermophilus*, formerly named *Bacillus stearothermophilus*) on a strip, and therefore are considered the most reliable level of testing available. Using biologic indicators during a sterilization cycle provides the only direct method of demonstrating lethality within that particular load. However, it is important to understand that a failure of the sterilization process may still occur even with a negative biologic indicator result. Reasons for failure can be due to any number of things, based on the sterilization method. Although the sterilant may have penetrated the location of the biologic indicator within the pack, it may not have penetrated the contents of the entire load. Additionally, a vacuum leak or air pocket may be present, the sterilant may be of poor quality or of inadequate volume, the pack itself may be wrapped too densely, or the load may have been packed so tightly that the sterilant could not adequately penetrate the load.[16]

Biologic indicators should be run with loads containing orthopedic implants, or after sterilizer failures and major repairs. A positive control should be analyzed in tandem with every post-sterilization biologic indicator to ensure that there were viable organisms present in the first place. There are biologic indicator kits that include an incubator and spore test kits, which can be analyzed on site, or mailout companies that incubate the positive control and sterilized spore strips and monitor results, including written quarterly reports.

Agent-specific biologic indicators are also be used during low-temperature sterilization, such as ethylene oxide, hydrogen peroxide gas plasma, and ozone sterilization processes. Nonetheless, it is possible to have a negative biologic indicator and still have a chemical indicator failure elsewhere in the load.[18]

Use of process challenge device containing a biologic indicator (± Class 5, e.g. Bowie–Dick test) ensures that the steam sterilizer is removing air efficiently in dynamic air removal (i.e. vacuum-assisted) steam sterilizers, or to detect trapped air within the sterilizer that will likely compromise sterility. In large facilities, process challenge devices are often run at the beginning of each day.[1,6]

LOW TEMPERATURE ETHYLENE OXIDE STERILIZATION

Ethylene oxide has been used worldwide by the healthcare industry for low temperature sterilization since the early 1940s.[21] Its advantages include economical, efficient, and reliable sterilization of delicate items such as fragile ophthalmic instruments, fiber optics, cameras, drills, electronics, scopes, and plastic or rubber items that would otherwise be damaged by heat and moisture. In fact, the only materials that cannot be sterilized using ethylene oxide are food, drugs, and liquids.

Ethylene oxide is an effective antimicrobial agent that should be handled with care, and all users should be properly trained to use it. The Andersen Anprolene® Key Operator Certification Program is designed to ensure that all operators are familiar with the ethylene oxide sterilization process, and the majority of information needed to obtain this certification is included in this document.[22]

Ethylene oxide has a boiling point of 10.7 degrees C (51.26°F). In its purest form, 100% ethylene oxide vapor is flammable and explosive,[23] but smaller entry-level Anprolene ethylene oxide sterilizers (1 load/day) use less than 18 g ethylene oxide per cycle, which meets state and US Environmental Protection Agency emission requirements without the need for additional abatement equipment.

Unheated cabinets operate at room temperature (recommended ≥ 20 degrees C; 68°F) with humidity level above 35%, and are capable of sterilizing and aerating the load. Depending on the items being sterilized, ethylene oxide exposure times are either 12 or 24 hours. Larger facilities (universities, hospitals, and device manufacturers) may employ larger sterilizers (up to 33 cubic feet in size), which feature a heated 50 degrees C (122°F), multi-oad cabinet capable of independent processing of multiple sterilization batches. These sterilizers utilize 5–11-g ampoules and a 16-hour cycle. Alternately, medical device manufacturers may use a system that combines a vacuum sealer with an ethylene oxide injector to sterilize individual items or kits.[22]

Proper preparation of items to be sterilized is also imperative for a successful outcome. Carefully follow the instructions for operating Andersen ethylene oxide sterilizer models AN74i, AN74ix, AN74j, and AN2000 (room-temperature ethylene oxide systems):[22]

Item Preparation for Ethylene Oxide Sterilization

- First scrub items surgically clean, using an approved instrument detergent and water. Residual dried protein such as blood, pus, serum, or other organic materials will protect microorganisms from the effect of ethylene oxide gas.
- Clean items can either be towel dried or allowed to drain (air) dry prior to packaging. Using heat (such as from a hair dryer) to facilitate the drying process will dehydrate spores, making them more resistant to ethylene oxide gas, and is not advised.
- Items with removable parts (e.g. syringes, plastic Poole tips), should be completely disassembled prior to packaging, to create an unobstructed path for ethylene oxide penetration. Caps, plugs, stoppers, plungers, valves, stylets or other obstructions should be removed, so as to provide unimpeded E ethylene oxide gas exposure to all surfaces and interior cavities.
- When sterilizing instruments containing batteries, the batteries should be removed and wrapped separately to prevent a spark that could ignite ethylene oxide. Food and drugs cannot be sterilized with ethylene oxide because it can cause changes in their chemical composition.
- Prehumidification of items is an important part of the ethylene oxide sterilization process, especially when items cannot be washed with water, or if the relative humidity level is below 35%.
    - If the nature of the item precludes water immersion, place it in 100% relative humidity for at least four hours prior to wrapping and sterilization.
    - An easy and effective way to humidify items is to dip a sponge in hot water and wring it out or use an Anprolene Humidichip humidity stabilizer, and place it with the item to be sterilized inside of an ethylene oxide gas sterilization bag that has been sealed shut with a twist tie. Once four hours have elapsed, remove the item from the humidification bag and wrap it for processing as outlined below.
- Items should be packaged in ethylene oxide approved gas permeable materials such as cloth, paper drapes, SMS polypropylene (3M), paper/plastic peel pouches or Seal and Peel® waterproof packaging, a transparent, peel open, extended shelf-life packaging material specifically designed for use with the Anprolene sterilization system.
- Consult each manufacturer's instructions to determine the storage shelf life using these materials. Other plastic films (e.g. nylon, polyester) are virtually impervious to ethylene oxide and are not advised. Other containers or sterilizers should not be used with Anprolene ethylene oxide gas.[22]

Ethylene Oxide Sterilization using Anprolene AN74i and AN74ix Sterilizer Operation (other model operations may vary)

1. Ensure the power cord is plugged into the wall outlet and the power switch is turned on. Wait until the SELF TEST and number of PUMP HOURS data appears in the digital display.
2. Contour a new plastic ethylene oxide gas sterilization bag inside the cabinet. Reusing sterilization bags is not advised due to the potential for punctures.

3. Arrange items to be sterilized inside the sterilization bag, together with one ampoule of ethylene oxide gas, one Humidichip, and one Dosimeter or AN80 Steritest®. The ethylene oxide ampoule should be unrolled while remaining inside its gas release bag, and should be placed on top of the middle of the load. Keeping the gas release bag intact helps to prevent accidental exposure to the user or cabinet contents and stops the gas from escaping too quickly to achieve sterilization. The dosimeter/AN80 Steritest should be situated in an area deemed most difficult for the gas to penetrate.
4. Insert the purge tube deep inside of the sterilization bag's load and securely seal it closed using the Velcro strap. Ensure the purge tube is attached to the quick-release connector.
5. Depress the PURGE button, and wait while excess air is evacuated from the sterilization bag and the display countdown reaches 00.00.00.
6. Once BREAK AMPOULE appears on the display, carefully crack the end of the ethylene oxide gas ampoule through the top wall of the sterilization bag until you feel a snap and hear a "pop," indicating release of the ethylene oxide gas and activation of the sterilization cycle. It is important to avoid puncturing the sterilization bag itself.
7. Close and lock the sterilizer door. Remove the key. Securing the load ensures that the liner bag is not punctured or accidentally ignited and facilitates the removal of exhausted gases.
8. Select the desired 12- or 24-hour CYCLE LENGTH. The usual cycle time is 14 hours, which includes a 12-hour sterilization cycle and a 2-hour purge cycle. However, when sterilizing a full load of gas absorbent items or tubing longer than three feet or with an inner lumen diameter of ≤ 1 mm, two gas ampoules and a 24-hour cycle may be required. The sterilization cycle should not be interrupted under any circumstances.
9. At the end of the sterilization cycle all items are sterile, and metal or glass items may be used immediately. Plastic and all other materials will require 24 additional hours of aeration time before the items can be safely used, regardless of the sterilization cycle length. Items may be aerated inside the sterilizer cabinet or in a well-ventilated area with a temperature of at least 20 degrees C (68°F) and at least 10–12 air changes per hour.
10. Record the appearance of the dosimeter. The color change must have reached the triangle marker to consider the contents of the sterilization bag as sterile. Discard the empty cartridge and the used Humidichip in the trash.

Ethylene Oxide Sterility Assurance

TheAN87 dosimeter is designed to integrate the effects of time, temperature and ethylene oxide concentration at one location in each load sterilized. The yellow material in the dosimeter column will turn blue in proportion to the dose of sterilizing gas detected, and provides immediate graphic evidence that the conditions necessary for sterilization to occur have, or have not, been met. It has been reported that at temperatures of 20 degrees C (68°F), 1500 mg/l-hours of exposure to ethylene oxide will sterilize instruments heavily contaminated with appropriately humidified spores. At least 2000 mg/l-hours of exposure has occurred once the blue color in the column exceeds the triangular pointer (▲) on the dosimeter, indicating that a dose higher than that required for sterilization has been delivered.[22]

Sterility verification for each individual item in the load can be assessed using either a class one (exposed vs not exposed) indicator or, for a better assessment, an integrating chemical indicator. Furthermore, biologic indicator challenges are advised on a routine basis, following the standard operating procedure, regulatory, or licensing agencies governing each organization.

The AN80 Steritest is a reliable bacterial challenge designed specifically for use with Anprolene. It consists of a prepackaged dosimeter and a bacterial spore preparation containing about 1 000 000 *B. atrophaeus*, (10 times the usual spore strip challenge), also known to be most resistant to sterilization.

Monitoring Ethylene Oxide Exposure

Ethylene oxide is toxic when inhaled, and can cause severe skin and eye irritation or burns and respiratory tract irritation or lung injury, and central nervous system damage; exposure effects may be delayed. Liquid contact may cause frostbite or allergic skin reactions, and any part of the body exposed to ethylene oxide liquid should be washed immediately for at least 15 minutes with water.

Monitoring personnel exposure to airborne ethylene oxide concentrations can be accomplished on-site by wearing an AirScan badge adjacent to the breathing zone. The AirScan badges meet US OSHA accuracy requirements for ethylene oxide monitoring methods. Aerating items sufficiently will reduce operator exposure sufficiently to meet OSHA's short-term exposure level of 5 ppm for any given 15-minute period, but 1 ppm is permissible for an 8-hour time-weighted average badge.[22]

HYDROGEN PEROXIDE GAS STERILIZATION

Hydrogen peroxide gas sterilization is another low-temperature sterilization method. Hydrogen peroxide is triggered to create a reactive plasma or vapor. The plasma cloud consists of ions, electrons, and neutral atomic particles that visibly glow. Free radicals in hydrogen peroxide clouds interact with the cell membranes, enzymes, or nucleic acids to disrupt the life of microorganisms. Hydrogen peroxide gas sterilization is highly sporicidal even at low concentrations and temperature.

SURGICAL HUCK TOWEL, GOWN AND CLOTH DRAPE CARE

The AAMI sets forth extensive guidelines and rationalizes recommended practices for the processing of reusable surgical textiles for use in healthcare facilities.[25] Relevant content from this preeminent resource is included below. Always wear PPE when handling infectious linens or contaminated professional garb; separate laundry facilities are advised. Presoak contaminated articles with diluted bleach (9 parts water: 1 part household bleach) for 10 minutes prior to machine washing with hot water.[2] However, avoid the use of bleach for laundering surgical textiles, as bleach can damage fabric threads and as such will decrease the usable life span of fabrics over time. When washing gowns, towels, and drapes, use as little laundry detergent as possible. Laundered textiles can retain soap particles and deposit them on the surface of the instruments during the sterilization process. It may be prudent to run all laundered surgical textiles through an extra rinse cycle to remove excess soap particles.[16] Furthermore, fabric softeners can also diminish the absorbency of cotton, which could contribute to wet packs post-steam sterilization.[16,24]

Single-use disposable gowns, drapes and towels eliminate the need for laundering, folding and reprocessing, and may be more cost effective and ecologically sound. Surgical gowns should meet AAMI/ANSI standards.

Folding Gowns for Sterilization

1. Lay a clean and lint-free gown onto the table with the front of the gown facing up. Bow tie the left chest string together with the back string coming from the right side (Figure 22.18a).
2. Bring both sleeves toward the center of the gown, and symmetrically flatten the outer surface of the gown (Figure 22.18b).
3. Fold each side panel in toward the center of the gown over the sleeves (Figure 22.18c).
4. Fold the sides of the gown toward the middle (Figure 22.18d).
5. Accordion the gown so that the gown's neck region is at the top (Figure 22.18d).
6. Add a fold surgical huck towel (Figure 12e) and place it on top of the folded gown.
7. Remember to include an internal chemical indicator.
8. Monitor the lifespan of the gown by checking the boxes on the usage grid located near the lower hem each time the garment is processed (washed, dried, and sterilized; Figure 22.19).

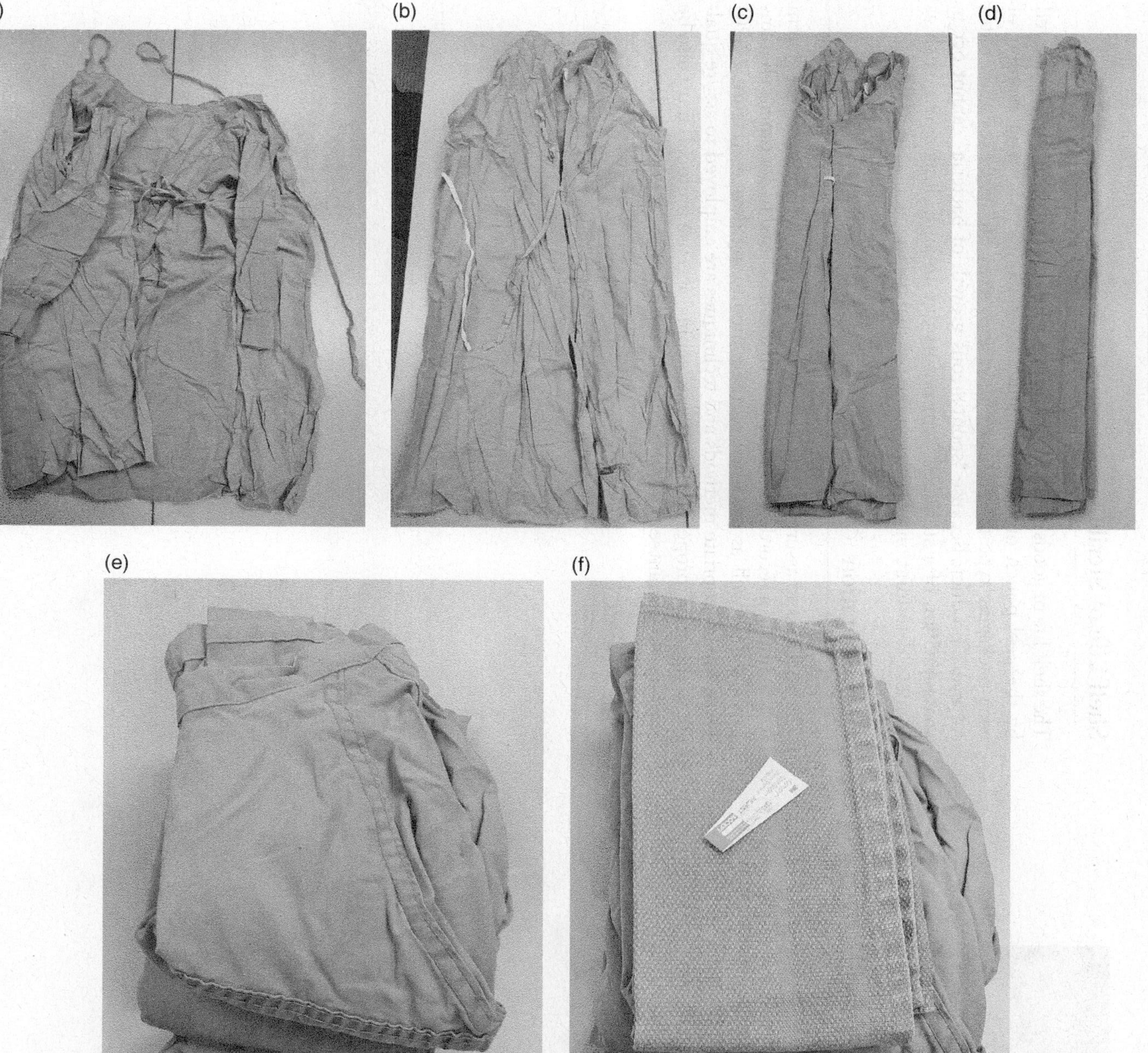

Figure 22.18 (a–e) Steps for folding gowns for sterilization.

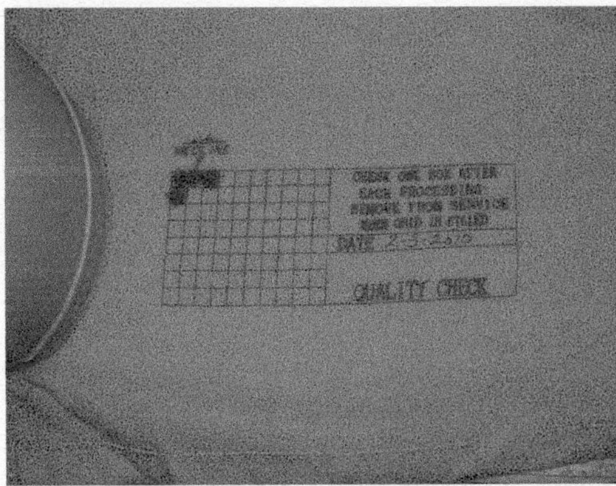

Figure 22.19 Some gown manufacturers provide a usage grid near the lower hem. The grid is designed so that one box is marked each time the gown is used. The gown should be removed from service once all of the grid boxes are filled. Source: photograph courtesy of author.

Shelf Life of Sterile Goods

The shelf life of goods sterilized in peel pouches or paper materials is dictated by the peel pouch or paper's manufacturer. Contact the manufacturer of each packaging type to establish the various shelf life (e.g. expiration date) for every product. Because "spontaneous growth of bacteria" cannot occur, contamination of a sterilized item occurs due to an inciting event, such as wetness, deterioration, or holes in the original packaging (Table 22.3).[19]

Documentation

The final step to assuring a successful sterilization process monitoring system is to maintain a record keeping system that can be used to document all items processed as well as evidence of their monitoring devices (Figure 22.20) Once the appropriate methods and techniques are employed to assure quality sterilization, proper storage, housekeeping, and use protocols must also be followed to guarantee the "probability of sterilization" at multiple levels.

AUTOCLAVE LOG

Use of this form is voluntary and not required by the Department of Health. The form is provided as a service to assist salons in complying with the record-keeping requirements of Chapter 64E-19, FAC.

DATE	LENGTH OF RUN		CHECK IF CLEANING DONE	CHECK IF SERVICING DONE	CHECK IF SPORE TESTING DONE	CHECK IF TEST RESULTS RECEIVED
	TODAY	CUMULATIVE TOTAL				

- There must be a sterilization indicator in each autoclaving to monitor the sterilization procedure. The indicator must indicate exposure to steam and 250 degrees Fahrenheit.
- Spore tests must be performed every 40 hours of autoclave operation, but not less than quarterly.
- Spore tests must be verified through an independent laboratory.
- The autoclave must be cleaned at the frequency recommended by the manufacturer.
- The autoclave must be serviced at the frequency recommended by the manufacturer, but not less than once a year.
- A copy of the manufacturer's instructions for cleaning and servicing the autoclave must be kept on file in the establishment.

Figure 22.20 Autoclave record.

ACKNOWLEDGEMENTS

The author would like to thank Victoria LaPerche, (CST), and Danielle Browning, LVMT, VTS (Surgery), for their assistance with this chapter.

REFERENCES

1. Association for the Advancement of Medical Instrumentation. (2017). *Comprehensive Guide to Steam Sterilization and Sterility Assurance in Health Care Facilities*. Arlington, VA: AAMI.
2. Stull, J., Bjorvik, E., Bub, J. *et al.* (2018). *2018 AAHA Infection Control, Prevention, and Biosecurity Guidelines*. Lakewood, CO: AAHA.
3. de Miguel Garcia C,C.K. (2018). Equipment cleaning and sterilization. In: *Veterinary Anesthetic and Monitoring Equipment* (ed. K.G. Cooley and R.A. Johnson), 377–389. Hoboken, NJ: Wiley.
4. Occupational Safety and Health Administration. (2012). *Occupational Safety and Health Regulations (Standards 29 CFR) Hazard Communication. 1910.1200.* Washington, DC: US Department of Labor. https://www.osha.gov/laws-regs/regulations/standardnumber/1910/1910.1200 (accessed 3 August 2021).
5. Occupational Safety and Hazard Administration. (2012). *Occupational Safety and Health Regulations (Standards 29 CFR) Bloodborne Pathogens. 1910.1030.* Washington, DC: US Department of Labor. https://www.osha.gov/laws-regs/regulations/standardnumber/1910/1910.1030 (accessed 3 August 2021).
6. Centers for Disease Control and Prevention. (2003). Appendix A: Regulatory Framework for Disinfectants and Sterilants. *MMWR Morb Mortal Wkly Rep* 52(RR17): 62–64.
7. Reuss-Lamky, H. (2017). Keys to successful high-level disinfection and sterilization processes. *Today's Vet Nurse* January. https://todaysveterinarynurse.com/articles/keys-to-successful-high-level-disinfection-and-sterilization-processes (accessed 3 August 2021).
8. Centers for Disease Control and Prevention. (2008). Chemical disinfectants: guideline for disinfection and sterilization in healthcare facilities. Alcohol. https://www.cdc.gov/infectioncontrol/guidelines/disinfection/disinfection-methods/chemical.html (accessed 3 August 2021).
9. National Institute for Occupational Safety and Health. *Glutaraldehyde: Occupational hazards in hospitals*. DHHS (NIOSH) Publication No. 2001–115. Cincinnati, OH: Centers for Disease Control and Prevention; 2001. https://www.cdc.gov/niosh/docs/2001-115/default.html (accessed 12 August 2021).
10. Association for the Advancement of Medical Instrumentation. (2013). *ANSI/AAMI ST58:2013 Chemical Sterilization and High Level Disinfection in Health Care Facilities*. Arlington, VA: AAMI.
11. Food and Drug Administration. (2019). FDA-cleared sterilants and high level disinfectants with general claims for processing reusable medical and dental devices. http://is.gd/vK7uV6 (accessed 3 August 2021).
12. Iowa State University, Center for Food Security and Public Health. Disinfection. http://www.cfsph.iastate.edu/Disinfection (accessed 3 August 2021).
13. Occupational Safety and Hazard Administration. (2012). *Occupational Safety and Health Regulations (Standards 29 CFR) Air Contaminants. 1910.1000.* Washington, DC: US Department of Labor. https://www.osha.gov/laws-regs/regulations/standardnumber/1910/1910.1000. (accessed 3 August 2021).
14. Shultz, R. (2005). *Inspecting Surgical Instrument: An Illustrated Guide*. Chicago, IL: International Association of Healthcare Central Service Material Management.
15. Kovachs, S.M. (2011). Understanding the Sonic Cleaning Process. http://www.crazy4clean.com/StudyGuideSC.pdf (accessed 3 August 2021).
16. Reuss-Lamky. (2011). Beating the "bugs": sterilization is instrumental. *Vet Tech J* November: E1–E9.
17. Rodriguez, P. (2008). The proper care and repair of surgical instruments. *Vet Pract News* April: 18 https://www.veterinarypracticenews.com/the-proper-care-and-repair-of-surgical-instruments (accessed 3 August 2021).
18. 3M Health Care. (2013). *Fundamentals of Sterilization Process Monitoring*. St. Paul, MN: 3M Health Care.
19. Ellis, A.M. (2017). Surgical instruments and aseptic technique. In: *McCurnin's Clinical Textbook for Veterinary Technicians*, 9e (ed. J.B. Bassert) 1094. St. Louis, MO: Elsevier Saunders.
20. AORN Recommended Practices Committee. (2006). Recommended practices of sterilization in perioperative practice setting. *AORN J*. 2006;83(3): 700–703, 705–708, 711–716.
21. Griffith, C.L. and Hall, L. (1943). Sterilization Process. US Patent No. Re 22,284.
22. Andersen Products. (2012). *Anprolene® Gas Sterilization Key Operator Training Kit*. Haw River, NC: Andersen Products, Inc.
23. Union Carbide. (1984). *1984 Flammability Data on EO-N2-Air Mixtures at 1 Atmosphere*. Danbury, CT: Union Carbide.
24. American National Standards Institute. (2008). *Processing Of Reusable Surgical Textiles For Use In Health Care Facilities*. ANSI/AAMI ST65:2008 (R2018). Washington, DC: ANSI.

Chapter **23**

Surgery

Heidi Reuss-Lamky, LVT, VTS, (Anesthesia/Analgesia), (Surgery), CFVP

Veterinary Technician and Nurse's Daily Reference Guide: Canine and Feline, Fourth Edition. Edited by Mandy Fults and Kenichiro Yagi.

Companion website: www.wiley.com/go/fults/veterinary

Abbreviations

CCL, cranial cruciate ligament
CNS, central nervous system
CPR, cardiopulmonary resuscitation
CRT, capillary refill time
CT, computed tomography
DIC, disseminated intravascular coagulation
DJD, degenerative joint disease
ECG, electrocardiogram
GDV, gastric dilation volvulus
IPPV, intermittent positive pressure ventilation
IV, intravenous
KCS, keratoconjunctivitis sicca
MRI, magnetic resonance imaging
Nd-YAG, neodymium-doped yttrium aluminium garnet
OHE, ovariohysterectomy
PPDH, peritoneopericardial diaphragmatic hernia
PCV, packed cell volume
PPV, positive pressure ventilation
SQ, subcutaneous
TPP, total plasma protein

Some of the listed surgical procedures may not be performed in the average clinical setting. However, at some point, technicians will be faced with having to explain a particular procedure to a client. These descriptions are not meant as directions on how to perform the procedure, but rather a quick synopsis that will allow the technician to prepare for the procedure, manage patient care, and explain the procedure and aftercare to a client whose pet may be undergoing these procedures.

With every surgical procedure, pain management needs to be addressed and handled (see Chapter 18: Pain Management).

INSTRUMENT PACKS

Basic Surgical Packs

The packs listed in Skill Box 23.1 are examples of the instruments included in common surgical packs. Each clinic will need to organize packs that best fit their surgery type and surgeon. Each surgeon has preferences on individual types of instruments for different surgeries. Each pack may include gauze, laparotomy pads, huck towels, bulb syringe and a saline bowl, or they may be wrapped separately. Often needles, sutures, and scalpel blades are prepared separately.

Skill Box 23.1 / Basic Instrument Packs

General surgical pack

- Grooved director
- Halstead hemostatic forceps (curved and straight)
- Crile or Kelly hemostatic forceps (curved and straight)
- Debakey thumb forceps
- Brown Adson thumb forceps
- Handheld retractors (army–navy or Senn)
- #3 Bard Parker scalpel handle – small animal
- #4 Bard Parker scalpel handle – large animal
- Tissue scissors (Mayo and Metzenbaum)
- Suture scissors
- Spay hook
- Thumb forceps
- Tissue forceps
- Towel clamps

Gastrointestinal pack

- Babcock forceps
- Pair of intestinal forceps (Doyens)
- Pair of Carmalt forceps
- Brown Adson thumb forceps

(*Continued*)

Skill Box 23.1 / Basic Instrument Packs (Continued)

Laceration pack

- Hemostatic forceps
- Needle holder
- Scalpel handle
- Scissors
- Thumb forceps

Ophthalmic pack (smaller more delicate instruments)

Eyelid forceps
- Eyelid retractor
- Hartman hemostatic forceps
- Lacrimal cannulas
- Derf or Castroveijo needle holders
- Beaver blade scalpel handle
- Iris or tenotomy scissors
- Bishop–Harmon thumb forceps

Neurology pack

- Bone wax
- Dental spatula
- Dural hook
- Rongeurs, single action (Lempert, Kerrison)

Orthopedic pack

- Bone drill
- Bone chuck and key
- Bone-cutting forceps
- Bone-holding forceps
- Bone rasps and files
- Periosteal elevator
- Gigli handles and wire
- Mallet
- Osteotome
- Orthopedic wire
- Pin cutter
- Retractors
- Senn retractor
- Volkman retractor
- Rongeurs
- Wire-cutting scissors

Thoracic pack

- General surgical pack
- Instruments with long handles
- Rib retractors
- Wilson rib spreader
- Bone-cutting forceps
- Right angle forceps
- Vessel clamps
- Bulldog clamp

Specialized Surgical Packs

Many instruments may be used only on occasion and should be set aside in separate packs. Instruments weaken with constant scrubbing and autoclaving, and should therefore not be subjected to unnecessary sterilization. The instrument type and number included in each of these packs will depend on surgeon preference:

- Biopsy/trephine pack
- Orthopedic implant set (compression set)
- Micro-surgery pack
- Bone curettes
- Bone holding forceps pack
- Screw set
- Wire pack
- Pin set
- Suction tips and tubing pack.

For details of how to pack instrument packs, see Chapter 22: Disinfection and Sterilization in Veterinary Healthcare.

PATIENT PREOPERATIVE PROTOCOL

Once a surgical procedure has been planned, a set of preoperative guidelines should be followed to ensure the safety of the patient (Skill Box 23.2). These guidelines evaluate the patient physically, correct underlying problems if possible, and prepare the patient for the actual procedure. They also ensure that the client is aware of the steps ahead and is comfortable with their decision. Specific details for a particular surgery are listed in that section.

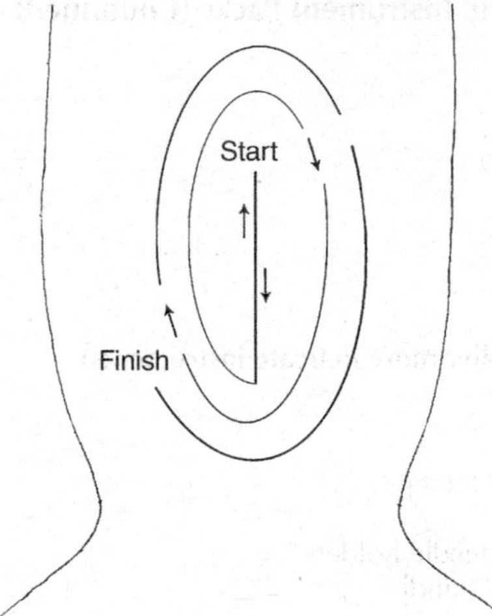

Figure 23.1 Typical surgical scrub pattern for an abdominal incision. Care must be taken to rotate sponges to maintain the same edge facing the intended incision location.

Skill Box 23.2 / Patient Preoperative Protocol

Client communication

- Ensure that the client is aware of the procedure, options, risks, postoperative care, and cost.
- The client should sign a consent understanding the risk of anesthesia and designate a CPR code status.

Preanesthetic evaluation

- Signalment
- History
- Current medications
- Weight
- Vital signs
- Fasting status
- Physical examination
- Laboratory workup
- Additional diagnostic tests
- ASA physical status
- Pain score
- Emergency drug sheet
- See also Table 20.1: Preanesthetic evaluation, page 858)

Patient stabilization

- Fluid therapy (see Chapter 14: Patient Care Skills in Clinical Practice, Fluid Therapy, page 673)
- Correct acid–base abnormalities.
- Pain management plan (see Chapter 18: Pain Management).
- Drug administration (see Skill Box 14.8: Injections, page 661).
- Stabilizing procedures (e.g. oxygen therapy, thoracocentesis, abdominocentesis; see Chapter 14: Patient Care Skills in Clinical Practice, Oxygen Therapy, page 689, and Chapter 16: Medical Procedures).
- Nutritional evaluation and administration (see Chapter 17: Nutrition).

(Continued)

Skill Box 23.2 / Patient Preoperative Protocol (Continued)

Patient preparation

- The owners may bathe the animal a day prior to surgery if necessary.
- Withhold food for 6–12 hours before surgery in healthy adults and continue to offer water. Fasting instructions for young animals and those prone to hypoglycemia should be determined by the veterinarian.
- Avoid all venipunctures near the surgical site when drawing blood for preoperative blood work (e.g. no jugular sticks prior to thyroidectomy).
- The patient should be allowed to urinate and defecate prior to induction.
- Use a surgical safety checklist:
  - Verify the correct patient, surgical procedure, and surgical site.
  - Have all necessary supplies and equipment sterile and in working order for the procedure.
  - Three checkpoints:
    - Before the induction of anesthesia.
    - Before the skin incision is made.
    - On conclusion of the surgery.
- Induce anesthesia (see Table 20.5: General anesthesia induction, page 872).
- Prepare the surgical site:
  - Clip the intended site with wide margins to allow for drape movement, additional incisions, and drain placement. If adequate hair is not removed from the patient, it may creep into the sterile field.
  - Use a clean, sharp and cool #40 electric clipper blade. Do not shave the hair the day before surgery. The hair should be removed no more than four hours before surgery to avoid the risk of surgical-site infection.
  - When using a hanging-leg preparation, the tie or tape used to hang the limb should be free from debris and hair, which could fall into the surgical field. An impervious layer (such as an exam glove) should be used to cover any remaining hair on distal limb.
  - After clipping, remove excess hair and debris with a vacuum.
  - Express the bladder.
  - Place perianal purse-string sutures or gauze packing in the anus to reduce fecal contamination for surgeries involving the perineal region. Make a note, both on the patient and in the medical record, to verify that the anal purse-string is to be removed post-surgery.
  - Cleanse the surgical site with an antiseptic soap (prewash the skin using a non-medicated soap, to remove any organic debris, before applying an antiseptic agent).
  - Move the patient into the surgical suite and perform the sterile skin preparation.
  - Begin scrubbing along the intended incision line and move in a circular pattern moving away from the center. Be sure not to return to the center as this may translocate bacteria back to the incision line. Follow recommended contact times for each antiseptic.
- Solutions used for cleaning are variable, a standard should be set for each hospital (e.g. povidone-iodine, chlorhexidine, alcohol).
- Depending on the product, rinsing with sterile saline or alcohol may be necessary.
- Prevent surgical fires by allowing the alcohol rinse to completely dry when using electrocautery and avoid the use of alcohol when using a laser.
- Note: Pooling of antiseptic solutions should be prevented or soaked up with a sterile sponge prior to draping the patient.
- One-step prep wands are an alternative to the traditional sterile scrub. A sterile wand combining alcohol and chlorhexidine or povidone iodine is painted on the skin and left to dry for around three minutes. Once dry, the patient may be draped as usual.
- The final sterile prep should be performed after all anesthesia monitoring have been connected.
- When using air warming devices, the blankets may be placed over the patient, but the unit should be not turned on until after they have been thoroughly draped in.
- The circulating nurse should inspect all packages prior to handing off to sterile personnel. The technician should verify proper packing and sterilization method was used, intact seals, no presence of holes, dried wet spots, rips or tears, and the chemical indicator color has appropriately changed on the sterile package.
- Moisten the electrocautery plates when using monopolar and have the foot pedal in position for bipolar cautery.
- Use non-penetrating towel clamps to secure suction hoses or electrocautery cords onto the sterile drape.
- When using an electrosurgical handpiece during surgery, the sterile scrub nurse should clean char from the electrode tip. This should be performed away from the incision, the char that accumulates and encourages bacterial proliferation.
- Conversations and traffic through the operating room should be kept to a minimum and no food or drink permitted.
- Non-sterile personnel should avoid passing between two sterile fields.
- Non-sterile personnel should use care to not touch or reach over a sterile field.
- Non-sterile personnel should maintain 12 inches from all parts of the sterile field to avoid accidental contamination.
- When pouring lavage solutions, the scrub assistant should place the bowl on the back corner of the table; the circulating nurse carefully pours the solution into the bowl, or the scrub assistant holds the receptacle away from the sterile table while the circulating nurse slowly pours the fluid to prevent splashing. Any remaining fluid in the bottle should be discarded.
- Laminar flow is recommended over conventional ventilation systems in the operating room.
- Positive pressure ventilation and 15 air exchanges per hour are recommended in the operating room.
- Operating doors should be shut while the operation is in progress.
- Dust on lights can shower down over the surgical wound, so light should be positioned prior to opening any surgical packs. The surgical lights are damp dusted each morning and wiped after each procedure with a hospital approved disinfectant.

SURGICAL PREPARATION

Surgical hand scrubs are performed to reduce the risk of nosocomial infections. The purpose of this is to remove debris and both transient and resident microorganisms from the nails, hands, and forearms. Scrubs begin in the expected cleanest area (e.g. hands) and end in the dirtiest area (e.g. elbow). All jewelry, watches, and nail polish should be removed. Nails should be cut short (2 mm) and subungual areas cleaned with a nail file.

Traditional hand scrubbing is accomplished with brushes or sponges. Brushes do not increase antimicrobial effectiveness and may damage the skin and increase bacterial counts. Brushes should only be used on the nails and cuticles. Before starting an aseptic surgical hand preparation, a routine washing of the hands and forearms should be performed using a non-medicated soap.

Hand Scrub

There are two methods for traditional hand scrubbing: timed and counted stroke.

Timed Scrub

- Generally, this method takes five to six minutes in total.
- To begin, cover the entire area to be scrubbed with antiseptic soap to help ensure adequate contact time on the skin.
- Starting at the fingertips, move to the hand and work your way along the forearm to the elbow.
- Each hand and arm should be scrubbed for a total of two to three minutes.

Counted Stroke Method

- To begin, cover the entire area to be scrubbed with antiseptic soap (hands to elbow).
- Strokes are counted per surface area of skin.
- Apply 20–30 strokes per area of skin.
- Scrub the nails and top of fingers, then the four sides of the fingers, hands, wrists, and forearms.

After completing the scrub, rinse hands under running water, using care not to touch the sink faucet. During and after the rinse, hold your arms above the waist and hands above the elbows. Warm water is recommended, but hot water should be avoided.

Hand Drying

- Pick up a sterile towel and dry one hand in a blotting fashion.
- Using the top half of the sterile towel, grasp the towel with one hand, and starting at the fingers of the opposite hand, work down the arm to dry. Using the dry hand, grab the bottom half of the towel and carefully rotate the towel to dry the opposite hand.
- Do not allow the bottom half of the towel to touch any non-sterile items (i.e. scrub top).
- Keep your hands held out in front of your body at chest level, with the hands higher than the elbows when walking to the gowning station.
- Note: take care not to drip water onto the sterile gown when grasping the towel.

Alternative to a Traditional Hand Scrub

Alcohol-based hand rubs (waterless rubs) are less drying to the skin, have a quicker onset of action over traditional methods and studies favor them as being more cost effective. These rubs combine alcohol with common antiseptics (chlorhexidine and povidone iodine). Read the manufacturers' instructions before use to be sure of the proper volume, contact time, and application process. When using waterless hand rubs:

- Hands must be *completely* dry before application.
- Skin should be free from organic debris.
- Generously apply the product on hands and forearms, rub into the skin and allow to air dry.
- Typically, one to two minutes contact time is needed.
- Note: if the hands contact a non-sterile object, the scrub should be lengthened or repeated for one minute.

Common clinic recommendations: perform a traditional five- to six-minute scrub first scrub of the day, then subsequently use antiseptic rubs solutions.

Surgical Gowning and Gloving

- After the surgical scrub has been completed and hands are dry, pick up the sterile gown and take a step back away from the counter.
- Slide your arms down into the sleeves while avoiding touching the front of the gown.
- Arms are held out and slightly up, have an assistant from behind reach under the gown at the shoulders to lift the gown into place and tie.
- Using a closed gloving technique don a pair of sterile gloves

Note: be cognizant of where people and equipment are so that accidental contamination of the sterile gown and gloves does not occur.

Skill Box 23.3 / Surgical Gloving

Step	Description	
Closed gloving		
1.	Open glove package with hands remaining *inside* the gown cuff.	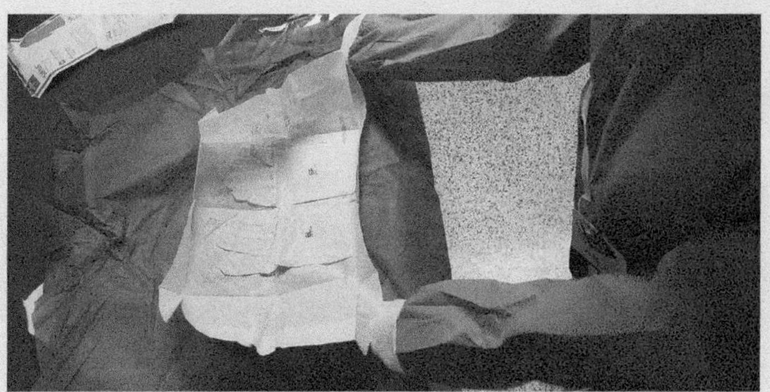

(Continued)

Skill Box 23.3 / Surgical Gloving (Continued)

Step	Description	
2.	Pick up the glove for your non-dominant hand.	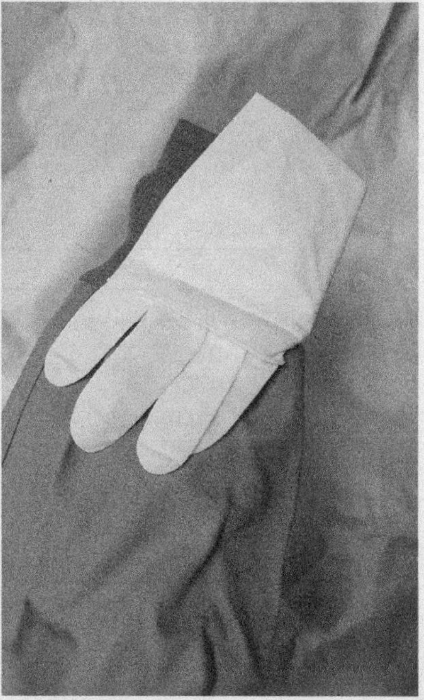
3.	Gloving your non dominant hand first, the hand remains inside the gown with palm facing up. Place the glove on top of the gown cuff with the thumb of the glove down (touching the gown) and the fingers toward the elbow (think "thumb to thumb, fingers to you").	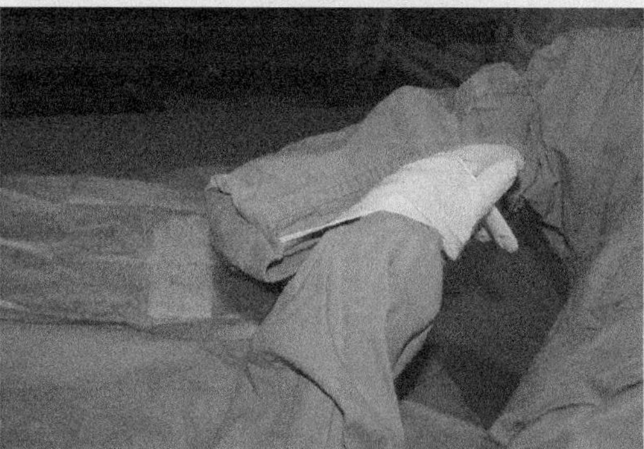

(Continued)

Skill Box 23.3 / Surgical Gloving (Continued)

Step	Description	
4.	Pull the glove over the cuff sleeve of the gown.	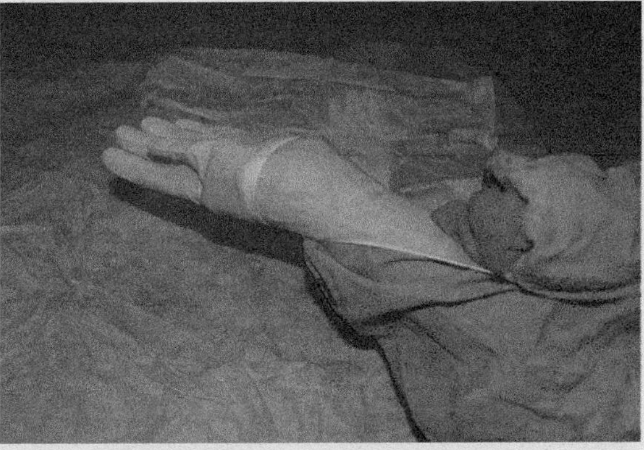
5.	Grab the top of the glove cuff and pull down over the sleeve of the gown, while pushing your hand through the cuff *into the glove*.	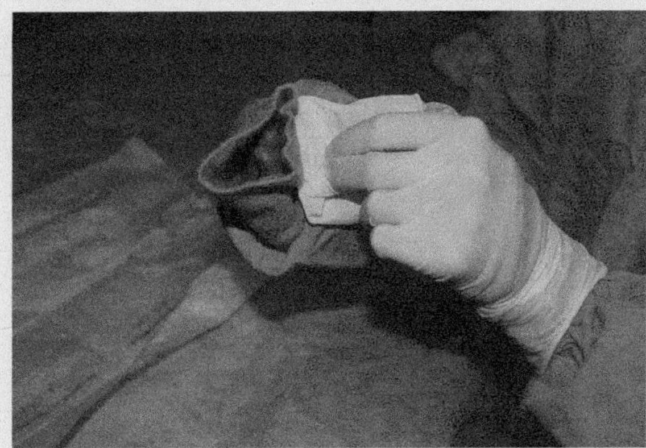
6.	Repeat steps 3–5 to glove the dominant hand, keeping the hand inside the cuff.	

(*Continued*)

Skill Box 23.3 / Surgical Gloving (Continued)

Step	Description	
*Open gloving**		
1.	To begin, pick up the folded cuff portion of the glove and slide the hand into the glove (do not unfold the cuff).	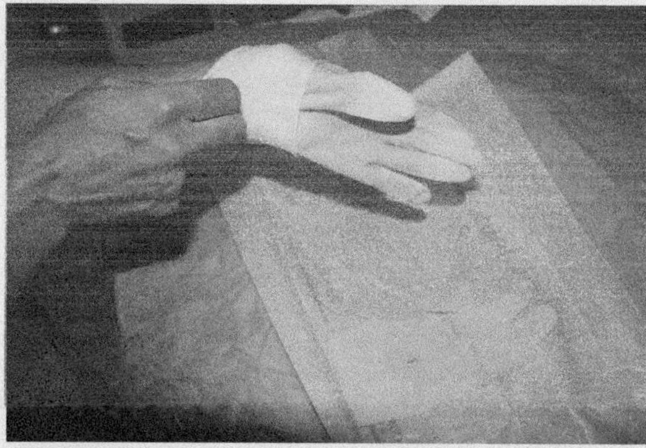
2.	Next, slide the sterile gloved fingers inside the opposite glove cuff.	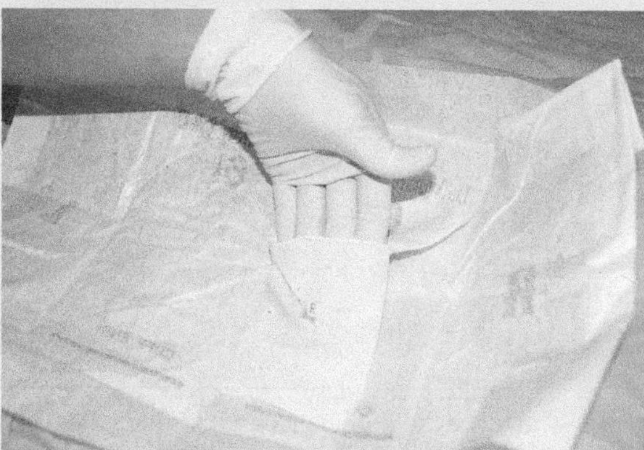

(*Continued*)

Skill Box 23.3 / Surgical Gloving (Continued)

Step	Description	
3.	**Lift glove off paper and slide non-sterile fingers into open cuff.**	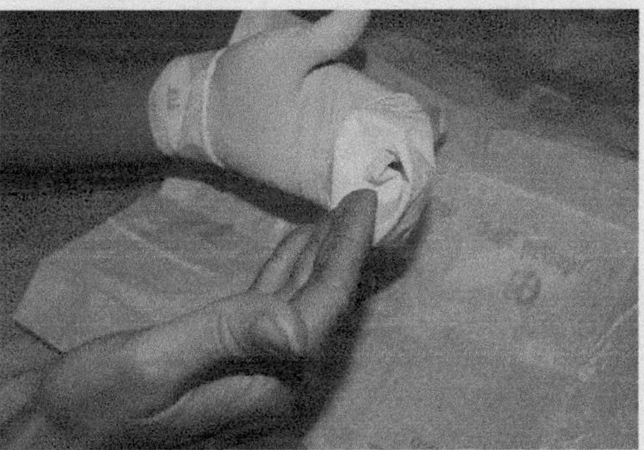
4.	**Slide the fingers under the cuff and unfold, repeat on opposite side.**	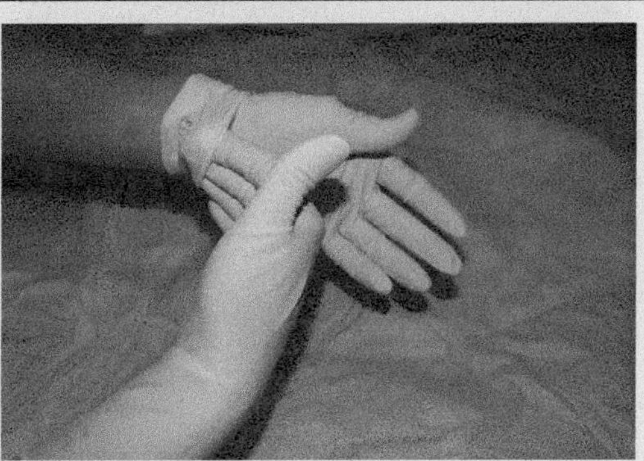

*This technique is used when sterile gloves are required without the use of a gown.

Skill Box 23.4 / Toweling and Draping the Patient

Step	Description
1.	Pick up and unfold one blue "huck" towel.
2.	Hold the towel horizontally in front of you, between your chest and waist level. 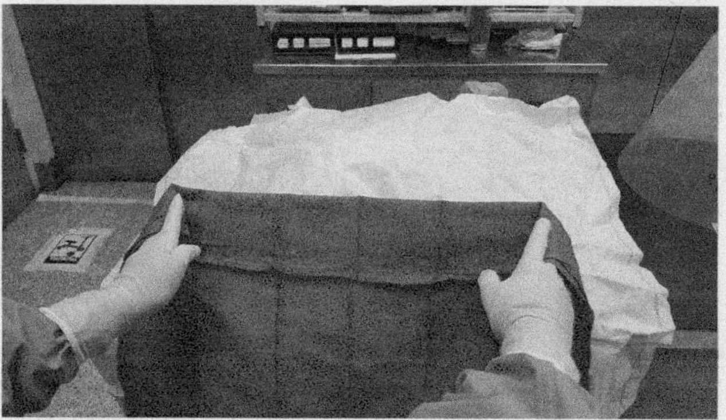
3.	Fold the top ¼ portion of the towel over and then grab both outside edges of the folded end with your fingers. 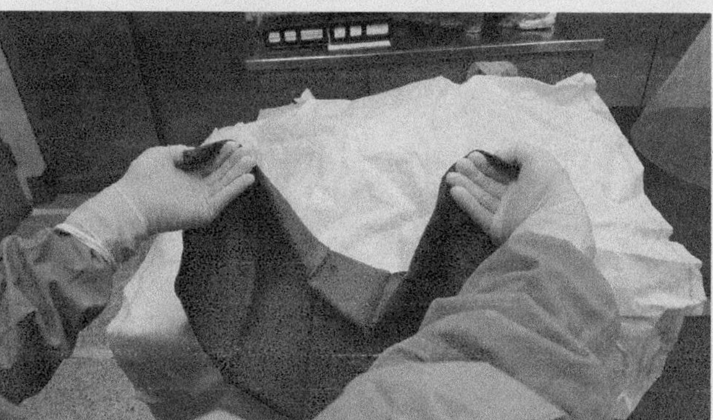

(*Continued*)

Skill Box 23.4 / Toweling and Draping the Patient (Continued)

Step	Description	
4.	Roll hands inward to protect your fingers from non-sterile areas during placement.	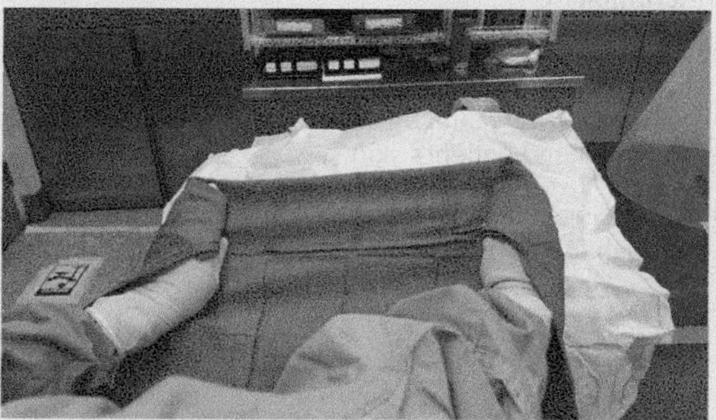
Placing the towels		
5.	• Lean your body away from the operating room table to ensure that the front of the gown is not contaminated. • Now reach over the patient to place the first towel in aseptic fashion. Repeat this step until all exposed hair surrounding the surgical field is covered. • Take care when placing the towel to not drag hands across non-sterile areas.	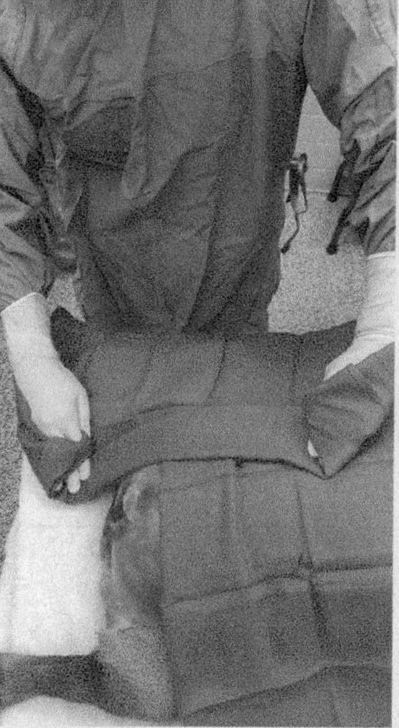

(*Continued*)

Skill Box 23.4 / Toweling and Draping the Patient (Continued)

Step	Description	
Placing the towel clamps		
6.	• Hold the towel clamp at a 90-degree angle, push down on the drape to secure a bite of both the towel and patient's skin. • Note: Once you pierce the towel clamp through the towel, the tips should never come back through the towel until the end of surgery.	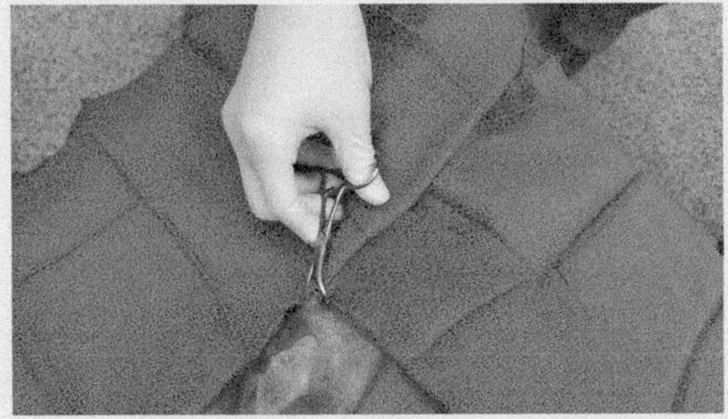
Placing the drape		
7.	• Place the fenestration hole over your surgical field, hold the center of the drape in place and drop the edge of the drape closer to you, first toward the floor. • *Do not* drop your hands lower than the table; allow the drape to fall toward the floor.	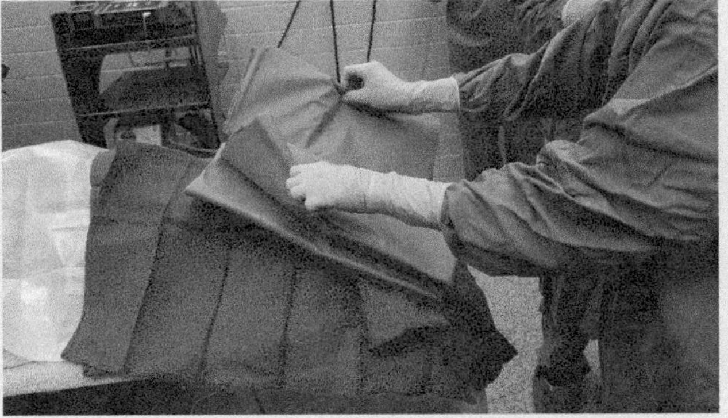

(*Continued*)

Skill Box 23.4 / Toweling and Draping the Patient (Continued)

Step	Description
	• Next, lean forward and open the remaining drape to cover the patient. • Always keep your sterile gloved hands protected under the layers of the fabric when opening the drape in an aseptic fashion.

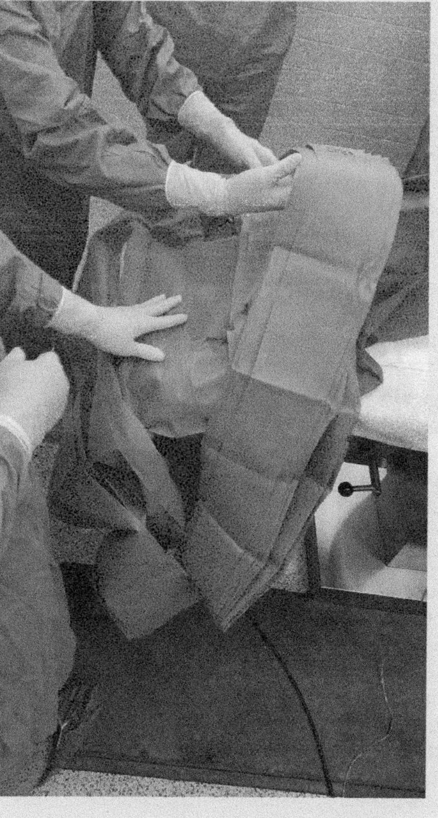

When moving through the operating room

STERILE personnel pass with BACK to FRONT of NON-STERILE personnel.

SURGICAL PROCEDURES

Abdominal Surgery

Table 23.1 / Abdominal surgery: celiotomy

Procedure	Abdominal surgery (celiotomy)
Instruments	• Abdominal pack • Electrocautery • Gauze sponges with a radio-opaque marker/laparotomy pads • General surgical pack • Self-retaining abdominal retractor (Balfour or Gosset retractor) • Saline bowl • Sterile saline, warmed • Suction tips and tubing pack
Patient preparation	• Surgical safety checklist • Preanesthetic evaluation • Preoperative protocol (including preemptive analgesics) • Empty the urinary bladder • Flush prepuce of male dogs with antiseptic solutions • See particular surgery
Surgical technique	1. Count sponges prior making an abdominal incision. 2. Open the abdomen along the ventral midline along the linea alba. 3. Exteriorize the organ or area to be examined and pack with saline-moistened gauze sponges. 4. Keep tissues consistently moist with warm saline. When placing moistened laparotomy pads under an abdominal retractor, only wet the portion on the pad should touch the viscera. 5. Handle the internal organs carefully to avoid further damage. For contaminated procedures, provide new sterile drapes, towels, gloves, and instruments for abdominal closure. 6. Routine abdominal closure in small animals: a. Two or three layers. b. Appose muscularis with external rectus sheath using a 0, 2-0, 3-0 monofilament, synthetic, absorbable suture on a taper needle, in a simple continuous pattern. c. Appose subcutaneous tissue using a 3-0 monofilament, synthetic, absorbable suture on a taper needle. d. Intradermal patterns 2-0,3-0,4-0 absorbable on a taper or cutting needle. e. Appose skin using a 3-0 nonabsorbable suture on a cutting needle. 7. Monitor the patient for excessive blood loss, contamination of peritoneal cavity, and an ↑ tendency to vomit with organ manipulation.
Complications:	
Procedural	• Abscess • Adhesions between visceral surfaces • Dehiscence • Failure of intended surgery • Gastric or intestinal perforation • Gossypiboma • Hemorrhage (e.g. poor hemostasis and inadvertent injury to vascular organs) • Ileus • Intestinal stricture • Pancreatitis • Peritonitis/sepsis (e.g. contamination with gastrointestinal contents)
Patient	• Abdominal pain • Fever • Hypothermia with prolonged procedures • Tenesmus/constipation/dyschezia • Vomiting and regurgitation
Patient care	• Continue analgesia postoperatively • Monitor frequency, appearance, and ability to defecate • Standard postoperative care • Confine and restrict activity until suture/staple removal 10–14 days or as directed by the veterinarian
Client education	• Postoperative care protocol • Follow the feeding guidelines of the veterinarian post-surgery • Importance of wearing the Elizabethan collar

Table 23.2 / Abdominal surgery: abdominal hernia, diaphragmatic hernia, hepatectomy

Procedure	Abdominal hernia	Diaphragmatic hernia	Hepatic lobectomy

Definition	• Ring or sac defect in the abdominal wall with possible protrusion of fat, omentum or part of an abdominal organ
	Common types of hernia:
	• Congenital
	  • blstUmbilical
	  • Substernal (PPDH)
	  • Scrotal
	  • Inguinal
	• Traumatic
	  • Paracostal
	  • Dorsal lateral
	  • prepubic
	  • femoral
	  • diaphragmatic
		Variably sized hole in the diaphragm allowing passage of the abdominal contents into the thoracic cavity	Partial: to remove a portion of a liver lobe
			Complete: removal of an entire liver lobe

Indications	• Symptomatic: patient discomfort, local tissue discoloration, or organ obstruction • Significant protrusion affecting the patient quality of life • Significant risk to hollow organ incarceration[1]	• Herniation of liver, spleen, gastrointestinal tract, pancreas, uterus or omentum into the thoracic cavity • 85% traumatic, blunt force trauma, most common cause is hit by car	• Biopsy, neoplasia, necrosis, nodule, abscess, or hemorrhage
Patient preparation	• Dorsal recumbency • Prepare xyphoid to pubis, including 3 inches on either side of the hernia	• Dorsal recumbency • Midline celiotomy • Position in reverse Trendelenburg • Prepare mid-chest to pubis	• Dorsal recumbency • Prepare mid-chest to pubis • Coagulation tests and thrombocyte count

(Continued)

Table 23.2 / Abdominal surgery: abdominal hernia, diaphragmatic hernia, hepatectomy (Continued)

Procedure	Abdominal hernia	Diaphragmatic hernia	Hepatic lobectomy
Surgical technique	1. Make an incision over the hernia and dissect down to the hernia orifice. 2. Remove any adhesion and return the organs and/or viscera to the peritoneal cavity. 3. Sharply freshen the edges of the hernial orifice and suture to close. 4. Perform routine closure of the abdomen. 5. Autologous (patient's own tissue) or non-autologous (surgical mesh) may be required to close the defect.	1. Make a ventral midline abdominal incision. 2. Examine any herniated structures for extended strangulation/obstructive damage and then place back into the abdominal cavity. 3. Examine the abdominal cavity contents, lungs, and pleural space for any further damage. 4. Examine the diaphragm for any other tears and then suture the defect(s) closed. 5. Place a chest tube and maintain for 8–12 hours to ensure control of the pleural space. 6. Air can also be aspirated as the last suture is tied, but this does not allow pleural space maintenance if needed. 7. Perform routine closure of the abdominal wall.	1. Make a ventral midline abdominal incision. 2. Place laparotomy pads between the liver and diaphragm for better visualization. 3. Examine the liver for biopsy areas or portions to be removed. 4. Perform a lobectomy using blunt dissection and suture ligation, staple (TA™ linear stapler) or seal vessel. 5. Observe the area for confirmation of adequate hemostasis, and perform routine closure of the abdominal wall after a sponge count.
Patient care	• Postoperative monitoring for infection, dehiscence or breakdown, that can result in peritonitis, evisceration, and strangulation	• Monitor pain, heart rate, CRT, mucous membrane color, pulse strength and character, respiratory rate, blood pressure, blood gases, and pulse oximetry	• Patient care: recovery from anesthesia should be closely monitored since delayed drug metabolism may result after hepatectomy
Client education	• Exercise restriction until healed		
Complications	• Hemorrhage • Visceral injury • Strangulated hernia • Contamination • Inability to close the abdominal wall without tension • Poor tissue strength	• Reexpansion pulmonary edema • Pneumothorax upon repair	
Expected pain	• Moderate	• Moderate to severe	• Moderate to severe
Notes	• Chronic or small hernias may not require surgical intervention	• IPPV is crucial to allow the surgeon to work while avoiding injury to pulmonary tissue	

Table 23.3 / Abdominal surgery: splenectomy

Procedure	Splenectomy
Definition	• Surgical removal of the spleen
Indications	• Splenic neoplasia, torsion, or severe trauma to the spleen
Patient preparation	• Shave and surgically prepare from mid-chest to the pubis • Administer preoxygenation • Administer fluids • Banked blood should be available for a potential transfusion
Surgical technique	1. Perform a ventral midline incision. 2. Apply suction to remove blood if there has been a prior hemorrhage. 3. Exteriorize the spleen and double ligate the vessels of the splenic hilus with sutures, an LDS™ stapling device, or a vessel-sealing device. 4. Flush with sterile saline and suction out. 5. Take a biopsy of the liver if appropriate. 6. In dogs with splenic torsion and large breeds, perform a gastropexy 7. Do a sponge count. 8. Carry out routine abdominal closure.
Complications	• Hemorrhage • Vascular compromise • Arrhythmias • DIC • GDV • Infection • Oxygen transport
Patient care	• Patient should be monitored for 24 hours post-surgery and PCV/total solids should be reviewed every few hours until the animal is stable
Expected pain	• Mild to moderate
Notes	• Check ECG to monitor for arrhythmias post-surgery • In surgery for splenic torsions, the spleen is not de-rotated before removal

Aural Surgery

Common surgeries of the ear, include aural hematoma, pinnectomy, total ear canal ablation, ventral bulla osteotomy, and lateral ear canal resection.

Table 23.4 / Aural surgery

Procedure	Aural surgery
Instruments	• Cartilage scissors • Electrocautery • Laceration pack or general surgical pack • Bone curette • Jacobs hand chuck and steinman pin • Hand-held and self-retaining retractors • Suction
Patient preparation	• Preanesthetic evaluation • Preoperative protocol • See particular surgery
Surgical technique	1. Electrocautery is an important part of ear surgery because of the highly vascular tissue and degree of hemorrhage. 2. CO_2 laser. 3. See Figure 23.2.
Complications:	
Procedural	• Hematoma formation • Hemorrhage
Patient	• Head shaking or scratching • Hearing loss • Head tilt • Horner syndrome
Patient care	• Bandage of ear against head and wrapped and secured with stockinette or tape • Standard postoperative care • Continue analgesia postoperatively • Ear medications • Confine and restrict activity until suture/staple removal or as directed by the veterinarian
Client education	• Postoperative care protocol • Caution when removing head bandages to not accidentally cut the off the pinna

Table 23.5 / **Aural surgery: aural hematoma, lateral ear canal resection**

Procedure	Aural hematoma	Lateral ear canal resection
Definition	• Hematoma of the pinna • Remove blood clots, prevent recurrence and retain the ear's natural appearance	• Removal of the lateral ear wall to allow proper drainage and exposure of the horizontal canal to increase ventilation • Must be performed early in the course of chronic otitis externa if success is to be achieved
Indications	• Irritations causing head shaking or scratching at ears	• Few indications • Trauma, or neoplasia involving the lateral canal • Anatomic due to breed (e.g. Shar Pei)
Patient preparation	• Lateral recumbency • Clean and treat underlying otitis externa if present • Place 1–2 cotton balls in ear canal to prevent fluid accumulation in deep canal • Prepare the entire pinna on both sides	• Lateral recumbency with head propped up on a towel • Clean the ear canal of all waxy material and debris • Prepare entire pinna and the external ear canal region (e.g. side of the face)
Surgical technique	Simple: 1. Prepare the ear aseptically. 2. Use a needle to drain hematoma at the most dependent area of the hematoma. 3. Passive drainage: insert a Penrose drain or teat cannula for two weeks. 4. Active drainage: insert a modified butterfly catheter. 5. Place a finger-trap suture to hold the fenestrated catheter in place. 6. Insert the needle portion into a blood vacutainer tube to provide negative suction. 7. This active technique provides a way of monitoring the quantity and nature of the hematoma fluid. Chronic hematoma: 1. Make an incision down the long axis of the pinna in an "S" shape. 2. Probe the pinna for and remove fibrin tags and blood clots and flush with saline. 3. Place a mattress pattern or simple interrupted sutures, using non-absorbable monofilament suture, along the surface of the pinna to remove any dead space and allow complete apposition of both sides of the ear cartilage. 4. Place a non-adherent pad over the incision and bandage the ear i over the top of the head. 5. CO_2 lasers can be used to create 2–5-mm drainage sites. Non-surgical treatment. 1. Aspirate the hematoma fluid and administer systemic and/or local infusion of corticosteroids.[2]	1. Two incisions are made parallel to the vertical ear canal margins and a transverse incision joining them. 2. The skin and SQ tissue are reflected, and two incisions are made through the cartilage to expose the inside of the vertical canal. 3. The reflected flap of cartilage is trimmed and sutured to the skin to make a drainboard ventrally.
Patient care	• Bandaging is an important part of treating aural hematomas • It can be a challenge to not put the head bandage on too tight or too loose (see Chapter 19: Wound Care and Bandaging) • Label the outside of the bandage *clearly* to avoid an accidental pinnectomy when cutting the bandage off	• Warm compress 3–4 times a day for 2–3 days if there is excessive swelling

(*Continued*)

Table 23.5 / **Aural surgery: aural hematoma, lateral ear canal resection (Continued)**

Procedure	Aural hematoma	Lateral ear canal resection
Client education	• Strict confinement is necessary to allow pinna to heal properly	• This procedure is not a cure, but will offer a temporary solution • Continuous medical management may still be required, but is made easier • Do not use any foreign object (e.g. cotton balls, cotton-tipped applicators) in the shortened ear canal, to avoid damage to the tympanic membrane
Expected pain	• Mild to moderate	• Severe to excruciating
Notes	• Laser surgery provides another technique requiring no sutures. • Even with appropriate treatment, disfiguration (cauliflower appearance) of the pinna may occur • Important to treat underlying ear disease	• Chronic otitis externa and media may require removal of the entire ear canal

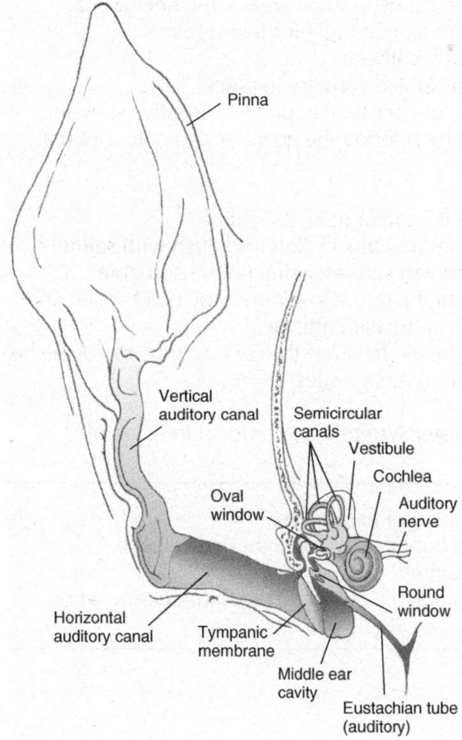

Figure 23.2 The ear.

Table 23.6 **Gastrointestinal Surgery: Anal Sacculectomy, Enterotomy**

Procedure	Anal Sacculectomy	Enterotomy
Definition	• Removal of one or both of the anal sacs and associated anal sac duct	• Incision made into the small intestines
Indications	• Correction of long-term anal sac infection, recurrent impaction, anal fistulae, and neoplasia	• Examination for ulcers, strictures, or neoplasia, full-thickness biopsy, obstruction (i.e foreign body), and feeding tube placement
Patient Preparation	• Perform caudal epidural • Ventral recumbency with rear legs draped over the end of the table and tail secured cranially • Prepare a 4-in. radius around the anus • Express anal sacs, evacuate as much of the feces from the colon as possible, and pack rectum with sponges or place anal purse-string (make notation on the patient about purse-string) • *Closed:* ±Instill self-hardening gel or resin into sac(s) to be removed	• Dorsal recumbency • Prepare entire abdomen, xiphoid to pubis
Surgical Technique	*Closed:* Place hemostat, self-hardening gel/resin, balloon-tip catheter into the gland to isolate the hardened sac; an incision is made over the sac. The surrounding tissue is gently dissected away from the sac, and the sac and duct are removed. The area is lavaged with warmed saline, and the remaining tissue is closed in a routine closure. *Open*: The anal sac orifice is visualized and a grooved director is placed into the sac orifice to the most ventral aspect. An incision is made along the grooved director, and the entire sac and duct are dissected out. The area is lavaged with warmed saline, and the remaining tissue is closed in a routine closure. • Remove packed sponges in the rectum and anal purse-string.	A midline abdominal incision is made. The entire length of intestines are examined, the affected area is then exteriorized and packed with saline-moistened gauze sponges. Stay sutures are placed, and the bowel contents are milked away from the intended incision site. Intestinal forceps or an assistant using a scissor-like grip with the index and middle finger occlude the intestines on either side of the enterotomy. An incision is made into the intestines to obtain biopsies or for obstruction removal. Resection and anastomosis is potentially performed based on the viability of the intestines. The abdomen is flushed with warm saline and the enterotomy is covered with a piece of omentum. Sponge count, contaminated instruments and gloves are replaced, and routine closure of the abdomen is performed.

Notes	• *Instruments:*
	  • *Closed:* self-hardening gel or resin and administration equipment, anal sac catheter
	  • *Open:* grooved director
	  • *Thick padding on operating room table*
	  • *Surgery:* Careful, atraumatic dissection with minimal muscle damage is essential to preserve nerve and sphincter function.
	• *Patient care:* Cold pack the surgical site immediately after surgery once the patient is normothermic; antibiotics for 7–10 days postoperatively if contamination occurs.
	• *Expected pain:* moderate
		• *Surgery:* Stay sutures may not be necessary, especially if a surgical assistant is present.
		• *Surgery:* Enterotomy incisions are usually made in the antimesenteric border directly distal to the obstruction.
		• *Expected pain:* moderate to severe

Table 23.7 / **Gastrointestinal Surgery: Gastric Dilation Volvulus and Gastrotomy**

Procedure	Gastric dilatation volvulus (gastric torsion, bloat)	Gastrotomy
Definition	• To reposition the stomach and the spleen to their correct location and restore blood circulation • Fix the stomach to the abdominal wall to prevent further torsion	• Incision made into the stomach
Indications	• A distended stomach rotated on the mesenteric axis	• Full-thickness biopsy, foreign body, and partial gastrectomy
Instruments	• Suction, electrocautery and laparotomy pads	
Patient preparation	• Orogastric decompression or needle trocarization • Dorsal recumbency • Prepare mid-chest to pubis • Supportive care of IV fluids, antibiotics, analgesics • Correct acid–base and electrolyte imbalances • ECG and coagulation profile • Large bore IV catheter in front limb	• Dorsal recumbency • Clip mid-thorax to pubis
Surgical technique	1. Make a midline abdominal incision. 2. Perform further orogastric decompression if necessary via an orogastric tube or suction. 3. Rotate the stomach back to its normal position and assess for necrotic tissue. 4. If necrosis is seen, perform a partial gastrectomy. 5. Evaluate the spleen for torsion and necrosis, and perform a splenectomy if necrosis is noted. 6. Perform a gastropexy is then performed on the right side of the animal. 7. Replace contaminated instruments and gloves, count sponges and perform routine closure of the abdomen.	1. Make a cranial midline abdominal incision. 2. Examine the entire length of the intestines, then exteriorize the stomach and pack with saline-moistened gauze sponges. 3. Place stay sutures. 4. Incise the stomach and suction free of liquid contents. 5. Remove the foreign body or take biopsy specimens. 6. Typically, close the stomach 2-0 or 3-0 absorbable monofilament suture on a taper needle, in a multilayer fashion, lavage with warmed saline, and possibly cover with omentum. 7. Perform single-layer closure for gastrotomies near the pylorus. 8. Replace contaminated instruments and gloves. 9. Count sponges and perform routine closure of the abdomen.
Complications	• Perioperative death in 10–27% of dogs with GDV[2]	• Esophagitis secondary to reflux and vomiting
Patient care	• Monitor electrolytes, blood gases, PCV, TPP, urinary output, ECG, and CVP as necessary • Begin feeding a soft, low-fat diet 12 hours postoperatively and monitor for vomiting	
Client education	• Water and food 12 hours after surgery if no vomiting	
Expected pain	• Moderate to severe	• Moderate
Notes		• Feeding tubes can be placed at the time of surgery if their use is expected • Prognosis is good when no evidence of perforation

Table 23.8 / Gastrointestinal surgery: intestinal resection and anastomosis

Procedure	Intestinal resection and anastomosis
Definition	• Removal of a diseased or non-viable section of the intestines with end-to-end bowel reattachment
Indications	• A non-functioning section of bowel possibly caused by obstruction, neoplasia, intussusception, bowel necrosis, trauma, pythiosis, infiltrative bowel disease, or mesenteric volvulus
Patient preparation	• Dorsal recumbency • Prepare from mid-thorax to the pubis • Clip and flush the prepuce of male dogs
Surgical technique	1. Make a ventral midline abdominal incision. 2. Exteriorize the area of the intestines to be resected, pack with saline-moistened gauze sponges, and ligate major vessels. 3. Milk the bowel contents away from the intended site. 4. Occlude the intestines on either side of the enterotomy, using intestinal forceps or an assistant using a scissor-like grip with the index and middle finger. 5. Remove the diseased portion, and use one of many types of suture patterns or staples to allow complete closure of the intestines. 6. Flush the entire abdomen with warmed saline if contamination is suspected. 7. Flush the site of anastomosis with saline and then cover with a piece of omentum. 8. Verify a sponge count, replace contaminated instruments and gloves, and perform routine closure of the abdomen.
Complications	• Dehiscence of anastomosis leakage 3–14% and is detected 2–5 days after surgery • Short-bowel syndrome • Ileus
Client education	• Low residue diets for patients that underwent large small bowel resection or ileocolectomy
Expected pain	• Moderate to severe

Integument Surgery

Table 23.9 / Integument surgery

Procedure	Integument surgery
Instruments	• Laceration pack or general surgical pack • Skin marker • ± Passive or active drain
Patient preparation	• Preanesthetic evaluation • Preoperative protocol • If multiple masses are set to be removed, verify location with the owner by using a permanent marker or shaving a small area over the masses • See particular surgery
Surgical technique	• See particular surgery
Complications	• Dehiscence, skin necrosis, and slough • Failure of intended surgery • Infection • Seroma
Procedural:	
Patient	• Fever • Drainage from the incision • Patient molestation of the incision • Pain or swelling from infection or SQ seroma
Patient care	• Monitor signs of infection: pain, swelling, redness and heat • Place a bandage drain material when a Penrose drain is placed • Pain management • Standard postoperative care • Confine and restrict activity until suture/staple removal or as directed by the veterinarian
Client education	• Postoperative care protocol

Table 23.10 / Integument surgery: abscess and laceration

Procedure	Abscess, superficial	Laceration, superficial
Definition	• Accumulation of purulent exudate under the skin, forming an isolated cavity in body tissue because of a pathogen	• A full-thickness disruption through the dermis and exposing the SQ
Indications	• Swelling and painful at the location • Sepsis	• To restore skin integrity and allow for epithelialization by primary intention healing
Patient preparation	• Positioned to allow access to the affected site • Prepare the site to include the location of swelling with an additional 2–6-inch margin of hair removed • Perform an antiseptic skin preparation	• Positioned to allow access to the affected site • Prepare the site to include the location of injury with an additional 2–4-inch margins. • Clipped hair and other debris must not enter the laceration site; fill with sterile lubricant or cover with a moistened gauze sponge
Surgical technique	1. Use a sterile sharp instrument or blade to make an opening into the abscess or to enlarge the tract's opening. 2. Drain accumulated exudate and fluid, and lavage the cavity with copious amounts of fluid (e.g. 0.05% chlorhexidine, diluted betadine, saline) to remove any additional contaminated fluid, bacteria, or debris. 3. Remove any devitalized tissue, and make an additional hole for drain placement. 4. Place a passive drain in a dependent area and suture into place for 3–5 days. 5. Cover the area with an absorbent bandage.	1. Clip and clean the area, and remove any foreign material. 2. Debride devitalized tissue and lavage the area (e.g. chlorhexidine, diluted betadine, saline) to remove any additional contaminated fluid, bacteria, or debris. 3. Close the dead space via sutures, and a place a drain if necessary. 4. Appose the skin edges and suture or staple closed.
Patient care	• Systemic broad spectrum antibiotics postoperatively for ≥ 1 week	• ± Bandage and immobilize for ↑ healing and to ↓ swelling
Client education	• Warm compress 2–3 times daily to keep drain open and draining for around 3–5 days • Elizabethan collars or other measures must be taken to avoid chewing at suture line or any drains placed • Keep the drain site covered with absorbent dressing; change daily	• Elizabethan collars or other measures must be taken to avoid chewing at suture line or any drains placed
Expected pain	• Mild to moderate	• Mild to moderate
Notes	• Abscesses should not be opened in sterile operating rooms to avoid contamination	• Suture line skin tension will delay healing and promote dehiscence

Table 23.11 / Integument surgery: mass removal and onychectomy

Procedure	Mass removal	Onychectomy (declaw)
Definition	• Surgical excision of a tumor, mass, growth, or cyst	• Removal of the nail and entire third phalanx
Instruments	• See Table 23.9	• Tourniquet, skin glue, sterile nail trimmers, electrosurgery, radiosurgery or CO_2 laser and protective eye-wear with proper laser optical density lenses
Indications	• Obstruction with function, neoplasia, or cosmetic	• Trauma, infection, or neoplasia • Owner with fragile skin, a clotting disorders or poor immunity • Prevent euthanasia
Patient preparation	• Positioned to allow access to the affected site • Prepare the site to include the tumor location with an additional 2–6-inch margin • Larger margins when neoplasia is suspected or confirmed • Local analgesic blocks may need to be avoided prior to excision of mass • Pre-medication with diphenhydramine when mast cell tumor is suspected or confirmed	• Lateral recumbency • Typically, clipping of the hair is not indicated; paws can be clipped if long hair is present • Scrub each toe with an antiseptic, rinse with saline • Avoid alcohol when using laser
Surgical technique	1. Varying techniques are employed for the varying sizes and shapes of specific tumors. 2. Perform excision as atraumatically as possible to avoid spread of tumor cells and protect adjacent tissue. 3. Make an elliptical incision around the tumor through all layers, assuring wide enough margins to prevent regrowth. 4. Dissect out the tumor while maintaining hemostasis to prevent tumor cells or other substances (e.g. histamine) from spilling into the area. 5. Close the dead space via sutures, and place a drain if necessary. 6. Appose the skin edges and suture closed. 7. Replace instruments, gloves, and drapes when removing tumors from multiple sites.	1. Place a ring block with opioid analgesics or lidocaine bupivacaine. 2. Traditional declaw: 3. Using a scalpel or guillotine nail trimmers, remove the entire third phalanx. 4. Milk the blood proximally, and a place a tourniquet below the elbow. 5. After excising the toe, appose the skin with sutures or tissue glue. 6. Place a secure bandage to prevent hemorrhage. Laser declaw: 1. Use a CO_2 laser to remove the entire third phalanx; 0.4 mm tip 5–8 watts in continuous wave mode. 2. With both techniques, take care to avoid cutting the digital pads.
Complications	• See Table 23.9	• Surgical: the third phalanx must be removed from each toe to avoid additional pain, nail regrowth, infection, "phantom" pain sensation, and/or occasional limping • Patient: patient biting as a substitute for clawing; recommendations may vary, but the owner should expect the animal to remain hospitalized for 1–2 days post-surgery

(*Continued*)

Table 23.11 / Integument surgery: mass removal and onychectomy (Continued)

Procedure	Mass removal	Onychectomy (declaw)
Patient care	• Incision care	
Client education	• Elizabethan collars or other measures must be taken to avoid chewing at the suture line	
Expected pain	• Moderate	• Moderate to severe
Notes	• Histopathology: odentify cut edges and deep layers with tissue ink and suture tags • Fix in 10% formalin 1 : 10	

Neurological Surgery

Table 23.12 / Neurological surgery

Procedure	Neurological surgery
Instruments	• General surgical pack • Orthopedic pack • Neurology pack • Burr air drill • Micro-instruments
Patient preparation	• Preanesthetic evaluation • Complete neurological evaluation radiographs, CT, MRI • Preoperative protocol • Patient with spinal instability should be put in braces or secured to a rigid surface to decrease further damage • Avoid dorsal flexion of the cervical region in atlantoaxial luxation • ± corticosteroid administration • Two venous catheters should be placed to allow rapid fluid and blood administration if hemorrhage were to occur • Patient positioning is determined for each procedure (e.g. linear traction, gentle flexion, extension, rotation) to facilitate visualization, reduce fractures, and/or decompress spinal cord
Surgical technique	• See particular surgery

(Continued)

Table 23.12 / **Neurological surgery (Continued)**

Procedure	Neurological surgery
Complications	• Venous sinus hemorrhage • Nerve or CNS damage • Spinal instability and/or collapse • Seroma • Infection
Procedural:	
Patient	• Decubital sores, urinary tract infection, urine scald • Joint stiffness and muscle atrophy • Pneumonia and gastrointestinal tract ulceration
Patient care	• Critical observation for the first 24 hours (e.g. pain management, respiratory depression, GDV, seizures) • Intensive patient care (e.g. frequent rotation, bladder expression, physical therapy, maintaining a clean and dry environment) • Use barrier film products to prevent skin damage from urine and feces
Client education	• Postoperative care protocol • Physical rehabilitation often required daily until healed and full function returns (days to weeks) • Frequent neurological exam over the first 12 months

Table 23.13 / **Neurological surgery: disk fenestration, dorsal laminectomy, and hemilaminectomy**

Procedure	Disk fenestration	Dorsal laminectomy	Hemilaminectomy
Definition	• Creation of a window in the ventral annulus to access and remove the nucleus pulposus that is calcified or may become calcified/degenerated	• Removal of dorsal lamina and supraspinous process to expose the spinal cord and correct the underlying problem	• Removal of right and/or left lateral lamina to expose the spinal cord and correct the underlying problem (e.g. removal of disk material or tumor, fracture stabilization)
Indications	• Disk rupture, spinal cord compression, nerve root entrapment	• Compressive lesions located in the dorsal or lateral vertebral canal (e.g. disk fragments, fracture segments, tumors)	• Lesions located in the lateral, dorsolateral or ventrolateral vertebral canal (e.g. disk material or tumor, fracture fragment)

(*Continued*)

Table 23.13 / **Neurological surgery: disk fenestration, dorsal laminectomy, and hemilaminectomy (Continued)**

Procedure	Disk fenestration	Dorsal laminectomy	Hemilaminectomy
Surgical technique	1. Make an incision based on the surgical approach (e.g. ventral, lateral or dorsolateral). 2. Dissect to the annulus fibrosus; make a window and remove the nucleus pulposus. 3. Changing the patient's position may facilitate the removal of the nucleus pulposus. 4. Close the incision routinely.	1. Make an incision in the dorsal midline along the spinous process. 2. Dissect down to the affected intervertebral body or space and enter the vertebral canal. 3. After the vertebral canal is entered, a durotomy may or may not be performed to relieve spinal cord swelling. 4. Remove the compressive lesion and irrigate with sterile saline. 5. Wire can be used to close the site with a layer of SQ fat placed over the site to prevent adhesions. 6. Close the remaining area routinely.	1. Make an incision in the dorsal midline along the length of the spinous processes. 2. Dissect down to the affected intervertebral body or space at the lateral aspect, and enter the vertebral canal. 3. After the vertebral canal is entered, a durotomy may or may not be performed to relieve spinal cord swelling. 4. Remove the compressive lesion and irrigate with sterile saline. 5. Place a layer of SQ fat over the site to prevent adhesions and close the remaining area routinely.
Complications	• See Table 23.12	• Venous sinus hemorrhage • Bone hemorrhage • CNS trauma	• Venous sinus hemorrhage • Bone hemorrhage • CNS trauma
Notes	• Most commonly performed in conjunction with laminectomy or hemilaminectomy		

Ophthalmic Surgery

Table 23.14 / **Ophthalmic surgery**

Procedure	Ophthalmic surgery
Instruments	• Ophthalmic surgical pack • Eyelid speculum • Operating microscope or magnification head loupe may be required for certain procedures • Focal light source • Beaver blade or #15 blade • Multifilament absorbable suture

(Continued)

Table 23.14 / **Ophthalmic surgery (Continued)**

Procedure	Ophthalmic surgery
Patient preparation	• Preanesthetic evaluation • Preoperative protocol • Ventral recumbency with the head propped up on a towel or cushion • Place a sterile ophthalmic ointment in the eye to protect from clipped hair and cleaning solutions • Prepare area immediately around the eye by clipping, brushing away, or using adhesive tape to clean the area; flush conjunctival sac with a diluted (0.2%)povidone iodine solution and gently wash surrounding area with cotton-tipped swabs or surgical sponges soaked in the diluted antiseptic; rinse with saline • Avoid using soaps, detergents, and alcohol as they may all cause damage to the delicate eye tissues • When preparing instruments for ophthalmic procedures avoid using detergents and enzymatic cleaners on instruments
Surgical technique	• See particular surgery
Complications:	
Procedural	• Failure of intended surgery • Infection • Tissue necrosis • Keratitis secondary to corneal drying or trauma • Scar tissue leading to chronic irritation
Patient	• Swelling • Pain and pruritus
Follow-Up	
Patient care	• Continue analgesia postoperatively • Standard postoperative care • Allow a quiet anesthetic recovery to prevent trauma upon waking • Prevention of self-trauma; confine and restrict activity until suture/staple removal or as directed by the veterinarian • Monitor daily for tearing, mucopurulent discharge, inflammation, blepharospasm
Client education	• Postoperative care protocol
Notes	• See Figure 23.3

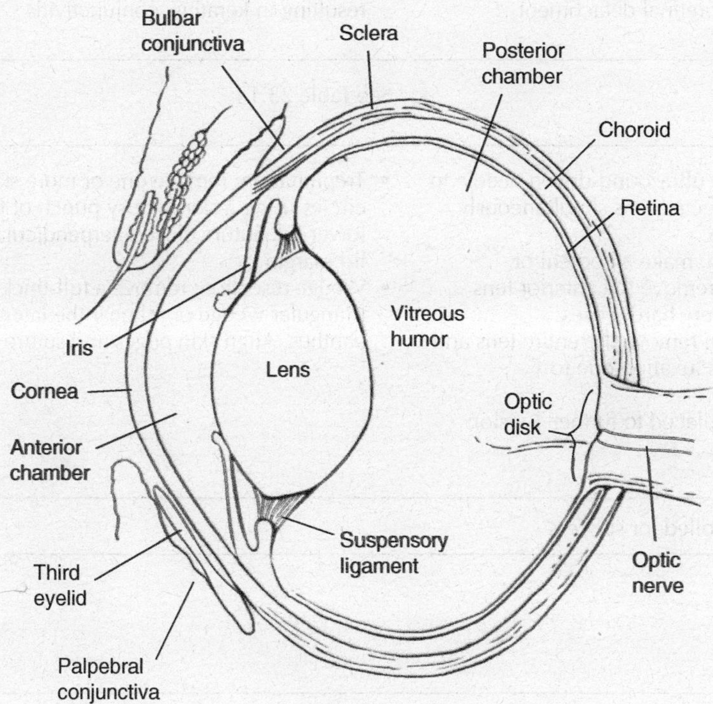

Figure 23.3 The eye.

Table 23.15 / **Ophthalmic surgery: cataracts, ectropion, and entropion**

Procedure	Cataracts	Ectropion	Entropion
Definition	• Removal of the lens through surgical removal or physical dissolution	• Removal of excess skin to decrease laxity and shorten and strengthen the lower eyelid	• Eversion of a section of eyelid skin, depending on the type of entropion
Indications	• Opacity of the lens, which could lead to uveitis, glaucoma, visual deficits, or retinal detachment	• Outward rolling (eversion) of the eyelid resulting in keratitis, conjunctivitis	• Inward rolling of the eyelid margin resulting in keratitis, corneal ulceration, and pain
Patient preparation	See Table 23.14	See Table 23.14	See Table 23.14
Surgical technique	• Phacoemulsification: use an ultrasound-driven needle to emulsify and remove the affected lens simultaneously and to irrigate the eye • Extracapsular lens extraction: make a corneal or corneoscleral incision, and remove the anterior lens capsule; typically used for very hard lenses • Intracapsular lens extraction: remove the entire lens and capsule; only used with lens luxation due to ↑ complications • An intraocular lens is often placed to further ↑ vision	• Trephination: remove one or more skin circles using a skin biopsy punch of the lower lid. Suture closed perpendicular to the lid margin • Wedge resection: remove a full-thickness triangular wedge of lid near the lateral canthus. Align skin edges and suture closed	• Modified Hotz–Celsus: remove an elliptical or crescent-shaped area of skin 1–3 mm below the margin of the lid, depending on the location of the entropion. Suture the area closed with a multifilament nonabsorbable suture, allowing lid eversion and for it to remain in a normal anatomic position • Temporary tacking: evert the eyelid margin and tack it in place with sutures
Patient care	• Inflammation must be controlled for success		
Client education			• Ectropion may be initially present until swelling has decreased; multiple procedures may be needed.
Expected pain	• Moderate	• Moderate	• Moderate
Notes	• Indications: must be distinguished from nuclear sclerosis	• Surgical complication: entropion may result with overcorrection	• Surgical: Everting sutures may be used temporarily in young dogs for correction without excision of eyelid.

Table 23.16 / Ophthalmic surgery: conjunctival flap and enucleation

Procedure	Conjunctival flap	Enucleation
Definition	• A conjunctival flap is secured over the site of a deep corneal ulcer to provide protection and a source of blood vessels, antibodies, and serum antiproteases	• Removal of the eye (e.g. globe, nictitating membrane, eyelid margins)
Indications	• Deep corneal ulcers, trauma, descemetoceles, ruptures, corneal diseases	• Glaucoma, trauma, neoplasia, endophthalmitis, panophthalmitis, congenital defects, severe infections
Surgical technique	1. Clean the ulcer of any necrotic tissue and corneal epithelium to ensure graft adherence. 2. Harvest a thin flap from the bulbar conjunctiva and place over the ulcer; suture into place. 3. Suture the harvested site closed. 4. Trim the flap after the ulcer has healed (4–6 weeks) without disturbing the conjunctiva from the former ulcer site.	Subconjunctival: 1. Make an incision at the lateral canthus, through and under the conjunctiva and stabilize the eye. 2. Dissect the eye through the muscle attachments, optic nerve, and blood vessels, and then remove. 3. Suture the tissues in a layered fashion. Transpalpebral: 1. Suture the eyelids closed. 2. Make an elliptical incision through the skin of the eyelid.
Complications	• Flap failure (e.g. bacterial infection, poor technique, flap necrosis, inadequate ulcer debridement)	• Hemorrhage (e.g. angularis oculi vein is severed), damage to the optic chiasm affecting vision in the remaining eye
Client education	• Elizabethan collar and activity restriction for 1 week	
Expected pain	• Moderate	• Moderate

Table 23.17 / Ophthalmic surgery: prolapse of the gland of the third eyelid and traumatic proptosis

Procedure	Prolapse of the gland of the third eyelid (cherry eye)	Temporary tarsorrhaphy (traumatic proptosis)
Definition	• Repositioning of the third eyelid gland and anchoring in a more normal position	• Sewing the eyelids together
Indications	• Hypertrophy and prolapse of the third eyelid gland	• Maintain eye in position after proptosis, protect the cornea, facial nerve paralysis, corneal ulcers

(*Continued*)

Table 23.17 / Ophthalmic surgery: prolapse of the gland of the third eyelid and traumatic proptosis (Continued)

Procedure	Prolapse of the gland of the third eyelid (cherry eye)	Temporary tarsorrhaphy (traumatic proptosis)
Surgical technique	Pocket technique: 1. Make an incision along the margins of the gland into the palpebral conjunctiva. 2. Form a pocket, and return the gland to its normal position by tucking with a conjunctival fold. 3. Appose the incision and then suture together over the gland. Anchoring technique: 1. Anchor suture distally in the palpebral surface. 2. Pass needle through the third eyelid, exiting near the start of the laceration. 3. Close laceration with a continuous suture pattern. At completion, pass the suture through the gland and gently anchor in the bulbar conjunctiva.	1. Suture eyelid closed using stents (tubing or rubber bands) to avoid pressure necrosis. 2. An area at the medial canthus is left open to allow application of medications. 3. 4-0 to 6-0 nylon or multifilament nonabsorbable suture on a micropoint needle, the use of an operating microscope helps to aid in accurate suture placement.[2]
Patient care	• Check tear production	• Wear Elizabethan collar
Client education	• Removal of the gland is no longer recommended due to future risks of KCS; suture abrasion of cornea • Eye medications 2–4 weeks post-surgery • Wear Elizabethan collar	• Keep the eye moist with sterile saline, viscous lubricating ointment, or antibiotic ointment
Expected pain	• Moderate	• Mild

Orthopedic Surgery

Table 23.18 / Orthopedic surgery

Procedure	Orthopedic surgery
Preparation	
Instruments	• Orthopedic pack • Pin set • Screw set • Implant set • Periosteal elevator set
Patient preparation	• Preanesthetic evaluation • Preoperative protocol • Lateral recumbency
Surgical technique	• See particular surgery
Complications:	
Procedural	• Failure of intended surgery • Infection (e.g. osteomyelitis) • Malunion or non-union from inadequate immobilization
Patient	• Gait alterations • Pain • Bandage molestation
Follow-up	
Patient care	• ± bandage • Physical therapy • Pain management • Standard postoperative care • Confine and restrict activity until suture/staple removal or as directed by the veterinarian.
Client education	• Postoperative care protocol

Table 23.19 / **Orthopedic surgery: cranial cruciate ligament rupture, femoral head and neck ostectomy, and fracture repair**

Procedure	Cranial cruciate ligament rupture	Femoral head and neck ostectomy	Fracture repair
Definition	• To stabilize the joint by ↓ or eliminating abnormal forces exerted on the stifle joint because of ligament loss, and thereby to prevent further injury and return the leg to normal function	• Removal of the femoral head and neck to form a fibrous false joint	• To provide stability so fracture healing may occur, with the least amount of disruption to the natural healing process
Indications	• Progressive lameness and degenerative joint disease • Positive cranial drawer	• Canines and felines with hip dysplasia or hip injury (fracture, septic arthritis, and neoplasia) • Pain as a result of bone-on-bone contact	• Any type of break in a bone, typically a long bone
Patient preparation	• Variable, surgeon preference • Dorsal or lateral recumbency, rotated to allow placement of the stifle flat on the table when flexed • Prepare hip to tarsus	• Lateral recumbency • Prepare dorsal midline to stifle	• Variable: dependent on fracture site
Surgical technique	There are many techniques, the following are just a few: 1. Tibial plateau leveling osteotomy: repositioning of the tibial plateau through osteotomy to allow surrounding muscles to provide stifle stability and neutralize cranial tibial thrust. 2. Extracapsular stabilization (lateral fabellotibial suture): extracapsular technique using heavy suture to pass from the lateral fabella to the tibial crest. 3. Tibial tuberosity advancement: move the tibial tuberosity cranially to modify the patellar tendon angle, neutralizing tibiofemoral shear force. 4. Stifle arthroscopy: provides an ideal view of the stifle joint and provides direct access to intra-articular structures.	1. Make a craniolateral incision. 2. Dissect the hip joint down and luxate the hip to allow ↑ visibility. 3. Remove the femoral head and the entirety of the neck with a combination of a drill, mallet and osteotome or with an oscillating drill. 4. Remove any irregularities of the cut bone with rongeurs to provide a smooth surface. 5. Suture the joint capsule closed over the acetabulum and return all tendons and muscles to their original location and suture. 6. Perform routine closure of the tissue in layers.	1. Cerclage wire: place wire around the bone fracture for stabilization, often used with other techniques. 2. Tension band wiring: place wire and intramedullary pins to fix and apply compression to the tension side of a fracture to counteract muscle traction at insertion of muscles. 3. Interlocking nail and intramedullary pin fixation: place pins down the intramedullary canal of long bones and fix at either end with screws or cross-locking bolts. 4. Stack pinning: place multiple intramedullary pins for internal fixation. 5. Bone plate and screw fixation: place screws through bone plates along fracture site for stabilization.

(*Continued*)

Table 23.19 / Orthopedic surgery: cranial cruciate ligament rupture, femoral head and neck ostectomy, and fracture repair (Continued)

Procedure	Cranial cruciate ligament rupture	Femoral head and neck ostectomy	Fracture repair
Client education	• A 4–5-month recovery period is often seen, but the patient should follow the veterinarian's postoperative instructions for optimal recovery • Physical rehabilitation is often required daily until healed and full function returns; restrictions on use vary between procedure choices	• Activity is started early helps to prevent muscle atrophy • Physical rehabilitation often required daily until healed and full function returns • Permanent limp may be present due to shortened leg length	• Physical activity should be restricted until given approval by the veterinarian • Physical rehabilitation often required daily until healed and full function returns • Some implants require retrieval later, especially with loosening
Expected pain	• Moderate to severe	• Moderate to severe	• Moderate to severe
Notes	• Surgical technique chosen is most often based on the surgeon's preference • Meniscus integrity is examined in each patient as 30–80% of dogs with CCL ruptures have a meniscal tear	• Pain management: multimodal analgesia	

Table 23.20 / Orthopedic surgery: patellar luxation, total hip replacement, and triple pelvic osteotomy (TPO)

Procedure	Patellar Luxation	Total Hip Replacement	TPO
Definition	• To stabilize the patella in the trochlea and allow movement of the limb without luxation	• Replacement of the femoral head and acetabular cup with artificial prostheses	• Rotation of the acetabulum portion of the pelvis to help prevent degenerative joint disease in hip dysplasia
Indications	• Patella that luxates spontaneously or with palpation	• Pain and loss of function from DJD, secondary to hip dysplasia	• Young dogs (5–18 months) with hip dysplasia and no signs of degenerative joint disease
Patient preparation	• Dorsal or lateral recumbency • Prepared from lumbar spine to tarsus • Regional block	• IV antibiotics are started the day before the procedure, and the surgery site is clipped to check for skin infections • Lateral recumbency • Prepared from lumbar spine to tarsus • Examine surgical site for pyoderma • Epidural • Verify all implants and instruments are available and sterilized	• Lateral recumbency • Prepared from lumbar spine to tarsus

(Continued)

Table 23.20 / **Orthopedic surgery: patellar luxation, total hip replacement, and triple pelvic osteotomy (TPO) (Continued)**

Procedure	Patellar Luxation	Total Hip Replacement	TPO
Surgical technique	1. Trochlear block recession: to deepen the trochlear groove by forming a flap of cartilage, removing underlying bone, and replacing the flap. 2. Trochlear wedge recession: to deepen the trochlear groove by cutting a wedge of cartilage out and replacing it further recessed into the groove. 3. Tibial tuberosity transposition: transplantation of the attachment of the patellar ligament to a more lateral position, using Kirschner wires and a tension-band wire for stabilization. 4. Medial fascial release: soft tissue technique, release of the medial retinaculum to allow the patella to stabilize in the deepened groove.	1. Make a craniolateral incision. 2. Remove the femoral head and a portion of the neck and replace with the prosthetic femoral stem. 3. Widen the location of the original acetabular cup, and cement the prosthetic acetabular cup to the medial pelvic wall. 4. Reduce the femoral head into the acetabular cup, and close the joint tightly. 5. Perform routine closure of the tissue in layers. 6. Cementless caps are also used, allowing bone growth into the shell of the cap. 7. Precise preparation of the femoral canal and acetabulum are required for a tight fit. Often chosen for younger animals.	1. Make three incisions into the wing of the ilium, pubis, and ischium around the acetabular cup. 2. The acetabulum is then free to be rotated to provide more dorsal coverage of the femoral head. 3. Place bone plates, wires, or screws to secure the acetabulum in its new position. 4. Perform routine closure of the tissue in layers.
Complications	See Table 23.18	• Infection of implants • Loosening, and weakening of cement • Luxation	• Infection and loosening of bone plates
Client education	At least 3 weeks of restricted activity necessary	• Physical rehabilitation is often required daily until healed and full function returns	• Restrict to leash walks for 6 weeks or until there is radiographic evidence of complete healing • Physical rehabilitation is often required daily until healed and full function returns
Expected pain	• Moderate to severe	• Moderate to severe	• Moderate to severe
Notes	• Surgery: warranted for grades 3 and 4 luxation		

Reproductive Tract Surgery

Table 23.21 / Reproductive tract surgery

Procedure	Reproductive tract surgery
Preparation	
Instruments	• General surgical pack • Spay hook • Carmalt forceps
Patient preparation	• Preanesthetic evaluation • Preoperative protocol • Dorsal recumbency • Flush prepuce of male dogs with antiseptic solutions
Surgical technique	• See particular surgery
Complications:	
Procedural	• Adhesions of uterine stump, bladder, or scrotal skin • Failure to remove all gonadal tissue completely (e.g. ovarian remnant syndrome) • Hemorrhage • Peritonitis/sepsis • Inadvertent damage to vital urinary structures (e.g. ureters)
Patient	• Inappetence • Pain • Incisional infection or dehiscence
Preparation	
Patient care	• Standard postoperative care • Confine and restrict activity until suture/staple removal (typically 10–14 days) or as directed by the veterinarian
Client education	• Postoperative care protocol

Table 23.22 / Cesarean section, orchiectomy, and ovariohysterectomy

Procedure	Cesarean section (C-section, hysterotomy)	Orchiectomy (alter, neuter, castration)	Ovariohysterectomy (spay)
Definition	• Removal of all fetuses from the uterus through the abdomen	• The removal of the testes	• The removal of the uterine body, horns, and ovaries
Indications	• Dystocia, uterine inertia, prolonged gestation, fetal distress or death, trauma, toxemia, or high-risk pregnancies	• Sterilization, reduction of aggressiveness, wandering and marking behavior, cancer, traumatic injury, infections, prostate gland problems	• Sterilization, uterine infections, cancer, uterine torsion, congenital abnormalities, ovarian-induced hormone imbalances, elimination of estrus, extensive injury

Patient preparation	• Dorsal recumbency
	• Prepare xiphoid to pubis
	• Prepare as much of the surgical site as possible before induction of anesthesia to limit depression of neonates
	• Safe protocol example: Induction with IV propofol, light plane of isoflurane inhalant and atropine to treat bradycardia
	• Caution: avoid narcotic premedications that might compromise fetal condition via placental blood flow
		• Verify that the patient is a male, has not previously been neutered, and has two palpable testicles
		• Canine:
		  • Dorsal recumbency
		  • Prepare the prepuce to the area surrounding and including the scrotum
		• Feline:
		  • Ventral recumbency
		  • Prepare the area surrounding and including the scrotum
			• Verify that the patient is a female and has not been previously spayed
			• Dorsal recumbency
			• Manually express the bladder in non -pregnant females
			• Prepare the entire ventral abdomen

Surgical technique	1. Make a ventral midline incision and exteriorize the horns of the uterus. 2. Pack the incision with moistened gauze or laparotomy pads to avoid abdominal contamination. 3. Make an incision into the uterus and, one by one, milk each fetus down to the incision and gently pull it out. 4. Remove the amniotic sac and place the fetus, with placenta attached, in a sterile towel and gently drop into a towel held firmly by a non-sterile assistant. 5. Clamp the umbilical cord 2–6 cm from the abdominal wall. 6. Once all the fetuses have been removed, check the uterine horns for any remaining fetuses or placentas. 7. Close the uterine incision, moisten with saline, cover with omentum, and return to the abdominal cavity. 8. Perform routine closure of the tissue in layers.	Canine: 1. Make a pre-scrotal incision over the testicle and expose it through the fascia. 2. Either ligate the entire spermatic cord to remove the testicle (closed), or incise the outer tunic to reveal the spermatic vessels and cord. 3. Ligate these structures or knot onto themselves (open). 4. Place gentle traction on the scrotum to allow the remaining tunic tissue to retract into the scrotum. 5. Repeat the procedure for the second testicle. Feline: 1. Make an incision into the scrotum over each testicle in a caudoventral position. 2. The open or closed technique may then be applied.	1. Make a ventral midline incision, and locate the left uterine horn. 2. Stretch or break the suspensory ligament, and ligate and detach the ovary. 3. Locate the right uterine horn, and break the broad ligament; ligate and detach the ovary. 4. Ligate the uterus at the stump, and remove the combined uterus and ovaries. 5. Count the sponges and perform routine closure of the tissue in layers.

(Continued)

Table 23.22 / **Cesarean section, orchiectomy, and ovariohysterectomy (Continued)**

Procedure	Cesarean section (C-section, hysterotomy)	Orchiectomy (alter, neuter, castration)	Ovariohysterectomy (spay)
	9. En bloc resection of the uterus (OVH before removal of the fetuses) results in shorter anesthesia time and less abdominal contamination. 10. Fetus need to be removed from the uterus within 60 seconds. 11. 11.Clamp the ovarian pedicles prior to the uterine body to minimize fetal hypoxia.[1]		
Complications	• Hemorrhage, peritonitis, endometriosis, mastitis, incisional infection • Copious amounts of clotted or foul-smelling vaginal discharge should be reported		
Patient care	• Bitches are monitored for hypothermia, hypotension hypocalcemia, neonatal resection and agalactia • An odorless bloody vaginal discharge is to be expected lasting several weeks • Avoid postoperative analgesics that will be passed into the milk	• Monitor for scrotal hematoma	• Monitor for extreme listlessness, persistent bleeding, urinary incontinence or obstruction, seroma and incisional infection
Client education		• Insemination is still possible for several weeks after neuter • Behavioral changes expected after neutering may take several months to show and no changes may be seen in animals altered later in life	• Dogs spayed early have ↑ risk of urinary incontinence, joint disease and obesity • Animals altered prior to their first estrus have a ↓ risk of mammary tumors (around 80%) • Spaying cats after 2 years and dogs 2.5–4 years of age has minimal effect on mammary tumor development[2]
Expected pain	Moderate	Mild to moderate	Mild to moderate
Notes	• OHE does not prevent the bitch from producing milk • Clean off all antiseptics from skin before puppies nurse		

Neonatal Resuscitation Post-Cesarean

There are many methods that can be employed to stimulate a neonate to begin spontaneous respirations. A delivered neonate should be immediately placed in a dry towel with an assistant. The placental membranes should all be removed and the oropharynx cleared of fluid and secretions. The neonate should be dried off by rubbing the chest vigorously with the towel to lessen the chances of hypothermia and to stimulate respirations. If spontaneous respirations do not begin, cardiopulmonary resuscitation procedures should be followed (see Chapter 10: Emergency Medicine).

Postoperative Care of Neonates and Dam

Skill Box 23.5 / Postoperative Care of Neonates and Dam

Neonatal care

1. Remove fetal membranes and verify that the umbilical cord is temporarily clamped 2–6 cm from the abdomen.
2. Assess the condition: whether a heartbeat can be palpated, clear the mouth and nose of fluid and mucus by gentle suction or cotton swabs.
3. Stimulate respiration:
   a. Rub the neonate briskly with a towel.
   b. Caution: strong force, such as swinging or slinging, should be avoided, because of the possibility of brain damage.
   c. Administer naloxone (0.01–0.04 mg/kg IV or 1 drop per neonate under tongue) to reverse opioids given preanesthesia.
   d. Doxapram is no longer recommended.
   e. Place an acupuncture needle or a small-gauge needle (< 25 g) between the upper lip and the nose to a depth of 2–4 mm while firmly holding the head extended and elevated above the heart.
4. If the above methods do not produce a neonate that is breathing and crying, emergency resuscitation must take place.
5. Once the neonates are stable, ligate and disinfect the umbilical cord and place them in a warm, confined location (e.g. incubator, box with towels, or circulating hot water pad).
6. Caution: neonates are often small enough to fall between the bars on a cage door.
7. Place them with the dam as soon as possible to nurse.
8. Verify that the neonates are free of congenital abnormalities and are nursing appropriately before discharge.

Note: see also Chapter 14: Neonatal and Pediatric Care, page 636.

Dam care

1. Mammary glands should be cleaned of surgical preparation solutions, blood, or fetal fluids.
2. The dam should be allowed to recover from anesthesia alone and then returned to her litter once there is no risk of injury to the neonates.
3. Monitor for the first few hours after surgery for relapses into shock due to uterine hemorrhage.
4. Continue to monitor for appropriate behavior signs of the dam, (e.g. grooming and allowing neonates to nurse).
5. Discharge dam and litter once she is able to stand and continues to show appropriate mothering instinct.

Thoracic Surgery

Table 23.23 / Thoracic surgery

Thoracic surgery	
Preparation	
Instruments	• Electrocautery • General surgical pack • Extra hemostats • Self-retaining retractor • Suction tips and tubing pack • Thoracic pack
Patient preparation	• Preanesthetic evaluation • Preoperative protocol • Oxygen support • Dorsal or lateral recumbency • See particular surgery
Surgical technique	• Ventilation support and circulation monitoring required throughout surgery • See particular surgery
Complications:	
Procedural	• Hemorrhage (e.g. hemothorax) • Pleuritis/sepsis • Pneumothorax • Ventricular arrhythmias
Patient	• Pain • Difficulty breathing
Follow-Up	
Patient care	• Monitor radiographs for signs of pleural effusion • Monitor for pain and discomfort • Pain management • Standard postoperative care • Confine and restrict activity until suture/staple removal or as directed by the veterinarian
Client education	• Postoperative care protocol

Table 23.24 / **Thoracic surgery: sternotomy, thoracotomy, intercostal**

Procedure	Sternotomy, median	Thoracotomy, intercostal
Definition	• To gain access to the thoracic cavity by splitting the sternum; structures in the dorsal mediastinum (e.g. esophagus and bronchial hilus) will not be accessible	• To gain access to one-third of the left or right side of the thorax and expose selected thoracic organs via an intercostal approach
Indications	• Cardiac and respiratory diseases, esophageal foreign body, neoplasia, correction of cardiovascular defects, and to obtain biopsy specimens	• Cardiac and respiratory diseases, neoplasia, correction of cardiovascular defects, and to obtain biopsy specimens
Instruments	• Oscillating saw • Osteotomes and mallet • Wire pack • Hemoclips	See Table 23.23
Patient Preparation	• Dorsal recumbency • Prepare entire thorax thoracic inlet to umbilicus • Patient is placed on a ventilator	• Lateral recumbency • Prepare lateral thorax shoulder to last rib, dorsal midline to ventral midline (including axillary region) • Patient is placed on a ventilator
Surgical Technique	1. Make an incision over the midline on the sternum. 2. Cut the sternum with an oscillating saw or sternal splitter. 3. Place retractors and perform the exploratory. 4. Place a chest tube before closure, if necessary. 5. Verify the sponge count. 6. Suture the thoracic wall closed in many layers. 7. Create a pleural vacuum through the chest tube, and place a light bandage over the tube entrance. 8. Remember to place clamp on chest tube prior to insertion.	1. Choose the correct intercostal space based on the location in the thorax desired. 2. Make an incision from the costovertebral junction to the sternum, and then dissect the muscles through to the thoracic cavity. 3. Warn the anesthetist that the pleural cavity is about to be punctured. 4. Access the organs once the cavity is punctured and the lungs have collapsed. 5. Before closure, place a temporary or permanent chest tube if necessary. 6. Suture the thoracic wall closed in many layers. 7. Create a pleural vacuum through the chest tube and place a light bandage over the tube entrance.
Complications	• Pneumothorax • Hemothorax • Pulmonary edema	• Pneumothorax • Hemothorax • Pulmonary edema
Patient care	• Monitor pain, heart rate, CRT, mucous membrane color, pulse strength and character, respiratory rate, blood pressure, blood gases, and pulse oximetry	• Monitor pain, heart rate, CRT, mucous membrane color, pulse strength and character, respiratory rate, blood pressure, blood gases, and pulse oximetry
Expected pain	• Severe	• Moderate to severe

Upper Respiratory Surgery

Table 23.25 / Upper respiratory: stenotic nares, elongated soft palate, everted laryngeal saccules

Procedure	Alar fold wedge resection	Elongated soft palate resection, staphylectomy	Everted laryngeal saccules excision
Definition	• Widening of stenotic nares	• Surgical shortening of the soft palate	• Removal of everted laryngeal saccules(grade I laryngeal collapse)
Indications	• Brachycephalic airway syndrome • Inspiratory dyspnea	• Dyspnea (open mouth breathing, prominent snoring, stressful breathing; seen mainly in brachycephalic breeds)	• Dyspnea • Observed everted saccules on oral exam
Instruments	• #11 surgical blade • Laceration pack • Cotton tipped applicators • 3-0 or 4-0 absorbable suture	• Long instruments (thumb forceps, needle holders and scissors) • Malleable retractor • Gauze • Cotton-tipped applicators • Absorbable suture	
Patient preparation	• Use anti-anxiolytics and/or sedatives as needed to minimize stress • Preoxygenation and rapid induction • IV access • ± anticholinergics • Gently wipe any gross debris from the nose • Sternal position with head propped up on a folded towel	• Use anti-anxiolytics and/or sedatives as needed to minimize stress • Preoxygenation and rapid induction • IV access • ± anticholinergics	• Kept in a calm environment to prevent additional stress to the animal • Preoxygenation and rapid induction • Excision may require extubating, to better visualize the saccules
Surgical technique	1. Perform a technique (vertical, lateral, or horizontal wedge resection, punch resection, laser ablation, alar wing amputation, alaplasty) to correct the nares. 2. Place sutures.	1. Positioning and adequate lighting are crucial. 2. Place the patient in sternal recumbency with the head suspended above the table. 3. Tie the tracheal tube and the tongue to the mandible with gauze. 4. Use stay sutures to apply traction to the palatial tissue. 5. Pack the pharynx with gauze. 6. Trim the soft palate using a cut and suture method or with a CO_2 laser. 7. When using a laser, protect the endotracheal tube with a moistened gauze and checked so no leaks are verified.	1. Patient is placed in sternal recumbency with the head suspended above the table. 2. The everted saccule is excised at its base using scissors or biopsy forceps.

(Continued)

Table 23.25 / Upper respiratory: stenotic nares, elongated soft palate, everted laryngeal saccules (Continued)

Procedure	Alar fold wedge resection	Elongated soft palate resection, staphylectomy	Everted laryngeal saccules excision
Patient care	• Post-surgery, the patient's respiration is monitored carefully	• Overnight monitoring in the clinic is suggested to watch for respiratory distress ± O_2 cage • Steroids may be dispensed to decrease swelling • Postoperatively, a temporary tracheostomy may be indicated if the patient is having a difficult recovery	• Post-surgery, the patient's respiration is monitored carefully • Overnight monitoring is suggested to watch for respiratory distress • Steroids may be dispensed to decrease swelling
Client education	• Early correction of the nares is recommended • Correction of the upper airway may resolve gastrointestinal signs • The patient should wear an Elizabethan collar to prevent self-inflicted trauma to the area	• Canned soft food is recommended for 1–2 weeks after surgery	
Notes		• Laser safety (eye protection and closed doors) at all times when operating the laser • Procedure recommended for pets between 4 and 24 months of age • May be necessary for adults with an elongated palate	

Table 23.26 / Upper respiratory surgery: laryngeal paralysis/tracheal collapse

Procedure	Laryngeal paralysis	Tracheal collapse
Definition	• Paralysis of the arytenoid cartilage preventing laryngeal adduction and abduction	• A progressive disease resulting in a loss of rigidity of the C-shaped tracheal rings and a redundant dorsal membrane, decreasing the diameter of the tracheal lumen • Placement of rings or a stent to support and alleviate the obstruction of the trachea from surrounding flaccid cartilage
Indications	• Respiratory distress, syncope or collapse, hyperthermia	• Dyspnea, exercise intolerance, coughing, gagging, collapse

(Continued)

Table 23.26 / Upper respiratory surgery: laryngeal paralysis/tracheal collapse (Continued)

Procedure	Laryngeal paralysis	Tracheal collapse
Patient preparation	• Lateral recumbency • Oxygen support • Laryngeal function exam ± dopram (1 mg/kg IV) • Prepare lateral neck determined by the surgeon; most often it will be the left lateral neck • Temporary tracheotomy may be indicated	• Oxygen support • Stent: no preparation, lateral recumbency • Rings: prepare the ventral cervical region, including cranial ventral chest, dorsal recumbency
Surgical technique	1. Unilateral arytenoid lateralization "tieback": incise into the lateral neck and dissect to the laryngeal area. 2. Place a nonabsorbable suture through the arytenoid cartilage and the cricoid cartilage to abduct the arytenoid cartilage laterally to widen. 3. Lavage the site with sterile saline. 4. Perform routine closure of the tissue in layers.	Extraluminal tracheal rings: 1. Make an incision along the ventral cervical midline. 2. Dissect to the cervical trachea. 3. Position a polyurethane ring around the circumference of the trachea and secure in place with 4-0 monofilament nonabsorbable suture. 4. Place an additional 4–5 rings 5–8 mm apart along the trachea. 5. Lavage the site with sterile saline and close the tissue in layers. Intraluminal nitinol tracheal stent: 1. Take radiographs of the trachea with PPV to measure the diameter of the trachea. 2. Place the patient in lateral recumbency. 3. Place the stent under fluoroscopic guidance or with the aid of a rigid endoscope.
Complications	• Postoperative aspiration pneumonia	Surgery: • Rings: nerve damage,(laryngeal paralysis), implant infection, continued collapse beyond ring, tracheal necrosis, pneumothorax • Stent: stent fracture, stent migration, excessive granulation tissue, tracheitis, persistent infection Patient: • Edema, laryngeal paralysis, respiratory distress, aspiration pneumonia, continued cough • Uncommon complications include perineal hernia and rectal prolapse
Patient care	• Oxygen support and corticosteroid treatment. Withhold food until the patient is fully awake • Offer 2–3 meatballs by hand to control feeding	
Client education	• Expect improvement in 90% of cases • Aspiration pneumonia has been reported in 8–21% of dogs that have undergone unilateral arytenoid lateralization	• Weight must be controlled and harnesses used instead of collars • Antitussives, sedatives, and anti-inflammatories
Expected pain	• Mild to moderate	

Urogenital Tract Surgery

Table 23.27 / Urogenital tract surgery

Procedure	Urogenital Tract Surgery
Preparation	
Instruments	• Abdominal pack • General surgical pack • Cystotomy spoon • Saline bowl • Saline, warmed • Suction tips and tubing pack • Syringe, 60-ml catheter tip • Urethral catheter(s)
Patient preparation	• Preanesthetic evaluation • Preoperative protocol • Flush prepuce of male dogs with antiseptic solutions • See particular surgery
Surgical technique	• See particular surgery
Complications:	
Procedural	• Urinary incontinence • Stricture formation • Hemorrhage • Urinary tract infection • Urine extravasation
Patient	• Stranguria • Urine scalding
Follow-Up	
Patient care	• Hematuria for 12–36 hours up to 5–7 days is normal • Monitor ease and amount of urine production • Standard postoperative care • Confine and restrict activity until suture/staple removal
Client education	• Postoperative care protocol

Table 23.28 / Urogenital tract surgery: cystotomy, urethrostomy and scrotal urethrostomy

Procedure	Cystotomy	Perineal urethrostomy	Scrotal urethrostomy
Definition	• An incision made into the urinary bladder	• To widen the distal urethra and create a permanent opening	• The creation of a permanent opening into the urethra at the level of the scrotum
Indications	• Cystic or urethral calculi, neoplasia, urethral reimplantation, repair of ectopic ureters	• Recurrent cystic calculi, trauma, urethral stricture, tumor • Most are performed in male felines	• Recurrent cystic calculi, trauma, urethral stricture, or tumor • Preferred method in male dogs
Patient preparation	• Dorsal recumbency • Place urinary catheter and retropulsion of urethral stones into the bladder, confirm with abdominal radiographs • Prepare entire abdomen and include vulva in females	• Positioning is surgeon dependent: ventral recumbency with rear legs draped over the end of the table and tail secured cranially, or dorsal recumbency with legs pulled cranially (this position is ideal for patients that require a cystotomy) • Place a purse-string suture in the anus • ± Place and secure a urinary catheter and empty the urinary bladder • Prepare the entire perineal area, including the base of the tail • Prepare the abdomen for cystotomy	• Dorsal recumbency with rear legs abducted and secured caudally • Place and secure a urinary catheter and empty the urinary bladder • Prepare the prepuce to the area surrounding and including the scrotum
Surgical technique	1. Make a caudal midline abdominal incision. 2. Examine the caudal abdomen for additional abnormalities. 3. Isolate and exteriorize the bladder, pack with saline-moistened gauze sponges, and place stay sutures. 4. Make a ventral cystotomy incision into the bladder away from the ureters, urethra, and between major blood vessels. 5. Examine the bladder for tumors, calculi, and a diverticulum. 6. Flush the bladder by retrograde propulsion via the urinary catheter, and remove any grit via spoon or suction. 7. Securely close the bladder wall and distend with saline to check for leakage. 8. Verify sponge count and perform routine closure of the abdominal wall.	1. Make an elliptical incision around the scrotum, starting halfway between the anus and scrotum. 2. If also neutering, proceed in the normal neuter procedure. 3. Dissect the area down to the urethra, and make an incision into the dorsal midline of the urethra and enlarge to 3 cm. 4. Suture the urethra mucosa and skin together to make a single edge around the elliptical incision, leaving a new urethral orifice. 5. Remove the penis caudal to the urethral incision and suture. 6. Remove the urinary catheter, and place a new one in the new urethral orifice and suture into place.	1. Make an elliptical incision over the base of the scrotum. 2. If the patient is not neutered, do this in the normal fashion. 3. Dissect the area down to the urethra, and make an incision into the ventral midline of the urethra and enlarge to 2.5–4 cm. 4. Suture the urethra mucosa and skin together to make a single edge around the elliptical incision, leaving a new urethral orifice.

(*Continued*)

Table 23.28 / Urogenital tract surgery: cystotomy, urethrostomy and scrotal urethrostomy (Continued)

Procedure	Cystotomy	Perineal urethrostomy	Scrotal urethrostomy
Complications	See Table 23.27	• Urethral stricture and urine extravasation	• Most common complication is persistent hemorrhage • Other complications include urocystitis and urethral stricture
Patient care	• Appropriate medical management started	See Table 23.27	• Apply petroleum jelly or a liquid barrier film around incision to ↓ urine scald
Client education	See Table 23.27	• Use shredded paper litter until suture removal • Stress to the owner the importance of the e-collar, cats must not groom the perineal site until fully healed	• Bleeding during urination may occur for 3–5 days • If bleeding persists longer than 14 days, may require a revision
Diagnostics	• Calculi must be sent out for analysis and culture of bladder wall or urine • Abdominal radiographs to confirm complete removal		

Table 23.29 / Endoscopy: flexible gastrointestinal and rigid

Procedure	Flexible endoscopy	Rigid endoscopy
Definition	• Flexible endoscopy is used to evaluate the internal surface of hollow structures through a natural opening. • Most commonly, it is used for gastroscopy, rhinoscopy, and bronchoscopy • Flexible endoscopes are a greater financial investment and require more extensive training to use properly when compared to the rigid endoscope	• As its name suggests, a rigid endoscope is a stiff tube that cannot change directions (e.g. turn corners), but with a lens at its tip, it is able to look back upon itself • It is most commonly used for arthroscopy, cystoscopy, laparoscopy, otoscopy, rhinoscopy, thoracoscopy, urethroscopy, and vaginoscopy
Indications	• Internal evaluation of the gastrointestinal tract, respiratory tract, nasal passages, urinary tract • Biopsies, brushes, washes, foreign body retrieval, polyp or tumor removal, esophageal stricture dilation, feeding tube placement	• Internal evaluation of the gastrointestinal tract, respiratory tract, nasal passages, urinary tract, joints, thoracic and abdominal cavities • Biopsies, foreign body retrieval, polyp or tumor removal, joint cartilage and bone fragment removal, chest tube placement • Tracheal stent placement • Assisted gastropexy • Assisted ovariectomy

(Continued)

Table 23.29 / **Endoscopy: flexible gastrointestinal and rigid (Continued)**

Procedure	Flexible endoscopy	Rigid endoscopy
Equipment	• Endoscope and variety of telescopes • Accessory instruments (e.g. biopsy forceps, cytology brushes, balloon dilating catheters) • Retrieval instruments (e.g. coin-retrieval device, rat's tooth forceps, four-wire basket)	• Endoscope and variety of telescopes • Trocar-cannula unit (e.g. arthroscopy sheath, cystoscopy sheath) • Accessory instruments (e.g. biopsy forceps, aspiration, cautery, CO_2 insufflators, motorized shavers, diode lasers)
Technique	1. Upper gastrointestinal : anesthetize the patient, place in left lateral recumbency, and insert a mouth gag. 2. Advance the scope into the gastrointestinal tract through the center of the lumen, while distending the lumen with air and observing the surrounding structures. 3. At completion, remove the endoscope while observing for hemorrhage and evacuating any infused air. 4. Recover the patient.	1. Depending on the procedure (e.g. laparoscopy), the patient should be nil by mouth for 6–12 hours beforehand. 2. Sedate or anesthetize the patient and surgically prepare the area to be examined. 3. Insert a cannula (e.g. insert laparoscopic cannula into the abdomen) to allow insertion of the endoscope and to avoid repeated trauma to tissues and leakage of insufflated gas. 4. Place additional instruments (e.g. light source, drainage needle) to form a triangle based on the endoscope placement. 5. At completion, remove the instruments, suture the incision sites closed, and recover the patient.
Precautions	• Iatrogenic trauma (e.g. perforations, organ laceration) • Hemorrhage (e.g. nasal, liver, kidney biopsies, coagulopathies), respiratory compromise (e.g. gastric distension with air), aspiration pneumonia (e.g. dilated esophagus, gastric distention with food), GDV (e.g. gastric distention with air), esophagitis (e.g. reflux)	
Biopsies	• Samples are immediately removed from the biopsy forceps carefully using a 25-gauge needle • Samples are unfolded and placed with the luminal side up on a tissue cassette sponge • Samples are allowed to adhere to the sponge, but are then promptly put in formalin to avoid drying out • Extremely important to follow manufacturer's instructions on handling, setup, cleaning, and maintenance • Endoscopes are handled by the ocular (eyepiece) and overflexion must always be avoided.	

SUTURE TECHNIQUES

Suturing provides the hemostasis and tissue support needed for wound healing. As technicians, suturing opportunities may present themselves as closing a surgical incision or necropsy, suturing lacerations, or suturing in drains, feeding tubes, or urinary catheters. The decision of the most appropriate type of suture pattern and knotting is important to the success of the suture line.

Skill Box 23.6 / Suture Patterns

Method	Suture patterns
Indications	• Traumatic wound closure • Surgical incision closure • To secure a catheter or drain
Contraindications	• Contaminated wound may be left open • Staples may be preferred to expedite closure or fixation
Setup	• Suture material • Needle holders • Scissors • Thumb forceps
Procedure:	
Simple interrupted	1. Place the suture by inserting the needle perpendicular to the plane of the tissue, with its ends emerging on opposite sides of the wound an equal distance from the wound edge on each side. The two sides of the suture should be symmetrically placed in terms of depth and width, while maintaining a greater width at the base. 2. Place a knot while pulling the skin edges together. 3. To remove: lift tags and cut one side of the suture loop and pull the tags to remove the suture. 4. Remove every other suture initially to ensure healing.
Simple continuous	1. Start the suture by placing a simple interrupted suture, which is tied but not cut. 2. Place a series of simple sutures without interruption while maintaining even spacing and tension. 3. Tie off the suture line by placing a knot using the tail end of the suture and place the last loop. 4. To remove: cut the end suture knot, and using thumb forceps, remove the entire suture line.
Continuous locking (blanket suture) or Ford interlocking	1. Follow the steps according to the simple continuous suture pattern, but pass the needle through the loop preceding it as each stitch is placed or pass the needle above the unused suture. 2. Removal: cut the end suture knot, and using thumb forceps, remove the entire suture line.
Chinese finger trap	1. Place an interrupted suture in the skin near the tube, or a purse-string suture around the tube (e.g. closed suction drain, thoracostomy tube or feeding tube) to be secure. 2. Do not cut the suture. Tie a surgeon's throw and take both ends of the suture and wrap around the tube and back, and then tie a surgeon's throw. 3. Continue this pattern 5–10 times and end with a square knot on top of the tube. The distance of each throw is equal to the width of the tube being sutured. 4. Removal: cut the suture connected to the stay sutures and see the instructions for simple interrupted sutures to remove the stay sutures.
Complications	• Tissue reaction • Wound infection • Suture line failure and dehiscence • Abscess (do not purse-string around esophagostomy tubes)
Maintenance	• Keep sutures clean and dry • Observe daily for redness, swelling, and discharge • Monitor patients for licking or chewing at the suture line, and place an Elizabethan collar

Knot Tying

Square Knot

Place the suture needle (A) on top of the suture end (B), then bring the suture needle (A) under the suture end (B) and pull, allowing skin edges to come together. Place the suture end (B) on top of the suture needle end (A), then bring the suture end (B) under the suture needle (A) and pull tight. The second half of the knot is always made in the opposite direction to the first part, to ensure that the knot lies flat. Failure to perform this step opposite to the first results in a granny knot, which is prone to slippage and knot failure.

Surgeon's Knot

Begin with the first step of the square knot, repeat, and then finish with the final step of the square knot.

Instrument Tie (Square or Surgeon's Knot)

For the first throw, the needle end of the suture is wrapped around the tip of the needle holders. The needle holders are then used to grasp the suture end on the opposite side of the suture line. The suture end is pulled through the loop and tightened to allow the edges to come together. The second throw is done in the same manner on the opposite side of the suture line.

Tip: All knots should be placed on the same side of the incision.

POSTOPERATIVE CARE PROTOCOL

The final success of each surgical procedure often lies in the patient care that follows the procedure. This care begins as the anesthetic gas is turned off and continues with the client at home. Communication is the key through the transition from surgery table to recovery, and finally, when the patient is discharged to the client. Written instructions should be sent home with the client, as often, the information is more than can be remembered from one conversation. Clients should be strongly encouraged to phone if any questions or concerns arise. Follow-up phone calls by the staff one to two days after a surgical procedure will also encourage client communication.

Skill Box 23.7 / Standard Postoperative Care Instructions

- Medication instructions (e.g. antibiotics, pain).
- Rehabilitation and activity instructions (e.g. massage, range of motion exercises, confined, leash walks).
- Nutrition:
  - Feed only half of the normal food and water the first evening after surgery.
  - Monitor for vomiting, inappetence, and nausea.
  - Diet change based on surgical findings (e.g. bladder calculi).
- Wound care:
  - Check incisions daily for redness, swelling, discharge, odor, warm to the touch.
  - Prevent licking, chewing, or rubbing at incision line, sutures, and staples.
  - Keep the animal and bandages dry and clean until suture or bandage removal.
  - Avoid bathing or swimming until suture removal or for 10–14 days with SQ sutures.
- Follow-up:
  - Appointments (e.g. rechecks, suture or drain removal, lab work, radiographs)
  - Phone if any of the following occurs:
    - Repeated vomiting
    - Extreme listlessness
    - Bleeding or discharge
    - Loss of appetite for >24 hours
    - Opened incision lines or unexplained swelling (e.g. seroma).

Preventing Self-Trauma

Rarely will an animal disturb an incision line out of boredom; more often, it is due to pain, irritation (e.g. tight sutures, cleaning solutions, clipper burn), infection, or rough tissue handling. When an animal begins to bother their incision line (e.g. licking, chewing, rubbing), investigation into why is warranted and possibly implementing the following ideas:

1. Use an E-collar (neck brace, etc.) at all times.
2. Apply a bandage (e.g. soft padded bandage, hobbles, or bodysuit)).
3. Apply a foul-tasting substance (e.g. bitter apple, atropine, Tabasco, or thumb-sucking preparations) around the area.
4. Cover the area with a sock, T-shirt, or stockinette.
5. Apply a body brace, side bar, or tail-tip protector.

ALTERNATIVE SURGICAL OPTIONS

Endoscopy, a minimally invasive procedure, includes visualization of the gastrointestinal tract, respiratory tract, peritoneal cavity, pleural cavity, urinary bladder, and joints. The examination of these structures can allow direct visualization of the structure to aid in further diagnosis (e.g., biopsies, brushings, washes), together with performing often curative procedures (e.g. foreign body retrieval, polyp or tumor removal, dilation of strictures, cartilage and bone fragment removal). Owing to the delicate nature of this specialized equipment and the potential patient complications with their use, only trained individuals should operate this equipment.

Arthroscopy is a specialized endoscopic procedure, but has become very common among specialty practices, and is therefore widely available. This procedure is performed with the use of a rigid endoscope and is used to evaluate diseases of the shoulder, elbow, hock, hip, and stifle joints of canines (size limitations). Evaluation can lead to a diagnosis and/or treatment.

Table 23.30 / Laser surgery

Procedure	Laser surgery (light amplification by stimulated emission of radiation)
Definition	• Laser surgery consists of light interaction (reflected, absorbed, scattered, transmitted) with tissue, causing certain effects • Surgical laser – class IV
Indications	• Surgery requiring precise incision, excision, photoablation, and hemostasis (e.g. perianal fistulas, soft palate, pinna) • Lithotripsy and angioplasty • Soft tissue procedures • Dermatology surgery (e.g. acral lick granuloma) • Ophthalmic surgery (e.g. glaucoma, tumors, retinal detachment) • Declaw
Equipment	• Several different lasers (e.g. CO_2 laser, Nd: YAG lasers, diode lasers) exist with varying wavelengths, delivery, and application techniques • Endotracheal tubes approved for laser surgery, or less desirably, a red rubber endotracheal tube wrapped in metal tape
Technique	• The laser tip is focused toward the tissue to be incised and discharged • Technique is variable depending on desired outcome (e.g. focused laser location for drilling a hole)
Precautions	• Exposure risk: ocular damage, burns, inhalation of viable tumor cells • Protective eyewear should always be worn and the patient's eyes should be shielded (use appropriate optical density) protection • Proper evacuation of noxious smoke • Use blackened or pitted instruments to absorb stray or reflected light • Combustion/fire • Approved endotracheal tubes to avoid explosion of flowing oxygen • A bucket of water and a CO_2 fire extinguisher should be within reach • Use moistened gauze sponges or drapes around the surgical area • Evacuate or pack the rectum to control methane gas release • Avoid use of excess iodine or any alcohol during skin preparation • Appropriate warning signs and window barriers should be available; signs must indicate the class of laser being used

(Continued)

Table 23.30 / Laser surgery (Continued)

ADJUNCTS TO SURGERY

Laser use in veterinary medicine continues to advance and additional new uses are explored. Despite its claim of reduced tissue trauma, pain, and healing time, safety must be of extreme importance. Many additional steps must be taken before laser equipment is used in the operating room to assure safety of the patient, surgeon, and support staff.

REFERENCES

1. Johnston, S.A. and Tobias, K.M. (2018). *Veterinary Surgery: Small Animal Expert Consult*, 2e. Elsevier.
2. Tobias, K. (2017). *Manual of Small Animal Soft Tissue Surgery*, 2e. Hoboken, NJ: Wiley Blackwell.

Section Seven

Complementary and Alternative Veterinary Medicine

Chapter 24

Regenerative Medicine

Nicole LaForest, MPH, LVT, RVT

Veterinary Technician and Nurse's Daily Reference Guide: Canine and Feline, Fourth Edition. Edited by Mandy Fults and Kenichiro Yagi.

Companion website: www.wiley.com/go/fults/veterinary

Abbreviations

AD-MSC, adipose-derived mesenchymal stem cells
bFGF, basic fibroblast growth factor
BM-MSC, bone marrow-derived mesenchymal stem cells
cGMP, current good manufacturing practices
IBD, inflammatory bowel disease
IGF1, Insulin-like growth factor 1
IV, intravenous
PGDF, platelet-derived growth factor
SVF, stromal vascular fraction
VEGF, vascular endothelial growth factor
TGF-β, transforming growth factor beta

STEM-CELL THERAPEUTICS

Stem cell therapeutics has become one of the largest areas of scientific research around the globe. It was first introduced into equine practice in 1995 with the injection of bone marrow derived cells into tendon injuries. The use of stem cells in canine bone marrow transplants date back as early as the 1960s. There has since been great interest in its use in small animals and humans for many different medical conditions, in particular osteoarthritis. It is estimated that 10–12 million dogs in the United States are affected with osteoarthritis, and it is the most common cause of chronic pain. As of 2019, there are over 9000 published papers on the efficacious use of regenerative medicine.

Stem cells are unspecialized cells capable of self-renewal and differentiation into a specialized cell, and perhaps any type of tissue in the body that is needed. Another term for regenerative medicine is "prolotherapy". Prolotherapy is a regenerative injection treatment used to stimulate the healing mechanism to repair damaged or injured areas in the spine and joints. This term may be inclusive of both stem cell therapy and platelet-rich plasma. Both treatment modalities can be used in conjunction to serve as a transport to the intended treatment area.

Regenerative medicine therapies should only be implemented or recommended following a thorough examination with a veterinarian. Diagnostic imaging and further treatment options should be discussed prior to starting prolotherapy as it is known to be contraindicated in the presence of cancer, infection, coagulopathies, non-steroidal anti-inflammatory drugs (NSAIDs) and steroids.

The patients are monitored closely before, during and after initiating treatment for any adverse effects. By routinely tracking our patients closely with examinations, surveys and all otherwise client communications; we are able to adjust their therapies as needed and determine the patients progress.

CELL DIFFERENTIAL

Culturing mesenchymal stem cells will prevent the cells from passing through the blood–brain barrier due to their engorged diameter.

Table 24.1 / Cell differential

Cell differential	Technique	Indications/Comments
Mesenchymal stem cells		
• Primarily found in abundance in adipose tissue. Can also be found in bone marrow, dental pulp (marrow) and placenta • Multipotent stem cells derived by culturing various biological tissues such as adipose and bone marrow • Contain osteoblasts, myocytes, adipocytes, chondrocytes	• Mesenchymal stem cells are found in excess in cultured adipose tissue and bone marrow • Sample size is system dependent ranging from 5–60 gauge + minimum • Culturing, cloning and storage is available through cGMP-certified laboratories • Processing in-house per manufacturer	• Induces anti-apoptosis (VEGF, TGF-β, bFGF) • Angiogenesis IGF1, interleukin 6, VEGF) • Chemoattractants induce leukocyte migration to injured tissue

(Continued)

Table 24.1 / **Cell differential (Continued)**

Cell differential	Technique	Indications/Comments
Bone marrow-derived mesenchymal stem cells		
• BM-MSCs form superior cartilage compared with AD-MSCs • Contain osteoblasts, myocytes, chondrocytes • Abundant in multipotent cells • Pluripotent cells present with the ability to regenerate as other cell lineage	• Collected from long bones such as the iliac crest, femur or humerus • Should be administered through a micron filter to prevent a systemic infection due to the higher count of neutrophils and debris that may be present in the sample if processed in-house • Culturing, cloning and storage is available through cGMP certified laboratories • Limited plasticity • General anesthesia needed to collect sample • BM-MSCs have a slower population doubling time than AD-MSCs • Processing in-house per manufacturer • 600 000 to 2 million stem cells per 1 g bone marrow can be expected with SVF processing based on the system	• Can be used for bone marrow transplantation following chemotherapy to regenerate the destroyed bone marrow • Used in conjunction with hematopoietic stem cells and platelet-rich plasma to recruit cells where needed • Tissue regeneration • Lineage priming • Heterogeneity • Osteoarthritis • Degenerative joint disease • Spondylosis • Sprains/strains • Ligament ruptures • Gastrointestinal diseases (IBD, Chrohn's, etc.) • Autoimmune disorders such as Lupus and multiple sclerosis • Diabetes • Cataracts • Self-renewing; may harvest samples multiple times if warranted • Will differentiate into a variety of mesodermal lineages
Adipose-derived mesenchymal stem cells		
• Contain osteoblasts, myocytes, adipocytes, chondrocytes • Abundant in multipotent, pluripotent and unipotent cells • Produces 100 times the amount of mesenchymal stem cells than BM-MSCs • Not a self-renewing harvest site	• Gonads will yield the highest number of cells. • Falciform ligament is the most commonly used site for harvesting adipose tissue • The scapula, flank and inguinal canal may also be used as a donor site • Culturing, cloning and storage is available through cGMP certified laboratories	• Liver disease • Corneal lesions • Articular lesions • Cutaneous lesions • Osteoarthritis • Degenerative joint disease • Spondylosis

(Continued)

Table 24.1 / **Cell differential (Continued)**

Cell differential	Technique	Indications/Comments
	• Adipose tissue has a particularly high concentration of regenerative cells due to the high density of microvascularization of this tissue • These regenerative cells can be isolated, concentrated and administered at the point of use in a single procedure within the operating room • Adipose tissue is not as essential as bone marrow • Adipose tissue can be harvested by a minimally invasive procedure under local anesthesia • 5–20 million stem cells per 1 g adipose can be expected with SVF processing	• Sprains/strains • Ligament ruptures • Gastrointestinal diseases (IBD, Chrohn's, etc.) • Other autoimmune disorders such as lupus and multiple sclerosis • Diabetes • Cataracts
Hematopoietic stem cells		
• Constantly repopulating all types of blood cells • Bone marrow or blood derived. • More prominent in platelet-rich plasma, serum therapy and interleukin-1 receptor antagonist protein • Multipotent stem cells derived by culturing bone marrow and whole blood • Contains a higher number of white and red blood cells than mesenchymal stem cells. • Not recommended by experts for IV or epidural use without filtration due to high counts of white and red blood cells. Perispinal injections are acceptable with caution • Abundant in omnipotent, multipotent pluripotent and unipotent cells • Used to treat a wide variety of hematological disorders • Found in cord blood, bone marrow and peripheral blood	• Limited plasticity • Collected from long bones such as the iliac crest, femur or humerus • Mechanically processed to separate from any mesenchymal stem cells present in the sample • Should be administered through a micron filter to prevent a systemic infection due to the higher count of neutrophils and debris that may present in the sample if processed in-house • Culturing, cloning and storage is available through cGMP certified laboratories • Found sparingly in platelet-rich and platelet-poor plasma • General anesthesia needed to collect sample • These regenerative cells can be isolated, concentrated and administered at the point of use in a single procedure within the operating room • 600 000 to 2 million stem cells per 1 g bone marrow can be expected with SVF processing based on system	• Skin laxity • Stimulation of hair growth • Acute myeloblastic leukemia • Chronic myeloid leukemia • Non-Hodgkin's lymphoma • Tay-Sachs disease. • Osteoarthritis • Sport injuries – ligament ruptures • Fractures • Can be complemented with the use of granulocyte-macrophage-colony stimulating factors to allow the hematopoietic stem cells present in the blood for recruitment • Similar to BM-MSCs in function, but are far less elastic

(*Continued*)

Table 24.1 / **Cell differential (Continued)**

Cell differential	Technique	Indications/Comments
Platelet-rich plasma		
• Commonly referred to as autologous conditioned plasma • A whole blood product that contains a high concentration of platelets • Contains various different cytokines and growth factors to treat a variety of deep and soft tissue injuries • Abundant in pluripotent and unipotent cells • Scarce in multipotent cells • Concentrated platelets in plasma • Platelets release growth factors IGF1, PDGF, VEGF	• Derived from whole blood • Can be processed in-house or at a cGMP certified laboratory • Processing varies depending on the system used • All in-house systems require whole blood to be collected under aseptic technique; 10–60 ml needed • Closed-system is highly encouraged to not contaminate the sample during processing and prior to injection • Platelet-poor plasma is considered the supernatant of platelet-rich plasma and the sample and is discarded during processing	• Ligament injuries • Sprains and strains • Burn wounds • Cataracts • Open wound • Degenerative joint disease • Stomatitis • Keratoconjunctivitis sicca • Bone graft healing (osteotomies, fracture repairs • The sample should be 3–4 × patient's baseline platelet levels. Complete blood count may be run on the final sample for quality control

POST-INJECTION CARE

- Therapeutic inflammation is often noted 2–7 days after the injection.
- Can be managed with pain medication (gabapentin or opioids)
- Avoid steroids and NSAIDs for one week before and two weeks after the injection.
- Hypothermic therapy to the area once or twice daily for 5–10 minutes where the injection was given can decrease platelet activation.
- The pet's activity should be restricted to mild/moderate activity for three to four weeks after a subcutaneous injection, so as to not cause a soft-tissue injury.
- Commit to rehabilitation programs for 8–12 weeks.
- Redness from the injection site is not a normal after effect of any injection.

OTHER FORMS OF REGENERATIVE MEDICINE

Other forms of regenerative medicine include:

- Interleukin-1 receptor antagonist protein
- Gene and genome therapy
- Tissue engineering
- Autologous cancer therapy
- Biomedicine.

WHEN IS REGENERATIVE MEDICINE INDICATED?

- Clearly defined diseases.
- Non-surgical candidate – surgery first, if needed.
- Can be used in conjunction with surgery.

- Limited intra-articular osteophytes.
- One or two joints maximum injected at a time to reduce the risk of sepsis if sample is contaminated.
- No other major systemic diseases such as cancer.
- No major spinal disease.
- NSAIDs – non-responsive or lack of tolerance.
- Owner has rational expectations.

RULES AND REGULATIONS

The US Food and Drug Administration (FDA) regulates regenerative therapies under TITLE 21 Federal Regulation 1271:

- Category I – whole blood, bone marrow, organ transplants.
- Category II – cell and tissue products not dependent on metabolic activity of living cells; require minimal manipulation.
- Category III – dependent on metabolic activity of living cells and include products that are cultured or more than minimally manipulated, not intended for homologous use, combined with a drug or device.

Currently, the US Food and Drug Administration (FDA) approves the use of autologous regenerative medicine therapy. Allogeneic and xenogeneic biological products may be used for organ and tissue transplantation, including blood-derived products such as with albumin and whole blood, plasma and platelets for emergent use only. Compassionate care use must be approved with the FDA prior to initiating treatment.

PRECAUTIONS AND CONTRAINDICATIONS

- Pets diagnosed with cancer should not be treated outside a controlled setting. Local injections of regenerative cells may be injected. It is discouraged to give stem cells intravenously if a cancer morphology has been detected.
- Not a compatible therapy with infection.
- Infection with *Pseudomonas*, *Enterococcus* or *Klebsiella*.
- Coagulopathies should be taken into consideration.
- Thrombocytopenia.
- Septicemia.
- NSAIDs use can still be considered (2 days).
- Do not use in conjunction with steroids (7 days) or immunosuppressants (14 days).
- Should not be used to replace emergent intervention procedures.
- Antibiotic and bacteriostatic drugs can inhibit the effects of both stem cell therapy and plasma-rich platelets.

Table 24.2 / Common injection sites

Anatomical landmark	Technique/Approach	Recommended volume (cc)*
Hind limb		
Stifle	• Flex stifle to 90-degree angle • Appreciate joint space medially or laterally to patella ligament • Insert 22 gauge needle	0.5–3
Hip	• Lateral recumbency • Abduct hip • Insert 22 gauge spinal needle cranial to the greater trochanter positioned medially and slightly dorsal into the joint	0.5–3

(Continued)

Table 24.2 / **Common injection sites (Continued)**

Anatomical landmark	Technique/Approach	Recommended volume (cc)*
Hock	• Lateral recumbency • Flex the hock and approach the joint space from the caudomedial aspect • 22 gauge needle recommended	0.5–1
Achilles tendon	• Lateral recumbency • Flex the hock and approach the tendon sheath from the caudal aspect; injecting directly into any lesions, adhesions or surgical repair site. • 22 gauge needle recommended	0.5–2
Thoracic limb		
Carpus	• Lateral recumbency • Dorsal approach of the carpal joint • Flex the carpus to expose joint • 22 gauge needle recommended	0.5–1
Elbow	• Medial aspect • Flexed or straightened • Insert 22 gauge needle distal to the medial epicondyle of the humerus	0.5–1.5
Shoulder	• Lateral recumbency • Abduct humerus • Lateral approach off acromion process, aim it slightly proximal • Use 22 gauge 1½-inch needle	0.5–3
Other		
Epidural	• Place the patient in sternal recumbency with hind limbs flexed • Locate the lumbosacral space caudal to L7. Redirect needle if CSF or blood is seen • Use 22 gauge spinal needle	0.5–1
Muscle/tendon injuries	• Ultrasound is highly recommended to appreciate the intended injection site • Patient may be placed in sternal dorsal, or lateral recumbency	0.5–6*
Pododermatitis, wound and skin grafting	• Dermal needle/insulin needle recommended	Dependent on treatment area*

* Dosing and volume administration will be dependent on the patient size, the treatment plan and area.

RECOMMENDATIONS AND STANDARDS OF CARE

Common Soft Tissue and Orthopedic Use

Brachii tenosynovitis, supraspinatus insertionopathy, infraspinatus contracture, teres minor myopathy, ossification, laxity, tendinopathy and instability, flexor carpi ulnaris tendinopathy/avulsion, digital flexor tendon elongation, medial and lateral collateral ligament rupture, abductor pollicis longus tenosynovitis, psoas, iliopsoas, popliteal muscle avulsion, gastrocnemius muscle avulsion, superficial digital flexor tendon luxation; acute and chronic fractures, luxation, osteoarthritis, osteophytes, hip dysplasia, myopathy, neuropathy, ligament ruptures, patellar and digital extensor tendonitis and Achilles tendon avulsion.

Platelet-Rich Plasma Dosing

- Current recommendations are for three to four doses above the patient's platelet baseline.
- One to two doses are not likely to produce a noticeable effect on the patient's condition.
- Five doses or more may lead to a systemic or local infection, because of the high number of white blood cells present in bone marrow-derived mesenchymal stem cells, hematopoietic stem cells, platelet-poor and platelet-rich plasma.
- + Platelet concentration.
- – Red blood cell concentration.
- + Monocyte concentration.
- – Neutrophil concentration.

Stem Cell Dosing

- Widely dependent on degree of injury or disease: more is not always better.
- Research shows that roughly a minimum of one million cells may be needed to elicit an efficacious response for a majority of injuries and illness.
- In-house systems support data ranging from one to five million stem cells with a stromal vascular fraction sample.
- Culturing cells with a current good manufacturing practice certified facility will yield the highest cell count.

Regenerative Cell Activation

It is widely speculated that the body's cells must be activated by the use of thrombin and calcium chloride to release various growth factors from the present alpha granules. A hemoglobin less than 10 g/dl and a platelet count less than 105/μl is recommended for platelet-rich plasma.

FURTHER READINGS

Alderman, D., Alexander, R. (2011). Advancements in stem cell therapy: applications to veterinary medicine. *Today's Vet Pract* July/August. https://todaysveterinarypractice.com/advances-in-stem-cell-therapy-application-to-veterinary-medicine (accessed 7 August 2021).

Black, L.L., Gaynor, J., Gahring, D. *et al.* (2007). Effect of adipose-derived mesenchymal stem and regenerative cells on lameness in dogs with chronic osteoarthritis of the coxofemoral joints: a randomized, double-blinded, multicenter, controlled trial. *Vet Ther* 8: 272–284.

Black, L.L., Gaynor, J., Adams, C. et al. (2008). Effect of intraarticular injection of autologous adipose-derived mesenchymal stem and regenerative cells on clinical signs of chronic osteoarthritis of the elbow joint in dogs. *Vet Ther* 9: 192–200.

Carr, B.J., Canapp, S. (2016). Regenerative medicine for soft tissue injury and osteoarthritis. *Today's Vet Pract* July/August. https://todaysveterinarypractice.com/regenerative-medicine-for-soft-tissue-injury-osteoarthritis/#:~:text=PLATELET%2DRICH%20PLASMA%20THERAPY&text=PRP%20is%20used%20in%20both,osteoarthritis%20and%20soft%20tissue%20injuries (accessed 7 August 2021).

Franklin, S.P. and Cook, J.L. (2013). Prospective trial of autologous conditioned plasma versus hyaluronan plus corticosteroid for elbow osteoarthritis in dogs. *Can Vet J* 54: 881–884.

Lopez, M.J. (2013). Stem cell therapies: reality in the making. *Clin Brief* June.

Murphy, M., Moncivais, K. and Caplan, I. (2013). Mesenchymal stem cells: environmentally responsive therapeutics for regenerative medicine. *Environ Mol Med* 45: e54.

Nixon, A.J., Dahlgren, L.A., Haupt, J.L. *et al.* (2008). Effect of adipose-derived nucleated cell fractions on tendon repair in horses with collagenase-induced tendinitis. *Am J Vet Res* 69: 928–937.

Silva, R.F., Carmona, J.U. and Rezende, C.M. (2013). Intra-articular injections of autologous platelet concentrates in dogs with surgical reparation of cranial cruciate ligament rupture: a pilot study. *Vet Comp Orthop Traumatol* 26: 285–290.

Tamimi, F.M., Montalvo, S., Tresguerres, I. *et al.* (2007). A comparative study of 2 methods for obtaining platelet-rich plasma. *J Oral Maxillofac Surg* 65: 1084–1093.

Webster, R., Herbert, B., Blaber, S. *et al.* (2011). Mesenchymal stem cells in veterinary medicine. *Vet Nurse* 2: https://doi.org/10.12968/vetn.2011.2.2.58.

Section Eight

Licensure and Certifications in Veterinary Technology and Nursing

Chapter 25

Veterinary Technician/ Nurse Specialist Certifications

Mandy Fults, MS, LVT, CVPP, VTS (Clinical Practice C/F) and Kenichiro Yagi, MS, RVT, VTS (ECC), (SAIM)

Veterinary Technician and Nurse's Daily Reference Guide: Canine and Feline, Fourth Edition. Edited by Mandy Fults and Kenichiro Yagi.

Companion website: www.wiley.com/go/fults/veterinary

Abbreviations

ACVIM, American College of Veterinary Internal Medicine
ACVR, American College of Veterinary Radiology
ACVTP, Academy of Veterinary Clinical Pathology Technicians
ADVT, Academy of Dermatology Veterinary Technicians
AEVNT, Academy of Equine Veterinary Nursing Technicians
AIMVT, Academy of Internal Medicine Veterinary Technicians
ALAVTN, Academy of Laboratory Animal Veterinary Technicians and Nurses
APRVT, Academy of Physical Rehabilitation Veterinary Technicians
AVBT, Academy of Veterinary Behavior Technicians
AVDT, Academy of Veterinary Dental Technicians
AVECCTN, Academy of Veterinary Emergency and Critical Care Technicians and Nurses
AVMA, American Veterinary Medical Association
AVNT, Academy of Veterinary Nutrition Technicians
AVOT, Academy of Veterinary Ophthalmic Technicians
AVST, Academy of Veterinary Surgical Technicians
AVTAA, Academy of Veterinary Technicians in Anesthesia and Analgesia
AVTCP, Academy of Veterinary Technicians in Clinical Practice
AVTDI, Academy of Veterinary Technicians in Diagnostic Imaging
AVZMT, Academy of Veterinary Zoological Medicine Technicians
CE, continuing education
CPR, cardiopulmonary resuscitation
CVPP, certified veterinary pain practitioner
CVTS, Committee on Veterinary Technician Specialties
DVM, Doctor of Veterinary Medicine
ECVDI, European College of Veterinary Diagnostic Imaging
NAVTA, National Association of Veterinary Technicians in America
VTS, veterinary technician specialist

Veterinary technician/nurse specialty academies began in the 1990s and are regulated under the National Association of Veterinary Technicians in America (NAVTA) Committee on Veterinary Technician Specialties (CVTS), formed in 1994. The CVTS has procedures, standards and guidelines set in place for each academy, to become accredited and maintain accreditation. The NAVTA specialty academies are recognized within the United States, Canada, and any other country with a recognized licensing or credentialing process.

All academy applicants must have graduated from an American Veterinary Medical Association (AVMA) approved veterinary technician/nursing school and/or are legally credentialed to practice as a veterinary technician/nurse in some state or province of the United States, Canada, or other country. Additionally, most academies require the applicant to be a NAVTA member.

OVERVIEW OF VETERINARY ACADEMY APPLICATION REQUIREMENTS

The information provided in Table 25.1 is a general overview of each academy's application requirements. Interested candidates must thoroughly review the application/credentialing guidelines provided by each academy for greater detail. Modifications to an academy's application process can occur annually; therefore, always check for updates.

Table 25.1 / Overview of veterinary academy application requirements

Institution	Accreditation established	Description	Requirements
Academy of Veterinary Emergency and Critical Care Technicians and Nurses	Provisional 1996 Full 2006	The AVECCTN was the first specialty academy formed for credentialed veterinary technicians/nurses. AVECCTN specialists have the knowledge and experience needed to work in an emergency or critical care facility. They are knowledgeable in a wide range of medical conditions related to this discipline. The AVECCTN specialist is proficient in performing CPR; they are quick to respond calmly and efficiently with technically driven tasks, such as obtaining venous and arterial access. They manage patients on ventilators, provide nutritional support via enteral and parenteral routes and much more. As a specialist additional career opportunities are available, such as publishing, lecturing, and/or becoming an instructor.	• Minimum work experience is 3 years and 5760 hours as a credentialed veterinary technician/nurse in the field of veterinary emergency and critical care medicine. This experience must be completed within 5 years prior to application. • Minimum of 25 hours of CE within veterinary emergency and critical care medicine, completed within the 5 years prior to application submission. • Completed skills list. • A case record log of 50 cases, maintained in the year prior to the application deadline. • 4 detailed case reports. • 2 letters of recommendations from a VTS (emergency and critical care, anesthesia, internal medicine) member, a diplomate of the American College of Veterinary Emergency and Critical Care, a Veterinary Emergency Critical Care Society veterinarian, or board-certified DVM specialist in anesthesia, internal medicine, or surgery.
Academy of Veterinary Dental Technicians	Provisional 2002 Full 2007	The AVDT was developed to promote excellence in the discipline of veterinary dentistry. The AVDT specialist has superior knowledge of the discipline, together with an advanced skill set. As a specialist, additional career opportunities open up, such as instructing, lecturing and publishing.	• Minimum work experience is 2 years and 6000 hours as a credentialed veterinary technician/nurse. • Minimum of 2000 contact hours in the practice of veterinary dentistry within 2 years prior to applying. • Must have access and ability to take intraoral dental x-rays. • Acceptance into a 2 year AVDT mentorship program. • Information on required case logs, case reports, CE, etc. will be provided after acceptance into the mentorship program. • Credentialing process takes approximately 2 years.

(*Continued*)

Table 25.1 / **Overview of veterinary academy application requirements (Continued)**

Institution	Accreditation established	Description	Requirements
Academy of Internal Medicine Veterinary Technicians	Provisional 2006 Full 2018	The AIMVT defines internal medicine as the branch of veterinary medicine concerned with non-surgical diseases in animals. AIMVT specialists have advanced knowledge and skill set for assisting veterinarians with complex acute and chronic disease states. They advocate for superior patient care, provide client education, and ensure consumer protection. Subspecialties: • Cardiology • Equine internal medicine • Large Animal internal medicine • Neurology • Oncology • Small Animal internal medicine.	• Submit your intent to apply. • Minimum work experience is at least 2 years and 6000 hours as a credentialed veterinary technician in the field of internal medicine. This experience must be completed within 5 years prior to application. • Minimum of 4500 contact hours in your specialty. • Minimum of 40 hours of CE within 5 years of the application date. A minimum of 70% of the continuing education must be within the subspecialty of application. • Completed skills and knowledge list specific to your subspecialty. • A record log of 50+ cases, maintained in the year prior to the application deadline. • 4 detailed case reports. • 2 letters of recommendation from a VTS of AIMVT, or a diplomate (if not available, see detailed information through website).
Academy of Veterinary Technicians in Anesthesia and Analgesia	Provisional 1998 Full 2019	The AVTAA was the second recognized specialty academy formed under NAVTA. Specialists demonstrate superior knowledge in the care and management of anesthesia cases. Anesthetic protocol development and patient monitoring requires extensive knowledge and an understanding of a multitude of emergency based and acute and chronic disease states. The veterinary technician/nurse specialist in anesthesia and analgesia promotes patient safety, consumer protection, professionalism, and excellence in anesthesia care.	• Preapplication submission. • Minimum work experience of 8000 hours as a credentialed veterinary technician, with 6000 contact hours in anesthesia care and management. This experience must be completed within 5 years prior to the application. • Minimum of 40 hours of CE within 5 years of the application date, presented by any veterinary diplomat or VTS on the topic of anesthesia and/or perioperative analgesia. • Letter of agreement signed by board certified doctor or VTS who will work with the applicant applying to AVTAA. • Completed skills and knowledge list. • A case record log of 50–60 cases, maintained in the year prior to the application deadline. • 4 detailed case reports. • 2 letters of recommendations.

(*Continued*)

Table 25.1 / **Overview of veterinary academy application requirements (Continued)**

Institution	Accreditation established	Description	Requirements
Academy of Laboratory Animal Veterinary Technicians and Nurses	Provisional 2016	The ALAVTN veterinary technician/nurse specialist promotes excellence in animal welfare and medical care in the distinct field of laboratory animal medicine. Categories of specialization: • Research clinical nursing • Research surgeon • Research anesthetist.	• Minimum work experience of 4000 hours as a credentialed veterinary technician, with 70% of time spent in the laboratory animal specific category of choice. This experience must be completed within 4 years prior to the application. • Minimum of 60 hours of CE within 5 years of the application date. • Completed skills and knowledge list. • A case record log of 50–60 cases, maintained in the year prior to the application deadline. • 4 case reports. • 2 letters of recommendation: one letter must be from a VTS or veterinary diplomate. The second letter from your supervising DVM or human medical doctor (if not available, see detailed information through website).

Academy of Veterinary Behavior Technicians	Provisional 2009	AVBT specialists demonstrate superior knowledge in scientifically and humanely based techniques of veterinary behavior, health, problem prevention, training, management, and behavior modification. The AVBT specialist have an advanced skillset within the discipline of animal behavior furthering their recognition as critical components of the veterinary behavior team in creating, maintaining, and strengthening the human-animal bond.
		Categories:
		• Clinical track
		• Research track
			• Minimum work experience of 4000 hours as a credentialed veterinary technician in the field of veterinary behavior. This experience must be completed within 5 years prior to application.
			• Minimum of 40 hours of CE within 5 years of your application, related to veterinary behavior.
			• Completed skills assessment form.
			• Case logs:
			  • Clinical track: a case record log of 50+ cases maintained for 1 year within the 3 years immediately preceding the submission of the application.
			  • Research track: cases consisting of behavior research or research using behavioral observations as a major portion of the study.
			• 5 case reports.
			• Publish a peer reviewed article.
			• 2 letters of recommendation from a VTS (behavior), a supporting veterinarian, or a diplomate of the American College of Veterinary Behavior

(Continued)

Table 25.1 / Overview of veterinary academy application requirements (Continued)

Institution	Accreditation established	Description	Requirements

Academy of Veterinary Clinical Pathology Technicians	Provisional 2011	The AVCPT was developed to advance the field and promote excellence in the discipline of veterinary clinical pathology. Specialists within this discipline conduct laboratory analysis to aid the clinician in determining a diagnosis. Career opportunities include employment within a clinical setting, diagnostic laboratory, academic, and research and government laboratories.	• Minimum work experience of 3 years and 4000 hours as a credentialed veterinary technician in clinical pathology. This experience must be completed within 6 years prior to application.
			• Minimum of 40 hours of CE within 6 years of your application date.
			• Statement of purpose.
			• Completed skills list.
			• Case log counts including a variety of laboratory testing. See specific details and provided log forms within the website. Three case reports:
			  • Case 1 – hematology
			  • Case 2 – serum clinical chemistry
			  • Case 3 – urinalysis.
			• 2 letters of recommendation from either a VTS, DVM, credentialed veterinary technician, and/or a member of the American Society of Veterinary Clinical Pathology.

Academy of Veterinary Technicians in Clinical Practice	Provisional 2010 Full 2021	The AVTCP is modeled after the American Board of Veterinary Practitioners. AVTCP specialists provide comprehensive, multidisciplinary care, demonstrating expertise in a range of clinical disciplines within their specie(s) specialty practice category. Practice categories: • Small animal (canine/feline) • Small animal (feline only) • Exotic companion animal • Production medicine.	• Letter of intent. • Minimum work experience of 5 years and 10 000 hours as a credentialed veterinary technician. This experience must be completed within 10 years prior to the application. • Minimum of 7500 contact hours within the selected practice category. • Minimum of 40 hours of CE within 5 years of your application date. 75% of CE must be within your practice category and needs to be diverse. CE must be presented by a veterinary diplomate, VTS, CVPP, or with a Certificate in Veterinary Practice Management (production medicine see specific requirements on website). • Completed skills and knowledge list specific to practice category. • A case record log of 50–70 cases, maintained in the year prior to the application deadline. • 4 detailed case reports. • 2 letters of recommendation: one letter must be from a VTS, veterinary diplomate, or CVPP. The second letter can be from the list above or a DVM.

(Continued)

Table 25.1 / Overview of veterinary academy application requirements (Continued)

Institution	Accreditation established	Description	Requirements
Academy of Dermatology Veterinary Technicians	Provisional 2015	The ADVT was developed to promote excellence in the discipline of veterinary dermatology. Becoming a specialist in dermatology requires advanced knowledge of the integumentary system, and additionally needs an interdisciplinary knowledge base of endocrinology, nutrition, clinical pathology, and pain management, to name a few that all play a role in the management of dermatological disorders. The ADVT specialist is proficient with performing dermatologic procedures and work with the veterinary team and client to advocate superior patient care.	• Minimum work experience of 3 years and 4000 hours as a credentialed veterinary technician/nurse in the field of veterinary dermatology. All experience must be completed within 5 years prior to the application. • A minimum of 40 hours of CE related to veterinary dermatology. The CE must be completed within 5 years prior to submitting the application. At least 10 hours of the CE must be completed within 2 years of application. • A case record log of 40 cases for 1 year within the 3 years immediately preceding the submission of the application. • 3 detailed case reports, each representing one of the following categories: allergic, autoimmune, infectious, parasitic, and endocrine. • 2 letters of recommendations written by VTS (dermatology), a supporting veterinarian, a veterinarian who is a member of the American Academy of Veterinary Dermatology, a veterinarian who is a member of the Canadian Academy of Veterinary Dermatology, a Diplomate of the ACVD, and other diplomates deemed appropriate by the regents.
Academy of Equine Veterinary Nursing Technicians	Provisional 2009	The AEVNT formed to promote excellence in the discipline of equine veterinary nursing. AEVNT specialist display excellence and dedication to providing superior nursing care to equine patients. Their knowledge is advanced and diverse in equine medicine and management, including topics covering nutrition, anatomy and physiology, preventive care, anesthesia, reproductive/genetics, nursing care, and more. Additionally, they advocate for educating the veterinary profession, industry and clients on equine nursing.	• Letter of intent. • Minimum work experience of 3 years and 5000 hours as a credentialed veterinary technician/nurse, with 3750 contact hours working within the specialized area of equine veterinary nursing. • Competed skills list. • Minimum of 50 hours of CE within 3 years prior to application. At least 10 hours must be obtained within 1 year prior to the application deadline. CE must be presented by a VTS, a veterinarian who is an AAEP member or a diplomate in practice. • A case record log of 50–75 cases, maintained in the year prior to the application deadline. • 5 detailed case reports. • 2 letters of recommendation that can be written by VTS, a licensed practicing veterinarian that is a current member of AAEP or a diplomat in equine practice.

(*Continued*)

Table 25.1 / **Overview of veterinary academy application requirements (Continued)**

Institution	Accreditation established	Description	Requirements
Academy of Physical Rehabilitation Veterinary Technicians	Provisional 2017	The APRVT was developed to further advance the practice of veterinary physical rehabilitation and promote public awareness. APRVT specialists have advanced knowledge of the musculoskeletal system, together with biomechanics. Orthopedic and neurological conditions, along with other medical concerns are routinely managed by these specialists. APRVT specialist have the experience and education to perform patient assessments, apply therapeutic exercises and modalities, and provide client consultations on a variety of medical cases.	• 1 year prior to application submission, must send: • Letter of intent • A completed curriculum vitae • 2 letters of reference • Documented current and future points (see website for detail). • Minimum work experience of 5 years and 10 000 hours as a credentialed veterinary technician/nurse with 2 years' experience in a general practice setting (additional detail within website). • Minimum of 3 years and 4500 contact hours in veterinary physical rehabilitation as a credentialed veterinary technician/nurse. • Have not earned a VTS in any recognized NAVTA specialty in the immediate 5 years prior to application submission. • Mentored by a DVM who has been certified in veterinary physical rehabilitation for a minimum of 5 years or is a diplomate of Veterinary Sports Medicine and Rehabilitation • Minimum of 40 hours of CE within 5 years of application date pertaining to veterinary physical rehabilitation or associated topics. • MUST be presented by a VTS member (in any of the specialty academies), a credentialed rehabilitation veterinarian or a veterinary diplomat of any American college. • Obtained required points (i.e. additional CE, published, lectured, Instructor, memberships, etc.) relating to veterinary physical rehabilitation. • A case record log of 40–60 cases in the year prior to the application deadline. • Completed knowledge form. • Completed equipment and modalities form. • 4 detailed case reports.

(*Continued*)

Table 25.1 / **Overview of veterinary academy application requirements (Continued)**

Institution	Accreditation established	Description	Requirements
Academy of Veterinary Nutrition Technicians	Provisional 2011	The AVNT was formed to develop and support the area of veterinary nutrition, develop the knowledge and expertise of veterinary technicians to become certified in the field of nutrition and endorse credentialed technicians as a vital part of the veterinary nutrition profession. The AVNT specialist has the ability, knowledge, skill set and education required to effectively assist veterinarians with nutritional case management for healthy and ill veterinary patients. Career opportunities may include clinical, research, industry, lecturing, instructing and publishing.	• Minimum of 4000 contact hours in veterinary nutrition, either clinical or researched based, as a credentialed veterinary technician. Must be completed within 3 years prior to application. • Minimum of 40 hours of CE related to veterinary nutrition, animal nutrition or nutrition research. At least 10 hours must be completed within the year the application is submitted. It is advisable that the CE comes from speakers who are VTS or diplomates of American College of Veterinary Nutrition, ACVIM, or the European College of Veterinary Emergency and Critical Care. • Completed skills list. Case logs: • Clinical track: a case record log of 40+ cases in the year prior to the application deadline. • Research track: a record log for 1 year within the 3 years immediately prior to the application deadline. Must consist of veterinary/animal research or research using veterinary nutrition technician observations as a major portion of the study. • 5 detailed case reports. • 2 letters of recommendation written from the following 4 categories: a VTS (nutrition) member, a supporting veterinarian, a veterinarian who is a member of the American Academy of Veterinary Nutrition, or a diplomate of the American College of Veterinary Nutrition, ACVIM, and other diplomates deemed appropriate by the Board of Regents.

(Continued)

Table 25.1 / **Overview of veterinary academy application requirements (Continued)**

Institution	Accreditation established	Description	Requirements
Academy of Veterinary Ophthalmic Technicians	Provisional 2016	The AVOT was created to advocate for ocular health, while working alongside a veterinary ophthalmologist. Specialists in this discipline have advanced knowledge and skills required to provide quality ophthalmic care. Additionally, they must have in-depth knowledge of non-ophthalmic disease states that can play a role in ocular health and management. As a specialist, additional career opportunities are possible, such as lecturing, instructing and publishing.	• Submit the AVOT VTS initial application. • Minimum work experience of 3 years and 6000 hours as a credentialed veterinary technician/nurse in the field of veterinary ophthalmology within 5 years prior to application Must work directly with a diplomate of the American College of Veterinary Ophthalmologists or the European College of Veterinary Ophthalmologists. • Must spend at least 75% of time in veterinary ophthalmology. • Minimum of 40 hours of CE related to veterinary ophthalmology. • Completed skills and knowledge list. • A case record log of 50–60 case, maintained in the year prior to the application deadline. • 4 detailed case reports. • 2 letters of recommendation: the first letter must be from a diplomate of the American College of Veterinary Ophthalmology. The second letter from a VTS (ophthalmology) or from a supporting veterinarian or diplomate of another veterinary college deemed appropriate by the Board of Regents (such as ACVIM, ACVS, or other).
Academy of Veterinary Surgical Technicians	Provisional 2010	The AVST was developed to increase the competence of those who perform specialty duties in the field of veterinary surgery. AVST specialists are knowledgeable in anatomy and physiology and have an advanced diverse surgical procedural skill set and knowledge for soft tissue, orthopedic and neurological procedures. The AVST specialist is skilled in bandaging and wound management, instrumentation care and sterilization, surgical equipment and aseptic technique, and much more.	• Minimum work experience of 5 years and 10 000 hours as a credentialed veterinary technician/nurse. • Minimum of 3 years and 6000 contact hours in the field of veterinary surgery, all within 5 years of beginning your application. 75% of time must be performing duties related to veterinary surgery. • A minimum of 40 hours of CE on topics related to veterinary surgery. • Completed skills list. • A case record log of 50–75 cases, maintained in the year prior to the application deadline. • 4 detailed case reports. • 2 letters of recommendation are required. One of the letters of recommendation must come from a VTS (surgery), or a diplomate of the American or European College of Veterinary Surgeons. Note: Until there are sufficient numbers VTS (surgery) technicians, letters of recommendation will be accepted from a VTS of any specialty. The second letter of recommendation must come from the candidate's supervising veterinarian.

(Continued)

Table 25.1 / **Overview of veterinary academy application requirements (Continued)**

Institution	Accreditation established	Description	Requirements
Academy of Veterinary Zoological Medicine Technicians	Provisional 2009	The AVZMT certifies credentialed veterinary technicians/nurses that have experience and superior knowledge in zoological medicine. The academy was founded to promote excellence in the discipline of zoo medicine through scientific and humane techniques.	• Minimum work experience of 5 years and 10 000 hours as a credentialed veterinary technician/nurse in the field of zoological medicine. All experience must be completed within 7 years prior to application and must be within a zoo setting. • Minimum of 40 hours of CE in zoological medicine or appropriate related topics within 5 years prior to application submission. • A case record log of 40 cases maintained within 3 years of application submission. • 5 detailed case reports. • 2 letters of recommendation from the following three categories (in order of desirability): an AVZMT member, a diplomate of the American College of Zoological Medicine, or a supervising zoo veterinarian.
Academy of Veterinary Technicians in Diagnostic Imaging	Provisional 2018	The AVTDI promotes excellence in the discipline of diagnostic imaging and comprises veterinary technicians/nurses knowledgeable in using a variety of diagnostic modalities including digital radiographs, fluoroscopic special procedures, computed tomography, magnetic resonance imaging, ultrasound and nuclear medicine imaging. AVTDI specialists know basic anatomy, are knowledgeable in radiation safety, use of personal protective equipment; and have the ability to assist or perform a variety of image-guided procedures and much more.	• Minimum work experience of 5 years and 10 000 hours as a credentialed veterinary technician/nurse in the field of veterinary medicine with 75% of that work experience (7500 hours) dedicated in the field of diagnostic imaging, clinical or research based. All work experience must be completed within 5 years prior to the application. • Minimum of 40 CE hours related to veterinary diagnostic imaging and advanced imaging modalities within 7 years of application. 10 hours of CE must be obtained within the year of application submission. • Completed skills list. • A case record log of 45–60 cases, maintained in the year prior to the application deadline. • 6 detailed case reports. • 2 letters of recommendation that can be written by AVTDI member, a diplomate of the ACVR, and/or a diplomate of the ECVDI, senior third-year ACVR/ECVD resident, a diplomate of an AVMA-recognized veterinary specialty college, or a member of another NAVTA VTS academy.

Chapter 26

Additional Certifications Obtainable by Veterinary Technicians

Caitlin Lewis, RVT and Kenichiro Yagi, MS, RVT, VTS (ECC), (SAIM)

In addition to being credentialed as a veterinary technician in their states, veterinary technicians have various opportunities to obtain additional certifications and credentials to validate their knowledge and competency in specific areas of practice. These certifications are often offered by private organizations which may be incorporations or non-profit associations and can be classified either as a certification or certificate program.

While this chapter attempts to list as many certifications with accuracy, please refer to each organization's official source of information for the most up-to-date details regarding their certification process as it can change over the course of time.

CERTIFICATION

The certification is obtained through non-profit associations following a strict set of requirements and certification application and evaluation process that establish standards in the area of practice. Typically overseen by an oversight organization recognizing the process.

CERTIFICATE PROGRAM

An educational program that offers coursework in the area of practice that do not have strict requirements to participate. Typically follows the format of online courses followed by an assessment.

Veterinary Technician and Nurse's Daily Reference Guide: Canine and Feline, Fourth Edition. Edited by Mandy Fults and Kenichiro Yagi.

Companion website: www.wiley.com/go/fults/veterinary

Table 26.1 / **Certifications veterinary technicians can pursue**

Organization	Certification	Certification abbreviation	Species	Website	Pathway
Behavior and training					
Animal Behavior Society	Certified Applied Animal Behaviorists	CAAB	Multiple	https://www.animalbehaviorsociety.org/web/applied-behavior-caab-application.php	• Doctoral degree with an emphasis in behavior • 2 years' experience • Presentations and letters of recommendation
Animal Behavior Society	Associate Certified Applied Animal Behaviorist	ACAAB	Multiple	https://www.animalbehaviorsociety.org/web/applied-behavior-caab-application.php	• Master's degree with an emphasis in behavior • 2 years' experience • Presentations and letters of recommendation
International Association of Animal Behavior Consultants	Certified Animal Behavior Consultant	CABC	Multiple	https://iaabc.org	
	Associate Certified Animal Behavior Consultant	ACABC	Multiple		
	Shelter Behavior Affiliate		Multiple		
Fear Free	Fear Free Certified Professional			https://fearfreepets.com	• Online course and assessment
Low Stress Handling University	Low Stress Handling Certified Professional		Multiple	https://lowstresshandling.com/low-stress-handling/certification-levels	
Association of Animal Behavior Professionals	Certified Parrot Behavior Technologist	CPBT	Avian	https://www.associationofanimalbehaviorprofessionals.com/membership	
	Certified Dog Behavior Technologist	CDBT	Canine		
	Certified Cat Behavior Technologist	CCBT	Feline		

(Continued)

Table 26.1 / **Certifications veterinary technicians can pursue (Continued)**

Organization	Certification	Certification abbreviation	Species	Website	Pathway
Karen Pryor Academy of Animal Training and Behavior	Karen Pryor Academy Certified Training Partner	KPA CTP	Canine	https://karenpryoracademy.com/ctp/choose-kpa-ctp	
Cannabis					
Veterinary Cannabis Education and Consulting	Veterinary Cannabis Counselor	VCC	Multiple	https://www.veterinarycannabis.org	• Online courses • written evaluation • case studies
Cardiopulmonary resuscitation					
American College of Veterinary Emergency and Critical Care	RECOVER Certified BLS Rescuer, RECOVER Certified ALS Rescuer		Multiple	https://recoverinitiative.org	• Online course followed by in-person workshop and practical assessment
	RECOVER Certified BLS Instructor, RECOVER Certified ALS Instructor		Multiple		• 3-day intensive workshop
Human–animal bond					
North American Veterinary Community	Human Animal Bond Certified		Multiple	https://www.vetfolio.com/courses/navc-the-human-animal-bond-certification?client=	• Online course
Laboratory animal care					
American Association of Laboratory Animal Science	Assistant Laboratory Animal Technician	ALAT	Lab Animal	https://www.aalas.org	• Application and exam
	Laboratory Animal Technician	LAT	Lab Animal		• Application and exam
	Laboratory Animal Technologist	LATG	Lab Animal		• Application and exam

(*Continued*)

Table 26.1 / **Certifications veterinary technicians can pursue (Continued)**

Organization	Certification	Certification abbreviation	Species	Website	Pathway
	Registered Assistant Laboratory Animal Technician	RALAT	Lab Animal		
	Registered Laboratory Animal Technician	RLAT	Lab Animal		
	Registered Laboratory Animal Technologist	RLATG	Lab Animal		• Online course
	Certified Manager of Animal Resources	CMAR	Lab Animal		
Nutrition					
North American Veterinary Community	Pet Nutrition Coach		Multiple	https://www.vetfolio.com/courses/navc-pet-nutrition-coach-certification	
Pain management					
International Veterinary Academy of Pain Management	Certified Veterinary Pain Practitioner	CVPP	Multiple	https://ivapm.org	• Application • CE • Competencies • Case studies • Examination
Practice management					
Veterinary Hospital Managers Association	Certified Veterinary Practice Manager	CVPM	N/A	https://www.vhma.org	• Experience • coursework • CE • letters of recommendation • examination

(Continued)

Table 26.1 / **Certifications veterinary technicians can pursue (Continued)**

Organization	Certification	Certification abbreviation	Species	Website	Pathway
Physical therapy and rehabilitation					
Animal Rehab Institute	Certified Equine Rehabilitation Assistant	CERA	Equine	https://animalrehabinstitute.com/certified-equine-rehabilitation-asssistant-cera-4375-00-for-registered-veterinary-technicians-ptas-bs-equine-science-graduates	• In-person and online coursework • Case presentations
	Certified Equine Kinesiology Taping Therapist	CEKTT	Equine	https://animalrehabinstitute.com/cektt-certified-equine-kinesiology-taping-therapist	• In-person and online coursework • Case presentations
	Certified Equine Massage Therapist	CEMT	Equine	https://animalrehabinstitute.com/courses/ceqm-certified-equine-massage-therapist	• In-person and online coursework.
Canine Rehabilitation Institute	Certified Canine Rehabilitation Veterinary Nurse	CCRVN	Canine	http://www.caninerehabinstitute.com/CCRVN.html	• In-person 5-day courses located in CO and FL plus online coursework • Take-home exam • Internship
	Certified Veterinary Acupuncture Therapist	CVAT	Canine	http://www.caninerehabinstitute.com/Certification_Programs_Acupuncture.lasso	• In-person and online coursework.
Healing Oasis Wellness Center	Certified Veterinary Massage and Rehabilitation Therapist	CVMRT	Canine and Equine	https://healingoasis.edu/veterinary-massage-rehabilitation-therapy-program	• In-person coursework
University of Tennessee	Certified Canine Rehabilitation Practitioner	CCRP	Canine	https://www.utvetce.com/canine-rehab-ccrp	• In-person and online coursework • Externship • Case reports • Exam

(Continued)

Table 26.1 / **Certifications veterinary technicians can pursue (Continued)**

Organization	Certification	Certification abbreviation	Species	Website	Pathway
	Certified Equine Rehabilitation Practitioner	CERP	Equine	https://www.utvetce.com/equine-rehab-cerp	• In-person and online coursework • Case presentations • Online exam
	Certified Canine Fitness Trainer	CCFT	Canine	https://www.utvetce.com/canine-fitness-ccft	• In-person and online coursework • Case presentations • Online exam
	Certified Canine Manual Therapist	CCMT	Canine	https://www.utvetce.com/canine-manual-therapy	• In-person and online coursework • Case presentations • Online exam
Feline					
American Association of Feline Practitioners'	Cat Friendly Veterinary Professional	CFVP	Feline	https://catvets.com/cfp/cat-friendly-certificate-program	• Application and exam
Surgical Research					
Academy of Surgical Research	Surgical Research Anesthetist	SRA	Multiple	https://surgicalresearch.org	• Application and exam
	Surgical Research Technician	SRT	Multiple	https://surgicalresearch.org	
Wildlife					
International Wildlife Rehabilitation Council	Certified Wildlife Rehabilitator	CWR	Wildlife	https://theiwrc.org/about-us/faq	Exam varies
	Locally licensed wildlife rehabilitator		Wildlife	Varies	Varies, but generally your state's Department of Fish and Game or Conservation and Natural Resources

(Continued)

Table 26.1 / Certifications veterinary technicians can pursue (Continued)

Organization	Certification	Certification abbreviation	Species	Website	Pathway
Hospice and Palliative Care					
International Association for Hospice and Palliative Care	Certified Hospice and Palliative Care Technician	CHPT	multiple	https://iaahpc.org/veterinary-certification	
Two Hearts Pet Loss Center	Certified Pet Loss Professional	CPLP	multiple	https://twoheartspetlosscenter.thinkific.com/collections?page=1	
Association for Pet Loss and Bereavement	Pet Loss Grief Specialist		multiple	https://www.aplb.org/pet-loss-grief-specialist-training	
Business					
North American Veterinary Community	Certified Veterinary Business Leader	CVBL	N/A	https://navc.com/certifications/cvbl	
Society of Human Resources Management	Society of Human Resources Management-Certified Professional	SHRM-CP	N/A	https://www.shrm.org/certification/about/Pages/default.aspx	
Mental/Emotional					
International Association of Trauma Professionals	Certified Compassion Fatigue Professional	CCFP	N/A	https://www.evergreencertifications.com/evg/detail/1007/certified-compassion-fatigue-professional-ccfp	
Institute for Social + Emotional Intelligence (ISEI)	Social + Emotional Intelligence Certified Coach		N/A	http://the-isei.com/seip_certification_program.aspx	

N/A, not applicable.

Chapter 27

Nursing Theory

Cristall Short, BSN, RN, CEN, CCRN, RVT, AAS

The credentialed veterinary technician role has evolved significantly over the past 10–15 years. Veterinary technicians are no longer merely assistants employed to restrain animals and/or perform diagnostic tests for the veterinarian. They have progressed into being degreed professionals, influential and highly valuable in their own right, evidenced by the contributions that they make to the overall quality of delivered care. The role now includes actively implementing scientifically based methodologies to optimize outcomes. The improved outcomes are not only related to direct patient care, but also such functions as improved administrative systems, education programs, and research development. Subsequently, the trend in the veterinary field to use the term "veterinary nurse" to describe the professional who participates alongside the veterinarian in practice is becoming more commonplace.

In support of the expanding role, NAVTA formed the Veterinary Nurse Initiative coalition (VNI) in 2017, which is seeking to unite the profession under a single title, credentialing requirements and scope of practice. Through the standardization and public awareness of the credential, the profession will make strides toward better recognition, mobility, and elevated practice standards, leading to better patient care and consumer protection.[1] Additionally, within the veterinary system's academic realm, educational programs are becoming increasingly sophisticated. As increasing numbers of baccalaureate and master's prepared veterinary personnel no longer fit into the traditional role of merely providing technical skills, academic programs are adapting by formally identifying themselves not as veterinary technology programs but as veterinary nursing programs.

Veterinary nursing can be viewed as the practice relating to the full professional scope of veterinary nursing care, requiring substantial knowledge of the biological, physical, and behavioral sciences, as well as the topic of nursing theory as it relates specifically to animal care. Veterinary nursing now goes beyond the former focus of providing practical or technical skills, now emphasizing the inclusion of scientific study and reasoning. By briefly examining the origin of nursing theory, it can be shown how its inclusion validates the vision for the standardization of contemporary professional veterinary nursing practice and a unified title.

Veterinary Technician and Nurse's Daily Reference Guide: Canine and Feline, Fourth Edition. Edited by Mandy Fults and Kenichiro Yagi.

Companion website: www.wiley.com/go/fults/veterinary

Historically, statistical mathematics became a defining attribute for establishing legitimacy in the nursing role, more specifically it proved the need for advanced education in professional nursing care. Florence Nightingale was highly educated, most notably in the field of mathematics. At the time she and her staff of trained nurses arrived at their assigned hospital on the battlefront of the Crimean war in 1854, the mortality rate for the injured soldiers was 60%. After studying the hospital's environmental conditions, Florence theorized that the principal cause of the appallingly high mortality rate was not related to the primary battle wounds, instead, she correlated her theory with substandard care and the unsanitary environment. Her work to improve sanitary conditions preceded the science surrounding germ theory, which was still in its formative stages. She outlined a formal plan for care based on her theories relating not only to improving sanitation but a variety of aspects for overall care that nursing could address. After some time, the statistical analysis revealed mortality had been reduced from 60% to 2%, thereby proving the effectiveness of the nursing care plan she had implemented.[2,3]

Before the addition of Florence and her trained nurses to the hospital setting, the doctors acting alone had not been able to remedy the appallingly high mortality rate. It was not evidence-based medicine that made the difference; it was evidence-based nursing that led to the significant reduction in mortality. Florence proved that nursing practice requires a specific educational base and that it is distinct and separate from medicine. She demonstrated how professional nursing practice can elevate overall care by addressing and resolving issues which the practice of medicine alone could not. Through her work, the foundation was laid for professional nursing and what would eventually become formally known in the academic arena as nursing theory and nursing science. Her work proved not only the effectiveness of the nursing process in direct patient care, but it proceeded to demonstrate the cost effectiveness of using highly trained nurses in hospitals over untrained, lesser educated staff.

As time went by, hospitals during the late 1800s once again began to return to the practice of hiring uneducated and unlicensed staff in order to save money. The statistical consequences related to patient morbidity and mortality were undeniable. In 1896, the Nurses Associated Alumnae of the United States and Canada was formed to protect the public from the danger of uneducated nursing personnel when very few of the people practicing nursing at the time had a formal nursing education. New requirements were established, mandating professional licensure. Hospital administrators feared the new requirements because they feared higher costs, but the result was quite the opposite. The better outcomes were proved to be supported by reduced costs.[4] In the modern nursing world, countless studies have shown that higher levels of scientific and theoretically based education within nursing not only improves care but also minimizes the cost of care considerably.

The argument that nursing principles are only applicable to human care is without foundation. General nursing concepts are equally applicable to the decisional process for professional veterinary nursing care. Nursing theory and nursing science are distinct areas of academic study; as with any academic field relating to science and theory, these topics are not owned by any one discipline (such as by human care providers), they are part of the intellectual domain. Nursing involves both practice and knowledge systems. An examination of systems science validates that systems are transdisciplinary entities.

Bibliography

3M Health Care. *Fundamentals of Sterilization Process Monitoring*. St. Paul, MN: 3M Health Care;2013.

Abu-Serriah M, Nolan AM, Dolan S. Pain assessment following experimental maxillofacial surgical procedure in sheep. *Lab Anim* 2007;41:345–352.

Academy of Veterinary Clinical Pathology Technicians. AVCPT Formula Guide. https://avcpt.net/candidate_packet/resources (accessed 27 June 2021).

Acierno M. Protein-losing nephropathy. Paper presented at the Pacific Veterinary Conference, July 2017, Long Beach, CA.

Acierno MJ, Brown S, Coleman AE, *et al.* ACVIM consensus statement: guidelines for the identification, evaluation, and management of systemic hypertension in dogs and cats. *J Vet Intern Med* 2018;32:1803–1822.

Ackermann AL, May ER, Frank LA. Use of mycophenolate mofetil to treat immune-mediated skin disease in 14 dogs – a retrospective evaluation. *Vet Dermatol* 2017;28:195–e44.

Adams LG. Diagnosis and treatment of refractory urinary incontinence. British Small Animal Veterinary Congress, 2011. April 2011, Birmingham, UK.

Adams V. Approach to the companion animal cancer patient part 1: an overview. *Vet Nurse* 2016;7:318–325.

Aguirre A, Darling T. (eds.). *Small Animal Internal Medicine for Veterinary Technicians and Nurses*. Ames, IA: Wiley Blackwell; 2012.

Alderman D, Alexander R. Advancements in stem cell therapy: applications to veterinary medicine. *Today's Vet Pract* 2011; July/August. https://todaysveterinarypractice.com/advances-in-stem-cell-therapy-application-to-veterinary-medicine (accessed 7 August 2021).

American Veterinary Dental College. AVDC abbreviations for use in case logs: equine and small animal. https://avdc.org/technician-services (accessed 3 August 2021).

Alleman AR. White Cell Responses in Disease I, Paper presented at Western Veterinary Conference 2003, Las Vegas, NV, 2003.

Allen DG, Pringle JK, Smith DA, *et al. Handbook of Veterinary Drugs*, 2e. Philadelphia, PA: Lippincott, Williams and Wilkins, 1998.

American Animal Hospital Association. Anesthesia Guidelines for Dogs and Cats. http://www.aahanet.org/PublicDocuments/Anesthesia_Guidelines_for_Dogs_and_Cats.pdf

American Animal Hospital Association. Nutritional Guidelines for Dogs and Cats. http://www.aahanet.org/PublicDocuments/NutritionalAssessmentGuidelines.pdf

American Animal Hospital Association. 2011 AAHA Canine Vaccination Guidelines. https://www.aahanet.org/PublicDocuments/CanineVaccineGuidelines.pdf

American Animal Hospital Association /AAFP. Pain Management Guidelines for Dogs & Cats. https://www.aahanet.org/PublicDocuments/CanineVaccineGuidelines.pdf

American Animal Hospital Association Canine Vaccine Task Force. 2006 AAHA canine vaccine guidelines. *J Am Anim Hosp Assoc* 2006;42(2):80–89.

American Association of Feline Practitioners. AAFP senior care guidelines. *J Feline Med Surg* 2021;23:613–638.

American Association of Feline Practitioners; Academy of Feline Medicine. Panel report on feline senior health care. *Compend Contin Educ Pract Vet* 1999;21: 531–539.

American College of Veterinary Anesthesiologists; American Veterinary Dental College. AVDC Nomenclature Committee. http://www.avdc.org/nomenclature.html

American Heartworm Society. *Current Canine Guidelines for the Prevention, Diagnosis, and Management of Heartworm* (Dirofilaria immitis) *Infection in Dogs*. Wilmington, DE: AHS; 2018.

American Heartworm Society. *Current Feline Guidelines for the Prevention, Diagnosis, and Management of Heartworm* (Dirofilaria immitis) *Infection in Cats*. Wilmington, DE: AHS; 2014.

American National Standards Institute. *Processing Of Reusable Surgical Textiles For Use In Health Care Facilities*. ANSI/AAMI ST65:2008 (R2018). Washington, DC: ANSI; 2008.

American Society of Anesthesiologists. *ASA Physical Status Classification System*. Schaumburg, IL: ASA. https://www.asahq.org/standards-and-guidelines/asa-physical-status-classification-system (accessed 31 July 2021).

American Veterinary Dental College. About AVDC. https://avdc.org/about (accessed 18 August 2021).

American Veterinary Dental College. AVDC abbreviations for use in case logs: equine and small animal. 2019. https://avdc.org/technician-services (accessed 3 August 2021).

Veterinary Technician and Nurse's Daily Reference Guide: Canine and Feline, Fourth Edition. Edited by Mandy Fults and Kenichiro Yagi.

Companion website: www.wiley.com/go/fults/veterinary

American Veterinary Dental College. Endodontic Disease and Root Canal Treatment http://avdc.org/rootcanaltreatment.html

American Veterinary Dental College. Standard Root Canal Therapy. http://www.avds-online.org/info/rootcanal.html

American Veterinary Medical Association. Authority of veterinary technicians and other non-veterinarians to perform dental procedures. https://www.avma.org/Advocacy/StateAndLocal/Pages/sr-dental-procedures.aspx (accessed 3 August 2021).

Anderson WD, Anderson BG. *Atlas of Canine Anatomy*. Philadelphia, PA: Lea & Febiger, 1994.

Andersen Products. *Anprolene® Gas Sterilization Key Operator Training Kit*. Haw River, NC: Andersen Products, Inc; 2012.

Andrews DA. Cytologic Features of Neoplastic Disease, Paper presented at Western Veterinary Conference 2002, Las Vegas, NV, 2002.

Angrimani DSR, Brito MM, Rui BR et al. Reproductive and endocrinological effects of benign prostatic hyperplasia and finasteride therapy in dogs. *Sci Rep* 2020;10:14834.

AORN Recommended Practices CommitteeRecommended practices of sterilization in perioperative practice setting. *AORN J.* 2006; 83(3): 700–703, 705–708, 711–716.

Arnold JE, Camus MS, Freeman KP, et al. (2019). ASVCP Guidelines: Principles of Quality Assurance and Standards for Veterinary Clinical Pathology (version 3.0). *Veterinary Clinical Pathology* 48: 542–618.

Association for the Advancement of Medical Instrumentation. *ANSI/AAMI ST58:2013 Chemical Sterilization and High Level Disinfection in Health Care Facilities*. Arlington, VA: AAMI; 2013.

Association for the Advancement of Medical Instrumentation. *Comprehensive Guide to Steam Sterilization and Sterility Assurance in Health Care Facilities*. Arlington, VA: AAMI; 2017.

Association of American Feed Control Officials. What is in pet food. 2021. https://www.aafco.org/Consumers/What-is-in-Pet-Food (accessed 12 August 2021).

Ateca LB, Reineke EL, Drobatz KJ. Evaluation of the relationship between peripheral pulse palpation and Doppler systolic blood pressure in dogs presenting to an emergency service. *J Vet Emerg Crit Care* 2018;28(3):226–231.

Atkins C, Bonagura J, Ettinger S, *et al.* Guidelines for the diagnosis and treatment of canine chronic valvular heart disease. *J Vet Intern Med* 2009;23:1142–1150.

Averill DR. Degenerative myelopathy in the aging German shepherd dog: clinical and pathologic findings. *J Am Vet Med Assoc* 1973;162:1045–1051.

Awano T, Johnson GS, Wade CM, *et al.* Genome-wide association analysis reveals a SOD1 mutation in canine degenerative myelopathy that resembles amyotrophic lateral sclerosis. *Proc Natl Acad Sci U S A* 2009;106:2794–2799.

Babyak JM, Sharp CR. Epidemiology of systemic inflammatory response syndrome and sepsis in cats hospitalized in a veterinary teaching hospital. *J Am Vet Med Assoc* 2016;249:65–71.

Bach E. *Bach Flower Essences for the Family*. London: Wigmore; 1996.

Balakrishnan A, Benasutti E. Pain assessment in dogs and cats. *Today's Vet Pract* 2012;2(3):68–74.

Baldwin K. Step-by-step placing an intraosseous catheter in the canine trochanteric fossa. *Vet Tech* 1999;20:656–659.

Baldwin K. Fluid Therapy for the companion Animal, Paper presented by Atlantic Coast Veterinary Conference 2001, Atlantic City, NJ, 2001.

Barger AM, Grindem CB. Analyzing the results of a complete blood cell count. *Vet Med* 2000;95:535–545.

Barker M. Local anaesthesia; part 1 regional anaesthesia of the head. *Vet Nurs J* 2013;28:396–399.

Bartels K. Surgical laser basics. *NAVTA J* 2005;Fall:29–34.

Bartels KE. Laser Basics, Paper presented at Western Veterinary Conference 2002, Las Vegas, NV, 2002.

Bartelt S. The art of tonometry. *Vet Tech* 2004;25:24–26.

Barter LS. Anesthesia: Debunking the Myths, Paper presented at Canine Medicine Symposium 2012. Davis, CA, 2011.

Bartges J. Management of urinary incontinence. Paper presented at the British Small Animal Veterinary Congress, April 2018, Birmingham, UK.

Bartges J. Oops, I did it again: urinary incontinence. Paper presented at the Southwest Veterinary Symposium, Sept 2018, San Antonio Texas.

Barthelemy A, Magnin M, Pouzot-Nevoret C, *et al.* Hemorrhagic, hemostatic, and thromboelastometric disorders in 35 dogs with a clinical diagnosis of leptospirosis: a prospective study. *J Vet Intern Med* 2017;31: 69–80.

Basilio P. Feline dentistry, a practical guide to oral health. *Vet Forum* 2008;February:50–57.

Bassert JM, McCurnin DM. *McCurnin's Clinical Textbook for Veterinary Technicians*, 2e. St. Louis, MO: Elsevier Saunders, 2017.

Bateman SW, Parent JM. Clinical findings, treatment and outcome of dogs with status epilepticus or cluster seizures: 156 cases (1990–1995). *J Am Vet Med Assoc* 1999;215:1463–1468.

Battaglia AM, Steele AM, Battaglia AM. *Small Animal Emergency and Critical Care for Veterinary Technicians*. St. Louis, MO: Elsevier; 2016.

Battaglia-Lawrence A. Shock: recognition, treatment and monitoring. *Vet Tech* 1997;18:167–178.

Battaglia-Lawrence A. Step-by-step placing a peripheral intravenous catheter. *Vet Tech* 1998;19:86–88.

Beckman B. Anatomical landmarks for nerve blocks for oral surgery. *Clinician's Brief* 2014;January:21–23.

Beckman B. Dental nerve blocks in dogs and cats enhance anesthesia safety. International Veterinary Dentistry Institute. https://veterinarydentistry.net/dental-nerve-blocks-dogs-cats (accessed 3 August 2021).

Beckman B. Gingival hyperplasia. *NAVC Clinician's Brief* 2010;January:11–14.

Beckman B, Legendre L. Regional nerve blocks for oral surgery in companion animals. *Compend Contin Educ Pract Vet* 2002;24:439–443.

Bednarski R, Grimm K, Harvey R, et al. AAHA Anesthesia Guidelines for Dogs and Cats. *J Am Anim Hosp Assoc* 2011;47(6):377–385.

Behrend E, Holford A, Lathan P, *et al.* 2018 AAHA diabetes management guidelines for dogs and cats. *J Am Anim Hosp Assoc* 2018;54:1–21.

Bellows J. *Feline Dentistry*. New York, NY: Wiley; 2011.

Bellows J. Tooth resorption in cats. *Veterinary Partner* 17 June. https://veterinarypartner.vin.com/default.aspx?pid=19239&id=4951295 (accessed 12 August 2021).

Bennett D, Kirkham D. The laboratory identification of serum antinuclear antibody in the dog. *J Comp Pathol* 1987;97:523–539.

Berendt M, Farquhar RG, Mandigers PJ, *et al.* International veterinary epilepsy task force consensus report on epilepsy definition, classification and terminology in companion animals. *BMC Vet Res* 2015;11:182.

Berentsen S, Sundic T. Red blood cell destruction in autoimmune hemolytic anemia: role of complement and potential new targets for therapy. *Biomed Res Int* 2015;2015:363278.

Berg M. A complete prophylaxis for the periodontal patient. *NAVTA J* 2005;Winter:53–58.

Berg M. Educating clients about preventative dentistry. *Vet Tech* 2005;February:102–111.

Bergerson WO. Golden opportunities: technical, economic, and professional aspects of urinalysis. *Vet Tech* 1998;19:574–583.

Bergman PJ. Side Effects of Chemotherapy: What You Should Know, Paper presented at ACVIM 2003, Charlotte, NC, 2003.

Bergman PJ. Chemotherapy Preparation, Administration and Disposal, Paper presented at ABVP 2004, New Orleans, LA 2004.

Bhat RA, Dhaliwal PS, Saini N, *et al.* Electrocardiographic evaluation in anemic dogs with blood parasitosis. *J Anim Res* 2017;7:205–207.

Bilbrough G, Evert B, Hathaway K, *et al.* IDEXX Catalyst SDMA Test for in-house measurement of SDMA concentration in serum from dogs and cats. 2018. https://www.idexx.com/files/catalyst-sdma-white-paper.pdf (accessed 22 July 2021).

Biller D. Understanding Contrast Studies, Paper presented at Atlantic Coast Veterinary Conference 2002, Atlantic City, NJ, 2002.

Biomedical Polymers. Instructions for BMP Leukochek. https://www.corelabsupplies.com/assets/pdf/BMP-LeukoChek-Procedural-Instructions.pdf (accessed 27 June 2021).

Birchard SJ, Sherding RG. *Saunders Manual of Small Animal Practice* 3e. Philadelphia, PA: Saunders; 2005.

Bistner SJ, Ford R, Raffe M. *Kirk & Bistner's Handbook of Veterinary Procedures and Emergency Treatment*, 9e. Philadelphia, PA: Elsevier Saunders; 2012.

Bizikova P, Burrows A. Feline pemphigus foliaceus: original case series and comprehensive literature review. *BMC Vet Res* 2019;15:22.

Black LL, Gaynor J, Gahring D. *et al.* (2007). Effect of adipose-derived mesenchymal stem and regenerative cells on lameness in dogs with chronic osteoarthritis of the coxofemoral joints: a randomized, double-blinded, multicenter, controlled trial. *Vet Ther* 2007; 8: 272–284.

Black LL, Gaynor J, Adams C. et al. Effect of intraarticular injection of autologous adipose-derived mesenchymal stem and regenerative cells on clinical signs of chronic osteoarthritis of the elbow joint in dogs. *Vet Ther* 2008; 9: 192–200.

Black V, Adamantos S, Barfield D, *et al.* Feline non-regenerative immune-mediated anaemia: features and outcome in 15 cases. *J Feline Med Surg* 2016;18: 597–602.

Blagburn BL. Ectoparasites in 2003, Paper presented at Western Veterinary Conference 2003, Las Vegas, NV, 2003.

Blunt MC, Young PJ, Patil A, Haddock A. Gel lubrication of the tracheal tube cuff reduces pulmonary aspiration. *Anesthesiology* 2001;95(2):377–381.

Bolette DP. Worming their way in: identifying cestodes, trematodes, and acanthocephala. *Vet Tech* 1998;19:510–517.

Bongura JD, Twedt DC. *Kirk's Current Therapy XV: Small Animal Practice*. St. Louis, MO: Saunders Elsevier; 2014.

Bongura JD, Twedt DC. *Kirk's Current Therapy XIV: Small Animal Practice*. St. Louis, MO: Saunders Elsevier; 2009.

Boon JA. *Manual of Veterinary Echocardiography*, 2e. Hoboken, NJ: Wiley-Blackwell; 2010.

Borjab JM, Ellison, GW, Slocum B. *Current Techniques in Small Animal Surgery*, 5e. Philadelphia, PA: Teton New Media; 2021.

Boswood A, Häggstrom J, Gordon SG, *et al.* Effect of pimobendan in dogs with preclinical myxomatous mitral valve disease and cardiomegaly: the EPIC study-a randomized clinical trial. *J Vet Intern Med* 2016;30:1765–1779.

Botsch V, Kuchenhoff H, Hartmann K, *et al.* Retrospective study of 871 dogs with thrombocytopenia. *Vet Rec* 2009;164:647–651.

Bougnoux, P. Omega-3 polyunsaturated fatty acids and cancer. *Curr Opin Clin Nutr Metab Care* 1999;2:121–126.

Bouhassira D, Lantéri-Minet M, Attal N. *et al.* Prevalence of chronic pain with neuropathic characteristics in the general population. *Pain* 2008; 136: 380–387.

Bowles D. Prostatic disease in the dog (proceedings). *dvm360*, November 2010. https://www.dvm360.com/view/prostatic-disease-dog-proceedings (accessed 16 July 2021).

Brady CA, Otto CM, Van Winkle TJ, *et al.* Severe sepsis in cats: 29 cats (1986–1998). *J Am Vet Med Assoc* 2000;217:531–535.

Brainard BM, Buriko Y, Good J, *et al.* Consensus on the rational use of antithrombotics in veterinary critical care (curative): domain 5 – discontinuation of anticoagulant therapy in small animals. *J Vet Emerg Crit Care (San Antonio)* 2019;29:88–97.

Braswell C, Crowe DT. Hyperbaric oxygen therapy. *Compend Contin Educ Vet* 2012;34:E1–E6.

Brearley MJ. Radiotherapy: When Should I Refer? Presented at the British Small Animal Veterinary Congress, 2006.

Breton A. Gastric dilatation and volvulus: diagnosis to recovery. *NAVTA J* 2009;Summer:36–42.

Brewer WG. Preventing and Treating Chemotherapy Toxicity, Paper presented at Western Veterinary Conference 2003, Las Vegas, NV, 2003.

Brisson BA. Intervertebral disc disease in dogs. *Vet Clin Small Anim* 2010;40: 829–858.

Brock N. *Veterinary Anesthesia Update: Guidelines and protocols for small animal anesthesia*, 2e. Gibson, BC: Veterinary Anesthesia Northwest; 2014.

Brondani JT, Mama KR, Luna SP. *et al.* Validation of the English version of the UNESP-Botucatu multidimensional composite pain scale for assessing postoperative pain in cats. *BMC Vet Res* 2013;9:143.

Brooks W. Dental home care for dogs and cats. *Veterinary Partner* 2019;15 February. https://veterinarypartner.vin.com/default.aspx?pid=19239&id=4951515 (accessed 13 August 2021).

Brooks W. Orphan puppy and kitten care. *Veterinary Partner* 2020;10 March. https://veterinarypartner.vin.com/default.aspx?pid=19239&id=4951456 (accessed 13 August 2021).

Brown DC. The Canine Brief Pain Inventory. https://www.vet.upenn.edu/research/clinical-trials-vcic/our-services/pennchart/cbpi-tool (accessed 29 July 2021).

Brown M, Brown L. *Lavin's Radiography for Veterinary Technicians*, 7e. St Louis, MO: Elsevier; 2021.

Browning DC. Alternative Therapies in Veterinary Wound Management (VT64), Paper Presented at Western Veterinary Conference 2012.

Bruyette D. Senior Wellness Programs, Paper presented at Atlantic Coast Veterinary Conference 2002, Atlantic City, NJ, 2002.

Bryant S. (ed.) *Anesthesia for Veterinary Technicians*. Ames, IA: Wiley-Blackwell, 2013.

Buback J. Surgical management of gastrointestinal foreign bodies. *DVM Magazine* 2011;April:8S–12S.

Budach SC, Mueller RS. Reproducibility of a semi quantitative method to assess cutaneous cytology. *Veterinary Dermatology* 2012; 23: 426–e80.

Buffington CAT. Pandora syndrome in cats: diagnosis and treatment. *Today's Vet Pract* 2018;30–39. https://todaysveterinarypractice.com/pandora-syndrome-in-cats (accessed 22 July 2021).

Burbidge HM, Pfeiffer DU, Blair HT. Canine wobbler syndrome: a study of the Doberman pinscher in New Zealand. *N Z Vet J* 1994;42:221–228.

Burkholder WJ. Age-related changes to nutritional requirements and digestive function in adult dogs and cats. *J Am Vet Med Assoc* 1999;215:625–629.

Burns KM. Avoiding the Consequences of Malnutrition: Applications of Parenteral & Enteral Nutrition. Paper presented at ACVIM 2010. Anaheim, CA, 2010.

Burns KM. FLUTD – using nutrition to go with the flow. *NAVTA J* 2014;Convention Issue:7–12.

Burns KM. Managing overweight or obese pets. *Vet Tech* 2006;June:385–389.

Burns KM. Why is Rocky so stocky? Obesity is a disease! *NAVTA J* 2013;Convention Issue:16–19.

Burns KM, Forrester SD. Feline lower urinary tract disease. *NAVTA J* 2007;July/August.

Burris P. It's the little things. . . Cryptosporidium. *Vet Tech* 2000;21:192–201.

Byard V. Case study: dentistry. *NAVTA J* 2005;Winter:32–34.

Canapp SO. Incorporating Nutraceuticals into Veterinary Sports Medicine and Rehabilitation. Paper presented at Western Veterinary Conference 2010, Las Vega, NV, 2010.

Cannon M. Feline chronic gingivostomatitis. *Comp Anim* 2015;20:616–623.

Capnography for Paramedics. 2010 AHA Capnography Guidelines. http://emscapnography.blogspot.com (accessed 12 August 2021).

Cappuccino JG, Welsh, CT. *Microbiology: A laboratory manual*, 12e. New York, NY: Pearson; 2019.

Carmichael DT. Dental corner: using intraoral regional anesthetic nerve blocks. *dvm360.com* 2004; 1 September. https://www.dvm360.com/view/dental-corner-using-intraoral-regional-anesthetic-nerve-blocks (accessed 12 August 2021).

Carmichael DT. Dental corner: how to perform a nonsurgical extraction. *dvm360.com* 2005; 1 May. https://www.dvm360.com/view/dental-corner-how-perform-nonsurgical-extraction (accessed 12 August 2021).

Carr AP, Michels G. Identifying noninfectious erosive arthritis in dogs and cats. *Vet Med* 1997;92:804–810.

Carr BJ, Canapp S. Regenerative medicine for soft tissue injury and osteoarthritis. *Today's Vet Pract* 2016; July/August. https://todaysveterinarypractice.com/regenerative-medicine-for-soft-tissue-injury-osteoarthritis/#:~:text=PLATELET%2DRICH%20PLASMA%20THERAPY&text=PRP%20is%20used%20in%20both,osteoarthritis%20and%20soft%20tissue%20injuries (accessed 7 August 2021).

Carroll GL. Pain Management in the Orthopedic Patient, Paper presented at Western Veterinary Conference 2004, Las Vegas, NV, 2004.

Cartee RE, Selcer BA, Hudson JA, et al. *Practical Veterinary Ultrasound*. Philadelphia, PA: Williams & Wilkins, 1995.

Carter GR, Chengappa, MM, Roberts, AW. *Essentials of Veterinary Microbiology*, 5e. Baltimore, MD: Williams and Wilkins, 1995.

Cassuto J, Sinclair R, and Bonderovic M. Antiinflammatory properties of local anesthetics and their present and potential clinical implications. *Acta Anaesthesiol Scand* 2006;50:265–282.

Cauzinille L. Fibrocartilaginous embolism in dogs. *Vet Clin Small Anim* 2000;30: 155–167.

Centers for Disease Control and Prevention. Appendix A: Regulatory Framework for Disinfectants and Sterilants. *MMWR Morb Mortal Wkly Rep* 2003; 52(RR17): 62–64.

Centers for Disease Control and Prevention. Chemical disinfectants: guideline for disinfection and sterilization in healthcare facilities. Alcohol. 2008. https://www.cdc.gov/infectioncontrol/guidelines/disinfection/disinfection-methods/chemical.html (accessed 3 August 2021).

Chabanne L, Fournel C, Rigal D, *et al.* Canine systemic lupus erythematosus. Part II. Diagnosis and treatment. *Comp Contin Educ* 1999;21:402–408.

Chaloub S, Langston CE, Farrelly J. The use of darbepoetin to stimulate erythropoiesis in anemia of chronic kidney disease in cats: 25 cases. *J Vet Intern Med* 2012;26: 363–369.

Chan DL. Nutrition Basics for Intensive Care Patients. Paper presented at World Small Animal Veterinary Association World Congress Proceedings 201. Geneva, Switzerland, 2010.

Chan DL. Intralipids in Parenteral Nutrition: Friend or Foe? Paper presented at International Veterinary Emergency and Critical Care Symposium 2011. Nashville, TN, 2011.

Chan DL. Critical Care Nutrition: Improving Patient Outcomes. Paper presented at World Small Animal Veterinary Association World Congress Proceedings 2012. San Antonio, TX, 2012.

Chan DL. Early Enteral Nutrition is Warranted in the Septic Abdomen. Paper presented at International Veterinary Emergency and critical Care Symposium 2012. San Antonio, TX, 2012.

Chan DL. Re-evaluation of Feeding Strategies in Critically Ill Patients. Paper presented at ACVIM 2012. New Orleans, LA, 2012.

Chan DL. Revisiting Nutritional Controversies. Paper presented at World Small Animal Veterinary Association World Congress Proceedings 2012. San Antonio, TX, 2012.

Chandler JC. Surgery STAT: Tie-over bandage: a solution for wounds in difficult locations. dvm360.com 2009; 1 June. https://www.dvm360.com/view/surgery-stat-tie-over-bandage-solution-wounds-difficult-locations

Chandler ML. Practical matters: desmopressin is safer than water deprivation to identify the cause of polyuria and polydipsia in dogs. *dvm360*. http://veterinarymedicine.dvm360.com/practical-matters-desmopressin-safer-water-deprivation-identify-cause-polyuria-and-polydipsia-dogs (accessed 27 June 2021).

Chandler ML, Guilford WG, Payne-James, J. Use of peripheral parenteral nutritional support in dogs and cats. *J AM VET MED ASSOC*, 2000;216:669–673.

Cherry B. The benefits of regional dental blocks. Veterinary Technician, May 2009:28–35.

Chew DJ, DiBartola SP, Schenk PA. Chronic renal failure. In: *Canine and Feline Nephrology and Urology*, 2e. St. Louis, MO: Elsevier; 2011.

Chew DJ, DiBartola SP. *Interpretation of Canine and Feline Urinalysis*. Wilmington, DE: Gloyd Group; 1998.

Chirek A, Silaghi C, Pfister K, *et al.* Granulocytic anaplasmosis in 63 dogs: clinical signs, laboratory results, therapy and course of disease. *J Small Anim Pract* 2018;59:112–120.

Chrisman CL. The neurological examination. *NAVC Clinician's Brief* 2006; January:11–16.

Christensen B. Canine prostate disease. *Vet Clin N Am Small Anim Pract* 2018;48: 701–719.

Christopher MM. Evaluation of Bone Marrow, Paper presented at WSAVA World Congress Proceedings 2004, Rhodes, Greece, 2004.

Church DB. When Hormones Fail: Managing Endocrine Emergencies. Paper presented at London Vet Show 2011, London, England, 2011.

Ciribassi J. Understanding behavior: feline hyperesthesia syndrome. *Compend Contin Educ Vet* 2009;31:E10.

Clare M, Hopper K. Mechanical ventilation: ventilator indications, goals, and prognosis. *Compend Contin Educ Pract Vet* 2005;27(3):195.

Clare M, Hopper K. Mechanical ventilation: ventilator settings, patient management, and nursing care. *Compend Contin Educ Pract Vet* 2005;27(4):269.

Coates JR, Jeffery ND. Perspectives on meningoencephalomyelitis of unknown origin. *Vet Clin Small Anim* 2014;44:1157–1185.

Coates JR, Wininger FA. Canine degenerative myelopathy. *Vet Clin Small Anim* 2010;40:929–950.

Coates JR, March PA, Oglesbee M, *et al.* Clinical characterization of a familial degenerative myelopathy in Pembroke Welsh Corgi dogs. *J Vet Intern Med* 2007;21: 1323–1331.

Cohn L, Côté E. *Côté's Clinical Veterinary Advisor, Dogs and Cats*, 4e. St. Louis, MO: Mosby; 2019.

Colmery I, Ben H. Diagnosing dental disease film vs. digital radiography. *Vet Tech* 2005;February:114–119.

Companion Animal Parasite Council. General guidelines for dogs and cats. 2020. https://capcvet.org/guidelines/general-guidelines (accessed 27 June 2021).

Comparative Pain Research Laboratory. Feline Musculoskeletal Pain Index. North Carolina State University; 2015. https://painfreecats.org/the-fmpi (accesssed 29 July 2021).

Congdon, J. At-home medications to smooth the "in-hospital" experience. In: Proceedings of the NAVC Conference, January 14–18, 2012, Orlando, Florida. Book 1: Small Animal and Exotics: Disciplines A-R. Gainesville, FL: North American Veterinary Conference; 2012.

Cooley K. The Ins and Outs of the Anesthesia Machine, Paper presented at Atlantic Coast Veterinary Conference 2001. Atlantic City, NJ, 2011.

Corbee RJ, Van Kerkhoven WJS. Nutritional support of dogs and cats after surgery or illness. *Open J Vet Med* 2014;4:44–57.
Cordell D, Duke A, Mack JD, et al. Delivering compassionate care: a roundtable discussion part II. Good medicine is only the beginning. *Vet Tech* 2000;21: 284–288.
Cornell C. Nursing Management of the Heart Failure Patient, Paper presented ACVIM 2003, Charlotte, NC, 2003.
Cornell University Animal Health Diagnostic Laboratory. Tests and submissions fact sheets. 2019. https://www.vet.cornell.edu/animal-health-diagnostic-center/programs/nyschap/modules-and-documents (accessed 27 June 2021).
Cornell University College of Veterinary Medicine. (2020). Hematology. *eClinPath* http://www.eclinpath.com/hematology (accessed 27 June 2021).
Cornick-Seahorn J, Marks, SL. Emergency! Treating patients in shock. *Vet Tech* 1998;19:355–369.
Corti L. Nonpharmaceutical approaches to pain management. *Top Companion Anim Med* 2014;29:24–28.
Côté E. (ed.). *Clinical Veterinary Advisor*. St. Louis, MO: Elsevier; 2015.
Cotter SM. Blood transfusions in animals. In: *Merck Veterinary Manual*. 2019. http://www.merckvetmanual.com/circulatory-system/blood-groups-and-blood-transfusions/blood-transfusions (accessed 26 July 2021).
Covey HL, Connolly DJ. Pericardial effusion associated with systemic inflammatory disease in seven dogs (January 2006–January 2012). *J Vet Cardiol* 2018;20: 123–128.
Crawford P, Connor, K. A breath of a chance: pleural effusions in small animals. Part I. *Vet Tech* 2000;21:455–461.
Creedon JMB, Davis H. *Advanced Monitoring and Procedures for Small Animal Emergency and Critical Care*. Chichester: Wiley-Blackwell; 2012.
Crisi PE, Aste G, Traversa D, *et al.* Single and mixed feline lungworm infections: clinical, radiographic and therapeutic features of 26 cases (2013–2015). *J Feline Med Surg* 2017;19:1017–1029.
Crook T, McGowan C, Pead M. Effect of passive stretching on the range of motion of osteoarthritic joints in 10 Labrador retrievers. *Vet Rec* 2007;160:545–547.
Crowe DT. Airway Access Technique: The Surgical Parachutes, Paper presented at Western Veterinary Conference 2002. Las Vegas, NV, 2002.
Crowe DT. On the Cutting Edge of Emergency and Critical Care, Paper presented at Western Veterinary Conference 2002. Las Vegas, NV, 2002.
Crowe DT. Procedures Involving Emergency Care of Fractures/Wounds, Paper presented at Western Veterinary Conference 2002. Las Vegas, NV, 2002.
Crowe DT Jr., Dennis T, Devey J. Oxygen, oxygen, oxygen: the wonder drug. *NAVTA J* 2004;Fall:45–47.
Crowe DT Jr., Devey J. Peel-away long venous catheter technique minimizes placement steps. *DVM Newsmagazine* 2000;15–35.
Crump K. Integrated Medicine: a Discussion of Flower Essence Therapy, Paper presented at the 2002 SAVMA Symposium, Fort Collins, CO, 2002.
Cuddon PA. Acquired canine peripheral neuropathies. *Vet Clin North Am Small Anim Pract* 2002;32:207–249.
da Costa RC. Cervical spondylomyelopathy (wobbler syndrome) in dogs. *Vet Clin Small Anim* 2010;40:881–913.
da Costa RC, Parent JM, Holmberg DL, *et al.* Outcome of medical and surgical treatment in dogs with cervical spondylomyelopathy: 104 cases. *J Am Vet Med Assoc* 2008;233:1284–1290.
Dalla Costa E, Minero M, Lebelt D. *et al.* Development of the horse grimace scale (HGS) as a pain assessment tool in horses undergoing routine castration. *PLoS One* 2014;9:e92281.
Dastan F, Jamaati H, Emami H, *et al.* Reducing inappropriate utilization of albumin: the value of pharmacist-led intervention model. *Iran J Pharm Res* 2018;17: 1125–1129.
Davis H. Triage in the Emergency Room, Paper presented at Atlantic Coast Veterinary Conference 20061 Atlantic City, NJ, 2001.
Davis H. Cardiopulmonary Resuscitation: an Overview, Paper presented at Western Veterinary Conference 2002. Las Vegas, NV, 2002.
Davis H. Critical Care Essentials, Paper presented at Atlantic Coast Veterinary Conference 2008. Atlantic City, NJ, 2008.
Davis H, Jensen T, Johnson A, *et al.* 2013 AAHA/AAFP Fluid therapy guidelines for dogs and cats. *J Am Anim Hosp Assoc* 2013;49:149–159.
Day MJ. Immunodiagnostic Tests for Autoimmune Disease, Paper presented at Western Veterinary Conference 2003, Las Vegas, NV, 2003.
De Lahunta A. Neurological examination. In: *Braund's Clinical Neurology in Small Animals: Localization, diagnosis and treatment* (ed. CH Vite CH). International Veterinary Information Service; 2001. https://www.ivis.org/library/braunds-clinical-neurology-small-animals-localization-diagnosis-and-treatment/neurological (accessed 12 August 2021).
de Miguel Garcia CCK. Equipment cleaning and sterilization. In: *Veterinary Anesthetic and Monitoring Equipment* (ed. K.G. Cooley and R.A. Johnson), 377–389. Hoboken, NJ: Wiley; 2018.
De Risio L, Adams V, Dennis R, *et al.* Association of clinical and magnetic resonance imaging findings with outcome in dogs suspected to have ischemic myelopathy: 50 cases (2000–2006). *J Am Vet Med Assoc* 2008;233:129–135.
De Risio L, Adams V, Dennis R, *et al.* Magnetic resonance imaging findings and clinical associations in 52 dogs with suspected ischemic myelopathy. *J Vet Intern Med* 2007;21:1290–1298.
Decker SD, Fenn J. Acute herniation of nondegenerate nucleus pulposus. Acute non-compressive nucleus pulposus extrusion and compressive hydrated nucleus pulposus extrusion. *Vet Clin Small Anim* 2018;48:95–109.

DeClue AE, Delgado C, Chang C, *et al.* Clinical and immunologic assessment of sepsis and the systemic inflammatory response syndrome in cats. *J Am Vet Med Assoc* 2011;238:890–897.

DeForge DH. Root canal therapy. *Vet Pract News* 2009;17 April. https://www.veterinarypracticenews.com/root-canal-therapy (accessed 12 August 2021).

Degan M. Pseudohyperkalemia in akitas. *J Am Vet Med Assoc* 1987;190:541–543.

DeStefano CJ. Applied Kinesiology in Anima Practice, Paper presented at the 2002 SAVMA Symposium, Fort Collins, CO, 2002.

Devey J. Coagulation Monitoring: Survival for the Critical Patient, Paper presented at Western Veterinary Conference 2002. Las Vegas, NV, 2002.

Devey J. Nutrition for the Debilitated Gut. Paper presented at Western Veterinary Conference 2012, Las Vegas, NV, 2012.

Dewey CW, Bailey CS, Shelton GD, *et al.* Clinical forms of acquired myasthenia gravis in dogs: 25 cases (1988–1995). *J Vet Intern Med* 1997;11:50–57.

Di Giminiani P, Brierley VLMH, Scollo A. *et al.* The assessment of facial expressions in piglets undergoing tail docking and castration: toward the development of the piglet grimace scale. *Front Vet Sci*, 2016;3:100.

Doan T, Melvold R, Viselli S, et al. *Immunology*, 2e. Baltimore, MD: Lippincott Williams & Wilkins; 2013.

Donohoe C. Fluid therapy for the VN: Evaluation and Monitoring. Paper presented at World Small Animal Veterinary Association World Congress Proceedings 2012. San Antonio, TX, 2012.

Dos Anjos LMJ, Salvador PA, de Souza da Fonseca A, *et al.* Modulation of immune response to induced-arthritis by low-level laser therapy. *Biophototonics* 2019;12(2): e201800120.

Douglas SW, Williamson HD. *Principles of Veterinary Radiography*, 4e. London: Bailliere Tindall; 1987.

Dowers KL, Tasker S, Radecki SV, *et al.* Use of pradofloxacin to treat experimentally induced *Mycoplasma hemofelis* infection in cats, *Am J Vet Res* 2009;70:105–111.

Dracz RM, Mozzer LR, Fujiwara RT, *et al.* Parasitological and hematological aspects of co-infection with *Angiostrongylus vasorum* and *Ancylostoma caninum* in dogs. *Vet Parasitol* 2014;200:111–116.

Drobatz K. Approach to the Emergency Patient, Paper presented at ACVIM 2003. Charlotte, NC, 2003.

Ducote JM, Dewey CW, Coates JR. Clinical forms of myasthenia gravis in cats. *Compend Contin Educ Pract Vet* 1999;21:440–448.

Ducote JM, Johnson KE, Dewey CW, *et al.* Computed tomography of necrotizing meningoencephalitis in 3 Yorkshire terriers. *Vet Radiol Ultrasound* 1999;40: 617–621.

Duke-Novakovski T, Seymour C. (eds.). *BSAVA Manual of Canine and Feline Anesthesia and Analgesia*, 3e. Gloucester: British Small Animal Veterinary Association; 2016.

Dunning D. Rehabilitation of Fracture Patients (VET-372), Paper presented at the Western Veterinary Conference 2004, Las Vegas, NV, 2004.

Dunning D. Rehabilitation of Neurological Patients (VET-371), Paper presented at the Western Veterinary Conference 2004, Las Vegas, NV, 2004.

Dunning D. Rehabilitation of Postoperative Joint Surgery Patients (VET-370), Paper presented at the Western Veterinary Conference 2004, Las Vegas, NV, 2004.

Dunning D. Rehabilitation of Postoperative Patients (T-13), Paper presented at the Western Veterinary Conference 2004, Las Vegas, NV, 2004.

Dunning D. Rehabilitation of the Osteoarthritic Patient (VET-369), Paper presented at the Western Veterinary Conference 2004, Las Vegas, NV, 2004.

Dunning D. Therapeutic Exercise and Weight Management in the Obese Orthopedic Patient (VET-373), Paper presented at the Western Veterinary Conference 2004, Las Vegas, NV, 2004.

Dyson D, Gaynor JS, Grimm KA, et al. *Managing Medical, Surgical, Chronic, and Traumatic Pain*. Wilmington, DE: Gloyd Group; 2004.

Easton S. *Practical Veterinary Diagnostic Imaging*, 12e. Ames, IA: Wiley Blackwell; 2012.

Edwards NJ. *Bolton's Handbook of Canine Electrocardiography*, 2e. Philadelphia, PA: Saunders; 1987.

Elliott DA. Nutritional management of kidney disease. In: *Applied Veterinary Clinical Nutrition* (ed. A.J. Fascetti and S.J. Delaney) 251–268. Ames, IA: Wiley-Blackwell; 2012.

Ellis AM. Surgical instruments and aseptic technique. In: *McCurnin's Clinical Textbook for Veterinary Technicians*, 9e (ed. J.B. Bassert) 1094. St. Louis, MO: Elsevier Saunders; 2017.

Ellis CJ. Getting to the root of the problem. *Vet Forum* 2009;February:14–18.

Emily P, Penman S. *Handbook of Small Animal Dentistry*. Oxford: Pergamon Press, 1990.

Engelkirk PG, Duben-Engelkirk J, Fader RC. *Burton's Microbiology for the Health Sciences*, 11e. Burlington, MA: Jones and Bartlett; 2020.

Epstein ME, Rodan I, Griffenhagen G. *et al.* AAHA/AAFP pain management guidelines for dogs and cats, *J Feline Med Surg* 2015;17:251–272.

Estrin MA, Wehausen CE, Jessen CR. *et al.* Disseminated intravascular coagulation in cats. *J Vet Intern Med* 2006;20:1334–1339.

Ettinger SJ, Feldman EC, Côté E. *Textbook of Veterinary Internal Medicine: Diseases of the dog and cat*, 8e. St Louis, MO: Elsevier; 2017.

Hermanson JW, De Lahunta A (eds.). *Miller's Anatomy of the Dog*, 5e. Philadelphia, PA: Saunders; 2019.

Evans HE, de Lahunta A. *Miller's Guide to the Dissection of the Dog*. Philadelphia, PA: Saunders; 1971.

Evans J, Levesque D, Kowles K, *et al.* Diazepam as a treatment for metronidazole toxicosis in dogs: a retrospective study of 21 cases. *J Vet Intern Med* 2003;17(3): 304–310,.

Fascetti AJ. Obesity Management in Dogs and Cats, Paper presented at Western Veterinary Conference 2004, Las Vegas, NV, 2004.

Fascetti AJ, Delaney SJ. *Applied Veterinary Clinical Nutrition*. Chichester, West Sussex: Wiley; 2012.

Brooks MB, Harr KE, Seelig D, et al. (eds.). *Schalm's Veterinary Hematology*, 7e. Amers, IA: Wiley-Blackwell; 2021.

Feldman EC, Nelson RW, Reusch C (eds.). *Canine and Feline Endocrinology and Reproduction*, 4e. St. Louis, MO: Elsevier; 2014.

Felumlee AE, Reichle JK, Hecht S, *et al.* Use of ultrasound to locate retained testes in dogs and cats. *Vet Radiol Ultrasound* 2012;53:581–585.

Fenn J, Drees R, Volk HA, *et al.* Comparison of clinical signs and outcomes between dogs with presumptive ischemic myelopathy and dogs with acute noncompressive nucleus pulposus extrusion. *J Am Vet Med Assoc* 2016;249:767–775.

Fenner WR. *Quick Reference to Veterinary Medicine*, 3e. Ames, IA: Wiley-Blackwell; 2000.

Fields SE. Hematologic reference ranges. *Merck Veterinary Manual*. Kenilworth, NJ: Merck Sharp & Dohme Corp; 2015. https://www.merckvetmanual.com/special-subjects/reference-guides/hematologic-reference-ranges (accessed 27 June 2021).

Fine DM, DeClue AE, Reinero CR. Evaluation of circulating amino terminal-pro-B-type natriuretic peptide concentration in dogs with respiratory distress attributable to congestive heart failure or primary pulmonary disease. *J Am Vet Med Assoc* 2008;232:1674–1679.

Fingeroth JM, Thomas WB. (eds.) *Advances in Intervertebral Disc Disease in Dogs and Cats*. Ames, IA: Wiley Blackwell; 2015.

Fiocchi EH, Cowgill LD, Brown DC, *et al.* The use of darbepoetin to stimulate erythropoiesis in the treatment of anemia of chronic kidney disease in dogs. *J Vet Intern Med* 2017;31:476–485.

Firth AM, Haldane SL. Development of a scale to evaluate postoperative pain in dogs. *J Am Vet Med Assoc* 1999;214:651–659.

Fletcher DJ, Boller M, Brainard BM. *et al.* RECOVER evidence and knowledge gap analysis on veterinary CPR. Part 7: clinical guidelines. *J Vet Emerg Crit Care* 2012;22(Suppl 1):S102–S131.

Food and Drug Administration. FDA-cleared sterilants and high level disinfectants with general claims for processing reusable medical and dental devices. 2019. http://is.gd/vK7uV6 (accessed 3 August 2021).

Ford RB. Vaccines and vaccinations: change is in the wind. *NAVTA J* 2005;Spring:31–35.

Foreyt WJ. *Veterinary Parasitology Reference Manual*, 5e. Ames, IA: Wiley-Blackwell; 2002.

Formenton MR, Pereira MAA, Fantoni DT. Small animal massage therapy: a brief review and relevant observations. *Top Companion Anim Med* 2017;32:139–145.

Fortney W. The Care and Feeding Orphaned Puppies and Kittens. Paper presented at Western Veterinary Conference 2010. Las Vegas, NV, 2010.

Fortney WD. "Painless" Vaccinations: How to Minimize Yipping, Paper presented at Western Veterinary Conference 2004, Las Vegas, NV, 2004.

Fortney WD. Neonatal Clinical Findings: Is It Normal or a Problem, Paper presented at the Western Veterinary Conference 2004, Las Vegas, NV, 2004.

Fortney WD. Triage and Diagnosis for Sick Neonates, Paper presented at Western Veterinary Conference 2004. Las Vegas, NV, 2004.

Fortney WD. The Care and Feeding of Orphan Puppies and Kittens, Paper presented at the Atlantic Coast Veterinary Conference 2006, Halifax, Nova Scotia, 2006.

Fossum TW. Proceedings from Veterinary Post Graduate Institute Seminar on Soft-Tissue Surgery. Texas A & M, 1997.

Fossum TW. *Small Animal Surgery*, 5e. Philadelphia, PA: Elsevier; 2019.

Fossum TW. Postoperative Care for Nurses/Technicians. Paper presented at World Small Animal Veterinary Association World Congress Proceedings 2013. Cancun, Mexico, 2013.

Fox PR, Sisson D, Moise NS (eds.). *Textbook of Canine and Feline Cardiology*, 2e. Philadelphia, PA: Saunders; 1999.

Fox SM. *Pain Management in Small Animal Medicine*. Boca Raton, FL: CRC Press; 2014.

Foy D. Acute renal failure (acute kidney injury). Paper presented at the AAHA Conference, 20 March 2014, Music City Center, Nashville, TN.

Franklin SP, Cook JL. Prospective trial of autologous conditioned plasma versus hyaluronan plus corticosteroid for elbow osteoarthritis in dogs. *Can Vet J* 2013; 54: 881–884.

Frazee EN, Leedahi DD, Kashani KB. Key controversies in colloid and crystalloid utilization. *Hosp Pharm* 2015;50:446–453.

Freeman LM. Beneficial effects of omega-3 fatty acids in cardiovascular disease. *J Small Anim Pract* 2010;51:462–470.

Freeman LM. Critical Care Nutrition. Paper presented at Convention of the Canadian Veterinary Medical Association 2012. Montreal, Quebec, 2012.

Freeman LM, Stern JA, Fries R, *et al.* Diet-associated dilated cardiomyopathy in dogs: what do we know? *J Am Vet Med Assoc* 2018;253:1390–1394.

Gandini G, Cizinauskas S, Lang J, *et al.* Fibrocartilaginous embolism in 75 dogs: clinical findings and factors influencing the recovery rate. *J Small Anim Pract* 2003;44:75–80.

Gasteiger G, D'Osualdo A, Schubert D, *et al.* Cellular innate immunity: an old game with new players. *J Innate Immun* 2017;9:111–125.

Gaynor JS. Is postoperative pain management important in dogs and cats? *Vet Med* 1999;94:254–257.

Gelens H. Intraosseous Fluid Therapy, Paper presented at Western Veterinary Conference 2003. Las Vegas, NV, 2003.

Gilbert SG. *Pictorial Anatomy of the Cat*, 9e. Seattle, WA: University of Washington Press; 1991.

Gingerich DA, Strobel JD. *Vet Ther* 2003;4:56–65. http://www.thek9rehabcenter.com/wp-content/uploads/2015/09/CODI.pdf (accessed 29 July 2021).

Giunti M, Troia R, Bergamini PF, *et al.* Prospective evaluation of the acute patient physiologic and laboratory evaluation score and an extended clinicopathological profile in dogs with systemic inflammatory response syndrome. *J Vet Emerg Crit Care (San Antonio)* 2015;25:226–233.

Glaze K. Treating a broken heart: congenital heart disease: Part I. *Vet Tech* 1998;19:169–179.

Glaze K. Treating a broken heart: congenital heart disease: Part II. *Vet Tech* 1998;19:339–347.

Glaze M. Management of Deep Corneal Ulcers, Paper presented at Atlantic Coast Veterinary Conference 2002, Atlantic City, NJ, 2002.

Gleerup KB, Andersen PH, Munksgaard L. *et al.* Pain evaluation in dairy cattle. *Appl Anim Behav Sci* 2015;171:25–32.

Goggs R, Mastrococco A, Brooks MB. Retrospective evaluation of 4 methods for outcome prediction in overt disseminated intravascular coagulation in dogs (2009–2014): 804 cases. *J Vet Emerg Crit Care (San Antonio)* 2018;28:541–550.

Goldberg ME. A look at chronic pain in cats. *Vet Nurs J* 2017;32:67–77.

Goldberg ME. A look at chronic pain in dogs, *Vet Nurs J* 2017;32:37–44.

Goldberg ME. Be the pain-attacking offensive midfielder – local anaesthetic blocks every practice can utilize. *Vet Nurs J* 2017;32:329–338.

Goldberg ME. The fourth vital sign in all creatures great and small. *NAVTA J* 2010; Winter:31–53.

Goldberg ME, Tomlinson J. *Physical Rehabilitation for Veterinary Technicians and Nurses*. Hoboken, NJ: Wiley Blackwell; 2018.

Gommeren K, Desmas I, Garcia A, *et al.* Inflammatory cytokine and C-reactive protein concentrations in dogs with systemic inflammatory response syndrome. *J Vet Emerg Crit Care (San Antonio)* 2018;28:9–19.

Goodale E. Pemphigus foliaceous. *Can Vet J* 2019;60:311–313.

Goodman RA, Breitschwerdt EB). Clinicopathologic findings in dogs seroreactive to Bartonella henselae antigens. *Am J Vet Res* 2005;66:2060–2064.

Goodwin C. Canine cilia disorders. *Vet Tech* 1998;19:115–124.

Gookin JL, Bunch SE, Rush LJ, et al. Evaluation of microcytosis in 18 shibas. *J Am Vet Med Assoc* 1998;212:1258–1259.

Gordon SG, Saunders AB, Roland RM, *et al.* Effect of oral administration of pimobendan in cats with heart failure. *J Am Vet Med Assoc* 2012;241:89–94.

Gourley IM, Vasseur PB. *General Small Animal Surgery*. Philadelphia, PA: Lippincott; 1985.

Graff L. *A Handbook of Routine Urinalysis*. Philadelphia, PA: Lippincott Williams and Wilkins; 1983.

Granger N, Smith PM, Jeffery ND. Clinical findings and treatment of non-infectious meningoencephalomyelitis in dogs: a systematic review of 457 published cases from 1962 to 2008. *Vet J* 2010;184:290–297.

Greiner EC, McIntosh A. Comparison of the efficacy of three fecal flotation media. *Vet Tech* 1997;18:283–287.

Griffin, B., Bushby, P.A., McCobb, E., et al. The Association of Shelter Veterinarians' 2016 veterinary medical care guidelines for spay-neuter programs. *J Am Vet Med Assoc* 2016;249(2):165–181.

Griffith CL, Hall, L Sterilization Process. US Patent No. Re 22,284; 1943.

Grimm KA, Lamont LA, Tranquilli WJ, et al. (eds.). *Veterinary Anesthesia: The fifth edition of Lumb and Jones*. Ames, IA: Wiley-Blackwell; 2015.

Grimm KA, Tranquilli WJ, Lamont LA. *Essentials of Small Animal Anesthesia and Analgesia*, 2e. Ames, IA: Wiley-Blackwell; 2011.

Grundy SA, Barton C. Influence of drug treatment on survival of dogs with immune-mediated hemolytic anemia: 88 cases (1989–1999). *J Am Vet Med Assoc* 2001;218: 543–546.

Guilford, W.G., Jones, B.R., Markwell, P.J. *et al.* Food sensitivity in cats with chronic idiopathic intestinal problems. *J Vet Int Med* 2001;15: 7–13.

Gultekin GI, Raj K, Foureman P, *et al.* Erythrocytic pyruvate kinase mutations causing hemolytic anemia, osteosclerosis, and secondary hemochromatosis in dogs. *J Vet Intern Med* 2012;26:935–944.

Hackett TB. Feline Fluid Therapy: Crystalloids, Colloids and Fluid Planning, Paper presented at Western Veterinary Conference 2002. Las Vegas, NV, 2002.

Hackett TB, Mazzaferro, EM. *Veterinary Emergency and Critical Care Procedures*, 2e. Ames, IA: Wiley-Blackwell; 2012.

Häggström J, Boswood A, O'Grady M, *et al.* Effect of pimobendan or benazepril hydrochloride on survival times in dogs with congestive heart failure caused by naturally occurring myxomatous mitral valve disease: the QUEST study. *J Vet Intern Med* 2008;22:1124–1135.

Hagman R. Pyometra in small animals. *Vet Clin N Am Small Anim Pract* 2018;8: 639–661.

Hamilton S. Therapeutic exercises for the canine patient. *NAVTA J* 2003;Fall:43–47.

Hancock R, Rashmir-Raven A. Principles and techniques of the Robert–Jones bandage. *Vet Tech* 2000;21:463–465.

Hand MS, Thatcher, CD, Remillard RL, et al. *Small Animal Clinical Nutrition*, 5e. Topeka, KS: Mark Morris Institute; 2010.

Hanks J, Spodnick, G. Wound healing in the veterinary rehabilitation patient. *Vet Clin North Am Small Anim Pract* 2005;35:1453–1471.

Hansen HJ. A pathologic-anatomical study on disc degeneration in dog, with special reference to the so-called enchondrosis intervertebralis. *Acta Orthop Scand Suppl* 1952;11:1–117.

Hanson B. Common Mistakes in Fluid Therapy, Paper presented at ACVIM 2003, Charlotte, NC, 2003.

Harari J. *Surgical Complications and Wound Healing in the Small Animal Practice*. Philadelphia, PA: Saunders; 1993.

Harvey CE. *Feline Dentistry*. Veterinary Clinics of North America, Vol. 22, No. 6. Philadelphia, PA: Saunders; 1992.

Harvey CE, Emily PP. *Small Animal Dentistry*. St. Louis: Mosby; 1993.
Harvey JW. Congenital erythrocyte enzyme deficiencies. *Vet Clin North Am Small Anim Pract* 1996;26:1003–1011.
Harvey JW. Erythrocyte Morphology in Disease, Paper presented at Western Veterinary Conference 2006, Las Vegas, NV, 2006.
Hawkins BJ. Down in the mouth: examining the feline oral cavity. *Vet Tech* 1997;18:671–678.
Heath D. Lifeline to recovery: intravenous catheterization techniques. *Vet Tech* 1998;19:614.
Heath D. Step-by-step placing an over-the-needle catheter in the cephalic vein. *Vet Tech* 1998;19:617.
Heath S, Rusbridge C, Johnson N. *et al.* Feline orofacial pain syndrome. In: Proceedings of the Australian Veterinary Association (AVA) Annual Conferences. Proceedings of the 3rd AVA/NZVA Pan Pacific Veterinary Conference, Dental Stream, Brisbane, Queensland, Australia, June 2010.
Heins AL. A new approach to treatment of periodontal disease. *Vet Tech* 1997;18:372–378.
Hellyer PW. Pain Assessment and Multimodal Analgesic therapy in Dogs and Cats, Paper presented at ABVP 2006, San Antonio, TX.
Hendrix CH, Robinson E. *Diagnostic Parasitology for Veterinary Technicians*, 5e. St. Louis, MO: Elsevier; 2017.
Hendrix CM, Robinson E. *Diagnostic Veterinary Parasitology*, 5e. St. Louis, MO: Mosby; 2016.
Henry CJ, Higginbotham ML. (eds.). *Cancer Management in Small Animal Practice*. Maryland Heights, MO: Saunders Elsevier; 2010.
Hickman A. Parenteral Nutrition. Paper presented at Spring Conference, Kansas State University (Spring 1997).
Hielm-Björkman AK, Rita H, Tulamo RM. Psychometric testing of the Helsinki chronic pain index by completion of a questionnaire in Finnish by owners of dogs with chronic signs of pain caused by osteoarthritis. *Am J Vet Res* 2009;70:727–734.
Hoffman KA. Magnetic resonance imaging as a localization tool. *Vet Tech* 2006;December:744–748.
Holden E, Calvo G, Collins M. *et al.* Evaluation of facial expression in acute pain in cats. *J Small Anim Pract* 2014;55:615–621.
Holloway C, Buffington T. Basic guidelines for dogs and cats. *Vet Tech* 1999;20:499–505.
Holloway C, Buffington T. A clinical problem: obesity and related health risks. *Vet Tech* 2000;21:281–283.
Holmstrom SE. *Veterinary Dentistry: A team approach*, 3e. St Louis, MO: Elsevier; 2019.
Holmstrom SE, Frost P, Fitch PF, Eisner ER. *Veterinary Dental Techniques for the Small Animal Practitioner*, 3e. Philadelphia, PA: Elsevier; 2004.
Hopper K. Shock: Causes, Diagnosis and Therapy, Paper presented at Canine Medicine Symposium 2011. Davis, CA, 2011.
Hoskins JD. *Veterinary Pediatrics: Dogs and Cats from Birth to Six Months*, 3e. Philadelphia, PA: Saunders; 2001.
Hoskins JD. Pediatric health care and management. *Vet Clin North Am Small Anim Pract* 1999;29:837–852.
Hoskins JD. Small Animal Pediatric Medicine, Paper presented at the Tufts Animal Expo 2002, Boston, MA, 2002.
Hoskins JD. Pediatric Critical Care, Paper presented at Western Veterinary Conference 2004. Las Vegas, NV, 2004.
Huang HP, Yang HL, Liang SL, *et al.* Iatrogenic hyperadrenocorticism in 28 dogs. *J Am Anim Hosp Assoc* 1999;35:200–207.
Hughes D. Triage and major body system evaluation. *World Small Animal Veterinary Association Proceedings*. https://www.vin.com/apputil/content/defaultadv1.aspx?id=3854120&pid=11196 (accessed 13 August 2021).
Hughes D. Cardiovascular Assessment and Haemodynamic Monitoring, Paper presented at ECVIM-CA/ESVIM Congress, Munich, Germany, 2002.
Humm K. How to Interpret Arterial Blood Gas. Paper presented at Paper presented at World Small Animal Veterinary Association World Congress Proceedings 2012. San Antonio, TX, 2012.
IDEXX Reference Laboratories. Directory of tests and services. 2019. https://www.idexx.com/en/veterinary/reference-laboratories/tests-and-services (accessed 27 June 2021).
Ikram M, Hill E. *Microbiology for Veterinary Technicians*. St. Louis, MO: Mosby; 1991.
International Renal Interest Society. IRIS Staging of CKD (modified 2019). http://www.iris-kidney.com/guidelines/staging.html (accessed 22 July 2021).
Iowa State University, Center for Food Security and Public Health. Disinfection. http://www.cfsph.iastate.edu/Disinfection (accessed 3 August 2021).
Ivens VR, Mark DL, Levine ND. *Principal Parasites of Domestic Animals in the United States: Biological and diagnostic information*, 2e. Urbana, IL: Colleges of Agriculture and Veterinary Medicine, University of Illinois at Urbana-Champaign; 1989.
Jack CM, Watson PM. *Veterinary Technicians Daily Reference Guide: Canine and Feline*, 3e. Ames, IA: Wiley Blackwell; 2014.
Jacob F, Polzin DJ, Osborne CA, *et al.* Clinical evaluation of dietary modification for treatment of spontaneous chronic renal failure in dogs. *J Am Vet Med Assoc* 2002;220:1163–1170.
Jaegger G, Marcellin-Little DJ, Levine D. Reliability of goniometry in Labrador retrievers, *Am J Vet Res* 2002;63:979–986.
Jandrey KE. Capnography: What is the Evidence? Paper presented at International Veterinary Emergency and critical Care Symposium 2006. San Antonio, TX, 2006.
Jasani S. *Small Animal Emergency Medicine*. Edinburgh: Elsevier Saunders; 2011.

Johnston SA, Tobias M. (*Veterinary Surgery: Small Animal Expert Consult*, 2e. Elsevier; 2018.

Joseph D. Step-by-step placement of jugular catheters in small animals. *Vet Tech* 2000;21:587–590.

Kara A. Pain, anxiety, or dysphoria – how to tell? A video assessment lab. *Proc Am Coll Vet Surg* 2011;2011:509–512.

Kass PH, Farver TB, Strombeck DR, *et al.* Application of the log-linear and logistic regression in the prediction of systemic lupus erythematosus in the dog. *Am J Vet Res* 1985;46:2340–2345.

Kathmann I, Cizinauskas S, Doherr MG, *et al.* Daily controlled physiotherapy increases survival time in dogs with suspected degenerative myelopathy. *J Vet Intern Med* 2006;20:927–932.

Kazacos KR. Diagnostic Methods for Internal Parasites, Paper presented at Western Veterinary Conference 2002, Las Vegas, NV, 2002.

Kealy JK, McAllister H, Graham JP. *Diagnostic Radiology of the Dog and Cat*, 5e. Philadelphia, PA: Saunders; 2010.

Keating SCJ, Thomas AA, Flecknell PA. *et al.* Evaluation of EMLA cream for preventing pain during tattooing of rabbits: changes in physiological, behavioural and facial expression responses. *PLoS One* 2012;7:e44437.

Kennedy MA. Diagnostic Methods for Feline Viral Pathogens, Paper presented at ACVIM 2003, Charlotte, NC, 2003.

Kenney EM, Rozanski EA, Rush JE, *et al.* Association between outcome and organ system dysfunction in dogs with sepsis: 114 cases (2003–2007). *J Am Vet Med Assoc* 2010;236:83–87.

Kent M, Platt SR, Schatzberg SJ. The neurology of balance: function and dysfunction of the vestibular system in dogs and cats. *Vet J* 2010;185:247–258.

Kerwin SC. Introduction to Arthroscopy, Paper presented at Western Veterinary Conference 2004, Las Vegas, NV, 2004.

Kesel ML. *Veterinary Dentistry for the Small Animal Technician*. Ames, IA: Iowa State University Press, 2000.

Khan FA, Gartley CJ, Khanam A. Canine cryptorchidism: an update. *Reprod Domest Anim* 2018;53:1263–1270.

King L, Boag A. *BSAVA Manual of Canine and Feline Emergency and Critical Care*, 3e. Quedgeley, Gloucester: British Small Animal Veterinary Association; 2018.

King LG. Fluid Therapy for Critically Ill Cats I, Western Veterinary Conference 2004. Las Vegas, NV, 2004.

King LM. Fluid Therapy for Critically Ill Cats II, Paper presented at Western Veterinary Conference 2004, las Vegas, NC, 2004.

Kirk CA. Top Nutraceuticals in Pet Foods and Practice. Paper presented at World Small Animal Veterinary Association World Congress Proceedings 2011. Jeju Island, Korea.

Kirk RW. *Kirk's Current Veterinary Therapy X: Small Animal Practice*. Philadelphia, PA: Saunders; 1989.

Kirk RW. *Kirk's Current Veterinary Therapy XI: Small Animal Practice. Small Animal Practice No. 11*. Philadelphia, PA: Saunders; 1992.

Kirk RW. *Kirk's Current Veterinary Therapy XII: Small Animal Practice*. Philadelphia, PA: Saunders; 1995.

Kirkby K. The Future in Wound Management, Presented Seattle Veterinary Specialists C.E. Symposium, Seattle, WA 3/13/11, 2011.

Klein S, Peterson M. Canine hypoadrenocorticism: part II. *Can Vet J* 2010;51: 179–184.

Ko J, Krimins, R. Anesthetic monitoring: your questions answered. *Today's Vet Pract* 2012;January/February:23–29.

Kornegay JN, Barber DL. Diskospondylitis in dogs. *J Am Vet Med Assoc* 1980;177: 337–341.

Kovachs SM. Understanding the Sonic Cleaning Process 2011. http://www.crazy4clean.com/StudyGuideSC.pdf (accessed 3 August 2021).

Kurita GP, Ulrich A, Jensen TS. *et al.* How is neuropathic cancer pain assessed in randomised controlled trials? *Pain* 2012; 153: 13–17.

Laflamme DP, Kealy RD, Schmidt DA. Estimation of body fat by conditioning score. *J Vet Intern Med* 1994;154:59–65.

LaFlamme D. Sweet success: managing diabetes mellitus. *Vet Tech* 2001;22:24–25.

Langford DJ, Bailey, A.L., Chanda, M.L. *et al.* (2010). Coding of facial expressions of pain in the laboratory mouse. *Nat Methods* 7: 447–449.

Lappin MR. Feline toxoplasmosis. *Vet Tech* 1997;18:298–299.

Lappin MR. Use of Rectal Cytology in Diagnosis of Feline Diarrhea, Paper presented at Western Veterinary Conference 2006, Las Vegas, NV, 2006.

Lavin LM. The imaging chain: links to high-quality radiography. *Vet Tech* 2001;22:230–241.

Leib MS. Introduction to Gastrointestinal Endoscopy, Paper presented at Western Veterinary Conference 2006, Las Vegas, NV, 2006.

Lemke KA, Dawson SD. Local and regional anesthesia. *Vet Clin North Am Small Anim Pract* 2000;30:839–857.

Levi M, Toh CH, Thachil J. Guidelines for the diagnosis and management of disseminated intravascular coagulation. *Br J Haematol* 2009;145:24–33.

Lewis DD, Hosgood G. Complications associated with the use of iohexol for myelography of the cervical vertebral column in dogs: 66 cases (1988–1990). *J Am Vet Med Assoc* 1992;200:1381–1384.

Lichtenberger M. Noninvasive Cardiac Output Monitoring, Paper presented at Western Veterinary Conference 2002. Las Vegas, NV, 2002.

Lisciandro, G.R. *Focused Ultrasound Techniques for the Small Animal Practitioner*. Hoboken, NJ: Wiley; 2014.

Litster A, Atwell R. Physiological and haematological findings and clinical observations in a model of acute systematic anaphylaxis in Dirofilaria immitis-sensitized cats. *Aust Vet J* 2006;84:151–157.

Little, S. *Successful Weight Loss: Finding the inner cat*. Lakewood, CO: American Animal Hospital Association; 2017.

Little S. Vaccination protocols for catteries. *Cat Fanciers' Almanac* 1998;15(2). https://cfa.org/vaccination-protocol-for-catteries (accessed 13 August 2021).

Littman MP. Protein-losing nephropathy in small animals. *Vet Clin Small Anim* 2011;41:31–62.

Littman MP, Goldstein RE, Labato MA, *et al*. ACVIM small animal consensus statement on Lyme disease in dogs: diagnosis, treatment, and prevention. *J Vet Intern Med* 2006;20:422–434.

Liu J, Cao X. Cellular and molecular regulation of innate inflammatory responses. *Cell Mol Immunol* 2016;13:711–721.

Lobprise H, Dodd J. *Wiggs's Veterinary Dentistry: Principles and Practice*, 2e. Hoboken, NJ: Wiley Blackwell; 2018.

Looney AL. Acupuncture and Physical Therapy Analgesic Modalities, Paper presented at the Tufts Animal Expo 2002, Boston, MA, 2002.

Lopez MJ. Stem cell therapies: reality in the making. *Clin Brief* 2013; June.

Lorenz MD, Coates JR, Kent M. *Handbook of Veterinary Neurology*, 5e. St Louis, MO: Elsevier Saunders; 2011.

Love L, Harvey R. Arterial blood pressure measurement: physiology, tools, and techniques. *Compend Contin Educ Pract Vet* 2006;June:450–460.

Lowrie M. Vestibular disease: diseases causing vestibular signs. *Compend Contin Educ Vet* 2012;34(7):E1.

Lucroy MD. Cancer pain management. In *A Color Handbook of Small Animal Anesthesia and Pain Management* (ed. J. Ko), 305–310. Boca Raton, FL: CRC Press; 2013.

Lynch G. About cataract surgery. *Veterinary Vision* 2017;July. https://www.sagecenters.com/veterinaryvision/for-veterinarians/clinical-forum/specific-disease-topics/cataract (accessed 12 August 2021).

McCarthy GC, Megalla SA, Habib AS. Impact of intravenous lidocaine infusion on postoperative analgesia and recovery from surgery: a systematic review of randomized controlled trials. *Drugs* 2010;70:1149–1163.

McClure RC, Dallman MJ, Garrett PD. *Cat Anatomy*. Philadelphia, PA: Lea & Febiger; 1973.

McCormick TS. *The Essentials of Microbiology*. Piscataway, NJ: Research and Education Association; 1995.

MacDougall LM, Hethey JA, Livingston A. *et al*. Antinociceptive, cardiopulmonary, and sedative effects of five intravenous infusion rates of lidocaine in conscious dogs. *Vet Anaesth Analg* 2009;36:512–522.

McEntee MC. Radiation Therapy Today: Options and Applications, Paper presented at Atlantic Coast Veterinary Conference 20061 Atlantic City, NJ, 2001.

Macgregor JM, Rush JE, Laste NJ, *et al*. Use of pimobendan in 170 cats (2006–2010). *J Vet Cardiol* 2011;13:251–260.

Macintire DK. Pediatric intensive care. *Vet Clin North Am Small Anim Pract* 1999;29:971–988.

Macintire DK. Pediatric Emergencies, Paper presented by Western Veterinary Conference 2002. Las Vegas, NV, 2002.

Macintire DK. Metabolic Derangements in Critical Patients, Paper presented by ACVIM 2003. Charlotte, NC, 2004.

Macintire DK. Reproductive Emergencies I: Dystocia, Acute Metritis, Eclampsia, Paper presented by Western Veterinary Conference 2004. Las Vegas, NV, 2004

Macintire DK. Reproductive Emergencies II: Mastitis, Pyometra, Prolapses, and Mismatching, Paper presented by Western Veterinary Conference 2004. Las Vegas, NV, 2004.

Macintire DK, Drobatz KJ, Haskins SC, Saxon WD. *Manual of Small Animal Emergency and Critical Care Medicine*, 2e. Ames, IA: Wiley-Blackwell; 2012.

McLennan KM, Rebelo CJB, Corke MJ. *et al*. Development of a facial expression scale using footrot and mastitis as models of pain in sheep. *Appl Anim Behav Sci* 2016;176:19–26.

McMichael M, Dhupa N. Pediatric critical care medicine: physiologic considerations. *Compend Contin Educ Pract Vet* 2000;22:206.

MacWilliams P. Profiling the Urinary System I, Paper presented at Western Veterinary Conference 2003, Las Vegas, NV, 2003.

MacWilliams P. Profiling the Urinary System II, Paper presented at Western Veterinary Conference 2003, Las Vegas, NV, 2003.

MacWilliams P. Cytologic Assessment of Abdominal and Thoracic Effusions I-II, Paper presented at Western Veterinary Conference 2006. Las Vegas, NV, 2006.

Madsen LM. Perioperative pain management. *Vet Tech* May 2005:359–367.

Magen L, Shaughnessy ML, Sample SJ, *et al*. Clinical features and pathological joint changes in dogs with erosive immune-mediated polyarthritis: 13 cases (2004–2012). *J Am Vet Med Assoc* 2016;249:1156–1164.

Maggs DJ, Miller PE, Ofri R. *Slatter's Fundamentals of Veterinary Ophthalmology*, 6e. St Louis, MO: Elsevier; 2018.

Maher J. Wakin' up is hard to do [blog post]. *VetBloom* 2016;6 September. http://blog.vetbloom.com/anesthesia-analgesia/wakin-up-is-hard-to-do (accessed 30 July 2021).

Maloney C. Fluid therapy in small animals. *Vet Tech* 2003;24(7):462–471

Mama K. New options for managing chronic pain in small animals. *Vet Med* 1999;94:352–357.

Markwell PJ, Buffington CA, Chew DJ, *et al*. Clinical evaluation of commercially available urinary acidification diets in the management of idiopathic cystitis in cats. *J Am Vet Med Assoc* 1999;214:361.

Marsden SP. Alternative Approaches to Cancer: Treatments, Paper presented at the Western Veterinary Conference 2002, Las Vegas, NV, 2002.

Marsden SP. An Integrated Approach to Holistic Physical Medicine, Paper presented at the Western Veterinary Conference 2002, Las Vegas, NV, 2002.

Marsden SP. Theory and Practice of Chinese Physical Therapies, Paper presented at the Western Veterinary Conference 2002, Las Vegas, NV, 2002.

Mathews K. Neuropathic pain in dogs and cats: if only they could tell us if they hurt. *Vet Clin N Am Small Anim Pract* 2008;38:1365–1414.

Mathews KA. Pain assessment and general approach to management. *Vet Clin North Am Small Anim Pract* 2000;30:729–755.

Mathews KA. Pain Management for the Critically Ill I and II, Paper presented at Western Veterinary Conference 2004, Las Vegas, NV, 2004.

Mathews KA, Kronen PW, Lascelles D. *et al.* WSAVA guidelines for recognition, assessment and treatment of pain, *J Small Anim Pract* 2014;55:E10–E68.

Mathews KA, Sinclair M, Steele AM, et al. *Analgesia and Anesthesia for the Ill or Injured Dog and Cat* Hoboken, NJ: Wiley; 2018.

Matteson V. Block that pain, local anesthesia in dogs and cats. *Vet Tech* 2000;21: 332–339.

Mauldin G. Practical Clinical Nutrition. Paper presented at a lecture at Buffalo Academy, 2000.

Mauragis D, Berry CR. Small animal abdominal ultrasonography, part 3: Basics of imaging optimization: how to obtain high-quality scans. *Today's Vet Pract* 2015; November/December. https://todaysveterinarypractice.com/small-animal-abdominal-ultrasonography (accessed 3 July 2021).

Mauragis D, Berry CR. Small animal radiography of the scapula, shoulder and humerus. *Today's Vet Pract* 2012; May/June. https://todaysveterinarypractice.com/1475 (accessed 3 July 2021).

Mazzaferro EM. Arterial catheterization. *Veterinary Key* 2016; 10 September. https://veteriankey.com/arterial-catheterization (accessed 13 August 2021).

Mazzaferro EM. Fluid therapy: the critical balance between life and death. *NAVC Clin Brief* 2006;November:73–75.

Meadows I, Gwaltney-Brant S. The 10 most common toxicoses in dogs. *Vet Med* 2006;92:142–148.

Melan T, Carrera-Justiz S. A review: emergency management of dogs with suspected epileptic seizures. *Topics Comp Ann Med* 2018;33:17–20.

Meleo KA. Clinical Radiation Therapy, Paper Presented at Western Veterinary Conference 2003, Las Vegas, NV, 2003.

Melzack R, Wall P. Pain mechanisms: a new theory. *Science* 1965; 150: 971–979.

Merola V, Dunayer, E. The 10 most common toxicoses in cats. *Vet Med* 2006;95: 339–342.

Merck, Sharpe & Dohme. *MSD Veterinary Manual*. Whitehouse Station, NJ; Merck; 2021. https://www.msdvetmanual.com (accessed 12 August 2021).

Merrill L. *Small Animal Internal Medicine for Veterinary Technicians and Nurses*. Ames, IA: Wiley-Blackwell; 2012.

Merskey H, Bogduk N. *Classification of Chronic Pain*. Seattle, WA: International Association for the Study of Pain Press; 1994.

Metzger FL, Rebar A. Three-minute peripheral blood film evaluation. *dvm360* 2004;1 December. http://veterinarymedicine.dvm360.com/three-minute-peripheral-blood-film-evaluation-preparing-film (accessed 27 June 2021).

Michel KE. Designing an Effective Weight Reduction Program, Paper presented at Atlantic Coast Veterinary Conference 2002, Atlantic City. NJ, 2002.

Michel KE. Optimizing Diets for Enteral Nutrition: What and Where to Feed. Paper presented at International Veterinary Emergency and Critical Care Symposium 2011. Nashville, TN, 2011.

Michel KE. Weight Reduction in Cats: Great Frustrations in Feline Nutrition, Paper presented at WASVA World Congress Proceedings, 2001, Vancouver, BC, 2001.

Michigan State University Veterinary Diagnostic Laboratory. Endocrinology Reference Ranges. Revision 20. https://cvm.msu.edu/vdl/laboratory-sections/endocrinology (accessed 27 June 2021).

Middleton C. Understanding the physiological effects of unrelieved pain. *Nurs Times* 2003; 99: 28–31.

Mihatov L. So what is Giardia anyway? *Vet Tech* 2000;21:188–190.

Miller E. Immunosuppressive therapy in the treatment of immune-mediated disease. *J Vet Intern Med* 1992;6:206–213.

Miller E. The use of cytotoxic agents in the treatment of immune-mediated diseases of dogs and cats. Semin. *Vet Med Surg (Small Anim)* 1997;12:157–160.

Millis DL, Levine D, Taylor RA. *Canine Rehabilitation and Physical Therapy*, 2e. St. Louis, MO: Elsevier Saunders; 2014.

Mills D. Introduction to Small Animal Physical Rehabilitation Presented at the Atlantic Coast Veterinary Conference 2002, Atlantic City, NJ, 2002.

Mills D. Therapeutic and Aquatic Exercises. Paper presented at the Atlantic Coast Veterinary Conference 2002, Atlantic City, NJ, 2002.

Mills D. Therapeutic Ultrasound and Neuromuscular Electrical Stimulation. Paper presented at the Atlantic Coast Veterinary Conference 2002, Atlantic City, NJ, 2002.

Mison MB. Topical Agents in Open Wound Management, Presented Seattle Veterinary Specialists C.E. Symposium, Seattle, WA 2011.

Mitchell DM. Emerging Medical Therapies: Homotoxicology. Paper presented at Western Veterinary Conference 2012. Las Vegas, NV, 2012.

Moore AH, Rudd S. *BSAVA Manual of Canine and Feline Advanced of Veterinary Nursing*, 2e. Quedgeley, Gloucester: British Small Animal Veterinary Association; 2008.

Moore AH. *Manual of Advanced Veterinary Nursing*. Quedgeley, Gloucester: British Small Animal Veterinary Association; 2000.

Moore AS, Frimberger AE. *Oncology for Veterinary Technicians and Nurses*. Ames, IA: Wiley-Blackwell; 2010.

Moore GE. Leptospirosis in dogs. *NAVC Clin Brief* 2011;25:28.

Moses L. Pain Management and Comfort of the Geriatric Hospitalized Patient. Paper presented at International Veterinary Emergency and Critical Care Symposium 2011. Nashville, TN, 2011.

Mueller RS, Krebs I, Power HT, *et al.* Pemphigus foliaceus in 91 dogs. *J Am Anim Hosp Assoc* 2006;42:189–196.

Muhlbauer MC, Kneller SK. *Radiography of the Dog and Cat: Guide to making and interpreting Radiographs*. Oxford: Wiley-Blackwell; 2013.

Muir WW, Woolf CJ. Mechanisms of pain and their therapeutic implications. *J Am Ved Med Assoc* 2001; 219: 1346–1356.

Muir WW III, Hubbell, JAE, Bednarski RM, Lerche P. *Handbook of Veterinary Anesthesia*, 5e. St. Louis, MO: Elsevier Mosby; 2013.

Mullane PA. Practical neonatal care: tube feeding. *Vet Tech* 1998;19:532–535.

Munana KR. Update seizure management in small animal practice. *Vet Clin Small Anim* 2013;43:1127–1147.

Muri K, Valle PS. Human–animal relationships in the Norwegian dairy goat industry: assessment of pain and provision of veterinary treatment (part II). *Anim Welfare* 2012;21:547–558.

Murphy K, Hibbert A. The flat cat: 1. A logical and practical approach to management of this challenging presentation. *J Feline Med Surg* 2013;15(3):175–88.

Murphy M, Moncivais K, Caplan I. Mesenchymal stem cells: environmentally responsive therapeutics for regenerative medicine. *Environ Mol Med* 2013; 45: e54.

Navarini L, Bisogno T, Margiotta DPE, *et al.* Role of the specialized proresolving mediatory resolving D1 in systemic lupus erythematosus: preliminary results. *J Immunol Res* 2018;2018:5264195.

National Institute for Occupational Safety and Health. *Glutaraldehyde: Occupational hazards in hospitals*. DHHS (NIOSH) Publication No. 2001–115. Cincinnati, OH: Centers for Disease Control and Prevention; 2001. https://www.cdc.gov/niosh/docs/2001-115/default.html (accessed 12 August 2021).

Nelson RW, Couto CG. *Small Animal Internal Medicine*, 6e. St. Louis, MO: Elsevier Mosby; 2014.

Niemiec B. *Small Animal Dental, Oral and Maxillofacial Disease: A color handbook*. Boca Raton, FL: CRC Press; 2011.

Niemiec, B. (ed.). *Veterinary Periodontology* Ames, IO: Wiley Blackwell; 2013.

Niemiec BA. The importance of dental radiology. *Today's Vet Pract* 2011;November/December:75–80.

Niemiec B, Gawor J, Jekl V. *Practical Veterinary Dental Radiography*. Boca Raton, FL: CRC Press; 2018.

Niemiec B, Gawor J, Nemiec A. *et al.* World Small Animal Veterinary Association Global Dental Guidelines. *J Small Anim Pract* 2020; 16: E36–E161.

Nixon AJ, Dahlgren LA, Haupt JL. *et al.* Effect of adipose-derived nucleated cell fractions on tendon repair in horses with collagenase-induced tendinitis. *Am J Vet Res* 2008; 69: 928–937.

Norkus CL. (ed.) *Veterinary Technicians Manual for Small Animal Emergency and Critical Care*. Hoboken, NJ: Wiley; 2019.

Novotny B. Nutritional assessment. Hill's HealthCare Connection, 1996;95: 139–149.

O'Brien TR. *Radiographic Diagnosis of Abdominal Disorders in the Dog and Cat: Radiographic interpretation, clinical signs, pathophysiology*. St Louis, MO: Saunders; 1978.

Occupational Safety and Hazard Administration. *Occupational Safety and Health Regulations (Standards 29 CFR) Air Contaminants. 1910.1000*. Washington, DC: US Department of Labor; 2012. https://www.osha.gov/laws-regs/regulations/standardnumber/1910/1910.1000. (accessed 3 August 2021).

Occupational Safety and Health Administration. *Occupational Safety and Health Regulations (Standards 29 CFR) Hazard Communication. 1910.1200*. Washington, DC: US Department of Labor; 2021. https://www.osha.gov/laws-regs/regulations/standardnumber/1910/1910.1200 (accessed 3 August 2021).

Occupational Safety and Hazard Administration. *Occupational Safety and Health Regulations (Standards 29 CFR) Bloodborne Pathogens. 1910.1030*. Washington, DC: US Department of Labor; 2021. https://www.osha.gov/laws-regs/regulations/standardnumber/1910/1910.1030 (accessed 3 August 2021).

O'Connell K, Wardlaw J. Unique therapies for difficult wounds. *Today's Vet Pract* 2011;July/August:10–16.

Ogilvie GK, Moore AS. *Managing the Veterinary Cancer Patient: A practice manual*. Trenton, NJ: Veterinary Learning Systems; 1995.

Ograin V, Burns KM. Kidney disease and nutrition: yes they will eat! *NAVTA J* 2017;Convention Issue:16–21.

Okano S, Yoshida M, Fukushima U, *et al.* Usefulness of systemic inflammatory response syndrome criteria as an index for prognosis judgment. *Vet Rec* 2002;150:245–246.

Olivry T. A review of autoimmune skin diseases in domestic animals I: superficial pemphigus. *Vet Dermatol* 2006;17:291–305.

Olivry T. Auto-immune skin diseases in animals: time to reclassify and review after 40 years. *BMC Vet Res* 2018;14:157.

Olsen JL, Ablon L, Giangrasso A. *Medical Dosage Calculations*, 6e. Menlo Park, CA: Addison-Wesley Nursing; 1995.

O'Marra SK, Delaforcade AM, Shaw SP. Treatment and predictors of outcome in dogs with immune-mediated thrombocytopenia. *J Am Vet Med Assoc* 2011;238: 346–352.

Osborne JN, Sharp NJH. Putting wobblers back on track: part II. *Vet Tech* 1998;19: 519–527.

Osborne CA, Stevens JB. *Handbook of Canine and Feline Urinalysis*. St. Louis, MO: Ralston Purina Company; 1981.

Osborne CA, Stevens JB. *Urinalysis: A Clinical Guide to Compassionate Patient Care*. Trenton, NJ: Veterinary Learning Systems; 2006.

Owen JL, Harvey JW. Hemolytic anemia in dogs and cats due to erythrocyte enzyme deficiencies. *Vet Clin North Am Small Anim Pract* 2012;42:73–84.

Owens JM, Biery DN. *Radiographic Interpretation for the Small Animal Clinician*, 2e. Ames, IA: Wiley; 1998.

Paes G, Paepe D, Meyer E, *et al.* The use of the rapid osmotic fragility test as an additional test to diagnose canine immune-mediated haemolytic anaemia. *Acta Vet Scand* 2013;55:74.

Paige CF, Abbott JA, Elvinger F, Pyle RL. Prevalence of cardiomyopathy in apparently healthy cats. *J Am Vet Med Assoc* 2009;234:1398–1403.

Paltrinieri S, Paciletti V, Zambarbieri J. Analytical variability of estimated platelet counts on canine blood smears. *Veterinary Clinical Pathology* 2018;47:197–204.

Papajeski BM. Diagnostic blood smear preparation. *Vet Team Brief* 2018;August: 37–41.

Parashar R, Sudan V, Jaiswal AK, *et al.* Evaluation of clinical, biochemical and haematological markers in natural infection of canine monocytic ehrlichiosis. *J Parasit Dis* 2016;40:1351–1354.

Pascoe PJ. Perioperative pain management. *Vet Clin North Am Small Anim Pract* 2000;30:917–932.

Pastor J. Applications of the Blood Smear in Emergency Medicine, Paper presented at WSAVA World Congress 2002, Granada, Spain, 2002.

Pavletic M. *Atlas of Small Animal Wound Management and Reconstructive Surgery*, 4e. Hoboken, NJ: Wiley Blackwell; 2018.

Peak R. Feline tooth resorption: extraction of retained premolar root. *NAVC Clin Brief* 2010;January:21–24.

Peak RM. Regional and Local Dental Nerve Blocks for cats and Dogs, Paper presented at Atlantic Coast Veterinary Conference 2006, Atlantic City, NJ, 2006.

Pinheiro D, Machado J, Viegas C, *et al.* Evaluation of biomarker canine-prostate specific arginine esterase (CPSE) for the diagnosis of benign prostatic hyperplasia. *BMC Vet Res* 2017;13:76.

Pitcairn RH, Pitcairn, SH. *Dr. Pitcarin's Complete Guide to Natural Health for Dogs and Cats*, 4e. Emmaus, NJ: Rodale Books; 2017.

Plumb DC. *Plumb's Veterinary Drug Handbook*, 9e. Ames, IA: Wiley-Blackwell; 2018.

Plumlee KH. Treatment of Insecticide Poisoning, Paper presented at Western Veterinary Conference 2004. Las Vegas, NV, 2004.

Plunkett SJ. *Emergency Procedures for the Small Animal Veterinarian*, 3e. Philadelphia, PA: Saunders; 2012.

Podell M, Volk HA, Berendt M, et al. 2015 ACVIM small animal consensus statement of seizure management in dogs. *J Vet Intern Med* 2016;30:477–490.

Polkinghorn A. Chlamydial conjunctivitis in animals. *MSD Veterinary Manual* 2020; December. https://www.msdvetmanual.com/eye-diseases-and-disorders/chlamydial-conjunctivitis/chlamydial-conjunctivitis-in-animals (accessed 13 August 2021).

Polzin DJ. 11 guidelines for conservatively treating chronic kidney disease. *Vet Med* 2007;102:788–799.

Poppenga RH. Zootoxins, Paper presented at Western Veterinary Conference 2002. Las Vegas, NV, 2002.

Poundstone M. Emergency medicine: CPR techniques. *Vet Tech* 1992;13:357–362.

Preziosi DE. Feline pemphigus foliaceus. *Vet Clin North Am Small Anim Pract* 2019;49:95–104.

Quandt JE, Lee, JA, Powell, LL. Analgesia in critically ill patients. *Compend Contin Educ Pract Vet* 2005;27(6):433–445.

Quantz JE, Miles MS, Reed AL, *et al.* Elevation of alanine transaminase and gallbladder wall abnormalities as biomarkers of anaphylaxis in canine hypersensitivity patients *J Vet Emerg Crit Care (San Antonio)* 2009;19:536–544.

Quimby J. Enhancing Appetite in the Feline Patient. Paper presented at ACVIM 2012. New Orleans, LA, 2012.

Quimby J. How to approach proteinuria. Paper presented at the Southwest Veterinary Symposium 2017, September 2017, San Antonio, TX.

Quinn PJ, Markey BK, Leonard FC, et al. *Veterinary Microbiology and Microbial Disease*, 2e. Ames, IA: Wiley-Blackwell; 2011.

Ralph AC, Brainard BM. Update on disseminated intravascular coagulation: when to consider it, when to expect it, when to treat it. *Top Companion Anim Med* 2012;27:65–72.

Ralphs SC, Beale BS, Whitney WO, *et al.* Idiopathic erosive polyarthritis in six dogs (description of the disease and treatment with bilateral pancarpal arthrodesis). *Vet Comp Orthop Traumatol* 2000;13:191–196.

Rand J (ed.). *Veterinary Clinics of North America: Small Animal Practice*. Philadelphia, PA: Elsevier; 2013.

Randall A. The (hook)worms crawl in: Ancylostoma infection in humans. *Vet Tech* 1999;20:189–197.

Randolph JE, Scarlett J, Stokol T, MacLeod JN. *et al.* Clinical efficacy and safety of recombinant canine erythropoietin in dogs with anemia of chronic renal failure and dogs with recombinant human erythropoietin-induced red call aplasia. *J Vet Intern Med* 2004;18:81–91.

Ratcliff CR. Wound exudate: an influential factor in healing. *Adv Nurse Pract* 2008; 16:32–36.

Reagan WJ, Irizarry RA, DeNicola DB, et al. *Veterinary Hematology: Atlas of common domestic and non-domestic species*, 3e. Hoboken, NJ: Wiley-Blackwell; 2019.

Rebar AH. *Handbook of Veterinary Cytology*. St. Louis, MO: Ralston Purina; 1980.

Rebar AH. Cytology of Effusions, Paper presented at World Small Animal Veterinary Association World Congress Proceedings 2006.

Rebar AH. Cytology of Effusions, Paper presented at Atlantic Coast Veterinary Conference 2009. Atlantic City, NJ, 2009.

Rebar AH, MacWilliams PS, Feldman BF, et al. *A Guide to Hematology*. Jackson, WY: Teton NewMedia; 2002.

Reid J, Nolan AM, Hughes JML. *et al.* Development of the short-form Glasgow composite measure pain scale (CMPS-SF) and derivation of an analgesic intervention score. *Anim Welfare* 2007;16:97–104.

Reid J, Scott EM, Calvo G. *et al.* Definitive Glasgow acute pain scale for cats: validation and intervention level. *Vet Rec* 2017;180:449.

Reijgwart ML, Schoemaker NJ, Pascuzzo R. *et al.* The composition and initial evaluation of a grimace scale in ferrets after surgical implantation of a telemetry probe. *PLoS One* 2017;12:e0187986.

Reina-Doreste Y, Stern JA, Keene BW, *et al.* Case–control study of the effects of pimobendan on survival time in cats with hypertrophic cardiomyopathy and congestive heart failure. *J Am Vet Med Assoc* 2014;245:534–539.

Reuss-Lamky H. Beating the "bugs": sterilization is instrumental. *Vet Tech J* 2011; November: E1–E9.

Reuss-Lamky H. Keys to successful high-level disinfection and sterilization processes. *Today's Vet Nurse* 2017; January. https://todaysveterinarynurse.com/articles/keys-to-successful-high-level-disinfection-and-sterilization-processes (accessed 3 August 2021).

Richards JR. Caring for the senior cat, American Association of Feline Practitioners/academy of feline medicine update Vol 3. *Vet Tech* 1999;20:438–441.

Richards JR. Caring for the senior cat, American Association of Feline Practitioners/academy of feline medicine update Vol 2. *Vet Tech* 1999;20:368–372.

Richards JR, Elston TH, Ford RB, et al. The 2006 American Association of Feline Practitioners Feline Vaccine Advisory Panel Report. *J Am Vet Med Assoc* 2006;229:1405–1441

Riel D. Bone Marrow Aspirates and Arthrocentesis, Paper presented at ACVIM 2002, Dallas, TX, 2002.

Rieser TM. Emergency Management of Heart Failure, Paper presented at Western Veterinary Conference 2003. Las Vegas, NV, 2003.

Rieser TM. Logical Fluid Therapy, Paper presented at Western Veterinary Conference 2003. Las Vegas, NV, 2003.

Rivera A. Clinical Importance of Triage and Vital Signs, Paper presented at ACVIM 2003. Charlotte, NC, 2003.

Rivera MJ. A pointed approach: the fundamentals of veterinary acupuncture. *Vet Tech* 2000;21:32–40.

Rivera MJ. Homeopathy: like cures like. *Vet Tech* 2000;21:681–684.

Rivera MJ, Rivera, PL. Veterinary chiropractic. *Vet Tech* 2000; 21:301–304.

Robertson J. A practical approach to using the IRIS CKD guidelines and the IDEXX SDMA test in everyday practice. 2017 Hill's Global Symposium, 6 May 2017, Washington, DC. https://files.brief.vet/migration/article/37636/robertson-proceedings_hgs2017_final_0-37636-article.pdf (accessed 22 July 2021).

Rochette J. Local Anesthetic Nerve Blocks and Oral Analgesia, Paper presented at WSAVA World Congress Proceedings 2001, Vancouver, BC, 2001.

Rodriguez P. The proper care and repair of surgical instruments. *Vet Pract News* 2008; April: 18 https://www.veterinarypracticenews.com/the-proper-care-and-repair-of-surgical-instruments (accessed 3 August 2021).

Romagnoli SE. Canine cryptorchidism. *Vet Clin N Am Small Anim Pract* 1991;21: 533–544.

Rose LJ, Dunn ME, Allegret V, *et al.* Effect of prednisone administration on coagulation variables in healthy beagle dogs. *Vet Clin Pathol* 2011;40:426–434.

Rosenfeld AJ. The True Nature of Triage: Concepts of Emergency Evaluation, Paper presented at the Atlantic Coast Veterinary Conference 2002, Atlantic City NJ, 2002.

Ross JA, Moses AGW, Fearon KCH. The anti-catabolic effects of omega-3 fatty acids. *Curr Opin Clin Nutr Metab Care* 1999;2:219–226.

Ross S, Osborne C, Kirk C, *et al.* Clinical evaluation of dietary modification for treatment of spontaneous chronic kidney disease in cats. *J Am Vet Med Assoc* 2006;229:949–957.

Rossmeisl JH. Vestibular disease in dogs and cats. *Vet Clin Small Anim* 2010;40:81–100.

Roudebush P, Davenport DJ, Novotny BJ. The use of nutraceuticals in cancer therapy. *Vet Clin North Am Small Anim Pract* 2004;34:249–269.

Royer N. Step by step, performing cystocentesis. *Vet Tech* 1997;18:298–299.

Rozanski E. The CRASH Cart, Paper presented at Tufts Animal Expo 2002, Boston, MA 2002.

Ruben D. Transfusion medicine. Blood products, blood-typing and preliminary testing. *Vet Tech* 2004;25:484–492.

Rudloff E. Clinical Signs of Respiratory Distress, Paper presented at Western Veterinary Conference 2002. Las Vegas, NV, 2002.

Rudloff E. Emergency Transport and Survey, Paper presented at Western Veterinary Conference 2002. Las Vegas, NV, 2002.

Rudloff E. The Rule of 20 in the ICU, Paper presented at Western Veterinary Conference 2002. Las Vegas, NV, 2002.

Ruess-Lamky, H. Purr-fect feline anesthesia, *Today's Vet Nurse* March/April 2016: 1–19.

Ruoff CM, Kerwin SC, Taylor AR. Diagnostic imaging of discospondylitis. *Vet Clin Small Anim* 2018;48:85–94.

Saker KE, Selting KA. Cancer. In: *Small Animal Clinical Nutrition*, 5e (ed. M.S. Hand, C.D. Thatcher, R.J. Remillard *et al.*), 587–607. Topeka, KS: Mark Morris Institute; 2010.

Sandman KM, Harari J. Canine cranial cruciate ligament repair techniques: is one best? *Vet Med* 2001;96:850–855.

Schaefer H, Kohn B, Schweigert FJ, *et al.* Quantitative and qualitative urine protein excretion in dogs with severe inflammatory response syndrome. *J Vet Intern Med* 2011;25:1292–1297.

Schebitz H, Wilkens H. *Atlas of Radiographic Anatomy of the Dog and Cat*, 3e. Philadelphia, PA: Saunders; 1978.

Schenck PA, Strombeck DR. *Home-Prepared Dog and Cat Diets*, 2e. Ames, IA: Wiley-Blackwell, 2010.

Schmuel DL, Cortes Y. Anaphylaxis in dogs and cats. *J Vet Emerg Crit Care (San Antonio)* 2013;23:377–394.

Schneider L. Hyperbaric Oxygen Therapy. Paper presented at Australian Veterinary Association Conference 2010.

Schnyder M, Di Cesare A, Basso W, *et al.* Clinical, laboratory and pathological findings in cats experimentally infected with *Aelurostrongylus abstrusus*. *Parasitol Res* 2014;113:1425–1433.

Schoen A. Companion Animal Chiropractic and Physical Manipulative Therapies, Paper presented at the WSAVA World Congress Proceedings, 2001, Vancouver, BC, 2001.

Schoen AM, Wynn, SG. *Complementary and Alternative Veterinary Medicine*. St. Louis, MO: Mosby; 1998.

Schoenherr WD. Management of Feline Obesity, Paper presented at Western Veterinary Conference 2004, Las Vegas, NV, 2004.

Schroeder, C. Regional anesthesia and pain management in veterinary medicine. American Society of Regional Anesthesia and Pain Medicine. https://www.asra.com/guidelines-articles/original-articles/article-item/asra-news/2020/04/30/regional-anesthesia-and-pain-management-in-veterinary-medicine (accessed 25 September 2021).

Sharp B. Feline physiotherapy and rehabilitation: 1. Principles and potential. *J Feline Med Surg* 2012;14:622–632.

Shelton GD, Lindstrom JM. Spontaneous remission in canine myasthenia gravis: implications for assessing human MG therapies. *Neurology* 2001;57:2139–2141.

Shelton GD, Schule A, Kass PH. Risk factors for acquired myasthenia gravis in dogs: 1154 cases (1991–1995). *J Am Vet Med Assoc* 1997;211:1428–1431.

Short JL, Diehl S, Seshadri R, *et al.* Accuracy of formulas used to predict post-transfusion packed cell volume rise in anemic dogs. *J Vet Emerg Crit Care (San Antonio)* 2012;22:428–434.

Scilowicz OD. Beyond drugs: pain management with alternative physical therapy modalities. *NAVTA J* 2013;January/February:32–35.

Scott DW, Miller WH, Griffin CE, Campbell K. *Muller and Kirk's Small Animal Dermatology*. St Louis, MO: Saunders; 2020.

Scott-Moncrieff JC. Update on Insulin Therapy of Dogs and Cats, Paper presented at Western Veterinary Conference 2012. Las Vegas, NV, 2012.

Secrest S. Basic principles of ultrasonography. *Vet Tech* 2006;December:756–763.

Seim HB, Withrow SJ. Pathophysiology and diagnosis of caudal cervical spondylomyelopathy with emphasis on the Doberman Pinscher. *J Am Anim Hosp Assoc* 1982;18:241–251.

Severin GA. *Severin's Veterinary Ophthalmology Notes*, 3e. Fort Collins, CO: American Animal Hospital Association; 1996.

Shaffran N. Blood gas analysis. *Vet Tech* 1998;19:95–103.

Shaffran N. Pain in critically ill small animals: ethical aspects. *Vet Tech* 1998;19:349–353.

Shaffran N. Pain management: the veterinary technician's perspective, *Vet Clin Small Anim* 2008;38:1415–1428.

Sharp S. Dental radiography. *Vet Tech* 2005;February:92–99.

Shaw LK, Henry JE. Radiographic positioning: head, shoulders, knees and toes, Part 1. *Today's Veterinary Nurse* 2016;November/December. https://todaysveterinarynurse.com/articles/radiographic-positioning-head-shoulders-knees-and-toes-part-1 (accessed 3 July 2021).

Shelton GD. Myasthenia gravis and disorders of neuromuscular transmission. *Vet Clin North Am Small Anim Pract* 2002;32:189–206.

Shipp AD, Fahrenkrug, P. *Practitioners' Guide to Veterinary Dentistry*. Glendale, CA: Griffin; 1992.

Shultz R. *Inspecting Surgical Instrument: An Illustrated Guide*. Chicago, IL: International Scilowicz OD; 2005. Silva RF, Carmona JU, Rezende CM. Intra-articular injections of autologous platelet concentrates in dogs with surgical reparation of cranial cruciate ligament rupture: a pilot study. *Vet Comp Orthop Traumatol* 2013; 26: 285–290.

Silverstein D. Shock States: Rapid Recognition & Treatment, Paper presented at ACVIM 2011. Denver, CO, 2011.

Silverstein DC, Hopper K. (eds.) *Small Animal Critical Care Medicine*, 2e. St. Louis, MO: Elsevier, Saunders; 2015.

Simpson K, Chapman P, and Klag A. Long-term outcome of primary immune-mediated thrombocytopenia in dogs. *J Small Anim Pract* 2018;59:674–680.

Sink AA, Feldman, BF. *Laboratory Urinalysis and Hematology for the Small Animal Practitioner*. Jackson, WY: Teton NewMedia; 2004.

Sink CA, Weinstein N, Marlowe A. *Practical Veterinary Urinalysis*. Chichester: Wiley-Blackwell.

Sirois M. *Laboratory Procedures for Veterinary Technicians*, 7e. St. Louis, MO: ElsevierMosby; 2020.

Sirios M, Anthony, E. Fluid Therapy, What, Why, and How, Paper presented by Atlantic Coast Veterinary Conference 2002, Atlantic City, NJ, 2002.

Sirios M, Anthony, E. Hematology, Paper presented by Atlantic Coast Veterinary Conference 2002, Atlantic City, NJ, 2002.

Sirois M, Anthony, A. In-House Coagulation Testing, Paper presented at Atlantic Coast Veterinary Conference 2002, Atlantic City. NJ, 2002.

Skarda RT. Anesthesia case of the month. *J Am Vet Med Assoc* 1999;214:37–39.

Slatter DH. *Textbook of Small Animal Surgery* 2e. 2 vols. Philadelphia, PA: Saunders; 1993.

Smee NM, Harkin KR, Wilkerson MJ. Management of serum antinuclear antibody titer in dogs with and without systemic lupus erythematosus: 120 cases (1997–2005). *J Am Vet Med Assoc* 2007;230:1180–1183.

Smith FWK, Tilley LP, Sleeper Mm, Brainard BM. *Blackwell's Five-Minute Veterinary Consult*, 7e. Ames, IA: Wiley-Blackwell, 2021.

Smith R. A case of ocular granulomatous meningoencephalomyelitis in a German Shepherd dog presenting as bilateral uveitis. *Aust Vet Pract* 1995;25:76–78.

Smith SA. The New Cell-Based Model of Coagulation. Paper presented at ACVIM 2008. San Antonio, TX, 2008.

Sobel DS. In Introduction to Rigid Operative Endoscopy, Paper presented at British Small Animal Veterinary Congress 2006, Birmingham, England, 2006.

Solano-Gallego L, Sainz A, Roura X, *et al.* A review of canine babesiosis: the European perspective. *Parasit Vectors* 2016;9:336.

Sorjonen DC. Clinical and histopathological features of granulomatous meningoencephalomyelitis in dogs. *J Am Anim Hosp Assoc* 1990;26:141–147.

Sotocinal SG, Sorge RE, Zaloum A. *et al.* The rat grimace scale: a partially automated method for quantifying pain in the laboratory rat via facial expressions. *Mol Pain* 2011;7: 55.

Sparkes A, Cannon M, Church D, et al. ISFM consensus guidelines on the Practical Management of Diabetes Mellitus in cats. *J Feline Med Surg* 2015;17: 235–250.

Spellane-Newman M. Laser surgery: the cutting edge. *Vet Tech* 2001;22:412–416.

Spotswood TC, Kirberger RM, Koma LM, *et al.* Changes in echocardiographic variables of left ventricle size and function in a model of canine normovolemic anemic. *Vet Radiol Ultrasound* 2006;47:358–365.

Spreng D. How To Prepare Emergencies, Paper presented at WSAVA World Congress 2002, Granada, Spain, 2002.

Stafford C. Enhanced radiographic studies. *Vet Tech* 2004;June:384–397.

Stafford D. The great mimic: canine Addison's disease. *Vet Tech* 1999;20:490–497.

Stanley B. Impaired wound healing challenges. *NAVTA J* 2007;Fall:39–45.

Steagall P, Robertson S, Taylor P. (eds.). *Feline Anesthesia and Pain Management*. Ames, IA: Wiley; 2017.

Stearns ED. Computed radiography in perspective. *NAVTA J* 2004;Summer:53–58.

Steele AM. Under Pressure: ABP, CVP, What are the Numbers Really Telling Us? Paper presented at IVECCS 2006, San Antonio, TX.

Stein D. *Natural Healing for Dogs and Cats*. Berkeley, CA: Crossing Press; 1993.

Stull J, Bjorvik E, Bub J. *et al. 2018 AAHA Infection Control, Prevention, and Biosecurity Guidelines*. Lakewood, CO: AAHA; 2018.

Summerfield NJ, Boswood A, O'Grady MR, *et al*Efficacy of pimobendan in the prevention of congestive heart failure or sudden death in Doberman Pinschers with preclinical dilated cardiomyopathy (the PROTECT study) *J Vet Intern Med* 2012;26:1337–1349.

Surgeon TW. Pain Management, Paper presented at Western Veterinary Conference 2004, Las Vegas, NV, 2004.

Swaim SF, Henderson, RA Jr. *Small Animal Wound Management*. Philadelphia, PA: Williams & Wilkins; 1997.

Swaim SF, Renberg, WC, Shike, KM. *Small Animal Bandaging, Casting, and Splinting Techniques*. Ames, IA: Wiley-Blackwell; 2011.

Swann JW, Szladovits B, Glanemann B. Demographic characteristics, survival and prognostic factors for mortality in cats with primary immune-mediated hemolytic anemia. *J Vet Intern Med* 2016;30:147–156.

Sykes J. *Greene's Infectious Disease of the Dog and Cat*, 5e. Philadelphia, PA: Elsevier; 2016.

Tamimi FM, Montalvo S, Tresguerres I. et al. A comparative study of 2 methods for obtaining platelet-rich plasma. *J Oral Maxillofac Surg* 2007; 65: 1084–1093.

Tams TR. Diarrhea Caused by Giardia and Clostridium perfringens Enterotoxicosis, Paper presented at Atlantic Coast Veterinary Conference 2001, Atlantic City, NJ, 2001.

Taylor PM, Robertson SA. Pain management in cats: past, present and future. Part 1. The cat is unique. *J Feline Med Surg* 2004;6:313–320.

Taylor R. Developing Protocols for Physical Therapy, Paper presented at the WSAVA World Congress Proceedings 2001, Vancouver, BC, 2001.

Taylor R. Physical Therapy in Veterinary Medicine, Paper presented at the WSAVA World Congress Proceedings 2001, Vancouver, BC, 2001.

Taylor S. Feline lower airway disease: asthma and beyond. *Vet Nurse* 2017;8(1): https://doi.org/10.12968/vetn.2017.8.1.17.

Tear M. *Small Animal Surgical Nursing: Skills and Concepts*, 3e. St. Louis, MO: Elsevier; 2016.

Terry B. Arterial catheter placement. *Vet Tech* 2005;July:439–441.

Texas A&M University Gastrointestinal Laboratory. Cardiac troponin: reference intervals – canine. http://vetmed.tamu.edu/gilab/service/assays/cardiac-troponin (accessed 27 June 2021).

Theriogenology Foundation. What is theriogenology? https://www.theriofoundation.org/page/Theriodefinition (accessed 16 July 2021).

Thomas J. *Anesthesia and Analgesia for Veterinary Technicians and Nurses*, 6e. St Louis, MO: Mosby; 2022.

Thomas WB. Diskospondylitis and other vertebral infections. *Vet Clin Small Anim* 2000;30:169–181.

Thomas WB. Idiopathic epilepsy in dogs. *Vet Clin North Am Small Anim Pract* 2000;30:183–206.

Thompson D. The pain process. Veterinary Anesthesia and Analgesia Support Group. http://www.vasg.org/the_pain_process.htm (accessed 30 July 2021).

Thompson NM. Injection-site sarcomas in cats. *Vet Tech* 2005;February:140–144.

Thompson RCA. Gastrointestinal Parasites of Dogs and Cats: Current Issues, Paper presented at Bayer Zoonosis Symposium 2003, Chicago, IL, 2003.

Thrall DE. Textbook of Veterinary Diagnostic Radiology, 7e. St Louis, MO: Elsevier; 2018.

Thrall MA. *Veterinary Hematology and Clinical Chemistry*. Ames, IA: Wiley-Blackwell; 2012.

Ticer JW. *Radiographic Technique in Veterinary Practice*. Philadelphia, PA: Saunders; 1984.

Tighe, M., Brown M. *Moby's Comprehensive Review for Veterinary Technicians*, 5e. St. Louis, MO: Saunders; 2020.

Tighe MM, Brown M. *Mosby's Comprehensive Review for Veterinary Technicians*, 4e. Baltimore, MD: Mosby; 2014.

Tilghman M. Chiropractic Theory, Paper presented at the Atlantic Coast Veterinary Conference 2002, Atlantic City NJ, 2002.

Tilley LP. *Essentials of Canine and Feline Electrocardiography Interpretation and Treatment*, 3e. Philadelphia, PA: Lippincott Williams & Wilkins; 1992.

Timmann D, Konar M, Howard J, *et al.* Necrotising encephalitis in a French Bulldog. *J Small Anim Pract* 2007;48: 339–342.

Tipold A, Jaggy A. Steroid-responsive meningitis-arteritis in dogs: long-term study of 32 cases. *J Small Anim Pract* 1994;35:311–316.

Tipold A, Schatzberg SJ. An update on steroid responsive meningitis-arteritis. *J Small Anim Pract* 2010;51:150–154.

Tizard I. *Veterinary Immunology*, 10e. St. Louis, MO: Elsevier; 2018.

Tobias K. *Manual of Small Animal Soft Tissue Surgery*, 2e. Hoboken, NJ: Wiley Blackwell; 2017.

Towell TL. *Practical Weight Management in Dogs and Cats*, 2e. Ames, IA: Wiley-Blackwell; 2011.

Tracy DL. *Small Animal Surgical Nursing*, 3e. St. Louis, MO: Mosby; 2000.

Tranquilli WJ, Grimm, KA. Pain Management Alternatives for Common Surgeries, Paper presented at Managing Pain Symposium 2003, Orlando, FL.

Tranquilli WJ, Grimm, KA, Lamont, LA. Pain Management for the Small Animal Practitioner. Jackson, WY: Teton NewMedia, 2004.

Tutt C. *Small Animal Dentistry: A Manual of Techniques*. Ames, IA: Blackwell; 2006.

Tvedten H. Urine Sediment Examination, Paper presented at Western Veterinary Conference 2004, Las Vegas, NV, 2004.

Twedt DC. Applications of Neutraceuticals in Veterinary Medicine. Paper presented at Western Veterinary Conference 2009. Las Vegas, NV, 2009.

Ummel C, Zody, K. Sparkle Technique and Other Bright Ideas in Radiographic Imaging VSPN Continuing Education, July, 2006.

Union Carbide. *1984 Flammability Data on EO-N2-Air Mixtures at 1 Atmosphere*. Danbury, CT: Union Carbide; 1984.

University of Glasgow. VetMetrica HRQL. https://www.newmetrica.com/vetmetrica-hrql (accessed 29 July 2021).

University of Liverpool. Liverpool Osteoarthritis in Dogs (LOAD) owner questionnaire for dogs with mobility problems. 2014. https://dspace.uevora.pt/rdpc/bitstream/10174/19611/2/liverpool%20OA%20in%20dogs%20-%20load.pdf (accessed 29 July 2021).

US Food and Drug Administration. Pet Food Labels – General. July 2020. https://www.fda.gov/animal-veterinary/animal-health-literacy/pet-food-labels-general#:~:text=Pet%20food%20labeling%20is%20regulated,and%20proper%20listing%20of%20ingredients (accessed 12 August 2021).

US Food and Drug Administration. Product regulation. https://www.fda.gov/animal-veterinary/animal-food-feeds/product-regulation (accessed 29 July 2021).

Valenciano AC, Cowell RL. *Cowell and Tyler's Diagnostic Cytology and Hematology of the Dog and Cat*, 5e. St. Louis, MO: Mosby; 2019.

Van Dyke JB. Physical Modalities and Their Application in Veterinary Rehabilitation. Paper presented at Western Veterinary Conference 2012, Las Vegas, NV, 2012.

Vemulapalli TH, Hammac KG. *Microbiology for Veterinary Technicians*. Bloomington, IN: Animalibris Publishing; 2015.

Verstegen-Onclin K. Infectious and congenital diseases in cats. British Small Animal Veterinary Congress 2008. https://www.vin.com/doc/?id=3862916 (accessed 16 July 2021).

Veterinary Vision. Glaucoma. Veterinary Vision 2021. https://www.sagecenters.com/veterinaryvision/for-veterinarians/clinical-forum/specific-disease-topics/glaucoma-3 (accessed 12 August 2021).

Vigano F, Galilei VG. Fluid Therapy: Choosing the Right Fluid, Paper presented at ECVIM-CA/ESVIM Congress, Munich, Germany, 2002.

Vilar-Saavedra P, Hosoya K. Thromboelastographic profile for a dog with hypocoagulable and hyperfibinolytic phase of disseminated intravascular coagulopathy. *J Small Anim Pract* 2011;52:656–659.

Volhard W, Brown, K. *The Holistic Guide for a Healthy Dog*, 2e. New York, NY: Howell Book House; 2000.

Waddell LS. Evaluation and Interpretation of Blood Gases, Paper presented at Western Veterinary Conference 2004, Las Vegas, NV, 2004.

Wagner AE. Is butorphanol analgesic in dogs and cats? *Vet Med* 1999;94:346–351.

Wallisch K, Tepanier LA. Incidence, timing, and risk factors of azathioprine hepatotoxicosis in dogs. *J Vet Intern Med* 2015;29:513–518.

Wanamaker BP, Massey KL. *Applied Pharmacology for the Veterinary Technician*, 5e. St Louis, MO: Elsevier Saunders; 2015.

Wardrop KJ, Birkenheuer MC, Blais MB, et al. Update on canine and feline blood donor screening for blood-borne pathogens. *J Vet Intern Med* 2016;30:15–35.

Webb AA, Taylor SM, Muir GD. Steroid-responsive meningitis-arteritis in dogs with noninfectious, nonerosive, idiopathic, immune-mediated polyarthritis. *J Vet Intern Med* 2002;16:269–273.

Webb CB. Use of Nutraceutical Antioxidants in Veterinary Medicine. Paper presented at Western Veterinary Conference 2010. Las Vegas, NV, 2010.

Webster R, Herbert B, Blaber S. et al. Mesenchymal stem cells in veterinary medicine. *Vet Nurse* 2011; 2: https://doi.org/10.12968/vetn.2011.2.2.58.

Weinkle TK, Center SA, Randolph JF, *et al.* Evaluation of prognostic factors, survival rates, and treatment protocols for immune-mediated hemolytic anemia in dogs: 151 cases (1993–2002). *J Am Vet Med Assoc* 2005;226:1869–1880.

Weinstein DA. The Effect of Body Position on Indirect Systolic Blood Pressure Measurement in Dogs. Paper presented at ACVIM 2012. New Orleans, LA, 2012.

Weiss DJ, Wardrop KJ (eds.). *Schalm's Veterinary Hematology*, 6e. Ames, IA: Wiley Blackwell; 2010.

Weisse C. Interventional Oncology: New Treatment Options for Pets with Non-Resectable or Metastatic Cancers. Paper presented at World Small Animal Veterinary Association World Congress Proceedings 2012. San Antonio, TX, 2012.

Welch JA, Gillette RL, Swaim SF. *Management of Small Animal Distal Limb Injuries*. Jackson, WY: Teton NewMedia; 2015.

Welsh E. (ed.). *Anaesthesia for Veterinary Nurses*, 2e. Ames, IA: Wiley-Blackwell, 2009.

Wetmore LA. Novel Delivery Systems of Opioids in Practice. Paper presented at International Veterinary Emergency and critical Care Symposium 2012. San Antonio, TX, 2012.

Whatmough C, Lamb, CR. Computed tomography: principles and applications. *Compend Contin Educ Pract Vet* 2006;November:789–798.

Wiinberg B, Jensen AL, Johansson PI, *et al.* Development of a model based scoring system for diagnosis of canine disseminated intravascular coagulation with independent assessment of sensitivity and specificity. *Vet J* 2010;185:292–298.

Wiinberg B, Jensen AL, Johansson PI, *et al.* Thromboelastographic evaluation of hemostatic function in dogs with disseminated intravascular coagulation. *J Vet Intern Med* 2008;22:357–365.

Williams JF, Zajac, A. *Diagnosis of Gastrointestinal Parasitism in Dogs and Cats*. St. Louis, MO: Ralston Purina; 1980.

Williams LT, Bagley, RS. Pot-bellied dogs? Diagnosing and managing canine hyperadrenocorticism. *Vet Tech* 1998;19:47–56.

Williard MD. GI Endoscopy, Paper presented at British Small Animal Veterinary Congress 2006, Birmingham, England, 2006.

Willis CE, Thompson SK, Shepard SJ. Artifacts and misadventures in digital radiography. *Appl Radiol* 2004; https://appliedradiology.com/articles/artifacts-and-misadventures-in-digital-radiography (accessed 5 July 2021).

Wilson HE, Jasani S, Wagner TB, *et al.* Signs of left heart volume overload in severely anaemic cats. *J Feline Med Surg* 2010;12:904–909.

Wilson M, Mauragis D, Berry CR. Small animal skull and nasofacial radiography including the nasal cavity and frontal sinuses. *Today's Vet Pract* 2015;November/December. https://todaysveterinarypractice.com/imaging-essentials-small-animal-skull-nasofacial-radiography-including-the-nasal-cavity-frontal-sinuses (accessed 3 July 2021).

Windsor RC, Vernau KM, Sturges BK, *et al.* Lumbar cerebrospinal fluid in dogs with type I intervertebral disc herniation. *J Vet Intern Med* 2008;22:954–960.

Wingfield SG, Wingfield, WE. Triage in trauma: nursing implications and initial assessment. *Vet Tech* 1997;18:183–190.

Wingfield WE. *Enteral Nutritional Support in Critically Ill Dogs and Cats: Making the Right Decisions*. Fort Collins, CO: Colorado State University; 1998.

Wischnitzer S, Wischnitzer E. Atlas and Dissection Guide for Comparative Anatomy, 6e. New York, NY: WH Freeman; 2006.

Wohl JS. Applications of Fluid Therapy in the Critical Patient, Paper presented at ACVIM 2003, Charlotte, NC, 2003.

Wong C, Koenig A. The colloid controversy: are colloids bad and what are the options? *Vet Clin North Am Small Anim Pract* 2017;47:411–421.

Wortinger A. Managing inflammatory bowel disease. *Vet Tech* 1998;19:689–695.

Wortinger A. Learning and teaching from pet food labels. *Vet Tech* 1999;19: 586–590.

Wortinger A. Nutritional support for hospitalized pets. *Vet Tech* 1999;20:316–323.

Wortinger A. Probiotics and Prebiotics. Paper presented at International Veterinary Emergency and critical Care Symposium 2012. San Antonio, TX, 2012.

Wortinger A, Burns K. *Nutrition for Veterinary Technicians and Nurses*, 2e. Ames, IA: Wiley-Blackwell; 2015.

Wright ZM. Palliative and Hospice Care for the Terminal Cancer Patient. Paper presented at Western Veterinary Conference 2012. Las Vegas, NV, 2012.

WSAVA Global Nutrition Committee. Body condition score tools for dogs and cats. https://wsava.org/global-guidelines/global-nutrition-guidelines (accessed 28 July 2021).

WSAVA Global Nutrition Committee. Guidelines on Selecting Pet Foods. Dundas, Ontario: World Small Animal Veterinary Association. https://www.wsava.org/WSAVA/media/Arpita-and-Emma-editorial/Selecting-the-Best-Food-for-your-Pet.pdf (accessed 28 July 2021).

WSAVA Global Nutrition Committee. Short Diet History Form. Dundas, Ontario: World Small Animal Veterinary Association. https://wsava.org/global-guidelines/global-nutrition-guidelines (accessed 28 July 2021).

WSAVA Nutritional Assessment Guidelines Task Force. Nutritional assessment guidelines. *J Small Anim Pract* 2011;52:385–396.

Wuestenberg K. *Clinical Small Animal Care: Promoting Patient Health through Preventative Nursing*. Ames, IA: Wiley-Blackwell, 2012.

Young JF. Advancement in imaging: digital radiography: PACS and kDICOM. *NAVC Clin Brief* 2005;October:44–45.

Yousef M, Mansouri P, Partovikia M, *et al*. The effect of low level laser therapy on pemphigus vulgaris lesions: a pilot study. *J Lasers Med Sci* 2017;8: 177–180.

Zajac AM, Conboy GA. *Veterinary Clinical Parasitology*, 8e. Chichester, West Sussex: Wiley-Blackwell; 2012.

Zambelli A. Caring for the Cancer Patient: It's More Than Just Drugs and Surgery. Paper presented at World Small Animal Veterinary Association World Congress Proceedings 2011. Jeju Island, Korea.

Zimbro MJ, Power DA, Miller SM, et al. *DifcoTM & BBLTM Manual of Microbiological Culture Media*, 2e. Sparks, MD: Becton Dickinson; 2009.

Zoff A, Bradbrook C. Constant rate infusions in small animal practice. *Comp Anim* 2016;21:516–522.

Zsombor-Murray E, Freeman, LM. Peripheral parenteral nutrition. *Compend Contin Educ Pract Vet* 1999;21:512–523.

Index

Note: Page numbers in *italics* denote figures.

Veterinary Technician and Nurse's Daily Reference Guide: Canine and Feline, Fourth Edition. Edited by Mandy Fults and Kenichiro Yagi.

Companion website: www.wiley.com/go/fults/veterinary